MANIC-DEPRESSIVE ILLNESS

MANIC-DEPRESSIVE ILLNESS

FREDERICK K. GOODWIN, M.D.
Administrator
Alcohol, Drug Abuse and Mental Health Administration
and
Senior Investigator
National Institute of Mental Health

KAY REDFIELD JAMISON, Ph.D.
Associate Professor of Psychiatry
The Johns Hopkins University School of Medicine

New York   Oxford
OXFORD UNIVERSITY PRESS
1990

Oxford University Press

Oxford   New York   Toronto
Delhi   Bombay   Calcutta   Madras   Karachi
Petaling Jaya   Singapore   Hong Kong   Tokyo
Nairobi   Dar es Salaam   Cape Town
Melbourne   Auckland

and associated companies in
Berlin   Ibadan

Library of Congress Cataloging-in-Publication Data
Goodwin, Frederick K., 1936–
Manic-depressive illness
by Frederick K. Goodwin, Kay Redfield Jamison.
p.   cm   Includes bibliographical references.
ISBN-13 978-0-19-503934-4
ISBN-10 0-19-503934-3
1. Manic-depressive psychoses.   I. Jamison, Kay Redfield   II. Title.
[DNLM: 1. Bipolar Disorder.   WM 207 G656m]
RC516.G66 1990   616.89'5—dc20   DNLM/DLC   for Library of Congress
89–16396   CIP

19   18

Printed in the United States of America
on acid-free paper

This book is dedicated to

My mother and father,
who taught me to respect learning,
and to Rosemary, Kathleen, Fred, Jr.,
and Dan

F.K.G.

My family,
Frances Lear,
and
Richard Jed Wyatt

K.R.J.

and to our patients

Foreword

Publication of this book is a major event—for psychiatry, for the study and treatment of manic-depressive disease, and for those who are afflicted with that illness.

The affective disorders do not suffer from lack of attention. Journal articles abound; multiauthor symposium proceedings and other edited volumes flourish. But complete handbooks are few and far between, and those written by a single author or jointly by a few authors are still rarer. In their introductory chapter, the present authors point to a book from 1953 as being the last comprehensive and interpretive review of manic-depressive illness.

The "interpretive" is significant since—in addition to offering a detailed, up-to-date, and loyal review of the literature—Drs. Goodwin and Jamison have thought through every aspect of this many-faceted disease, and they present with candor their own interpretations and recommendations. For the reader this challenges and kindles constant interest, particularly because the authors take pains to point out what we still do not know or do not know with certainty. The book should become a treasure trove of ideas for young researchers.

The authors come well equipped to their task, and they complement each other admirably. Dr. Goodwin, formerly Scientific Director of the National Institute of Mental Health and presently Administrator of the Alcohol, Drug Abuse and Mental Health Administration, is a psychiatrist whose expertise in biological psychiatry is complemented by his commitment to psychotherapy. Dr. Jamison is a clinical psychologist, the co-founder and formerly Director of the Affective Disorders Clinic at the University of California, Los Angeles. She presently holds an appointment as Associate Professor of Psychiatry at the Johns Hopkins University School of Medicine. Both Dr. Goodwin and Dr. Jamison have extensive personal experience with the treatment of manic-depressive patients, and this lends relevance to their interpretations and practical usefulness to their advice.

The book is called *Manic-Depressive Illness*, but readers, especially those from Europe, should be informed that the emphasis is on bipolar disorder, although with comments, when relevant, on recurrent unipolar affective disease. The introductory chapter explains the reasons for this and gives an interesting account of how and why American and European psychiatrists diverge in their concept of unipolar illness. The authors are remarkably well versed in the European literature, including classical studies. Kraepelin is quoted frequently.

Reflecting the two authors' joint orientation and different backgrounds, biological and psychological issues are given even weight, the latter including topics scantily treated in handbooks, such as manic-depressive illness and creativity, combined drug therapy and psychotherapy, and medication compliance.

This book is a broad one. Although I am not usually a patient person, I relished its length and did not mind a certain redundancy, because repetition has been employed for clarity and cohesion. The book is anything but reductionistic; problems are described in their full complexity, and the clear exposition makes arguments easy to follow. I have learned a lot.

A distinguishing feature of the book is its ardor and compassion; time and again I was moved when I read it. That has to do with the authors' obvious fascination with the disease and with their deep respect for and understanding of those who suffer from it. As in no earlier comparable treatise, the patient's point of view has come to the fore, and I hope many patients and their relatives will study it. The book is filled with fantastically apt and illuminating (and sometimes wryly humorous) quotes from patients with the insight of personal experience—some of them famous authors, some just human beings intensely alive. They will be cited often in the future, as will the book as a whole.

Finally, and importantly, the book is written in exquisite language: rich and precise, supple and poignant. I congratulate those who are embarking on its study.

Mogens Schou, M.D.
Emeritus Professor of Biological Psychiatry
Aarhus University
Denmark

Preface

By any standard, *Manic-Depressive Illness* is a monumental work. It is monumental in its size, its breadth of vision, its insight into the nature of affective disorders, and its mastery of the scientific basis for understanding and treating them. Drs. Goodwin and Jamison have produced an extraordinarily comprehensive volume that is likely to become a classic esteemed by researchers and practitioners alike.

The authors have reviewed, freshly analyzed, and interpreted the world literature on manic-depressive illness, a literature that has grown in two decades from a small assortment of anecdotal clinical reports into a dauntingly vast collection of research reports from the fields of psychiatry, psychology, social work, nursing, biology, molecular genetics, pharmacology, neuroscience, and the arts. Equally important, they have created a sophisticated guidebook for practitioners. It is grounded in research but reflects a sensitivity to the practitioner's need to act—even in the face of imperfect scientific knowledge. Drawing on their extensive clinical and research expertise, Drs. Goodwin and Jamison offer a wealth of well-reasoned and useful advice for the acute and chronic management of manic-depressive patients. I cannot recall a better example of the creative integration of scientific knowledge with the realities of applying new concepts to patient care.

Manic-Depressive Illness is a unique synthesis, reflecting not only the clinical judgment and scientific skills of its two authors, but those of many other talented professionals as well. As noted by the authors in their acknowledgments, the National Institute of Mental Health (NIMH) played a considerable role, fostering both the field and this volume. NIMH sponsorship of the book is consistent with the Institute's original mandate from the U.S. Congress to conduct research on mental illness, disseminate information, provide national leadership for services, and ultimately improve the mental health of this nation's people. *Manic-Depressive Illness* fulfills many of these goals by offering a multidisciplinary readership a new appreciation of the dramatic scientific and clinical progress possible when extensive resources and systematic research are devoted to understanding affective disorders.

The advances documented in this book count among the most exciting in all of medicine. No longer are depression and manic-depressive illness considered rare conditions with few long-term consequences. Now they are recognized as widespread, usually recurrent mental illnesses that affect millions of people in the United States at any one time and approximately 1 of every 11 individuals at some time in their lives. No more are major depression and manic-depressive illness considered "personal" problems, secrets to be guarded within the tightest of family circles. Rather, they are now known to be treatable disorders that result from the interactions of an individual's biology with psychological, social, and environmental factors. More importantly, with proper management, they carry a promising prognosis for full recovery.

But they are still among the major untreated illnesses of our time. Fewer than one of three individuals with diagnosable affective illness now receive treatment in the United States. These disorders account for millions of dollars annually in lost productivity and tragic loss of life. The severe, recurrent forms dealt with in this book exact an especially heavy toll. As Drs. Goodwin and Jamison indicate throughout their book, the task of understanding and conquering manic-depressive illness is far from complete. Despite enormous scientific progress, much work remains to be done to enhance our understanding of the fundamental etiology of affective disorders, our capacity for primary prevention, and our ability to enhance the safety and efficacy of treatment. In addition, there are still wide gaps between the diagnostic and treatment capabilities of specialists and those of many clinicians on the front lines of medical and mental health service delivery. This book should go a long way toward meeting that educational challenge.

NIMH will continue to give high priority to advancing the scientific study of affective illness, disseminating important findings to lay and professional audiences, and improving the care of the mentally ill. It is our hope that *Manic-Depressive Illness* will, through its example, inspire its readers to make their own special contributions to the field, whether as researchers, clinicians, or mental health advocates.

Lewis L. Judd, M.D.
Director
National Institute of Mental Health

Acknowledgments

A decade has passed since we began this book, a decade marked by great change in the understanding and treatment of manic-depressive illness. Because this book evolved along with this maturation of the field, we trace its development and our reasons for undertaking such a project in some detail in Chapter 1. Here, we simply note that our conception of the work expanded rapidly as we tried to keep pace with the astonishing growth in the knowledge base. Translating our evolving aspirations into reality would not have been possible, however, without the help of others. We wish to acknowledge these generous and important contributions.

The National Institute of Mental Health (NIMH), through its intramural research program, provided most of the technical support throughout this long project, particularly during the work's acceleration over the last 3 years. This book simply would not have been possible without the NIMH involvement. One intention in providing this assistance was to make a virtually finished product available to Oxford University Press, thereby reducing the publisher's costs and allowing it to price the book within the reach of a broad audience, especially students, patients, and their families.

Along with the substantial material support has come the sustaining personal support from our scientific colleagues in the Institute. Two pillars of the intramural program's administrative structure deserve special mention. Hazel W. Rea, the program's deputy director, and Susan B. Thompson, program analyst, have been especially sustaining for Dr. Goodwin. Their unflagging, unambiguous, and uncompromising belief in the project kept it alive on more than one occasion. Dr. Goodwin also would like to acknowledge his first mentor, Dr. William E. Bunney, Jr., and his longtime colleague, Dr. Dennis L. Murphy, who together contributed so much to the emergence of manic-depressive illness as a major focus of NIMH research advances. In addition to the support of colleagues, the unceasing encouragement and help of Rosemary P. Goodwin has been, as always, a mainstay.

During most of the time she worked on the book, including sabbatical leaves, Dr. Jamison was provided generous financial and institutional support by the University of California, Los Angeles. Over the last 3 years, her salary support was largely provided by Frances Lear's North Star Fund. Dr. Jamison is deeply indebted to three of her former colleagues at the University of California—Professor Louis Jolyon West, Dr. Michael Gitlin, and Dr. Robert Gerner—for their professional and personal support. Dr. Raymond DePaulo, Jr., of the Johns Hopkins Department of Psychiatry, has been both a friend and the best of what a Hopkins physician–teacher is all about. Professor Mogens Schou and Dr. Anthony Storr provided singular understanding and friendship to Dr. Jamison, for which she is enormously grateful. The wit, patience, and intellectual contributions from Dr. Richard Jed Wyatt made completion of this book possible.

No other person, except the authors themselves, was more responsible for the successful completion of the project than Bette L. Runck, senior science writer and editor at NIMH, whose skill, intelligence, writing abilities, and sensitivity are reflected throughout the book. Ms. Runck's contribution went well beyond what one traditionally expects from an editor. By drawing on an unusually broad background in mental health issues, she was able to influence the book's content and tone in many important ways. Moreover, she managed and coordinated the entire production, including much of the preliminary searching of the literature necessary for the substantial revisions made in the last few years. She also introduced us to technology that made it possible to incorporate new research findings into the last stages of the book's production.

Ms. Runck's two principal assistants were C. David Missar, an NIMH research assistant, and Kathleen K. Goodwin, M.S.W., whose efforts were supported by contributions to the Foundation for Advanced Education in the Sciences (FAES) at the National Institutes of Health (NIH), including grants from the Commonwealth Fund and Oxford University Press. Mr. Missar and Ms. Goodwin, both of whom brought an unusual degree of organizational ability to the project, spent literally years tracking down materials in the library. Insofar as the book serves as an accurate bibliographic reference source, they are largely responsible. In addition, as graduate students in clinical psychology and social work, Mr. Missar and Ms. Goodwin were able to make important contributions of their own, including some preliminary literature reviews, the design of the tables, and the drafting of some text segments and tables.

At earlier phases of the book's development, similar help was provided by Marion H. Webster and Marcia D. Minichiello, both NIMH senior research assistants. The graphic production of the tables and figures was done by David R. Powell and Kenneth A. Weeks of the intramural Research Services Branch. Many others contributed to the production of the book. Anne H. Rosenfeld and Anne W. Cooley brought their superb editorial skills to bear at several stages, as did Paul J. Sirovatka at a late stage. Harriet Sirovatka coordinated much of the secretarial work on the book during its early phases for Dr. Goodwin, and Paula Stoessel worked in a similar capacity for Dr. Jamison. Other research and secretarial assistance was provided by Betty J. Alaish, Loretta Alexander, Roberta L. Holcomb, Arlene I. Jaffe, Zula Melup, Eloise Orr, Nancy Scheff, Barbara Shidler, Maxine F. Steyer, and Trudy C. Welsh.

The NIH Library and its staff deserve special mention for their dependable services. Dr. Jamison also wishes to acknowledge the research and library support from the UCLA Biomedical Library, St. George's Medical School in London, the University of Oxford, the British Library, the Johns Hopkins University Library, and especially the staff of the London Library for providing an exceptionally pleasant working environment.

Dr. Goodwin wishes to acknowledge the invaluable contributions of his intramural NIMH colleagues and friends, who, in addition to reviewing chapters, generously offered to assist with early drafts in the areas of their expertise. Specifically, Dr. Peter Roy-Byrne contributed to an early draft of Chapter 6. Drs. Jacqueline N. Crawley and Robert M. Post provided parts of the literature review in Chapter 16. For Chapter 17, Dr. William Z. Potter contributed substantially to the review of the amine hypotheses, the neurotransmitter bridge, and clinical-biological correlates, Drs. Philip W. Gold and Mark Smith to the section on neuroendocrine studies, and Dr. Steven M. Paul to drafts of the receptor and neuroendocrine sections. One part of Chapter 18 was aided by the efforts of Drs. Dilip V. Jeste and James B. Lohr, who, together with Dr. Goodwin, published a 1988 review of neuroanatomical studies. Dr. T. Peter Bridge assisted in another part of the review of neuroanatomy. Chapter 19 was greatly influenced by hours of discussion with Dr. Thomas A. Wehr, who also carefully reviewed and improved the chapter. We also thank Dr. Elliot Gershon for agreeing to write Chapter 15.

Additional review of specific chapters, which resulted in substantial improvements, included those from Drs. Nancy C. Andreasen, Jules Angst, Marie Åsberg, Daniel Auerbach, Wade H. Berrettini, Gerald L. Brown, M. Audrey Burnam, Paula J. Clayton, Rex W. Cowdry, J. Raymond DePaulo, Jr., David L. Dunner, William Flynn, Ellen Frank, Daniel X. Freedman, Robert H. Gerner, Michael J. Gitlin, Constance L. Hammen, Stephen Hinshaw, Thomas R. Insel, Dean Jamison, David C. Jimerson, Marvin Karno, David J. Kupfer, Markku Linnoila, Morris A. Lipton, Giovanni Muscettola, Dennis L. Murphy, John I. Nurnberger, Jr., Barbara L. Parry, E.S. Paykel, David Pickar, Arthur J. Prange, Robert F. Prien, Darrel A. Regier, Ruth L. Richards, Norman E. Rosenthal, Alec Roy, David A. Sack, Harold A. Sackeim, Mogens Schou, Anthony Storr, Herman M. vanPraag, Detlev von Zerssen, Myrna M. Weissman, Jeremy Waletzky, Robert Winter, and Richard J. Wyatt, and from Rosemary P. Goodwin, M.S.W.

Finally, we would like to acknowledge the sustained faith of Jeffrey House of Oxford University Press. Over the course of a decade, Mr. House firmly but gently prodded the book to completion, providing the necessary counterweight to the incessant demands of the authors' other responsibilities and to the pull of the literature to ever deeper and more obsessive probing. It would have been much easier on all of us, especially Mr. House, if we had spent a sustained period of time working on the book exclusively, but that simply was not feasible. Once the manuscript was final, others at Oxford University Press saw it through production. We wish especially to thank Susan Hannan, development editor, for her expert and careful attention during this phase.

Manic-Depressive Illness is the product of the authors' collaboration over many years, during which we had extensive discussions about the major biological, psychological, artistic, treatment, and philosophical issues associated with manic-depressive illness. We brought to this work different educational and professional backgrounds, as well as different intellectual and perceptual styles, which, we believe, have complemented and stimulated one another's thinking. Although the book as a whole is truly collaborative, each of us took responsibility for writing individual chapters, which were then reviewed and revised collaboratively. Dr. Goodwin wrote Chapters 3, 5, and 6, and 16 through 23. Dr. Jamison wrote Chapters 2, 7 through 14, and 24 through 27. We jointly wrote Chapters 1 and 4 and the epilogue.

We wish to note that all authors' royalties from this book go directly to two foundations, the Foundation for Advanced Education in the Sciences for the support of NIMH intramural research and the Manic-Depressive Illness Foundation for the support of public education about the nature and treatment of manic-depressive illness.

F.K.G.
K.R.J.

Contents

MANIC-DEPRESSIVE ILLNESS

1

Introduction

Mania is sickness for one's friends, depression for one's self. Both are chemical. In depression, one wakes, is happy for about two minutes, probably less, and fades into dread of the day. Nothing will happen, but you know twelve hours will pass before you are back in bed and sheltering your consciousness in dreams, or nothing. It isn't danger; it's not an accomplishment. I don't think it a visitation of the angels but a weakening in the blood.

—Robert Lowell[1]

Manic-depressive illness magnifies common human experiences to larger-than-life proportions. Among its symptoms are exaggerations of normal sadness and fatigue, joy and exuberance, sensuality and sexuality, irritability and rage, energy and creativity. In its diverse forms, manic-depressive illness afflicts a large number of people—the exact number depending on how the illness is defined and how accurately it is ascertained. First described thousands of years ago, found in widely diverse cultures, manic-depressive illness always has fascinated medical observers, even while it baffles and frightens most others. To those afflicted, it can be so painful that suicide seems the only means of escape; one of every four or five untreated manic-depressive individuals actually does commit suicide.

Over the past three decades, research has yielded effective treatments that have radically altered clinical work in manic-depressive illness. Principally, it was the discovery of lithium that galvanized the treatment community, instilling new hope among clinicians, their patients, and the public. Also important, the emergence of lithium and the antidepressants gave birth to whole new fields of scientific investigation. Studies of the illness have dominated biological psychiatry, which has itself begun to lead the profession. Manic-depressive illness has been an increasingly important focus of work in other disciplines also. Insights gained from the study of an illness that is biological in origin yet psychological in expression have underscored the urgency and inevitability of paradigms of mental illness that give balanced attention to biology, psychology, and the environment. Methodologies developed expressly for studies of manic-depressive illness have been incorporated as standard tools of clinical investigation in other areas of biomedical and behavioral research of psychopathology. Because symptoms of the illness shade over into normal human experience, it provides a model for the study of normal states as well.

Extraordinary accomplishments notwithstanding, manic-depressive illness remains a study in paradox, as evidenced by the persistent stigma attached to it. Despite our ability to treat the illness, patients and their physicians often either fail to recognize it or are reluctant to acknowledge it. Consequently, not even one in three receives treatment. Overly narrow conceptions of the illness contribute further to inappropriate and inadequate treatment. The most recent epidemiological data indicate that the proportion of bipolar patients in treatment—a mere 27 percent despite the effectiveness of available treatments—is the lowest of all major psychiatric disorders.

MANIC-DEPRESSIVE ILLNESS DEFINED

The title of this book and its table of contents make it clear that we see manic-depressive illness as a medical condition, an illness to be diagnosed, treated, studied, and understood within a medical context. This position is the prevailing one now, as it has been throughout history. Less universal is our diagnostic conception of manic-depressive illness, which evolved in the course of writing this book. Derived from the work of the "great classifier," Emil Kraepelin, it encompasses roughly the same group of disorders as the term *manic-depressive illness* does in European usage. It differs, however, from contemporary American concepts of bipolar disorder. Kraepelin built his observations on the work of a small group of 19th century European psychiatrists who, in their passion for ever finer distinctions, had cataloged abnormal human behavior into hundreds of classes of disorder. More than any other single individual, Kraepelin brought order and sense to this categorical profusion. He constructed a nosology based on careful description, reducing the categories of psychoses to two: manic-depressive illness and dementia praecox, later renamed *schizophrenia*.

Kraepelin's model consolidated most of the major affective disorders into one category because of their similarity in core symptoms, family history of illness, and, especially, the pattern of recurrence over the course of the patients' lifetime, with periods of remission and exacerbation and a comparatively benign outcome without significant deterioration. He saw mania as one manifestation of the illness, not as the distinguishing sign of a separate bipolar disorder, as it is in today's American diagnostic practice.

The European and American concepts of manic-depressive illness began to diverge almost immediately after Kraepelin's ideas became widespread in the early years of the 20th century. Europeans, adhering to a traditional medical disease model, emphasized the longitudinal course in both research and clinical work. Ever pragmatic, Americans wanted to treat the illness with the techniques at hand, which at that time were derived from the "moral treatment" movement in mental hospitals and the emerging dynamic therapies based on psychoanalytic theory. Research and clinical efforts in the United States thus slighted clinical description and genetics and turned instead to the psychological and social contexts in which the symptoms occurred.

On the continent, explorations of linkage between clinical typology and family history led to the formulation of the bipolar–unipolar distinction, by which manic-depressive patients were grouped according to the presence or absence of a prior history of mania. First proposed by a German, Karl Leonhard, the distinction was elaborated by other Europeans, such as Jules Angst and Carlo Perris, and by the Washington University group in St. Louis, Missouri, the neo-Kraepelinians who gave impetus to the new concern for an etiology-free, description-based diagnostic system in the United States.

The bipolar–unipolar distinction represented a logical refinement of the already well-defined Kraepelinian model, with its emphasis on recurrence and endogeneity. As useful as it is in both research and clinical contexts, it proved to be problematic when applied to the much broader American conception of affective disorders. The bipolar subgroup was clearly defined, but the other component of Kraepelinian manic-depressive illness—endogenous, recurrent unipolar depression—was obscured by its confusion with other affective disorders. In American usage, *unipolar* disorder encompassed any mood disorder that was not bipolar, regardless of its severity or course. Although the third edition of the *Diagnostic and Statistical Manual of Mental Disorders* (DSM-III) clarified the situation somewhat by requiring that criteria for major affective disorder be met before the bipolar–unipolar distinction is drawn, a diagnosis of unipolar disorder was still broader than the Kraepelinian concept, since it did not require a prior course of illness.

Our own struggle to confine and limit the focus of this book has followed a course similar to the larger historical one. We started with a framework of Kraepelinian manic-depressive illness, that is, recurrent major affective illness with and without mania. Later, we focused more exclusively on bipolar illness as a way of imposing workable boundaries on the scope of this project. Once thoroughly immersed in the subject, however, we became more and more convinced that isolating bipolar illness from other major depressive disorders prejudges the relationships between bipolar and unipolar illness and diminishes appreciation of the fundamental importance of recurrence. By the end, we had returned to a position close to where we began, convinced of the value of the original unified concept of manic-depressive illness, albeit with a special emphasis on the bipolar form.

DIMENSIONS OF THE ILLNESS

The presence or absence of mania, in addition to depression, is but one critical aspect of manic-depressive illness. The other is cyclicity, which may ultimately prove to be as useful as polarity in differentiating forms of affective illness. The classic European focus on longitudinal studies has provided an ample database for redirecting the emphasis of pathophysiology to mechanisms of cyclicity—that is, the biology of recurrence. To do such research, an investigator must analyze each patient's biological functioning over time and relate it to the natural course of illness. Such data are still uncommon. The priority that American clinicians are beginning to assign to recurrence is a tribute to the persuasiveness of our European colleagues' meticulous longitudinal clinical observations. Kraepelin's descriptions have had a lasting quality: Again and again during our study of the contemporary literature, we returned to his original writings to rediscover modern ideas.[2] To a remarkable degree, his work anticipated, explicitly and implicitly, contemporary theoretical developments. One example is the spectrum concept—the continuity of manic-depressive symptoms with normal fluctuations in mood, energy patterns, and behavior.

The longitudinal view provided by Kraepelin and many others both before and since persuaded us to survey the literature on recurrent unipolar illness along with that on bipolar illness, our primary focus. If we had confined ourselves to the bipolar literature, we would have excluded enormous amounts of potentially relevant data and insights. This recognition of the essential unity of major recurrent affective illness is evident throughout the book. In Chapter 23 on lithium prophylaxis, for example, we point out that similarities between recurrent unipolar and bipolar illness constitute firm ground for speculating about common neurobiological substrates.

The issue of cyclicity opens many new areas of inquiry. Manic and depressive episodes can be predicted to revert to normal at some finite time, either spontaneously or in response to effective treatment. The opportunity to compare biological measures during the illness with the same measures in the recovered state is essential in psychobiological research, since it permits longitudinal studies that can circumvent the problem of interindividual variability. The recurrent pattern—that of recovery to normal or change to an opposite state—makes the illness an unsurpassed paradigm for separating state and trait variables in mental illness. The regularity of recurrence in some patients permits the clinical investigator to anticipate the onset of an episode and, thus, to schedule data collection at critical points. The frequent rapidity of the switch from one state to another, especially the switch into mania, allows intensive efforts to understand the relationships between stress and biological changes in the onset of illness by looking at the temporal sequence of events—one approach to the ultimate question of causality.

The illness also is an interesting study in the coexistence of opposites or, more precisely, deviations from normal in opposite directions. Even lay observers may recognize that the illness is at times accompanied by periods of creativity, productivity, and high energy but at other times by profound fatigue and apparent indifference. Clinicians see a more subtle manifestation of this Janus-like illness in the effects of lithium in preventing its apparently opposite expressions. The dual action, perhaps diminishing some of the silver lining along with the cloud, challenges the clinician's psychotherapeutic skills in managing the issue of treatment acceptance, especially medication compliance.

THE SCIENCE OF THE ILLNESS

For the biological investigator, the presence of distinct and, in many respects, opposite states poses interesting questions about the mechanism of action of drugs. Medications now in use produce six discrete clinical responses: increases or decreases in depression, in mania, and in the frequency of episodes. This range of outcomes provides scientists with a rich array of correlations between drug effects and behavior, correlations that suggest underlying pathophysiological mechanisms. The exploration of these correlations has been a key component in the maturing of modern neurobiology. More than 40 years have passed since the initial clinical observation of lithium's effectiveness in manic-depressive illness and more than 20 years since the exhaustive, mandatory clinical trials were performed so that lithium could be approved for general clinical use throughout the world. New research reports on this single agent continue to be generated at a rate exceeding 1,000 per year.

More recently, research on manic-depressive illness has played a central role in efforts to apply new and emerging technologies, such as molecular genetics, to the study of psychiatric conditions. The application of these techniques depends on sensitive and reliable epidemiological and diagnostic case-finding methodologies to identify family pedigrees with a high incidence of the illness. Preliminary results suggest that several genotypes may underlie different forms of the illness. It is also possible that, like the multiple genetic forms of diabetes, several genotypes are expressed in common clinical phenomena.

Research on manic-depressive illness also has contributed new, empirically based theories about the pathophysiology of psychiatric disorders, including the influence of the physical environment—light and temperature in particular—on their course and expression. Of equal interest are the efforts to describe mechanisms by which the psychosocial environment interacts with the individual's biology to produce symptoms. One of the most promising lines of inquiry grew out of longitudinal observations: external stress appeared to activate or precipitate some initial episodes of illness, but eventually the illness seemed to take on a life of its own, since later episodes began without obvious precipitating stress. Robert Post drew an analogy between this process (initial activation giving way, over time, to a self-driven process) and the phenomenon of *kindling* in the central nervous system. Kindling is a process in which a highly regulated system, such as the limbic system in the brain, shows an escalating response to a repetitive stimulus, reaching a point where the stimulus is no longer needed for the disturbance to continue. The anticonvulsants, including carbamazepine, were shown to prevent kindling in animals and, in fact, had been used by several Japanese clinicians in manic-depressive patients. Post and his

colleagues reasoned that the increasingly endogenous character of some forms of manic-depressive illness might be analogous to kindling. As predicted by this hypothesis, carbamazepine was found in controlled studies to be particularly effective in rapid-cycling bipolar patients who had been resistant to lithium. Studies of kindling underscore the importance of early detection and treatment, which by interrupting the process may reduce the frequency of later recurrences.

OVERVIEW

In a book of this size and scope, a certain amount of redundancy is inevitable. Issues pertaining to the dimensional aspects of manic-depressive illness, for example, severity, polarity, and cyclicity, are introduced in clinical descriptions in Chapter 2, are then formally discussed in Chapter 4, and come up again in considerations of cycle length in Chapter 6. Where an issue could logically be discussed in more than one chapter, decisions occasionally were made on a somewhat arbitrary basis. For example, biological predictors of suicide are covered in Chapter 17, which reviews biochemical and pharmacological studies, rather than in Chapter 10, which focuses on suicide.

Clinical Description and Diagnosis

The book is divided into five sections, the first of which focuses on clinical phenomenology and diagnosis. In a reversal of common textbook practice, we begin with patients' own descriptions of their experience of the illness, followed by the classic descriptions of early clinical observers who were working in the era before effective medications altered the natural expression of the illness (Chapter 2). Although the formal diagnostic criteria, presented in Chapter 5, are essential for designing a common language for researcher and clinician, they fail to convey either the richness of the illness or the variability of its expression.

A separate chapter traces the evolution of the concept of the illness, which has remained remarkably consistent since the times of Hippocrates (Chapter 3). The spectrum of the illness, covered in Chapter 4, highlights the fact that diagnostic and subgroup boundaries represent somewhat arbitrary distinctions, with individual patients often falling in a gray area. Also emphasized is the spectrum of manic states, which, unlike the well-described depressive spectrum, is often overlooked.

Despite its importance, the spectrum concept should not obscure the reliable, predictive, diagnostic categories that can be shaped from clusters of symptoms, which do exist. Chapter 5 guides the clinician through the problems of diagnosis. Most important is the differential diagnosis of manic-depressive illness and schizophrenia, organic brain disorders, substance abuse, and borderline personality disorders.

Clinical Studies

The second section covers various clinical aspects of manic-depressive illness. Appropriately, in Chapter 6 we begin with a discussion of course and outcome, fundamental characteristics of the illness that provided the basis for differentiating it from schizophrenia. In addition to the obvious importance of natural course for clinicians who are assessing prognosis and planning treatment, it is important to scientists as well, since it offers many useful clues to pathological processes. Historical observations on course and outcome are considered together with data gathered in contemporary large-scale studies.

Chapter 7 on epidemiology argues that manic-depressive illness, especially its bipolar forms, is more common than is usually thought. Among the most important recent observations are the early age of onset documented in careful community surveys and the surprisingly high prevalence of manic-depressive illness in homeless populations.

The next three chapters highlight special clinical aspects of the illness. Chapter 8 deals with manic-depressive illness in children and adolescents, in whom often and tragically the illness goes unrecognized. Although rare in prepubertal children, manic-depressive illness often begins in adolescence. Indeed, well over one third of all cases begin before the age of 20. If the kindling hypothesis is substantiated, early recognition and immediate, vigorous treatment would be expected to reduce subsequent pathology. At the very least, early treatment would reduce the tragic psychological scarring caused by untreated illness. All too typical is the individual, initially treated in his or her mid-to-late 20s, who has

already lived with the illness for more than a decade, a period critical for life's major beginnings in relationships, education, and career.

The focus on the young highlights the frequent coexistence of drug and alcohol abuse among young manic-depressive patients. Growing recognition of the frequent coexistence of the illness with substance abuse prompted us to devote an entire chapter (Chapter 9) to describing these problems and another to treating them (Chapter 26). Recent analyses of data obtained through the National Institute of Mental Health Epidemiological Catchment Area program indicate that the presence of a depressive or anxiety disorder can double the chance of subsequent substance abuse. Conversely, illicit drugs and alcohol can adversely affect the course and treatment of manic-depressive illness by altering the same brain mechanisms that regulate mood, including the potential for kindling.

Like substance abuse, the importance of suicide in manic-depressive illness is reflected in the assignment of two chapters to it, one describing its clinical correlations (Chapter 10), one considering its prevention (Chapter 27). Throughout the 1960s and the 1970s, suicide hotlines, prevention centers, and school-based educational programs proliferated as well-intentioned efforts to prevent suicide. What they tended to overlook, even to obscure, was the fact that the presence of an affective disorder, especially manic-depressive illness, is the single most important risk factor for actual completed suicide. With as many as 25 percent of all untreated manic-depressive individuals killing themselves, major suicide prevention could be achieved by increasing the recognition and treatment of manic-depressive illness. The lethal nature of this illness cannot be overemphasized.

Psychological Studies

Manic-depressive illness has been a rich source of theory and data for investigators interested in psychological mechanisms. The third section of the book considers these developments. Manic-depressive illness has contributed to the general study of psychology by serving as a paradigm for explorations of state and trait differences. It also has been a model for the general psychological assessment of cognition and the more specific differentiation of cognition in manic and depressive states from those in schizophrenia. Chapter 13 is devoted to methods for assessing manic and depressive states, thus adding the perspective of formal psychological assessment to the discussion of differential diagnosis in Chapter 5. Also pertinent to differentiating manic-depressive illness from other psychiatric illness, especially schizophrenia, are the distinguishing characteristics of hallucinations and delusions found in psychoses. The section opens with a survey of what is known about formal thought disorder, perception, and cognition in manic-depressive illness (Chapter 11), a chapter that also reviews the neuropsychological literature.

The psychological manifestations of manic-depressive illness, observable in personality and behavior as well as cognitive patterns, can result in profound discord in family life and other social relationships. Studies of personality functioning in manic and depressed states are described and compared with normal states in the patients themselves and in the general population in Chapter 12. Personality disorders that commonly coexist with manic-depressive illness also are covered, as are the effects of lithium on personality. The chapter then considers interpersonal aspects of the illness.

Widespread interest in creativity has made this aspect of the study of manic-depressive illness well known. The age-old link between "madness" and creativity has been studied with increasingly sophisticated methods in recent years. Research has demonstrated that it is manic-depressive illness, not schizophrenia, that is most often associated with creative accomplishment. Among the most interesting developments in this field is the hypothesis that the genetic predisposition for manic-depressive illness also confers a creative edge to affected individuals and their close relatives. Explorations into the characteristics that go toward making some individuals more creative than others should have implications for the general population. Among the features of the illness being considered are the heightened energy level and speed of cognition of hypomania, associated with a global, inclusive associative process. In addition to raising important psychological, social, and ethical issues, this and related positive features of the illness can play a key role in reducing the burden of stigma borne by patients. Understanding these positive aspects is, of

course, a necessary preparation for dealing with one of the most sensitive and difficult issues in treatment—medication compliance.

Pathophysiology

The size of the fourth section of the book, the largest, testifies to the wealth of biological knowledge that has accrued through research on manic-depressive illness. This disorder has come to represent an extraordinarily rich source of information about interrelationships of behavioral and biological phenomena. Certainly, it has stimulated fascinating and productive theories about brain–behavior relationships. Particularly fruitful have been studies employing animal models and the pharmacological bridge, the link between the effects of drugs in animals and their clinical effects in human beings, and vice versa.

The section opens with a survey of the literature on genetics (Chapter 15). Wishing to ensure that the chapter carefully and accurately reflects this important area, we invited Elliot Gershon, a renowned leader in the field, to write it. Although we worked closely with him in shaping the chapter, it remains his contribution, the only one in the book to be written by a guest author. It reviews early developments in the study of genetic epidemiology, which lead Gershon to the conclusion that the twin-study data continue to be the most clinically persuasive of the genetic evidence in manic-depressive illness. The newer developments in the field are then explored, beginning with an explanation of new technologies and what can be expected to be learned from each. Among the techniques now being used in this field are pedigree analysis and analysis by restriction fragment length polymorphisms to identify specific chromosomal locations as potential genetic markers.

Chapter 16, on biochemical models, provides the conceptual base necessary to an appreciation of the biochemical and pharmacological studies that follow. Much of modern neurobiology and neuropharmacology has been driven by attempts to understand the effects of mood-altering drugs. Indeed, attempts to understand why certain drugs affect mood have inspired major hypotheses about the neurobiology of behavior. The chapter also describes animal models that have attempted to simulate affective illness. Chapter 17, on biochemistry and pharmacology, reviews the formidable literature on neurotransmitter and neuroendocrine function, along with neuropeptides, electrolytes, and membrane function. The first portion of the chapter is organized by biological system. The second re-examines the biochemical data in terms of important clinical correlates, such as phasic changes, well-state studies, and response predictors.

In Chapter 18, we consolidate three areas of contemporary inquiry—anatomy, physiology, and medical aspects—that traditionally are not included with the literature on pathophysiology. The unifying theme of the chapter is the novelty and sense of uncharted waters that these various fields bring to the study of manic-depressive illness. Neuroanatomy has not been in the mainstream of thinking about the biology of the illness, largely because fixed lesions do not seem to be compatible with the tendency of the illness to remit. With the emergence of the new brain-imaging technologies, it becomes important to review the anatomical correlates of mania and depression critically, if only to help guide the application of imaging approaches. Electrophysiology, a field historically more concerned with schizophrenia than manic-depressive illness, has produced some evidence supplementing what has been learned about brain laterality in anatomical studies. The concluding portion of the chapter includes the new and interesting leads in the areas of immunological, viral, and medical factors that may be implicated in manic-depressive illness. Although this literature is sparse, it will undoubtedly increase in importance.

Chapter 19 covers sleep and biological rhythms, reflecting our judgment that these two fields, which developed independently of one another, have found a natural point of convergence in the pathophysiology of manic-depressive illness. It is increasingly clear that sleep physiology is an important part of circadian physiology and that sleep disturbances found in affective illnesses may reflect disturbances in circadian rhythms. This area of study has, in our estimation, yielded some of the most interesting new developments in the understanding of the illness. The recent description of seasonal affective disorder, for example, represents a systematic, quantitative rediscovery of classic observations of seasonality in mood disorders. The speed with which the initial observation of seasonal mood disorder

was incorporated into DSM-III-R testifies to the responsiveness of our current diagnostic system. It demonstrates that a new concept can be evaluated, replicated or rejected, and if replicated, incorporated into standard diagnostic systems with dispatch.

Research on biological rhythms has spawned the development of three novel physiological but nonpharmacological treatments for mood disorders—partial sleep deprivation, phase advance, and high-intensity light—that are described in Chapter 22 on the treatment of acute bipolar depression. At a more general level, the contemporary focus on biological rhythms has given rise to environmental psychiatry, and thus the chapter emphasizes the subtle environmental influences on manic-depressive illness and offers relevant clinical suggestions.

Chapter 20, the last of the section, represents an attempt at synthesizing the pathophysiological evidence, but we realize that such an ambition is premature. Nevertheless, the chapter represents our effort to evaluate critically several of the major hypotheses reviewed in the section and to suggest what they may tell us about future directions for research. We offer these speculations about the future while being fully aware that predicting directions in research is always a hazardous, somewhat foolhardy undertaking. In thinking about the future, we emphasize biological findings that relate to recurrence and to underlying state-independent differences rather than to the state of mania or depression. Thus, we give high priority to the need for longitudinal approaches, as opposed to the cross-sectional approaches so prominent in many areas reviewed in this section.

Treatment

The final section of the book covers all aspects of the treatment of manic-depressive illness. It is traditional in its organization, separating acute from prophylactic treatment and medical from psychological treatment. Despite this division, we wish to emphasize the profound importance of integrating medical and psychological approaches. Although the structure of the section is traditional, the organization of each chapter is not. The first part of Chapters 21, 22, and 23 contains practical recommendations on clinical management. In the subsequent review of the treatment research literature in each of these chapters, we highlight areas inadequately explored in existing reviews. These areas include the efficacy of lithium in depression as well as mania and the quality of the prophylactic response. We discuss treatment controversies, for example, lithium versus tricyclics in preventing unipolar depression, the use of adjunctive treatments for breakthrough episodes during lithium prophylaxis, and the use of alternative or adjunctive approaches for patients who do not respond to lithium.

The two chapters on psychotherapy and compliance (Chapters 24 and 25) should be read together. Our purpose here is not to provide a general psychotherapy primer but to focus on issues of special importance to the psychotherapy of manic-depressive illness. These issues include fears of recurrence, dealing with psychological scars left by the illness, and concerns about genetic vulnerability. The central issue in the psychological management of bipolar patients is medication compliance, and recent studies suggest substantial enhancement of treatment outcome associated with adjunctive psychotherapy, no doubt reflecting the contribution of improved compliance. In the discussion of compliance in Chapter 25, we return to the core issue of the paradox of a very effective drug, which nevertheless can have an impact on aspects of the illness that might have been valued by the patient. Given the all-too-common tendency on the part of clinicians to be unaware of subtle compliance problems, we believe that this is an issue warranting a separate chapter. Another, Chapter 26, is devoted to the special treatment issues that arise in manic-depressive patients who abuse alcohol and drugs.

As bears repeated mention, manic-depressive illness is lethal. We have underscored this fact by summarizing what is known about suicide rates and clinical correlates in Chapter 10, and in the treatment section we emphasize clinical methods we think are most useful in reducing the risk of suicide among acutely ill patients (Chapter 27). We also emphasize again the fundamental premise that the best approach to the prevention of suicide lies in the effective and aggressive treatment of the underlying illness.

THE DEVELOPMENT OF THE BOOK

The awesome size of the literature on manic-depressive illness makes it all but impossible for clinicians and researchers to keep up and to see the broader clinical, human, and scientific picture. The National Library of Medicine's Medline file on bipolar disorder alone grows at a rate of more than 300 new citations a year; nearly 1,400 citations on other depressive disorders are added yearly. We were somewhat aware of the problem before we began this book. Over the past decade, as we struggled through that literature, we became increasingly concerned that the very magnitude of the new, scattered evidence is threatening a coherent overall view of the illness. In recent decades, research on the illness contributed to a geometric expansion of the knowledge base in increasingly specialized fields. The productivity of the research enterprise has generated diverse points of focus, which are often appreciated only by individuals in a given subfield. An unfortunate outgrowth of such specialization is that the wealth of new information typically has been made available only in the form of individual research reports or reviews of selected areas; at best, these occasionally are published in edited volumes.

Working during this period of extraordinary productivity and ferment in the study of manic-depressive illness, we saw the need for a comprehensive book that would attempt to impose order on a rich but vast and disparate literature. We were convinced that goal could be accomplished only by seeing the subject through from beginning to end—in other words, by writing a book rather than editing a collection. The only such comprehensive, interpretive review of bipolar manic-depressive illness available was John D. Campbell's *Manic Depressive Disease*, published in 1953 and clearly outdated. He was, after all, writing before the psychopharmacological revolution, which ushered in the era of biological psychiatry and the maturation of quantitative epidemiology, followed by molecular genetics, brain imaging, and other new technologies. Much the same can be said of the 1952 book *Manic-Depressive Illness and Allied Conditions* by Leopold Bellak and his colleagues, who approached the subject from a psychoanalytical frame of reference. More contemporary is the excellent monograph *Manic-Depressive Illness*, written by George Winokur, Paula Clayton, and Theodore Reich in 1969, which was less a review than an in-depth discussion of their study of 100 patients with manic-depressive illness.

Our own frustration with the rapidly enlarging literature was crystallized for us in a 1982 review of the highly regarded *Handbook of Affective Disorders,* edited by E. S. Paykel.[3] The reviewer praised the publication, but expressed his longing to know what Professor Paykel himself thought of the myriad aspects of the problem—that is, to see it through a single frame of reference. Joined by common interests, we presumed to undertake the task of offering a unified perspective that would attempt to integrate rather than merely juxtapose the extraordinary array of information that exists.

In the 10 years since we began this book, we have developed a profound respect for the judgment of the many talented scholars in our field who refrained from similar presumption. Yet, although the task has been far more difficult than we anticipated, writing this book has rewarded us personally and professionally. Our intention was to go beyond a review of the literature—to assess the nodal points in the knowledge of the illness, to integrate them in a way that would enhance the quality of clinical care available, and to suggest opportunities for future research. In the late 20th century, manic-depressive illness continues to present new challenges and questions that extend from the realm of basic neurobiological science to those of clinical and social ethics. The skill that the field brings to identifying these questions will determine the strategies formulated to answer them and, in turn, will bear directly on future gains in treatment and prevention.

Throughout the writing of this book, we have been impressed time and again by the excellent science, imaginative clinical research, and profoundly important treatments generated by so many of our colleagues. We are delighted to acknowledge our debt to them, both for their science and for the hundreds of thousands of lives that they have saved. Our debt to our patients is immeasurable.

NOTES

1. From *Collected Prose*, p. 286.
2. The contemporary rediscovery of Kraepelin has been well documented by Schorer (1982). For example, he notes that it was Kraepelin who first associated a relatively poor prognosis with rapid cycles, mixed states, and coexisting substance abuse, who noted the decreasing well intervals with time, and who developed the spectrum concept.
3. Crammer, 1982.

PART ONE

CLINICAL DESCRIPTION
AND DIAGNOSIS

It is not manic *and* depressive psychosis, but manic-depressive, indicating an entity
with varying mood reactions, one merging into another, not always by sudden re-
versals or changes in mood, but frequently by gradual transformations, often so
slight as to be imperceptible to the casual observer. Likewise, with the other emotional reactions in this disease, there is a pathologic *distortion* characterized by a
ceaseless undulation. (pp. 83-84)   —Campbell, 1953

The clinical manifestations of manic-depressive illness are exceptionally diverse. Expressed through
widely disparate temperaments, its symptoms, course, severity, and amenability to treatment differ
from individual to individual. Mood and behavior fluctuate in any one patient as well, waxing and
waning from one episode to another, one day to another. This variability calls to mind Winston
Churchill's injunction that "Things hardly ever happen the same way twice over, or if they seem to do
so, there is some variant which stultifies undue generalizations." Yet manic-depressive illness is among
the most consistently identifiable of all mental disorders, and it is one of the oldest, discernible in
descriptions of the Old Testament and recognized in clinical medicine almost 2,000 years ago.

This section (Chapters 2 through 5) presents the fundamental clinical concepts of manic-depressive
illness: the phenomenology of the disorder and its formal diagnostic structure and boundaries. For this
we turn first, in Chapter 2, to the description made by the earlier, classic clinicians who left their mark
by their extraordinary ability to capture in words the rich and vivid reality of their clinical observations.
We then supplement these medical views with those from patients, whose writings portray the fascinating, chaotic, and devastating personal experiences of this illness. We close by shifting to the structure of
data-based phenomenological studies, which complement and tie together the clinical description.

The three chapters that follow all pertain to diagnosis. Chapter 3 traces the evolution of the concept of
manic-depressive illness from the ancient Greco-Roman idea that mania is an end-stage of depression to
the seminal consolidation and synthesis at the beginning of this century and to Leonhard's splitting of
Kraepelin's unity into bipolar and unipolar forms. In re-examining this dichotomy, we focus on the need
to consider both cyclicity and polarity. We conclude that the more recurrent and serious forms of
unipolar disorder have much in common with bipolar illness.

Chapter 4 surveys the spectrum of manic-depressive illness in all its various dimensions. These
include the spectrum within the depressed and manic states, the range of severity from cyclothymia to
core bipolar illness, and the variations in the degree of polarity, the rapidity of cycling, the duration of
episodes, and the stability of changes in the affective state. The chapter opens with a discussion of the
compatibility of a dimensional view of these aspects of the illness, on the one hand, with the categorical
approach necessary for diagnostic structure, on the other.

The formal categories for manic-depressive illness found in the most widely used diagnostic systems are enumerated and evaluated in Chapter 5. Compared with the systems from which they evolved, contemporary taxonomies for classifying mental disorders are reliable, relatively easy to use, and remarkably free of etiological assumptions. Yet they have shortcomings: The criteria of contemporary systems sacrifice specificity in their focus on cross-sectional presenting signs and symptoms, without a means of incorporating prior course and family history. Further, the separation of bipolar disorders from depressive disorders at the outset seems to prejudge the complex issue of subgroup relationships. Also problematic is the treatment of mild forms of mania, which are given less diagnostic prominence than warranted by clinical reality. Returning to the positive side, present-day diagnostic systems have standardized and clarified approaches to differentiating manic-depressive illness from schizophrenia and organic brain disorders.

Three concerns have determined the scope and substance of these chapters. First, the requirements of sound research have produced operational criteria for selecting homogeneous groups of clinical subjects. Extended into clinical diagnostic systems, the criteria, as noted, have made diagnoses more objective and reliable. Commendable as they are, these achievements have been purchased at a price. Rarely does one encounter discussions of mental illness in current journal articles that fully represent the varieties and texture of experience. Traditional psychiatric literature is filled with descriptions that make today's accounts seem arid.

Second, we believe that the relationship between bipolar and unipolar forms of affective illness has become somewhat obscured, especially in American usage. When the polarity distinction was introduced in the 1960s from the European studies of Leonhard, Angst, and Perris and the European-style studies of the Washington University group in St. Louis, the universe of patients was bound by the Kraepelinian concept of manic-depressive illness: It encompassed "endogenomorphic" affective illness with a prior course, that is, recurrent depressive disorders. However, as the bipolar–unipolar distinction was applied to the broader American category of affective illness, unipolar depression became diffuse, since it incorporated a wide range of depressive states and conditions that had in common only one unifying characteristic—they were not bipolar.

A third concern that has shaped these chapters is comprised of two conflicting parts. In marking out the territory encompassed by manic-depressive illness, we believe it essential to include so-called bipolar-II disorder, that is, illness characterized by a pattern of depressive and hypomanic episodes. Indeed, it is the underdiagnosis of hypomania that explains why the frequency of bipolar illness has been so underestimated. This is scarcely just an academic issue, since the inappropriate treatment of bipolar-II patients can lead to full-blown mania. Originally, the bipolar-II pattern was described in patients who had been hospitalized for their depression. Now, appropriately, it encompasses patients whose hypomania alternates with depressive episodes of varying severity. As this practice expands, it raises questions about differentiating manic-depressive illness from normal variants in personality or personality disorders. Although, if carried too far, this could lead to overdiagnosis, we believe that, by and large, the underdiagnosis of bipolar disorder is still a major problem.

In summary, this section of the book describes the wide varieties of temperament, experience, and pathological states that comprise manic-depressive illness. It also reviews the diagnostic systems that have sought to establish categories and borders. Although we remain impressed by the diversity of illness, we also acknowledge the stable coherence of the diagnostic concept.

2

Clinical Description

. . . notwithstanding manifold external differences certain common fundamental features yet recur in all the morbid states mentioned. Along with changing symptoms, which may appear temporarily or may be completely absent, we meet in all forms of manic-depressive insanity a quite definite, narrow group of disorders, though certainly of very varied character and composition. Without any one of them being absolutely characteristic of the malady, still in association they impress a uniform stamp on all the multiform clinical states. (p. 2)

—Emil Kraepelin, 1921

To understand manic-depressive illness—to diagnose it accurately and to treat it effectively—requires close familiarity with what Kraepelin called "the common fundamental features of the disease." This chapter gives a general description of hypomanic and manic states, depressive states, and mixed states, as well as the cyclothymic features that often underlie these states.[1] Clinical description is approached from three perspectives: that of uniquely experienced and observant classic clinicians, such as Professor Emil Kraepelin, that of manic-depressive patients themselves, and that of clinical investigators who have conducted data-based studies. By combining these perspectives (at the unavoidable cost of some redundancy), we hope to capitalize on the descriptive and heuristic strengths of each while avoiding the limitations of any one alone.

We have chosen to quote from the classic clinical literature, often predating pharmacotherapy, for several reasons: First, descriptions found in these sources are powerful and have not been superseded; Kraepelin, particularly, remains without peer. Second, the lack of effective treatments and a tendency to take care of patients over many years, often lifetimes, allowed prepharmacotherapy clinicians to observe the relatively unimpeded course of the illness, as well as its severity. Third, modern diagnostic systems, al-

though vital in advancing treatment and research, have resulted in less emphasis on clinical description and proportionately more emphasis on data-based articles. Few psychiatric residents, graduate students, scientists, and clinicians now read Kraepelin and Bleuler. Fewer still have read Aretaeus, Griesinger, Falret, Campbell, or Henderson and Gillespie. We believe that the clinical writings of these individuals provide both historical perspective and a singular understanding of the nature of manic-depressive illness.

The quotations from manic-depressive patients provide the subjective dimension missing from clinicians' and researchers' reports, however astute their observations. These descriptions, which vary widely, reflect both the nature of the illness and the nature of people. In the scientific literature, relatively scant attention is paid to firsthand accounts of manic-depressive illness. The clinical sciences more often have relied on taxonomic systems, clinical description, and diagnostic and objective observer ratings as a basis for studying and describing psychotic illnesses. One reason for this virtual exclusion of experiential information is that it is highly subjective and possibly distorted. Thus, patients may remember with clarity some aspects of their disorder and forget or ignore others; they may verbalize what is easiest to describe and say nothing about aspects less readily articulated. They may relate only those experiences most novel to them, giving disproportionate weight to out-of-the-ordinary events, or they may describe what they think the observer wishes to hear. Further, people most able to discuss their experiences articulately may be, by virtue of this fact, atypical. In addition, moods can radically alter memory and perceptions and can result in state-dependent distortions.

These are legitimate concerns to anyone wishing systematic, clear-cut, and reducible data. Clinicians have long been aware, however, that experiential data are vital to an understanding of individuals and their illnesses. Likewise, the heuristic value of hypotheses generated from patients' descriptions of their feelings, thoughts, and behaviors is well established. Good clinical management of manic-depressive illness, both pharmacological and psychotherapeutic, depends on recognizing the concerns of patients and the positive and negative consequences it has for them. Descriptive information gathered from patients also has been important in clinical research studies, such as those describing the switch process (Bunney et al., 1972a, b, c) or unraveling the paradoxical effects of lithium as both an antidepressant and antimanic agent (Goodwin et al., 1969).

There are strong limitations on the effective use of language to describe unusual events, such as extreme moods, gross cognitive and perceptual distortions, and both subtle and profound changes in sensory experience. Lowe (1973) has noted that "ordinary language does not describe subjective experiences equally well in different sense modalities (cf. visual or auditory experiences as against gustatory, olfactory, or kinaesthetic experiences)." Yeats (1962), in discussing the idiosyncrasies of the language of moods, put it somewhat differently in his remarks about a mystic: "The poems were all endeavors to capture some high, impalpable mood in a net of obscure images . . . these were often embedded in thoughts which have evidently a special value to his mind, but are to other men the counters of an unknown coinage."

Despite the shortcomings of language and the highly personalized vocabulary often used by patients in describing their manic-depressive illness, certain words, phrases, and metaphors are chosen time and again, forming a common matrix of experiences. Often these images center on nature, weather, the day/night cycle, and the seasons; often, too, they convey unpredictability, periodicity, tempestuousness, or a bleak dearth of feelings. Religious themes and mystical experiences pervade the language, again conveying an extraordinary degree and type of experience, one beyond control, comprehension, or adequate description.

At a narrower conceptual level, certain individual words and phrases are heard repeatedly by clinicians treating patients with manic-depressive illness. Depression carries with it common language fragments: The patient is "slowed down," "in a fog," or "tired" and describes life as having "lost its color," "dull, flat, and dreary." Everything is "hopeless," "heavy," "too much of an effort," "drab, colorless, pointless." Life is a "burden," and things just "drag on and on."

Hypomania and mania elicit descriptions of a much livelier and more energetic kind. Life is "effortless," "charged with intensity," and filled with "special meaning." The patient is "racing," "speeded up," "wired," "hyper," "high as a kite," "moving in the fast lane," "ecstatic," "full of energy," "flying." Other people are described as "too slow" and "can't keep up."

The clinical descriptions derived from data-based studies compensate, in part, for the selective attention of both clinicians and patients. They provide a more objective view of the frequency and character of symptoms in manic-depressive illness. In selecting such studies for this chapter, we have to some extent emphasized manic states, partly because differential diagnosis is more problematic in mania and partly because far more systematic studies of symptoms and their profiles have been carried out on mania than on bipolar depression, mixed states, or cyclothymia. The relative scarcity of data-based studies on bipolar depression is a cause for both surprise and concern. There is, however, an exceedingly large general literature on depression, which, unfortunately, seldom parcels out bipolar depression from the many nonbipolar forms. Recent data-based clinical studies, although using standardized diagnostic criteria and making the necessary distinctions between bipolar and unipolar depression, have not tended to focus on clinical patterns of bipolar depression but rather on such issues as psychotic (or delusional) versus nonpsychotic (or nondelusional) status. Usually, bipolar patients have been excluded from these samples.

The same caveats about methodology apply here as apply in all discussion of research findings about manic-depressive illness: First, diagnostic criteria and expertise vary across studies. Second, investigators often fail to specify the stage, severity, or duration of the affective state. Third, measurement techniques lack sophistication; there is a tendency, for example, to measure only the presence or absence of a symptom, rather than its intensity, constancy, and duration. Other problems exist as well. For instance, the interesting and illuminating clinical study done by Winokur and his colleagues (1969), although an invaluable contribution to the literature, suffers from having analyzed data based on multiple episodes (e.g., 100 episodes of mania in 61 patients). To the extent that a given individual shows a similar symptom pattern from one affective episode to another, a contaminating element is introduced.

We present in this chapter only those aspects of symptom presentation relevant to clinical description. These include the observable patterns of mood, thought, and behavior typically used in clinical diagnosis. (Detailed discussion of related topics are found in Chapters 4, 5, 11, 12, and 18.)

Many generalizations can be made from the clinical descriptions of manic-depressive illness, but individuals are bound to differ widely in an illness that is genetically based, environmentally influenced, and psychologically expressed. Kraepelin (1921), although committed to the idea and practice of classification, also was sensitive to the infinite capacity for individual expression in the illness. Referring to the subclassifications proposed by earlier writers, he wrote: "I am convinced that that kind of effort . . . must of necessity wreck on the irregularity of the disease" (p. 139). Clinical differences across individuals can be striking (as are, more often, their similarities), but it remains unclear how much one episode resembles another in a given individual. Anecdotal accounts, but little systematic data, support some constancy of psychotic and non-psychotic features in the same patient across time.[2]

Finally, although much of the clinical description emphasizes differences across clinical states, we stress from the start that the oscillation into, out of, and within the various forms and states of

the disease is, in its own right, a hallmark of manic-depressive illness. Manic and depressive symptom patterns clearly have a polar quality, but the overlapping, transitional, and fluctuating aspects are enormously important in describing and understanding the illness as a whole. Thus, Kraepelin (1921) wrote:

The delimitation of the individual clinical forms of the malady is in many respects wholly artificial and arbitrary. Observation not only reveals the occurrence of gradual transitions between all the various states, but it also shows that within the shortest space of time the same morbid case may pass through most manifold transformations. (p. 54)

Campbell (1953) emphasized this fundamentally dynamic nature of manic-depressive illness by comparing the illness with a movie:

The fluidity, change, and movement of the emotions, as they occur in the ever-changing cyclothymic process, may be compared to the pictures of a cinema, as contrasted with a "still" photograph. Indeed, the psychiatrist, observing a manic-depressive patient for the first time, or as he undergoes one of the many undulations in mood, from melancholia to euphoria or from hypomania to a depression, is reminded of the experience of entering a movie during the middle of the story. No matter where one takes up the plot, the story tends to swing around again to the point where it started. The examiner may observe the manic-depressive patient first in a manic reaction, later in a depression, but eventually, if followed long enough, in another manic reaction. Like the movie, which is a continuous but constantly changing process, the cyclothymic process is also continuous even though for the moment the observer is attracted by the immediate cross-section view. This conception of change, or constant undulation of the emotions, is much more accurate than a static appraisal. (pp. 112-113)

For each of the clinical states and patterns discussed—mania, depression, mixed states, and cyclothymia—clinical description in three general areas of functioning is presented: mood, cognition and perception, and activity and behavior. First, however, we introduce the disorder with a general description drawn from the experience of patients.

THE PATIENT'S EXPERIENCE: AN OVERVIEW

There is a particular kind of pain, elation, loneliness, and terror involved in this kind of madness. When you're high it's tremendous. The ideas and feelings are fast and frequent like shooting stars and you follow them until you find better and brighter ones. Shyness goes, the right words and gestures are suddenly there, the power to seduce and captivate others a felt certainty. There are interests found in uninteresting people. Sensuality is pervasive and the desire to seduce and be seduced irresistible. Feelings of ease, intensity, power, well-being, financial omnipotence, and euphoria now pervade one's marrow. But, somewhere, this changes. The fast ideas are far too fast and there are far too many; overwhelming confusion replaces clarity. Memory goes. Humor and absorption on friends' faces are replaced by fear and concern. Everything previously moving with the grain is now against—you are irritable, angry, frightened, uncontrollable, and enmeshed totally in the blackest caves of the mind. You never knew those caves were there. It will never end. Madness carves its own reality. It goes on and on and finally there are only others' recollections of your behavior— your bizarre, frenetic, aimless behaviors—for mania has at least some grace in partially obliterating memories. What then, after the medications, psychiatrist, despair, depression, and overdose? All those incredible feelings to sort through. Who is being too polite to say what? Who knows what? What did I do? Why? And most hauntingly, when will it happen again? Then, too, are the annoyances—medicine to take, resent, forget, take, resent, and forget, but always to take. Credit cards revoked, bounced checks to cover, explanations due at work, apologies to make, intermittent memories of vague men (what *did* I do?), friendships gone or drained, a ruined marriage. And always, when will it happen again? Which of my feelings are real? Which of the me's is me? The wild, impulsive, chaotic, energetic, and crazy one? Or the shy, withdrawn, desperate, suicidal, doomed, and tired one? Probably a bit of both, hopefully much that is neither. Virginia Woolf, in her dives and climbs, said it all: "How far do our feelings take their colour from the dive underground? I mean, what is the reality of any feeling?" —Patient with manic-depressive illness

This description of manic-depressive illness was written by a patient who, by the age of 30, had been through two violently psychotic manic episodes, countless hypomanias and mixed states, several incapacitating and lengthy depressions, and a nearly lethal suicide attempt. Alluded to are many of the same fears and worries common to most individuals with manic-depressive illness: the frightening, tumultuous, and extremely damaging aspects—to self and others—of manias and depressions, the powerful effects of the illness on subsequent functioning, ongoing and potential relationships, and general expectations of the future, the inherent unpredictability of the course of the disease, and the ongoing fear, often terror, of recurrence of illness. Practical consequences of mania and depression usually include, among others, the alienation of friends, lovers, and family members, the inability to move forward or naturally in a career, and major financial problems stemming from overspending, ill-considered investments, substantial and often uninsurable medical expenses, and foregone production.

Additionally, many manic-depressive individuals find it difficult to adjust to the idea of having a serious, chronic, and life-threatening illness, one generally requiring lifelong maintenance medication, with side effects, for its control. Subtle features pervade this illness, including a fundamental, if usually transitory, inability to perceive reality with accuracy and to judge a course of action with prudence. Once an acute episode is over, the person is left with palpably shaken self-confidence. For a considerable period following a manic or depressive episode, many patients continue to question their judgment, their ability to assess situations, and their capacity to understand their relationships with other people.

Etiological assumptions made about the illness deeply affect the highly individualized experience of manic-depressive illness. Despite the compelling arguments that can be made for the biological origins of the illness—and despite their potential for alleviating its associated guilt and stigma—patients often find these explanations intuitively unpersuasive, especially in the early stages of illness. Thus, although some patients do experience profound depression as biologically rooted, others interpret it as a spiritual ordeal, and still others as psychological in origin. Hypomania is often perceived as highly intoxicating, powerful, productive, and desirable. Patients find it difficult to think of it as a sickness or as part of the same illness as depression and mania.

Common themes appear repeatedly in patients' descriptions of their illness. They are fearful of recurrence, they are concerned about transmitting it to their offspring, they feel shame and humiliation, they suffer the havoc wrought by each episode on their relationships with others, they confront disturbing psychological issues during recovery, and they reflect on the long-term meaning of the illness in their lives.

Fears of Recurrence

Fears that the illness will return are common and often form the crux of patients' concerns about work and personal relationships (see Chapter 24). For example, Robert Lowell (1977) wrote, with morbid wit, in his poem, "Since 1939": "if we see a light at the end of the tunnel,/it's the light of an oncoming train."

A physician, hospitalized several times for mania, described his fears of recurrence (especially of mania), as well as the damaging effects his illness had on his career:

Two years is a long time out of professional medical circulation—things forgotten, things not learned or heard of, but the most daunting problem is the prospect of further episodes of mania. The depression if it occurs is a more private feature of the syndrome. Mania is very public with a multitude of interested parties. . . .

Questions remain: will there be further episodes; how frequently; and will they be as debilitating? No-one can offer guarantees or even reliable answers yet. Meanwhile what about my capacity to work, earn a living, to occupy myself, and fulfil my responsibilities? The qualities for a doctor are vastly different from those of a poet. A hospital consultant is nothing if not reliable. My unreliability is already manifest. (Anonymous, *Lancet*, 1984, p. 1268)

Fears of Inheritance

Another typical concern derives from the heritable component in manic-depressive illness. Many patients, having grown up in an environment of extreme mood swings, express fear they will end up like the affected parent, especially when that parent has been severely disabled, repeatedly hospitalized, or alcoholic. The fear is even greater if the parent committed suicide. The daughter of a manic-depressive woman described her fear of inheriting the illness and her difficulty in establishing an independent identity:

Ever since I was small, I have been told that I was just like my mother. I was named after her, and very soon I took to thinking that I was going to be committed when I was 21, like she was. . . . I was sure that they were going to come and haul me away. . . . I felt that the only way I could separate my thoughts and feelings from her would be for her to die, and I often hated her and wished for her death, especially when she was manic. (Anthony, 1975b, p. 292)

Often, too, patients (and their spouses) agonize over the possibility of passing on the illness to children. Joshua Logan, in his autobiography, wrote about this fear, expressed in a conversation between Logan and his first wife:

I asked her if she wanted to have children with me. She said no.
I asked why, but she refused to answer. . . . she

would never have children by me, and that I should know why. I looked at her blankly, and she added:
"I have no wish to bring insane children into this world." (Logan, 1976, p. 153)

Shame

Manic-depressive individuals experience acute shame and humiliation for many reasons: because of psychosis (particularly manic) and shame for bizarre and inappropriate behavior, violence, financial irregularities, and sexual indiscretions, to name a few of the common problems. One patient stated, "No one who has not had the experience can realize the mortification of having been insane" (Reiss, 1910). Robert Lowell, in "Home," described the indignities of psychiatric hospitalization: "we might envy museum pieces/that can be pasted together or disfigured/and feel no indignity" (1977). And Graves (1942) wrote:

While the intoxication of mania lasts, I for one have no disposition to embrace death. After the intoxication is over, my chief emotional reaction is shame and disgust with myself, and a wonder that my fear of death could be so wonderfully and idiotically twisted. That the facing humiliation, of despair, or deprivation should produce a desire for death is quite natural.

Joshua Logan, in turn, described his chagrin in the wake of a manic episode:

How can I go back to the theatre after all I've put my friends through, after all the galloping whispers and all the people who've seen me in this strange state? How will anybody, as long as I live, believe that I'm well again? (Logan, 1976, p. 180)

In portions of two letters to T. S. Eliot, Robert Lowell wrote of his embarrassment following two different manic episodes:

[June 1961] The whole business has been very bruising, and it is fierce facing the pain I have caused, and humiliating [to] think that it has all happened before and that control and self-knowledge come so slowly, if at all.

[March 1964] I want to apologize for plaguing you with so many telephone calls last November and December. When the "enthusiasm" is coming on me it is accompanied by a feverish reaching to my friends. After it's over I wince and wither. (Robert Lowell, cited in I. Hamilton, 1982, pp. 286, 307)

Interpersonal Problems

The widely varying reactions of others to the person who has manic-depressive illness include anger, concern, withdrawal, unrealistically high or low expectations, rejection, and denial of the illness.[3] Robert Lowell (1977) wrote of the isolation, pain, and misunderstanding experienced during one of his hospitalizations for mania:

> At visiting hours, you could experience
> my sickness only as desertion. . . .
> Dr. Berners compliments you again,
> "A model guest . . . we would welcome
> Robert back to Northamptom any time,
> the place suits him . . . he is so strong."
> I am on the wrong end of a dividing train—
> it is my failure with our fragility.

John Custance, a British writer and former naval intelligence officer, described the denial of others after his release from a psychiatric hospital. He also depicted his own denial and the gradual sealing-over process so characteristic of the recuperation period:

> But once I get out of a Mental Hospital all this changes. I find myself in a totally different "atmosphere". I cannot, however hard I try, get even my most intimate relatives and friends to understand or take any interest in what may or may not have happened to me during my "madness". Gradually the vividness of my memory fades; like my relatives, I try to put the whole experience out of my mind, and in fact it does to a certain extent disappear into "lower levels of my Unconscious". Then I find myself genuinely wondering whether these memories so far as they are conscious at all, are not "delusions", "hallucinations", as "unreal" as the actual technical hallucination I know I have had and have described earlier. (Custance, 1952, p. 115)

A different kind of denial, a "conspiracy of silence," is described by Norman Endler, a Canadian psychologist writing about his illness (depression with hypomania) and the effect it had on those around him:

> In April 1977, when I first started getting depressed, not only did I deny it to myself but so did my friends and colleagues. My secretary and administrative assistant, as indicated earlier, asked me what was wrong. My gradual withdrawal from interaction, my lack of cheerfulness, and my quietness were interpreted by them as anger at something done wrong. After about four weeks my wife insisted that I should see a doctor. My children said nothing to me. My colleagues at York said nothing to me, and the professionals (psychiatrists, psychologists, and social workers) in the Department of Psychiatry, Toronto East General Hospital, said nothing to me. I'm sure that some, if not most of them, must have noticed that something was wrong with me. (If they had not, they shouldn't be working in the mental health field.)
>
> Why did my colleagues participate in an unintended "conspiracy of silence"? There are a number of factors

to consider. First, suppose they commented on my depression and they were wrong. Suppose I wasn't really depressed but only very tired. This would have been most embarrassing for them. Second, some people do not like to interfere or intrude in the lives of others. Third, suppose it were true that I was depressed. How could they handle it without embarrassing me? The fact that I was chairman might have been another factor. Because the "show" was running smoothly, there was not need to question the chief executive officer. My guess is that my friends didn't say anything because they probably couldn't believe that it was true . . . when I was hypomanic, none of my colleagues confronted me. Here, again, they were following the social norm of not interfering. Because I had previously been depressed, they probably perceived it as a recuperative period and gave me the benefit of the doubt. (Endler, 1982, pp. 148-149)

Recovery

The postpsychotic or recovery phase is an important but seldom discussed aspect of manic-depressive illness. The recovery to normal thinking and feeling and the adjustment to the interpersonal, medical, professional, and financial consequences of mania and depression are usually slow, exhausting, frustrating, and partially futile experiences for patients. In the following passage, one patient describes the stages in her recovery from a manic episode:

> The first symptom of recovery was a gradually increasing power to direct my thoughts into desired channels. I discovered that what seemed to be facts were in many cases delusions. Suddenly one day a feeling of self-control returned. The rapidity of thought seemed greatly lessened, and I was once more able to concentrate my mind on one subject for more than a few minutes at a time. Then came the feeling that I was well and must go home. Previous to this I realized my abnormal mental condition, and had no desire to see or be seen by my friends. Now I was seized with an eager longing to see my relatives and friends. It was like coming back from the dead. I overcame my restlessness by cleaning, scrubbing, mending and writing. My brain seemed unusually active and clear. I wrote for hours at a time; essays, poems, aphorisms, etc., flowed from my pen with great rapidity. I again began to take an interest in my personal appearance, and gradually returned to my normal mental health state. (Reiss, 1910)

Virginia Woolf, in a letter written in 1910 from a hospital while she was confined for mania, described the slowness and subtlety of psychological recovery: "I have been out in the garden for 2 hours; and feel quite normal. I feel my brains, like a pear, to see if its [sic] ripe; it will be exquisite by September" (Woolf, 1975). She also described the gradual return from depression to normality: "I think the blood has really been getting into my brain at last: It is the oddest feeling, as though a dead part of me were coming to life" (cited in Love, 1977).

The recovery period typically is filled with anxieties about things done, or left undone, during the preceding mania or depression, concerns about the future, and fears about the completeness of recovery. Robert Lowell, in his poem, "Home," articulated an apprehension expressed by many manic-depressive individuals: the denial by physicians and family members of painful chinks in the patient's psychological armor, as well as the erosive nature of the cumulative effects brought about by repeated episodes: " 'Remarkable breakdown, remarkable recovery' "—/but the breakage can go on repeating/once too often" (see also Chapter 24).

Uncertainty about the future, as well as confusion about the origins and meaning of the illness, were expressed by Joshua Logan (1976):

Still, none of that shook off the dreariness of having an illness that didn't seem like one, of not knowing how or when I'd be rid of it, of not knowing even why it had happened to me, of having iron bars on the windows—even though those bars were fashioned like curlicued decorative devices. Was I ever, ever, going to get out? And if I did—what would I do? Where would I go? (p. 178)

Inevitable ruminations about behavior when ill, especially when manic, are part of the recovery phase:

I've been out of my *excitement* for over a month, I think, now, and am in good spirits, though I don't feel any rush of eloquence to talk about the past. It's like recovering from some physical injury, such as a broken leg or jaundice, yet there's no disclaiming these outbursts—they are part of my character—me at moments. . . . The whole business was sincere enough, but a stupid pathological mirage, a magical orange grove in a nightmare. I feel like a son of a bitch. (Lowell, cited in I. Hamilton, 1982, p. 218)

Lowell, born into an old-line Boston family, where "Lowells talk only to Cabots and Cabots talk only to God," wrote poignantly of his fall from "pedigreed tulip to weed" in his painful recovery:

Recuperating, I neither spin nor toil.
Three stories down below,
a choreman tends our coffin's length of soil,
and seven horizontal tulips blow.

Just twelve months ago,
these flowers were pedigreed
imported Dutchmen; now no one need
distinguish them from weed.
Bushed by the late spring snow,
they cannot meet
another year's snowballing enervation.
I keep no rank nor station.
Cured, I am frizzled, stale and small.

Long-Term Perspectives

Manic-depressive illness summons up in those who have it strong, often ambivalent feelings (see Chapters 24 and 25). Here we present the reflections of a few patients about the general influence of manic-depressive illness on their lives. John Custance (1952) described the relationship between his illness and his ethical and religious beliefs:

Manic-depression brought to me—as it does to nearly all who suffer from it—an intense emotional religious experience, very foreign to the temper of staid Anglicanism in which I was brought up. Is it true? Perhaps the question is wrongly put, and so unanswerable. But I cannot set it down as meaningless and go on as though it had never been. It is far too intimately a part of me; it is the unforgettable and inescapable. On my strange journey there were giddy heights as well as depths. (p. 13)

In a letter to poet John Berryman, also manic-depressive (see Chapter 14), Robert Lowell discussed their chaotic lives:

All winter I've had an uncomfortable feeling of dying into rebirth. Not at all the sick, dizzy allegorized thing such words suggest and which I've felt going off my rocker. But the flat prose of coming to an end of one way of life, whittled down and whittled down and picking up nothing new though always about to. . . .
What queer lives we've had even for poets! There seems something generic about it, and determined beyond anything we could do. You and I have had so many of the same tumbles and leaps. We must have a green old age. We both have drunk the downward drag as deeply as is perhaps bearable. (Lowell, 1962, cited in I. Hamilton, 1982, p. 298)

The following essay written by a manic-depressive patient touches on many of the issues mentioned earlier and brings into focus a few of the positive aspects of the illness that many patients, once stabilized on medication, report having experienced (see Chapters 14, 24, and 25):

I have often asked myself whether, given the choice, I would choose to have manic-depressive illness. If lithium were not available to me, or didn't work for me, the answer would be a simple No—and it would be an answer laced with terror. But lithium does work for me and therefore I suppose I can afford to pose the question. Strangely enough I think I would choose to have it. It's complicated. Depression is awful beyond words or sounds or images; I would not go through an extended one again. It bleeds relationships through suspicion, lack of confidence and self-respect, the inability to enjoy life, to walk or talk or think normally, the exhaustion, the night terrors, the day terrors. There is nothing good to be said for it except that it gives you the experience of how it must be to be old, to be old and sick, to be dying; to be slow of mind, to be lacking in grace, polish, and coordination; to be ugly; to have no belief in the possibilities of life, the pleasures of sex, the exquisiteness of music, or the ability to make yourself and others laugh.

I get enraged when others imply they know what it is like to be depressed because they have gone through a divorce, lost a job, or broken up with someone. Those experiences carry with them feelings. Depression, instead, is truly flat, stale, and unprofitable. It is also true, absolutely so, that people cannot abide being around you when you are depressed. They might think they ought to, and they might even try, but you know and they know that you're a pain in the ass: you're irritable and paranoid and humorless and lifeless and critical and demanding and no reassurance is ever enough. You're frightened, and you're frightening, and you're "not at all like yourself but will be soon," but you know you won't.

So why would I want anything to do with this illness? Because I honestly believe that as a result of it I have felt more things, more deeply; had more experiences, more intensely; loved more, and been more loved; laughed more often for having cried more often; appreciated more the springs, for all the winters; worn death "as close as dungarees," appreciated it—and life—more; seen the finest and the most terrible in people, and slowly learned the values of caring, loyalty, and seeing things through. I think I have seen the breadth and depth and width of my mind and heart, and seen how frail they both are, and how ultimately unknowable they both are. Depressed, I have crawled on my hands and knees in order to get across a room, and have done it for month after month. But, normal or high, I have run faster, thought faster, loved faster than most I know. And I think much of this is related to my illness—the intensity it gives to things and the perspective it forces on me. I think it has made me test the limits of my mind (which, while wanting, is holding), and the limits of my upbringing, family, education, and friends.

The countless hypomanias, and mania itself, all have brought into my life a different level of sensing and feeling and thinking. Even when I have been most psychotic—delusional, hallucinating, frenzied—I have been aware of finding new corners in my mind and heart. Some of those corners were incredible and beautiful and took my breath away and made me feel as though I could die right then and the images would

sustain me. Some of them were grotesque and ugly and I never wanted to know they were there or ever to see them again. But, always, there were those new corners and—when feeling my normal self—I cannot imagine becoming jaded to life, because I know of those limitless corners, with their limitless views.

HYPOMANIC AND MANIC STATES

Classic Descriptions

Manic states are characterized typically by heightened mood, more and faster speech, quicker thought, brisker physical and mental activity levels, and more energy (with a corresponding decreased need for sleep), irritability, perceptual acuity, paranoia, heightened sexuality, and impulsivity. In hypomania, the less severe form of mania, these changes are generally moderate and may or may not result in serious problems for the individual experiencing them. As the episode intensifies, however, they profoundly disrupt the lives of manic patients, their families, and society. The degree, type, and chronicity of cognitive, perceptual, and behavioral disorganization determine the subclassifications or stages of mania: hypomania, acute mania, delirious mania, and chronic mania. The first three forms of mania correspond, with some exceptions, to the stages of mania delineated in more recent, data-based investigations (e.g., Carlson and Goodwin, 1973). Thus, hypomania is roughly equivalent to stage-I mania, acute mania to stage-II, and delirious mania to stage-III. Detailed quantitative descriptions of these more recently conceptualized stages of mania are presented in Chapter 4.

Hypomania

Mood, cognitive, and behavioral changes in hypomania can be pronounced or subtle, and they lend themselves well to astute and interesting clinical description.

Mood. Mood in hypomania is usually ebullient, self-confident, and exalted, but with an irritable underpinning. Most clinical investigators emphasize the elevated, volatile, and fluctuating nature of hypomanic mood. Campbell (1953) describes, on the one hand, the euphoric aspect of mood:

Associated with the euphoria there is a genuine feeling of well-being, mentally and physically, a feeling of happiness and exhilaration which transports the individual into a new world of unlimited ideas and possibilities. . . . When a 19-year-old manic was advised that he was indeed ill, he replied, "if I'm ill, this is the most wonderful illness I ever had." (pp. 151, 153)

Kraepelin (1921) described the euphoric aspect of hypomanic mood but also emphasized the quick changes, irritability, and rage that are integral to it:

Mood is predominantly exalted and cheerful, influenced by the feeling of heightened capacity for work. The patient is in imperturbable good temper, sure of success, "courageous," feels happy and merry, not rarely overflowingly so. . . .

On the other hand there often exists a great emotional irritability. The patient is dissatisfied, intolerant, fault-finding . . . he becomes pretentious, positive, regardless, impertinent and even rough, when he comes up against opposition to his wishes and inclinations; trifling external occasions may bring about extremely violent outbursts of rage. (p. 56)

Cognition and Perception. Cognition and perception, especially the former, are, like mood, strongly altered in hypomania. Falret (1854, cited in Sedler, 1983) wrote that "profusion of ideas is prodigious," and most authors emphasize that, to a point, associations of thinking can be furthered by mild hypomania. They also comment that thought is relatively intact in the less severe forms of mania:

The *thinking* of the manic is flighty. He jumps by by-paths from one subject to another, and cannot adhere to anything. With this the ideas run along very easily and involuntarily, even so freely that it may be felt as unpleasant by the patient. . . .

Because of the more rapid flow of ideas, and especially because of the falling off of inhibitions, artistic activities are facilitated even though something worth while is produced only in very mild cases and when the patient is otherwise talented in this direction. The heightened sensibilities naturally have the effect of furthering this. (Bleuler, 1924, pp. 466, 468)

Activity and Behavior. Activity and behavior are greatly increased and diversified in hypomania. Patients become seemingly indefatigable, firmly opinionated, and interpersonally aggressive. Additionally:

The manic patient may expend a considerable amount of his energy and pressure of ideas in writing. His writing is demonstrative, flashy, rhetorical and bombastic. He insists that the physician must read every word, even though the content is biased, full of repetition, rambling and circumstantial. Capital letters are used unnecessarily, sentences are underscored and flight of ideas and distractibility destroy the coherence of the theme. The subject of the manic's writing often pertains to the correction of wrongs, religious tangents, gaining his freedom, institution of lawsuits. . . .

One patient made three visits to Washington to obtain a patent on a cotton-chopping machine; another attempted to speak to the President by long-distance telephone to warn him that the Russians might land on the coast of Florida. Urged on by the pressure of ideas as well as an excess of physical energy the manic patient has an inner drive which will not allow him to rest. (Campbell, 1953, pp. 152, 154-155)

The following case history of hypomania is taken from the excellent clinical descriptions of Henderson and Gillespie (1956):

The patient . . . had been an extraordinarily capable man . . . and had reached a position of great distinction. He was always of an aggressive type, very much a leader, described by some as too independent, by others as an agitator, and, by his son, as one who could not brook opposition. . . .

After arrival he stated that it seemed as if he had entered Paradise after escaping from Hell, but he immediately wished to alter the domestic arrangements to meet his own whims. . . . When asked by the nurse not to disturb the others, he abused and cursed her. At breakfast he talked incessantly, and made offensive personal remarks. He pointed out that one of the Matrons did not look well—that no doubt she had "spent the night on the tiles". . . . He called on the local lawyer, and wasted his time, telling him of all the actions he intended to bring. He troubled the doctor, who in consequence tried to avoid him, but this could not be done, as the patient stood beside his motor until the doctor was forced to appear and listen to his rambling talk. (pp. 239-240)

Acute Mania

Acute mania is strikingly different from both normal and hypomanic states in cognition, perception, and behavior. In contrast, mood differs little from that seen in hypomania, although subjective distress is heightened palpably.

Mood. Mood in acute mania is not described well by the classic writers, perhaps because psychotic cognition and behavior are more obvious. Kraepelin (1921), however, did write that:

Mood is unrestrained, merry, exultant, occasionally visionary or pompous, but always subject to frequent variation, easily changing to irritability and irascibility or even to lamentation and weeping. (p. 63)

Cognition and Perception. Cognition and perception become fragmented and often psychotic in acute mania. Coherence gives way to incoherence; rapid thinking proceeds to racing and disjointed thinking; distractibility becomes all-pervasive. Paranoid and grandiose delusions are common, as are illusions and hallucinations. In Kraepelin's description (1921), the patients:

. . . show themselves sensible and approximately oriented, but extraordinarily distractible in perception and train of thought. Sometimes it is quite impossible to get into communication with them; as a rule, however, they understand emphatic speech, and even give isolated suitable replies, but they are influenced by every new impression; they digress, they go into endless details. (p. 62)

Kraepelin (1921) then goes on to describe the progressively worsening clinical state, *delusional mania:*

The Delusions and Hallucinations, which in the morbid states hitherto described are fugitive or merely indicated, acquire in a series of cases an elaboration which calls to mind paranoid attacks. His surroundings appear to the patient to be changed; he sees St. Augustine, Joseph with the shepherd's crook, the angel Gabriel, apostles, the Kaiser, spirits, God, the Virgin Mary. . . .[4]
The delusions, which forthwith emerge, move very frequently on religious territory. . . . He preaches in the name of the holy God, will reveal great things to the world, gives commands according to the divine will. (pp. 68-69)

Activity and Behavior. Particularly dramatic and extreme among the clinical features of acute mania are the patients' frenetic, seemingly aimless, and occasionally violent activities. Bizarre, driven, paranoid, impulsive, and grossly inappropriate behavior patterns also are typical. In the following passage, Campbell (1953) describes the relationship between the cognitive distortions and behavior:

In the more acute manic reactions the patient, driven by a greater pressure of activity, terror and excitement, becomes violent, attacks his neighbors or begins to shout all kinds of accusations against his alleged persecutors. . . . Distortions, misinterpretations and ideas of reference are now elaborated into delusions of persecution accompanied by violence and panic. The patient runs down the street nude, sets fire to the house, starts an argument with the police, shoots a gun on the street or starts suddenly to preach the gospel in a frenzied manner. . . . If crossed or interfered with in any way he becomes abusive, destructive, homicidal. Suicide is also a danger in this phase. (pp. 159-160)

Delirious Mania

Delirious mania, or Bell's mania, is a relatively rare, grave form of mania characterized by severe clouding of consciousness. When Bell described the syndrome in the mid-19th century, he noted its sudden onset, severe insomnia, loss of appetite, disorientation, paranoia, and extremely bizarre hallucinations and delusions (Bell, 1849).[5] Kraepelin also observed the acute onset and noted that patients were "stupefied, confused, bewildered," in addition to being completely disoriented for time and place. At the core of the illness he found a "dreamy and profound clouding of consciousness, and extraordinary and confused hallucinations and delusions." Bond (1980), in a systematic diagnostic article, states that acute delirious mania can be distinguished by (1) acute onset with or without premonitory signs of irritability, insomnia, or emotional withdrawal, (2) presence of the hypomanic or manic syndrome (DSM-III) at some point during the illness, (3) development of signs and symptoms of delirium, (4) personal history of either mania or depression, (5) family history of major affective disorder, and (6) responsivity to standard treatments for mania.

Mayer-Gross, Slater, and Roth (1960) give a general overview of manic excitement, emphasizing the medical gravity of the untreated clinical situation.

Manic excitement in its most severe form leads to *confusion,* in which the typical symptoms of mania are obscured. Consciousness, which is clear in the less severe states, becomes clouded, illusions and hallucinations may be observed, and the condition may resemble a delirium. These states are seriously debilitating and may endanger life. *Sleep* is severely disturbed in these graver psychoses, but it is also shortened in the milder forms. Another bodily symptom is the exhaustion which supervenes on months of hyper-activity and reduced sleep. The intake of food may be seriously interfered with, for the manic may never take an uninterrupted meal, being constantly diverted to something else. *Body-weight,* which increases in the milder stages, rapidly drops, and very careful nursing is required. . . .
The possibility that the atypical features in manic confusion or delirium are due to nutritional deficiencies of the same kind as those sometimes causing delirium in infective illness, cannot be excluded. (pp. 213-214)

Mood. Mood during delirious mania is described by Kraepelin (1921) as:

. . . very changing, sometimes anxiously despairing ("thoughts of death"), timid and lachrymose, distracted, sometimes unrestrainedly merry, erotic or ecstatic, sometimes irritable or unsympathetic and indifferent. (p. 71)

Cognition and Perception. The extreme cognitive and perceptual changes during delirious mania are primarily manifested through clouding of consciousness, hallucinations, and delusions:

This state is accompanied by a dreamy and profound clouding of consciousness, and extraordinary and confused hallucinations and delusions. . . . Consciousness rapidly becomes clouded; the patients become stupefied, confused, bewildered, and completely lose orientation for time and place. . . .
At the same time dreamy, incoherent delusions are developed. (Kraepelin, 1921, pp. 70-71)

Activity and Behavior. The extremely disturbed and psychotic behavior of delirious mania underscores the origin of the phrase "raving maniac." Kraepelin (1921) graphically recounts this:

At the beginning the patients frequently display the signs of senseless raving mania, dance about, perform peculiar movements, shake their head, throw the bedclothes pell-mell, are destructive, pass their motions under them, smear everything, make impulsive attempts at suicide, take off their clothes. A patient was found completely naked in a public park. Another ran half-clothed into the corridor and then into the street, in one hand a revolver in the other a crucifix. . . . Their linguistic utterances alternate between inarticulate sounds, praying, abusing, entreating, stammering, disconnected talk, in which clang-associations, senseless rhyming, diversion by external impressions, persistence of individual phrases, are recognized. . . . Waxy flexibility, echolalia, or echopraxis can be demonstrated frequently. (p. 72)

Chronic Mania

Chronic mania was observed and described by many early clinicians, including Pinel (1801), Esquirol (1838), Griesinger (1865), Schott (1904), Kraepelin (1921), and Wertham (1929). According to Schott, only the lack of recovery distinguished the chronic from the acute form of the illness (see also Chapter 6). A first manic episode after the age of 40 was thought to put the patient at much higher risk than if it occurred earlier (Henderson and Gillespie, 1956). Wertham (1929) outlined the central features of chronic mania: reduced intellectual productivity and general activity levels, increased behavioral stereotypy, and an overall intellectual weakening. Hare (1981), in an excellent historical review of the concept of mania, discusses the declining interest in the subject of chronic mania after the 19th century. He attributes this in part to the decreasing morbidity of manic illness, and he maintains that improvements in general health and hygiene resulted in significant changes in the manifestation, severity, and consequences of mania.

Hare (1981) acknowledges, however, that there still exists:

. . . the ghost as it were, of a process of mental enfeeblement which can occur in affective psychosis and which generally *did* occur, to a more severe degree, until towards the end of the nineteenth century. (p. 97)

Kraepelin (1921) provides an overview of the intellectual and emotional blunting in chronic mania and the chronicity of its effects, and he draws distinctions between chronic mania and extreme, continuous, rapid cycling, and a few of the possible contributory factors:

Here manic features dominate the picture. The patients are in general sensible and reasonable, and perceive fairly well; memory and retention are also fairly well preserved. On the other hand there exist increased distractibility, wandering and desultoriness of thought, a tendency to silly plays on words, poverty of thought. The patients have no understanding of their state, consider themselves perfectly well and capable of work.
Mood is exalted, but no longer exultant, enjoying activity, but silly and boastful; occasionally it comes to flaring up without strength or durability. The finer emotions are considerably injured. . . . Only the coarser enjoyments, eating, drinking, smoking, snuffing, still arouse in them vivid feelings, further the satisfaction of their personal wishes and wants; everything else has become to them more or less indifferent. . . .
At this point we have to mention in a few words another group of cases, in which the psychic decline reveals itself in continual, abrupt fluctuation between lachrymose anxiety, irritability, and childish merriment. States of this kind sometimes appear to be developed from a continuous accumulation of short circular attacks. (pp. 161-162)

Subjective Experiences of Patients

Mood

John Custance (1952) described the mood of well-being at the beginning of his manic episodes:

First and foremost comes a general sense of intense well-being. I know of course that this sense is illusory and transient. . . . Although, however, the restrictions of confinement are apt at times to produce extreme irritation and even paroxysms of anger, the general sense of well-being, the pleasurable and sometimes ecstatic feeling-tone, remains as a sort of permanent background of all experience during the manic period. (p. 30)

Another patient also described this general sense of well-being: "There is a delicious feeling of physical fitness and well-being throughout the whole body, and great joy and elation. Both physical and mental energy seem inexhaustible" (cited in Tredgold and Wolff, 1975). As it progresses, this sense of well-being often is accompanied by a sense of benevolence and communion with nature; frequently it relates to what Henderson and Gillespie (1956) have called a "heightened sense of reality." These experiences, analogous to the beatific and mystical experiences of saints and other religious leaders, share certain features with contemporary experiences of "universal communion" induced by mescaline, LSD, and other hallucinogenic substances. The interaction among emotional, cognitive, and sensory–perceptual changes is complex, as we see in the following passages and later in the section on hyperacusis:

It is actually a sense of communion, in the first place with God, and in the second place with all mankind, indeed with all creation. It is obviously related to the mystic sense of unity with the All. . . .
A feeling of intimate personal relationship with God is perhaps its paramount feature. . . .
The sense of communion extends to all fellow-creatures with whom I come into contact; it is not merely ideal or imaginative but has a practical effect on my conduct. Thus when in the manic state I have no objection to being more or less herded together—as is inevitable in public Mental Hospitals—with men of all classes and conditions. Class barriers cease to have any existence or meaning. (Custance, 1952, pp. 37, 40)

Religiosity is pronounced in many manic episodes. It ranges from the experiences of communion with God and the universe to mystical and religious experiences expressed in a delusional extreme. The sense of moral imperative and certainty of moral beliefs is closely related to, and dependent on, mood:

Of late years my excitements have grown more severe. I begin by taking an over-active interest in everything going on around me. Everything seems rosy. I feel happy and nothing depresses me. I feel propelled by some unknown force to constant action. I am possessed with the idea of righting wrongs and straightening out things in general. All the faults in the administration of the ward, the hospital and the government must be corrected. (Reiss, 1910)

Cognition

During hypomanic and manic states, thinking becomes very fluid and productive—to the point of loosening of normal patterns of association and racing thoughts and flight of ideas. Paranoid ideation and delusions (especially of power, grandeur, and persecution, which are described later) also can occur. One patient described the ease and fluidity of hypomanic thinking (Tredgold and Wolff, 1975) as follows:

The memory is complete. One idea calls up a host of related ideas without effort. The man cannot but consider every question of judgment or conduct in all its aspects simultaneously, and he sees the right answer at once. . . .

Perhaps most pathognomonic of hypomanic and manic cognitive patterns are the flight of ideas and the subjective experience of racing thoughts. The following poem by a manic-depressive patient was written, without pause and in a few minutes' time, during a hypomanic episode. Its infectious cadence, tangential and occasionally loose language, frequent punning, fast and flowing rhythm, and recurrent sexual references are characteristic of the hypomanic state.

God Is a Herbivore

Thyme passes, mixed with long grasses of herbs in the field.
Rosemary weeps into meadow sweeps
While curry is favored by the sun in its heaven.
The glinting scythe cuts the mustard twice
And the sage is ignored on its rock near the shore.
Hash is itself: high by being.
Laws says shallots shall not — so they shan't
    But . . .
The coriander meanders, the cumin seeds come
While a saffron canary eats juniper berry
Ignoring opened sesame seeds on the ground.

The overwhelming and ultimately exceedingly unpleasant nature of racing thoughts is expressed below in one patient's account of manic illness. Grandiosity of delusional proportions and a compelling sense of moral and social awareness also are described:

The condition of my mind for many months is beyond all description. My thoughts ran with lightning-like rapidity from one subject to another. I had an exaggerated feeling of self importance. All the problems of the universe came crowding into my mind, demanding instant discussion and solution—mental telepathy, hypnotism, wireless telegraphy, Christian science, women's rights, and all the problems of medical science, religion and politics. I even devised means of discovering the weight of a human soul, and had an apparatus constructed in my room for the purpose of weighing my own soul the minute it departed from my body. . . .

Thoughts chased one another through my mind with lightning rapidity. I felt like a person driving a wild horse with a weak rein, who dares not use force, but lets him run his course, following the line of least resistance. Mad impulses would rush through my brain, carrying me first in one direction then in another. To destroy myself or to escape often occurred to me, but my mind could not hold on to one subject long enough to formulate any definite plan. My reasoning was weak and fallacious, and I knew it. (Reiss, 1910)

Grandiosity of thinking, delusions of power and grandeur, and the highly personalized and psychotic meaning acquired by ordinary events are described by professional golfer Bert Yancey (*Los Angeles Times,* 1978) in his account of a manic episode:

I was a Messiah. I was going to the Orient to bring an end to the evil of Communism and bring the religions of the Orient into line with Christianity. I was saying, "All right, all the whites over here, all the blacks over there, we're going to have us a Chinese fire drill," or something like that.

Which meant a great deal to me at the time. And people were laughing, right? That's high, right? Literally and figuratively. That's a natural high. That's manic-depressive illness. You're uninhibited. You do things that have a great deal of meaning to you, but they don't have any meaning to other people. They don't understand your meaning.

So in comes the Security and takes me into the quiet room. And down there I was spitting on a light bulb, thinking if I watched the saliva burn, the different colors and shapes, I could find the key to the cure for cancer.

Finally, one patient describes the extreme mental anguish often experienced during mania: the terrifying thoughts and feelings associated with racing thoughts, delusions, and auditory hallucinations. The simultaneous existence of severe suicidal ideation and mania also is clearly portrayed.

I have felt infinitely worse, more dangerously depressed, when manic than when in the midst of my worst depressions. In fact, the most awful I have ever felt in my entire life—one characterized by chaotic ups and downs—was the first time I was manic. I had been high many times before, but they had never been frightening experiences—ecstatic at best, confusing at worst. In fact, I had learned to accommodate quite well to

them. I developed mechanisms of self-control to keep down the peals of otherwise singularly inappropriate laughter, and rigid limits on my irritability. I learned to avoid situations that might otherwise trip or jangle my hypersensitive wiring, and I learned to pretend I was paying attention or following a logical point when my mind was off chasing rabbits in a thousand directions. My work and professional life flowed. But nowhere did this, or my upbringing, or my intellect, or my character, prepare me for insanity. Although I had been building up to this for weeks, and certainly knew something was seriously wrong, there still was a definite point when I knew I was insane. My thoughts were so fast that I couldn't remember the beginning of a sentence halfway through. Fragments of ideas, images, sentences raced around and around in my mind like the tigers in Little Black Sambo. Finally, like those tigers, they became meaningless melted pools. Nothing once familiar to me was familiar. I wanted desperately to slow down but could not. Nothing helped—not running around a parking lot for hours on end or swimming for miles. My energy level was untouched by anything I did. Sex became too intense for pleasure, and during it I would feel my mind encased by black lines of light that were terrifying to me. My delusions centered on the slow painful deaths of all the green plants in the world—vine by vine, stem by stem, leaf by leaf they died and I could do nothing to save them. Their screams were cacophonous. Increasingly, all of my images were black and decaying.

At one point I was determined that if my *mind*—by which I made by living and whose stability I had assumed for so many years—did not stop racing and begin working normally again, I would kill myself by jumping from a nearby, twelve-story building. I gave it 24 hours. But, of course, I had no notion of time and a million other thoughts—magnificent and morbid—wove in and raced by. Endless and terrifying days of endlessly terrifying drugs—thorazine, lithium, valium, and countless injections of sodium amytal—finally took an effect. I could feel my mind being reined in, slowed down, and put on hold. But it was a very long time until I recognized my mind again, and much longer until I trusted it.

Perception and Sensation

The perceptual and somatic changes that almost always accompany hypomania and mania often reflect the close and subtle links among elevated mood, a physical sense of well-being, expansive and grandiose thought, and heightened perceptual awareness. John Custance (1952) described the temporal ordering of somatic, mood, and cognitive symptoms during the initial phases of his manic episodes:

Thus at the onset of phases of manic excitement I have sometimes noticed the typical symptoms, the pleasurable tingling of the spinal chord [sic] and warm sense of well-being in the solar plexus, long before any reaction in the mental sphere occurred. The same thing happens with the sinking feeling of fear and horror which accompanies extreme depression. (p. 16)

Clearly, as with virtually all signs and symptoms of manic-depressive illness, perceptual and somatic changes vary in degree and kind—from mild increases in awareness of objects and events actually present in the individual's environment to total chaotic disarray of the senses, resulting in visual, auditory, and olfactory experiences completely unrelated to existing physical phenomena. At the milder end of perceptual change, one patient described the relationship of heightened awareness, strongly charged but normal emotional reactions, and psychotic perceptions:

In normal life at times of strong emotion, and especially at moments of great fear, we find that we are more keenly aware than usual of the external details of our world. The sunshine on wet roofs across the way, the faded edge to the blue window curtain, a scent of pipe tobacco in the room, the way the man in the armchair clasps and unclasps his hands—all is more clearly etched in consciousness because of the feeling aroused by the nearness of enemy bombers, or the gravity of an operation taking place next door, or the tenseness of waiting until an expected person, acutely loved or deeply hated, will walk in. In psychotic states, where the fate of the whole universe may be at stake, awareness of material objects and of trivial events can be heightened to an extent that is outside the range of sane experience. (Coate, 1964)

Another patient described auditory changes experienced during hypomania, including the intensification and progression of sensations, from mildly heightened musical awareness to hyperacusis and, finally, sensory confusion.

Almost always when I start to get manic I notice the change in the way I experience music. Gradually I am aware of an incredible intensity of feelings. Each note from a horn, an oboe or a cello becomes unbearably poignant. I hear each note alone, all notes together, each and all with piercing beauty and clarity. And then, after drugged and magical time spent as if in the orchestra's pit, a totally different world of music seduces. Classical work seems too slow, too painfully sad, I become impatient with the pace. Rock music played far too loud is what satisfies. I go from cut to cut, album to album matching mood to music, music to mood. Soon my rooms are strewn with records and album jackets and tapes. It is a search for the perfect sound. I cannot begin to process it all and become completely confused, disoriented and overwhelmed.

John Custance wrote of his sensory experiences while in the preliminary stage of a manic episode. Because he was not yet psychotically fragmented or delusional, he was able to concentrate intensely and to keep in order a wide diversity of ideas and sensations. This ability is not uncommon in hypomania, although many manic-depressive patients who experience scattered thinking early in their episodes never go through this hyperalert but concentrated phase. Those who do and who also possess creative ability find this stage an exceptionally productive one (see Chapter 14).

The first thing I note is the peculiar appearances of the lights—the ordinary electric lights in the ward. They are not exactly brighter, but deeper, more intense, perhaps a trifle more ruddy than usual. Moreover, if I relax the focusing of my eyes, which I can do very much more easily than in normal circumstances, a bright star-like phenomenon emanates from the lights, ultimately forming a maze of iridescent patterns of all colours of the rainbow, which remind me vaguely of the Aurora Borealis. . . . Connected with these vivid impressions is a rather curious feeling behind the eyeballs, rather as though a vast electric motor were pulsing away there.

All my other senses seem more acute than usual. Certainly my sense of touch is heightened; my fingers are much more sensitive and neat. . . .

My hearing appears to be more sensitive, and I am able to take in without disturbance or distraction many different sound-impressions at the same time. (Custance, 1952, pp. 31-32)

The same author also described specific physical sensations he experienced during his manic episodes. His perceived imperviousness to pain and cold, as well as his delusional beliefs about electrical and other influences, occur in many manic patients:

Metabolism is rapid. I can stand cold without difficulty or discomfort; an inner warmth seems to pervade me. I can, for example, walk about naked out of doors on quite cold nights—to throw off my clothes is incidentally a strong impulse and presumably symbolises the freedom from restraint which is a feature of the whole condition. My skin seems peculiarly resistant; I have walked barefooted on stony and thorny ground, squeezed myself naked through furze fences and so on without suffering discomfort. Perhaps this is akin to the strange feats of fire walkers or dancing Dervishes. It certainly seems to show the influence of mind over matter. I fear nothing—freedom from fear is another notable symptom—so nothing seems to hurt me. (Custance, 1952, p. 59)

Activity and Behavior

Behavioral changes during mania include increases in psychomotor activity and in the pressure and rate of speech, heightened irritability and aggressive behaviors, increases in spending and other impulsive behaviors, hypersexuality, and frenzied, bizarre, often aimless activity. Detailed descriptions of these behavioral changes were given earlier in this chapter, especially by Kraepelin, and specific discussions of hypomanic and manic behavior can be found elsewhere in the book. We present here descriptions of only a few of the behavioral changes common or especially interesting in manic states. In the first two passages, Coate and Custance describe their increased enthusiasm for, and involvement in, a wide variety of creative interests and activities. Coate's description (1964) reflects the clear influence of mood and grandiosity on her thinking and behavior. The sense of time urgency and the special significance of events and objects also are evident in her writing:

. . . I must record everything and later I would write a book on mental hospitals. I would write books on psychiatric theory too, and on theology. I would write novels. I had the libretto of an opera in mind. Nothing was beyond me. My creative impulse had found full outlet and I had enough now to write to last me for the rest of my life.
I made notes of everything that happened, day and night. I made symbolic scrap-books whose meaning only I could decipher. I wrote a fairy tale; I wrote the diary of a white witch; and again I noted down cryptically all that was said or done around me at the time, with special reference to relevant news bulletins and to jokes which were broadcast in radio programmes. The time, correct to the nearest minute, was recorded in the margin. It was all vitally important. The major work which would be based on this material would be accurate, original, provocative, and of profound significance. All that had ever happened to me was now worthwhile.

For Custance (1952), both creativity and learning were heightened:

In some forms of insanity, including especially mania, this ripening of the instinct, this eager readiness to absorb and learn new things, to become interested in fresh games, sports and forms of work, seems to recur. It certainly does in my own case. I have, in actual fact, learnt more while confined in Mental Hospitals than anywhere else, including my School and University. I have learnt drawing, shorthand, some languages, studied philosophy and psychology as deeply as I was able, collected and systematically written down and filed innumerable scraps of information on all sorts of subjects, and, above all, read in the book of human nature, which is as it were exposed in the raw. I know the

history, background and medical diagnosis of many of the patients in the wards I have been in. Finally I have written this book. (pp. 244-245)

A common aspect of the illness is impulsive and irrational financial behavior. The psychological and interpersonal consequences, as well as the economic ones, can be devastating and potentially life threatening. It is relevant to keep in mind the frequency of financial themes and content in depressive delusional systems (see Chapter 11). The return of postmanic reason and subsequent awareness of financial extravagances and other painfully embarrassing actions often occur in the harsh context of severe postmanic depression. The humorous aspects of many manic purchases, unfortunately, often obscure the acute shame felt by patients:

When I am high I couldn't worry about money if I tried. So I don't. The money will come from somewhere, I am entitled, God will provide. Credit cards are disastrous, personal checks worse. Unfortunately, for manics anyway, mania is a natural (if unnatural) extension of the economy. What with credit cards and bank accounts there is little beyond reach. So, I bought twelve snake bite kits, with a sense of urgency and importance. I bought precious stones, elegant and unnecessary furniture, three watches within an hour of one another (in the Rolex rather than Timex class: champagne tastes bubble to the surface, are the surface, in mania), and totally inappropriate siren-like clothes. During one spree I spent several hundreds on books having titles or covers that somehow caught my fancy: books on the natural history of the mole, twenty sundry Penguin books because I thought it could be nice if the penguins could form a colony, five Puffin books for a similar reason, on and on and on it went. Once I shoplifted a blouse because I could not wait a minute longer for the woman-with-molasses feet in front of me in line. I imagine I must have spent far more than $30,000 during my two manic episodes, and God only knows how much more during my frequent hypomanias. I haven't any idea where most of the money went.
Anyway, it's terrific fun at the time: money flows, objects accumulate. But then, back on lithium and rotating on the planet at the same pace as everyone else, you find the piper needs paying. Your credit is decimated, your mortification complete: mania is not a luxury one easily affords. It's aggravating enough to have the illness and certainly aggravating to have to pay for medications, blood tests and psychotherapy. They, at least, are deductible. But money spent while manic doesn't fit into the Internal Revenue Service concepts of medical expense or business loss. So, after mania, when most depressed, you're given excellent reason to be even more so.

Data-Based Studies

The form and ways which mania manifests are manifold. Some are cheerful and like to play . . . others passionate and of destructive type, who seek to kill others as well as themselves. —Aretaeus, ca. 150 AD[6]

Mania is a complicated, volatile, and fluctuating cauldron of symptoms. Although classically described as a state of extraordinary energy and activity, it can occur clinically as manic stupor and catatonia. Manic mood, frequently characterized as elated and grandiose, as often as not is riddled by depression, panic, and extreme irritability. For years, mania was mistakenly differentiated from schizophrenia because it reputedly lacked a thought disorder. It now is recognized as an often floridly psychotic condition (see Chapter 11). Manic episodes differ from person to person and in the same individual from time to time. Kraepelin (1921) and Falret (1854, cited in Sedler, 1983) noted a tendency for constancy in symptom patterns across episodes in the same individual, however. Although few systematic data are available on this point, Wellner and Marstal (1964), in a study of 279 manic episodes in 221 patients, concluded that "atypical attacks are followed by atypical, and typical by typical significantly more often than not ($p = 0.002$), indicating the patients' inclination to reproduce the type of their psychoses" (p. 176). Likewise, Beigel and Murphy (1971a) found that patients with multiple manic attacks tended to exhibit similar behavior and mood patterns during subsequent episodes. Whatever the constancy of clinical picture across attacks, it is clear that symptoms vary widely in any one manic episode as it progresses through its various stages. These stages, characterized by Carlson and Goodwin (1973) and discussed more fully in Chapter 4, begin with elation or irritability, move into a more severe form as arousal and hyperactivity escalate, and culminate in floridly psychotic disorganization.

Mood Symptoms

Research on mood symptoms in mania, summarized in Table 2-1, demonstrates that most patients are depressed, labile, or expansive as often as they are euphoric; they are irritable even more often. The depression, irritability, and mood lability are generally seen less often in early stages, although few studies clearly specified the stage level or severity of mania at the time of observation.

Winokur and his colleagues (1969) observed depressed mood in 68 percent of their manic patients, as well as more severe depressive symptoms (including depressive delusions and psychomotor retardation) in a significant subgroup. They found that "short depressive contaminations in the manic episode" were significantly more common in women (79 percent) than in men (49 percent). They, like many investigators, were particularly impressed by the volatility of mood during the manic episode:

In our series of patients, the degree of mood elevation varied from patient to patient and from time to time during the same episode. The changes in mood were capricious, responding to internal as well as external stimuli and so very changeable that they defied measurement. . . . In only 5% was the mood unchanging over a period of hours or days. (p. 62)

Carlson and Goodwin (1973), as noted earlier, observed mood changes as a function of the stage of mania and divided the longitudinal course of their patients' illness into three stages as a function of the predominant mood: Stage I was characterized by euphoria, stage II by anger and irritability, and stage III by severe panic and delirium. Kotin and Goodwin (1972), in their study of depression during mania, found depressive affect to be pervasive. Indeed, in 10 of their 20 manic patients, the mean depression rating was significantly higher during the manic episode than during nonmanic, depressed periods in the hospital. They noted that mania and depression ratings correlated positively in a majority of patients both during manic periods and for the entire hospital stay. These findings, observed the authors, "are contrary to the common view that a patient is either manic or depressed" (p. 683).

Murphy and Beigel (1974), who earlier used mood and cognitive symptoms to distinguish manic subtypes (Beigel and Murphy, 1971a), reiterated the criticism of simple, polar opposite mood states:

It would appear that the traditional conception of mania and depression as representing "opposite" pathologic extremes of affective expression is simplistic and reductionistic in several ways. While most depressive states share the common affect of sadness, mania appears to be not as well characterized by elation but rather by a state of heightened overall activation, with enhanced affective expression together with la-

Table 2-1. Mood Symptoms During Mania: Frequency of Symptoms per Episode

Study	Patients N	Irritability %	Euphoria %	Depression %	Lability %	Expansiveness %
Clayton et al., 1965	31		97			
Winokur et al., 1969	100[a]	85	98	68[b]	95	
Beigel & Murphy, 1971a	12		67	92		
Kotin & Goodwin, 1972	20			100		
Carlson & Goodwin, 1973	20	100	90	55	90	
Taylor & Abrams, 1973b	52	81	31			66
Murphy & Beigel, 1974	30			90		
Winokur & Tsuang, 1975a	94	70	92[c]			
Abrams & Taylor, 1976	78	76	44		59	
Leff et al., 1976	63		97			
Loudon et al., 1977	16	75	81[d]	63[e]	56	44
Taylor & Abrams, 1977	123[f]	81	39		52	60
Carlson & Strober, 1979	9[g]	100	89			
Prien et al., 1988	103			67[h]		
Weighted Mean		80	71	72	69	60

[a]100 episodes, 61 patients
[b]Depressive delusions in 24%, suicidal ideation in 7%
[c]Irritable only (8%), euphoric only (30%), irritable and euphoric (62%)
[d]"Hypomanic affect"
[e]Suicidal ideation in 25%
[f]Calculations based on N = 119
[g]Adolescents
[h]Mild depression (45%) moderate to severe depression (22%)

bility of affect. The co-occurrence of severe depressive thought content and behavior (eg, crying) with elation and heightened anger and other affects in varying intensities in the same manic individual suggests that the equation of elated mood with mania represents an oversimplification of the varied phenomena of mania. (p. 647)

Cognitive Symptoms

Nonpsychotic cognitive symptoms are common during mania. Grandiosity and flight of ideas—subjectively experienced as racing thoughts—were observed in approximately three-quarters of the manic patients described in studies summarized in Table 2-2. Less clearly and more variably defined were distractibility, poor concentration, and confusion, a fact that might partially account for the wider range of results on these variables—16 to 100 percent for distractibility, for example, and 8 to 58 percent for confusion. Definitions were especially wide-ranging for *confusion*, meaning anything from "somewhat

confused and unable to follow the gist of a conversation" to the more severe clinical usage of the term, that is, disorientation and serious memory difficulties.

Psychotic Features

An extensive series of studies and reviews clearly documents the existence and importance of psychotic features in both mania and depression.[7] These studies documented what earlier clinical observers had described in detail.[8]

Definitions of what constitutes a *psychotic feature* vary from investigator to investigator. Here we use the general definition—the presence of hallucinations and/or delusions—unless otherwise specified. (Chapter 11 develops specific definitions for thought disorder and discusses in detail its rate and nature in manic-depressive illness.) Abrams and Taylor (1981) have provided systematic definitions and criteria. Endicott and colleagues (1986) included, in addition to delu-

Table 2-2. Cognitive Symptoms During Mania (Excluding Psychotic Features)

Study	Patients N	Grandiosity %	Flight of Ideas/ Racing Thoughts %	Distractibility/ Poor Concentration %	Confusion[a] %
Lundquist, 1945	95				23
Clayton et al., 1965	31	79	100	97	58
Winokur et al., 1969	100[b]	86	93	100	8
Carlson & Goodwin, 1973	20	100	75	70	35
Taylor & Abrams, 1973b	52		77		33
Abrams & Taylor, 1976	78	71	41		26
Leff et al., 1976	63		49	16	
Loudon et al., 1977	16	50	25[c]	75	
Taylor & Abrams, 1977	123[d]				27
Carlson & Strober, 1979	9	67	56	67	
Braden & Ho, 1981	11		91[e]	55	
Weighted Mean		78	71	71	25

[a]Disorientation and memory lapses; unclear criteria in some studies
[b]100 episodes, 61 patients
[c]Combined symptoms = 56%
[d]Calculations based on N = 119
[e]Persistent = 55%

sions and hallucinations, "marked formal thought disorder, accompanied by either blunted or inappropriate affect, delusions or hallucinations of any type, or grossly disorganized behavior."

Problems in the assessment of psychotic features are many and troublesome (see Chapters 11 and 13). Orvaschel and colleagues (1982) found that family reports of affective delusions identified only 18 percent of probands who admitted such symptoms on direct interview with the Schedule for Affective Disorders-L (SADS-L). Rosen and co-workers (1983a), in a study of psychosis in 89 bipolar patients, found that 49 patients (55 percent) emerged as psychotic on the basis of interviews (SADS) alone. After a review of all interviews and prior records, however, 63 were identified as psychotic. Price and co-workers (1984b), like Orvaschel and colleagues (1982), found a lack of reliability in reports from family members. Yet, as Pope and Lipinski (1978) observed in their key review of the literature, the findings of all these studies, despite wide differences in time, setting, and sample selection, are strikingly consistent.

Table 2-3 summarizes findings from 26 studies

of psychotic features in mania. Approximately two thirds of manic-depressive patients were reported to have a lifetime history of at least one psychotic symptom (phase of illness unspecified, but more usually manic). The range of rates over seven studies was 47 to 75 percent. This result is consistent with Carlson and Goodwin's finding (1973) that 30 percent of their bipolar-I patients (i.e., those who have a history of mania) never went into stage-III mania. Rosenthal and colleagues (1979) also observed that 33 percent of their bipolar-I patients never became psychotic during mania.

The presence or history of any delusion was more than three times as likely as the history or presence of any hallucination. One in five manic patients was reported to have a formal thought disorder, and a similar proportion demonstrated first-rank Schneiderian symptoms. It remains unclear what percentage of patients experiencing delusions also experience hallucinations. Whether a patient having hallucinations of one type (e.g., visual) is more, less, or equally likely to have hallucinations of another type (e.g., auditory) also is still unknown.

Evidence suggests that early age of onset in manic-depressive illness is more likely to be associated with an increased rate of psychotic symptoms. Carlson and Strober (1979) found that manic-depressive illness first appearing during adolescence was characterized by especially florid psychotic symptoms. Rosenthal's group (1980b) observed that those bipolar-I patients who also met Research Diagnostic Criteria (RDC) for schizoaffective illness had a younger age of onset and more non-Schneiderian delusions and hallucinations. Rosen and colleagues (1983b) found a negative correlation of 0.4 between age at onset and psychotic symptom score. This relationship is illustrated in Figure 2-1. The findings suggest that bipolar-I patients who become ill at a young age are more likely to be floridly psychotic than are those with a later age of onset. Rosen and colleagues also point out that their findings raise the possibility that RDC schizoaffective disorders are really a form of bipolar-I disorder. Age-specific issues relevant to delusions and hallucinations are more fully discussed in Chapter 8.

Some, but far from conclusive, evidence relates the presence of psychotic symptoms to severity of illness. Abrams and Taylor (1981) found "only a trend" toward an association between severity of manic syndrome and "schizophrenic features," including delusions and hallucinations. Carlson and Goodwin (1973), however, reported covariance between ratings of psychosis and ratings of manic severity. Likewise, R.C. Young and co-workers (1983) found a positive relationship between the total score on the Mania Rating Scale and the presence of psychotic symptoms.

R. C. Young and associates (1983) also examined the relationship between psychotic features and other manic symptoms. They found no relationship between psychotic features and language–thought disorder, insight, disruptive–aggressive behavior, appearance, rate and amount of speech, or demographic variables, such as age, sex, and race. They did find, however, that psychotic patients were significantly more likely than nonpsychotic patients to have elevated mood, increased psychomotor activity and energy, and increased sexual interest, and they were more likely to endorse sleep-disturbance items.

Finally, Endicott and her colleagues (1986) studied 1,084 first-degree relatives of 298 probands with schizoaffective, psychotic, and nonpsychotic major depressive disorder. They found that, over the course of a lifetime, bipolar disor-

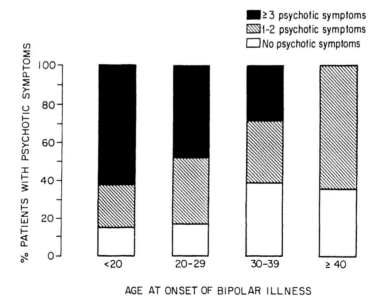

Figure 2-1. Number of psychotic symptoms as a function of age of onset in bipolar patients (adapted from data in Rosen et al., 1983b).

Table 2-3. Psychotic Symptoms

Study	Patients N	Delusions			
		Any %	Grandiose %	Persecutory/ Paranoid %	Passivity %
Lange, 1922	700				
Bowman & Raymond, 1931–32a,b	1009			20	
Rennie, 1942	66	24			
Lundquist, 1945	95				
Astrup et al., 1959	96			18	9
Clayton et al., 1965	31	73			47
Winokur et al., 1969	100[b]	48		19	22
Beigel & Murphy, 1971a	12			33	
Carlson & Goodwin, 1973	20	75		65	20
Carpenter et al., 1973	66				
Taylor & Abrams, 1973b	52		60	42	
Murphy & Beigel, 1974	30			23	
Guze et al., 1975	19				
Abrams & Taylor, 1976	78			55	
Leff et al., 1976	63	67			
Loudon et al., 1977	16		43	25	
Taylor & Abrams, 1977	123[d]		52	65	
Carlson & Strober, 1979	9	56			
Rosenthal et al., 1979[a]	66		35[c]	35[c]	
Brockington et al., 1980a	32			53	
Rosenthal et al., 1980b	71		41	30	
Rosen et al., 1983a	89				
Rosen et al., 1983b	71				
Winokur, 1984	122	54			4
Endicott et al., 1986	298[e]				
Black & Nasrallah, 1989	467	44			
Weighted Mean		48	47	28	15

[a]Lifetime or course of illness
[b]100 episodes, 61 patients
[c]Phase of illness not specified
[d]Calculations based on N = 119
[e]Bipolar fraction unclear
[f] 38 reported psychotic symptoms during manic phase only, 6 during both manic and depressed phases, and 5 during depressed phase only
[g](71) refers to total % psychotic (only 55% were considered psychotic on the basis of interview alone)

der and psychosis were positively associated in both probands and relatives. Bipolar illness in a proband did not predict psychosis in a relative, however, whereas psychosis in a proband was related to increased risk of psychosis but not to bipolarity in relatives. These findings suggest that, although bipolarity and psychosis often oc-cur in the same individuals, they may not reflect the same genetic influence, according to Endicott and colleagues. They speculate that "the risk for the 'expression' of psychotic symptoms is increased in individuals who also have had a bipolar disorder" (p. 11). Findings from this major study led them to argue for a "typological division"

During Mania

	Hallucinations			History of Psychotic Symptoms[a] %	Thought Disorder %	First-rank Schneiderian Symptoms %
Any %	Auditory %	Visual %	Olfactory %			
	7				8	
	17	9				
22						
13						
	24					9
	21	9				
40						
						23
	48	27	15			12
				53[b]		
	44					
	47				84	11
	33				44	
	30[c]	21[c]		67[c]		
	34				9	34
	30	25		74[c]		34
				55(71)[f,g]		
				75[c]		
	14	9		64[c]		
				47[c]		
14	13	6				
15	18	10	17	58	19	18

between psychotic and nonpsychotic forms of affective syndromes.

Activity and Behavior Symptoms

Studies of activity and behavior during mania, summarized in Table 2-4, showed that sleep and speech symptoms are common in manic patients. About four of five patients were observed to have insomnia or a decreased need for sleep. Virtually all exhibited hyperverbosity and rapid or pressured speech. A majority was also hyperactive. Although about two of three were hypersexual, only 29 percent actually exposed themselves or were nude in a public situation.

Table 2-4. Activity and Behavior

Study	Patients N	Hyper-activity %	Decreased Sleep[a] %	Violent/ Assaultive Behavior %	Rapid/ Pressured Speech %	Hyperver-bosity %
Lange, 1922	700					
Allison & Wilson, 1960	24					
Clayton et al., 1965	31		94		100	
Winokur et al., 1969	100[b]	76	90		99	
Carlson & Goodwin, 1973	20	100		75	100	100
Taylor & Abrams, 1973b	52	100		48	100	
Abrams & Taylor, 1976	78	100		46	100	
Leff et al., 1976	63	81	63			86
Loudon et al., 1977	16	56	69		75	
Taylor & Abrams, 1977	123[c]			46		
Carlson & Strober, 1979	9	100	78			89
Abrams & Taylor, 1981	111					
Weighted Mean		87	81	49	98	89

[a]Includes decreased need for sleep and insomnia

[b]100 episodes, 61 patients

[c]Calculations based on N = 119 (except for catatonia rating)

DEPRESSIVE STATES

Classic Descriptions

The bipolar depressive states, in sharp contrast to the manias, are usually characterized by a slowing or decrease in almost all aspects of emotion and behavior: rate of thought and speech, energy, sexuality, and the ability to experience pleasure. As with the manic states, severity varies widely. Symptoms can range from mild physical and mental slowing, with very little distortion in cognition and perception, to profound depressive stupors, delusions, hallucinations, and clouding of consciousness. Of the three major symptomatic groups we have been examining—mood, cognition and perception, activity and behavior—mood is perhaps the least variable across the depressive states. Cognition and perception, on the other hand, change profoundly, as do activity and behavior. We first present extensive clinical descriptions of depressive mood, then emphasize cognitive, psychomotor, and behavioral changes in various depressive states (i.e., nonpsychotic, psychotic, and stuporous depressions). Cognition

and perception are discussed most extensively in the section on psychotic depression, whereas activity and behavior figure more importantly in the discussion of depressive stupor.

Mood

Mood, in all of the depressive states, usually is bleak, pessimistic, and despairing. A deep sense of futility is often accompanied, if not preceded, by the belief that the ability to experience pleasure is permanently gone. The physical and mental worlds are experienced as monochromatic, as shades of grays and blacks. Heightened irritability, anger, paranoia, emotional turbulence, and anxiety are common correlates of depressive mood. The frightening lack of color and the inability to experience meaningful emotional responses were described by Campbell (1953):

General impairment in emotional feeling is another symptom often described by the manic-depressive patient in a depressive episode. In addition to distortions in sensing impressions, such as a queer, odd or unreal feeling, the patient may complain of a universal dulling of the emotional tone. This symptom, like the feeling of unreality, frightens the patient because it tends to

Symptoms During Mania

Nudity/ Sexual Exposure %	Hyper- sexuality %	Extrava- gance %	Religi- osity %	Head Decoration %	Regression (pronounced) %	Cata- tonia %	Fecal Incontinence Smearing %
					27		
	70						
	74						
	65	69					
	80		50		45		
23				33		14	19
33				38			14
	27	32					
	25		25				
29				32		28	10
	78				56		
						19	
29	57	55	39	34	28	22	13

alienate him from his environment. Indeed, it is an important constituent of the patient's fear of insanity. It is bad enough not to speak the same language as other people—it is worse not to feel the same emotions. (p. 106)

Mayer-Gross, Slater, and Roth (1960) emphasized the negative cognitive and affective tone of such patients:

There is a diminished capacity for normal affective response to sad as well as happy events, a phenomenon which is merely one aspect of a *generalized insufficiency of all mental activities.* . . . Whatever is experienced seems to be painful. Even enjoyable experiences have this effect, partly by making the patient more acutely aware of his incapacity for normal appreciation, partly because he is at once sensible of any unfortunate aspect they may have; he may in fact show considerable ingenuity in seeing the bad side of everything. Past, present, and future are alike seen through the same dark and gloomy veil; the whole of life seems miserable and agonizing. The depth of the affect cannot easily be measured from its *outward expression.* The silent shedding of tears may be seen in an otherwise expressionless face; another patient will mock at himself and at his complaints with a grim and sardonic but surprising humour or call himself a fraud or a fool: in another a sudden smile or expression of gaiety will deceive the physician about the severity of the underlying emotion. (p. 209)

Kraepelin (1921), typically, gives a graphic description of the profound despair and hopelessness of depression:

Mood is sometimes dominated by a profound inward dejection and gloomy hopelessness, sometimes more by indefinite anxiety and restlessness. The patient's heart is heavy, nothing can permanently rouse his interest, nothing gives him pleasure. . . .

He feels solitary, indescribably unhappy, as "a creature disinherited of fate"; he is sceptical about God, and with a certain dull submission, which shuts out every comfort and every gleam of light, he drags himself with difficulty from one day to another. Everything has become disagreeable to him; everything wearies him, company, music, travel, his professional work. Everywhere he sees only the dark side and difficulties; the people round him are not so good and unselfish as he had thought; one disappointment and disillusionment follows another. Life appears to him aimless, he thinks that he is superfluous in the world, he cannot restrain himself any longer, the thought occurs to him to take his life without his knowing why. He has a feeling as if something had cracked in him, he fears that he may become crazy, insane, paralytic, the end is coming near. (p. 76)

Nonpsychotic Depression

Kraepelin's *melancholia simplex* (nonpsychotic depression) is characterized by moderate to severe symptoms. Mood usually is severely depressed, and suicidal thinking and behavior are not uncommon. Mental and physical slowing are almost always present and can exist as pronounced psychomotor retardation. Somatic preoccupations, self-denigration and guilt, confusion and indecision, marked fatigue, ruminative thinking, morbid obsessions, and irrational fears are also part of the clinical picture. The depression is "simple," as Kraepelin uses the word, primarily in the sense that it is uncomplicated by delusions or hallucinations.

Cognition and Perception. Virtually all mental activity is markedly slowed in depression. By definition, patients with nonpsychotic depression do not manifest clouding of consciousness, nor do they experience delusions or hallucinations. Suicidal thinking, however, is often of extraordinary and dangerous proportions, and morbidly ruminative and hypochondriacal thinking is common. The profoundly slowed but nonpsychotic nature of this type of depressive thought and its indecisive and ruminative quality are portrayed in the following passage[9]:

Thinking is difficult to the patient, a disorder, which he describes in the most varied phrases. He cannot collect his thoughts or pull himself together; his thoughts are as if paralyzed, they are immobile. . . . He is no longer able to perceive, or to follow the train of thought of a book or a conversation, he feels weary, enervated, inattentive, inwardly empty; he has no memory, he has no longer command of knowledge formerly familiar to him, he must consider a long time about simple things, he calculates wrongly, makes contradictory statements, does not find words, cannot construct sentences correctly. (Kraepelin, 1921, p. 75)

Activity and Behavior. Like thought and verbal expression, activity and behavior are almost always slowed in bipolar depression. Fatigue, lack of activity, impairment in the volition of will, and profoundly altered sleep and eating patterns are hallmarks of this type of depression (see Chapter 19 for detailed discussion of altered sleep and activity patterns). Campbell (1953) described the fatigued, retarded appearance of depressed patients:

Depressed mood is often suggested by the bearing, gait or general appearance of the patient. The depressed individual usually walks slowly and reacts sluggishly. He appears to push himself along, as if he were being held back, rather than propelling himself with normal agility. There are no unnecessary movements with the hands or feet, the patient sitting in a languorous but not restful posture. The shoulders sag, the head is lowered and the entire body seems to droop; loosely hanging clothes sometimes suggest the weight loss often present in the melancholic individual. Everyone is acquainted with the tendency of the angles of the mouth to turn down in the saddened person; a smile, when it occurs, must be forced, and even then there is something sickly or distorted in its expression. The facial musculature of the depressed individual lacks tone, giving the face an inert, myasthenic appearance. The upper eyelids also manifest this careworn expression. . . .

The eyes, which normally portray the spark, vitality and curiosity of the personality, are dull and lustreless. In some individuals the eyes have a faraway, unnatural stare, which even the layman recognizes as a mark of extreme pre-occupation or mental illness. (p. 85)

As Mayer-Gross, Slater, and Roth (1960) characterized the somatic symptoms of depression:

The patient may come to the physician with any of many *complaints,* the number of which correspond to the manifold ways in which the illness is experienced subjectively. The complaint may be one of sudden and complete loss of interest and enjoyment in usual pursuits; of an uncomfortable realization of diminishing quickness of thought and action; of difficulty with customarily easy mental activities; of inability to reach any decision, even in trifling matters; of "loss of will power"; or of a feeling of incapacity, only abolished by taking increasing quantities of alcohol or coffee. Bodily symptoms may be to the fore, e.g. a general feeling of fatigue, of pressure in the head or chest, of heaviness of all limbs, of sleeplessness, loss of appetite, and constipation. . . .

Retardation, as may clearly be discerned from the descriptions of intelligent patients, is not the same as the absorption of energy and interest by grief. Although some patients, devoid of other spontaneous activity, talk freely about their personal preoccupations, in others the whole mental life shows a uniform retardation, and they may mistakenly be regarded as slothful, stupid or demented, until with approaching recovery retardation recedes and mental activity is regained. Especially in the higher functions of will, purpose and decision is the retardation experienced as an almost intolerable burden. The patient feels incapable of initiating or following any complex sequence of thought; the power of imagination fails; ideas and images lose their vividness; memory does not respond promptly to attempts at recollection; the capacity for self-expression diminishes, and speech is an effort. . . .

Disturbance of sleep is the most important of the bodily symptoms. Insomnia sometimes precedes all other psychological symptoms, and restoration of sleep may be the first sign of approaching recovery. The patients may have difficulty in getting to sleep, but most typically wake early or several times during the night, and the sleep is unrefreshing and not infrequently disturbed by horrible dreams.

Anorexia is but one aspect of inertia of the whole digestive and metabolic system. Food may be resolutely refused for this reason, but other motives, such as desire for death and belief in an utter unworthiness, even of being fed and supported by others, not infrequently play a part. Constipation is very common, sometimes fairly severe, and is of great moment to the patients, so much so that slight constitutional depressives are sometimes treated for years for *"nervous dyspepsia"* . . . . Loss of weight may occur very early and may be out of proportion to the diminished intake of food. Increase of body-weight is a common herald of recovery. Menstruation may diminish, not infrequently ceases during a depressive phase, and sexual desire and potency are reduced. The general bodily appearance indicates a lowering of all bodily activities. The skin is dry, the vasomotor responses are sluggish, and the patient looks years older than he does when in health. (pp. 208-211)

Suicidal ideation and behavior, which can occur in the absence of delusions, hallucinations, and psychomotor retardation, are a serious and all-too-frequent component of nonpsychotic depression, described by Kraepelin (1921):

The torment of the states of depression, which is nearly unbearable, according to the perpetually recurring statements by the patients, engenders almost in all, at least from time to time, weariness of life, only too frequently also a great desire to put an end to life at any price. . . .
The extraordinarily strong tendency to suicide is of the greatest practical significance. Sometimes it continually accompanies the whole course of the disease, without coming to a serious attempt owing to the incapacity of the patients to arrive at a decision. . . . Sometimes the impulse to suicide emerges very suddenly without the patients being able to explain the motives to themselves. . . .
Occasionally after indefinite prodromata the first distinct morbid symptom is a suicidal attempt. Only too often the patients know how to conceal their suicidal intentions behind an apparently cheerful behaviour, and then carefully prepare for the execution of their intention at a suitable moment. (pp. 25, 87-88)

Psychotic Depression

Psychotic depression (Kraepelin's *melancholia gravis*) is characterized by the same signs and symptoms as those present in nonpsychotic depression, usually in worsened form, with the addition of delusions and hallucinations. (Systematic studies of manic-depressive thought disorder are discussed in detail in Chapter 11.) Here we

present Bleuler's descriptions (1924) of the nature and extent of depressive delusions, hallucinations, and paranoia, as well as their primary content areas of expression (somatic, religious, and financial).

In the severer cases delusions are invariably present and may stand in the foreground. At the same time the hallucinations usually but not always increase. . . . The devil appears at the window, makes faces at the patients. They hear themselves condemned, they hear the scaffold erected on which they are to be executed, and their relatives crying who must suffer on their account, or starve or otherwise perish miserably.
But the *delusions* especially are never absent in a pronounced case and always as delusions of economic, bodily, and spiritual ruin. The patients think that they became poor, and it does no good to show them their valuables or their balance in the bank; that has no significance for them. Debts are there anyway, or demands are to be expected that will wipe out everything. . . .
Not at all rare are compulsive fears, transitory or lasting throughout the entire phase, e.g. doing some harm to the loved one, or compulsive thoughts, often of a coprolalic or sacrilegious nature. Unjustifiable self-reproaches may assume a compulsive form before belief in their correctness comes in and transforms them into delusions. (pp. 475-476)

A more severe form of psychotic depression, although still less severe than delirious depression, is termed by Kraepelin *fantastic melancholia* (equivalent to Griesinger's *melancholia with delusions* or what many investigators have called *depressive insanity*). Delusions and hallucinations are more pronounced, some clouding of consciousness usually occurs, and violent excitement can alternate with mild stuporous states.

A further, fairly comprehensive group of cases is distinguished by a still greater development of *delusions*. We may perhaps call it "fantastic melancholia." Abundant *hallucinations* appear. . . . there are also multifarious delusional interpretations of real perceptions. The patient hears murderers come; some one is slinking about the bed; a man is lying under the bed with a loaded gun; an electro-magnet crackles. . . . The trees in the forest, the rocks, appear unnatural, as if they were artificial, as if they had been built up specially for the patient, in fact, even the sun, the moon, the weather, are not as they used to be. . . .
Hypochondriacal delusions usually reach a considerable development; they often completely resemble those of the paralytic. . . .
Consciousness is in this form frequently somewhat clouded. The patients perceive badly, do not understand what goes on, are not able to form clear ideas. They complain that they cannot lay hold of any proper

thought, that they are beastly "stupid," confused in their head, do not find their way, also perhaps that they have so many thoughts in their head, that everything goes pell-mell. . . .

The Volitional Disorders are also not quite uniform. The activity of the patients is frequently dominated by volitional inhibition; they are taciturn, even mute, cataleptic; they lie with vacant or strained expression of countenance in bed. . . .

Anxious restlessness, however, seems to me to be more frequent, occasionally alternating with slight stuporous states. . . .

At times more violent states of excitement may be interpolated. The patients scream, throw themselves on the floor, force their way senselessly out, beat their heads, hide away under the bed, make desperate attacks on the surroundings. . . . Serious attempts at suicide are in these states extremely frequent. (Kraepelin, 1921, pp. 89-95)

Delirious Melancholia

Delirious melancholia represents the most severe stage of cognitive and perceptual distortion and disorientation. Delusional thought becomes progressively unclear and fragmented, and hallucinations are particularly vivid, bizarre, and frightening. It is a depressive state predominantly characterized by clouding of consciousness. Kraepelin (1921) more than anyone has written about the mental and physical aspects of this stage of depression:

Gradual transitions lead to a last, delirious group of states of depression, which is characterized by *profound visionary clouding of conscience*. Here also numerous, terrifying hallucinations, changing variously, and confused delusions are developed. . . .

During these changing visionary experiences the patients are outwardly for the most part strongly inhibited; they are scarcely capable of saying a word. They feel confused and perplexed; they cannot collect their thoughts, know absolutely nothing any longer, give contradictory, incomprehensible, unconnected answers, weave in words which they have heard into their detached, slow utterances which they produce as though astonished. . . .

For the most part the patients lie in bed taking no interest in anything. (pp. 95-97)

Depressive Stupor

Depressive stupor, the most severe form of psychomotor retardation, often constitutes an acute medical emergency. Stupor is described here by Henderson and Gillespie (1956).

This condition may be defined as a state of intense psychic inhibition during which regression may occur to an infantile, if not more primitive level. The patient,

usually, is confined to bed, is mute, inactive and uncooperative. His bodily needs require attention in every way; he has to be fed, washed and bathed. Precautions have to be taken to prevent the retention of faeces, urine and saliva. In some cases all attempts at movement are strongly resisted. In other cases the muscles are more flaccid, and the body and limbs can be moulded into any position. On the surface it may seem as if there was a total absence of feeling or emotion, but that is often more apparent than real, for, after recovery, many patients give a vivid account of the distress which they have experienced. The idea of death is believed by some to be almost universal in stupor reactions, and may be regarded as a form of expiation for the wickedness for which they hold themselves responsible. Some patients may have a clear appreciation of their position and surroundings throughout the whole period of the stupor, but in the majority a considerable dulling of consciousness occurs.

During all these stages of depression the *physical health* suffers greatly. The patient becomes weak, loses weight, has a poor appetite, a coated tongue, and constipation. The circulation is enfeebled, and there is cyanosis, especially of the extremities. (p. 258)

Subjective Experiences of Patients

Since then I have led, truly, the existence of a frog and not even that of a living one, but that of a galvanized frog. To be sure, I appear at times merry and in good heart, talk, too, before others quite reasonably, and it looks as if I felt, too, God knows how well within my skin; yet the soul maintains its deathly sleep and the heart bleeds from a thousand wounds.
—Hugo Wolf, 1891[10]

Mood

Mood associated with bipolar depression tends to be dominated by a dull, flat, and colorless sense of experience; despair, hopelessness, and pessimism, often fueled by marked physical and mental lethargy; and a sharp decrease in the pleasure obtained from ordinarily gratifying events and people. The 19th century French composer Hector Berlioz, although never committed to an insane asylum (as was Austrian composer Hugo Wolf), suffered from severe cyclothymia. Berlioz described in his memoirs the two types of depressions, or "spleen," he had experienced: an active, painful, tumultuous, and cauldronous one (almost certainly a mixed state), and another type, characterized by ennui, isolation, lethargy, and a dearth of feeling:

What can I say that will give some idea of the action of this abominable disease?. . . .

There are moreover two kinds of spleen; one mocking, active, passionate, malignant; the other morose and wholly passive, when one's only wish is for silence and solitude and the oblivion of sleep. For anyone possessed by this latter kind, nothing has meaning, the destruction of a world would hardly move him. At such times I could wish the earth were a shell filled with gunpowder, to which I would put a match for my diversion. (Berlioz, translated by Cairns, 1969, pp. 227-228)

One patient described the difference between feeling normal and being depressed in this way:

It is so hard to explain how at different times you can do the same things, see the same people, go to the same places, and yet everything is so totally different. When I am my normal self I feel active, alive, able to enjoy things and to participate easily with other people; I eagerly seek them out. There is no question but that life and these experiences have great meaning to me. But when depressed it seems as though my friends require much more from me than I can ever possibly give, I seem a drain and burden on them; the guilt and resentment are overwhelming. Everything I see, say, or do seems extraordinarily flat and pointless; there is no color, there is no point to anything. Things drag on and on, interminably. I am exhausted, dead inside. I want to sleep, to escape somehow, but there is always the thought that if I really could sleep, I must always and again awake to the dullness and apathy of it all.

Hugo Wolf's account of his depression focuses, as do many descriptions written by depressed or formerly depressed individuals, on the painful contrast between the subjective experience of an arid, sterile reality and a perception of the external world as an unobtainable, visible but not habitable world of light, warmth, and creation:

What I suffer from this continuous idleness I am quite unable to describe. I would like most to hang myself on the nearest branch of the cherry trees standing now in full bloom. This wonderful spring with its secret life and movement troubles me unspeakably. These eternal blue skies, lasting for weeks, this continuous sprouting and budding in nature, these coaxing breezes impregnated with spring sunlight and fragrance of flowers . . . make me frantic. Everywhere this bewildering urge for life, fruitfulness, creation— and only I, although like the humblest grass of the fields one of God's creatures, may not take part in this festival of resurrection, at any rate not except as a spectator with grief and envy. (Quoted in Walker, 1968, p. 322)

The sense of lost vitality and energy is of singular importance in understanding the subjective experience of depression. The ebb and flow of life's force or vigor and its painful absence in depression are described by F. Scott Fitzgerald in *The Crack-Up* (1956, first published in 1936), an autobiographical account of his nervous breakdowns:

. . . of all natural forces, vitality is the incommunicable one. In days when juice came into one as an article without duty, one tried to distribute it—but always without success; to further mix metaphors, vitality never "takes." You have it or you haven't it, like health or brown eyes or honor or a baritone voice.

"Ye are the salt of the earth. But if the salt hath lost its savour, wherewith shall it be salted?" —Matthew 5:13 (p. 74)

Cognition

Cognitive changes during depression can be subtle or profound and often are a combination of both. Depressed patients frequently complain that their process of thinking has slowed down. They are confused, ruminative, cannot concentrate, and feel inadequate and useless. These changes are described in different ways by two individuals with manic-depressive illness:

I doubt, completely, my ability to do anything well; it seems as though my mind has slowed down and burned out to the point of being virtually useless. The wretched convoluted thing works only well enough to torment me with a dreary litany of my inadequacies and shortcomings in character, and to haunt me with the total, the desperate hopelessness of it all. What is the point in going on like this; it is crazy. I am crazy, I say to myself. Others say "It's only temporary, it will pass, you will get over it," but of course they haven't any idea how I feel although they are certain they do. If I can't feel, move, think, or care then what on earth is the point? (Patient with manic-depressive illness)

I seem to be in perpetual fog and darkness. I cannot get my mind to work; instead of associations "clicking into place" everything is inextricable jumble; instead of seeming to grasp a whole, it seems to remain tied to the actual consciousness of the moment. The whole world of my thought is hopelessly divided into incomprehensible watertight compartments. I could not feel more ignorant, undecided, or inefficient. It is appallingly difficult to concentrate, and writing is pain and grief to me. (Custance, 1952, p. 62)

Irrational fears, which can range from fear and panic to obsession and delusion, are common in depression. F. Scott Fitzgerald summed up the experience as "the dark night of the soul":

Now the standard cure for one who is sunk is to consider those in actual destitution or physical suffering—this is an all-weather beatitude for gloom in general and fairly salutary day-time advice for everyone. But at three o'clock in the morning, a forgotten package has the same tragic importance as a death sentence, and the cure doesn't work—and in a real dark night of the soul it is always three o'clock in the morning, day after day. (1956, p. 75)

Robert Schumann was more explicit about his terror:

I was little more than a statue, neither cold nor warm; by dint of forced work life returned gradually. But I am still so timid and fearful that I cannot sleep alone. . . . Do you believe that I have not courage to travel alone to Zwickan for fear that something might befall me? Violent rushes of blood, unspeakable fear, breathlessness, momentary unconsciousness, alternate quickly. (Quoted in Niecks, 1925, p. 142)

The extraordinary magnification of ordinary fears obsessed Custance (1952):

I was utterly miserable and wanted to die, but my fears, troubles and worries were of normal human mischances which might happen to anybody. I feared poverty, failure in life, inability to educate my children, making my wife miserable, losing her, ending up in the gutter as the most revolting type of beggar and so on. My fears had in fact become so overpowering as to appear to me like certainties, but they were only earthly, human fears. Beyond the ridge bordering this ordinary universe of common human experience unending horrors awaited me. But I did not know; I had not crossed it, at any rate in that direction.

Preoccupation with sin and perceived religious transgressions are not uncommon in severe depression, and many deeply depressed patients would empathize with Cowper's "strong sense of God's wrath, and a deep despair of escaping it." William James has written definitively of this, as well as of religious ecstasies, in *The Varieties of Religious Experience* (1902).

Finally, thoughts of suicide often accompany the despair, apathy, guilt, and feelings of inadequacy associated with depression. Extensive subjective descriptions of suicidal thoughts and feelings are presented in Chapter 10.

Behavior and Sleep

Although social isolation, psychomotor retardation or agitation, and other behavioral changes accompany depression, changes in sleep patterns are among the most pervasive, quantifiable, and pathognomonic symptoms. They are also highly distressing for patients. (Research on sleep disturbances is discussed in detail in Chapter 19.) Bell, in his 1972 biography of Virginia Woolf, describes her sleepless nights and their aftermath: "After such nights the days brought headaches, drilling the occiput as though it were a rotten tooth; and then came worse nights, nights made terrible by the increasing weight of anxiety and

depression." Bell continues with Woolf's own description of such nights from her novel *The Voyage Out,* thought to be drawn in part from her own experience with manic-depressive illness:

. . . those interminable nights which do not end at twelve, but go on into the double figures—thirteen, fourteen, and so on until they reach the twenties, and then the thirties, and then the forties . . . there is nothing to prevent nights from doing this if they choose. (Quoted by Bell, 1972, Vol. II, p. 11)

Sylvia Plath—probably manic-depressive, certainly hospitalized and treated for severe depression—described her experience in *The Bell Jar* (1971):

I hadn't washed my hair for three weeks. . . .
I hadn't slept for seven nights.
My mother told me I must have slept, it was impossible not to sleep in all that time, but if I slept, it was with my eyes wide open, for I had followed the green, luminous course of the second hand and the minute hand and the hour hand of the bedside clock through their circles and semicircles, every night for seven nights, without missing a second, or a minute, or an hour.
The reason I hadn't washed my clothes or my hair was because it seemed so silly.
I saw the days of the year stretching ahead like a series of bright, white boxes, and separating one box from another was sleep, like a black shade. Only for me, the long perspective of shades that set off one box from the next had suddenly snapped up, and I could see day after day after day glaring ahead of me like a white, broad, infinitely desolate avenue.
It seemed silly to wash one day when I would only have to wash again the next.
It made me tired just to think of it.
I wanted to do everything once and for all and be through with it. (pp. 142-143)

For F. Scott Fitzgerald, too, sleep and the night became sources of terror:

. . . every act of life from the morning toothbrush to the friend at dinner had become an effort . . . hating the night when I couldn't sleep and hating the day because it went towards night. I slept on the heart side now because I know that the sooner I could tire that out, even a little, the sooner would come that blessed hour of nightmare which, like a catharsis, would enable me to better meet the new day. (1956, pp. 72-73)

Data-Based Studies

Surprisingly little has been done to describe quantitatively the clinical features of bipolar depression per se. The vast depression literature seldom differentiates bipolar from unipolar depression, and when it does, it usually excludes bipolar depression from study and discussion. For detailed clinical description of bipolar depression (of a data-based nature) we have relied primarily on the monograph of Winokur's group (1969).[11] In this section we present data-based studies of bipolar depression, bipolar–unipolar differences in depressive symptomatology, and psychotic features in bipolar depression.

Clinical Features

Clinical description of 21 bipolar depressed patients (5 men and 16 women, with a combined total of 33 separate depressive episodes) was given by Winokur and colleagues (1969). The investigators describe the onset of depression as abrupt in five episodes (15 percent) and gradual in 28 (85 percent). Further details of the symptoms of illness are given in Tables 2-5 and 2-6. Mood was observed to be melancholic or tearful in virtually all patients, with approximately half of them displaying hopelessness. Fully three fourths of bipolar depressed patients were described as irritable, almost as high a percentage as found by the same authors (85 percent) and others (80 percent) in manic patients (Table 2-1).

Table 2-5 summarizes nonpsychotic cognitive and perceptual changes during bipolar depres-

Table 2-5. Mood Symptoms and Nonpsychotic Cognitive and Perceptual Symptoms During Bipolar Depression[a]

Symptom	%	
Mood Symptoms		
Melancholy	100	
Tearfulness	94	
Irritability	76	
Hopelessness	52	
Cognitive and Perceptual Symptoms		
Self-deprecatory	97	
Insight present on admission	91	
Self-accusatory	91	(66)[b]
Poor concentration	91	(83)[b]
Diminished clarity of thought	91	
Diminished speed of thought	91	
Suicidal thoughts	82	(83)[b]
Poor memory	52	
Fear of losing mind	48	
Excessive concern with finances	45	
Fear of death	33	
Obsessions	6	

[a]Thirty-three depressive episodes in 21 bipolar patients
[b]Comparable figures from Carlson and Strober (1979) are given in parentheses

Adapted from Winokur et al., 1969

sion. Self-deprecatory and self-accusatory thoughts were present in almost all patients. With few exceptions, patients also reported substantially impaired cognitive ability; 91 percent reported poor concentration, diminished clarity of thought, and diminished speed of thought. One half complained of poor memory. Suicidal thoughts were very common (82 percent), a figure in close agreement with the rate (83 percent) found in a study of bipolar depressed adolescents (Carlson and Strober, 1979).

Activity, behavior, and somatic symptoms during bipolar depression are summarized in Table 2-6. Comparison figures from Carlson and Strober (1979) and Casper and colleagues (1985) also are given. Sleep difficulties were pronounced and pervasive. Fatigue and psychomotor retardation were seen in approximately three fourths of the bipolar depressed patients; loss of appetite and sexual drive also were common. Most patients had somatic complaints and the majority reported a diurnal mood variation (the majority felt worse in the morning and better in the evening).

Bipolar–Unipolar Differences in Depression

Compared with unipolar patients, depressed bipolar patients have a younger age of onset and a higher rate of significant suicide attempts and appear clinically to be less physically active and more likely to sleep excessively. Other reported differences include lower ratings of anxiety, anger, and physical complaints, more psychomotor retardation, and a greater likelihood of experiencing depressive delusions or hallucinations. This evidence remains problematic, however, because much of it is based on observations made of heterogeneous groups of unipolar patients. Further discussion of this issue and detailed descriptions of bipolar–unipolar differences are found in Chapter 3 (see especially Table 3-3).

Psychotic Features in Bipolar Depression

Delusions and hallucinations often occur in bipolar depression, but they are less frequent than psychotic symptomatology in mania. It can be seen in Table 2-7 that delusions were present in 12 to 66 percent of bipolar depressive episodes and in 44 to 96 percent of manic episodes. Hallucinations, less common in both mania and depression, were relatively more frequent in manic epi-

Table 2-6. Activity, Behavior, and Somatic Symptoms in Bipolar Depression

Category of Symptoms	Patients %		
	Winokur et al., 1969[a]	Carlson & Strober, 1979	Casper et al., 1985
Sleep Disorder			
Insomnia	100		
Global sleep disturbance			85
Difficulty falling asleep	58		
Early morning awakening	27		77
Hypersomnia	23		
Activity			
Fatigue	76		
Psychomotor retardation	76	83	
Social withdrawal	100		
Weight and Appetite			
Loss of appetite	97	50	45
Increase in appetite			23
Loss of weight			26
Libido			
Loss of sexual interest	73		77
Somatic Complaints	67		
Diurnal Mood Variation	64		72

[a]100 episodes, 61 patients

sodes. Several investigators have demonstrated a constancy in the presence or absence of psychotic symptoms across depressive episodes,[12] although the generalizability from unipolar to bipolar depression has not been demonstrated.

MIXED STATES

Because mixed states represent a complicated and confused part of manic-depressive illness, they can be conceived of as transitional states from one phase of illness to another or as independent clinical states combining various mixtures of mood, thought, and activity components (Table 2-8). To a considerable extent, mixed states are even more vulnerable to the inadequacies of modern diagnostic systems than are other types or stages of affective illness. Mixed states can be broadly defined as the simultaneous presence of depressive and manic symptoms. Yet we know, for example, that mania frequently is accompanied by moderate to severe depression. Should depres-

Table 2-7. Comparison of Psychotic Features During Mania and Bipolar Depression

Category of Symptoms	Patients %			
	Winokur et al., 1969[a]	Carlson & Strober, 1979	Rosenthal et al., 1980[b]	Black & Nasrallah, 1989
Delusions				
Mania	48	56	96[c]	44
Depression	33	66	28	12
Hallucinations				
Mania	21[b]	33	66	14
Depression	6[b]	50	24	8

[a]100 episodes, 61 patients
[b]Episodes of auditory hallucinations only
[c]Includes delusions during euthymic states

sion during mania be conceptualized as a mixed state, a typical mania, an atypical mania, or a severe (stage-related) form of mania? Until systematic, discriminating definitions and criteria are developed, the pragmatism of the immediate clinical or research issue will decide such questions.

Classic Descriptions

Mixed states, in which symptoms of depression and mania combine, are important for both theoretical and clinical reasons. The implications of mixed states for pathophysiology are discussed in Chapter 20. Relevant data-based studies are presented later in this chapter. Systematic diagnostic criteria, impressively standardized for most other types and phases of the affective disorders, are least well developed for the mixed states. Differential diagnosis—especially between mixed states, agitated depressions, and borderline conditions—can be a difficult clinical problem (see Chapter 5). The existence of mixed states, however, has been observed for centuries. A 17th century physician described the alternating and combining qualities of mania and melancholy in one of his patients, Lady Grenville. Characterizing the illness as "her Ladyship's annual raving," he wrote to her husband:

For there are twin symptoms, which are her constant companions, Mania and Melancholy, and they succeed each other in a double and alternate act; or take each other's place like the smoke and flame of a fire; so that the noble patient is first melancholy, while her animal spirits are unable to disentangle themselves from the dense cloud of fumes which surround them; and then maniacal, when the saline and sulphureous atoms of the blood are stirred up and loosened by the immoderate heat of their surroundings. (Dr. Claude Brouchier, 1679, cited in Dewhurst, 1962, p. 122)

Falret (1854, cited in Sedler, 1983) noted the strong depressive quality often occurring before, during, and after manic episodes, as well as *melancolie anxieuse,* "characterized by constant pacing and inner turmoil, which incapacitates these patients so they cannot concentrate, and this state sometimes ends up as manic agitation." Kraepelin (1921) described mixed states, and their similarities and dissimilarities to manic and depressive states:

We observe also clinical *"mixed forms,"* in which the phenomena of mania and melancholia are combined with each other, so that states arise, which indeed are composed of the same morbid symptoms as these, but cannot without coercion be classified either with the one or with the other. . . . The mixed states frequently fall outside the limits of the ordinary states in a very conspicuous way. . . . Our customary grouping into manic and melancholic attacks does not fit the facts, but requires substantial enlargement, if it is to reproduce nature. At the same time it turned out that this enlargement ran out in the direction not of the fitting in of fresh morbid symptoms, but only of the different combination of morbid symptoms known for long. Further, it was seen that the mixed states, even when they appeared not as interpolations but as independent attacks, behaved with regard to their course and issue quite similarly to the usual forms, and lastly, that they might in the same morbid course simply take the place of the other attacks especially after a somewhat long duration of the malady. (pp. 4, 191-192)

Kraepelin conceptualized mixed states as primarily transitional phenomena but recognized their existence as individual attacks that frequently occur in later stages of the illness, often associated with poor outcome. We have summarized Kraepelin's classification (Table 2-8) and description of mixed states as different combinations of the manic and depressive symptoms of mood, activity, and thought. Campbell (1953), with his characteristic and important emphasis on the fluctuating nature of moods, reiterated the mixed nature of most emotional states, especially manic-depressive illness:

There are more mixed reactions of this disease than is generally realized. It could truly be stated that, to some extent, all manic-depressive reactions are "mixed" types, in that the symptomatology is anything but static.

The mixed type of manic-depressive psychosis epitomizes the entire cyclothymic process, in that it contains the symptoms characteristic of the various phases. Whether it is a sustained reaction or represents a phase of metamorphosis between the major forms, the mixed type emphasizes the underlying similarities between the depressive and hypomanic, the fact that the manic and depressive reactions may be superimposed, and that the same individual possesses the potentialities for either form. . . . Manic-depressive is a dynamic, constantly changing process which, at times, may manifest symptoms of both phases simultaneously. It is in the mixed form that the observer graphically realizes the homogeneity of the entire process. (pp. 144, 146)

Data-Based Studies

To date, the best theoretical and clinical discussions of mixed states—their clinical course, presentation, and correlates, as well as hypotheses

Table 2-8. Kraepelin's Classification of Mixed States

	I Depressive or Anxious Mania	II Excited or Agitated Depression	III Mania With Poverty of Thought
Mood	**Anxiety** Anxiously despairing	**Anxiety** Anxious, despondent, lachrymose, irritable, occasional self-irony	**Elation** Cheerful, pleased, unrestrained; somewhat irritated, repellent, or afterwards breaking into a merry laugh
Activity	**Overactivity** Great restlessness; wholly senseless pressure of activity	**Overactivity** They run hither and thither, wring their hands, pluck at things, loud rhythmic cries; monotonous lamenting	**Overactivity** Excitement is often limited to making faces, dancing about, throwing things, changes in dress; many...conduct themselves so quietly and methodically that superficial excitement does not appear at all; incapable of regular occupation, very abrupt, short-lived, impulsive outbursts of violence
Thought	**Flight of Ideas** Distractible, absent-minded; incapable of systematic observation; veritable passion for writing with disorderly effusions; thoughts come of themselves	**Inhibition of Thought** Delusions are frequently present; extraordinary poverty of thought; extraordinarily monotonous in utterances; perceive well, understand what goes on, apart from delusional interpretation	**Inhibition of Thought** Perceive slowly and inaccurately; cannot immediately call things to mind. Their conversation is monotonous, not infrequently making an impression of weak-mindedness; state is subject to great fluctuation
Summary Mood Activity Thought	Depressed Manic Manic	Depressed Manic Depressed	Manic Manic Depressed

	IV Manic Stupor	V Depression with Flight of Ideas	VI Inhibited Mania
Mood	**Elation** Cheerful; smile without recognizable cause; supportive, erotic	**Depression** Cast-down and hopeless; anxiety; sad and moody	**Elation** More exultant, occasionally irritable, distractible, inclined to jokes
Activity	**Gross Motor Retardation** Usually inaccessible; lie quiet in bed …decorate themselves…without sign of restlessness or excitement. Not infrequently catalepsy can be demonstrated. Unexpectedly give utterance to loud and violent abuse… throw their food, suddenly take off their clothes, and immediately sink back into inaccessibility	**Motor Retardation** They read much, show interest in, and understanding of their surroundings…. although almost mute, and rigid in their whole conduct	**Motor Retardation** In outward behaviors, conspicuously quiet, appears, however, as if a great inward tension existed, as the patients may suddenly become very violent
Thought	**Inhibition of Thought** Occasionally isolated delusions of changing content find utterance; for the most part they prove themselves fairly sensible and well oriented	**Flight of Ideas** Incited by delusions; occasionally the patients, who cannot give utterance in speech, are capable of writing…often desultory, full of ideas of sin and delusional fears; the heaping up of synonymous phrases, the jumping off to side thoughts, show flight of ideas… recognizable only in writings	**Flight of Ideas** They easily fall into chattering talk with flight of ideas and numerous clang associations
Summary Mood Activity Thought	Manic Depressed Depressed	Depressed Depressed Manic	Manic Depressed Manic

Summarized from Kraepelin, 1921

Table 2-9. Rates of Mixed States

Study	Patients	
	N	%
Winokur et al., 1969	61	16[a]
Kotin & Goodwin, 1972	20	65
Himmelhoch et al., 1976a	84	31
Akiskal & Puzantian, 1979	60[b]	25
Nunn, 1979	112	36
Secunda et al., 1985	18	44
Prien et al., 1988	103	67
Post et al., 1989	48	46
Total N	506	Pooled 40.1

[a]10/61 patients observed with mixed states; a total of 18 episodes occurred, 14 of which were directly observed in hospital. Noted 68% of manic episodes characterized by depressive periods lasting from minutes to days, but these were not conceptualized as mixed states and occurred far more frequently

[b]60 bipolar patients (total sample: 100 psychotic affectively ill patients)

regarding their existence and nature (including the relationship of mixed states to the continuum hypothesis of affective illness, kindling and rapid cycling, and mixed heredity hypotheses)—are those of Kraepelin (1921), Campbell (1953), Winokur and colleagues (1969), and Himmelhoch (1979, Himmelhoch et al., 1976a).

Reported rates of mixed states vary as a function of inclusion criteria, as reflected in the eight studies summarized in Table 2-9. An average of 40 percent of affectively ill patients had mixed states across these studies, although the overall average rises up to 48 percent if the lowest figure, that from Winokur and colleagues (1969), is changed to the higher figure they report when using less stringent, albeit more typical, criteria (68 percent). By any standard, mixed states are clearly not as rare as they were once reputed to be.

Symptomatic presentations of mixed states are mixed to various degrees, ranging from a single opposite-state symptom found in the midst of an otherwise "pure" manic or depressive syndrome (such as depressive mood during mania or racing thoughts during depression), to more complicated mixtures of mood, thought, and behavior. Documentation for the frequent occurrence of depressive mood during mania was presented in Table 2-1. Kotin and Goodwin (1972) systematically investigated the relationship of depression to mania in 20 hospitalized patients. Through an

analysis of nurses' and physicians' behavioral ratings and notes, they found a statistically significant positive association between mania and depression in the majority of cases. One of these cases is illustrated in Figure 2-2.

Racing thoughts during depression are another type of mixed state, one observed by earlier clinicians (Kraepelin, 1921; Lewis, 1934). More recently it has been examined by Ianzito and colleagues (1974) and by Braden and Qualls (1979). Ianzito's group found a relatively low rate of racing thoughts in their 89 depressed inpatients (5 percent), but they used the Present State Exam, which emphasizes the pleasurable and exciting quality, as well as the rapidity, of thought. Braden and Qualls, on the other hand, found that one third to one half of their depressed inpatients reported racing thoughts, with a definite diurnal variation (worsening in the evening, greatest severity at bedtime). They concluded that:

In bipolar patients and cyclothymics, the racing thoughts may occur in both "high" and "low" states. The symptom may thus be related more to the underlying pathology of the affective illness than to the characteristics of either "pole." (pp. 17-18)

The symptomatic presentation of mixed states has been characterized by Himmelhoch and associates (1976a) and by Akiskal (1983a) as dysphoric mood, alternating with elevated mood, racing thoughts, grandiosity, suicidal ideation, persecutory delusions, auditory hallucinations, severe insomnia, psychomotor agitation, and hypersexuality. Kotin and Goodwin (1972) summarized their clinical impressions of the mixed states as follows:

Mania was nevertheless clearly identifiable by pressure of speech, increased motor activity, anger, intrusiveness, grandiosity, and mood instability. Depression during mania was frequently evidenced by expressed feelings of helplessness and hopelessness and thoughts of suicide. Sleep disturbance, irritability, anorexia, and many other symptoms are common to both conditions. (p. 60)

Winokur and colleagues (1969) very carefully documented the course and symptoms of mixed states; the quantitative results of their work are given in Table 2-10. They concluded that the single most striking feature of mixed states was the variability and lability in mood: "It is this panoply of varying and contrasting emotions which makes these patients difficult to diagnose" (p. 81).

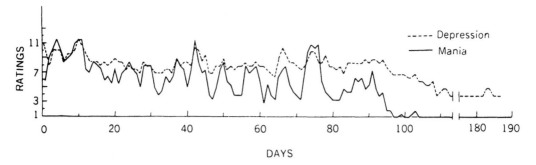

Figure 2-2. Mania and depression ratings during the hospital course of Patient F (Kotin and Goodwin, 1972), a 30-year-old unmarried woman with a long history of psychiatric hospitalization for mania and depression. She remained manic for more than 3 months during her hospitalization at the National Institute of Mental Health. Her level of mania fluctuated between ratings of 3 and 11, and her depression ratings varied from 6 to 10 (both on a 15-point scale). The highest depression ratings were those during periods of manic elation.

Winokur's group observed that mixed states tended to resemble mania in the push of speech, physical activity, and hyperactivity. Delusions, on the other hand, tended to be depressive in nature, as did mood and the vegetative signs and symptoms.

Table 2-10. Symptoms of Mixed Manic-Depressive Psychosis

Category of Symptoms	Patients[a] %
Mood	
Depressed	100
Euphoric	100
Irritable	100
Labile	100
Hostile	79
Cognitive and Perceptual	
Distractibility	100
Grandiosity	57
Flight of ideas	43
Delusions (depressive)	36
Delusions (nondepressive)	21
Auditory hallucinations	14
Visual hallucinations	7
Disorientation	7
Activity and Behavior	
Increased psychomotor activity	100
Insomnia	93
Pressure of speech	93
Decreased sexual interest	63
Suicidal threats or attempts	43
Increased alcohol intake	43
Anxiety attacks	43
Extravagance	14

[a] 14 episodes in 10 patients of mixed manic-depressive psychosis

Adapted from Winokur et al., 1969

They found that 79 percent of the onsets of mixed states were gradual, that there was prior depression of appreciable clinical proportions in 71 percent of patients, that diurnal variation occurred in 64 percent, that the average period from onset to euthymia was 24 days, and that more than half (57 percent) of mixed episodes were followed by a depression.

Women comprised 60 percent of Nunn's sample (1979) of patients with mixed states, consistent with the finding by Himmelhoch and co-workers (1976a) that 55 percent of their sample were women. Winokur and colleagues (1969), on the other hand, found that 9 of their 10 patients with mixed episodes were women and that 13 of the 14 episodes analyzed were experienced by women. This discrepancy almost certainly is due to the more stringent criteria they used in defining mixed states. Himmelhoch and co-workers (1976) found no correlation between mixed states and the severity of illness or with the rapidity of mood swings. They did find, however, that patients with mixed states were far more likely to have a history of drug abuse.

CYCLOTHYMIA AND MANIC-DEPRESSIVE TEMPERAMENTS

Classic Descriptions

Cyclothymia and related personality types form a large part of the manic-depressive spectrum. The relationship of predisposing personalities (or temperaments) and cyclothymia to the subsequent development of manic-depressive psychosis is a fundamental one. (It is discussed further below, as well as in Chapters 4, 7, 8, and 12.) Cycloid temperament, a generic term for the spectrum of manic-depressive personality types, is manifested in several ways: as predominantly depressive, manic or hypomanic, irritable, or cyclothymic.[13] Campbell (1953) describes these personality types and their relationship to manic-depressive illness and to one another:

> The term *cycloid personality* is an overall or general appellation, indicating all forms of the prepsychotic manic-depressive personality. The cycloid personality may occur in one of three forms, with innumerable gradations and mixtures between the three. First, is the hypomanic personality, the overactive, jovial, friendly, talkative and confident individual who, if he becomes psychotic, *usually* develops the manic form of manic-depressive psychosis. . . . Second, is the depressive type, the worried, anxious, thoughtful, sorrowful, individual who, if he becomes psychotic, *usually* develops the depressive form of manic-depressive psychosis. The third form of the cycloid personality is the cyclothymic personality who may have mixed traits, or be euphoric and friendly at one time, and depressed and pessimistic at another, and who may develop either a manic or depressive reaction, or swing from one into the other. It is important to realize that the manic reaction, melancholia, hypomanic reaction, cyclothymic personality, cycloid personality, depressive personality and periodic insanity, are all a part of the same disease process, and that any one of these may change into any other. (pp. 25-26)

Kretschmer's generic term *cycloid personality* (1936) encompassed all types of prepsychotic personality in manic-depressive patients; he stressed the overlap among these personality types:

> Men of this kind have a soft temperament which can swing to great extremes. The path over which it swings is a wide one, namely between cheerfulness and unhappiness. . . . Not only is the hypomanic disposition well known to be a peculiarly labile one, which also has leanings in the depressive direction, but many of these cheerful natures have, when we get to know them better, a permanent melancholic element somewhere in the background of their being. . . . The hypomanic and melancholic halves of the cycloid temperament relieve one another, they form layers or patterns in individual cases, arranged in the most varied combinations. (Quoted by Campbell, 1953, pp. 26-27)

Clearly, not all cyclothymic or cycloid personalities go on to develop the full manic-depressive syndrome, and we concern ourselves here primarily with the clinical description of cycloid temperaments and cyclothymic disorders.

Kraepelin described a *depressive temperament,* which is characterized by a "permanent gloomy emotional stress in all the experience of life," and its antithesis, *manic temperament:*

> Patients, as a rule, have to struggle with all sorts of internal obstructions, which they only overcome with effort; . . . they lack the right joy in work. . . . From youth up there exists in the patients a special susceptibility for the cares, the difficulties, the disappointments of life . . . in every occurrence feel the small disagreeables much more strongly than the elevating and satisfying aspects. . . . Frequently . . . a capricious, irritable, unfriendly, repellent behaviour is developed. The patients are occupied only with themselves, do not trouble themselves about their surroundings. . . .
> Every task stands in front of them like a mountain; life with its activity is a burden which they habitually bear . . . without being compensated by the pleasure of existence. (pp. 119-120)

In manic temperament, the patients' "understanding of life and the world remains superficial," their "train of thought is desultory, incoherent, aimless," and their mood is "permanently exalted, careless, confident." Patients are also:

> . . . convinced of their *superiority* to their surroundings. . . . Towards others they are haughty, positive, irritable, impertinent, stubborn. . . . *unsteadiness and restlessness* appear before everything. They are accessible, communicative, adapt themselves readily to new conditions, but soon they again long for change and variety. Many have belletristic inclinations, compose poems, paint, go in for music. . . . Their mode of expression is clever and lively; they speak readily and much, are quick at repartee, never at a loss for an answer or an excuse. . . .
> Their life is invariably a chain of thoughtless and extraordinary, not infrequently also nonsensical and doubtful activities. . . .
> Many patients join new movements with fervent zeal which rapidly flags. . . . make purchases far beyond their circumstances. . . .
> With their surroundings the patients often live in constant *feud.* (pp. 126-128)

Kraepelin goes on to discuss a milder form of manic temperament within the "domain of the normal," but still a "link in the long chain of manic-depressive dispositions," a form that progressed to what he called *irritable temperament.* In Kraepelin's words (1921):

> It concerns here brilliant, but unevenly gifted personalities with artistic inclinations. They charm us by their intellectual mobility, their versatility, their wealth of ideas, their ready accessibility and their delight in adventure, their artistic capability, their good nature,

their cheery, sunny mood. But at the same time they put us in an uncomfortable state of surprise by a certain restlessness, talkativeness, desultoriness in conversation, excessive need for social life, capricious temper and suggestibility, lack of reliability, steadiness, and perseverance in work, a tendency to building castles in the air. . . periods of causeless depression or anxiety. . . .

The *irritable temperament,* a further form of manic-depressive disposition, is perhaps best conceived as a *mixture of the fundamental states* . . . in as much as in it manic and depressive features are associated. . . . The patients display from youth up extraordinarily great fluctuations in emotional equilibrium and are greatly moved by all experiences, frequently in an unpleasant way. While on the one hand they appear sensitive and inclined to sentimentality and exuberance, they display on the other hand great irritability and sensitiveness. They are easily offended and hot-tempered; they flare up, and on the most trivial occasions fall into outbursts of boundless fury. "She had states in which she was nearly delirious," was said of one patient; "Her rage is beyond all bounds," of another. It then comes to violent scenes with abuse, screaming and a tendency to rough behaviour. . . . The patients are positive, always in a mood for a fight, endure no contradiction, and, therefore, easily fall into disputes with the people round them, which they carry on with great passion. . . .

The colouring of mood is subject to frequent change. . . .

Their power of imagination is usually very much influenced by moods and feelings. It, therefore, comes easily to delusional interpretations of the events of life. The patients think that they are tricked by the people round them, irritated on purpose and taken advantage of. (pp. 129-131)

Cyclothymic temperament is characterized, in Kraepelin's words (1921), by "frequent, more or less regular fluctuations of the psychic state to the manic or to the depressive side." Kraepelin described cyclothymic individuals in these words:

These are the people who constantly oscillate hither and thither between the two opposite poles of mood, sometimes "rejoicing to the skies," sometimes "sad as death." To-day lively, sparkling, beaming, full of the joy of life, the pleasure of enterprise, and pressure of activity, after some time they meet us depressed, enervated, ill-humoured, in need of rest, and again a few months later they display the old freshness and elasticity. (p. 132)

Kretschmer (1936) pointed out a tendency of these individuals to drift toward either mania or depression:

The temperament of the cycloids alternates between cheerfulness and sadness, in deep, smooth, rounded waves, only more quickly and transitorily with some,

more fully and enduring with others. But the mid-point of these oscillations lies with some nearer the hypomanic, and with others nearer the depressive pole.

Finally, Slater and Roth (1969) provide a general description of the "constitutional cyclothymic," emphasizing the natural remissions and seasonal patterns often inherent to the temperament. The alternating mood states, each lasting for months at a time, are continuous in some individuals but subside, leaving periods of normality, in others. In Slater and Roth's words, the cyclothymic constitution:

. . . is perhaps less frequent than the other two "basic states", but its existence in artists and writers has attracted some attention, especially as novelists like Björnsen and H. Hesse have given characteristic descriptions of the condition. Besides those whose swings of mood never intermit, there are others with more or less prolonged *intervals of normality.* In the hypomanic state the patient feels well, but the existence of such states accentuates his feeling of insufficiency and even illness in the depressive phases. At such times he will often seek the advice of his practitioner, complaining of such vague symptoms as headache, insomnia, lassitude, and indigestion. . . . In typical cases such alternative cycles will last a lifetime. In cyclothymic artists, musicians, and other creative workers the rhythm of the cycles can be read from the dates of the beginning and cessation of productive work.

Some cyclothymics have a *seasonal rhythm* and have learned to adapt their lives and occupations so well to it that they do not need medical attention. (pp. 206-207)

Data-Based Studies

Compelling evidence argues for including cyclothymia as an integral part of the spectrum of bipolar manic-depressive illness.[14] The data presented here, primarily from Akiskal and his colleagues (1977, 1979a), describe several aspects of cyclothymia: its clinical presentation, symptomatic patterns of mood, cognition and behavior, and subsequent development of full affective episodes in cyclothymic patients. (Related issues are discussed in Chapters 4, 8, 12, 13, and 15.)

Waters (1979), in his review of the literature, cited widespread agreement that mood and energy swings often precede clinical illness by years. In a study of 33 patients with definite bipolar illness, he found that one third reported bipolar mood swings or hypomania predating the actual onset of their illness. These subsyndromal mood

Table 2-11. Operational Criteria for Cyclothymia

General
Onset in teens or early adulthood
Clinical presentation as a personality disorder (patient often unaware of "moods" per se)
Short cycles, usually days, which are recurrent in an irregular fashion, with infrequent euthymic periods
May not attain full syndrome for depression and hypomania during any one cycle, but entire range of affective manifestations occurs at various times
"Endogenous" mood changes, i.e., often wake up with mood

Biphasic Course
Hypersomnia alternating with decreased need for sleep (although intermittent insomnia can also occur)
Shaky self-esteem which alternates between lack of self-confidence and naive or grandiose overconfidence
Periods of mental confusion and apathy, alternating with periods of sharpened and creative thinking
Marked unevenness in quantity and quality of productivity, often associated with unusual work hours
Uninhibited people-seeking (that may lead to hypersexuality) alternating with introverted self-absorption

Behavioral Manifestations
Irritable-angry-explosive outbursts that alienate loved ones
Episodic promiscuity; repeated conjugal or romantic failure
Frequent shift in line of work, study, interest, or future plans
Resort to alcohol and drug abuse as a means for self-treatment or augmenting excitement
Occasional financial extravagance

From Akiskal et al., 1979a

swings were characterized by (1) onset in early adulthood, (2) occurrence most often in spring or fall, (3) occurrence on an annual or biennial basis, (4) onset unrelated to current life events (with the exception of the first episode), (5) persistence of symptoms for 3 to 10 weeks, (6) a change in energy level, rather than the experience of dysphoria, and (7) sensitivity to lithium treatment (comparable to that for manifest bipolar illness).

Akiskal and his colleagues have further described and quantified these "subsyndromal" mood swings. Table 2-11 presents operational criteria for cyclothymia, and Table 2-12 summarizes findings on the clinical presentation of cyclothymic temperament. Their sample of 50 cyclothymic patients was characterized by the following: a female/male rate of 3:2, young age of onset, which is consistent with other data suggesting an onset of first symptoms between ages 12 and 14 (Akiskal et al., 1977; Depue et al., 1981), and a tendency for the first clinical presentation to be perceived as a personality rather than

Table 2-12. Clinical Presentation of Cyclothymic Temperament

Sample Characteristics	
Number of females	30
Number of males	20
Incidence	
Ambulatory population with *repeated* interpersonal and conjugal conflicts	10%
Unselected mental health clinic population with neurotic and personality disorders	3-4%
Age of Onset	
Brought to clinical attention in late teens or early 20s; actual onset often earlier	86%
Clinical Subtypes of Cyclothymia[a]	
Pure cyclothymia	40%
Predominantly depressed cyclothymia	50%
Hyperthymia	10%
Common Descriptions of Patients by Parents, Siblings, and Friends	
Explosive, sensitive, moody, high-strung, hyperactive	

[a]Irritable-mixed periods predominated in 14% of the patients

Adapted from Akiskal et al., 1979a

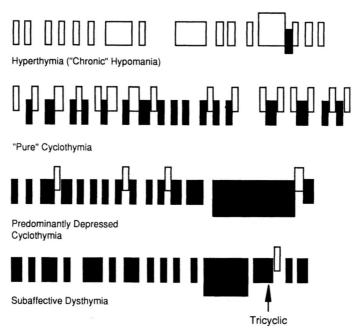

Hyperthymia ("Chronic" Hypomania)

"Pure" Cyclothymia

Predominantly Depressed
Cyclothymia

Subaffective Dysthymia

Tricyclic

Figure 2-3. The spectrum of affective temperamental disorders. This figure depicts the four types of overlapping subaffective disorders: predominantly hyperthymic disorder, where depressive swings rarely occur, "pure" cyclothymia, with an equal proportion of depressive and hypomanic swings, predominantly depressed cyclothymia, where syndromal depressive episodes are common and therefore designated as bipolar-II disorder; and subaffective dysthymia, where the natural (drug-free) course is that of subsyndromal depression, often complicated by syndromal depressions, but brief hypomanic switches on tricyclic challenge occasionally occur (reproduced from Akiskal, 1983c).

mood disorder, with family members and friends describing the patient as "high-strung," "explosive," "moody," "hyperactive," or "sensitive."

The most frequent subtypes of cyclothymia, illustrated in Figure 2-3, are *pure cyclothymia* (equal proportion of depressive and hypomanic swings, alternating with each other in an irregular fashion), *predominantly depressed cyclothymia* (depressive periods dominate the clinical picture, interspersed by "even," "irritable," and occasional hypomanic periods), and, *hyperthymia* (hypomanic traits dominate—decreased need for sleep, expansive behavior, "wild lifestyle"—with occasional depressive and irritable episodes).

Mood, cognitive, and behavioral patterns in cyclothymia are shown in Table 2-13. Although no comparison figures are available for either the general population or other clinical populations, the percentages given here are helpful in providing an overall view of cyclothymia. As might be expected, the mood and cognitive aspects parallel, in milder form, those for mania and depres-

sion. It would be interesting to have more detailed studies of changes in cognition and perception across cyclothymic state changes. Particularly interesting, however, are the measured frequencies of quite specific behavior patterns, although, again, comparison population figures would be especially illustrative. Three fourths of the patients met criteria for alternating patterns of sleep disorder, fluctuating levels in the quality and quantity of work or school productivity, and financial disinhibition. One half of the patients reported patterns of frequent shifts in interests or plans, drug or alcohol abuse, and fluctuating levels of social interaction. Episodic promiscuity or extramarital affairs were reported by 40 percent of the sample, and joining new movements with zeal, then disillusionment, by 25 percent.

Table 2-14 presents data on the natural course or progression of cyclothymia, that is, the relationship of cyclothymic states to the subsequent development of bipolar affective episodes. Approximately one third (36 percent) of the

Table 2-13. Mood, Cognitive, and Behavioral Patterns
in 46 Cyclothymic Patients

	Patients %
Mood	
Irritable periods lasting a few days	50
Explosive, aggressive outbursts (ego-dystonic)	50
Cognitive	
Shaky self-esteem alternating between lack of self-confidence and naive or grandiose overconfidence	75
Periods of mental confusion and apathy alternating with periods of sharpened creative thinking	50
Activity and Behavior	
Hypersomnia alternating with decreased need for sleep	75
Marked unevenness in quantity and quality of work, often associated with unusual self-imposed working hours	75
Repeated buying sprees, financial extravagance, or financial disasters	75
Repeated shifts in work, study, interest, or future plans	50
Drug and alcohol abuse	50
Uninhibited people-seeking alternating with introverted self-absorption	50
Episodic or unexplained promiscuity or extramarital affairs (ego-dystonic)	40
Joining new movements with zeal, rapidly changing to utter disillusionment	25

Adapted from Akiskal et al., 1977

cyclothymic patients, in contrast to only 4 percent of the nonaffective controls, developed full syndromal depression, hypomania, or mania. Of the 25 cyclothymics requiring antidepressant medication for their depressive illness, 11 (44 percent) became hypomanic. This rate was comparable to the switch rate in bipolar controls (35 percent), but since none of the nonaffective group received antidepressants, to make a comparison here is meaningless.

Table 2-14. Affective Episodes in Cyclothymic and Nonaffective Personalities
Over a One- to Two-Year Period of Follow-up

Clinical Affective Episode	Cyclothymic Group Patients % (N = 50)	Nonaffective Group Patients % (N = 50)
1 **Drug-Free Course**		
Depression	26	4
Hypomania	16	0
Mania	6	0
Total[a]	36	4
2 **Course on Tricyclics[b]**		
Hypomania	44	0

[a]The total number of patients is less than the number of episodes shown in the first rows of both columns because several patients suffered both depressive and hypomanic episodes. The overall difference in the risk to develop clinical affective episodes for the cyclothymic and nonaffective personality groups was significant by the chi-square test at the $p < 0.001$ level.

[b]Tricyclics were used, when clinically warranted, on 25 of 50 cyclothymic patients and 11 (44%) developed hypomania. This was very similar to the rate of 35% seen in bipolar controls and both were very significantly different from the nonaffective personalities by chi-square analysis ($p < 0.001$).

Adapted from Akiskal et al., 1979a

SUMMARY

The clinical reality of manic-depressive illness is infinitely varied, far more complex than the preferred term of the day, *bipolar affective disorder*, might suggest. The pathognomonic cycles of mood and activity serve as a background to ever-changing thought, behavior, and feeling. The illness encompasses the extremes of human experience: Cognition ranges from psychosis to a pattern of fast, clear, and occasionally creative associations to retardation so profound that consciousness is clouded. Behavior can be hyperactive, expansive, and seductive, or it can be seclusive, sluggish, and suicidal. Mood swings between euphoria and despair, irritability and vulnerability. The rapid undulations and combinations of such extremes result in an intricately textured clinical picture: Manic patients are depressed and irritable at least as often as they are elated, for example. The highs associated with mania are generally only pleasant and productive during the milder stages.

Examining manic-depressive illness from several perspectives gives the truest appreciation of the experience. The exhaustively detailed descriptions of classic psychiatric writing focus on the subject with more care and patience in observation than is found in the contemporary literature. With its emphasis on systematic measurement and analysis, the research that is now most highly valued can objectively examine well-defined, specific questions related to the illness—although weighing the results of that research requires the leaven of wisdom that comes from intense clinical interchange. Accounts by patients themselves add another dimension, perhaps biased in their own way, yet enriching understanding of the illness as only subjective experience can.

NOTES

1. More detailed descriptions of symptoms and their course can be found in Chapters 3 through 12, 18, and 19.
2. Falret, 1854 [translated by Sedler, 1983]; Kraepelin, 1921; Campbell, 1953; Wellner and Marstal, 1964; Beigel and Murphy, 1971a.
3. Many of these reactions are discussed further in Chapter 12.
4. Kraepelin continues:
   Statues salute him by nodding; the moon falls down from the sky; the trumpets of the day of judgment are sounding. He hears the voice of Jesus, speaks with God and the poor souls, is called by God dear son. There are voices in his ears; the creaking of the floor, the sound of the bells take on the form of words. The patient has telepathic connection with an aristocratic fiancée, feels the electric current in the walls, feels himself hypnotized; transference of thought takes place.
5. As discussed later in this chapter, Carlson and Goodwin (1973), in their systematic study of the stages of mania, found that mania evolves gradually. In their hospitalized patients, the early stages of mania could be discerned in nurses' recordings of mood and behavior reviewed after the apparently sudden onset of manic episodes.
6. Translated by Jelliffe, 1931, p. 20.
7. Clayton et al., 1965; Winokur et al., 1969; Carlson and Goodwin, 1973; Taylor and Abrams, 1973b; Abrams and Taylor, 1976; Pope and Lipinski, 1978; Abrams and Taylor, 1981.
8. Kraepelin, 1921; Campbell, 1953; Henderson and Gillespie, 1956.
9. Suicidal behavior, discussed in the next section, is covered more fully in Chapter 10.
10. Quoted in Walker, 1968, p. 361.
11. More specialized reviews of related clinical topics can be found in Chapters 2, 3, 10, 11, 12, 13, and 19.
12. Charney and Nelson, 1981; Frangos et al., 1983; Helms and Smith, 1983; Winokur, 1984.
13. Reiss, 1910; Kraepelin, 1921; Bleuler, 1924; Kretschmer, 1936; Campbell, 1953; Slater and Roth, 1969.
14. Kraepelin 1921; Akiskal, 1981, 1983a; Akiskal et al., 1977, 1978b; Depue and Monroe, 1978.

3

Evolution of the Bipolar–Unipolar Concept

There is a certain category of patient who continually exhibits a nearly regular succession of mania and melancholia. This seemed sufficiently important to us to serve as a basis for a specific mental disorder, which we call circular insanity because these patients repeatedly undergo the same circle of sickness, incessantly and unavoidably, interrupted only by rather brief respites of reason.

—Jean Pierre Falret, 1854[1]

Manic-depressive insanity . . . includes on the one hand the whole domain of the so-called periodic and circular insanity, on the other hand simple mania, the greater part of the morbid states termed melancholia and also a not inconsiderable number of cases of amentia. (p. 1)　　　　　—Emil Kraepelin, 1921

It was the work of Angst and Perris that helped spread my theory that unipolar and bipolar diseases . . . have different clinical pictures. The bipolar form displays a considerably more colorful appearance; it varies not only between the two poles, but in each phase offers different pictures. The unipolar forms . . . return, in a periodic course, with the same symptomatology. (pp. 3-4)

—Karl Leonhard, 1979

Medical conceptions of mania and depression are as old as secular medicine itself. From ancient times to the present, an extraordinary consistency characterizes descriptions of these conditions. Few maladies in medical history have been represented with such unvarying language. Although the essential features are recognizable in the medical literature through the centuries, the boundaries that define mania and depression and the relationship between them have changed during that time. Not surprisingly, the evolution of the concept has gone from a broader to a narrower definition. As we shall see, this trend may have gone further than the evidence warrants.

HISTORICAL ROOTS

Pre-19th Century Ideas[2]

The medical writers of ancient Greece conceived of mental disorders in terms that sound remarkably modern. They believed that melancholia was a psychological manifestation of an underlying biological disturbance, specifically, a perturbation in brain function. In documents dating back to the fifth and fourth centuries BC, Hippocrates and his school[3] describe melancholia as a condition "associated with 'aversion to food, despondency, sleeplessness, irritability, restlessness,' and they stated that fear or depression that is prolonged means melancholia" (Jackson, 1986, p. 30). Early conceptions of *melancholia* and *mania* were, however, broader than those of today. The two terms, together with *phrenitis*, which roughly corresponds to an acute organic delirium, comprised all mental illness throughout most of the ancient period. As Jackson (1986) points out, "disorders similar to our mania and our melancholia constituted significant portions of the larger groupings of mental disorders that were subsumed under those rubrics in ancient times." (p. 249).

56

As they did with other illnesses, the Hippocratic writers argued forcefully that mental disorders were not due to supernatural or magical forces, beliefs that characterize most primitive societies and that have resurfaced from time to time throughout history. In Greece, "Hippocrates did not encounter excessive resistance in the magical sphere because these diseases had long been interpreted as phenomena deriving from an underlying humoural disturbance" (Roccatagliata, 1986, p. 170). This essentially biological explanation for the cause of melancholia, which survived until the Renaissance, was part of the prevailing understanding of all health as an equilibrium of the four humors—blood, yellow bile, black bile, and phlegm—and all illness as a disturbance of this equilibrium. First fully developed in the Hippocratic work *Nature of Man* (ca. 400 BC), the humoral theory linked the humors with the seasons and with relative moistness. An excess of black bile was seen as the cause of melancholia, a term that literally means "black bile." Mania, by contrast, was usually attributed to an excess of yellow bile.

Aristotle, who differed with the Hippocratic writers by seeing the heart rather than the brain as the dysfunctional organ in melancholy, introduced the notion of a "predisposition" to melancholy. The "marker" of that predisposition was a relative excess of black bile, which he thought was common in small amounts in all people. As Whitwell points out, Aristotle thought those with the excess had melancholic temperaments that were associated with being gifted:

Aristotle appears to have been the first to draw attention to the problem of the frequent occurrence of melancholia, or at least a degree of mental depression in the case of philosophers, statesmen, artists and poets, and he gives as examples Plato, Socrates and Empedocles. This is a question which is constantly recurring in later literature, the explanation of which is attempted by Marsilius Ficinus.[4] (Whitwell, 1936, p. 59)

Deliberations on the relationship between melancholia and mania date back at least to the first century BC, as noted by Soranus of Ephesus: "The followers of Themison, as well as many others, consider melancholy a form of the disease of mania" (Jackson, 1986, p. 250). Soranus himself (*fl.* 100 AD) believed that melancholia and mania were two distinct diseases but with similar prodromal symptoms and requiring similar treatments:

For Soranus, mania involved an impairment of reason with delusions; fluctuating states of anger and merriment, although sometimes of sadness and futility and sometimes "an overpowering fear of things which are quite harmless"; "continual wakefulness, the veins are distended, cheeks flushed, and body hard and abnormally strong"; and a tendency for there to be "attacks alternating with periods of remission." Melancholia involved being "downcast and prone to anger and . . . practically never cheerful and relaxed"; "signs . . . as follows: mental anguish and distress, dejection, silence, animosity toward members of the household, sometimes a desire to live and at other times a longing for death, suspicion . . . that a plot is being hatched against him, weeping without reason, meaningless muttering, and again, occasional joviality"; and various somatic symptoms, many of them gastrointestinal. (Jackson, 1986, p. 250)

Aretaeus of Cappadocia, who lived in the second century AD, appears to have been the first to suggest that mania was an end-stage of melancholia, a view that was to prevail for centuries to come. Roccatagliata (1986), who refers to Aretaeus as "the clinician of mania," notes that he "isolated cyclothymia as a form of mental disease presenting phases of depression alternating with phases of mania," and reports Aretaeus's characterization of the illness:

"Some patients after being melancholic have fits of mania . . . so that mania is like a variety of being melancholy." He described a kind of cyclothymia which presented only intermittent stages of mania: "It arises in subjects whose personality is characterised by gayness, activity, superficiality and childishness." The mania was expressed in "furor, excitement and cheerfulness." Other types of mania, he said, had delirious manifestations of an expansive type, so that the patient "has deliriums, he studies astronomy, philosophy . . . he feels great and inspired." So he identified a bipolar cyclothymia, a monopolar one consisting only of manic phases, and a paranoid psychosis which he considered akin to schizophrenic mania. (p. 229)

Although Aretaeus included syndromes that today would be classified as schizophrenia, his clear descriptions of the spectrum of manic conditions influenced Pinel and are impressive even today:

According to Aretaeus, the classical form of mania was the bipolar one: the patient who previously was gay, euphoric, and hyperactive suddenly "has a tendency to melancholy; he becomes, at the end of the attack, languid, sad, taciturn, he complains that he is worried about his future, he feels ashamed." When the depressive phase is over, such patients go back to being gay, they laugh, they joke, they sing, "they show off in public with crowned heads as if they were returning victorious from the games; sometimes they laugh and dance all day and all night." In serious forms of mania, called furor, the patient "sometimes kills and slaughters the servants"; in less severe forms, he often exalts himself: "without being cultivated he says he is a philosopher . . . and the incompetent [say they are] good artisans . . . others yet are suspicious and they feel that they are being persecuted, for which reasons they are irascible." (Roccatagliata, 1986, pp. 230-231)

Aretaeus believed that mania originated in the heart, which secondarily heated the mind, and this heat inflamed the brain and "depraved its imaginative functions" (Roccatagliata, 1986, p. 229). Melancholy, similarly, had an endogenous etiology; melancholic delirium arose:

. . . "without motive, like the loss of reason, insomnia, and despair." The vital tone was subject to typical circadian variations, which in melancholy were inverted with respect to the normal person, so that the patients "wake up suddenly and are seized by a great tiredness." (Roccatagliata, 1986, p. 231)

The next important medical writer, Galen of Pergamon (131-201 AD), firmly established melancholia as a chronic and recurrent condition. His few comments on mania included the observation that it can be either a primary disease of the brain or secondary to other diseases. Galen's "contribution" was, in the opinion of most medical historians, his brilliant, all-encompassing elaboration of the humoral theory, a system so compelling that it dominated—and stifled—medical thought for more than a millennium.

Medical observations in succeeding centuries continued to subscribe to these conceptions of depression and mania laid down in classical Greece and Rome. As Jackson (1986) observes, most authors wrote of the two conditions as separate illnesses, but usually in adjoining chapters and ascribing them to humoral causes that suggested a close connection between them. Yet where mania and depression are considered in the historical medical literature, a link is almost always made, as can be seen in the timeline below:

LINKING MANIA AND DEPRESSION THROUGH HISTORY[5]

ca. 150   In my opinion melancholia is without any doubt the beginning and even part of the disorder called mania. The melancholic cases tend towards depression and anxiety only . . . if, however, respite from this condition of anxiety occurs, gaiety and hilarity in the majority of

cases follows, and this finally ends in mania. Summer and autumn are the periods of the year most favourable for the production of this disorder, but it may occur in spring.—Aretaeus of Cappadocia[6]

ca. 575   Those affected with such a condition are not suffering from melancholia only, for they tend to become maniacal periodically and in a cycle. Mania is nothing else but melancholia in a more intense form.—Alexander of Trallus[7]

ca. 1000   Undoubtedly the material which is the effective producer of mania is of the same nature as that which produces melancholia.—Avicenna[8]

ca. 1300   Mania and melancholia are different forms of the same thing.—Joh. Gaddesden[9]

ca. 1500   [Melancholia] manifestly differs from what is properly called mania; there is no doubt, however, that at some time or other, authorities agree that it replaces melancholia.—Joan Manardus[10]

1549   Most physicians associate mania and melancholia (truly dreadful diseases) as one disorder, because they consider that they both have the same origin and cause, and differ only in degree and manifestation. Others consider them to be quite distinct.—Jason Pratensis[11]

ca. 1600   Perturbation of the spirit of the brain when mixed with and kindled by other matter can produce melancholia, or if more ardent, mania.—Felix Platter[12]

1672   [Manics and melancholics] are so much akin, that these Distempers often change, and pass from one into the other; for the *Melancholick* disposition growing worse, brings on *Fury;* and *Fury* or *Madness* [mania] growing less hot, oftentimes ends in a *Melancholick* disposition. These two, like smoke and flame, mutually receive and give place to one another.—Thomas Willis[13]

1735   If Melancholy increases so far, that from the great Motion of the Liquid of the Brain, the Patient be thrown into a wild Fury, it is call'd *Madness* [mania]. Which differs only in Degree from the sorrowful kind of Melancholy, is its Offspring, produced from the same Causes, and cured almost by the same Remedies.—Herman Boerhaave[14]

ca. 1744   There is an absolute Necessity for reducing Melancholy and Madness to one Species of Disorder, and consequently of considering them in one joint View. . . . We find that melancholic Patients, especially if their Disorder is inveterate, easily fall into Madness, which, when removed, the Melancholy again discovers itself, though the Madness afterwards returns at certain Periods.—Robert James[15]

1751   Medical writers distinguish two kinds of Madness, and describe them both as a constant disorder of the mind without any considerable fever; but with this difference, that the one is attended with audaciousness and fury, the other with sadness and fear: and that they call mania, this melancholy. But these generally differ in degree only. For melancholy very frequently changes, sooner or later, into maniacal madness; and, when the fury is abated, the sadness generally returns heavier than before.—Richard Mead[16]

1806   [Mania is] often no other than a higher degree of melancholia. . . . it does not appear to me any wise difficult to suppose, that the same state of the brain may in a moderate degree give melancholia; and in a higher, that mania which melancholia so often passes into.—William Cullen[17]

1845   Several distinguished masters, Alexander de Tralles, and Boerhaave himself, were of the opinion, that melancholy . . . was only the first degree of mania. This is in some cases true. There are in fact, some persons who, before becoming maniacs, are sad, morose, uneasy, diffident and suspicious.—Jean-Etienne-Dominique Esquirol[18]

1854   There exists a special type of insanity characterized by two regular periods, the one of depression and the other of excitement. . . . This type of insanity presents itself in the form of isolated attacks; or, it recurs in an intermittent manner; or, the attacks might follow one another without interruption.—Jules Baillarger[19]

1892   By circular insanity, or *folie à double forme*, we understand a special form of mental derangement, the attacks of which are characterised by a regular sequence of two periods—one of depression, and another of excitement, or inversely.—Antoine Ritti[20]

From classical Greece until the middle ages, mental and physical afflictions were primarily the concern of medical doctors. As illness gradually became the responsibility of the monasteries, the early insights were submerged. The period that followed was, in retrospect, a dark age, when mental illness was generally attributed to either magic or sin and possession by the devil.

By the late middle ages, empirical science had attracted interest and the beginnings of acceptance, engendered by the ascendancy of Baconian philosophy. At that point, however, in the realm now covered by psychiatry, scientific interpretations were limited to anatomical, physiological, and pathological studies of the brain.

Empirical clinical observations without religious overtones did not reappear until the beginning of the 17th century. A key figure in this descriptive renaissance was Felix Platter, who, in 1602, published his systematic observations and classifications of mental disorders. Although his descriptions of mania and melancholia were extensive and methodical, there was little to suggest the longitudinal or recurrent nature of the illness, or the distinctions between manic-depressive illness and schizophrenia. As noted previously, the subsequent literature of the 17th and 18th centuries is replete with clinical observations of manic and depressive phenomena. There are literally thousands of such observations, for the most part disconnected from one another. Many are accompanied by hastily erected classification systems and etiological speculations, which sometimes anticipate contemporary theory to a fascinating extent. As Jelliffe (1931) wrote, the "epidemic of classification" was further spread by the powerful influence of Linnaeus's work on the classification of plants. Even more new empirical observations were added when the advent of autopsies opened the door for neuropathological observations and their attendant speculations. This evidence was gathering in a conceptual climate still dominated by the traditional separation of the mind ("soul") from the body. The era was not yet ready for a new synthesis or unifying insights, despite its increasing need of them.

19th Century Ideas

The explicit conception of manic-depressive illness as a single disease entity dates from the mid-19th century. Falret and Baillarger, French "alienists," independently and almost simultaneously formulated the idea that mania and depression could represent different manifestations of a single illness. Students of Esquirol and, therefore, intellectual descendants of Pinel, they had been strongly influenced by Pinel's sharp disdain for the "classification epidemic" as well as by contemporary arguments for a unitary concept of general paresis. In 1854, Falret described a circular disorder (*la folie circulaire*), which for the first time expressly defined an illness in which "this succession of mania and melancholia manifests itself with continuity and in a manner almost regular." The same year, Baillarger (1854a) described essentially the same thing (*la folie à double forme*), emphasizing that the manic and depressive episodes were not two different attacks but rather two different stages of the same attack. Although clearly anticipating Kraepelin's later synthesis, these descriptions focused on chronic illness with poor prognosis; the relationship of these "forms" to other varieties of mania or melancholia was not mentioned. Other valuable contributions were made by Griesinger (1867), who provided rich clinical descriptions of melancholia and mania, although he described primarily chronic states with poor prognosis. As Aretaeus had centuries before, Griesinger conceived of mania as an end-stage of a gradually worsening melancholia and both as different stages of a single, unitary disease (Jackson, 1986).

Although mild cases of mania had been described by Falret, Esquirol, and other observers, Mendel (1881) was the first to define *hypomania* as "that form of mania which typically shows itself only in the mild stages abortively, so to speak." Kahlbaum (1882) described circular disorders (*cyclothymia,*) which were characterized by episodes of both depression and excitement but which did not end in dementia, as chronic mania or melancholia could. Despite these contributions, most clinical investigators continued to regard mania and melancholia as separate entities, chronic in nature and following a deteriorating course.

THE KRAEPELINIAN SYNTHESIS

It was left to Kraepelin[21] to segregate psychotic illnesses from each other and clearly draw the perimeter around manic-depressive illness. The early editions of his textbook of psychiatry held the seeds of his later synthesis, particularly his special emphasis on careful diagnosis based on *both* longitudinal history and the pattern of current symptoms. Nevertheless, these early editions were still struggling with the then-traditional categories of melancholia and circular psychosis. In the sixth edition, published in 1899, the term *manic-depressive* encompassed the circular psychoses and simple manias. Kraepelin expressed doubt that melancholia and the circular psychoses were really separate illnesses, but he was still reluctant to take a definite stand.

By 1913, in the eighth edition of Kraepelin's text, virtually all of melancholia had been subsumed under manic-depressive illness. Only a few forms of involutional melancholia remained separate. Kraepelin placed special emphasis on the features of the illness that most clearly differentiated it from dementia praecox: the periodic or episodic course, the more benign prognosis, and a family history of manic-depressive illness.

In a relatively short time, Kraepelin's views were widely accepted, thus bringing some unity to European psychiatry. His was the first fully developed disease model in psychiatry backed by extensive and carefully organized observations and descriptions. It did not exclude psychological or social factors, and, in fact, Kraepelin was one of the first to point out that psychological stresses could precipitate individual episodes. By including "slight colourings of *mood,*" which "pass over without sharp boundary into the domain of *personal predisposition,*" he also provided the basis for the later development of spectrum concepts (see Chapter 4).

Wide acceptance of Kraepelin's broad divisions led to further explorations of the boundaries between the two basic categories of manic-depressive illness and dementia praecox, the delineation of similarities across them, and the possibility that subgroups could be identified within the two basic categories. Kraepelin's extraordinary synthesis is important not because it draws the ultimately "correct" picture of nature, but rather because it builds a solid and empirically anchored base for future developments. This was his major accomplishment.

POST-KRAEPELINIAN DEVELOPMENTS

After Kraepelin, evolution of the concept of manic-depressive illness proceeded differently in Europe than it did in the United States (Pichot, 1988). Europeans continued to place primary emphasis on the traditional medical disease model of mental illness, whereas psychiatrists in the United States were profoundly influenced by the new perspectives of psychoanalysis and other theories emphasizing psychological and social factors. During the first half of this century, the views of Adolf Meyer (Meyer, 1950–1952) gradually assumed a dominant position in American psychiatry, a position maintained for several decades. Meyer believed that psychopathology emerged from interactions between an individual's biological and psychological characteristics and his social environment. Although not incompatible with Kraepelin's descriptions of manic-depressive illness, Meyer's approach implied a somewhat different conceptual framework. The Meyerians, although allowing for the operation of biological and genetic factors, understood them as part of an individual's vulnerability to specific psychological and social influences. This perspective was symbolized by the rubric "manic-depressive *reaction*" in the first official American Psychiatric Association diagnostic manual published in 1952.

The disease model, by contrast, is based on the premise that clinical phenomena in a given patient are understandable (and, therefore, potentially predictable) in terms of a given disease with a specific natural history and pathophysiology. European psychiatry in the 19th and early 20th centuries had successfully employed this traditional medical disease model in the definition and treatment of general paresis secondary to syphilis of the central nervous system and organic syndromes associated with vitamin deficiencies (especially pellagra). Failure to identify mechanisms of pathophysiology in the major so-called functional psychoses, including manic-depressive illness, stimulated doubts about the continued usefulness of the model, particularly since the prevailing biological hypotheses emphasized infectious agents and neuropathological lesions. Consistent with this pessimism was the failure of the biologically based treatments of the time. In this climate, it is not surprising that American psychiatrists, manifesting the national penchant for pragmatism, were drawn to treatment approaches that emphasized psychological and social factors. When the Meyerian focus, considerably influenced by psychoanalysis,[22] turned to manic-depressive illness, the individual and his environment were the natural focus, and clinical descriptions of symptoms and the longitudinal course of the illness were given less emphasis.

Until relatively recently, the American nosological systems for affective disorders reflected these competing sets of etiological assumptions. Depression was divided into several dichotomies: reactive-endogenous, neurotic-psychotic, and more recently, primary-secondary. Forgotten in these conceptions is the fact that a single parameter cannot differentiate aspects of illness that are at least partially independent of one another: severity, neurotic features, thought disorder, precipitating events, physiological symptoms, and genetic vulnerability. Dichotomous systems thus founder on their a priori assumptions about etiol-

ogy. Even the primary-secondary distinction, although free of assumptions about severity, quality of symptoms, and precipitating events, is based on another supposition: It assumes that depression or mania associated with other illnesses is relatively free of genetic influence, an assumption that has not been supported by the data (Andreasen et al., 1988).

In Europe, the post-Kraepelinian evolution of the concept of manic-depressive illness took a different turn. The European psychosocial and psychoanalytical traditions continued to develop in relative isolation from the mainstream of psychiatry, which largely retained its medical or disease orientation; psychoanalytic thinking per se did not have as important an influence on the European concept[23] of manic-depressive illness as it did on the American one. Although Kraepelin's fundamental distinction between manic-depressive illness and dementia praecox endured (Mayer-Gross et al., 1955), nosological disputes soon arose.

Eugen Bleuler, in his classic contributions to descriptive psychiatry (1924), departed from Kraepelin by conceptualizing the relationship between manic-depressive (affective) illness and dementia praecox (schizophrenia) as a continuum without a sharp line of demarcation. To Bleuler, a patient was predominantly schizophrenic or predominantly manic-depressive. Patients were distributed all along this spectrum, and an individual patient could be at different points on the spectrum at different times. Bleuler believed that a patient's location on the spectrum depended on the number of schizophrenic features he demonstrated. In that sense, Bleuler considered the affective symptoms to be nonspecific. These issues are explored more fully in Chapters 4 and 5.

Bleuler also broadened Kraepelin's concept of manic-depressive illness by designating several subcategories and using the term *affective illness*. The influence of his modifications of Kraepelin's taxonomy could be seen in the *International Classification of Diseases* (8th and 9th editions) and the closely related early versions of the *Diagnostic and Statistical Manual* of the American Psychiatric Association (DSM-I and II). Bleuler's subcategories of affective illness anticipated the principal contemporary subdivision of the classic manic-depressive diagnostic group—the bipolar–unipolar distinction.

THE BIPOLAR–UNIPOLAR DISTINCTION

From its inception, Kraepelin's unitary concept of manic-depressive illness was criticized for being too inclusive, but it was not until 1957 that Leonhard proposed a classification system that went beyond clinical description alone. Leonhard observed that, within the broad category of manic-depressive illness, some patients had histories of both depression and mania, whereas others had depressions only. He then noted that patients with a history of mania (whom he termed *bipolar*) had a higher incidence of mania in their families when compared with those with depressions only (whom he termed *monopolar*). In 1966, Angst and Perris independently provided the first systematic family history data to support Leonhard's distinction, a distinction validated by an independent criterion—family history. As discussed in Chapter 15, some of the subsequent family history studies are consistent with a model in which bipolar and unipolar are variants of the same fundamental disorder, with bipolar representing the more severe end of the spectrum. The bipolar–unipolar subdivision was not formally incorporated into the World Health Organization *International Classification of Diseases* (through ICD-9), although it appears that "circular" manic-depressive psychosis is equivalent to bipolar illness and that manic-depressive illness, depressed type, represents unipolar depression. The bipolar–unipolar distinction was formally incorporated into the American system (DSM-III) in 1980, and it becomes explicit in the upcoming revision of the ICD, ICD-10 (see Chapter 5).

Before the mid-1970s, the scientific literature on manic-depressive illness typically did not include information on the number of patients with or without a history of mania. Even the contemporary literature frequently lacks this information. Nevertheless, during the past decade, the bipolar–unipolar distinction has been examined in more than 100 studies covering family history, natural course, clinical symptoms, personality factors, biological measures, and response to various pharmacological treatments. The question of bipolar–unipolar differences in clinical features of depression is reviewed in this chapter; these as well as other reported bipolar–unipolar differences (e.g., biological, pharmacological, psychological) are summarized in Table 3-1 and

further detailed in the relevant chapters. Our purpose in outlining these reported differences here is to introduce a framework helpful to understanding them.

Differentiating Features

The criteria that distinguish bipolar from unipolar illness have changed over the years, at least among American investigators. In the original descriptions of Leonhard and the subsequent studies of Angst, Perris, and Winokur, both *bipolar* and *unipolar* were used to describe patients with a phasic course of recurrent episodes, characterized by autonomous "endogenous" features and clear functional impairment. In some American settings, however, *unipolar* came to mean all depressed patients without a history of hypomania or mania (i.e., *unipolar* meaning simply nonbipolar)—a heterogeneous population that could include at least a few patients who might have been classified as "neurotic," "reactive," "characterological," or "atypical" in other diagnostic systems. As Roth (1983) has expressed it:

> The significant point in this context is that Leonhard intended that bipolar–unipolar dichotomy for endogenous states alone. . . . When the endogenous syndrome is discarded, unipolar disorders become a large and compendious bag to be commingled with a wide variety of disorders of affect, including neuroses of different kinds. (pp. 47-48).

This problem of heterogeneity in the unipolar group is perpetuated by DSM-III-R. Criteria for unipolar major depression in this newest American diagnostic system do not include an item concerning prior history or course, despite evidence suggesting a clear distinction between family history and course in different subtypes (Winokur, 1979b). Winokur divides his primary unipolar patients[24] (none of whom has a family history of mania) into *familial pure depressive disease* (FPDD), *sporadic pure depressive disease* (SPDD), and *depression spectrum disease* (DSD). The two pure types have no other preceding psychiatric diagnoses and no alcoholism among first-degree relatives. The distinction between them is that FPDD patients have a first-degree relative with primary depression, whereas SPDD patients do not. DSD patients are those with alcoholism or antisocial personality among first-degree (male) relatives; they are predominantly female patients with early onset. Winokur

Table 3-1. Overview of Reported Bipolar–Unipolar Differences[a]

	Bipolar	Unipolar
Phenomenology of Depression		
Natural Course		
Age of onset	Younger	Older
	Narrower range	Broader range
Number of episodes	Higher	Lower
Cycle length	Shorter	Longer
Precipitants of episodes	More important at illness onset	Relation to illness onset not clear
Marital status	Single status not a risk factor	Single status is a risk factor
Epidemiology		
Lifetime risk	1.0%	5%
Proportion of major affective illness	20-50%	50-80%
Sex ratio	F = M	F > M
Substance abuse	More frequent	Less frequent
Suicide	Higher rate?	Lower rate?
Cognition and Perception		
Psychosis	More?	Less?
Perceptual approach	Global	Differentiated, integrated
Personality/Interpersonal		
Depression/introversion	Less	More
Social desirability	More	Less
Impulse control	Less	More
Stimulus seeking	More	Less
Personality profile (e.g., MMPI)	More normal	Less normal
Divorce rate	Higher	Lower
Family History/Genetics		
Monozygotic twin concordance rates	Higher	Lower
Mania among first-degree relatives	More	Less
Biological/Physiological		
Noradrenergic function (peripheral?) (metabolites, receptors, neuroendocrine response)	Less	More
Serotonergic function	Lower?	Higher?
Pain sensitivity	Less	More
Hemispheric function dysfunction	More nondominant	?
Regional metabolism: Fronto-occipital ratio	Lower	Higher
Sleep/Rhythms		
Sleep duration	Longer	Shorter
Phase advance	Less frequent?	More frequent?
Seasonal patterns	Fall/winter depression Spring/summer mania?	Spring depression Fall depression?
Pharmacological Response		
Antidepressant response to tricyclics	Less?	More?
Antidepressant response to lithium	More	Less
Manic/hypomanic response to tricyclics/MAOIs	More frequent	Less frequent
Prophylactic response to lithium	Equivalent when bipolar and unipolar cycle length are comparable	
Prophylactic response to tricyclics	Poor	Good

[a]See individual chapters for details. Not all of the reported differences have been replicated uniformly. The sequence of the table follows that of the chapters.

(1980a) suggested that genetically the FPDD subtype is closely related to bipolar illness. This aspect of unipolar heterogeneity—unipolar patients with certain bipolar characteristics—is discussed in Chapter 4 under the spectrum of polarity.

Bipolar groups may also be heterogeneous. Most studies, particularly those first to use the distinction, did not specify criteria for bipolar beyond indicating a "history of mania." Presumably, in many studies, *bipolar* included only patients with frank mania requiring hospitalization, whereas in others, the bipolar group no doubt included patients with milder symptoms (hypomania). Then, Dunner and colleagues (1976d) suggested that bipolar patients could be more meaningfully classified as either bipolar I or bipolar II. They based their recommendation on their studies of hospitalized depressed patients who met criteria for primary major affective disorders, that is, no prior history of another psychiatric diagnosis. Bipolar-I patients were defined as those with a history of mania severe enough to have resulted in treatment (usually hospitalization). Such full-blown mania usually was accompanied by psychotic features. Bipolar-II patients, by contrast, had (in addition to major depression requiring hospitalization) a history of hypomania—that is, specific symptoms of sufficient magnitude to be designated as abnormal by the patient or the family and to result in interference in normal role functioning but not severe enough to result in hospitalization. This original distinction between bipolar-I and bipolar-II disorder is different from that made in more recent studies, notably those of Akiskal (1981, 1983a), Endicott and colleagues (1985), and Coryell and associates (1985), who also use the bipolar-II terminology. Whereas the work of Dunner and colleagues (1976d) emerged from studies of seriously depressed patients without other psychiatric diagnoses, the later studies were done, by and large, in patients in whom neither the depressed nor the hypomanic phase was severe enough to require hospitalization[25] and in whom concomitant diagnoses (principally borderline personality disorder and substance abuse disorder) were not uncommon. Such definitional confusion has contributed to certain curiosities in contemporary diagnostic systems.

Having earlier recognized the problem of the range of meanings that could confuse the application of the bipolar-II category, Angst (1978) proposed a nomenclature that would account for milder forms of both depression and mania. He divided bipolar patients into Md and mD, with M and D indicating an episode requiring hospitalization, and m and d designating episodes clearly different from normal but not of sufficient severity to necessitate hospitalization (Figure 3-1). Although Angst's mD group is analogous to bipolar-II, as originally defined by Dunner and

his colleagues, other systems have no subcategory analogous to his Md group. This is unfortunate, since Angst has reported interesting differences among these subgroups; for instance, the ratio of females to males is substantially higher in the predominantly depressed subgroups (unipolar and Dm), whereas males are more frequent in the predominantly manic subgroups (MD and Md).

Angst's dm category refers to patients whose episodes of moderate depression and hypomania are not severe enough to make the clinician consider hospitalization. They are similar to some of the bipolar-II patients in the studies of Akiskal, Endicott, Coryell, and their colleagues and would meet criteria for "cyclothymia" in DSM-III-R (see Chapter 5). These patients represent a very important group, and, as discussed in Chapter 4, both family history and pharmacological response data indicate that they should be considered as part of the manic-depressive spectrum (Akiskal et al., 1977, 1979a; Egeland, 1983; Depue et al., 1981). One problem complicating research on bipolar-II disorders is the poor reliability of the diagnosis, which is caused principally by the difficulty in establishing a history of hypomania (Andreasen et al., 1981). Depressed patients are especially poor at recalling prior episodes of hypomania; family members do better. The sensitivity of the diagnostic process to hypomania also can be increased by multiple interviews over time (Rice et al., 1986).

Judging from its treatment in standard textbooks, there has been a clear tendency to underdiagnose the bipolar forms of manic-depressive illness. Recent data require revision of the more traditional view of bipolar as substantially less common than unipolar illness. In a longitudinal study with sensitive methods of ascertainment (Egeland, 1983), the incidence of cyclothymia was greater than that of the bipolar-I pattern, an observation made more than 100 years earlier by Falret. In this contemporary study, when cyclothymia, bipolar-II, and bipolar-I were considered together, the incidence of bipolar illness was approximately equal to that of unipolar illness—that is, it accounted for 50 percent of major affective illness.[26] Angst and colleagues (1978) also found that the ratio of bipolar to unipolar illness was about 1:1 in patients followed for up to 16 years. Initial diagnoses of monopolar (unipolar) illness changed to bipolar in 10 percent

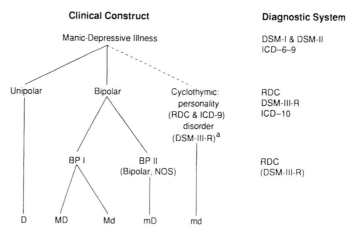

Figure 3-1. The evolution of the bipolar–unipolar distinction.
[a]Before DSM-III, cyclothymia was classified as a personality disorder. In DSM-III-R, cyclothymia is classified as an affective disorder, assumed to be related to the bipolar disorders.

of the 254 patients studied when hypomania was ascertained; those with three or more depressive episodes were especially likely to be rediagnosed. Unfortunately, many studies of recurrent affective illness employ relatively insensitive methods of ascertainment and correspondingly rigid criteria for an episode. Although such rigid criteria are useful for certain research purposes, they exclude many patients from consideration. Egeland (1983) has referred to the bipolar illness typically represented in the literature (i.e., bipolar I) as the "tip of the iceberg" of bipolarity. Weissman and Myers (1978) found that the prevalence of bipolar-II disorder at any point in time is 0.6 percent, although the small sample size of this study dictates caution. For a further discussion of the impact of diagnostic boundaries on incidence data, see Chapter 7.

Despite the heterogeneity in both the bipolar and unipolar groups, the breadth of reported bipolar–unipolar differences is impressive. They include four separate spheres of data—genetic, clinical, biological, and pharmacological. Bipolar and recurrent unipolar disorders, nevertheless, appear to be very similar in some important respects (e.g., prophylactic response to lithium). Taken together, the data suggest that they are best considered as two subgroups of manic-depressive illness rather than separate and distinct illnesses. The available data also support a continuum model, with "pure" bipolar illness on one end and unipolar illness on the other.

Implicit in the foregoing review of the bipolar–

unipolar distinction is the need for a more explicit focus on the relationship between cyclicity and polarity. To what extent do differences in cyclicity contribute to or obscure reported bipolar–unipolar differences? In other words, how are we to know if a given bipolar–unipolar difference is a function of the presence or absence of a history of mania or occurs because the bipolar group is more cyclic or recurrent than the unipolar group? Unfortunately, these important questions have yet to be systematically evaluated (see Chapter 4). The issue could be clarified if bipolar–unipolar comparisons were made between groups matched for cyclicity, that is, for episode frequency or average cycle length.

The relationship between polarity per se and other dimensions of affective illness—family history, age of onset, severity, psychotic features, response to treatment, and biological markers—generally has been studied one dimension at a time. A more comprehensive understanding of these interrelationships awaits studies that employ simultaneous weighing of multiple dimensions.

Unipolar Mania

The classic studies of Leonhard (1957), Perris (1966a), Angst (1966), and Winokur and colleagues (1969) note the relatively rare occurrence of manic patients with no apparent history of depression. In Leonhard's series, "pure mania" represented 9 percent of the bipolar group, whereas in the others, it made up less than 5 percent.

Although Leonhard initially considered patients with pure mania a separate group, subsequent studies indicated that they could not be distinguished from bipolar patients by either family history, course, treatment, or clinical features of mania. Thus, pure mania has generally been considered a variant of bipolar illness. Present knowledge suggests the likelihood that patients so identified have either had unreported depressions (Angst's Md form) or have not been followed long enough to rule out future depressions. For some unipolar manic patients, the diagnosis of depressive episodes is missed because they lack a prominent mood component, occurring primarily as episodes of increased sleep, decreased energy, and slowed thinking. There is as yet no compelling evidence that the few unipolar manias that have been reported represent a valid separate category.

Earlier, Abrams and colleagues (Abrams and Taylor, 1974b; Abrams et al., 1979) prompted a reevaluation of this question by reporting a 28 percent and an 18 percent incidence of unipolar mania among two relatively large independent samples of manic patients (n=127 for two samples). Among the problems with these two studies is the method of ascertaining a history of depression. The method relied on reports of the manic patients themselves at or near admission, presumably while they were still ill. Davenport and her colleagues (1979) at the National Institute of Mental Health (NIMH) have shown (as common sense would suggest) that manic patients report substantially fewer past depressive episodes than their families remember. Like previous authors, Taylor and Abrams found that their "unipolar manics" did not fundamentally differ from the bipolar patients in demographic characteristics, family history variables, symptoms, or in response to "doctor's choice" treatment.[27] Nurnberger and colleagues (1979) surveyed 241 bipolar-I patients in a lithium clinic and found 16 percent who had not been somatically treated for depression, although most of them did show depressive features on a systematic interview. These authors also concluded from their review of phenomenological and family history data that unipolar mania is a variant of bipolar illness, not a separate entity.

Future studies attempting to evaluate the validity of the concept of unipolar mania will have to employ careful diagnostic criteria, sensitive methods of ascertainment, and extensive follow-up periods. As the evidence now stands, we would agree with most authorities in the field that the existence of true unipolar mania as a separate entity is questionable. In our discussions here, they are included in the bipolar group.

False Unipolar Patients

Patients classified as unipolar who subsequently go through a manic or hypomanic episode—the so-called false unipolars—pose another problem (intermediate forms, i.e., unipolar patients with some bipolar characteristics—sometimes and somewhat misleadingly called *pseudounipolar*—are discussed in Chapter 4). Obviously, substantial numbers of such patients in a unipolar sample could either distort or conceal bipolar–unipolar differences.

Data from three longitudinal studies (Angst et al., 1978; Grof, unpublished; Perris, 1968) have been analyzed and are displayed in Table 3-2. The number of false unipolars is expressed as a percentage of the total unipolar group and as a function of numbers of depressive episodes without a mania. One might have expected the percentage of false unipolar patients to decrease as the group was "purified" by requiring more episodes of depression, that is, allowing more and more opportunity for latent bipolarity to express itself. In fact, however, the denominator (i.e., the number of true unipolar patients) also decreases as patients with more episodes are selected, since the unipolar patients who have only one, two, or three episodes are dropped. Thus, the actual percentage of false unipolar patients in the apparent unipolar population is relatively stable beyond

Table 3-2. Estimates of Percent False Unipolar Using Different Cutoff Points for "Unipolar Depression"

Required Number of Depressive Episodes	False Unipolar %		
	Grof (Unpublished)	Perris (1968)	Angst et al.[a] (1978)
1	18.5		28.4
2	15.3	13.1	26.2
3	11.9	11.4	22.5
4	13.2	12.5	22.9
5	7.8	10.7	25.0

[a]The larger percentages from the Angst data may reflect a sampling bias toward more recurrent forms of the illness

the second episode. These data indicate that the convention of requiring more than two episodes of depression before diagnosing unipolar illness is not only ineffective in reducing the percentage of false unipolars but may make the unipolar group less representative by biasing toward patients with relatively more episodes. On the other hand, the requirement of multiple episodes might be worthwhile when examining differences between the most recurrent forms of unipolar illness and bipolar illness. Since one of the important differences between unipolar and bipolar forms is that, on average, bipolar patients have a greater number of episodes over any given period, there is some value in selecting the more recurrent forms of unipolar depression to compare with bipolar illness—that is, to match the two populations for episode frequency. Perris' bipolar–unipolar studies come closest to this in that his unipolar patients had all had at least three depres-

sions. The median number is still significantly below that of his bipolar group, however.

Clinical Differences between Bipolar and Unipolar Depression

In his early observations, Leonhard noted that his bipolar patients showed more symptomatic variability from episode to episode than did the recurrent unipolar patients, whose depressive symptoms he characterized as "stereotyped." To our knowledge, no systematic study has been done to follow up this interesting observation, which may reflect the potential among the bipolar patients to experience more combinations of symptoms, such as is seen with mixed states. In his initial study, Perris (1966a) found no significant difference between bipolar and unipolar depressed patients on a profile of items from a depression rating scale. However, other studies, the results of which are summarized in Table 3-3, found

Table 3-3. Clinical Differences Between Bipolar and Unipolar Depressions

Anxiety	UP > BP	Greenhouse & Geisser, 1959; Beigel & Murphy, 1971a; Brockington et al., 1982a
Overt expressions of anger	UP > BP	Beigel & Murphy, 1971a
Physical complaints	UP > BP	Greenhouse & Geisser, 1959; Beigel & Murphy, 1971a;
Psychomotor retardation	BP > UP	Beigel & Murphy, 1971a; Dunner et al., 1976a; Himmelhoch et al., 1972; Kotin & Goodwin, 1972; Katz et al., 1982
Psychomotor agitation	UP > BP	Greenhouse & Geisser, 1959; Beigel & Murphy, 1971a; Kupfer et al., 1974; Katz et al., 1982
Level of measured physical activity	UP > BP	Kupfer et al., 1974
Symptomatic variability across episodes	BP > UP	Leonhard, 1957
Mood lability within episode	BP > UP	Brockington et al., 1982a
Total sleep time	BP > UP	Hartmann, 1968; Kupfer et al., 1972
"Shut down" depressions	BP > UP	Greenhouse & Geisser, 1959; Beigel & Murphy, 1971a; Kupfer et al., 1974; Katz et al., 1982
Postpartum episodes	BP > UP	Reich & Winokur, 1970; Kadrmas et al., 1979
Pain sensitivity[a]	UP > BP	Davis & Buchsbaum, 1981
Fragmented REM sleep	BP > UP	Duncan et al., 1979; Mendelson et al., 1987
Weight loss	UP > BP	Abrams & Taylor, 1980

[a]Refers to experimental pain stimulation

differences over a wide range of clinical features.[28] Since these studies employ a variety of criteria for the unipolar group, generalizations are difficult. Some do not control for differences in severity of depression or patient age. Some compare bipolar patients with nonbipolar patients, clearly suggesting greater heterogeneity in the latter group. Indeed, many of these apparent differences might be accounted for on that basis. Even in the study by Katz and his colleagues (1982), which employed prior screening by the Research Diagnostic Criteria (see Chapter 5), greater heterogeneity in the unipolar group is plausible, since the research criteria allow for sleep and appetite changes in either direction. In fact, Kupfer and his group (1975), examining unipolar depressed patients with a variety of clinical and personality measures, described a subgroup with symptoms similar to those of bipolar depression. Like bipolar patients, these unipolar depressed patients were more retarded, had lower levels of anxiety, and ate and slept more. They, like the bipolar patients, had been hospitalized more often in the past than the unipolar patients, although the incidence of past depressive episodes, suicide attempts, and substance abuse was similar for all the patients. Kupfer suggests that this subgroup of unipolar patients may share some common biological and pharmacological response characteristics with bipolar patients. Overlapping with this grouping are the unipolar patients described by Winokur and Clayton (1967) as familial pure depressive disease and by Mendels (1976) as "pseudounipolar."[29] Both of these research teams emphasized other similarities to bipolar disorder—early age of onset, high episode frequency, positive family history of mania, and bipolar-like responses to pharmacotherapy (see Table 4-3).

Bipolar patients appear to have shut down depressions when compared with unipolar patients. Studies of differential clinical characteristics seem to point to a lower level of externally observable activation and a greater frequency of delusions and hallucinations in the bipolar subgroup,[30] but it is not known whether all of these differences would be apparent if the bipolar and unipolar groups were matched for episode frequency.

Earlier, NIMH investigators reported a series of clinical, genetic, pharmacological, and biological studies of bipolar–unipolar differences in which bipolar-I and bipolar-II patients were analyzed separately (Dunner et al., 1976d; Dunner, 1980). On some measures (a family history of mania, family history of suicide, augmenter pattern on the evoked response, antidepressant response to lithium), the bipolar-I and bipolar-II groups were similar to one another and dissimilar to the unipolar patients. On other measures, the bipolar-II group appeared to be intermediate between the bipolar-I and unipolar groups (age of onset, behavioral response to L-dopa and to tricyclics), and finally, on some measures, the bipolar-II patients were more similar to the unipolar patients than to the bipolar-I group (symptoms of anxiety, agitation during depression, lack of antidepressant response to tryptophan, normal platelet MAO). Perhaps the major problem limiting the interpretation of this interesting series of studies is the fact that the initial diagnosis of depressive illness was made prior to the availability of formal diagnostic criteria, and, thus, even though all of the patients had depressions severe enough to require hospitalization, the unipolar groups were probably heterogeneous.

In a comparison of bipolar-I and bipolar-II patients with major depressive disorder as diagnosed by DSM-III, Coryell and colleagues (1985) found more severe depressions among the bipolar-I patients, who had longer episodes, were more likely to have received medication, were more frequently hospitalized, had greater incapacity when depressed, and made more suicide attempts. Using the Research Diagnostic Criteria, Endicott and colleagues (1985) compared 122 bipolar-I, 66 bipolar-II, and 104 recurrent unipolar depressed patients (two or more episodes of major depressive disorder) on several illness and family history variables. Significant differences between the bipolar-I and bipolar-II subgroups and between the bipolar and unipolar groups are summarized in Table 3-4. When compared with unipolar patients, bipolar-I and bipolar-II patients had a younger age of onset and, among the females, a higher rate of significant suicide attempts and more depressive delusions or hallucinations. On the other hand, bipolar-II and unipolar patients were similar in that they both had higher rates of chronic affective symptoms than had bipolar-I patients (see Chapter 6). Bipolar-II females had higher rates of

Table 3-4. Bipolar I-Bipolar II and Bipolar-Unipolar Differences[a]

	BP I vs BP II		BP I/BP II vs UP[b]	
	Males	Females	Males	Females
Age at onset of first significant affective symptoms	NS	NS	UP > BP	UP > BP II
Tendency to cycle within episodes	NS	NS		
Lifetime suicide attempt with at least moderate intent to die	NS	NS	NS	BP I & BP II > UP
Lifetime diagnosis				
Affective illness				
Psychotic major depression	NS	NS	NS	BP I > UP
Chronic depressive disorder	NS	BP II > BP I	UP > BP I	UP > BP I
Nonaffective illness				
Prior history of other affective disorders	NS	BP II > BP I	UP > BP I	NS
Alcoholism	NS	BP II > BP I	NS	BP II > UP
Antisocial personality	BP II > BP I	NS	BP II > UP	NS
Premenstrual dysphoria		BP II > BP I		BP II > UP

Family history of affective illness[c]	BP I vs BP II males & females	BP vs UP males & females
Mania/hypomania	NS	BP I > UP
BP I	BP I > BP II	BP I > UP
BP II	BP II > BP I	BP II > UP
Manic only	BP I > BP II	BP I>UP
UP major depression	NS	NS

[a]Differences noted are at 0.05 level

[b]Recurrent (more than 2 episodes) major depression

[c]Percentage of index patients with at least one first-degree relative who met criteria for specific RDC affective disorders

Summarized from Endicott et al., 1985

---

alcoholism than unipolar or bipolar-I females. Bipolar-II females also were more likely to suffer from premenstrual dysphoria. Most important, Coryell and colleagues (1984) and Endicott and associates (1985) found that bipolar-I and bipolar-II patients tended to breed true; that is, bipolar-I patients tended to have bipolar-I relatives, and bipolar-II patients tended to have bipolar-II relatives, a finding that is in agreement with the data of Fieve and colleagues (1987)[31] and partly with that of Gershon and associates (1982a). There is, of course, overlap in all of the family history data, suggesting that bipolar-I and bipolar-II disorders are on a continuum. (These genetic issues are discussed more thoroughly in Chapter 15.) It is important to note again that, unlike the original cohort of bipolar-II patients

described by Dunner and his colleagues at the NIMH (1976d), the Coryell and the Endicott studies were done using samples made up largely of outpatients, whose depressions were generally less severe than those described by Dunner's group. Finally, it also bears repeating that the position of this important diagnostic subgroup is somewhat obscured by the existing structure of DSM-III-R, which includes it in a residual category, "bipolar disorder not otherwise specified" (see Chapter 5).

SUMMARY

Although a surprisingly contemporary concept of manic-depressive illness can be found in ancient descriptions, these early roots became obscured by later ideas and beliefs. The modern re-emergence of a scientific concept can be traced to a multitude of observations made in the 17th and 18th centuries. Kraepelin, following 19th century pioneers who recognized that mania and depression were two expressions of a single illness, brought order to the plethora of classification systems that had emerged. In 1899, he used the term *manic-depressive* for the first time, and by 1921 he had taken the decisive step of separating it from dementia praecox. Kraepelin described manic-depressive illness as having a periodic or episodic course, a relatively benign prognosis, and a family history of the same illness. His quickly accepted disease model continued to dominate contemporary European conceptions of psychiatric illness. American ideas about the nature and etiology of manic-depressive illness, by contrast, detoured through psychoanalytic and Meyerian schools of thought, which gave greater weight to psychological and social factors. This emphasis, in turn, led to a focus on the presenting episode, with relatively less attention to longitudinal course.[32]

American nosological systems for affective disorders have, until recently, reflected mutually exclusive etiological assumptions.[33] The assumptions are evident in the reactive-endogenous, neurotic-psychotic, and primary-secondary dichotomies. Bleuler's modifications to Kraepelin's system, a subdividing and renaming of manic-depressive illness as *affective illness*, also were reflected in nosological systems used worldwide and anticipated the bipolar–unipolar distinction.

In 1957, Leonhard described that distinction, basing his separation of bipolar illness on the presence of mania in the personal and family history of manic-depressive patients. DSM-III reflected the distinction, and the upcoming ICD-10 will as well. In its original conception, unipolar illness was a disorder with a phasic course, like bipolar illness but without the mania. This emphasis on a disorder with a course did not take hold in the United States, so that the term *unipolar illness* came to mean any nonbipolar affective illness. The resulting heterogeneity has tended to obscure similarities and differences between bipolar and unipolar groups.

Heterogeneity among bipolar patients themselves has clouded interpretation of research results. One useful distinction—between a form of illness with full-blown manias (bipolar I) and one with hypomania only (bipolar II)—has been further confused by different usage of the term by different investigators. Perhaps the most useful subclassification of the bipolar group was proposed by Angst, who created four subtypes, based on the different levels of severity of both the depressive and manic phases.

The Kraepelinian notion of manic-depressive illness was unitary; all recurrent affective illness was included, although he anticipated the later bipolar–unipolar subdivision. Unfortunately, the DSM-III-R, by structurally separating bipolar illness from major depressive illness, by relegating bipolar-II disorder to a residual category, and by not including the course of the illness and the history of the patient as criteria, has tended to prejudge the question of the relationship between bipolar and recurrent unipolar forms. At the very least, these systems, for all their advantages, make it awkward to examine the bipolar-unipolar question. In addition, the DSM-III-R treatment of bipolar categories, together with its ignoring of prior course of illness, may reinforce two unfortunate knowledge gaps among some clinicians: They tend to underestimate how fundamental recurrence is to the major affective disorders, and they tend to underdiagnose bipolarity.

The bipolar–unipolar distinction has represented a major advance in the classification of affective disorders primarily because it provides a basis for evaluating genetic, pharmacological, clinical, and biological differences rather than representing a purely descriptive subgrouping. Considerable ambiguity concerning the boundary between bipolar and unipolar illness and the relationship between polarity and cyclicity still exists, however. As noted earlier, there is evidence that individual patients exhibit varying degrees of loading for mania or depression—evidence that strongly suggests a continuum or spectrum model (see Chapter 4). An optimal classification system would allow designation of these varying degrees of loading. At the moment, the system devised by Angst comes closest to this ideal.

NOTES

1. Quoted from Sedler and Dessain's translation of Falret's 1854 article (Sedler, 1983, p. 1129).

2. For the material in this section we are indebted to the historians in our field, especially to Jackson (1986) and Roccatagliata (1986) for their extensive scholarship. Whitwell, in his modestly titled *Historical Notes on Psychiatry* (1936), provides translations of ancient manuscripts and insights into the apparent manic-depressive symptoms of literary and historical figures, such as Orestes, Saul, and Herod the Great. Although not as sharply focused on affective illness, other sources have proved valuable in understanding the historical context in general medicine and psychiatry; they include Ackerknecht (1959, 1982), Zilboorg (1941), Alexander and Selesnick (1966), and Wightman (1971).

3. Medical historians believe that the works attributed to Hippocrates probably represent the work of his school. Ackerknecht, for example, states:

   From fifty to seventy books were later attributed to Hippocrates, and in the third century B.C. they were collected in Alexandria into the *Corpus Hippocraticum*. It is not known which of these books, if any, were actually written by the great physician. As a matter of fact, none of them contains the ideas attributed to him in the writings of Plato and Menon. (Ackerknecht, 1982, p. 55)

4. According to Jackson (1986), Marsilius Ficinus (Marsilio Ficino) was a 15th century philosopher, physician, and priest, who revitalized Aristotle's views "with far-reaching effects on his own and later times" (p. 100).

5. Although the idea for this timeline was ours, locating the quotations would have been next to impossible without the excellent historical sources cited for each. We are especially indebted to Whitwell (1936), Jackson (1986), and Roccatagliata (1986). The quotations, particularly those from the middle ages, do not always represent prevailing thought, but they do illustrate the thread of this theme through history. Also, when the conditions we would characterize as manic-depressive illness were interpreted as medical rather than philosophical or religious problems, a relationship between mania and depression was almost always suggested, explicitly or implicitly.

6. Cited by Whitwell, 1936, pp. 163-164. From: *De acut, et diut, morborum, causis, signis, et curatione* (Paris), 1554. R. Transl Moffatt, R.

7. Quoted by Whitwell, 1936, p. 175, who gives Trallianus's birth and death dates as 525–605, from Trallianus Alexander: *Medici libri duodecim*, interpret. Guintherius (Basil), 1556. Italics in original.

8. Quoted by Whitwell, 1936, p. 181, who gives Avicenna's birth and death dates as 980–1037. Whitwell cites as a source, *Opera*, ed. Alpagus et Benedictus (Venet.), 1582, and *Morb. Ment.* (Paris), 1659. Italics in original.

9. Quoted by Whitwell, 1936, p. 196, who gives Gaddesden's birth and death dates as 1280–1361. Source cited is Gaddesden Joh.: *Practica Johanni*

Anglica—Rosa medicina nuncupata. (Papiae), 1492. Transl. (Wulff.)

10. Cited by Whitwell, 1936, p. 205, who gives Manardus's birth and death dates as 1462–1536. Citation given is Manardus Joan: *Epist. Med.* Venet., 1542. Italics in original.

11. Quoted by Whitwell, 1936, p. 212, from Pratensis Jason: *De cerebri morbis.*. Basil 1549.

12. Quoted by Whitwell, 1936, p. 98, who gives Platter's birth and death dates as 1536–1614. Although it is not clear which of Platter's works is the source of this quotation, Whitwell later quotes from: *Praxeos medicae Tomi tres*. (Basil), 1656. *Histories and Observations*. London: Culpeper and Cole, 1664.

13. Quoted by Jackson (1986, p. 255) from Willis T: *Two Discourses Concerning the Soul of Brutes. . . .* Trans. S Pordage. London: Thomas Dring, Ch. Harper and John Leigh, 1683, pp. 201, 205.

14. Quoted by Jackson (1986, p. 256) from [Boerhaave H]: *Boerhaave's Aphorisms: Concerning the Knowledge and Cure of Diseases, Which is That of a Vital and Sensitive Man. The First is Physiological Shewing the Nature, Parts, Powers, and Affections of the Same. The Other is Pathological, Which Unfolds the Diseases Which Affect It and Its Primary Seat; to Wit, the Brain and Nervous Stock, and Treats of Their Cures: with Copper Cuts*. London: W and J Innys, 1735, pp. 323-324.

15. Quoted by Jackson (1986, p. 257) from: Robert James, *A Medicinal Dictionary; Including Physic, Surgery, Anatomy, Chymistry, and Botany, in All Their Branches Relative to Medicine. Together with a History of Drugs*. 3 vols. 2: *Mania*. London: T Osborne, 1743-1745.

16. Quoted by Jackson (1986, p. 258) from: Mead, Richard: Medical precepts and cautions. In: *The Medical Works of Richard Mead, M.D.* London: C Hitch et al., 1762, pp. 485-486.

17. Quoted by Jackson (1986, p. 259) from Cullen W: *First Lines of the Practice of Physic*. 2 vols., in 1. Edited by J Rotheram. New York: E Duyckinck, 1806, p. 497.

18. Quoted by Jackson (1986, p. 262) from Esquirol E: *Mental Maladies: A Treatise on Insanity*. Translated by EK Hunt. Philadelphia: Lea and Blanchard, 1845, pp. 381-382.

19. Quoted by Jackson (1986, p. 263) from Baillarger, 1854, p. 352.

20. Quoted by Jackson (1986, p. 268) from Ritti A: Circular insanity. In: *A Dictionary of Psychological Medicine Giving the Definition, Etymology and Synonyms of Terms Used in Medical Psychology, with the Symptoms, Treatment and Pathology of Insanity and the Law of Lunacy in Great Britain and Ireland*, edited by D Hack Tuke, 2 vols. Philadelphia: P Blakiston, 1892, p. 214.

21. The great German psychiatrist Emil Kraepelin, the son of an actor, was born in 1856 in Neustrelitz, near the Baltic Sea. His older brother Karl, a biol-

ogy teacher, influenced Emil's decision to become a doctor and an academician. Interested in psychiatry while still at the Wuerzburg Medical School, Emil Kraepelin, upon graduation in 1878, studied with the neuroanatomists Bernard von Gudden and P.E. Flechsig. He then turned to experimental psychophysiological research, under the tutelage of Wilhelm Wundt. He held mental hospital appointments in Munich, Leubus, and Dresden. In 1886, he became professor of psychiatry in Dorpat, then moved to the same position in Heidelberg in 1890 and to Munich in 1904 [or 1903?]. In 1922, he retired from teaching and became head of the Research Institute of Psychiatry in Munich.

According to Alexander and Selesnick (1966), Kraepelin's training, personality, and dedication were well suited to the task of classifying and generalizing the myriad clinical observations made during the 19th century:

He learned early to respect authority, order, and organization. . . . "Imperial German psychiatry" was said to have gained its prominence under the "chancellorship" of Kraepelin, one of Bismarck's admirers. (pp. 162-163)

As Bismarck unified Germany, Kraepelin brought order to the balkanized psychiatry of the turn of the century. The first edition of his textbook, which he continued to revise throughout his life, was published in 1883. In succeeding editions, he refined and expanded the textbook from the brief outline of the first edition to the 2,425 pages of the ninth edition, published in 1927, a year after his death. The textbook was notable for its division of major mental illness into two categories and for its emphasis on prognosis. The third and fourth parts of the eighth edition, covering manic-depressive "insanity" and paranoia, were published separately in 1921, and it is that monograph that is cited throughout this book.

Zilboorg (1941), from his psychoanalytical perspective, summarizes the personal observations of Kraepelin from those who knew him personally:

[They] tell of his rather pleasant, responsive personality, of his tactful ability in bringing people together to work as an organized group, and of his great gifts as a teacher; yet it is curious that his scientific personality was so very detached, almost distant from the inner life of the patient. To Kraepelin a mentally sick person seems to have been a collection of symptoms. He was a true son of the great, energetic, and creative age that was interested greatly in humanity but comparatively little in man. Perhaps this trait in Kraepelin as a psychiatrist, which today would be considered a defect, was the very characteristic which helped rather than hindered him in the creation of his great system and school. He was able to collect and to study thousands of case histories, covering not only the story of each illness, but the history of each patient's life before the illness and a follow-up history of his life after he left the hospital. Dealing with such large masses of data, Kraepelin was able to sort out everything these many individuals had in common, leaving out of consideration the purely individual data. He thus arrived at an excellent general picture, at a unique perspective of a mental illness as a whole. But he seems to have been

almost unaware that in his careful study he lost the individual. (p. 452)

Berrios and Hauser (1988) take issue with this assessment, noting the "great depth and beauty" of Kraepelin's late conceptual writing. They quote from a 1920 work: "If these observations approximate the truth we will have to look for the key to the understanding of the clinical picture primarily in characteristics of the individual patient. . .his expectations play a decisive role."

22. Some psychoanalytic writers implied that different phases of manic-depressive illness were linked through some underlying mechanism. Prominent here is the conception of mania as a defense against depression (see Chapter 12). This analytical formulation, reminiscent of the earliest observations that mania grew out of melancholia, could be said to have anticipated the current continuum model.

23. This would apply most clearly to German and British psychiatry, perhaps less so to French psychiatry (Leff, 1977).

24. *Primary* is defined as depression in the absence of any preexisting or antecedent psychiatric or medical disorder.

25. The widespread use of effective pharmacological treatments, along with earlier recognition, probably accounts for the fact that contemporary studies of manic-depressive illness are more dependent on outpatient samples, whereas earlier studies were predominantly of inpatients.

26. It is possible that the high BP/UP ratio in Egeland's Amish data reflects special genetic factors limited to that population. However, as noted, Angst's group (1978) also found a 1:1 ratio of bipolar to unipolar illness when the sample was followed for many years and hypomania was ascertained.

27. In their second study, however, Abrams and colleagues (1979) found a higher morbid risk for unipolar depression in the unipolar manic patients compared with the bipolar patients.

28. Compared with unipolar patients, bipolar depressed patients were reported to have lower ratings of anxiety, anger, and physical complaints (Beigel and Murphy, 1971b); more psychomotor retardation (Beigel and Murphy, 1971b; Himmelhoch et al., 1972; Katz et al., 1982; Kotin and Goodwin, 1972; Dunner et al., 1976a), lower levels of measured physical activity (Kupfer et al., 1974), and more total sleep time (Kupfer et al., 1972; Hartmann, 1968; Duncan et al., 1979).

29. As used in this context, *pseudounipolar* overlaps with, but is not identical to, the term *false unipolar* previously discussed. The latter term describes patients currently designated as unipolar but who will go on to become bipolar; it is in effect a probability statement. On the other hand, *pseudounipolar* describes patients whose symptoms, course of illness, family history, and treatment response suggest that they have, at least in part, the bipolar

diathesis. However, the diathesis need not be expressed symptomatically.

30. Some investigators (e.g., Weissman et al., 1988b; Strober and Carlson, 1982) have suggested that clinical, family history, and natural history data show a possible relationship between delusional unipolar depression and the bipolar spectrum.

31. Unpublished data cited by Dunner, 1987.

32. This emphasis on presenting episode rather than course was somewhat ironic, because Meyer's own writings emphasized a longitudinal perspective.

33. In this respect, the American nosological systems had departed from Adolf Meyer's unitary conceptual framework.

4

The Manic-Depressive Spectrum

Manic-depressive insanity . . . [includes] certain slight and slightest colourings of *mood*, some of them periodic, some of them continuously morbid, which on the one hand are to be regarded as the rudiment of more severe disorders, on the other hand pass without sharp boundary into the domain of *personal predisposition*. In the course of the years I have become more and more convinced that all the above-mentioned states only represent manifestations of a *single morbid process*. (p. 1)
—Emil Kraepelin, 1921

Manic-depressive illness occurs in multiple forms and degrees of severity. The classic descriptions cited in Chapter 2, systematic observations reported in the literature, and our own research and clinical experience and that of our colleagues all convince us that the cardinal features of the illness are dimensional, that is, distributed along a spectrum. We explore the spectrum issue here because it introduces concepts that shaped the formal diagnostic systems reviewed in Chapter 5, and it clarifies our own conceptions of bipolar illness, implicit in discussions throughout this volume.

Kraepelin observed that many individuals in the families of bipolar patients demonstrated labile mood and a cyclothymic temperament. Recent research is consistent with his observation. Patients diagnosed as cyclothymic have far more bipolar patients in their family histories than would be expected by chance (Akiskal et al., 1977; Depue et al., 1981; Dunner et al., 1982). Even more convincing are data from monozygotic twin pairs showing that when one twin is diagnosed as manic-depressive, the co-twin, if not actually manic-depressive, very frequently is cyclothymic (Bertelsen et al., 1977).[1]

Although diagnosis is central to all of medicine, the assumptions underlying its various meanings are seldom examined. The most common medical classification model—the *categorical* approach—posits discrete diagnostic entities or discrete subtypes within a larger diagnostic group. *Dimensional* approaches, the most common competing model, characterize the individual patient according to where he or she falls on a number of separate dimensions. In this model, each individual represents the point of intersection of multiple parameters. Both models have gained support from studies using discriminate function analysis and other statistical techniques. Clearly, though, the categorical approaches always prevail, not because they are more compellingly supported by the empirical evidence but because they are much easier to grasp conceptually and to deal with statistically. Multi-dimensional approaches, however eloquently descriptive of an individual patient, will remain essentially unhelpful if they cannot test generalizations—that is, be applied to prediction.

Contrary to common assumption, the categorical approach does not preclude the concept of a *continuum* (Grayson, 1987). A diagnostic category need not have absolutely discrete and discontinuous boundaries. Let us suppose for the moment that individuals with depressive disorders do distribute more or less evenly along a continuum with self-limiting grief reactions on one end and severe, disabling major depressive illness on the other end (Kendell, 1968; Goodwin, 1977a). Even if discontinuity (i.e., clustering at discrete points along the spectrum) is not demonstrable, a useful category can still be defined by establishing a minimum (or maximum) threshold of symptoms for inclusion in the category. And the pattern of illness characteristics—symptoms, course, family history, treatment response, for example—reflects a convergence of several dimensional variables. Such a model should be acceptable to those who are comfortable with large, internally variable categories—the so-called lumpers—as well as to those who want to create a new category for every variant—the splitters. Diagnostic issues are discussed in Chapters 3 and 5 in terms of groups and subgroups. This is simply a convenience, not a conviction that any particular group has discrete, discontinuous boundaries. On the contrary, we are impressed with the subtlety of the shadings.[2]

Exploration of spectrum models of manic-depressive illness is important for several reasons. The reliable characterization and validation of subsyndromal states similar to bipolar illness would (1) enhance research on genetic markers and modes of genetic transmission, as discussed in Chapter 15, (2) provide an approach for identifying individuals at risk for the development of bipolar illness, and (3) permit the evaluation of treatments for milder forms, including the question of whether early intervention could lessen the chance of progression to bipolar illness. Existing prospective and retrospective data indicate that approximately one third of the individuals with subsyndromal states phenomenologically related to bipolar illness (i.e., cyclothymia) will go on to develop the full syndrome of bipolar illness (Akiskal et al., 1979a; Depue et al., 1981, 1989a). The possibility that this progression may be hastened by treatment with antidepressant drugs (see Chapter 22) gives further urgency to identifying subsyndromal cases.

The concepts of secondary depression and secondary mania have received considerable attention because of their importance to differential diagnosis (see Chapter 5) and because they may shed light on the pathophysiology of mood states (see Chapters 16 and 17). Re-examined in light of spectrum models, secondary mania and depression, like their primary counterparts, also appear to be expressions of an underlying diathesis, but a

Table 4-1. Spectrum Concepts of Individual Features of Manic-Depressive Illness

- Severity of depressive states
- Severity of manic states
- Severity of mixed states
- Polarity
- Cyclicity
- Duration of episodes
- Instability or rapidity of state changes (switches)
- Responsivity to treatment

weaker one, which therefore requires a greater perturbation to be expressed clinically. This possibility is most certain in the case of pharmacologically induced manias. Family history data suggest a vulnerability for these effects, but one that is less severe than that associated with spontaneous manic episodes. Similarly, Goodwin and Bunney (1971), in reviewing the reports of depression occurring in patients on the antihypertensive (and amine-depleting agent) reserpine, noted that the occurrence of true depressive symptoms was associated with a personal or family history of affective illness. From this they concluded that reserpine is more accurately considered a precipitant rather than a de novo inducer of the depressive state.

The major cross-sectional and longitudinal intrinsic features of manic-depressive illness are shown in Table 4-1.[3] They provide the best framework for considering the relative merits of dimensional and categorical approaches. As we shall see, the relationship between these different perspectives is not always straightforward.

STATE

The Depressive Spectrum

The debate about whether depressive disorders should be divided into categories or arrayed along a continuum has gone on for decades, without resolution (Kendell, 1968, 1976). In our view, there is more evidence consistent with the spectrum concept than there is with the idea that depressive disorders constitute discrete clusters marked by relatively discontinuous boundaries (Kendell, 1968; Goodwin, 1977a). Kraepelin came to the same conclusion in his classic 1921 treatise on manic-depressive illness:

There is actually an uninterrupted series of transitions to "periodic melancholia," at the one end of which those cases stand in which the course is quite indefinite with irregular fluctuations and remissions, while at the other end there are the forms with sharply defined, completely developed morbid picture and definite remissions of long duration. (p. 124)

The continuum or spectrum concept can be evaluated by correlating quantitative ratings of depressive items (e.g., on the Newcastle Scale) with independent measures, such as response to biological treatment or measures of genetic vulnerability.[4] Patients who would fit the older definitions of *neurotic* or *reactive* depression, for example, can be shown to have more major depressive disorder among first-degree relatives than do normal controls, but they have fewer ill relatives than patients with major depressive disorder (Robins and Guze, 1972).

Evidence gathered in the 1970s suggests that the concept of a depressive spectrum also applies to bipolar illness. Akiskal and colleagues (1978a) studied 100 outpatients with mild depressive states, variously referred to as "neurotic," "reactive," or "situational." During the prospective follow-up of 3 to 4 years, 40 percent of the 100 patients developed major affective disorder, and nearly half of these (45 percent) were bipolar. The terminology applied to the so-called soft bipolar spectrum (Akiskal and Mallya, 1987) can be somewhat confusing. Dunner and colleagues (1982) described a group of patients, termed *bipolar, other,* who had received outpatient treatment for their depression (and sometimes for their hypomania) but had never been hospitalized. Although they would meet the broad DSM-III-R criteria for major depression (see Chapter 5), they are not as seriously ill and would be classified in the residual category, *bipolar disorder, not otherwise specified.*[5] This group seems to be similar to Angst's dm category as described in Chapter 3. Like Akiskal's cyclothymic patients, the family history of Dunner's "bipolar, other" patients is similar to that of bipolar-I patients, as is their positive response to lithium. Using both clinical and nonclinical populations of college students, Depue and colleagues developed a systematic approach to the evaluation of subsyndromal affective states, focusing particularly on bipolar

forms. The touchstone of this elegant series of studies was the development of the General Behavioral Inventory (GBI), a self-report measure of traits that can assess the pattern of cyclothymia over time (Depue et al., 1981; Depue and Klein, 1988). Each of its 73 items, drawn from clinical descriptions of hypomania and depression and focused on lability, incorporates the dimensions of intensity, duration, and frequency. (The GBI is described in more detail in Chapter 13.) GBI scores for depression distribute across normal, cyclothymic, and bipolar-II populations; each group merges imperceptibly into the other, consistent with the concept of a spectrum.[6] These studies imply that the concept of a depressive spectrum applies equally to bipolar and unipolar depression, challenging Klerman's view (1974) that neurotic depression should be subsumed entirely in the unipolar spectrum.

Manic States

A spectrum concept was implicit in the classic descriptions of mania from the late 19th and early 20th centuries, as is evident in the quotation from Kraepelin that opens this chapter. After a hiatus of more than half a century, attention is once again being paid to this issue. In their longitudinal analysis of untreated manic episodes, Carlson and Goodwin (1973) described three stages of mania progressing from mild hypomania to delirious psychotic mania. The principal features of the three stages are outlined in Table 4-2, and the relationship among these stages and daily behavioral ratings is illustrated in Figure 4-1. The stages were inferred from a study of 20 hospitalized manic-depressive patients, who had a complete manic episode at some time during hospitalization.[7] Manic episodes were identified by global mania ratings made twice a day by consensus of the nursing research team, and they were corroborated by the psychiatrists' and nurses' written descriptions of the patient's affect, psychomotor activity, and cognitive state. The sequence of the affective, cognitive, and behavioral symptoms over the course of the episode was recorded. Based on analysis of these recordings, the patient's longitudinal course was divided into three stages, with predominant mood as the primary criterion—from the euphoria of stage I, to the anger and irritability of stage II, to the severe panic of stage III. In some of their patients, the

Table 4-2. Stages of Mania

	Stage I	Stage II	Stage III
Mood	Lability of affect; euphoria predominates; irritability if demands not satisfied	Increased dysphoria and depression, open hostility and anger	Clearly dysphoric; panic-stricken; hopeless
Cognition	Expansivity, grandiosity, overconfidence; thoughts coherent but occasionally tangential; sexual and religious preoccupation; racing thoughts	Flight of ideas; disorganization of cognitive state; delusions	Incoherent, definite loosening of associations; bizarre and idiosyncratic delusions; hallucinations in 1/3 of patients; disorientation to time and place; occasional ideas of reference
Behavior	Increased psychomotor activity; increased initiation and rate of speech; increased spending, smoking, telephone use	Continued increased psychomotor acceleration; increased pressured speech; occasional assaultive behavior	Frenzied and frequently bizarre psychomotor activity

Adapted from Carlson and Goodwin, 1973

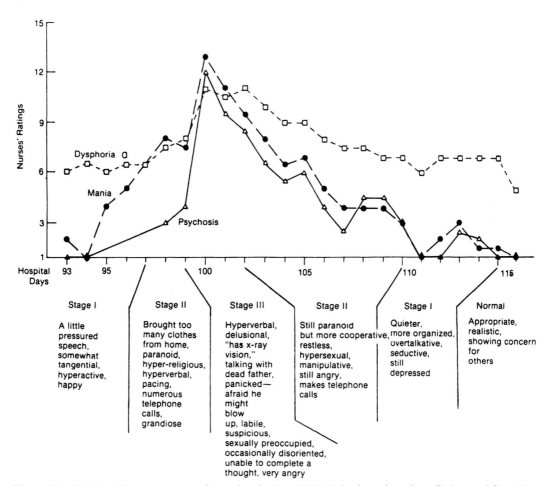

Figure 4-1. Relationship among stages of a manic episode and daily behavior ratings (from Carlson and Goodwin, 1973).

onset of mania (the switch) was gradual, clearly unfolding in a sequence until the full syndrome developed. In others, however, the onset was sudden and dramatic, but even in these cases, the earlier stages were present, if transient.

As Carlson and Goodwin elaborate, the initial phase of mania (stage I) typically is characterized by increased activity, by a labile mood that can be euphoric, irritable, or both, and by expansive, grandiose, and overconfident thoughts. Thinking remains coherent but is often tangential. Patients describe this change as "going high" and frequently report racing thoughts. In some instances, the "high" does not go beyond stage I, which corresponds to hypomania.

Many episodes progress to the next stage, however. Psychomotor activity increases—evident in the even more rapid speech—and the mood state becomes more labile, characterized by an admixture of euphoria and dysphoria. Irritability turns into open hostility and anger, and the accompanying behavior often is explosive and assaultive. As racing thoughts progress to a definite flight of ideas, cognition becomes increasingly disorganized. Preoccupations intensify, with grandiose and paranoid trends that are apparent as frank delusions. This level, which corresponds to frank mania, has been designated stage II.

In some patients, the manic episode can progress even further to an undifferentiated psychotic state (stage III), experienced by the patient as clearly dysphoric, usually terrifying, and accompanied by frenzied movement. Thought processes that earlier had been only difficult to follow become incoherent, and definite loosening of associations often is seen. Although delusions commonly are bizarre and idiosyncratic, some patients in this phase even experience ideas of reference, disorientation, and a delirium-like state. This phase of the syndrome is difficult to distinguish from other acute psychoses, at least superficially. In general, as the manic episode unfolds, stage I is dominated by elation (or irritability) and grandiosity, stage II by increasing hyperactivity and arousal, and stage III by florid psychotic disorganization.

In the 1973 Carlson and Goodwin study, many of the rated items showed graded continuous distributions, whereas others evidenced definite thresholds involving apparently qualitative shifts. The level of psychomotor activity continu-

ously escalated through all three stages, and ratings for manic mood continuously increased through stages I and II. On the other hand, ratings of psychoses were clearly not distributed along a continuum. This is illustrated by the case example presented in Figure 4-1. As can be seen, stage-III mania was characterized by the relatively abrupt and initial appearance of hallucinations, formal thought disorder in the Schneiderian sense, and organic delirium.

The stages of mania reflect the range of symptoms seen in hospitalized bipolar patients. Since that study was published in 1973, the focus has shifted to a milder portion of the mania spectrum typically seen in outpatients—a rediscovery of many of Kraepelin's classic observations. Kraepelin described a "manic temperament," which he originally termed *constitutional excitement*. The antithesis of the "depressive temperament," the manic temperament, at its most severe, was a handicapping condition marked by desultory, incoherent, and aimless thought, hasty and shallow judgment, restlessness, and exalted, careless, and confident mood—all of which resulted in a life that was "invariably a chain of thoughtless and extraordinary, not infrequently also nonsensical and doubtful activities." Kraepelin (1921) described the manic temperament as a "link in the long chain of manic-depressive dispositions," which in its least severe form could still be considered normal:

It concerns here brilliant, but unevenly gifted personalities with artistic inclinations. They charm us by their intellectual mobility, their versatility, their wealth of ideas, their ready accessibility and their delight in adventure, their artistic capability, their good nature, their cheery, sunny mood. But at the same time they put us in an uncomfortable state of surprise by a certain restlessness, talkativeness, desultoriness in conversation, excessive need for social life, capricious temper and suggestibility, lack of reliability, steadiness, and perseverance in work, a tendency to building castles in the air. . . . periods of causeless depression or anxiety. (pp. 129-130)

In his discussion of the issue, Klerman (1981) described a progression from normal happiness or joy through cyclothymic personality, nonpsychotic hypomania, psychotic mania, and delirious mania. It is clear, however, that this string of states does not reflect a spectrum of ever-increasing happiness and joy, since these pleasant emotions are replaced by qualitatively very dif-

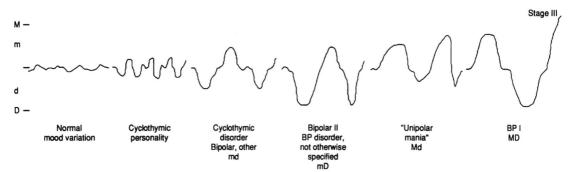

Figure 4-2. The spectrum of bipolarity.

ferent moods and sensations as one crosses the line from hypomania into mania. Klerman's recommendation that the term *elations* be used to encompass the spectrum of mania emphasizes mood over other important features, such as energy level, activity, behavior, and cognition. As noted earlier, the terminology can be confusing. In Klerman's spectrum, cyclothymic personality falls between normal happiness and hypomania. In DSM-III-R, a diagnosis of cyclothymia requires hypomanic episodes. In this diagnostic system, cyclothymia is differentiated from bipolar-II major affective disorder on the basis of its less severe depressions, which do not meet criteria for major depressive disorder. Using elation as the criterion for the manic spectrum also is reminiscent of older formulations in which depression and mania were at opposite ends of a continuum, with normal in the middle. Such a continuum is quite limited as a model primarily because it cannot account for *mixed states,* which, as we have seen in Chapter 2, are by no means rare. In general, it is best to consider the depressive spectrum and the manic spectrum as independent and capable of interacting in a variety of combinations and permutations.

BIPOLAR ILLNESS

If we integrate the depressive and manic spectrums, we can construct an overall spectrum of bipolar illness. At one end is cyclothymic personality, then cyclothymic disorder (*bipolar, other* in Dunner's terms and *md* in Angst's terms), followed by bipolar-II disorder (*mD, bipolar disorder, not otherwise specified* in DSM-III-R), then Md (often misdiagnosed as *unipolar mania*), and

finally MD, which is core bipolar illness. Figure 4-2 illustrates this spectrum by displaying the mood variation characteristic of each subgroup. Note that in this spectrum we implicitly consider mania to be more severe than depression, since the Md form is closer than the mD (bipolar II) to the severe end of the spectrum.

Differential vulnerabilities are discernible within the broad categories of hypomania-mania and depression. Whereas some individuals experience an episode spontaneously, others require nonspecific activating factors (stress), and still others require more specific activators, such as antidepressant drugs or electroconvulsive therapy (ECT).

As given, the spectrum is only descriptive. It does not necessarily imply a progression, nor does it require that all these states share some unitary relationship. There may be some individuals fitting the description of cyclothymic personality, for example, whose family history or response to treatment may not be related to bipolar-I disorder. Available data suggest, however, that a large percentage of individuals with the so-called soft or subsyndromal states apparently analogous to bipolar disorder do indeed belong in the bipolar spectrum by virtue of their positive family histories and their tendency to progress to full clinical disorder. Once we move beyond the temperaments into cyclothymic disorder,[8] the evidence compellingly argues for the inclusion of cyclothymic disorder in the bipolar spectrum. Cycles of mood and energy can continue indefinitely, constituting a mild form of manic-depressive illness, or they can progress to a more severe expression of it, sometimes after years.

Kraepelin (1921) assumed that cyclothymia is

part of the manic-depressive spectrum, and modern-day investigators[9] have argued persuasively for its inclusion on the basis of (1) family history data linking cyclothymia with the more severe forms of bipolar illness, (2) overlap and similarity of symptom patterns between cyclothymia and bipolar manic-depressive illness, (3) comparability of rates for pharmacologically induced hypomania, and (4) the subsequent development of full syndromal illness in many patients diagnosed initially as cyclothymic. In some instances, cyclothymia can be regarded as a milder expression of manic-depressive illness and, in others, as a precursor to the full syndrome of bipolar illness. (Further discussion of the literature on the phenomenology of cyclothymia can be found in Chapter 2.)

ILLNESS FEATURES

Polarity

The relationship between unipolar and bipolar illness is of interest both practically and theoretically. This issue was discussed in Chapter 3 and is summarized here. Observation of subtleties in family history and responses to different drugs suggests that a substantial number of unipolar patients are very closely related to bipolar patients and may represent an intermediate place on a polarity spectrum. We are referring here to the bipolar characteristics of some unipolar patients, not to the common clinical mistake of overlooking a prior hypomanic episode and thus failing to diagnose bipolar illness or to the problem of unipolar patients requiring reclassification to bipolar when mania develops later (see discussion of false unipolar diagnoses in Chapter 3). Winokur and Clayton (1967) described a group of unipolar patients with familial pure depressive disease (see Chapter 3) as being closely related to the bipolar subgroup. This and similar observations have been extended by Akiskal and colleagues (1985b), who described unipolar patients with an early age of onset, a high episode frequency, and a family history of bipolar illness as "pseudounipolar." Depue and Monroe (1978) referred to these patients as "unipolar II," and Cassano and colleagues (1988) as "bipolar III." Likewise, in a longitudinal study of successfully treated unipolar patients, Giles and colleagues (1989) found

that an early age of onset was the most powerful predictor of recurrence. The concept of atypical depression (Davidson et al., 1982) may also overlap with the pseudounipolar group.

This group of patients may share some pharmacologic response characteristics with the bipolar group. Thus, Akiskal and colleagues (1985b) and Cassano and associates (1988) found that such patients were at risk for developing hypomania on antidepressant medications. Further, in the initial controlled trial reporting antidepressant effects of lithium, the response rate among the cyclic unipolar patients was equivalent to that of the bipolar patients (Goodwin et al., 1969).

In his review of the double-blind controlled prophylactic trials of lithium, Schou (1979b) noted that unipolar patients with cycle lengths between 12 and 24 months (i.e., in the range of the typical bipolar patient) responded to prophylactic lithium as well as bipolar patients, and their lithium response was superior to that obtained with tricyclics (see Chapter 23). Taken together, these genetic and pharmacological data (summarized in Table 4-3) suggest that the more recurrent forms of unipolar depression are very closely related to bipolar illness (Akiskal, 1983a; Cassano et al., 1988). Another facet of the polarity spectrum, already alluded to in Chapter 3, is the relationship between polarity and severity of depression. Thus, several investigators have pointed out that differences between bipolar and unipolar groups diminish as the unipolar category includes more seriously ill, hospitalized patients (Winokur, 1980a; Tsuang et al., 1985; Stancer et al., 1987). These severity indices probably overlap considerably with the more recurrent forms of unipolar illness. Klein and colleagues (1988) have made the interesting observation that a higher proportion of unipolar patients with coexisting dysthymia (double depression) experience hypo-

Table 4-3 Pseudounipolar Depression
(Unipolar II or Bipolar III)

• Bipolar family history
• Hypersomnic-retarded
• Early onset
• High episode frequency
• Pharmacological hypomania
• Lithium responsive

Adapted from Akiskal, 1983a

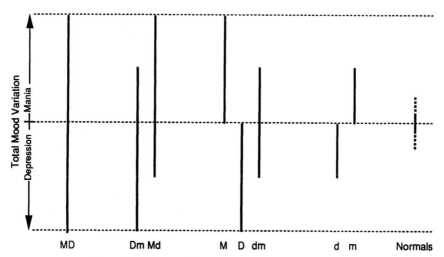

Figure 4-3. Range of total mood variation by subgroup.

manic episodes at follow-up, and their first-degree relatives have higher rates of bipolar-II disorder than unipolar patients without dysthymia. They suggest that double depression is heterogenous, with one subset linked to bipolar illness. This observation awaits replication.

Figure 4-3, which schematically illustrates the total mood variation possible within each subgroup, represents another way to express a spectrum of polarity.

Cyclicity

As reviewed in Chapter 6, individual bipolar patients vary considerably in their average length of time between episodes, ranging from less than every 48 hours to many years. Although considerable intraindividual variability in cycle length also is evident in bipolar patients, on average it is less than the interindividual variability. Cycle lengths among unipolar patients, which on the average are substantially longer than those for bipolar patients, also vary over a considerable range. Figure 4-4, illustrating typical patterns of cyclicity, emphasizes the enormous variability of the inherent cyclicity of bipolar illness.

We examined cycle length in the patients studied by Grof (Zis et al., unpublished data; Goodwin and Jamison, 1984), a sample not affected by prophylactic treatment (Figure 4-5). A continuum of cycle lengths is discernible in these data, although there were clusters at 12-month intervals that may (in part) reflect reporting bias. This phenomenon could reflect the impact of an-

nual (seasonal) rhythms on the inherent cyclicity of the illness. These data included too few short cycles to determine whether rapid cycling (defined as four or more episodes per year) exists on a continuum with longer cycles or whether it represents a discontinuity, that is, a separate subgroup. A similar question can be raised about the apparently rare phenomenon of ultrarapid cycles (such as every 48 hours). In this case, a distinct subgroup seems especially likely.

Related to ultrarapid cycling is the phenomenon of mood instability, in which moods shift sharply within the same day or even hour. Although this phenomenon is a common feature of stage-III mania, it also can be encountered outside of the context of typical bipolar illness. This form of rapid mood lability is probably heterogeneous diagnostically. Some patients meet criteria for borderline disorder, others for complex partial seizure, and still others for cyclothymia. We will return to this issue in Chapter 5 when we discuss differential diagnosis.

Finally, it is necessary to distinguish rapid cycling from continuous cycling, in which there is no free interval between episodes (see Chapter 6). Although many continuous cycles are indeed rapid, the two are not necessarily synonymous.

Duration of Episodes

As outlined in Chapter 6, episode length is widely variable from patient to patient, but it tends to be relatively constant within a given patient. Whether episode duration can be said to correlate posi-

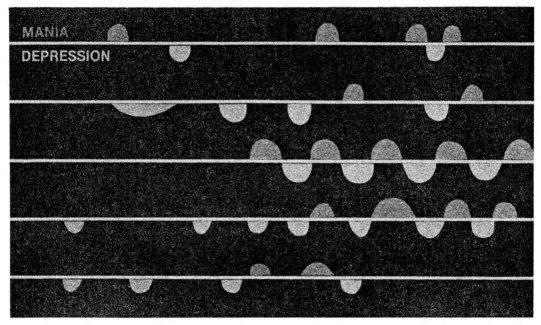

Figure 4-4. Representative patterns of cyclicity.

tively with overall illness severity is not clear. Some patients experience brief but severe episodes (micropsychoses), for example, and the relatively mild episodes of cyclothymia also are characteristically brief. On the other end of the spectrum are the episodes that go on to become chronic—that is, of indefinite length—and therefore no longer episodic at all. On the other hand, in the literature of the era before the use of lithium, many of the single-episode patients represented the chronically hospitalized who were

cycling but without free intervals of sufficient length to allow discharge.

Instability of State Changes

The rate at which state changes occur is a variable that is related to cyclicity but independent of it. Clearly, some patients can switch rapidly from one state to the other, whereas others change much more gradually. Whether this phenomenon exists on a continuum or in clusters is not known. The propensity to undergo shifts in mood, level of activation, or other changes associated with state may be a relatively constant characteristic throughout the entire bipolar spectrum (Depue et al., 1987). This characteristic appears to be independent of episode severity.

Treatment Responsivity

Response to treatment is an important variable that, in general, is independent of the severity of the illness. For some patients, it even appears to be inversely related to severity. Patients who experience clear-cut but serious episodes of mania and depression against a personality of stable maturity often can respond completely to pharmacological intervention. In contrast, some bipolar-II patients show considerable character pathology, interepisode lability, and the related problems of substance abuse. Although their

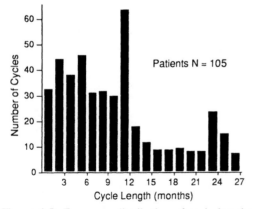

Figure 4-5. Frequency distribution of cycle lengths among 105 bipolar patients studied longitudinally (data from Zis et al., 1981, unpublished observations).

mood episodes are less severe and disruptive, the overall treatment outcome can be limited by the associated features. Such patients often lead chaotic lives, have poor or unpredictable social support systems, and comply poorly with medications.[10]

SUMMARY

A spectrum or continuum concept provides a useful way to integrate a variety of observations concerning manic-depressive illness. The identification of subsyndromal forms of bipolar illness itself enhances the study of genetic factors and also provides an approach to identifying individuals at risk for the development of full clinical bipolar illness. Spectrum models have been most useful in helping us understand the continuity between bipolar and unipolar forms of affective illness. This continuum has to do in part with issues of cyclicity. It also helps to conceptually accommodate the increasingly recognized subtle forms of hypomania that merge into personality and temperament. Still unexplored are questions of individual differences in certain characteristics, which, although independent of the illness, nevertheless interact with it. Here we might include general reactivity to environmental events, the extent of which would contribute to the threshold necessary to trigger a manic or depressive episode in an individual patient.

NOTES

1. These issues are discussed more thoroughly in Chapter 15.
2. Even within categories, variation always occurs. Cantor and Genero (1986) point out that the "natural" categories into which human beings organize their perceptual experiences do not have "obvious necessary and sufficient *criterial* properties, so that boundaries between closely related categories are ill-defined." People find it extraordinarily difficult or impossible to specify criteria for common object categories, such as furniture, birds, fruit, or clothing. Instead, they identify correlated features that imply a continuum of category membership, ranging from a prototype (an apple is a very typical fruit, for example) to a more atypical member (a tomato is a fruit often thought to be a vegetable). Assigning such atypical members to one category or another can be difficult, and the overlap of characteristic features from one category to another also "runs counter to the intuitive notion of well-defined, orthogonal categories with clearly demarcated boundaries" (p. 236).
3. Some of the differences among individual manic-depressive patients reflect differences in the illness per se, whereas others reflect the interaction of the illness with individual characteristics, some of which certainly involve genetic differences unrelated to manic-depressive illness.
4. The reactive-endogenous or the neurotic-psychotic dichotomies (or spectra) should not be taken simply as a reflection of differential severity, that is, from mild to severe in the consequences for the patient. As observed by Sir Aubrey Lewis in 1936:

   It may be said, simply, that severe emotional upsets ordinarily tend to subside, but that mild emotional states, when often provoked or long maintained, tend to persist, as it were, autonomously. Hence the paradox that a gross blatant psychosis may do less damage in the long run than some meagre neurotic incubus: a dramatic attack of mania or melancholia, with delusions, wasting, hallucinations, wild excitement and other alarms, may have far less effect on the course of a man's life than some deceptively mild affective illness which goes on so long that it becomes inveterate. The former comes as a catastrophe, and when it has passed the patient takes up his life again, active, cheerful, normal in every way, while with the latter he may never get rid of his burden. (p. 998)
5. The DSM-III-R category *bipolar disorder, not otherwise specified* was originally meant for bipolar-II patients, but many such patients meet DSM-III-R criteria for bipolar major affective disorder, given that the criteria for major depression are broad enough to include a wide range of severity. On the other hand, cyclothymia in DSM-III-R reflects a milder state referred to by Dunner as "cyclothymic personality" that is also milder than the cyclothymia described by Akiskal.
6. With appropriate cut-off scores, the GBI can be used for case identification in either nonclinical or clinical populations. It may be particularly useful in family studies. For example, when evaluated against clinically determined DSM-III diagnoses, the GBI was found to have a sensitivity of 90 percent and a specificity of 98 percent when used with adolescent offspring of bipolar-I parents and parents with nonaffective major psychiatric diagnoses (Klein et al., 1986b). Originally structured to identify only bipolar affective states, a broadened GBI has been applied to the separation of bipolar from unipolar subjects with considerable success (Depue et al., 1989a).
7. Despite the presence of schizophrenic-like symptoms during the manic episodes, the diagnosis of manic-depressive illness was confirmed on follow-up. Demographic data suggested that the patients in this study were like manic-depressive patients in other studies in relapse frequency, duration of illness, and other features.
8. Some investigators (e.g., Kukopulos et al., 1983; Akiskal and Akiskal, 1988; Cassano et al., 1988) focus on the opposite temperaments—depressive

and hyperthymic—and propose that a fundamental characteristic of bipolarity is the shift from one temperamental state into the opposite *extreme* in the form of an episode. Thus, depressive temperaments are vulnerable to a swing into hypomania or mania, whereas those with hyperthymic temperaments are likely to swing into depressions.

9. Akiskal, 1981, 1983a,b; Akiskal et al., 1977, 1978a, 1979a, 1983b; Depue and Monroe, 1981; Depue et al., 1978; Waters, 1979.

10. As detailed in Chapter 25, medication compliance is a major problem for both bipolar-I and bipolar-II patients, although the factors that contribute to it may be different in each group.

5

Diagnosis

The history of psychiatric diagnosis has been notable for its confusion, reflected in the myriad overlapping systems for classifying and subdividing depressive disorders. In the midst of this disarray, bipolar manic-depressive illness has remained a relatively consistent and stable diagnostic category. The consensus from the 1983 Dahlem Conference on the Origins of Depression confirmed the impression that, among the various subgroups of affective disorders, only bipolar illness emerges as undisputed. Characterizing patients as bipolar leads to valid predictions about family history, course, prognosis, and treatment response. In this chapter, we review the formal criteria for the diagnosis of manic-depressive illness, focusing on the bipolar form. With the category thus defined, we then reexamine the boundaries it shares with other major diagnostic categories, the majority of which have already been considered briefly in the discussion of spectrum concepts. Here the focus is on clinical decision making.

A careful reading of the relevant literature leads to the inescapable conclusion that reliable diagnosis requires a longitudinal as well as a cross-sectional view of the patient.[1] This literature also charts a course for clinicians, underscoring the need to meet repeatedly with the patient and to seek out other people, particularly family members, who can give a clearer picture of the patient's history, symptoms, and behavior. Such practices decrease the clinician's dependence on cross-sectional data and increase the reliability of diagnoses.

It is often assumed uncritically that the complexities and subtleties of our diagnostic endeavors will vanish as soon as the true causes of psychiatric disorders are uncovered. This notion probably stems from nostalgia for the relative clarity of the early days of the infectious disease era and a wish for a straightforward causal link, such as that found between inborn errors of metabolism and clinical disease. Without disparaging the importance of those discoveries, we should recognize that they have created unrealistic expectations. Compared to that early cause–effect paradigm, far more complex models now guide the study and treatment of common infectious diseases, models that account for the interactions between the immune system and influences on the individual's response to the etiologic agent. The direct link between inborn errors of metabolism and disease also is undependable as a prototype, since such diseases are rare and frequently are associated with early death. Identifying an association between a primary causal factor (such as an abnormal gene) and a particular clinical picture would not automatically resolve diagnostic confusion in psychiatry any more than it would in the rest of medicine. On the other hand, such advances can help immeasurably in clarifying the nature and meaning of heterogeneity. A good example is Huntington's disease. Although caused by a defect in a single autosomal dominant gene, its clinical manifestations are enormously varied and heterogeneous: In some patients, the disease leads to early severe debilitation, whereas in others it follows a chronic course; some patients endure severe mood symptoms and contemplate or commit suicide, whereas others experience motor dysfunction without psychological symptoms. Clearly, in each patient the specific gene defect interacts with highly individualized factors—genetic and environmental—and the disease in all of its heterogeneity is the outcome of the interaction.

THE DEVELOPMENT OF CONTEMPORARY DIAGNOSTIC SYSTEMS

Successive versions of the *International Classification of Diseases,* now undergoing its tenth revision (ICD-10), represent the official diagnostic systems used by clinicians throughout most of the world. The major exception, of course, is the United States, where clinicians use the American Psychiatric Association's (APA) *Diagnostic and Statistical Manual,* the third edition of which was revised in 1987 (DSM-III-R).[2] The relationship of these diagnostic systems to each other is illustrated in Figure 3-1 (see also Van Praag, 1982a,b). Two European systems of classification are also important—the Present State Examination, or (PSE)/CATEGO (Wing et al., 1974), and the system developed by the Association for Methodology and Documentation in Psychiatry (AMDP) (Guy and Ban, 1982).

ICD-6 Through ICD-9 and DSM-I and DSM-II

The first effort to establish a universal diagnostic system for psychiatric illnesses was made by the World Health Organization (WHO) in its 1948 International Classification of Diseases (ICD-6), formerly the International Classification of Causes of Death. As Andreasen (1982a) has pointed out, the ICD was designed as a system that could be applied throughout the world, and

thus it attempted to encompass a great variety of conceptual backgrounds, which in turn resulted in many of the categories overlapping. The 16 different subtypes of affective disorder in the ICD-9, grouped under eight different main headings, cannot readily be compared with the descriptive diagnostic systems that have evolved recently from systematic research on these disorders.

The APA's first diagnostic manual (DSM-I) was published in 1952. Although developed independently of the ICD, like it, the American system was not derived from systematic research. In DSM-I, *manic-depressive reaction* appeared along with *psychotic depressive reaction* as subcategories of *affective reactions,* which, in turn, comprised one of four categories of psychosis.

In 1968, the eighth revision of the ICD appeared, as did the revised APA manual (DSM-II), and they generally paralleled each other. *Manic-depressive reaction* became *manic-depressive illness* and, with *involutional melancholia,* was classified under *major affective disorders. Psychotic depressive reaction* was pulled out of the affective disorders category and became a separate class. ICD-9, which appeared in 1978, remains, at this writing, the official diagnostic system outside the United States. The ICD-9 categories for affective psychosis are outlined in Table 5-1 and displayed in parallel with those of DSM-III-R and ICD-10. As was true of its predecessors, the categories in ICD-9 overlap conceptually. Since they still do not incorporate clear descriptive criteria, they frustrate empirical solutions to the vexing problem of cross-national differences in diagnosis—a problem that must be solved before comparative epidemiological studies can be done properly (see Chapter 7). It is true that, compared to some diagnostic constructs, Kraepelin's formulation of a unitary illness involving recurrent episodes of depression with or without mania enjoyed relatively more cross-national agreement (Roth and Barnes, 1981; Faravelli and Pole, 1982; Klerman, 1984). Differences were still considerable, however, as evidenced in the U.S.–U.K. study of diagnosis described later, as well as in the comparisons between the more narrow German and French view of manic-depressive illness and that of the British (Kendell et al., 1974).

Table 5-1. Classification of Affective Disorders and Related Conditions

ICD-9	DSM-III-R (DSM-III)	ICD-10
Mood (Affective) Disorders	Mood Disorders (Affective Disorders)	Mood (Affective) Disorders

ICD-9 column:

Mood (Affective) Disorders

296.0 MDP, manic

296.1 MDP, depressed

296.2 MDP, circular, currently manic

296.3 MDP, circular, currently depressed

296.4 MDP, circular, mixed

296.5 MDP, circular, condition not specified

296.6 MDP, other and unspecified

Schizophrenic disorders, schizoaffective

Personality disorders, affective

Neurotic disorders, neurotic depression

Depressive disorder not elsewhere classified

DSM-III-R (DSM-III) column:

Mood Disorders (Affective Disorders)

Bipolar Disorders
296 Bipolar Disorder
  296.4x manic
  296.5x depressed
  296.6x mixed
301.13 Cyclothymia (Cyclothymic Disorder)
296.70 Bipolar Disorder not Otherwise
  Specified (Atypical Bipolar Disorder)
Depressive Disorders
296 Major Depression
  296.2x single episode
  296.3x recurrent (recurrent episode)
300.40 Dysthymia (or Depressive neurosis)
  (Dysthymia Disorder)
  Specify: primary or secondary type
  Specify: early or late onset
311.00 Depressive Disorder not Otherwise
  Specified (Atypical Depression)
Psychotic Disorders not Elsewhere Classified
298.80 Brief reactive psychosis
295.40 Schizophreniform disorder
  Specify: with or without good prognostic
  features (not in DSM-III)
295.70 Schizoaffective disorder
  Specify: bipolar or depressive type
  (not in DSM-III)

ICD-10 column:

Mood (Affective) Disorders

Manic Episode
Depressive Episode
  Severe
  Mild
Bipolar Affective Disorder
  Manic
  Depressed
  Mixed
  In remission
Recurrent Depressive Disorder
  Severe
  Mild
  Variable
Persistent Affective States
  Cyclothymia
  Dysthymia
Other Mood (Affective) Episodes
  Other affective episodes
  Other recurrent affective
    disorders
  Other persistent affective states
Schizoaffective Disorders
  Schizomanic
  Schizodepressive
Affective Disorders not Otherwise
  Specified

MDP = Manic-depressive psychosis

87

Empirically Based Systems: The Research Diagnostic Criteria, DSM-III-R, and ICD-10

ICD-9 and DSM-II were fundamentally flawed, despite their greater use of descriptive material and implicit recognition of the bipolar–unipolar distinction. They were essentially compromises constructed around isolated, mutually exclusive belief systems about etiology. In DSM-II, it appears that each school of psychiatric thought was assigned its own category, which reflected its own etiological assumptions. For example, a presumed psychosocial etiology was the defining characteristic for depressions not associated with physiological disturbances or major functional impairment. Depressions associated with these latter features were presumed to be endogenous—biological in origin. In both the ICD-9 and DSM-II, manic-depressive illness stayed in the "endogenous" column. *Neurotic (reactive) depression* and *psychotic depressive reaction* (or *reactive depressive psychosis*) were excluded from the manic-depressive illness category, implying that the presence of precipitating factors was incompatible with such a diagnosis.

Clearly, what was desperately needed was a nosological system that was etiologically neutral, a system that allowed the independent assessment of types and severity of symptoms, presence of precipitating events, extent of functional impairment, personality characteristics, and the presence of other psychiatric diagnoses. Without such a system, the long-standing debate pitting biological imperatives and predispositions against psychological forces and social influences would remain an exercise in polemics. Likewise, attempts to foster understanding of manic-depressive illness by bridging these insular schools of thought would continue to founder, as would efforts to clarify the relationship between affective illness and schizophrenia.

Starting with a series of studies by the Washington University group in St. Louis, such a system began to evolve during the early 1970s (Robins and Guze, 1970; Winokur et al., 1969; Feighner et al., 1972). This approach was based on the fundamental premise that a diagnostic category should be supported by *specific descriptive criteria*. The criteria would specify both which characteristics would lead to making that diagnosis (inclusive criteria) and which would lead to not making it (exclusive criteria). To be incorporated, a criterion must first prove to be reliable—that is, independent observers applying it in actual clinical situations must be able to agree on its meaning. These requirements marked a pivotal departure from psychiatry's past efforts to establish a standardized diagnostic system. It is no exaggeration to say that the empirical approach initiated by the St. Louis group, and carried forward by its fruitful collaboration with Robert Spitzer and his colleagues at the New York State Psychiatric Institute in the development of the Research Diagnostic Criteria (RDC) (Spitzer et al., 1978a,b), represented a fundamental advance in clinical psychiatry, providing a diagnostic instrument with a reasonably high level of interobserver reliability and stability.[3] The RDC formed the basis for the DSM-III (1980). Various approaches to the estimation of the validity of the affective diagnoses are reviewed elsewhere.[4]

The systems as they have so far evolved are by no means ideal. For example, as illustrated in Figure 5-1, the organization of the RDC and DSM-III-R[5] implies that bipolar disorder is distinct from major depression. This division discourages considerations of underlying unifying relationships between bipolar and unipolar patterns of disorder, including the possibility of a continuum between them (see Chapter 4). Further obscuring contemplation of a bipolar–unipolar continuum is the awkward placement of bipolar-II disorder as a residual category, under *bipolar disorder, not otherwise specified*. This classification is, nonetheless, a marginal improvement over DSM-III, where the residual category was referred to as *atypical*. Another drawback of the DSM-III and DSM-III-R is that they lack some of the rich clinical descriptiveness of the ICD-9.

Other criticisms can be made of the system in general, not just the bipolar category. First, natural course, longitudinal patterns, and family history in recurrent affective illness are not included in the DSM-III-R criteria, despite their clear importance. The lack of attention to course means that the DSM-III-R can define the episode more reliably than the disorder. For example, in their longitudinal studies of patients with mixed affective and schizophrenic symptoms, Angst and associates (1980b), Marneros and colleagues

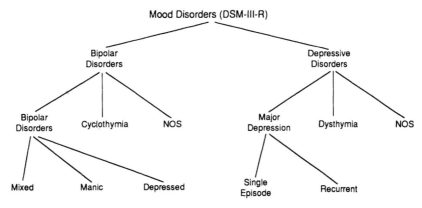

Figure 5-1

(1988), and Maj (1989) noted a high proportion who undergo syndrome shifts—that is, at one point in their history they can be diagnosed schizophrenic, at another as having an affective disorder. Second, since all criteria are equally weighted, a DSM-III-R diagnosis (or one made by the related RDC) cannot by itself replicate the complex process of pattern recognition by which the experienced clinician arrives at a diagnosis. These limitations are summarized by Himmelhoch (1984):

The diagnosis of the affective disorders is in danger of becoming a formula. Descriptors of depression or mania are selected from one diagnostic system or another as if from a Chinese menu. . . . Diagnosis turns into simple description, and diagnostic categories into neoplatonic Procrustean beds into which heterogeneous affective syndromes are forced to fit regardless of their obvious differences from one another regarding premorbid development, course, and outcome. Diagnosis as description, therefore, displaces the notion of diagnosis as hypothesis. (p. 271)

Although the RDC and DSM-III-R are very similar, the RDC criteria are more stringent and slightly more detailed because the RDC serves a different purpose than the DSM-III-R (see Table 5-2 for the principal differences in criteria for mood disorders between the two systems). Primarily a research instrument, the RDC was designed to help investigators select pure populations for research, excluding potential subjects who do not clearly fall within a given diagnostic category. DSM-III-R, in contrast, is used clinically, and criteria must be sufficiently inclusive to keep the number of undiagnosed patients to a minimum. Both the RDC and the DSM-III-R descriptors are criteria—inclusionary and exclusionary—whereas the ICD-9 descriptions are not, strictly speaking, empirically derived criteria; nor have the individual items been evaluated for reliability.

The ICD-10, now undergoing field trials, will become official by 1993. Heavily influenced by the development of DSM-III, it groups all of the mood disorders together. *Manic-depressive psychosis* is to be replaced by *bipolar affective disorder* and *recurrent depressive disorders. Neurotic depression, reactive depressive psychosis,* and *affective (cyclothymic) personality disorder* have been relocated to the major groups of affective disorders. The tentative classification scheme for ICD-10 is reviewed in Table 5-1.

We now turn to the specific diagnostic criteria as defined by DSM-III-R. For mania, depression, and mixed states, the criteria define episodes, and for cyclothymia and schizoaffective disorders, they also define the disorder. The role of biological measures in diagnosis is reviewed in Chapter 17.

DIAGNOSTIC CRITERIA

When making a diagnosis, the clinician ideally assesses presenting signs and symptoms and weighs them together with the patient's history and prior response to treatment and the family's history. Individual symptoms—even clusters of symptoms—viewed at one point in time often lack diagnostic specificity, although such cross-sectional views are sometimes all that are available. In the following section, we use the relevant DSM-III-R categories as a framework for discussing diagnoses.

Table 5-2. Principal Differences Between RDC and DSM-III-R
(Organized According to the RDC Categories)

General
RDC more stringent, (i.e., DSM-III-R criteria generally correspond to the probable level in RDC)

Manic Disorder
This is "Bipolar Disorder, Manic" in DSM-III-R (i.e., unipolar mania is folded into bipolar category)

Like DSM-III-R (but unlike DSM-III), the RDC include marked impairment in functioning (i.e., now both systems can differentiate mania from hypomania)

RDC exclude Schneiderian first-rank symptoms; DSM-III-R does not, as long as a full manic syndrome is present

Hypomanic Disorder
This is part of "Bipolar Disorder, Not Otherwise Specified" (NOS) in DSM-III-R (i.e., hypomania without depression is folded into a bipolar category)

Bipolar Depression with Mania (BPI)
and Bipolar Depression with Hypomania (BPII)
The difference between BPI and BPII disorders is awkward in DSM-III-R, since BPII is relegated to being part of the residual category, "Bipolar Disorder, NOS"

Major Depressive Disorder
As with mania, RDC exclude Schneiderian first-rank symptoms; DSM-III-R does not, as long as a full depressive syndrome is present

RDC require that the patient be functionally impaired or has sought help; DSM-III-R has no such requirements except for the "severe" level, coded in the 5th digit

Some of the RDC subtypes (primary, secondary, agitated, retarded, situational) are not carried over in the DSM-III-R; others (i.e., psychotic, endogenous, incapacitating) are expressed in 5th digit specifications

Schizoaffective Disorder   **— Manic Type**
                                  — Depressed Type
RDC require a full affective syndrome, plus either Schneiderian first-rank symptoms or psychotic symptoms before or after the affective episode

Patients meeting RDC criteria for schizoaffective disorder would be diagnosed by DSM-III-R as having a mood disorder

DSM-III-R requires the coexistence of all the acute symptoms of schizophrenia (See Table 5-8), plus at least two weeks of psychosis without prominent mood symptoms. (Key is the duration of the mood symptoms relative to the psychotic symptoms.)

DSM-III-R classifies as either "Bipolar Type" or "Depressive Type"

Mania and Hypomania

DSM-III-R defines a *manic episode* as follows:

The essential feature of a Manic Episode is a distinct period during which the predominant mood is either elevated, expansive, or irritable, and there are associated symptoms of the Manic Syndrome. The disturbance is sufficiently severe to cause marked impairment in occupational functioning or in usual social activities or relationships with others, or to require hospitalization to prevent harm to self or others. The associated symptoms include inflated self-esteem or grandiosity (which may be delusional), decreased need for sleep, pressure of speech, flight of ideas, distractibility, increased involvement in goal-directed activity, psychomotor agitation, and excessive involvement in pleasurable activities which have a high potential for painful consequences that the person often does not recognize. (pp. 214-215)

In DSM-III-R, diagnostic criteria for manic episode (Table 5-3) include psychotic features, even the Schneiderian first-rank symptoms that some investigators have thought to be pathognomonic of schizophrenia. The framers of DSM-III-R departed from earlier diagnostic systems because evidence had accumulated confirming the presence of considerable thought disorder and gross psychotic content in patients clearly defined as manic by all other indicators. Although the classic literature also supports the observation that mania has psychotic features (see Chapters 2 and 11), some observers believe that the DSM-III-R definition of mania is overly inclusive, which leads to diagnosing many schizoaffective patients as manic (see, e.g., Angst, 1986c). Specific exclusionary criteria are used to rule out other psychotic or organic mental disorders, a point that is developed in the section on differential diagnosis.

DSM-III-R defines a *hypomanic episode* less specifically than it does a manic one:

The essential feature of a Hypomanic Episode is a distinct period in which the predominant mood is either elevated, expansive, or irritable and there are associated symptoms of the Manic Syndrome. By definition, the disturbance is not severe enough to cause marked impairment in social or occupational functioning or to require hospitalization (as required in the diagnosis of a Manic Episode). The associated features of Hypomanic Episodes are similar to those of a Manic Episode except that delusions are never present and all other symptoms tend to be less severe than in Manic Episodes. (p. 218)

Although some symptoms of hypomania and mania are on a continuum, the psychotic disorganization of mania is not as clearly dimensional (see Chapter 4). Embedded in the DSM-III-R criteria for mania (Table 5-3) are the criteria for hypomania, that is, the same symptoms (A and B) without marked impairment (C). The RDC, on the other hand, are more precise in defining hypomania by requiring at least two associated symptoms (three if the mood is irritable rather than elated). Some clinical investigators continue to prefer these more detailed RDC criteria.

Bipolar-II disorder—that is, bipolar depression with hypomania—is called *bipolar disorder, not otherwise specified* in DSM-III-R. To be diagnosed with this disorder, the patient must have met the criteria for hypomania and major depressive disorders but never those for manic disorder or cyclothymia.[6] If a patient meets criteria for hypomania and has a history of depressions

not severe enough to be designated as major depression, the appropriate DSM-III-R diagnosis is cyclothymia.

Depression

As is true for mania and hypomania, the DSM-III-R criteria for depression are more precise than the descriptors in ICD-9, although the latter scheme does contain highly descriptive clinical language. DSM-III-R criteria for *major depressive episode* are outlined in Table 5-4. As with the criteria for mania, the boundaries of major depressive disorder were considerably broadened by incorporating additional psychotic features, including mood-incongruent delusions. We will return to this issue later when we discuss differential diagnosis. The requirement of at least 2 weeks' duration is regarded as too short by many clinicians, who prefer the 1 month originally in the Feighner criteria (Feighner et al., 1972).

Perhaps the most important difference between ICD-9 and DSM-III-R is that the former, under the rubric of *manic depressive psychoses, depressed type,* emphasizes the recurrent nature of endogenous forms of depression and implies that such depressions are closely related to bipolar illness (i.e., circular manic-depressive illness). DSM-III-R, on the other hand, separates bipolar depression from major depression (single episode or recurrent), thereby reinforcing the bipolar–unipolar dichotomy, as discussed in Chapter 3.

Within the DSM-III-R framework, there is no attempt to differentiate bipolar from unipolar depression on any grounds other than the presence or absence of a prior history of mania. Clinical features reported to differentiate bipolar from unipolar depression (see Chapter 3) are not incorporated into the DSM-III-R system.

Mixed States

DSM-III-R and ICD-9 do not provide separate empirically derived criteria for mixed states but instead refer to the criteria for mania and for depression. DSM-III-R criteria for *bipolar disorder, mixed* are:

A. Current (or most recent) episode involves the full symptomatic picture of both Manic and Major Depressive Episodes (except for the duration requirement of two weeks for depressive symptoms) . . . intermixed or rapidly alternating every few days.

Table 5-3. DSM-III-R Criteria for Manic Episode *(Compared with DSM-III)*

Note: A "Manic Syndrome" is defined as including criteria A, B, and C below.
         A "Hypomanic Syndrome" is defined as including criteria A and B but not C. *(DSM-III-R has*
         added criterion C to the definition of "Manic Syndrome," thereby differentiating it from
         "Hypomanic Syndrome." In DSM-III, criteria for Hypomania were listed under Cyclothymia)

A.   A distinct period of abnormally and persistently elevated, expansive, or irritable mood. *(DSM-III*
     called for one or more distinct periods; mood must be a prominent part of the illness and might
     alternate with depressive mood)

B.   During the period of mood disturbance, at least 3 of the following symptoms have persisted (4 if
     only irritable) and have been present to a significant degree
     1.   inflated self-esteem or grandiosity *(DSM-III noted that grandiosity may be delusional)*
     2.   decreased need for sleep, e.g., feels rested after 3 hours
     3.   unusually talkative or pressure to continue talking
     4.   flight of ideas or subjective experience that thoughts are racing
     5.   distractibility, i.e., attention too easily drawn to unimportant or irrelevant external stimuli
     6.   increase in goal-directed activity (social, work, school, sex) or psychomotor agitation
     7.   excessive involvement in pleasurable activities which have a high potential for painful
          consequences, e.g., buying sprees, sexual indiscretions, or foolish investments

C.   Mood disturbance sufficiently severe to cause marked impairment in occupational functioning or
     in usual social activities or relationships with others, or to necessitate hospitalization to prevent
     harm to self or others. *(DSM-III-R has added this criterion)*

D.   At no time during the disturbance have there been delusions or hallucinations for as long as 2
     weeks in the absence of prominent mood symptoms (i.e., before development or after remission)
     (DSM-III also excluded bizarre behavior)

E.   Not superimposed on Schizophrenia, Schizophreniform Disorder, Delusional Disorder *(Paranoid*
     Disorder in DSM-III), or Psychotic Disorder NOS *(DSM-III-R has added Psychotic Disorder*
     NOS)

F.   It cannot be established that an organic factor initiated and maintained the disturbance. Note:
     Somatic antidepressant treatment (e.g., drugs, ECT) that apparently precipitates a mood
     disturbance should not be considered an etiologic organic factor *(DSM-III-R has added this note)*

Manic Episode codes: 5th-digit code numbers and criteria for severity of current state of Bipolar
Disorder, Manic or Mixed
     1.   Mild: meets minimum symptom criteria (or almost meets symptom criteria if a previous
          episode)
     2.   Moderate: extreme increase in activity or impairment in judgment
     3.   Severe, without Psychotic Features: almost continual supervision required in order to
          prevent harm to self or others

                                                                                            Continued

Table 5-3 Continued. DSM-III-R Criteria for Manic Episode *(Compared with DSM-III)*

(DSM-III-R has added these 3 specifications)
4. With Psychotic Features: delusions, hallucinations, or catatonic symptoms. If possible, specify if mood-conguent or mood-incongruent

   Mood-congruent psychotic features: delusions or hallucinations whose content is entirely consistent with the typical manic themes of inflated worth, power, knowledge, identity, etc. *(DSM-III also included flight of ideas and unawareness that speech is not understandable)*

   Mood-incongruent psychotic features: Either A or B:
   A. delusions or hallucinations whose content does not involve the typical manic themes mentioned above. Also included are persecutory delusions, thought insertion, and delusions of being controlled
   B. catatonic symptoms, e.g., stupor, mutism, negativism, and posturing
5. In Partial Remission: full criteria were previously, but are not currently, met; some signs or symptoms have persisted
6. In Full Remission: full criteria were previously met, but there have been no signs or symptoms for at least 6 months

(DSM-III-R has divided and clarified the DSM-III "In Remission" category)

0. Unspecified

B. Prominent depressive symptoms lasting at least a full day. (p. 226)

The ICD-9 definition is vague and spotty:

Manic-depressive psychosis, circular type, mixed: An affective psychosis in which both manic and depressive symptoms are present at the same time. (p. 420)

By the DSM-III-R criteria, patients with rapid cycles would be included under mixed states if their episodes last less than 2 weeks. Other diagnostic systems are, for the most part, equally nonspecific in their treatment of mixed states. The Vienna Research Criteria are an exception, and we include them here for their descriptive value (Table 5-5).

The following case history demonstrates the extreme variability in the clinical picture of a patient with a mixed state:

The patient was a 21-year-old woman . . . hospitalized after her behavior had turned bizarre, with rapid speech, flight of ideas, rhyming, punning, outbursts of anger, and physical aggressiveness. . . . There was considerable evidence of depression admixed with typically manic behavior and at times this would break through to overt expressions accompanied by outbursts of crying. . . . In the midst of grandiose and confident statements she gave the suicidal message: "I felt so low last night that if someone had given me a gun or knife,

POW. I have to cover up my depression, that's part of the reason why I can't sleep". . . . Later, following successful treatment with lithium, the patient said, "My high mood is like rushing up excess energy and becoming extra active in order to lift myself out of depression. Depression is really the basic mood and the highness is a cover—a holding operation. I've always been so afraid of people knowing what I'm really thinking or feeling. I haven't wanted anyone to know I'm depressed because I had no reason to be depressed and I was ashamed of it." (Bunney et al., 1968, pp. 499, 500, 504, 505)

Cyclothymia

Consistent with our discussion of cyclothymia in Chapter 4, the DSM-III-R description notes that the boundaries between this disorder, *bipolar disorder,* and *bipolar disorder, not otherwise specified* are not well defined and that many investigators believe that it is a mild form of bipolar illness. The description continues with the associated features of cyclothymia, which are:

. . . similar to those of Manic Episode and Major Depressive Episode except that, by definition, there is no marked impairment in social or occupational functioning during the Hypomanic Episodes. In fact, in some cases the person is particularly productive in occupational situations and socially effective during Hypo-

Table 5-4. DSM-III-R Criteria for Major Depressive Episode *(Compared with DSM-III)*

Note: A "Major Depressive Syndrome" is defined by criterion A below.

A. At least 5 of the following symptoms have been present for 2 weeks and represent a change from previous functioning; at least 1 must be either (1) depressed mood or (2) loss of interest or pleasure. (Do not include symptoms due to physical condition, mood-incongruent hallucinations, incoherence, or marked loosening of associations.) *(DSM-III describes that for children under 6 these symptoms may be manifested in a sad facial expression)*

1. depressed mood (irritability in children and adolescents) almost all day of every day, as indicated subjectively or by others
2. marked diminished interest in pleasure in all or almost all activities, most all of the day, nearly every day, as indicated subjectively or by others
3. significant weight loss or gain without dieting (>5% of body weight a month) or decrease or increase in appetite (in children, consider failure to make expected weight gains)
4. insomnia or hypersomnia nearly every day
5. psychomotor agitation or retardation nearly every day (observable by others, not merely subjective feelings of restlessness or being slowed down) *(DSM-III notes that for children less than 6 this is hyperactivity)*
6. fatigue or loss of energy nearly every day
7. feelings of worthlessness or excessive or inappropriate guilt (may be delusional) nearly every day (not merely guilt or self-reproach about being sick) *(DSM-III add this latter distinction)*
8. diminished ability to think or concentrate, or indecisiveness, nearly every day, as indicated subjectively or by others
9. recurrent thoughts of death (not just fear of dying), recurrent suicidal ideation without a specific plan, or a suicide attempt or a specific plan for committing suicide
(DSM-III-R has clarified each symptom to some extent)

B. 1. It cannot be established that an organic factor caused disturbance
    2. The disturbance is not a normal reaction to death of a loved one (Uncomplicated Bereavement)
        Note: Morbid preoccupation with worthlessness, suicidal ideation, marked functional impairment, psychomotor retardation, or prolonged duration suggest bereavement complicated by Major Depression *(DSM-III-R has added this note)*

C. At no time during the disturbance have there been delusions or hallucinations for as long as 2 weeks without prominent mood symptoms (i.e., before development or after remission) *(DSM-III also included bizarre behavior)*

D. Not superimposed on Schizophrenia, Schizophreniform Disorder, Delusional Disorder *(Paranoid Disorder in DSM-III)*, or Psychotic Disorder NOS *(DSM-III-R has added Psychotic Disorder NOS)*

Continued

Table 5-4 Continued. DSM-III-R Criteria for Major Depressive Episode *(Compared with DSM-III)*

Major Depressive Episode codes: 5th-digit code numbers and criteria for severity of current state of Bipolar Disorder, Depressed, or Major Depression:

(DSM-III notes that when psychotic features and Melancholia are present, the coding system requires that the most clinically significant characteristic is recorded)

1. Mild: few, if any, symptoms in excess of those required for diagnosis, and symptoms result in only minor impairment in occupational functioning, social activities, or relationships with others

2. Moderate: symptoms or functional impairment between "Mild" and "Severe"

3. Severe, without Psychotic Features: several symptoms in excess of those required for diagnosis, and symptoms markedly interfere with occupational functioning, social activities, or relationships with others

(DSM-III-R has added these 3 specifications)

4. With Psychotic Features: delusions or hallucinations *(DSM-III also included depressive stupor).* If possible, specify whether the psychotic features are mood-congruent or mood-incongruent

>   Mood-congruent psychotic features: delusions or hallucinations whose content is entirely consistent with the typical depressive themes of personal inadequacy, guilt, disease, death, nihilism, or deserved punishment. *(DSM-III also included depressive stupor.)*

>   Mood-incongruent psychotic features: delusions or hallucinations whose content does not involve the typical depressive themes mentioned above. Included here are such symptoms as persecutory delusions (not directly related to depressive themes), thought insertion, thought broadcasting, and delusions of control

5. In Partial Remission: intermediate between "In Full Remission" and "Mild," and no previous Dysthymia. (If Major Depressive Episode was super-imposed on Dysthymia, the diagnosis of Dysthymia alone is given once the full criteria for a Major Depressive Episode are no longer met.)

6. In Full Remission: During the past 5 months, no significant signs or symptoms of the disturbance

(DSM-III-R has divided and clarified the DSM-III "In Remission" category.)

0. Unspecified

(DSM-III had "Without Melancholia" and "With Melancholia" as the 2 nd and 3 rd digits. DSM–III–R has replaced them with a list of criteria for "Melancholic Type" of a Major Depressive Episode)

Specify chronic if current episode has lasted 2 consecutive years without a period of 2 months or longer during which there were no significant depressive symptoms. *(DSM-III-R has added this specification)*

Specify if current episode is Melancholic Type. *(DSM-III-R has added this specification — see above)*

(DSM-III-R has added diagnostic criteria for seasonal patterning of Major Depressive Episodes)

Table 5-5. Vienna Research Criteria for Mixed States

Endogenomorphic — axial syndrome of unstable mixed states

A and B Obligatory

A. Appearance of rapidly alternating swings in affectivity, emotional resonance, or drive following a period of habitual functioning

    At least one of the following symptoms required
    1. Rapidly alternating swings between depressive and/or anxious, euphoric/expansive, or hostile mood
    2. Rapidly alternating and exaggerated emotional resonance touching various affective states (depressive, anxious, manic, hostile)
    3. Rapid change between inhibition, agitation, increased drive, and occasionally aggression. (The rapid swinging can bring about "concordant" or "discordant" changes in affectivity and drive — for example, manic mood combined with decreased drive — because each element may swing in a different rhythm)

B. Appearance of biorhythmic disturbances

    Symptoms 1 and 2 are required
    1. Diurnal variations of one or more of the symptoms under A
    2. Sleep disturbances
        At least one of the following symptoms required
        a. Early awakening
        b. Interrupted sleep

Adapted from Berner et al., 1983

---

manic Episodes. However, many people experience social difficulties in their interpersonal relationships and academic and occupational pursuits because of the recurrent cycles of mood swings.

Psychoactive Substance Abuse is common as a result of self-treatment with sedatives and alcohol during the depressed periods and the self-indulgent use of stimulants and psychedelic substances during the hypomanic periods. (pp. 226-227)

The DSM-III-R diagnostic criteria for cyclothymia are given in Table 5-6.

Schizoaffective Disorder

In DSM-I and -II, schizoaffective illness was included as a subtype of schizophrenia, reflecting the broad Bleulerian concept of schizophrenia as discussed later in this chapter. Subsequent research documented the frequent occurrence of Schneiderian first-rank[7] and related schizophrenic symptoms (e.g., catatonic features, paranoia, bizarre behavior, and formal thought disorder) in individuals whose family history, natural course, other symptoms, and treatment outcome clearly place them in the manic spectrum. American psychiatry departed significantly from the Bleulerian tradition when, in DSM-III, it substantially broadened the scope of affective ill-

nesses to include nonaffective psychotic symptoms. Schizoaffective illness was moved in DSM-III from schizophrenia to an intermediate category labeled *psychotic disorders not elsewhere classified.*

Although the original DSM-III did not provide criteria for schizoaffective disorder, the RDC and DSM-III-R do (Table 5-7). These criteria essentially restate the acute symptoms required for a diagnosis of schizophrenia (Table 5-8) but without continuous signs of illness for 6 months or more. The schizoaffective category is thus reserved for patients who meet the acute symptomatic criteria for mania (or depression) and for schizophrenia and who have had delusions or hallucinations in the absence of prominent mood symptoms for more than 2 weeks. (If the delusions or hallucinations are present for less than 2 weeks, the patient would meet criteria for a primary affective disorder.)

Some controversy persists over whether this newly delineated category is closer to affective illness or to schizophrenia. (These issues are discussed extensively in Marneros and Tsuang, 1986.) Some investigators believe that since patients with mood-incongruent symptoms are now

Table 5-6. DSM-III-R Criteria for Cyclothymia *(Compared with Cyclothymic Disorder in DSM-III)*

A. At least 2 years (1 for children and adolescents) of numerous hypomanic episodes (all of the criteria for Manic Episode except marked impairment) and numerous periods of depressed mood or loss of interest in pleasure (not meeting criterion A of Major Depressive Episode)

B. Never without hypomanic or depressive symptoms for more than 2 months at a time during a 2-year period (1 year for children and adolescents) *(DSM-III lists symptoms characteristic of hypomanic and depressive episodes)*

C. No clear evidence of a Major Depressive Episode or Manic Episode during the first 2 years (1 year for children and adolescents). Note: If, after this minimum period, there are Manic or Major Depressive Episodes, the additional diagnosis of Bipolar Disorder or Bipolar Disorder NOS should be given

D. Not superimposed on a chronic psychotic disorder, such as Schizophrenia or Delusional Disorder. *(DSM-III specified absence of psychotic features related to these disorders, e.g., delusions, incoherence, etc.)*

E. An organic cause cannot be established, e.g., repeated drug or alcohol intoxication. *(DSM-III-R has added this criterion. However, DSM-III did specify, not caused by other mental disorder)*

(DSM-III-R has generally simplified the criteria for Cyclothymia and has recognized different criteria for children and adolescents)

included under mood disorders in DSM-III-R, the remaining individuals with mixtures of schizophrenic and affective symptoms (particularly depressive symptoms) are closer to the schizophrenic end of the schizoaffective spectrum (Kendler et al., 1986). As outlined in Chapter 15, family history studies support an association between DSM-III-R (or RDC) schizoaffective disorder and manic-depressive illness, and probably also schizophrenia.[8] There is no reason, how-

Table 5-7. DSM-III-R Criteria for Schizoaffective Disorder *(Compared with DSM-III)*

A. A disturbance during which, at some time, there is either a Major Depressive or a Manic Syndrome concurrent with symptoms that meet the A criterion of Schizophrenia (see Table 5-8)

B. During an episode of the disturbance, there have been delusions or hallucinations for at least 2 weeks, but no prominent mood symptoms

C. Schizophrenia has been ruled out, i.e., the duration of all episodes of a mood syndrome has not been brief relative to the total duration of the psychotic disturbance

D. It cannot be established that an organic factor caused the disturbance

Specify: bipolar type (current or previous Manic Syndrome) or
depressive type (no current or previous Manic Syndrome)

(DSM-III-R has given this category specific diagnostic criteria. DSM-III was limited to examples of schizoaffective episodes.)

Table 5-8. DSM-III-R Criteria for Schizophrenia

Differences from DSM-III:

The A criterion has been reorganized to make it simpler, and slightly modified to take into account changes in the criteria for Delusional (Paranoid) Disorders. Furthermore, to exclude transient psychotic disturbances, the symptoms in A must be present for at least 1 week. The B criterion has been revised to take into account onset in childhood and to avoid the term "deterioration," which suggests that recovery never occurs. The requirement that the illness begin before age 45 has been eliminated since several studies have not supported the validity of this DSM-III criterion. However, to facilitate further study of this issue, a specification is provided for cases with late onset (after 45).

A. Presence of characteristic psychotic symptoms in the active phase: either 1, 2, or 3, for at least 1 week (unless the symptoms are successfully treated):
    1. 2 of the following:
        a. delusions
        b. prominent hallucinations (throughout the day for several days or several times a week for several weeks, each hallucinatory experience not being limited to a few brief moments)
        c. incoherence or marked loosening of associations
        d. catatonic behavior
        e. flat or grossly inappropriate affect
    2. bizarre delusions (i.e., involving a phenomenon that the person's culture would regard as totally implausible, e.g., thought broadcasting, being controlled by a dead person)
    3. prominent hallucinations (as defined in 1b above) of a voice with content having no apparent relation to depression or elation, or a voice keeping up a running commentary on the person's behavior or thoughts, or two or more voices conversing with each other

B. During the course of the disturbance, functioning in such areas as work, social relations, and self-care is markedly below the highest level achieved before onset of the disturbance (or, when the onset is in childhood or adolescence, failure to achieve expected level of social development).

C. Schizoaffective Disorder and Mood Disorder with Psychotic Features have been ruled out, i.e., if a Major Depressive or Manic Syndrome has ever been present during an active phase of the disturbance, the total duration of all episodes of a mood syndrome has been brief relative to the total duration of the active and residual phases of the disturbance.

D. Continuous signs of the disturbance for at least six months. The six-month period must include an active phase (of at least 1 week, or less if symptoms have been successfully treated) during which there were psychotic symptoms characteristic of Schizophrenia (symptoms in A), with or without a prodromal or residual phase, as defined below.

    Prodromal phase: A clear deterioration in functioning before the active phase of the disturbance that is not due to a disturbance in mood or to a Psychoactive Substance Use Disorder and that involves at least 2 of the symptoms listed below.

Continued

Table 5-8 Continued. DSM-III-R Criteria for Schizophrenia

Residual phase: Following the active phase of the disturbance, persistence of at least 2 of the symptoms noted below, these not being due to a disturbance in mood or to a Psychoactive Substance Use Disorder.

Prodromal or Residual Symptoms:
1. marked social isolation or withdrawal
2. marked impairment in role functioning as wage-earner, student, or homemaker
3. markedly peculiar behavior (e.g., collecting garbage, talking to self in public, hoarding food)
4. marked impairment in personal hygiene and grooming
5. blunted or inappropriate affect
6. digressive, vague, overelaborate, or circumstantial speech, or poverty of speech, or poverty of content of speech
7. odd beliefs or magical thinking, influencing behavior and inconsistent with cultural norms, e.g., superstitiousness, belief in clairvoyance, telepathy, "sixth sense," "others can feel my feelings," overvalued ideas, ideas of reference
8. unusual perceptual experiences, e.g., recurrent illusions, sensing the presence of a force or a person not actually present
9. marked lack of initiative, interests, or energy

Examples: 6 months of prodromal symptoms with 1 week of symptoms from A; no prodromal symptoms with 6 months of symptoms from A; no prodromal symptoms with 1 week of symptoms from A and 6 months of residual symptoms

E. It cannot be established that an organic factor initiated and maintained the disturbance.

F. If there is a history of Autistic Disorder, the additional diagnosis of Schizophrenia is made only if prominent delusions or hallucinations are also present.

Classification of course. The course of the disturbance is coded in the 5th digit:
1. Subchronic: the time from the beginning of the disturbance, when the person first began to show signs of the disturbance (including prodromal, active, and residual phases) more or less continuously, is less than 2 years, but at least 6 months
2. Chronic: same as above, but more than 2 years
3. Subchronic with Acute Exacerbation: reemergence of prominent psychotic symptoms in a person with a subchronic course who has been in the residual phase of the disturbance
4. Chronic with Acute Exacerbation: reemergence of prominent psychotic symptoms in a person with a chronic course who has been in the residual phase of the disturbance
5. In Remission: when a person with a history of Schizophrenia is free of all signs of the disturbance (whether or not on medication), "In Remission" should be coded. Differentiating Schizophrenia In Remission from No Mental Disorder requires consideration of overall level of functioning, length of time since the last episode of disturbance, total duration of the disturbance, and whether prophylactic treatment is being given
0. Unspecified.

ever, to assume a priori that family history is a more valid basis for forming categories than is treatment response or outcome. The position that schizoaffective illness ultimately will occupy on the spectrum of schizophrenia and affective illness may depend on whether one is referring to schizomanic conditions or schizodepressive ones. The schizomanic condition clearly seems more closely associated with affective illness (T. Reich, personal communication, 1985), and genetic data from the NIMH collaborative study (Rice et al., 1987b) strongly support the close relationship between bipolar-I disorder and schizoaffective manic illness. Schizoaffective depressed patients, on the other hand, differ considerably from each other in outcome, a substantial proportion of them close to the schizophrenic pole (Brockington et al., 1980b).[9]

Conceptual issues are the source of the debate over the relationship between affective illness and schizophrenia. Akiskal and Puzantian (1979) emphasize this confusion about schizophrenic symptoms in affective illness and point to problems in eliciting these symptoms:

An affirmative answer to the question, "Do people put thoughts in your head" does not necessarily mean that the patient is reporting thought insertion. It is the actual *experience* that one's ego is permeable—e.g., that thoughts are oozing out and alien influences are penetrating the mind—that is so characteristic of the Schneiderian criteria. Therefore, Schneider's *first rank* symptoms are most reliable when elicited through spontaneous report by the patient rather than by direct questioning. . . . the occasional presence of one or two first rank symptoms does not rule out the diagnosis of an affective psychosis made on the basis of the overall clinical picture, family history, response to treatment, and follow-up criteria. . . . [A] female patient, in a state of psychotic depression, complained that she was completely devoid of any energy and will, that voices had taken over her actions, and that they described every step before she took them. . . . such feelings of somatic passivity have long been described to occur in otherwise classical affective psychoses. (pp. 430-431)

Other diagnostic concepts that have been associated with schizoaffective mixtures of symptoms—schizophreniform disorder, brief reactive psychosis, cycloid psychosis, and atypical psychosis—are discussed individually below.

Problems in Applying the DSM-III-R Criteria

We have discussed conceptual problems inherent in the DSM-III-R system, including those engendered by the separation of bipolar disorder from the depressive disorders. Here we note the practical problems that arise when applying this system in clinical practice.

DSM-III-R lists bipolar disorder first, then assigns depressive disorders to a totally separate category. This separation of categories at the outset is incompatible with the reality of clinical practice, where assessing patients with depressive symptoms is the most common diagnostic decision faced. The clinician's first task is to determine if the patient meets criteria for major depressive disorder or dysthymia and then to review the history for evidence of bipolar or unipolar illness. Compounding the problems caused by separating bipolar and unipolar major affective disorders, milder depressive states are listed only under the depressive disorders—that is, the nonbipolar disorders. A patient who is mildly or moderately depressed and also has a history of mania finds a niche in this system only by some awkward fitting. The system implies more homogeneity and separateness for the bipolar category than is justified by the data.

Another practical problem stems from the fact that the DSM-III-R has dropped the ICD-9 *circular* category, presumably because bipolar disorders are circular by definition. This omission creates a practical difficulty in coding bipolar patients in remission. Since they must be coded as either manic, depressed, or mixed, it is difficult to know which fourth-digit state designation to choose.

Clinical Summary

The nosological systems that have evolved during this century are in many respects superior to those used earlier. They are, for the most part, etiologically neutral, allowing for independent assessment of types and severity of symptoms, presence of precipitating events, extent of functional impairment, personality characteristics, and the presence of other psychiatric diagnoses. Problems remain in the classification of manic-depressive illness, however. The RDC and DSM-III-R, for example, imply a greater separation of bipolar and unipolar affective illness than the evidence supports. The placement of bipolar-II as a residual category obscures its relationship to other affective illness. Also troubling is the absence of criteria concerning long-term course of illness from all categories of affective illness and the failure to provide for a mild form of depression in bipolar illness. These and other features are problematic for clinical as well as conceptual reasons.

THE PSYCHOSES—SEPARATE OR CONTINUOUS?

We have in front of us a fruit called psychosis, and we don't know whether it's a citrus that will divide itself into separable sections or an apple that we must divide along arbitrary lines. —Belmaker and Van Praag, 1980a

Clinicians frequently encounter patients with psychotic symptoms and must decide whether to diagnose affective illness, schizophrenia, or a schizophrenic-like condition. The classification of psychotic behavior has implications that reach beyond the care of individual patients, however. Interpreting the results of research from different points in history and different locations in the world rests on an understanding of how psychotic entities are defined. Evidence cited throughout this book must be seen through the diagnostic lens used at a given time and place. Because of the importance of this issue for differential diagnosis, epidemiology, genetics, and an understanding of the biological and psychological evidence, we digress for a brief survey of the traditional approaches to diagnosing psychosis.

As noted in Chapter 3, Kraepelin's deft structuring of his empirical observations has framed nosological considerations for the better part of this century. It is, however, a legacy not without problems, since dividing psychotic illness into two entities leaves many patients in a diagnostic no-man's-land. As Kendler (1986) points out, in the last several generations "no area in psychiatric nosology has been as controversial." Like many diagnostic dilemmas, this one has been magnified by too much reliance on presenting symptoms, too little on the history of the patient and his or her family. The formal definition and measurement of psychosis is discussed in Chapter 11 and is noted more briefly in Chapter 2.

The Two-Entities Tradition

Kraepelin's lucid discrimination of pattern in a mass of confusing clinical phenomena led him to propose a dichotomy of fundamentally different classes of psychotic illness (Kraepelin, 1896). Lacking knowledge of etiology or pathophysiology, he based the distinction on family history, age of onset, course, and outcome. In his original formulation, dementia praecox was marked by a steady downhill course into chronic dementia, and manic-depressive illness followed an episodic course with intermittent recovery. Kraepelin, "always aware of the provisional nature of his system" (Jablensky, 1981), later tempered his views (1919), acknowledging that features of the two illnesses were at times indistinguishable and that some dementia praecox patients appeared to recover, whereas some manic-depressive illness followed a progressive chronic course. Nosological hypotheses, especially those of such seductive simplicity, have a way of becoming dogma, however. When clinical realities—variable outcome, overlapping and, at times, indistinguishable presenting signs and symptoms—cast doubt on the concept of two basically different psychoses, modifications were proposed.

The major revision, of course, came from Bleuler (1911), who renamed dementia praecox *schizophrenia* and extended its boundaries. In Bleuler's hierarchical diagnostic order, certain schizophrenic symptoms were specific and pathognomonic—namely, those symptoms that defined the splitting of thought from feeling and behavior: formal thought disorder, blunted affect, autism, and ambivalence. The presence of any of these "fundamental symptoms" required a diagnosis of schizophrenia. Symptoms of affective illness, by contrast, were considered to be nonspecific; manic-depressive illness was diagnosed only after schizophrenia was excluded. Although Bleuler's system prevailed in the United States over the next several decades, many other countries, including the United Kingdom, followed different practices and defined affective disorder as encompassing a broader spectrum (Leff, 1977). The formal diagnostic systems used throughout the world before the 1980s by and large reflected either the Kraepelinian or Bleulerian conceptions of psychosis,[10] modified and confounded by etiological theorizing.

In clinical practice, the loose and redundant definitions of successive diagnostic systems encouraged idiosyncratic interpretations of diagnostic constructs. Manic-depressive illness, even the circumscribed entity Kraepelin defined, was not always diagnosed as such, especially in some parts of the United States. This point was demonstrated by Cooper and colleagues (1972), who initially tried to identify patient differences that would account for wide discrepancies in hospital admission rates for various mental disorders in the United States and the United Kingdom. In fact, using a cross-national team of diagnosticians, they found few differences in the patient samples between the two countries. But the chart diagnoses differed sharply: 62 percent of the New York patients had been diagnosed schizophrenic, compared with only 34 percent of the London sample. In London, psychotic depression had been diagnosed 5 times more often and mania 12 times more often than in New York (see Chapter 7).

Clearly, the New York concept of schizophrenia was so broad that it described virtually anyone with psychotic symptoms—what was then called "functional" mental illness. Cooper and colleagues point out that in the hubbub of the clinic, this need for a loosely defined category is understandable:

> Because many patients do not fit neatly into well-defined diagnostic categories, every classification has to have, in practice if not in theory, at least one category which is only loosely defined and can act as a "rag bag" for patients who do not fit in elsewhere. The dictum that "even a trace of schizophrenia is schizophrenia" . . . obviously lays the ground for a very loose definition of schizophrenia, enabling it to be used as a handy label for patients who do not possess the classical features of any other stereotype. It is our impression that patients with nondescript symptoms tend to be diagnosed as schizophrenics by New York psychiatrists at least in part because other diagnoses like manic-depressive illness are ruled out by the very close correspondence they require between the patients' symptoms and those of this stereotype before the diagnosis can be made. (1972, p. 129)

This broad definition of schizophrenia was able to survive into the early 1970s because a full appreciation of the specific treatments for manic-depressive illness had not yet been firmly established in the United States.

The U.S.–U.K. study was among the first to alert American psychiatrists to the possibility that they were diagnosing some affective patients as schizophrenic.[11] Subsequent research confirmed this impression (see, e.g., Silverstein et al., 1982). The adoption of DSM-III, along with growing appreciation of the treatment implications, appears to have modified American diagnostic practices. Andreasen (1987b) notes this change:

> The introduction of Schneiderian concepts to Great Britain in the late 1960's tightened up and narrowed British ideas [about schizophrenia], leading to a diver-

gence between British and American thinking. . . . By the 1980's, the pendulum in America had swung back to a narrower definition, largely through the influence of the St. Louis criteria, and American concepts are now narrower than British concepts. . . . American psychiatrists in 1960 were identifying very different patients as schizophrenic from those so identified in 1985, and a cross-national study conducted in 1985 would almost certainly indicate that Americans are using narrower concepts than are the British. (p. 10)

She concludes, "the boundary between schizophrenia and affective disorders must remain flexible, depending on whether the goal is research or patient care."[12]

A Schizophrenia–Affective Continuum

An alternative to choosing between two categories of psychosis is, obviously, to postulate a hybrid, which is what Jacob Kasanin did in 1933 when he coined the term *schizoaffective psychosis* to describe a group of relatively young patients with good premorbid adjustment who, in response to stress, developed the rapid onset of a psychosis characterized by "marked emotional turmoil," "false sensory impressions," but without "passivity." Most of Kasanin's patients went on to have subsequent episodes. Initial interest in schizoaffective symptoms grew out of curiosity about a relatively favorable outcome in some cases of schizophrenia—those with rapid onset, identifiable precipitating factors, good premorbid adjustment, and clear manic or depressive symptoms. This early conception of schizoaffective disorder as good-prognosis schizophrenia reflects one end of the current spectrum of views concerning patients whose characteristics place them somewhere between schizophrenia and manic-depressive illness.[13]

Uncertainty and disagreement continue over schizoaffective illness: Is it a separate disorder or a subtype of affective disorder? Are there varieties that are a subtype of schizophrenia? Or do most patients characterized as schizoaffective actually have a mixture of both illnesses? When Brockington and Leff (1979) applied eight different published definitions of schizoaffective illness to a sample of patients, they found virtually no agreement among the various definitions. As Taylor (1984) noted in his comprehensive review of this subject:

> Despite numerous studies of the diagnostic validity of schizoaffective psychosis or atypical psychosis, there

is no reliable, operationally defined set of criteria generally accepted by researchers and clinicians. (p. 136)

In the 1969 revision of the Mayer-Gross *Clinical Psychiatry,* Slater and Roth contended that the patient with a mixture of affective and schizophrenic symptoms who is observed long enough can usually be confidently diagnosed as having either affective illness or schizophrenia. They imply in this assertion that, by and large, the category has reflected incomplete or imperfect diagnoses rather than a meaningful diagnostic entity.

The family of diagnoses that have been associated with the concept of schizoaffective disorder includes *atypical psychosis, cycloid psychosis,* and *brief reactive psychosis. Schizophreniform disorder* was originally coined by Langfeldt (1937) to describe patients who today would probably be referred to as *schizoaffective* (although *schizophreniform* in DSM-III-R is not synonymous with *schizoaffective*).[14]

The existence of schizoaffective admixtures is compatible either with a two-disease model, which assumes discontinuity of symptoms, or a continuum model of psychotic illness, in which affective and schizophrenic symptoms represent different dimensions of vulnerabilities interacting to produce a spectrum of states from pure schizophrenia to pure manic-depressive illness. Such a position is favored by Meltzer (1984), who considered phenomenological, genetic, biological, outcome, and treatment response evidence concerning schizoaffective illness. "Current evidence appears most consistent with the idea that schizoaffective disorder is usually a variant of affective psychosis and sometimes a variant of schizophrenia," he concluded (p. 12). He believes, however, that a unitary conception of psychotic illness is far more interesting:

The overlap between the psychoses in regard to biological abnormalities, treatment response and course, if not inheritance patterns, would seem to argue for the interaction model. . . .

If this model is correct, the basis for deciding what diagnostic categories to use becomes very different. Whether the mixed phenomenological state, schizoaffective disorders, should be retained as a unique category, along with the phenomenological ends of the continuum, affective disorders and schizophrenia, would depend upon a variety of clinical considerations as much as anything. It might, for example, lead to groups of patients diagnosed as affective disorder or schizophrenia who are more homogeneous in regard to

a specific biological marker or treatment response. (Meltzer, 1984, p. 12)

Moldin and colleagues (1987) reached a similar conclusion in their high-risk studies, as did Strik and associates (1989) in a theoretical paper. Crow (1986) has also argued for a continuum model, from which he draws interesting etiological inferences; these are discussed in Chapter 20.

In their review of the phenomenology of schizoaffective disorder, Tsuang and Simpson (1984) also note the attractiveness of a unitary concept of psychosis. Nevertheless, after cataloging the empirical evidence supporting several mutually exclusive hypotheses about the nature of schizoaffective disorder, they conclude that no one concept of the illness emerges as any more supportable than any of the others. This apparently conflicting evidence may simply reflect the reality of a heterogeneous disorder, according to Tsuang and Simpson. They propose that research be directed at identifying homogeneous subgroups of schizoaffective patients. This strategy should not only further understanding in the long run but also benefit patients participating in the studies, since treatment choices—lithium or neuroleptics—would be better if they were predicated on more precise diagnoses.

DIFFERENTIAL DIAGNOSIS

The most commonly encountered problems in making a differential diagnosis in bipolar illness involve the overlapping boundaries with schizophrenia and schizoaffective illness and with personality disorders, especially borderline disorders. Bipolar illness must be distinguished from schizophreniform disorder, brief reactive psychosis, cycloid psychosis, atypical psychosis, organic brain disorders, and the epilepsies. The overlap between primary affective diagnoses and substance abuse is discussed in Chapter 9.

Schizophrenia and Schizoaffective Disorder

The clinician should be able to assign the great majority of patients a diagnosis of either affective illness or schizophrenia by carefully applying the diagnostic criteria introduced in Table 5-8. Schizoaffective disorder can sometimes be excluded by considering previous episodes; a history of either clear affective illness or clear schizophrenia cautions against diagnosing the present episode as schizoaffective.

Family history is important to consider in making a differential diagnosis. In a study of patients diagnosed as schizophrenic by DSM-III criteria, Kendler and Hays (1983) found that patients with a bipolar first-degree relative were more depressed during the period just before a psychotic episode than were those without such a close bipolar relative. Further, they showed more elated affect and more catatonic symptoms during the psychotic episode. Not surprisingly, Kendler and Hays caution against diagnosing schizophrenia in a patient with a first-degree relative with bipolar illness.

The sequence of symptoms is also important. In manic-depressive illness, delusions or hallucinations generally follow a period of more specific manic or depressive symptoms (e.g., changes in mood, activity, sleep). Age is another factor to consider in differentiating manic-depressive illness from schizophrenia. As reviewed in Chapter 8, when mania occurs in adolescence, schizophreniform symptoms tend to be especially prominent (Ballenger et al., 1982; Rosen et al., 1983b; Joyce, 1984a).

Mania versus Schizophrenia or Schizoaffective Disorder

Differentiating mania from schizophrenia or schizoaffective illness is a diagnostic challenge the clinician often faces. Limited epidemiological data indicate that schizomanic conditions are somewhat more common than schizodepressive ones (Rice et al., 1987b). Viewed cross-sectionally, acute symptoms of irritability, anger, paranoia, and catatonic-like excitement cannot distinguish mania from schizophrenia. Campbell (1953) described the confusing overlap in the presenting symptoms between acute mania and schizophrenia:

> The impulsive, combative and irrational behavior of the maniacal patient not infrequently is confused with . . . schizophrenia, particularly if the patient's delusional trend is at all bizarre or paranoid in nature. Spasmodic or apparently inappropriate laughter, which results from euphoria and exultation, should not be confused with the silly, irrelevant behavior of the schizophrenic. (p. 160)

Because presenting symptoms can be similar in mania and schizophrenia, the clinician must give equal attention to the level of premorbid function-

ing, family history, natural course, and the character of any prior episodes. This diagnostic decision has been made more rational and straightforward by the previously discussed broadening of the criteria for mania to include a range of psychotic features.

A key DSM-III-R criterion for diagnosing psychotic mania in the presence of schizophrenic symptoms is the more or less continuous prominence of the affective symptoms. Thus, bizarre mood-congruent delusions or hallucinations (including Schneiderian first-rank symptoms) are not inconsistent with a diagnosis of mania as long as they have been substantially accompanied by affective symptoms most of the time (the DSM-III-R criteria for mania allow up to 2 weeks of delusions or hallucinations free of other prominent manic symptoms, whereas the RDC allow 1 week).

If the period of quiet (i.e., affect-free) delusions or hallucinations is substantial (by criterion, exceeding 2 weeks), the diagnosis of either schizophrenia or schizoaffective illness should be considered. Schizophrenia would be diagnosed if, in addition, the patient continuously manifests overt signs of a psychotic illness for at least 6 months and the manic symptoms are brief relative to the duration of the schizophrenic symptoms. On the other hand, schizoaffective illness, manic type, would be diagnosed when the criterion of 6 months of continuous psychotic illness is not met but there have been more than 2 weeks of quiet delusions or hallucinations.

Scales that rate individual symptoms can show significant differences between diagnostic groups, but in general they have not been evaluated as instruments for differential diagnosis. One exception is the Activity-Withdrawal Scale of Venables (1957), shown by Klein (1982) to have correctly classified 83 percent of a group of acutely psychotic patients as either manic or schizophrenic. The Minnesota Multiphasic Personality Inventory (MMPI) is another exception, having been applied to the question of differentiating mania from schizophrenia by two groups of investigators. Using a discriminant function analysis, Post and colleagues (1986) were able to classify correctly 74 percent of the manic patients in their cross-validation sample. Two high-point pairs (Sc-Ma/Ma-Sc and Pa-Ma/Ma-Pa) were found in half of the manic patients but almost none of the schizophrenic patients. Walters and Greene (1989) were less successful in using the MMPI in differential diagnosis, but did note that certain scales, for example, 8 (Sc), 0 (Si), or a scale-8 high-point code, could be helpful in differential diagnosis if combined with other clinical data.

Strict application of the Bleulerian concept of thought disorder as pathognomonic of schizophrenia can result in misdiagnoses of manic-depressive patients (see Chapters 2 and 11). The markedly accelerated thinking of mania can lead to loosening of associations.[15] As Kraines (1957) points out, some schizophrenic-like "thought disorder" may result from the frenzy of mania. Thoughts tumble after each other so rapidly that they remain uncompleted, and the response to sensory impressions is so great that it results in distractibility. This rapid response to the stimulus of uncompleted thoughts can be mistaken for the thought disorder of schizophrenia. Lipkin and colleagues (1970) have suggested a therapeutic trial of lithium for some patients diagnosed as schizophrenic or schizoaffective, especially those who are negativistic, paranoid, excited, and hyperactive.

The following case history reported by Pope (1983) illustrates the devastation that can follow the misdiagnosis of manic-depressive illness as schizophrenia:

Ms. B, a 28-year-old woman, had been a psychiatric inpatient in a state hospital for the greater part of nine years. She had first been admitted at the age of 19 when she developed psychotic symptoms. . . . A history taken at that time by the admitting psychiatrist elaborately described her delusions and hallucinations but gave no information about whether Ms. B displayed mood change, activity change, an increase or decrease in energy level, or other affective symptomatology. No family history data were elicited. . . . Ms. B had been treated with virtually every antipsychotic drug available but had never been treated with lithium or ECT. . . . [Her] hospital records revealed that she had had periods of unusual irritability, coupled with increased activity and talkativeness . . . [and] had also displayed distractibility, grandiosity, and interpersonal intrusiveness. However, during most of her hospitalization, she was described as apathetic, with hypersomnia of ten to 11 hours a night, lacking in energy and concentration, eating poorly, and displaying little interest in social contact. She was also markedly self-deprecating and was described as having long guilty ruminations on religious themes. She had made two suicide attempts during these periods.

During Ms. B's ninth year in the hospital, her 21-year-old brother was admitted to a private psychiatric hospital. He was suffering from a relatively typical manic episode . . . [and] responded relatively well to lithium carbonate. When the brother's psychiatrist learned of Ms. B's illness, he elicited more information about the family and discovered that a maternal aunt and the maternal grandmother had had major depressive episodes. This evidence seemed to support his theory that Ms. B was suffering from a chronic form of bipolar disorder. . . . the brother's psychiatrist made further inquiries about the possibility of the sister's being given a trial of lithium carbonate. The doctors at the state hospital refused, saying that the patient was "clearly schizophrenic,". . . . However, after a great deal of pressure from Ms. B's mother, [they] reluctantly agreed to start Ms. B on lithium.

Within about three weeks Ms. B became markedly less agitated, less irritable, and more cooperative with staff. Shortly thereafter she was discharged to the quarterway house. Within two months, she transferred to a halfway house setting and was able to engage in a productive job with only a modest degree of supervision. However, she then became somewhat more depressed, and shortly thereafter stopped both her lithium and her antipsychotic drugs. Within a week, she had become sleepless, hyperactive, irritable, distractible, and grandiose. She was readmitted to the state hospital where she was treated with antipsychotic drugs but not with lithium. In spite of the clear temporal association between use of lithium and clinical response, the doctors claimed that the patient's "schizophrenic" symptoms ruled out a diagnosis of manic-depressive illness, and were unwilling to resume lithium therapy. At last report Ms. B's mother was still battling with the state hospital to reinstitute lithium. (pp. 326-327)

Bipolar Depression versus Schizophrenia or Schizoaffective Disorder

Just as was true with mania, the DSM-III-R criteria for differentiating bipolar depression from schizophrenia and schizoaffective disorder also focus on the prominence of the affective symptoms, their temporal relationship to the psychotic or schizophrenic symptoms, and the length of time the patient is continuously delusional or hallucinatory. (Like the differential for mania, the DSM-III-R criteria for major depression allow up to 2 weeks of "mood free" delusions or hallucinations, whereas the RDC allow 1 week.) These criteria reemphasize classic descriptions that include considerable psychosis among the affective disorders. As Akiskal and Puzantian (1979) have observed:

Vigorous and early outpatient treatment appears . . . to be preventing, to some extent, the emergence of the stuporous and agitated-psychotic melancholias . . . of Kraepelin's era. In brief, the present decade may well be witnessing epidemiological changes in the relative proportions of different clinical subtypes of affective disorder. . . . Some clinicians today seem to have reluctance in recognizing the psychotic forms of depression. . . . (p. 421)

Depressive symptoms commonly occur in schizophrenic patients, and catatonic stupor can be confused with the psychomotor retardation of bipolar depression. A diagnosis is more likely to be accurate if the overall course of illness is emphasized rather than the depressive symptoms alone. As noted earlier in the discussion of schizoaffective illness, the schizoaffective depressed patient (without a history of mania) is closer to schizophrenia (by outcome and family history criteria) than is the schizomanic patient.

Mixed Bipolar States versus Schizophrenia or Schizoaffective Disorder

Mixed bipolar states can present special differential diagnostic problems because of their instability, the often confusing mixture of manic and depressive symptoms, and the fact that they most characteristically occur in association with the more severe stages of mania (stage III).

Frequently associated with mixed states is the presence of alcohol or drug intoxication, which can further mask pure affective symptoms and confuse the differential diagnosis. The following case history illustrates this problem:

A 32 year old housewife was admitted to the psychiatric unit of a general hospital following a barbiturate overdose. This was her second agitated depressive episode in 5 years. The current episode was precipitated by the death of her 1 year old infant from pneumonia. She suffered from profound insomnia—initial, middle, and terminal—expressed ideas of guilt about minor sexual "transgressions" in her adolescence, saw no way out of her troubles, and felt she deserved to be tortured to death by violent means because she had failed as a wife and as a mother. Amitriptyline was rapidly raised to 200 mg at bedtime, providing partial relief from insomnia and restlessness. After this initial improvement in 6 days, the patient began to experience increasing agitation, complained of frightening dreams where two attendants were attacking her sexually, felt that "eyes" were looking at her when she took showers, experienced being "watched" in the dayroom and talked about on television, hallucinated "electrical" sensations on her skin, and heard indistinct noises, especially at night. These symptoms were controlled by thioridazine, 50 mg four times a day for one week. When she fully recovered from her depressive episode, she reluctantly revealed that she had used various combinations of sedative-hypnotics over a six month period to obtain relief from chronic insomnia. She had received these drugs from several physicians and was too ashamed on admission to admit this. Since nothing else

pointed to schizophrenia, the paranoid-hallucinatory phase of her illness was most parsimoniously explained as sedative-hypnotic withdrawal psychosis superimposed on the primary affective disorder. (Akiskal and Puzantian, 1979, p. 428)

Akiskal and Puzantian outlined 14 common "diagnostic pitfalls" that lead clinicians to misdiagnose affective illness as schizophrenia. Listed in Table 5-9, they serve as a practical anchor for our discussion of the differential diagnostic challenges existing with schizophrenia and related disorders.

Clinical Summary

The clinician can distinguish manic-depressive illness from schizophrenia or schizoaffective disorder in most cases by careful attention to the patient's personal and family history, premorbid functioning, age of onset, and the sequence of symptoms. In manic-depressive illness, delusions or hallucinations generally follow a period of either manic or depressive symptoms, and affective symptoms are prominent almost continuously.

Brief Reactive Psychosis

Brief reactive psychosis is a DSM-III-R category (Table 5-10) reserved for individuals who experience a psychotic episode lasting from a few hours to a month with "essential return to premorbid level of functioning." The psychotic symptoms follow immediately after a major psychological or social stress. If the criteria for mania or major depressive episode are met, the affective diagnosis takes precedence. Often, individuals initially placed in this category eventually will show symptoms that permit a diagnosis of either manic-depressive illness or schizophrenia. In their review of reactive psychoses, Jauch and Carpenter (1988a) note that known long-term and cross-sectional features of brief psychotic reactions do not distinguish the illness from acute, stress-associated affective psychoses.[16]

Cycloid Psychosis

The concept of cycloid psychosis, like schizoaffective disorder, is a hybrid rooted in the overlapping symptoms of schizophrenia and affective illness. It emerged from the work of Kleist (1947),[17] was later elaborated by Leonhard (1961), and was studied extensively by Perris

Table 5-9. Fourteen Common "Diagnostic Pitfalls" Leading to the
Misdiagnosis of Affective Disorder as Schizophrenia

1. Mistaking anhedonia and depressive depersonalization for schizophrenic emotional blunting
2. The superimposition of a manic or depressive psychosis on the substrate of an introverted personality
3. Affective psychosis in mentally retarded individuals
4. Incomplete interepisodic recovery
5. Rapid-Cycling bipolar affective disorder (see Chapter 6)
6. The predominance of irritability, hostility, and cantankerousness
7. Mistaking paranoid ideation for schizophrenia
8. Mixed states
9. Sleep deprivation and metabolic disturbances secondary to reduced caloric and fluid intake
10. The superimposition of unsuspected alcohol and drug withdrawal states
11. Difficulty in distinguishing formal thought disorder from flight of ideas
12. Lack of familiarity with the phenomenology of affective delusions and hallucinations
13. The equation of "bizarre" ideation with schizophrenia
14. Heavy reliance on incidential Schneiderian criteria in making differential diagnostic assignment of psychotic patients

Adapted from Akiskal and Puzantian, 1979

Table 5-10. DSM-III-R Criteria for Brief Reactive Psychosis

A. Presence of at least one of the following symptoms indicating impaired reality testing (not culturally sanctioned) *(DSM-III-R has clarified the exclusion of culturally sanctioned reactions)*:
   1. incoherence or marked loosening of associations
   2. delusions
   3. hallucinations
   4. catatonic or disorganized behavior

B. Emotional turmoil, i.e., rapid shifts in intense affects, or overwhelming perplexity or confusion

C. Appearance of A and B shortly after one or more events *(DSM-III-R has recognized the cumulative effects of several events)* that would be considered markedly stressful to most others in that person's culture

D. Absence of the prodomal symptoms of schizophrenia, and failure to meet criteria for Schizotypal Personality Disorder before onset

E. Duration of an episode is a few hours to one month *(DSM-III: maximum is 2 weeks)*, with eventual return to premorbid level of functioning. (When diagnosis must be made before recovery, it should be qualified as "provisional")

F. Not due to psychotic Mood Disorder (i.e., no full mood syndrome present, and an organic cause cannot be established)

(1974, 1988a). It thus achieved a place in Scandinavian and German psychiatry but has never been accepted as a category in formal diagnostic systems. As described by Leonhard and Perris, cycloid psychosis is a recurrent bipolar disorder, separate from either manic-depressive illness or schizophrenia; it is found predominantly among females and has a good prognosis. Leonhard, who described the psychosis most extensively, divided it into three subgroups:

- *Motility psychosis,* which has a "hyperkinetic pole" and "akinetic pole." "Whereas manic-depressive illness affects thinking, affectivity, and psychomotor activity, in the same way motility psychosis is a pure psychomotor illness" (Leonhard, 1961).
- *Confusion psychosis,* which Leonhard described as a condition affecting thinking but not psychomotor activity or affectivity. Leonhard described excited, confused thinking, which is less distractible and more disoriented than manic thinking, with pressured speech being common to both disorders.
- *Anxiety/elation psychosis,* which involves only mood. One pole is represented by anxiety, the other by ecstasy. Leonhard differentiated this psychosis from manic-depressive illness by stating that, although the patient's affect is either "cheerful or sad" in both disorders, ideas of reference, extreme grandiosity, and religious ecstasy are more characteristic of this cycloid psychosis.

As described by Leonhard, some of the symptoms of cycloid psychosis are typical of schizophrenia, others of affective disorders, especially those with mixed states, and still others of organic disorders, especially the prominence of confusional states. Outcome is somewhere between schizophrenia and affective illness (Brockington et al., 1982b), although family history data suggest more association with affective illness than with schizophrenia (Perris, 1974). The phenomenology of cycloid psychosis is further described in a review by Jamison (1982). In the absence of formal criteria, for purposes of differential diagnosis, it is best to treat cycloid psychosis as analogous to, or a type of, schizoaffective illness.

Atypical Psychosis

Classically, the atypical psychoses included patients who have schizophrenic symptoms but show rapid fluctuations in emotional state, an episodic course, and generally favorable outcome. Mitsuda (1965) concluded from his study of monozygotic twins that atypical psychosis could be distinguished genetically from schizophrenia and, to a lesser extent, from manic-depressive illness. The relationship between this disorder and the cycloid psychosis of Leonhard and Perris is not clear.

In the DSM-III-R, *psychotic disorders, not otherwise specified* (atypical psychosis), is a residual category for patients with psychotic symptoms who do not meet criteria for any other DSM-III-R disorder. For purposes of differential diagnosis, it would seem that such patients would fall in the schizoaffective spectrum.

Borderline Personality Disorder

The evolution of contemporary diagnostic systems has tended to somewhat reduce the heterogeneity of borderline personality disorder (see Chapter 12). DSM-III-R criteria for schizophrenia eliminate the earlier concepts of *latent* or *pseudoneurotic* schizophrenia, the individuals often considered to exist on the borderline. In the DSM-III-R, the traditional meanings of borderline are best captured by two axis-II diagnoses: *schizotypal personality disorder* and *borderline personality disorder.* Evidence from family history and outcome studies indicates that schizotypal personality disorder is part of the schizophrenia spectrum (McGlashan, 1983, 1987), whereas borderline personality disorder appears more related to the affective disorders (Stone, 1980).[18] Some think that this borderline–affective disorder relationship is best understood by conceiving of the personality disorder as part of the affective spectrum—that is, a subsyndromal form of affective illness (Akiskal et al., 1985c; Gunderson and Elliott, 1985), whereas others maintain that the personality disorder is independent, albeit frequently coexisting with affective disorder (McGlashan, 1983; Pope et al., 1983b). Some modern descriptions of borderline disorders are occasionally reminiscent of Kraepelin's characterization of the *manic-*

Table 5-11. DSM-III-R Criteria for Borderline Personality Disorder *(Compared with DSM-III)*

A pervasive pattern of *instability* of mood, interpersonal relationships, and self-image, beginning by early adulthood and present in a variety of contexts, as indicated by at least 5 of the following: *(DSM-III-R has changed this introduction. DSM-III noted here that the following criteria are current and long-term, are not limited to episodes, and significantly impair social or occupational functioning or subjective distress)*

1. a pattern of *unstable* and intense interpersonal relationships characterized by *alternating between extremes* of overidealization and devaluation

2. *impulsiveness* in at least two areas that are potentially self-damaging, e.g., spending, sex, substance abuse, shoplifting, reckless driving, binge eating (do not include suicidal or self-mutilating behavior covered in 5) *{DSM-III-R has added this exclusion and deleted physically self-damaging acts)*

3. *affective instability*: marked shifts from baseline mood to depression, irritability, or anxiety, usually lasting a few hours and only rarely more than a few days

4. inappropriate, intense anger or *lack of control* of anger, e.g., frequent displays of temper, constant anger, recurrent physical fights

5. *recurrent* suicidal threats, gestures, or behavior, or self-mutilating behavior *(DSM-III includes physically self-damaging acts such as recurrent accidents or physical fights)*

6. marked and persistent identity disturbance manifested by uncertainty about at least 2 of the following: self-image, sexual orientation, long-term goals or career choice, type of friends desired, preferred values

7. chronic feelings of emptiness or boredom

8. frantic efforts to avoid real or imagined abandonment (do not include suicidal or self-mutilating behavior covered in 5) *(DSM-III-R has added this exclusion)*

DSM-III included the criterion, "if under 18, does not meet criteria for identity disorder"

---

depressive temperament (see Chapters 2 and 4). Differential diagnosis focuses on whether the individual patient is manifesting borderline personality disorder alone, bipolar affective disorder alone (which may be subsyndromal), or both. How frequently the two disorders actually coexist (as opposed to overlap) is controversial (Baxter et al., 1984).

DSM-III-R borderline personality disorder (see Table 5-11) and major mood disorder coexist somewhat more frequently than would be expected by chance. Although much of the literature would suggest that the overlap is more likely to involve unipolar disorder (see Chapter 12), Akiskal and colleagues (1985a) have emphasized the close linkage to bipolar disorder. In a series of 100 outpatients diagnosed by DSM-III as borderline, 25 percent met criteria for bipolar-II disorder or cyclothymia on follow-up. Other studies of the coexistence of bipolar disorder and bor-

derline personality disorder unfortunately do not differentiate between bipolar-I and bipolar-II disorders.[19] Clinical experience suggests that the main overlap is with bipolar-II patients.

The differential diagnosis between bipolar *depression* and the depressive affect associated with borderline personality disorder involves attention to the issues of lability, reactivity, and the overall symptom cluster. The depressive affect associated with borderline personality disorder is marked by considerable day-to-day or even hour-to-hour variability, whereas the depressive mood associated with the bipolar episode is experienced as discrete episodes with a clear onset and termination and a relatively stable course during the episode.[20] The mood of the borderline patient is more likely to remain reactive to the environment and, even though intensely dysphoric, change quickly with the appropriate stimulation or intervention. As noted earlier, the symptom cluster of bipolar depression generally involves pervasive changes in the regulation of sleep and appetite (usually hyperphagia and hypersomnia). These features are not as prominently associated with the depressive mood in the borderline patient unless bipolar disorder also is present.

In evaluating elevated mood, the duration is also important. Given the extreme lability of mood in borderline disorder, mood elevation would probably not last long enough to meet the criteria for mania, although on duration alone, it could overlap with hypomania or cyclothymic disorder. The usual associated symptoms of hypomania, such as racing thoughts or decreased need for sleep, would not generally be part of the mood lability of the borderline patient, however. The absence of events that either precipitate or terminate the hypomanic mood would also suggest a true bipolar disorder, as would a positive family history of bipolar disorder, although the latter would not be conclusive. In practical terms, emphasis on the link between borderline and bipolar diagnoses is important because all too often the diagnosis of bipolar disorder is missed when borderline features are also present, especially in adolescents. As discussed in Chapter 8, bipolar disorder can be especially difficult to diagnose in this age group, since a wide range of apparently nonspecific symptoms is common. Not infrequently, individuals rediagnosed as bipolar on follow-up experienced their first manic or hypomanic episode after exposure to an antidepressant drug. The possibility of this outcome argues for considerable care in ruling out a bipolar diathesis before treating depressive syndromes in adolescents with presumed borderline features.

Organic Brain Disorders

Since manic-depressive illness has its own underlying biological foundation, differentiating it from the so-called organic brain disorders can be semantically and diagnostically confusing. DSM-III-R is not helpful on this matter. It recommends applying the term *organic* to disorders in which psychological and behavioral abnormalities are "associated with transient or permanent dysfunction of the brain." Wells (1985) pointed out that *organic* is used in three ways: (1) as representing symptoms that can be attributed directly to abnormalities of brain structure or brain chemical or electrical dysfunction, (2) as applied to specific, identified brain diseases associated with a well-described etiology and pathophysiology (e.g., Alzheimer's dementia and alcohol-withdrawal delirium), (3) as applied to specific syndromes with particular combinations of behavioral and neuropsychological symptoms. It is in this third sense that we will use the term organic to define syndromes, each of which can involve a wide variety of etiological factors.

The relevant organic syndromal clusters defined by DSM-III-R are Delirium, Dementia, Amnestic Syndrome, Organic Delusional Syndrome, Organic Hallucinosis, Organic Mood Syndrome, Organic Anxiety Syndrome, Organic Personality Syndrome, Intoxication and Withdrawal, and Organic Mental Syndrome, not otherwise specified. Delirium, Dementia, and Organic Personality Syndrome overlap with some of the associated symptoms of mania or depression, principally cognitive dysfunction, whereas Organic Mood Syndrome overlaps with the core mood symptoms of manic-depressive illness. In some cases, of course, these organic syndromes and manic-depressive illness involve not only overlapping symptomatology but perhaps also overlapping pathophysiology, as discussed in Chapter 18.

The absence of specific pathognomonic neuropsychiatric manifestations of organic brain disorders means that differentiating these disorders from manic-depressive illness requires understanding of the variety of conditions that can be associated with them. Some behavioral features are relatively more prominent in most of these disorders than in bipolar illness, principally changes in cognitive function, including impairment of orientation, memory, general intellectual function, and judgment. Of comparable importance in making a differential diagnosis is a history of manic-depressive illness. The absence of such a history does not rule out primary manic-depressive illness, especially when the patient is still within the age of risk for onset of the disorder.

A standard neurological examination usually does not aid in differential diagnosis, since in most organic psychiatric syndromes it remains normal until the disease is far advanced. The so-called soft neurological signs often thought to mark organic brain disease have not proven to be specific.

Neuropsychological testing can be helpful in quantifying the extent of impairment but is not particularly useful in the initial differential diagnosis. This is so because, as detailed in Chapter 11, both depression and mania can be associated with substantial disturbances in a wide variety of neuropsychological tests designed to measure cognitive changes.[21] Procedures such as computed tomography (CT) scans and electroencephalograms may be helpful, but unless they can identify a localized lesion, they do not prove to be reliable in differentiating organic brain disorder from manic-depressive illness.

The Concept of Secondary Affective Episodes

A brief digression is in order to review the concepts of secondary mania and depression (for a more complete discussion of this issue, see Chapter 18). Krauthammer and Klerman (1978) made an important conceptual contribution by reviewing the literature for reports of manic syndromes occurring shortly after medical, pharmacological, or other somatic dysfunctions.[22] They examined the phenomenology of the individual case reports, applying criteria similar to but somewhat less stringent than the RDC.[23] The cases included syndromes that occurred after ingestion of certain drugs, metabolic disturbances, infections, and central nervous system lesions. To insure that they were not dealing simply with a variant of toxic psychosis, Krauthammer and Klerman excluded cases in which frank confusion was present. Critical to the concept of secondary mania was the fact that the cases selected had no history of affective illness. The question of family history was less clear: Only half the case reports included data on relatives; among those there was no history of affective illness.[24]

The concept of secondary mania was not recognized in DSM-III. DSM-III-R, however, does note that organic factors may induce mania and divides them into those not induced by a substance (classified under Organic Affective Syndrome) or substance induced (categorized under Substance Use Disorders). The role of alcohol and drug abuse in the onset of affective episodes is discussed in Chapter 9, and the possibility that postpartum mania is a form of secondary mania is discussed in Chapter 6. Table 5-12 lists conditions that have been associated with secondary manic or hypomanic symptoms.

Krauthammer and Klerman concluded that patients with secondary mania are phenomenologically indistinguishable from patients with primary mania, with the exception of a later age of onset among the secondary cases (the median was 41). According to this view, a patient with a late onset of manic symptoms and with no personal or family history of affective illness might be suspected of having a disorder with an organic etiology.[25] Taylor and Abrams (1980), however, failed to find any clinical differences between familial and nonfamilial manic patients, nor could they find any higher incidence of potential medical or organic precursors in the nonfamilial group. They remind us that a negative family history in first-degree relatives by no means precludes genetic transmission, and they note that polygenic disorders often occur with this pattern. Their caution is important to keep in mind since the concept of secondary mania is based on uncontrolled case reports, which makes it impossible to rule out a chance association between a medical condition and true manic-depressive illness without a family history.

Secondary depression is not a recognized category in DSM-III-R, but the possible role of organic or medical predisposing factors is acknowledged. As originally formulated by Robins and Guze (1972), a diagnosis of primary depression excluded patients with a preexisting or concomitant psychiatric condition, including "schizophrenia, anxiety neuroses, phobias, neurosis, obsessive-compulsive neurosis, hysteria, alcoholism, drug dependency, antisocial personality, homosexuality and other sexual deviations, mental retardation, or organic brain syndrome." Patients with an incapacitating medical illness preceding and paralleling the depression also were considered to have a secondary, rather than a primary, depression. Attempts to validate the primary-secondary distinction by biological or treatment response criteria have not been successful (Carroll, 1982; Liebowitz et al., 1984a; Grove et al., 1987), and the distinction, when based on a history of the broad range of psychiatric disorders, is no longer used.

Nevertheless, for our purposes, the concept may still have some meaning, ambiguous though it may be. Goodwin and Bunney (1971), in their review of reported reserpine-induced depressions, found that the great majority of reserpine

Table 5-12. Organic Causes of Manic and Hypomanic Symptoms

Drug-related
- Isoniazid[a]
- Procarbazine[a]
- Levodopa[a]
- Bromide[a]
- Decongestants
- Bronchodilators
- Procyclidine
- Calcium replacement
- Phencyclidine
- Metoclopramide
- Corticosteroids and ACTH[a]
- Hallucinogens
- Sympathomimetic amines
- Disulfiram (Antabuse)
- Alcohol
- Barbiturates
- Anticholinergics
- Anticonvulsants
- Benzodiazepines

Metabolic disturbance
- Postoperative states[a]
- Hemodialysis[a]
- Vitamin B_{12} deficiency
- Addison's disease
- Cushing's disease
- Postinfection states
- Dialysis
- Hyperthyroidism

Neurological conditions
- Right-temporal seizure focus[a]
- Multiple sclerosis
- Right-hemisphere damage
- Epilepsy
- Huntington's disease
- Postcerebrovascular accident

Infection
- Influenza[a]
- Q fever[a]
- Neurosyphillis
- Post-St. Louis type A encephalitis[a]
- "Benign" herpes simplex encephalitis
- AIDS (HIV)

Neoplasm
- Parasagittal meningioma[a]
- Diencephalic glioma[a]
- Suprasellar craniopharyngioma[a]
- Suprasellar diencephalic tumor[a]
- Benign spheno-occipital tumor[a]
- Right-intraventricular meningioma
- Right-temporoparietal occipital metastases
- Tumor of floor of fourth ventricle

Other conditions
- Postisolation syndrome
- Right-temporal lobectomy
- Posttraumatic confusion
- Postelectroconvulsive therapy
- Deliriform organic brain disease

[a]Meets criteria of Krauthammer and Klerman for secondary mania

Adapted from Lazare, 1979, and Stasiek and Zetin, 1985

"depressions" were, in fact, pseudodepressions that did not mimic the full natural syndrome. Those with full endogenous or melancholic symptoms generally had a personal or family history of affective illness. These authors inferred that reserpine merely uncovered a vulnerability rather than inducing depression de novo (see Chapter 17).

As discussed in Chapter 4, an alternative to dichotomizing mania and depression into primary and secondary categories is a spectrum model reflecting varying levels of vulnerability. The greatest vulnerability would be expressed as a *primary* case, in which little or no external stress is required, and lower levels of vulnerability might only show up as *secondary* cases, that is, requiring the operation of external factors for the episode to appear.

With that necessary digression, we now return to the discussion of specific organic conditions, which we introduce with two related but nonaffective organic states—delirium and dementia—followed by the organic affective syndromes, which, because of their symptomatic overlap, present a different sort of diagnostic problem.

Delirium

The DSM-III-R diagnostic criteria for *delirium* are given in Table 5-13. Severe (stage-III) mania can involve clouding of consciousness, occasionally rendering it difficult to differentiate from organic delirium (see Chapter 2). The absence of the preceding stages of mania or of a history of mania is sometimes helpful in this differential diagnosis. Perceptual disturbances usually are

Table 5-13. DSM-III-R Criteria for Delirium
(Compared with DSM-III)

A. Reduced ability to maintain attention to external stimuli and to appropriately shift attention to new external stimuli

B. Disorganized thinking: rambling, irrelevant, or incoherent speech

C. At least two of the following:
  1. reduced level of consciousness
  2. perceptual disturbances: misinterpretations, illusions, or hallucinations
  3. disturbance of sleep-wake cycle with insomnia or daytime sleepiness
  4. increased or decreased psychomotor activity
  5. disorientation to time, place, person
  6. memory impairment *(In DSM-III this was a required symptom)*

D. Clinical features develop quickly (hours to days) and tend to fluctuate over the course of a day

E. Either 1 or 2:
  1. evidence from history, physical exam, or lab tests of an organic factor(s) judged to be etiologically related to the disturbance
  2. in the absence of such evidence, and without any nonorganic mental disorder, an etiologic organic factor can be presumed. *(DSM-III-R has added this 2nd alternative)*

more sudden in onset in organic delirium than in stage-III mania. On the other hand, the sustained euphoria (or irritability) characteristic of mania would not be likely in delirium.

As with all diagnoses of organic brain disorders, indications (from the history, physical examination, or laboratory data) of a specific organic etiological factor are important to the diagnosis. As noted in Chapter 9, manic episodes are commonly associated with substance abuse, particularly in young patients, and here the challenge is to differentiate a pure organic delirium from a manic episode precipitated and colored by alcohol or drugs.

Dementia

The DSM-III-R criteria for *dementia*, given in Table 5-14, overlap somewhat with delirium. The considerable attention that has been given to differentiating between true dementia and *depressive pseudodementia* is altogether justified, since the pseudodementia associated with depression is very treatable. As discussed in Chapter 11, bipolar patients, in particular, often experience profound deficits in cognition and memory and consequently are sometimes misdiagnosed as

having primary dementia. This differential diagnosis is encountered most frequently in elderly patients, in whom clinicians tend to neglect affective symptoms and focus instead on somatic and cognitive symptoms. Although a history of manic or depressive episodes is very helpful in this differential, it cannot be used absolutely: On the one hand, a small percentage of bipolar patients do not have their first episode until they are in their 50s or 60s; on the other hand, a few bipolar patients independently develop dementia later in life. Since a high proportion of the late-onset bipolar patients have frequent cycles (see Chapter 6), the clinical picture may convey chronicity and, therefore, may seem to be associated with an organic etiology. The following case report by Cowdry and Goodwin (1981b) illustrates late-onset bipolar disorder, originally misdiagnosed as dementia:

Mr. A, a 63-year-old retired craftsman, had gradually become nervous and withdrawn 3 years earlier after a series of changes at his place of employment. He began missing work and staying in bed. His wife noted that he had become preoccupied and that his memory was somewhat impaired. . . . A trial of amitriptyline resulted in urinary retention at low dosages, and the drug was discontinued. Significant impairment of at-

Table 5-14. DSM-III-R Criteria for Dementia
(Compared with DSM-III)

A. Demonstrate evidence of impairment in short- and long-term memory. Impairment in short-term memory may be indicated by inability to remember three objects after 5 minutes. Impairment in long-term memory may be indicated by inability to remember past personal information or facts of common knowledge. *(DSM-III-R has given greater detail for this criterion)*

B. At least one of the following:
    1. impairment in abstract thinking, e.g., inability to find similarities, differences between related words, difficulty in defining words and concepts, etc.
    2. impaired judgment, e.g., inability to deal reasonably with interpersonal, family, and job-related issues
    3. other disturbances of higher cortical function, e.g., aphasia, apraxia, agnosia, and "constructional difficulty"
    4. personality change, i.e., alteration or accentuation of premorbid traits

C. The disturbance in A and B significantly interferes with work or usual social activities or relationships with others *(DSM-III-R has added this criterion)*

D. Not occurring exclusively during the course of Delirium *(DSM-III said, "does not meet criteria for Delirium or Intoxication, although these may be superimposed")*

E. Either one or two:
    1. evidence from history, physical exam, or lab tests of an organic factor(s) judged to be etiologically related to the disturbance
    2. in the absence of such evidence, and without any nonorganic mental disorder, an etiologic organic factor cannot be presumed

Criteria for severity of Dementia:
    Mild: Although work or social activities are significantly impaired, capacity for independent living remains, i.e., adequate personal hygiene and judgment capabilities
    Moderate: Independent living is hazardous, some degree of supervision is necessary
    Severe: Daily functioning is so impaired that continual supervision is required, e.g., unable to maintain minimal personal hygiene; largely incoherent or mute

(DSM-III-R has added these criteria of severity)

---

tention and memory was noted, and a tentative diagnosis of dementia was made.

Mr. A was unable to return to work and spent most of his time in bed. Eight months after the onset of his symptoms he had a 2-week period of decreased sleep and increased activity; he was excessively talkative and wrote copious notes about his childhood memories. However, he remained distracted and forgetful. Mr. A experienced a period of confusion, during which time he repeatedly turned the lights on and off, and he was hospitalized for a neurological evaluation.

In the hospital a neurologist could find no focal signs. Results from a spinal fluid examination, glucose tolerance test, and EEG were normal. A CT scan of the skull showed moderate cortical atrophy without ventricular dilation. . . . The overall impression from the Halstead-Reitan battery was that Mr. A suffered from depression and cognitive impairment, "presumably the result of presenile deterioration."

When Mr. A was discharged, his family was advised that he was becoming demented and that he might need nursing home care. Mr. A remained in bed for most of the day during the next 4 months. He had profound anergia and anhedonia with marked deficits in attention and memory, and he felt hopeless, helpless, worthless, and guilty.

When Mr. A was first seen by us in outpatient consultation 3 years after the onset of this episode, he was quiet and withdrawn. His answers to questions had long pauses and were brief. He blamed himself for his current state and said he should be more active, but he had no interest. Mr. A described suicidal thoughts, which he had previously kept secret. No delusions or hallucinations were present. During formal testing Mr. A gave concrete replies to proverbs and showed marked impairment of short-term memory, but his memory for distant events remained intact. Careful interviewing of Mr. A and his wife disclosed that he had no history of any depressive episode before he was 60 years old and that he had no family history of depression, alcoholism, or sociopathy.

Because Mr. A's symptoms were suggestive of a bipolar mood disorder masquerading as senile dementia, antidepressant medication was considered. As noted, Mr. A had developed urinary retention on low doses of a tricyclic; therefore, lithium was chosen to avoid anticholinergic side effects. By day 8 of Mr. A's treatment (lithium level, 0.6 mEq/liter) he was feeling his "normal self," and his wife confirmed a dramatic improvement. Mr. A was out of bed all day doing tasks, saying he felt energetic and hopeful. His sleep and appetite were normal. He had no significant memory deficits during formal testing or in his daily living. (p. 1118)

Even if clear evidence of a prior episode is lacking, the temporal sequence of the affective and organic symptoms can be helpful in differentiating pseudodementia from organic dementia with secondary depression. In primary affective disorder, the onset of symptoms is more brisk, whereas in organic dementia, onset is more insidious. Furthermore, affective symptoms generally precede the cognitive impairments in pseudodementia, whereas the reverse is true for organic dementia accompanied by secondary depression.

Other aspects of the depressive syndrome, such as sleep and appetite dysregulation, are not especially helpful in differentiating bipolar illness from dementia. Neuropsychiatric testing can be useful, especially if a focal lesion is involved, but it cannot be relied on to make a clear differential, since bipolar depression can also be associated with profound cognitive impairment. As with other differential diagnostic questions, it is important to look for atypical forms of mania in the history, particularly episodic irritability or agitation in the absence of euphoria. The periods of secondary affective lability sometimes associated with primary dementing illnesses do not appear as discrete episodes. Obviously, a definitive diagnosis can be made if an organic cause for the dementia can be uncovered.

Because of its enormous public health importance, the issue of AIDS dementia deserves special attention. The human immunodeficiency virus (HIV) belongs to a class of retroviruses that are neurotrophic, that is, they have a special affinity for the nervous system. By the time the acquired immune deficiency syndrome (AIDS) has reached its peak, CNS involvement is almost universal. More important to the issue of differential diagnosis, however, is the finding that among 20 to 25 percent of AIDS patients, the presenting symptoms originate in the central nervous system. These early AIDS symptoms may be difficult to distinguish from depression (Price et al., 1986; Bridge et al., 1988). Mania has also been reported as an early symptom (Gabel et al., 1986). As the condition progresses, memory, concentration, and rapid alternating movements are impaired. Other indications include pyramidal tract signs, ataxia, leg weakness, and tremor. AIDS dementia becomes the presumptive diagnosis when the antibody test is positive. In addition, neuropsychological tests and magnetic resonance imaging (MRI) scans may be helpful in making the differential diagnosis.

Table 5-15 lists diseases or conditions that have been associated with dementia.

Organic Mood Syndrome

Some cases of organic mood syndrome share or mimic features of mania or depression, and consequently the borderline between this syndrome and manic-depressive illness can be difficult to distinguish (Shukla et al., 1988a). Hendrie (1978) suggested that, conceptually at least, organic mood syndrome can be differentiated from "true" mania or depression precipitated by organic precursors—syndromes that are phenomenologically identical to classic manic-depressive episodes. This conceptual distinction is often not easy to make in practice, of course. Both disorders could be included under the rubric of secondary manic or depressive episodes discussed earlier.

The DSM-III-R criteria for organic mood syndrome are listed in Table 5-16. In the organic *manic* syndrome, the predominant disturbance is the manic mood rather than clouding of consciousness. By definition, an organic manic syndrome cannot be distinguished from true functional mania on the basis of cross-sectional phenomenology; hence the differential is made on the basis of positive evidence (from the history, physical examination, or laboratory tests) of a specific organic factor judged to be etiologically

Table 5-15. Conditions Associated with Dementia

Parenchymatous diseases of the central nervous system
    Alzheimer's disease (primary degenerative dementia)
    Pick's disease (primary degenerative dementia)
    Huntington's disease
    Parkinson's disease

Systemic disorders
    Endocrine and metabolic disorders
        Thyroid disease
        Parathyroid disease
        Pituitary-adrenal disorders
    Liver disease
        Chronic progressive hepatic encephalopathy
    Urinary tract disease
        Chronic uremic encephalopathy
        Progressive uremic encephalopathy (dialysis dementia)
    Cardiovascular disease
        Cerebral hypoxia or anoxia
        Multi-infarct dementia
        Cardiac arrhythmias
        Inflammatory diseases of blood vessels
    Pulmonary disease
        Respiratory encephalopathy

Deficiency states
    Cyanocobalamin deficiency
    Folic acid deficiency

Drugs and toxins

Intracranial tumors

Infectious processes
    Creutzfeldt-Jakob disease
    Cryptococcal meningitis
    Neurosyphilis

Miscellaneous disorders
    Hepatolenticular degeneration
    Hydrocephalic dementia
    Sarcoidosis

The majority of these conditions require specific therapeutic intervention

Adapted from Wells, 1985

---

related to the syndrome.[26] Reported organic causes of manic and hypomanic symptoms were listed in Table 5-12.

The organic *depressive* syndrome is also phenomenologically indistinguishable from primary depression. Again, the differential diagnosis depends on the identification of organic factors that reasonably can be assumed to cause the depressive symptoms. The organic factors commonly associated with depressive syndromes are listed in Table 5-17.

Organic Personality Syndrome

Organic personality syndrome generally is associated with some structural brain damage, secondary to neoplasm, trauma, or cerebrovascular disease (see Chapter 18). The DSM-III-R criteria, listed in Table 5-18, often represent long-standing patterns of behavior; symptoms have an episodic character and affect is unstable. Although the mood disturbances are not dominant, the episodic nature and the associated lack of control over behavior render them important in the differential diagnoses of manic-depressive disorder.

As with the organic mood syndromes, the organic personality syndrome might be suspected in an individual over the age of 40 without a history of prior affective episodes, especially if there has been a recent history suggestive of brain damage. Indeed, closed head injuries are the most common cause of organic personality syndromes. When a lesion or injury involves the frontal lobes, personality changes predominate over neurological symptoms.

Epilepsies

Epilepsies are another group of disorders of the CNS that, like other organic disorders, must be differentiated from bipolar illness. The difficulty of this task is underscored by growing evidence of considerable overlap between some forms of epilepsy and manic-depressive illness.

Epilepsy, or primary seizure disorder, affects approximately 1 percent of the population and is the most common chronic neurological disease. More than half of patients with epilepsy have nonconvulsive forms rather than grand mal seizures. Principal among these is temporal lobe epilepsy, which is roughly synonymous with psychomotor epilepsy or complex partial seizures. The primary seizure disorders are, of course, recurrent. Associated organic mental syndromes can be divided into those occurring during actual seizure activity (ictal manifestations) and those manifested only during interictal periods.

This association between epilepsy and mood disorders has been a recurrent theme in the literature since the time of Hippocrates. As cited by Himmelhoch (1984), the unknown author of *Epidemics* stated:

Table 5-16. DSM-III-R Criteria for Organic Mood Syndrome
(Compared with Organic Affective Syndrome in DSM-III)

A. Prominent and persistent depressed, elevated, or expansive mood

B. Evidence from history, physical exam, or lab tests of an organic factor(s) judged to be etiologically related to the disturbance

C. Not occurring exclusively during the course of delirium

Specify: manic, depressed, or mixed *(DSM-III-R has added these specifications)*

DSM-III also included as a criterion absence of some of the symptoms associated with Delirium, Dementia and Organic Delusional Syndrome, or Organic Hallucinosis

Most melancholics usually also become epileptics, and epileptics melancholics. One or the other [condition] prevails according to where the disease leans: if towards the body, they become epileptics, if towards reason, melancholics. (p. 272)

Epidemiological surveys of large numbers of patients with epilepsy (see, e.g., Gibbs and Gibbs, 1952) indicate that psychotic symptoms are about 10 times more likely to occur in association with temporal lobe than with generalized epilepsy (reviewed by McKenna et al., 1985). The psychoses associated with temporal lobe epilepsy were initially described at a time when the broad Bleulerian concept of schizophrenia prevailed. It is thus not surprising that they tended to be described as schizophrenic, less frequently as affectively ill. Clinically, these psychoses are generally mixed syndromes with a prominence of visual and olfactory hallucinations, rapid fluctuations of mood, catatonic features, and dreamlike states—all of which occur in an episodic course. In his studies of patients with temporal lobe epilepsy, Flor-Henry (1969) found that 40 percent had either manic-depressive or schizoaffective features, and 42 percent had predominantly schizophrenic symptoms. Further frustrating attempts to understand the association between psychosis and temporal lobe epilepsy is the fact that patients can at times manifest predominantly affective symptoms and at other times predominantly schizophrenic symptoms.

Nonconvulsive seizure disorders may coexist with manic-depressive illness, or they may mimic it. This overlap is of theoretical importance, but it also influences treatment decisions. Monroe (1982) has defined a group of patients with "epileptoid episodic disorder," whose symptoms overlap manic-depressive illness, schizophrenia, and temporal lobe epilepsy. The affective episodes associated with this disorder are strikingly brief, usually less than 2 weeks, and always less than 6 weeks, in duration. In fact, the duration of the affective episodes is the principal criterion differentiating this disorder from manic-depressive illness.

In a series of 12 patients who met DSM-III criteria for bipolar disorder, Lewis and co-workers (1984) found 6 who had a cluster of temporal lobe symptoms having the quality of an

Table 5-17. Organic Causes of Depressive Symptoms

- Hypokalemia
- Hypercalcemia
- Reserpine-induced reactions
- Steroid psychosis
- Hypothyroidism
- Organic brain syndromes
- Hepatitis
- Cirrhosis
- Infectious mononucleosis
- Postviral-infection syndrome
- Cessation of amphetamine or cocaine use
- Carcinoma of the pancreas
- Degenerative diseases of the nervous system

Table 5-18. DSM-III-R Criteria for Organic Personality Syndrome
(Compared with DSM-III)

A. A persistent personality disturbance, lifelong or a change in or accentuation of a previously characteristic trait, involving at least one of the following:
   1. affective instability, e.g., marked shifts from normal mood to depression, irritability, or anxiety. *(DSM-III-R has added this symptom)*
   2. recurrent outbursts of aggression or rage that are grossly out of proportion to any precipitating psychosocial stressors
   3. marked impairment of social judgment, e.g., sexual indiscretions
   4. marked apathy and indifference
   5. suspiciousness or paranoid ideation

B. Evidence from history, physical exam, or lab tests of organic factor(s) judged to be etiologically related to the disturbance

C. This diagnosis is not given to a child or adolescent if the clinical picture is limited to the features that characterize Attention-deficit Hyperactivity Disorder

D. Not occurring exclusively during the course of Delirium, and does not meet criteria for Dementia *(DSM-III also excludes symptoms of Organic Affective Syndrome and Organic Delusional Syndrome)*

   Specify explosive type if outbursts of aggression or rage are the predominant feature *(DSM-III-R has added this specification)*

---

aura: olfactory hallucinations, metamorphopsia (visual misperception), déjà vu or mystical experiences, spontaneous anxiety, fear or rage, ideational viscosity,[27] driven speech, forced thoughts, memory blanks, and depersonalization.

Himmelhoch (1984) surveyed a large number of patients from an affective disorders clinic and found that 10 percent met criteria for what he has called *subictal affective disorder* (Table 5-19). Most of these patients were bipolar. The following case history is typical of Himmelhoch's patients:

SC was a 21-year-old white female college student who came to the Affective Disorders Clinic after treatment for depression and irritability with tricyclics,

Table 5-19. Criteria for "Dysthymic" Subictal Mood Disorders

1. Chronic depressive baseline

2. Brief "euphorias," often with beatific religious coloration

3. Brief severe depressive dips with impulsive suicide attempts (frequently wrist cutting)

4. Unusual amount of irritability and hostile outbursts

5. Marked premenstrual exacerbation in women

6. Paradoxical reactions to standard mood-active drugs

7. Severe cases often diagnosed as severe and/or rapid-cycling bipolar affective disorder, schizoaffective disorder, or, rarely, delusional depression; milder cases often diagnosed as dysthymic disorder, atypical or hysteroid depression, or cyclothymia

8. Range from frank temporal lobe epilepsy to behavioral disorders with paroxysmal EEG; or EEG may be normal, but patients fit above clinical descriptors

From Himmelhoch, 1984

chlordiazepoxide, and psychotherapy had failed. Indeed, she complained that her high-strung irritability and her labile mood became worse, testified to by a 22-lb weight loss during treatment. Relationships with family and friends had deteriorated under the assault of her impulsive irritability. Particular difficulty arose around her family's disapproval of her boyfriend, and stressful telephone calls from her family were followed by self-destructive behavior on two occasions: the first time by superficial wrist cutting; the second by slamming her fist ferociously into a wall, resulting in a Colles' fracture. Her moodiness became worse during each premenstrual period.

Her developmental history revealed she had been delivered 1 month prematurely after a very difficult pregnancy, that she was left-handed, and that she had great trouble separating from her mother to go to school. All this settled down by the age of 13, at which time she became a driven overachiever. During her senior year, her dysphoria, impulsivity, and irritability became chronic, interrupted only briefly by 3- to 4-day periods of outgoing, overachieving cheerfulness. One of her sisters had experienced Devic's multiple sclerosis and thyroid cancer but had seemingly recovered from both. A second sister had been successfully operated on for a chondrosarcoma.

Her mood lability, developmental history of soft neurologic signs, family history of neurologic illness, and paradoxic response to antidepressants all suggested the presence of a subictal dysthymia. EEG confirmed this impression, showing a bilateral grade II temporal dysrhythmia. Treatment with phenytoin stabilized her mood, but left her chronically mildly depressed. Changing her treatment to carbamazepine 600 mg daily produced a complete remission. A year after graduation, she left for Houston, Texas, where she has developed a successful career as an advertising executive. (pp. 278–279)

Silberman and colleagues (1985) studied 44 affective patients (34 of whom were bipolar) and compared them with 37 patients who had complex partial seizures and 30 controls. Twelve items thought to reflect temporal lobe dysfunction (i.e., transient sensory, cognitive, and affective phenomena), although absent in the control group, occurred with high frequency in the two patient groups, and there was substantial overlap. Some symptoms were predominantly confined to the epileptic patients: motor automatisms, vestibular, gustatory, and tactile hallucinations, and disorientation for time. Others, an altered rate of thinking and unexplained affective bursts, occurred exclusively in the manic-depressive patients. More interesting are the phenomena that overlapped the two groups: visual, auditory, and olfactory hallucinations and illusions, including illusions of significance and derealization,

jumbled thoughts, and amnesia. The symptoms were state dependent in both groups. Among the bipolar patients, the frequency and type of symptoms were similar during manic and depressive phases.

Himmelhoch views the mood lability associated with these temporal lobe disorders as existing on a spectrum with rapid-cycling affective illness. As discussed in Chapter 4, it is not clear if these patients with very short cycles do indeed form a continuum with the patients Dunner described, who have typical rapid cycles measured in several weeks to a few months. Himmelhoch emphasizes the mixed states, extreme mood lability, irritability, and poor response to standard mood-altering drugs in discussing these disorders, just as Monroe did. Some patients on the spectrum that includes complex partial seizures and subictal mood disorders are diagnosed as borderline or as emotionally unstable character disorder. Obviously, the differential diagnosis between borderline disorder and manic-depressive illness (see previous discussion) presupposes that organic factors had been ruled out initially.

Affective versus Organic: Clinical Summary

Given the possibility that the pathophysiology of manic-depressive illness may overlap with some organic disorders, differentiating between them cannot be reduced easily to simple formulas. For practical purposes, however, a differential diagnosis is critical to making an accurate treatment selection and prognosis. Thus, the clinician's first task when presented with manic or depressive symptoms is to consider other factors that might be corrected. The absence of a personal or family history of affective illness, and poor response to traditional treatments for manic-depressive illness are important clues suggesting an organic etiology.[28] Although no single medical screening test is definitive, certainly a neurological examination, formal neuropsychiatric testing, EEG, CT scan, and chemical screen for metabolic and toxic disturbances should supplement the careful history. Where the evidence points to a possible commingling of manic-depressive illness with a seizure disorder diatheses, anticonvulsants with a primary effect on temporal lobe disorders (e.g., carbamazepine) should become the treatment of choice. Patients with an underlying seizure diathesis expressed as mood disturbance will, of course, do poorly on many of the standard mood-altering drugs, since many of these drugs can lower seizure thresholds (see Chapters 21, 22, and 23). Biological tests that may be helpful in differential diagnosis are discussed in Chapters 17 and 18.

CLINICAL SUMMARY

To make an accurate diagnosis, careful exploration of the patient's past history is at least as important as a full description of the presenting episode. Whenever possible, the onset, duration, and treatment response of all past episodes should be recorded on a life chart, along with important life events. Much of this information can be obtained before the initial appointment by having the patient and family members fill out a life chart form.

When manic-like symptoms characterize the presenting picture, the clinician may face difficult questions of differential diagnosis. If a patient is in the hyperactive psychotic state described as stage-III mania in Chapters 2 and 3 and a complete history or family history is not available, the clinician must rely on an analysis of the presenting symptoms. (If there is a history of manic or depressive episodes, especially with well intervals, manic-depressive illness is the presumptive diagnosis, despite the atypical presenting symptoms.)

Principal diagnoses that should be ruled out are acute schizophrenia and organic and drug-induced psychoses, although the latter can, and often do, occur in an individual with manic-depressive illness. The presence of delusions (including paranoid delusions), hallucinations, and thought disorder does not support a diagnosis of schizophrenia over mania. Schizophrenia should be suspected, however, if the delusions are organized into a formal and stable system that has continued for a considerable time.

As a practical issue, differentiating acute stage-III mania from schizoaffective illness and schizophrenia is not absolutely critical, since the initial treatment, antipsychotic (neuroleptic) medication, often is essentially the same for all three.[29] If an affective component is suspected, lithium should be added. When the acute psychotic episode is under control, differential diag-

nosis often becomes clearer, even if information on the patient's personal or family history is still missing. If delusions or hallucinations persist in the absence of manic mood or hyperactivity (i.e., the patient is quietly delusional), schizophrenia or schizoaffective disorder is the more appropriate diagnosis. If the patient meets criteria for both schizophrenia and affective illness in the present episode or by history, schizoaffective illness is the appropriate diagnosis. Distinguishing between manic-depressive illness and schizophrenia can be particularly difficult in an adolescent, since at that age psychotic features are especially common in manic syndromes.

When vivid hallucinations (especially visual ones) or delusions dominate the clinical picture, particularly in a young person, a drug-induced state should be suspected, and a urine screen becomes especially important. Indeed, it is sensible to employ a urine screen routinely. True mania may be present even if these suspicions are borne out because it is not at all uncommon for initial manic episodes to be precipitated by drugs of abuse. In such cases, differential diagnosis can be difficult during the acute phase.

When presented with milder manic-like symptoms (or a history of them), the clinician must differentiate between clinical hypomania and normal elevated mood. Here it is important to recall the spectrum concepts outlined in Chapters 2 and 4. The threshold for a diagnosis of manic-depressive illness is reached when:

- Elation, excitement, or irritability cluster in discrete episodes lasting at least a week
- The symptomatic criteria outlined previously are met
- Symptoms are out of proportion to any environmental precipitant
- The symptoms seriously interfere with relationships
- Episodes have resulted in negative social, professional, or financial consequences for the individual.

We cannot overstate the importance of obtaining corroborating information from a spouse or other family member in evaluating the presence (or history) of hypomanic symptoms.

When presented with severe depressive symptoms, the clinician faces a somewhat different diagnostic challenge. Again, assuming that no history is available, one must rule out schizo-phrenia and schizoaffective illness, drug-induced states, and dementia. If delusions are present, they should be depressive in content in order to support an affective diagnosis. Otherwise, the differential criteria are similar to those noted previously for excited manic-like states.

The most important differential diagnostic issue in evaluating depression is to determine whether the patient has a unipolar or bipolar form of the illness. Obviously, this distinction must rest on knowledge of the patient's history, especially any prior episodes of mania or hypomania. Again, we wish to emphasize the importance of information from the family. If the patient has had two or more previous depressions without evidence of mania or hypomania, it is reasonably safe to assume a unipolar diagnosis, even though about 10 percent of such patients will later develop a manic episode and be reclassified as bipolar. A family history of mania can provide an important clue to a possible bipolar diathesis and may be helpful in choosing lithium over tricyclics for the prophylactic treatment of recurrent depression that initially appears to be unipolar.

With more moderate depressive symptoms, the differential diagnostic question is whether the patient meets criteria for a unipolar major depressive illness or cyclothymia. The spectrum concept outlined in Chapter 4 is again useful. A diagnosis of major depressive illness ultimately requiring pharmacological intervention is increasingly appropriate as depressive symptoms become more pervasive, cluster in discrete episodes lasting at least a few weeks, involve physiologic dysregulation (sleep, appetite, energy), and interfere with normal functioning. If a history of mania or hypomania is uncovered in the course of evaluating a patient with mild depressive symptoms, a manic-depressive diagnosis is clearly justified.

Sometimes patients whose acute symptoms do not meet criteria for manic-depressive illness have a history of relentless recurrences—that is, their atypical symptoms occur in discrete episodes. In such cases, the clinician should give special consideration to the diagnosis of manic-depressive illness. Here, differential diagnosis should include special attention to the boundaries between manic-depressive illness and certain personality disorders.

NOTES

1. Tsuang et al., 1981; M.B. Keller et al., 1981; Andreasen et al., 1981, 1986; Andreasen and Grove, 1982.
2. Both DSM-III and the Research Diagnostic Criteria (RDC), described later, are widely used by investigators throughout the world, however.
3. The RDC, together with the Schedule for Affective Disorders and Schizophrenia, proved to be reliable diagnostic instruments when used by interviewers from different centers around the country to rate past psychiatric symptoms and lifetime diagnoses in patients who were mentally ill at the time of assessment. However, the lifetime diagnoses of hypomania and recurrent unipolar depression were not as reliable as other categories (M.B. Keller et al., 1981). The stability of DSM-III affective diagnoses has been reviewed by Rice and colleagues (1986, 1987a).
4. Brockington et al., 1983; M.A. Young et al., 1983; Gershon et al., 1986; Fabrega et al., 1986; Tsuang et al., 1987; Breslau and Meltzer, 1988.
5. In the formal discussion of diagnosis to follow, we refer to DSM-III-R as our basic frame of reference, pointing out those few instances where it differs from DSM-III.
6. Studies of the relative reliability of specific diagnoses indicate that the bipolar-II category is not as reliable or stable as bipolar I, given the problems in ascertainment of a history of hypomania (Andreasen et al., 1981; Rice et al., 1986). This should be considered in evaluating the literature in bipolar–unipolar differences.
7. The Schneiderian first-rank symptoms that most often overlap between schizophrenia and manic-depressive illness include thought broadcasting, thought insertion, experiences of influence, delusional perceptions, and incomplete auditory hallucinations (Schneider, 1959). Descriptive data suggest that manic patients with first-rank and/or catatonic symptoms cannot be distinguished from those without such symptoms on the basis of family history or treatment response (Taylor, 1984). Jampala and colleagues (1985) reported that manic patients with so-called emotional blunting—"a constricted, inappropriate, unrelated affect of diminished intensity, with indifference or unconcern for loved ones, lack of emotional responsivity, and a loss of social graces"—had family histories suggestive of schizophrenia but with a pattern of treatment response more closely related to mania without emotional blunting.
8. Kendler et al. (1985) note that their patients with DSM-III schizoaffective disorder bore a familial relationship with schizophrenia. However, the study is difficult to interpret, since it did not include probands with affective disorder.
9. Schizoaffective depressed patients do not have a history of mania; that is, they are unipolar.
10. For a more complete discussion of the history of

this difficult dichotomy, see Ollerenshaw, 1973; Procci, 1976; Pope and Lipinski, 1978; Taylor and Abrams, 1980; Pope, 1983; and Andreasen, 1983.

11. Deficiencies in the practice of diagnosing schizophrenia or a manic-depressive illness with cross-sectional assessments of symptoms have been shown in several studies (e.g., Carlson and Goodwin, 1973; Carpenter et al., 1978; Kendell et al., 1979).

12. In his discussion of DSM-III, Meehl (1986) also advocates flexibility, pointing out the dangers of adhering too religiously to any conceptual entity in psychiatry:

   A disease entity, as delineated in the early stages of clinical experience and scientific study, at the level of mere syndrome description when there is as yet no (or minimal and conjectural) knowledge of the etiology or pathology underlying it, is an open concept. . . . It is neither philosophically rigorous nor scientifically sophisticated to make a literal identification of a disease entity with its currently accepted signs and symptoms. . . . Nothing but dogmatism on the one hand, or confusion on the other, is produced by pretending to give operational definitions in which the disease entity is literally identified with the list of signs and symptoms. Such an operational definition is a fake. (pp. 221-222)

13. Patients with a mixture of affective and schizophrenic symptoms were described by Kraepelin and his predecessors (Bell, 1849) and have been a major focus of the ongoing interest in the problem of differentiating schizophrenia from manic-depressive illness (Bleuler, 1911; Schneider, 1959).

14. The DSM-III-R definition of schizophreniform disorder departs from Langfeldt's concept and is no longer related to affective disorder. Now this category is reserved for patients who meet the acute symptomatic criteria for schizophrenia but who do not show continuous signs of the illness for 6 months or longer. Although a close relationship to schizophrenia is implied by the fact that the two diagnoses share many of the same criteria, schizophreniform disorder has a favorable outcome, with a return of normal functioning—an outcome more consistent with an affective diagnosis. The diagnostic criteria do not include affective symptoms, however. Taylor and Abrams (1984) found that 12 percent of 111 manic patients met the DSM-III criteria for schizophreniform disorder. The only variable on which they differed from other manic patients was in depressive symptoms. The morbid risk for alcoholism among their relatives was twice as great as for the other manic patients.

15. This point is illustrated by the following case history:

   The speech of this 30 year old medical technologist was so quick that nobody could follow him. Even when his speech was taped, we could not easily connect his thoughts, although some relationship can be seen between the various grandiose ideas: ". . . I can write up or down. I can call the jolly folks and the sad folks. I have one church on Madison Avenue, another in downtown. You don't go around messing with churches. No, I wasn't asleep. I just disappeared. Nobody even knew where I was. I was on a spaceship, man. I went up to the tombs. I was my own incarnation and the Egyptians were talking to me. Just check it with Alexander the Great. I am not a slave. I am from Africa. There are superhuman people, you know. I don't operate indoors, I operate outdoors. You cannot mix orange juice with bananas. I am simply disciplined. I have studied medicine in Egypt, not in the States. If I want, I can turn Italian. There is purpose, man, purpose. It's my secret. (Akiskal and Puzantian, 1979, pp. 429-430)

16. In a companion paper, Jauch and Carpenter (1988b) criticize DSM-III and DSM-III-R criteria for brief reactive psychosis as being much more restrictive than the original concept of the disorder. The practical result has been to curtail the study of the so-called third psychosis by severely limiting potential study cohorts. They suggest new criteria to use in testing the validity of the diagnosis.

17. Leonhard also cites Wernicke (1900) as source of this category.

18. In a prospective study of 180 inpatients with DSM-III-R borderline personality disorder, Fyer et al. (1988) found no greater association with affective disorder than they found between other personality disorders and affective disorder. These authors suggest that the previous reports of significant comorbidity may simply reflect high base rates of the relevant psychopathology.

19. Gaviria et al., 1982; Baxter et al., 1984; Friedman et al., 1982; Val et al., 1983.

20. Bipolar depression occurring simultaneously with manic symptoms—that is, a mixed state—would show considerable variability.

21. Although global neuropsychological improvement is not especially helpful in differentiating organic syndromes from manic-depressive illness, at times some of these techniques can pinpoint localized dysfunction, and obviously such information can be helpful to differential diagnosis.

22. The use of the term *secondary* in the Krauthammer and Klerman review does not include psychosocial precipitants of affective episodes. The topic of precipitating events is discussed in Chapter 6.

23. Only two, rather than three, symptoms were needed in addition to the mood and duration criteria.

24. Unfortunately, in the Krauthammer and Klerman study, the medication-related cases comprised the bulk of those without family history data. Also, negative family history may reflect problems of ascertainment.

25. Limited treatment evidence (mostly case reports) suggests, however, that secondary manic episodes also respond to antimanic treatments.

26. Shukla and colleagues (1988a) have shown that the organic factors are often missed by psychiatrists who misdiagnose the patients as having primary bipolar illness. In their study, the diagnosis of organic mood syndrome was associated with

older age of onset, lower frequency of manic episodes, shorter duration of symptoms, and more personality changes.

27. *Ideational viscosity* is defined as perseveratory thoughts, either grandiose or self-deprecatory in nature.

28. It is, of course, possible for a patient with manic-depressive illness to develop an organic brain syndrome secondary to some independent problem.

29. As discussed in Chapter 21, carbamazepine and clonazepam are increasingly used as alternatives to the neuroleptics in the initial management of psychotic mania.

PART TWO

CLINICAL STUDIES

Diverse clinical topics concerning manic-depressive illness comprise the five chapters in this section. Although each covers a separate topic with its own clear boundaries, the issues presented in this section cut across the entire book—that is, they are directly relevant to diagnoses, psychological issues, pathophysiology, and, of course, treatment.

In Chapter 6, we consider the natural course and outcome of bipolar illness, features that include age of onset, the number, patterning, and frequency of episodes, rapid cycling, duration and distribution of manic and depressive episodes, precipitants, and long-term outcome. These issues are critical not only as a foundation for the understanding of the illness itself and its pathophysiology (and, therefore, for the planning of future research) but also for treatment planning. The undeniably recurrent nature of manic-depressive illness is perhaps its most important characteristic.

We review the epidemiology of bipolar illness in Chapter 7. The very fact that manic-depressive illness is a relatively common illness and one that carries with it an exceptionally high morbidity makes it an important public health issue. We consider the many approaches available to epidemiologists and their associated problems in design and interpretation. Results of major studies of incidence, lifetime risk, and prevalence are presented, as are associated features, such as demographic correlates, prevalence rates among the homeless, cross-cultural studies, findings in immigrant populations, and seasonality.

Manic-depressive illness frequently first occurs in childhood or adolescence. In Chapter 8, we discuss the clinical presentation in young patients, issues in differential diagnosis, and predictors of bipolarity and prognosis. High-risk studies are beginning to provide valuable insights into the understanding of manic-depressive illness. The second half of Chapter 8 presents the personality, social, cognitive, and diagnostic findings derived from this paradigm.

Alcohol and substance abuse are frequent in bipolar illness and can complicate its diagnosis, course, and treatment. In Chapter 9, we explore what is known about rates of alcoholism and drug abuse in manic-depressive illness, as well as the relationships between abuse patterns, the illness, and genetic factors, phase of illness, self-medication, course, and precipitation of illness. The treatment issues surrounding dual-diagnosis patients are covered in Chapter 26.

Suicide is more closely associated with the affective illnesses than it is with any other disease or circumstance. In Chapter 10, after reviewing rates of suicide, we discuss clinical correlates of suicide in manic-depressive illness, including phenomenological features, treatment history, course of illness, and clinical states preceding suicide and suicide attempts. This discussion lays the groundwork for clinical management issues presented later in Chapter 27.

6

Course and Outcome

The universal experience is striking, that the attacks of manic-depressive insanity
. . . never lead to profound dementia, not even when they continue throughout life
almost without interruption. . . . As a rule the disease runs its course in isolated attacks more or less sharply defined from each other or from health, which are either
like or unlike, or even very frequently are [the] perfect antithesis. (p. 3)

—Emil Kraepelin, 1921

Emil Kraepelin's central insight, the one that continues as an organizing principle in modern descriptive psychiatry, was his division of the major
psychoses into two groups based largely on
course and outcome. He observed that whereas
dementia praecox (schizophrenia) tends to be
chronic and follow a deteriorating course, manic-
depressive illness is episodic and ultimately exacts a less devastating toll from those affected.[1]
Today we face a paradox: Although the discovery
of lithium's prophylactic potential has revived
interest in the natural course of manic-depressive
illness, widespread use of it and other prophylactic agents has substantially altered that course.
Investigators must confront the fact that "natural"
course now includes the unquantified effects of
routine prophylaxis. This chapter discusses contemporary studies of outcome in the community,
although those that assess the impact of prophylactic treatment are reviewed in Chapter 23.
Biological correlates of natural course are covered in Chapter 17.

As with most fields of inquiry, studies of
course and outcome are accompanied by methodological complexities that should be kept in
mind when interpreting the data. Two especially
important issues involve patient selection and diagnosis. The index hospitalization required in
most outcome studies can produce either under-

estimations or overestimations of recurrence. Underestimates can result when, during a single hospitalization, the patient has multiple rapid cycles
that are counted as a single episode. On the other
hand, overestimates can result from basing recurrence rates on hospital admission data because
they fail to include patients who experience a
single episode, recover without hospitalization,
and never have a recurrence. The retrospective
studies that dominate the available literature commonly produce underestimates because they are
more likely to miss episodes than to overcount
them.

Many of the classic studies of natural course do
not distinguish between the bipolar and unipolar
subgroups. Numerous interpretive problems result, particularly in studies from the United
States, where diagnostic criteria for unipolar illness (i.e., depressions that are not bipolar) allow
for considerable heterogeneity. For this reason
we emphasize the literature on bipolar patients,
although some conclusions may be relevant to the
more recurrent forms of unipolar illness as well.
Most classic studies of bipolar patients were done
with patients hospitalized for mania and thus do
not include the bipolar-II subgroup. The extent to
which patients with schizoaffective features were
included in the sample is another diagnostic issue
to be considered (see later discussion).

A common methodological problem is the lack of a generally accepted convention for collecting data on course or for defining recovery and relapse. This situation may be improving, however. Methods for charting the course of illness have been proposed for both retrospectively derived data (Post et al., 1988a) and prospectively derived data (Keller et al., 1987). These methods might well have clinical as well as research uses. For example, detailed description of prior course of illness may reveal that medications, such as lithium, given to the patient in the past were mistakenly judged ineffective when they had actually improved the course of the illness. Conversely, charting may uncover instances in which drugs exacerbated the course of illness. In addition, previously unrecognized associations of episode onsets with anniversaries, life events, or other stressors may aid in psychotherapeutic and behavioral management. These standardized methods are all the more important in industrialized countries where population mobility is increasing, a situation that leaves fewer opportunities for a single clinic or clinician to follow a cohort of patients over a lifetime.

A final consideration in reviewing this literature is its largely retrospective nature, a troublesome aspect given the problem inherent in recalling the past, especially for depressed patients. Future prospective studies need to focus on patients in naturalistic treatment settings.

AGE OF ONSET

The age when manic-depressive illness most often begins is intrinsically important to genetically vulnerable individuals and their clinicians, and it may offer clues to future course. Here we examine the age of onset literature in general. Chapter 8 focuses on studies of early onset in adolescence and perhaps even before puberty, and Chapter 15 examines how differences in age of onset relate to estimates of the degree of genetic vulnerability. Pooling the data from 22 studies reporting average onset age in bipolar affective illness (Table 6-1), the weighted mean is 28.1 years. Because the data are not normally distributed, however, the figure may be misleading. Averages can be raised by a relatively small number of patients with late onset, for example. When median age of

onset has been reported, it is generally in the mid-20s. The most recent comprehensive survey of age of onset comes from the National Institute of Mental Health (NIMH) Epidemiologic Catchment Area (ECA) study (Weissman et al., 1988a; discussed in greater detail in Chapter 7), which found a median age of onset of 18 years for bipolar-I patients (Christie et al., 1988). As noted below, this relatively low age may reflect in part a cohort effect.

Some of the variance across individual studies in Table 6-1 is related to the different criteria for onset.[2] The age when symptoms first appear generally is younger than the age when treatment is first sought, and first hospitalization is usually still later. Sometimes age at first treatment has been chosen on the assumption that dating of initial symptoms would be too imprecise. However, Egeland and colleagues (1987a) have shown that, by using age at "first impairment associated with affective symptoms," they could obtain a reliable indicator that, as expected, yielded a younger age of onset for bipolar patients (mean age = 15.5 years) than if they waited for full RDC to be fulfilled (mean age = 18.7 years), or first treatment (mean age = 22 years) or first hospitalization (mean age = 25.8 years). It is important to note that all of the individuals identified by this more sensitive indicator went on to meet RDC criteria for bipolar disorder.

To gauge the distribution of the published ages of onset more accurately in the bipolar patient population, we pooled data from 10 studies that specified the number of patients with first episodes beginning in each decade (a total of 1,304 patients). Divided this way (Figure 6-1), the peak onset period appears to be in the 20s. However, greater specificity is obtained by pooling data from six studies giving age of onset in 5-year intervals (Figure 6-2). This finer grained analysis results in a peak age of onset in the 15 to 19 age range, followed closely by the 20 to 24 range. Note that the age of onset distribution is generally similar for men and women.

Some investigators suggest that there are two primary patterns of onset—early and late. As discussed in Chapter 15, however, it is not yet clear to what extent separating these patterns really identifies distinct subgroups with differential phenomenology, pathophysiology, family history, outcome, or treatment response (James,

1977). One phenomenological association that is clear is that between psychotic (or schizoaffective) features and early age of onset among bipolar patients. In an extensive review of the literature, Angst (1986c) cites 10 studies reporting this relationship, a conclusion that has been extended by Blumenthal and colleagues (1987) in their study of the Amish. A secondary peak of late onset in women has been found (Angst, 1978; Zis et al., 1979) and is reflected in the small increase in onset frequency among women in the 45 to 50 age range in Figure 6-2. Such a subgroup, if it exists, might be considered analogous to onset of involutional melancholia. Although very late onset (i.e., over age 60) generally has been considered rare (Winokur et al., 1969; Loranger and Levine, 1978; Carlson et al., 1974), some data suggest that it may be more common than thought[3] (Spicer et al., 1973; Shulman and Post, 1980; Stone, 1989). Very late onset patients are less likely to be genetically vulnerable and more likely to be organically impaired.[4] These observations highlight the importance of differential diagnosis of primary mood disorders and the mood disorders secondary to specific neuropathology (see Chapter 5).

Diagnostic criteria that include a minimum age of onset can affect estimates of the prevalence of the illness. As detailed in Chapter 8, most studies of early onset report about one fourth of the patients with a first episode before age 20. Although adolescent onset is not at all uncommon, the question of whether full-blown bipolar illness can start before puberty remains controversial, despite several case reports of early childhood onset. These issues are discussed in Chapter 8, along with observations that many adolescents who later develop clear bipolar illness were troubled by lability of mood and behavior for several years before a definitive episode began. Although these illness precursors can be difficult to distinguish from normal storminess, it is important to do so because there is reason to believe that aggressive early treatment can diminish later morbidity (see Chapters 16, 20, and 23). Another issue affecting the interpretation of this literature is the cohort effect. As noted by Weissman and Klerman (1978, 1988) and by Gershon and colleagues (1987b), the age of onset for affective disorders (both unipolar and bipolar) appears to have been getting younger, beginning with the

cohort born in 1940. This issue is discussed further in Chapter 15. The relationship between age of onset and episode frequency is discussed later in this chapter.

NUMBER OF EPISODES

In his classic 1921 monograph, Kraepelin wrote that, of 459 manic-depressive patients he had studied (which included unipolar patients), only 55 percent experienced more than one episode and only 28 percent had more than three. A careful reading of his clinical descriptions suggests, however, that many of Kraepelin's ostensibly single-episode patients were, in fact, severely and chronically ill with multiple episodes, which at that time required continuous hospitalization.

Considered together, the longitudinal studies of manic-depressive patients not taking prophylactic medication (Table 6-2), which include both bipolar and unipolar forms, indicate that most patients—particularly those studied in the past 25 years—had more than one episode.[5] Table 6-2 also suggests that most patients with major affective disorder (i.e., Kraepelinian manic-depressive illness) have a recurrent illness. Many textbooks, apparently relying on older data, fail to emphasize this point sufficiently.

Angst (1980) subdivided his patients into three categories according to their pattern of recurrence: MD, Md, and Dm. As described in Chapter 4, MD represents the core illness, with both major manic and major depressive episodes; Md patients have full manic episodes, but their depressive episodes do not require hospitalization; Dm patients have been hospitalized for depression, but their manic episodes are not severe enough for hospitalization (i.e., they have histories of hypomania).[6] Angst's MD patients show a tendency toward the most episodes, but in the larger cohort sudied in the NIMH collaborative study, the Dm (bipolar-II) patients had the most prior episodes, although this number was not significantly different from the bipolar-I patients (Coryell et al., 1989b).

In their 1979 review of the literature on the natural course of manic-depressive illness (both unipolar and bipolar, with the index episode usually a hospitalization), Zis and Goodwin divided studies that showed low rates of relapse from

Table 6-1. Age of Onset

Study	Patients N	Mean (Range)	Male (N)	Female (N)	Criteria	Comments
Swift, 1907	67	50% < 30	40% < 30 (20)	55% < 30 (47)	First episode	Of the 105 manic-depressive patients studied, 67 were BP
Wertham, 1929	2,000	32.0			First hospitalization	All manic. 20% < 20 years, peak between 20 and 25 years. Longer duration is associated with later onset
Clayton et al., 1965	28	28.0			First symptoms	22% > 50 years
Perris, 1968	131	31.4	32.9 (56)	30.3 (75)	First treatment	Male onset significantly lower (<.01) if 1st episode mania, female lower (<.001) if 1st episode is depression. 40% had 1st episode between ages 15 and 25
Winokur et al., 1969	61	24.0 (15-67)	29.1 (26)	27.1 (35)	First symptoms	34% had 1st episode before age 20 24 years median
Baastrup et al., 1970	50	31.0 (12-72)			First episode	
Woodruff et al., 1971a	19	29.0			First episode	11% > 40 years
Mendlewicz et al., 1972a	60	29.9			First treatment	45% < 25 years 35% 25-40 years 20% > 40 years
Taylor & Abrams, 1973a	50	56% < 30	68% < 30 (19)	48% < 30 (31)	First episode	UP mania onset more frequent > 30 years. Less family history when onset > 30 years
Carlson et al., 1974	53	30.0			First treatment	58% < 30 years 10% > 60 years
Taschev, 1974	160	35.8	35.7 (91)	36.0 (69)		Follow-up of deceased patients

Study	N	Mean age (range)			Criterion	Comments
Dunner et al., 1976b	152	30.6	31.1 (83)	29.8 (69)		2/3 1st hospitalization, 1/3 1st symptoms
Petterson, 1977a	123	33.0	33.3 (54)	32.7 (69)	First symptoms	
Angst, 1978	95	34.7 (10-69)			First episode	Bimodal in females: 20-29 years and 40-49 years
Loranger & Levine, 1978	200	32.3 (8-74)	33.0 (100)	31.6 (100)	First symptoms	20% onset in adolescence, 33% hospitalized before age 25
Peselow et al., 1982a	238	28.9 (< 16-64)	31.1 (101)	27.3 (137)	First consultation	Patients divided into BP I & II and CT groups
Shan-Ming et al., 1982	108	24 (20-30)				All manic, all Chinese. Subsequent analysis (Shan-Ming & Luxi, 1985) suggested early and late onset subgroups (21.4 and 39.9) The early group had equal sex distribution but males predominated in the late group
Akiskal et al., 1983b	41	31.4 (14-67)			First depressive episode	
Baron et al., 1983b	142	26.3 (< 9 & 60-64)	25.6 (61)	26.9 (81)	First treatment or hospitalization	Onset 2% < 15 years, 11% in adolescence, 28% < 24 years, 43% < 30 years
Glassner & Haldipur, 1983	46	30.0			First episode	Mode = 20
Joyce, 1984a	200	28.3 (< 9 & 70-74)	28.4 (83)	28.2 (117)	First episode	23 years median (M&F) 42% 15-19 years
Weissman et al., 1988a	186	21.2 (17.9-26.3)	20.7 (76)	21.5 (110)	First symptoms	Data from the ECA study
Total N Patients for whom a mean was given	**4,210**	28.1[a]	30.3[a] (770)	28.7[a] (940)		

a The weighted means include studies that measured onset as first treatment but excluded the one study that reported only first hospitalizations. Obviously the mean age of onset would be younger if the first appearance of clinically significant symptoms were uniformly used as the criterion.

Update of Goodwin & Jamison, 1984

131

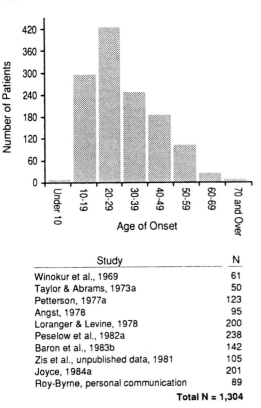

Study	N
Winokur et al., 1969	61
Taylor & Abrams, 1973a	50
Petterson, 1977a	123
Angst, 1978	95
Loranger & Levine, 1978	200
Peselow et al., 1982a	238
Baron et al., 1983b	142
Zis et al., unpublished data, 1981	105
Joyce, 1984a	201
Roy-Byrne, personal communication	89
Total N = 1,304	

Figure 6-1. Age of onset.

those that showed high rates. They found that those with low relapse rates were marred by five methodological limitations, the most frequent of which are listed in Table 6-3. For example, studies with low relapse rates tend to include only hospitalized episodes, introducing a bias toward patients with longer and more severe episodes. Thus, in Perris' 1968 study, only 40 percent of the patients had four or more hospitalized episodes, but when all episodes were included, more than 80 percent had four or more. Obviously, excluding episodes preceding the index hospital admission also leads to underestimation. When, for instance, Bratfos and Haug (1968) included preadmission episodes, the proportion of patients with single episodes dropped to 13 percent.

As noted previously, early studies often found a high proportion of single-episode patients because they included in that single-episode count the many chronic patients who, in fact, had multiple (but uncounted) episodes while hospitalized. Cutler and Post (1982a) traced the long-term course of illness in a group of bipolar patients chronically hospitalized in a state institution. Their detailed analysis indicated that each of these patients displayed a pattern similar to what

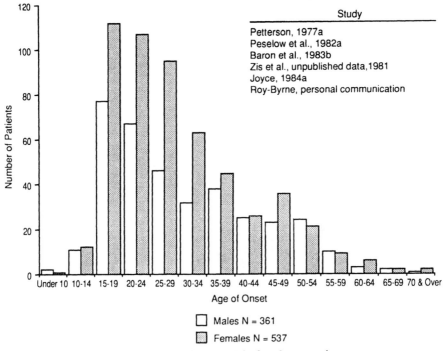

Study
Petterson, 1977a
Peselow et al., 1982a
Baron et al., 1983b
Zis et al., unpublished data,1981
Joyce, 1984a
Roy-Byrne, personal communication

☐ Males N = 361
▨ Females N = 537

Figure 6-2. Age of onset: Male/female comparison.

Table 6-2. Total Number of Episodes

Study	Patients N	Years of Observation R = Retrospective P = Prospective	Total Episodes %				Comments
			1	2-3	4-6	7+	
Kraepelin, 1921	459	Variable, up to a lifetime R	45	27		28	Many "single episode" patients were chronically hospitalized with continuous cycling
Pollock, 1931	5,739	11 R	55	35	8	2	Excluded episodes prior to index admission
Rennie, 1942	66	26 R	8	29	26	37	"Several" had 20 or more episodes
Lundquist, 1945	103	20%, <10 38%, 10-20 R 42%, 20-30	50	25		25	28% were chronic and are included in the "single episode" category; excluded episodes prior to index admission
Stenstedt, 1952	62	1.2-20+ R	26	42		32	Included non-recovered patients as single episode
Bratfos & Haug, 1968	42	1-12 P	13	42		45*	"Not free of symptoms for any length of time;" half of these were "chronic"
Perris, 1968	131	19.6 R	0	17	40	43	Average number of episodes, BP = 7, UP = 4
Carlson et al., 1974[a]	53	10 P	4	17	32	47*	*1/3 of these were rapid cyclers (4 or more episodes / year)
Angst, 1978, and Angst et al., 1979b[a]	95	26 P, R	0	8	22	69	16% had > 20 episodes. "New episode" required > 4 weeks asymptomatic interval
Zis et al., 1980	105	—P, R	6	13	33	48	
Fukuda et al., 1983	96	18-28 R	15	40	20	25	Hospitalized, questionnaire and chart review; no treatment with lithium, but other drugs used
Total number of patients 6,951			Range: 0-55	13-42	8-40	2-69	

[a] These studies included some patients treated prophylactically. Most of the other studies include patients treated acutely.
Update of Goodwin & Jamison, 1984

133

Table 6-3. Methodological Limitations Associated
with Low Relapse Rates in Affective Disorders

• Short duration of observation
• Focus on hospitalized episodes
• Exclusion of episodes preceding index admission
• Inclusion of nonrecovered patients
• Combined episodes treated as single episodes
• High UP/BP patient ratio

Kraepelin had observed more than half a century earlier—multiple, discrete episodes embedded in one single long-term hospitalization. Estimates of relapse rates probably were lower than justified in the older studies, even when based on patients who were not chronically hospitalized. In those cases, combined episodes (e.g., a mania followed by a depression, perhaps interspersed with a brief well interval) might have been counted as a single episode. The presence of a continuously circular course (Kukopulos et al., 1980) or rapid cycles (Dunner et al., 1976b) makes it more likely that multiple episodes will be counted as one.

On the other hand, two factors might be expected to increase reported relapse rates—treatment with antidepressants and selection of lithium clinic patients for study. Since the highest relapse rates generally are the most recent, it is conceivable, as suggested by Kukopulos and co-workers (1980), that the use of antidepressants for acute episodes might have influenced the results. Indeed, in his analysis of the incidence of manic switches in one hospital studied over six decades, Angst (1985) noted a fourfold increase when the pretreatment era was compared with the decades after ECT and antidepressant drugs became widely used. Although other explanations are possible, such as better diagnostic detection of mania, these data also are consistent with the possibility that effective antidepressant treatments may have altered the course in some manic-depressive patients toward more frequent recurrences. The evidence for and against this possibility is reviewed extensively in Chapter 22. A bias toward higher relapse rates would be likely when an outcome study draws all of its subjects from patients referred to a lithium maintenance clinic. The studies of Angst and of Grof cited elsewhere in this chapter, however, included all patients who came to the clinic for treatment of an

episode without regard to previous episodes (i.e., not just those deemed eligible for maintenance treatment). Thus, both underestimations and overestimations of true natural recurrence rates undoubtedly have occurred in the literature. It appears that the more frequent methodological problems are those that lead to underestimations of recurrence. The availability of effective antidepressant treatments may be one factor accounting for the higher relapse rates in recent studies.

Finally, a chart review of bipolar patients from the prepharmacology era (Winokur and Kadrmas, 1989) suggests that certain clinical features may be associated with the illness' natural tendency to recur. Winokur and Kadrmas found that, compared with patients who had only one or two episodes during a follow-up period averaging 2.4 years, patients with a polyepisodic course (more than three episodes) were more likely to have had an early age of onset, a finding that replicates an earlier report by Okuma and Shimoyama (1972). Winokur and Kadrmas also found that a polyepisodic course was associated with a more insidious onset of the index episode and a greater frequency of bipolar illness in first-degree relatives. The authors speculate that this last finding may indicate that it is cyclicity more than polarity that is genetically transmitted: The more total episodes, the greater the likelihood of manic episodes.

FREQUENCY OF EPISODES (CYCLE LENGTH)

Cycle length is defined as the time from the onset of one episode to the onset of the next. Variation in cycle length primarily reflects variation in the length of the symptom-free interval, since the duration of episodes tends to be relatively constant in a given individual. Onset is used to calculate cycle length because it is generally easier to pinpoint than the termination of an episode. In addition, treatment can easily obscure the natural length of an episode. Virtually all investigators agree that cycle length tends to get shorter with each recurrence; that is, episodes become more frequent.[7] But after three to five episodes, the extent of shortening slows down considerably and approaches a leveling off, that is, a maximum frequency of episodes.

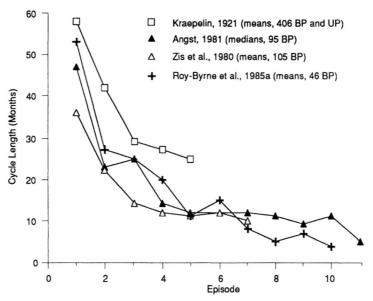

Figure 6-3. Relationship between cycle length and episode number (update of Goodwin and Jamison, 1984).

Common Cycle Length Patterns

Figure 6-3 illustrates the relationship between average cycle length and episode number. This graph is based on four independent studies with a total of 677 patients. Despite substantial individual variability, the averages show a remarkably consistent pattern across the studies. For example, note the pattern in the average of the 105 bipolar patients of Zis and colleagues (1979): The average cycle length between the first and the second episode is 36 months, then diminishes to about 24 months, then to 12 months. In 46 bipolar patients studied by Roy-Byrne and colleagues (1985a), the mean cycle lengths for the first seven episodes were 53, 28, 25, 20, 12, 15, and 9 months. In 95 bipolar patients from Angst's Zurich clinic, the median first cycle length was 48 months compared with 22 months for the second cycle, 24 months for the third, 14 months for the fourth, and 12 months for the fifth (Angst, 1981b). The longer average cycle length in the Kraepelin material reflects the inclusion of unipolar patients, whose cycles are longer (Angst, 1981b; Fukuda et al., 1983). The four studies illustrated in Figure 6-3 are consistent with the retrospective data of Taschev (1974), who found the average second cycle to be as long as the first but the fourth cycle half as long as the second. A prospective study of patients in the 1980s (Keller et al., 1982) also documented an increasing probability of relapse with each episode, a finding that suggests that some fundamental characteristics of the illness course may persist despite treatment.[8]

The considerable individual variability in patterns of relapse was pointed out by Kraepelin (1921):

> If we give no more examples, that is not because those already given represent adequately the multiplicity of the courses taken by manic-depressive insanity; it is absolutely inexhaustible. (p. 149)

This variability was examined in the 105 patients studied by Zis and colleagues (1979), who noted that many had prolonged intervals between the first and second episodes, the so-called latency period most frequently seen in patients whose first episode occurs before age 30. Angst (1984) estimated that 14 percent of his bipolar patients had latency periods longer than 5 years. (The implications of this latency for prophylactic management are discussed in Chapter 23.)

The relationship between frequency of episodes and age of onset remains somewhat unclear. Several older studies[9] found an increasing frequency of relapse as age of onset increased, but more recent studies do not. Two studies failed to show that association (Dunner et al., 1980; Roy-Byrne et al., 1985a), and two found the opposite (Okuma and Shimoyama, 1972; Winokur

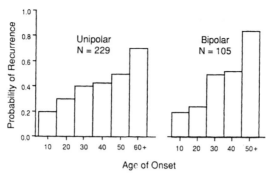

Figure 6-4. Probability of a relapse within 24 months following the initial episode (from Zis et al., 1979).

and Kadrmas, 1989).[10] A multiple regression analysis of the 105 bipolar patients studied by Grof showed that the patient's age and the age of onset each contributed independently to the prediction of relapse (Zis et al., 1979). Keller's prospective study of treated patients also showed that the probability of relapse increased with age. Figure 6-4, taken from the study of Zis and colleagues, shows that onset in the 20s is associated with a 20 percent probability of recurrence within 24 months, onset in the 30s with a 50 percent probability, and late onset (age 50 or older) with a very high (80 percent) probability of recurrence. However, only the first cycle length (the time between the first and second episode) was related to age of onset. On the other hand, Dunner and associates (1979b) did not find this association.

Another question is whether episodes come in bursts or clusters, as originally described by Kraepelin in his studies of predominantly chronic patients with frequent relapses. As discussed in Chapter 23, this issue is important in assessing prophylactic treatment, and indeed in making treatment decisions. If episodes of manic-depressive illness characteristically occur in clusters, then it may be difficult to interpret prophylactic trials of lithium in which a pretreatment period is compared with a period on the drug (mirror-image design). Saran (1970) compared episode frequencies in six untreated bipolar patients for 2 years preceding and 3 years following an arbitrary point in time. Even in such a small number of patients there was some suggestion of episode clustering. In a 2- to 20-year follow-up (mean 5.6 years) of patients admitted for manic episodes, Winokur (1975) found that 91 percent of the first episode patients had another episode during follow-up, compared with only 53 percent

of those with a history of previous episodes, a result interpreted as evidence of episode clustering. Further, when Cutler and Post (1982a) studied six chronically hospitalized manic-depressive patients with multiple in-hospital episodes, they also found clustering. As with Kraepelin's patients, however, it is not clear how broadly the findings in these very ill patients can be generalized.

Finally, in patients selected for lithium therapy because they had had two or more episodes during the preceding 2 years, Schou and colleagues (1970b) and Angst and co-workers (1970) found no evidence of clustering—that is, no difference in relapse rates in the periods before and after lithium treatment. Although further study of the clustering phenomenon would be useful, it is unlikely that sufficient numbers of untreated patients will be available for study.

A final question about the pattern of cycles in bipolar affective illness is whether burnout occurs. Kraepelin observed that the illness tends to decline after the fourth decade, although he did not elaborate on his observation. In a prospective follow-up study of 215 bipolar patients (150 bipolar I, 65 bipolar II) over a period of 17 to 21 years, Angst (1986d) reported no age-related decrease in frequency of episodes; 26 percent of the bipolar patients (vs 42 percent of the unipolar patients) were free of relapses over 5 or more years, although most patients were still actively ill through their 60s, when the follow-up generally ended.[11]

Rapid Cycling

The operational definition and general characteristics of rapid cycling are outlined in Table 6-4. Although most of the cases studied have repre-

Table 6-4.
Characteristics of Rapid-Cycling Patients

- At least 4 affective episodes per year
- 13–20% of all bipolars
- Initial onset 20%, later onset 80%
- Predominantly in females
- Majority begin the illness with a depressive episode

sented the bipolar-I pattern, bipolar-II cycling is not rare,[12] and indeed rapid-cycling unipolar depression has been reported (see, e.g., Zisook, 1988). The fact that rapid cycling generally develops later in the course of the illness may reflect underlying pathophysiological mechanisms, such as the progressive kindling or sensitization described by R.M. Post and colleagues (1984e, 1986a) (Figure 6-5; see Chapter 16). Late rapid cycling could also reflect the impact of certain treatments accelerating the natural course of the illness (see Chapter 22). The great majority of rapid cycling occurs in female patients,[13] a finding possibly related to the suggestion that a suboptimal thyroid function may be involved (Cho et al., 1979; Cowdry et al., 1983);[14] that is, females are more susceptible to the antithyroid effects of lithium. Both older age and later age of onset independently contribute to shorter cycle lengths, including rapid cycling, but the role of treatment in these associations is not clear. Reports of a

very high rate of rapid cycling among the mentally retarded with major affective disorder (Reid and Naylor, 1976; Glue, 1989) hint that organic factors may be involved in permitting the rapid cycles to occur.

The phenomenon of rapid cycling among bipolar patients (and some unipolar patients as well) is of considerable importance both theoretically and practically. At the theoretical level, rapid-cycling patients, for obvious reasons, make up a disproportionate share of those studied longitudinally—for example, in studies of the switch process from depression to mania, including biochemical comparisons of the two states. If such data are to have any generalizability, it is critical to know whether patients with rapid cycles, defined arbitrarily as having four or more episodes per year, make up a separate subgroup, a separate illness, or are fully part of the manic-depressive group but at one extreme of the cycle length continuum (see Chapter 4). This same question is also important to treatment. If rapid cycling and normal cycling involve wholly different pathophysiological mechanisms, treatment might need to be fundamentally different.

Table 6-5 highlights what is known about the relationship between rapid and non-rapid cycling in bipolar patients. The principal reason to consider a separate subgroup is the evidence for differences in pharmacological response. Patients without rapid cycles are more likely to respond to prophylactic lithium than are those with them,

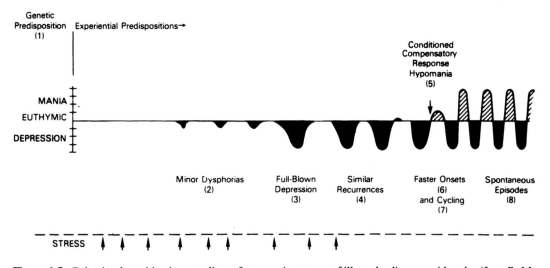

Figure 6-5. Behavioral sensitization paradigm of progressive course of illness leading to rapid cycles (from R. M. Post et al., 1986a).

Table 6-5. Rapid-Cycling Affective Disorder: Relationship to "Normal" Bipolar Affective Disorder

1. There are insufficient data to determine whether cycle length is distributed normally or bimodally

2. In general, rapid-cycling patients appear to be genetically and phenotypically related to non-rapid-cycling patients (Wehr et al., 1988; Nurnberger et al., 1988b)

3. Course of illness in rapid-cycling patients can include nonrapid-cycling phases

4. Rapid cycling could be viewed as an extreme development of tendencies inherent in nonrapid-cycling course
   - Increasing frequency of episodes[a] (Grof et al., 1974)
   - Switches between episodes with no normal interval[a] (Winokur et al., 1969)
   - Circularity of episodes (Kukopulos and Reginaldi, 1973)

5. Rapid cycling may exhibit a somewhat different pharmacological response profile

[a]Potentiated by antidepressants, which are also capable of inducing rapid cycling (Wehr and Goodwin, 1979, 1987a)

whereas anticonvulsants are effective in rapid-cycling patients, but their role in patients without rapid cycles is not yet as clear. These pharmacological differences may, however, be secondary to the effects of antidepressants on the course of illness. In one study of prophylaxis among rapid-cycling patients who had never been exposed to antidepressants (a rarity), Kukopulos and colleagues (1983) found a very high rate of response to lithium. Likewise, preliminary data on the prophylactic efficacy of carbamazepine in patients without rapid cycles are encouraging.

A study of the frequency distribution of cycle lengths could answer the question of whether rapid cycling represents a separate subgroup or is simply one end of a continuum. Cycle length data of Zis and colleagues (unpublished data), do not support a separable low cycle length group, although a larger sample would be needed to answer this issue definitively (see Figure 4-5). The existing family history data also are more consistent with the continuum notion in that the families of rapid-cycling patients have the same frequency of non-rapid-cycling affective disorders as do families of non-rapid-cycling patients (Nurnberger et al., 1988b; Wehr et al., 1988). The

question of whether ultrarapid cyclers (e.g., 48 hour cyclers) are also part of the continuum is unsettled. Taken together, the data outlined in Table 6-5 tend to favor the concept that rapid cycling represents one extreme of a manic-depressive spectrum.

ONSET AND DURATION OF EPISODES

In Chapters 4 and 21, we describe the way in which the onset of manic episodes can progress through identifiable stages, starting with mild hypomania (referred to by Jacobsen, 1965, as the "hypomanic alert"), through moderate manic symptoms, including grandiose or paranoid delusions, to severe mania accompanied by profound psychosis and even delirium. Although the time frame for the unfolding of these changes is quite variable, on an average, manic episodes begin more abruptly than depressive ones, the former often developing over a few days or even a few hours. Bipolar depressive episodes, on the other hand, often take weeks to develop fully (Rennie, 1942; Winokur, 1976). The onset of bipolar depressive episodes is still more abrupt than it is in unipolar depression, however (Winokur, 1976; Kendell, 1968; Hays, 1964). Post and associates (1981), studying the variability in the onset of manic episodes in the hospital, found a tendency toward a bimodal distribution, that is, separable patterns of slow onset and rapid onset. One source of this variation is the number of previous episodes. They found an increasing abruptness of manic onset with each successive episode, a phenomenon they believe has important biological implications (see Chapter 20). Molnar and colleagues (1988) also found a great deal of variation in prodrome duration, but, unlike the previous studies, their bipolar sample reported significantly longer manic than depressive prodromes.[15]

Estimates of the average duration of episodes in manic-depressive illness range from 4 to 13 months, the longer time generally from studies before drugs were available. Swift (1907), Kraepelin (1921), and Rennie (1942) noted that episodes generally lengthen as the illness progresses—a conclusion carried over into many textbooks—but Lundquist (1945) noted a shortening of later episodes.[16] In general, the more comprehensive studies of this issue actually find episode duration to be stable through the course of the illness, perhaps decreasing slightly after the first 10 or so episodes (Angst, 1981b; Pollock, 1931). The relationship of age to episode length may confound these findings, however, since MacDonald (1918), Wertham (1929), and Lundquist (1945) noted that the first episode of illness was longer in older than in younger patients. Roy-Byrne and colleagues (1985a), who found the same thing, suggested that it may indicate that older patients were slower to seek or receive treatment.

For most patients, bipolar depressive episodes are longer than manic ones,[17] a difference that is also found in patients treated using contemporary methods (Keller et al., 1986a).[18] Angst (1978) analyzed episode duration as a function of illness type and found that the longest episodes were associated with the core form of the illness (MD, i.e., bipolar I), whereas episodes of the Dm (bipolar II) form were shorter; the NIMH collaborative study (Coryell et al., 1989b) failed to replicate this observation.[19] Grof and co-workers (1979b) noted that episode length was substantially more likely to vary from one individual to another than from one time to another in a given patient. They suggested that for an individual patient, the length of previous episodes could, to some extent, predict length of subsequent episodes. In the NIMH collaborative study, a strong intraindividual correlation was noted only for manic episodes.[20]

PATTERN AND DISTRIBUTION OF MANIC AND DEPRESSIVE EPISODES

Estimates of the proportion of bipolar patients who begin the illness with a manic episode range from 34 to 79 percent, averaging just over 50 percent.[21] The studies with the highest estimates of manic onset use first hospitalization as the onset criterion. It is possible that the high estimates of manic onset result from the underestimation of depressive onsets not requiring hospitalization. Nevertheless, in Angst's study (1978) of 95 bipolar patients, in which onset was defined as the first occurrence of symptoms requiring treatment, 65 percent of the first episodes were manic (or hypomanic), whereas only 35 percent were depressive. On the other hand, Roy-Byrne and colleagues (1985a), defining onset as the first

symptoms meeting RDC criteria for an affective episode, found that 60 percent of 71 bipolar patients had a depressive first episode. Perris and d'Elia (1966) reported that among patients with a manic first episode, 62 percent went on to have a predominantly manic course, whereas only 25 percent had a predominantly depressive course. The reverse was true for those whose illness started with a depression. Perris and d'Elia's patients were not on prophylactic treatment, but Roy-Byrne and colleagues found the same trend in a treated population of bipolar patients. The relative distribution of manic and depressive episodes does not appear to change over the course of the illness (Angst, 1978) (Figure 6-6).

Gender differences in the frequency of the different course patterns as defined by Angst (1978) are also evident in Figure 6-6. Among his male patients, the predominantly manic forms (MD or Md) are most frequent, whereas among female patients, the predominantly depressive form (mD) is most frequent, a trend that was also observed in the NIMH collaborative study (Coryell et al., 1989b). Angst (1978), Taschev (1974), and Roy-Byrne and associates (1985a) all found that depressive and manic or hypomanic episodes occur with equal frequency in men, but depressive episodes clearly predominate in women. Angst's data on sex distribution are illustrated in Figure 6-7. In a longitudinal study[22] of 434 bipolar patients treated in an outpatient clinic in Rome (59 percent women, virtually the same proportion as in the Angst study), Kukopulos and colleagues (1980) reported a lower proportion with the core MD form (22 percent vs 45 percent of Angst's patients), a somewhat higher proportion with the Dm (bipolar II) (52 percent vs Angst's 38 percent) and the Md forms (26 percent vs 17 percent), and no significant sex differences in the distribution of the patterns.[23] The difference between Kukopulos' results and those of the others may be due to the fact that he studied outpatients, whereas the other samples included some inpatients.

Angst also noted a sex difference in the tendency to cycle immediately to an episode of opposite polarity (Table 6-6). Examining single depressive or manic episodes, he noted that women more often cycled from mania to depression than from depression to mania, whereas men were equally likely to cycle in either direction. This

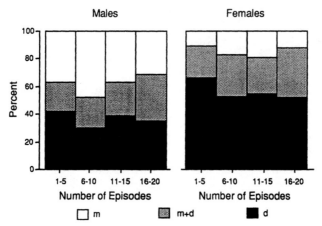

Figure 6-6. Frequency of disease course pattern by sex and number of episodes (adapted from Angst, 1978).

finding appears to be independent of the observation that women are more likely than men to switch from depression into mania while taking antidepressants (see Chapter 22).

The literature has been inconsistent in the relationships reported between predominantly manic or predominantly depressive episodes and age of onset or family history of affective disorder. Three studies (Mendlewicz et al., 1972a; Taylor and Abrams, 1973a; Stone, 1989) found a positive family history of affective disorder to be associated with an earlier age of onset, but this

Table 6-6. Patterns of Episodes: Frequency of Syndrome Patterns in Bipolar Disorder by Sex (95 Patients, 1,176 Episodes)

Pattern of Syndromes[a]	Males		Females		Males	Females
	N	%	N	%	%	%
D	80	18.3	194	26.3		
d	75	17.2	246	33.7	35.5	60.0
M	127	29.1	75	10.1		
m	27	6.2	26	3.5	35.3	13.6
DM	5	1.1	15	2.0		
Dm	23	5.3	66	8.9		
dM	7	1.6	4	0.5	15.3	16.6
dm	32	7.3	39	5.2		
MD	2	0.5	11	1.5		
Md	19	4.3	18	2.4		
mD	3	0.7	11	1.5	12.6	9.2
md	31	7.1	28	3.8		
Q	6	1.4	6	0.8		

The episodes, whether D, M, DM, or MD, are preceded and followed by well intervals. The percentages reflect the proportion of episodes across all patients, not the proportion of patients in which a particular pattern predominates

D = Severe depression (requiring hospitalization)
d = Mild depression (not requiring hospitalization)
M = Mania (requiring hospitalization)
m = Hypomania (not requiring hospitalization)
Q = Questionable, unknown

[a] Pattern reflects the sequence of episodes in the natural course

Adapted from Angst, 1978

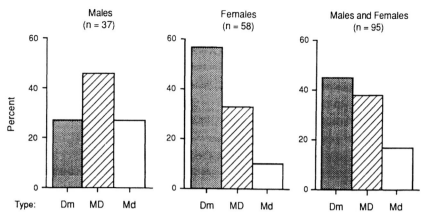

Figure 6-7. Typology of bipolar patients. *Type MD.* The patient suffered at least once from a severe manic and a severe depressive syndrome—the bipolar type. *Type Md.* The patient suffered at least once from a severe manic syndrome but showed only mild depressive symptomatology—the prevailing manic type. *Type Dm.* The patient suffered at least once from a severe depressive syndrome but showed only hypomanic symptoms—the prevailing depressed type (adapted from Angst, 1987).

finding was not replicated by Winokur (1975). An association between earlier age of onset and a higher proportion of manic episodes in the course of illness was reported by Mendlewicz and colleagues (1972a) and Angst (1978) but not by others (Taylor and Abrams, 1973a; Carlson et al., 1977; Roy-Byrne et al., 1985a).

To our knowledge, very few investigators have considered the issue of episode patterning. How often does a manic or depressive episode occur by itself—that is, preceded and followed by a normal period? How often do episodes occur in immediate conjunction with episodes of opposite polarity—that is, a biphasic or triphasic pattern? Winokur's group (1969) examined 100 separate manic episodes in 61 hospitalized bipolar patients and noted that 51 percent of the manic episodes had been immediately preceded by a depressive episode and 58 percent were immediately followed by a depression; triphasic episodes were not uncommon. Looking at depressive episodes, they found that 45 percent were preceded by a manic episode, whereas only 24 percent were followed by mania. Compared to manic episodes, depressive episodes were more likely to be uniphasic, that is, preceded and followed by a well interval.[24] Winokur and colleagues stressed that "the psychiatrist must be prepared to treat both poles of the illness during each episode" (1969, p. 85).

Others have found a higher proportion of uniphasic episodes. For example, in a sample of both inpatients and outpatients, Angst (1978) scored most episodes (71 percent in men and 73 percent in women) as uniphasic, with the well interval defined as at least 4 weeks (Table 6-6). Twenty-six percent of the episodes were biphasic, and, in most, the depression preceded the mania. Working with a hospitalized population, Roy-Byrne and co-workers (1985a) found a similarly high incidence of uniphasic episodes (60 percent) but, like Winokur, an equal incidence of each sequence in biphasic episodes.

Since most of Angst's patients were treated with drugs, the predominance of the depression-mania-interval pattern (DMI) over the MDI pattern may reflect pharmacologically induced mania or hypomania, although Roy-Byrne's patients, who were also treated, did not show this predominance. In the previously noted longitudinal outpatient study of Kukopulos and colleagues (1980), by the end of the observation period, the patterns of recurrence included no uniphasic episodes and 39 percent with a "continuous circular course," that is, essentially no free interval. The distribution of patterns is displayed in Table 6-7. The proportions of biphasic episodes that started with a depression and evolved to mania or hypomania (DMI course) were roughly the same as the reverse pattern (MDI course), in agreement with Roy-Byrne and colleagues (1985a). As noted in the Kukopulos data (Table 6-7), those with the continuous circular course were equally divided between long cycles and short cycles (i.e., rapid cyclers). The continuous circular course evolved during treatment, usually not until antidepres-

Table 6-7. Distribution of Patients According to Patterns of Illness Course

Course	Patients N	Patients (%)	M %	F %	BP I N	BP I (%)	BP II N	BP II (%)
Mania-depression-interval	119	(27)	45	55	101	(85)	18	(15)
Depression-mania-interval	106	(24)	39	61	23	(22)	83	(78)
Irregular[a]	39	(9)	38	62	31	(79)	8	(21)
Continuous circular - Long cycles	83	(19)	52	48	36	(43)	47	(57)
Continuous circular - Rapid cycles	87	(20)	30	70	16	(18)	71	(82)
Total	434		178 (41)	256 (59)	207	(48)	227	(52)

[a]Patients had no regular sequence of episodes. 31 had severe manias, 8 had hypomanic episodes, and 3 had recurrent mania.

Adapted from Kukopulos et al., 1980

sants had been used to treat episodes. The authors observed:

With time the course tended to change from monopolar to bipolar, and the frequency of recurrence increased. Concurrent treatments, especially antidepressants, contributed to these changes, while female sex, middle age and menopause, along with antidepressant drugs, contributed to the establishment of rapid cyclicity. The depression-hypomania course was the one which was most prone to rapid cyclicity. (p. 156)

Keller and colleagues (1986a), in the NIMH collaborative study of depression, found that 27 percent of bipolar-I patients with pure mania or pure depression had no free interval. In other words, they were likely to switch to an episode of the opposite polarity (i.e., to cycle) before recovering from the index episode.

Kraepelin (1921) observed that a given patient's symptoms during manic attacks were so strikingly similar from one episode to another that they often seemed virtual carbon copies of one another. To our knowledge, this common clinical observation has only seldom been studied systematically (see Chapters 2 and 11).

PRECIPITANTS OF EPISODES

The possible role of psychosocial or physical stress in precipitating illness, a subject of considerable interest in medicine and health,[25] also has been explored in manic-depressive illness. Although some theories assign primary causal

importance to psychosocial environmental forces, it is now generally accepted that environmental conditions—psychosocial or physical—contribute more to the timing of an episode than to underlying vulnerability, which is likely to be largely genetic.[26] Thus modern biological theory reaffirms the classic position of Kraepelin (1921):

We must regard all alleged injuries as possibly sparks for the discharge of individual attacks, but that the real cause of the malady must be sought in *permanent internal changes*, which at least very often, perhaps always, are innate. . . . Unfortunately, the powerlessness of our efforts to cure must only too often convince us that the attacks of manic-depressive insanity may be to an astonishing degree *independent of external influences*. (pp. 180-181)

However, the independence from external influences appears to develop over time, as illustrated in Figure 6-5. It was, in fact, Kraepelin who first noted that precipitating events play an important role in the onset of the first few episodes, but then, as the illness unfolds, the process driving the onset of new episodes seems to become more autonomous, with stressful events contributing little or nothing. This pattern was subsequently noted by others (Kinkelin, 1954; Angst, 1966) and has been replicated in recent studies that find significantly more stressful life events preceding early episodes than later ones (see Table 6-8). Early precipitating events, rather than merely influencing the timing of an episode, may actually activate the preexisting vulnerability, thereby making the individual more vulnerable to the next episode. The theoretical significance of this possibility, proposed by R.M. Post and co-workers (1986a), is elaborated in Chapters 16 and 20.

As discussed in the treatment section, awareness of the usual course of illness is essential to sound clinical management. Knowing that certain experiences do trigger episodes of mania or depression or that certain times of the year are associated with increased vulnerability (see seasonality discussion in Chapter 19), the clinician can help patients avoid or learn to cope better with high-risk situations (Silverstone and Romans-Clarkson, 1989). Indeed, if the illness becomes more endogenous with time, clinical prevention efforts might usefully focus on psychosocial or pharmacological strategies to attenuate the impact of early stress among individuals who are highly vulnerable genetically, such as those with bipolar illness on both sides of the family. However, we should keep in mind that the literature on precipitating events is largely retrospective; it is possible that patients are more likely to search for life events to explain their first episode, whereas once they adapt to the idea of having an illness, they may tend to expect episodes and consequently pay less attention to potential stressors.

Most studies of diagnostically heterogeneous groups of depressed patients suggest that stressful life events, such as losing a loved one, changing jobs, or moving, are more frequent during the 3 to 12 months preceding the onset of a depression. Although the literature on precipitating events in depression is extensive, that specifically pertaining to bipolar patients is more modest. It is comprised primarily of interesting but ultimately inconclusive case reports (reviewed by Ellicott, 1988), an intriguing report on increased relapses among bipolar patients after a hurricane (Aronson and Shukla, 1987), and 14 systematic studies, all but 3 of which are retrospective. These studies are outlined in Table 6-8, and conclusions are summarized in Table 6-8a. Taken together, they provide considerable support for the importance of stressful events in the onset of episodes in bipolar patients.

Interpreting this literature is complicated by the many methodological limitations outlined in Table 6-9. Controlled studies that use medical or surgical controls, for example, do not isolate the impact of the precipitating event from differences in genetic vulnerability between the comparison populations. Another pervasive problem in this literature is the difficulty distinguishing independent events from life situations that are a consequence of the illness, such as mood instability leading to job loss or marital separation. These issues are discussed in Chapter 12. Only a few of the studies outlined in Table 6-8 have adequately separated events from the consequences of illness.

A specific life event that deserves separate mention is childbirth. It not only affects the mother psychologically but also produces major changes in her internal hormonal milieu. Kraepelin (1921), as well as others (Bratfos and Haug, 1968; Kendell et al., 1976, 1987), noted that affective episodes occurred in the postpartum period more frequently than would be expected by chance, usually within several months of the birth. Reich and Winokur (1970) reported that 20 percent of bipolar women suffered postpartum mania. Women in this group had significantly more episodes during their postpartum period than at other times in their childbearing years, and those who had already had several episodes were more susceptible than those with one or few. Kadrmas and associates (1979) reported that bipolar women with postpartum episodes were less likely to have an affective recurrence outside the postpartum period. However, in a careful prospective study, Platz and Kendell (1988) found only a nonsignificant difference in this direction for bipolar patients, but they did find that unipolar patients with postpartum depression fared better during follow-up than a matched unipolar group. Thus, in some women, hormonal changes associated with childbirth may be sufficiently powerful to overcome relatively low vulnerability. Pregnancy also was a significant precipitating life event for fathers in one study. Davenport and Adland (1982) found a 50 percent incidence of affective episodes among 40 bipolar males during or immediately after their wives' pregnancies.

Manic or depressive episodes precipitated by drugs or physical illness, unlike those triggered by life events, pose a conceptual problem: Is the episode a true one, reflecting an endogenous vulnerability that was simply triggered by the antecedent factor, or a false one, reflecting a manic-like state resulting from the cerebral effects of the drug or illness? This question is often difficult to

Table 6-8. Precipitants of Episodes in Manic-Depressive Illness

Study	Patients N	Method	Results
Perris, 1966	145 BP 150 UP	Retrospective; no control; events 3 months prior to episode	34% of BP, 39% of UP; "psychic" and somatic factors equally common
Thomson & Hendrie, 1972	74 depressed (19 BP, 55 UP)	Retrospective; patients and controls (1 control group well, other medical patients) administered the Rahe Social Readjustment scale for the year prior to onset	Depressed patients had significantly higher mean life-change scores than either control group No significant BP/UP differences
Clancy et al., 1973	100 BP 225 UP 200 Schiz-ophrenic	Retrospective chart review; events counted within 3 months prior to onset	39% of UPs had precipitant, 27% of BPs, and 11% of schizophrenics. No significant BP/UP differences for type of precipitant
Hall et al., 1977	38 BP I	Prospective; all on lithium; 10 mo. follow-up with monthly contact; life events scored if questionnaire followed by interview; independent assessment of clinical state	45% relapsed; life events not significantly ↑ among relapsers, but hypomanic relapsers had ↑ work-related events than non-relapsers
Ambelas, 1979	67 BP (manic or hypomanic)	Retrospective; surgical controls; rapid cyclers and those with ≤10 episodes excluded; events counted 4 wk prior to admission, introducing possible bias[a]	28% of BP, 7% of controls had a precipitating event
Dunner et al., 1979b	79 BP (11 rapid cyclers)	Retrospective; interview and questionnaire; events counted 3 mo prior to episode; events during episode excluded	50% had at least 1 event prior to initial episode vs only 7% prior to subsequent episodes; no difference between rapid cyclers and non; not related to age or age of onset; ↑ work and interpersonal difficulties with manic vs depressed onset
Glassner et al., 1979	25 BP	Retrospective; patients and family interviewed; controls from community; Holmes and Rahe Life Events Scale	74% had stressful event(s) within 1 yr of initial episode, 56% following subsequent episodes compared to 16% for controls; most within 2-14 days after onset; role loss was central feature
Glassner & Haldipur, 1983	48 BP	Identical to 1979 study	Significantly more early onset (>20 yr) patients report stress preceding 1st and subsequent episodes than late onset (61% vs 23%); age at event not controlled

Continued

Table 6-8 Continued. Precipitants of Episodes in Manic-Depressive Illness

Study	Patients N	Method	Results
Kennedy et al., 1983	20 manic	Retrospective; studied in remission; 4 mo pre-admission vs 4 mo post-admission (2 mo after discharge); orthopedic control group; negativity of event quantified	Significantly more events prior to admission for manic patients before discharge than after, also more than in controls, especially work related
Bidzinska, 1984	97 (BP & UP)	Retrospective; studied in remission; interview and structured life event questionnaire; illness-related events excluded; age-matched community controls; events counted 3 mo prior to episode onset	Significantly more patients reported stress than controls; no BP/UP difference overall, although BP reported more work-related stressors
Perris, 1984	16 BP 58 UP	Retrospective; neurotic-reactive comparison group; events counted 1 yr prior to episode onset	For number of events, reactive depressive > BP > UP (highly significant); slightly fewer events prior to recurrent episodes compared to individual episodes (significant for only "undesirable" events)
Goplerud & Depue, 1985	31 CYC 24 NC	Prospective; 4 wk of daily self-ratings of mood, behavior, and level of subjective stress associated with specific events	Relative to the NC, the CYC showed prolonged duration of recovery of behavioral level following highly stressful events
Aronson & Shukla, 1987	30 BP	Retrospective	Significant ↑ in relapse among BPs in a lithium clinic 2 wk after a major hurricane, comprising 14% of patient pop.; no difference in relapse rates for age, duration of illness or lithium level, but relapses had significantly shorter period of prior stability
Hammen et al., 1989	23 BP 20 UP	Prospective; minimum follow-up of 6 mo; independent assessment of personality, symptoms, medication compliance, and stressful life events	6 BPs and 5 UPs had relapses during follow-up; the UPs but not the BPs displayed specific vulnerability to those life events which matched their personality type (autonomous-achievement vs sociotropic-interpersonal)

CYC = cyclothymics, NC = normal controls
[a]Presumably psychiatrists would be more likely to explore life events among their patients than would surgeons. The true differences between the groups could only be determined if the same team interviewed all the patients in both groups.

Update of review in Ellicott, 1988

Table 6-8a. Precipitants of Episodes in
Bipolar Illness: Conclusions

- Compared to the various control groups, all studies
  report significantly more stress prior to manic
  episodes

- Only one study involved a within-patient comparison
  (Kennedy et al., 1983), i.e., controlling for inherent
  stress vulnerability. It found significantly more
  stressful events preceding a manic episode

- The onset of initial (or early) episodes is more likely
  to be associated with stress than later episodes (5 out
  of 6 studies)

- Although bipolar-unipolar differences have been
  observed in some studies, there is no consistent
  pattern

- Work-related events may be particularly important
  precipitating factors for manic or hypomanic relapses

- Cyclothymia is associated with an increased response
  to stress, consistent with its being part of the bipolar
  spectrum (Depue et al., 1981)

resolve, although prompt resolution of the episode once the drug is removed or the physical
illness treated suggests the presence of a pseudo
illness. This conceptual issue is more fully developed in Chapter 18 under secondary mania. The
drugs and conditions frequently associated with
manic episodes are described in Table 6-10. The
special situation of mania precipitated by antidepressant treatment is discussed in Chapter 22.

Table 6-9. Methodological Limitations to
Precipitating-Event Studies

1. Objective vs subjective assessment
2. Questionnaire vs interview methods
3. Reliability and validity of life event measures
4. Contamination of the stress and illness variables
   (importance of assessing independent events)
5. Controllability of life events
6. Retrospective vs prospective methods
7. The criteria for and type of events that are
   sampled
8. Treatment and compliance, personality and social
   support not generally examined in studies of life
   stress and relapse
9. Differentiating acute and chronic stress

Adapted from Ellicott, 1988
O'Connell (1986) reviews and discusses some of these issues

Wehr and colleagues (1987a) proposed that
sleep reduction may be the common denominator
of several disparate events and stresses that reportedly precipitate mania. Indeed, this suggestion is
well supported by our clinical experience. Reports of manic episodes following (1) various
stressful events, such as bereavement (e.g.,
Krishnan et al., 1984), (2) the postpartum state,
and (3) jetlag associated with flying across time
zones, all have one thing in common: sleep loss
(see Figure 22-7). Because of the importance of
this issue, in Chapter 22 we outline specific approaches designed to minimize sleep loss in bipolar patients.

LONG-TERM OUTCOME

The literature on long-term outcome in bipolar
illness overlaps considerably with studies reviewed earlier in the discussion of course variables. Outcome studies can be difficult to interpret because, more often than not, the impact of
treatment is not explicitly evaluated. Also, many
studies include both bipolar and recurrent unipolar patients and span time periods before and after
drugs came into use, and the more recent studies
depend heavily on patients referred to research
centers after failing to respond to treatment in the
community. Earlier studies of outcome tended to
focus on whether patients recovered or went on to
a chronic course. More recently, the quality of
interepisode functioning also has been examined
as an outcome measure.

Most individual studies that have produced estimates of chronicity (Table 6-11) were based on
follow-up of patients hospitalized for mania, that
is, bipolar-I patients. To some extent the wide
variability in rates can be explained by differences in the definition of chronicity and recovery.
For example, Poort (1945) and Bratfos and Haug
(1968) both define chronic in such a way that it
includes patients with multiple relapses relatively
close together. Of the chronic patients in the latter
study, 38 percent were, in fact, described as "free
from symptoms" at the time of discharge. Likewise, all the patients Poort classified as chronic
had recovered from their first episode.

Wertham's study (1929) deserves attention not
only because of its large number of patients
(2,000) but also because, by including all hospitalized patients in a given geographical area, it

Table 6-10. Conditions and Drugs Reported to Precipitate Manic Episodes

General Category	Specific Factor	Study
Endocrine States or Substances	Cushings: Corticosteroid	Glaser, 1953; Goolker & Schein, 1953
	Hyperthyroidism: Thyroid	Corn & Checkley, 1983
	Androgens	Freinhar & Alvarez, 1985b
	Steroid & Steroid withdrawal	Pope & Katz, 1988; Venkatarangam et al., 1988; Goldstein & Preskorn, 1989; Viswanathan & Glickman, 1989
Drugs	Antidepressants[a]	
	Isoniazid	Jackson, 1957; Kane & Taylor, 1963; Chaturvedi & Upadhyaya, 1988
	Procarbazine	Mann & Hutchinson, 1967
	Levodopa	O'Brien et al., 1971; Ryback & Schwab, 1971; Van Woert et al., 1971; Brodie, 1973
	Methyldopa withdrawal	Labbatte & Holzgang, 1989
	Hallucinogens (e.g., LSD, PCP and Mescaline)	
	Cocaine[b]	
	Alcohol[b]	
	Bromide	Sayed, 1976
	Sympathomimetic amines	Waters & Lapierre, 1981
	Cimetidine; Amantadine	Hubain et al., 1982; Lazare, 1979; Rego & Giller, 1989
	Tolmetin	Sotsky & Tossell, 1984
	Iproniazid	Crane, 1956
	Methylphenidate	Koehler-Troy et al., 1986
	Triazolam	Weilburg et al., 1987
	Zidovudine[c]	Maxwell et al., 1988; O'Dowd & McKegney, 1988; Schaerf et al., 1988; Wright et al., 1989
	Buspirone	Liegghio & Yeragani, 1988; Price & Bielefeld, 1989
	Alprazolam	France & Krishnan, 1984
	Lorazepam	Rigby et al., 1989
Metabolic Conditions	Postoperative state	Muncie, 1934
	Hemodialysis	Cooper, 1967
Infections[d]	Influenza	Steinberg et al., 1972; Maurizi, 1985
	Q Fever	Schwartz, 1974
	Post - St. Louis type A encephalitis	Weisert & Hendrie, 1977
CNS Pathology Neoplasms[d]	Suprasellar diencephalic tumor	Guttman & Hermann, 1932; Greenberg & Brown, 1985
	Head trauma	Stern & Dancey, 1942; McKeown & Jani, 1987
	Parasagittal meningioma	Oppler, 1950
	Benign spheno-occipital tumor	Bourgeois & Campagne, 1967
	AIDS	Kermani et al., 1985; Gabel et al., 1986; Dauncey, 1988

Continued

Table 6-10 Continued. Conditions and Drugs Reported to Precipitate Manic Episodes

General Category	Specific Factor	Study
Vascular Lesions[d]	Aneurysm Infarction	Jampala & Abrams, 1983 Cummings & Mendez, 1984; Goldschmidt et al., 1988

Other	Epilepsy - right
	   temporal focus
	Vitamin B_{12} deficiency
	L - Glutamine
	Aspartame
	Metrizamide as a contrast
	   agent in myelography
		Rosenbaum & Barry, 1975
		
		Goggans, 1984
		Mebane, 1984
		Walton, 1986
		Kwentus et al., 1984

[a]Tricyclic, heterocyclic and MAO inhibitors
[b]The impact of alcohol and illicit drug abuse on manic-depressive illness is detailed in Chapters 9 and 26
[c]Used for treatment of AIDS
[d]A comprehensive review of secondary mania in association with CNS pathology can be found in Chapter 18
This table is based on the definition of secondary mania provided by Krauthammer and Klerman, 1978; the data have been updated by our own review and those of Lazare, 1979, Yassa et al., 1988a, and Sultzer & Cummings, 1989

probably reflects the total percentage of patients who required chronic care (i.e., longer than 5 years). It is interesting that this study produced by far the lowest estimate of chronicity—less than 1 percent. As we noted earlier in the chapter, the shorter follow-up periods, although associated with a lower total number of episodes, also are associated with higher estimates of chronicity because they include patients while still in the episode who would eventually recover if followed long enough. Thus five of the six studies involving a follow-up of less than 12 years showed chronicity rates of greater than 25 percent.

In a report of a 35-year follow-up of the original 100 patients initially admitted for mania in the Iowa-500 study, Tsuang and colleagues (1979) found that, when marital, residential, occupational, and psychiatric (symptomatic) status were combined, outcome was good in approximately 64 percent of patients, fair in 14 percent, and poor (i.e., chronic) in 22 percent. Compared with a well-matched group of patients admitted for minor surgical procedures and a group of schizophrenic patients, the manic group was intermediate in outcome, better than the schizophrenic patients but not as successful as the surgical patients. The comprehensiveness of the rating categories, the duration of follow-up, and the use of comparison groups make these data particularly valuable.

Some investigators have defined chronicity as the presence of prominent affective symptoms for more than 2 years without a remission, which in turn is defined as a relatively symptom-free period of a specified duration. Using this standard, chronicity figures for manic-depressive illness (both bipolar and unipolar) have ranged from 18 percent (Angst, 1984) to 6 percent (Fukuda et al., 1983). In the NIMH collaborative study of bipolar-I patients treated acutely for depression (either as inpatients or outpatients) and then followed for 5 years under naturalistic treatment conditions (Coryell et al., 1989b), the chronicity rate was quite low (11 percent), whereas the risk for the unipolar patients was twice that (24 percent). Cassano and colleagues (1988) also found a low chronicity rate for bipolar-I patients, but the rate among their recurrent unipolar patients was also low. Findings from the NIMH collaborative study (Keller et al., 1986a; Coryell et al., 1989b) and others (Himmelhoch et al., 1976b; S. Cohen et al., 1988) indicate that recovery, assessed over the short term (18 months in the NIMH study), is least likely for patients with mixed episodes, including those who cycle continuously from one phase to the other without a well interval. This finding suggests either that these episodes naturally lasted the longest or were the most resistant to treatment.

Another issue in interpreting chronicity estimates is the extent to which patients with schizoaffective features are included in the sample; such patients would shift the averages toward a less favorable outcome.[27] Even more clearly, the in-

Table 6-11. Estimates of Chronicity in Bipolar Manic-Depressive Illness

Study	Patients N	Length of Follow-up in Years	Not Recovering %	Comments
Wertham, 1929	2000	12[a]	0.8	"Chronic" included only patients who required chronic hospitalization for 5 years or more
Rennie, 1942	66	26[a]	11	"Chronic" not defined
Lundquist, 1945	103	14-32	8	Criterion was "social recovery"
Poort, 1945	39	10-15	56	All patients recovered from first episode "Chronic" includes many incapacitated by high relapse frequency
Stenstedt, 1952	162	1.16-20	1.2	
Hastings, 1958	67	6-12	46	Poor social adjustment in 19%, continuous incapacitation in 27%
Bratfos & Haug, 1968	42	1-12	45	Chronic referred to not symptom-free for any extended period of time; most socially incapacitated, but only 11% did not recover from the index hospitalization
Shobe & Brion, 1971	15	17[a]	53	"Unable to work or to function socially some or most of the time." Role of treatment is unclear
Morrison et al., 1973	87	.08-20 2.2[a]	0-73	Recovery estimates increase with longer follow-up; recovery defined as partially productive, i.e., social recovery with some residual symptoms
Carlson et al., 1974	53	1-10 3.2[a]	12	Community follow-up
Taschev, 1974	122* 38**		8.2 12	*Cyclothymic depression **Recurrent mania Postmortem study
Winokur, 1975	75	1-20	25	
Tsuang et al., 1979	100	35	22	Percentage represents "severe" psychiatric disability at follow-up, assessed by marital, employment, residential, physical, and mental health status.
Fukuda et al., 1983	1066	12	6.2	"Chronic" defined as patients without remission for more than 2 consecutive years. 18% were dead at follow-up. None received lithium

Continued

Table 6-11 Continued. Estimates of Chronicity in Bipolar Manic-Depressive Illness

Study	Patients N	Length of Follow-up in Years	Not Recovering %	Comments
Keller et al., 1986a[b]	155	1.5[a]	7* 32** 22***	* Index episode purely manic (N = 63) ** Index episode mixed or cycling (N = 67) *** Index episode purely depressed (N = 25)
Harrow et al., 1990	73	1.7±1.2[a]	42	Manic patients on lithium did not show better outcome than those not on lithium (p > .20)
Coryell et al., 1989b	53 BP I 64 BP II	5	11 11	No evidence of overall psychosocial deterioration or "downward drift" among BPs. Chronicity rates were twice as high among UPs (24%)
Total Patients	4,177	.08-35 yrs	0-73	

10 of the 17 studies are explicitly limited to BPs, the remainder are described only as "manic-depressive"
[a]Value represents the mean length follow-up
[b]Most of the patients in these studies were initially admitted for a manic episode (but see Taschev and Keller et al.)

Update of Goodwin and Jamison, 1984; also see the review by Silverstone and Romans-Clarkson, 1989

clusion of schizophrenic patients would bias the sample toward worse outcomes, but, in most follow-up studies,[28] only 5 percent or less of cases initially diagnosed as manic-depressive are later diagnosed as schizophrenic.[29] Recovery also can be compromised by concomitant medical (Black et al., 1988a) or neurological disorder (Hoff et al., 1988) or by substance abuse (see Chapter 9).

Aside from what we know about the efficacy of prophylactic treatment under study conditions (see Chapter 23), the question of how often bipolar-I illness becomes fully chronic will probably remain somewhat unsettled. In addition to differences in diagnosis and in the definition of chronicity, the considerable variation in findings also results from a high ratio of retrospective/prospective data and variable length of follow-up. True chronicity, in the form of an unremitting full-blown illness, is a relatively rare outcome for manic-depressive patients. However, a small but appreciable proportion of untreated and treated patients do develop rapid or continuous cycling (Dunner et al., 1977b; Fukuda et al., 1983), whereas some remain substantially impaired at least during short-term follow-up under prevailing conditions of available treatment in the community.

A final important measure of chronicity is the subtle quality of the "well interval" among those who are deemed to have "recovered." Kraepelin (1921) observed that "when the disease has lasted for some time and the attacks have been frequently repeated, the psychic changes usually become more distinct during the intervals also." This form of partial chronicity has not been adequately described. It can be difficult to sort out manifestations of ongoing illness from the social and occupational consequences of disruptive manic or depressive episodes—the scars of the illness. Some of these problems are discussed by Welner and colleagues (1977) in a critical review of the course and outcome of manic-depressive disorder. Three groups (Winokur et al., 1969; Carlson et al., 1974; Dion et al., 1988) differentiated symptomatic recovery from social recovery—for example, family stability and job status—and found that the former was more common than the latter. At 6-month follow-up, Dion and colleagues (1988) found that of those initially admitted for mania, 80 percent were essentially free of symptoms but only 43 percent were employed, with only 21 percent "working at their perceived level of employment." These differences may reflect the damaging impact of previous episodes, issues discussed further in Chapter 12.

If we include social incapacitation and diminished functioning between episodes, more than one third of bipolar patients seem to have some chronic (i.e., continuous) symptoms. Some of this pathology no doubt represents scars of the episodes themselves, and much of it reflects the absence of prophylactic treatment or poor treatment. Although estimating the incidence of partial chronicity under conditions of optimum treatment is impossible, it would certainly be substantially below one third. It is clear that some untreated or inadequately treated manic-depressive patients suffer a gradual downward drift as the illness progresses, traceable to the illness itself and to the social and occupational consequences of individual episodes. The extent of the deterioration that can occur is perhaps reflected in Angst's finding of a 15 percent incidence of organic brain syndrome among manic-depressive patients, an incidence that is even higher (23 percent) among elderly patients with the illness.

Compared to what we know about the bipolar-I subgroup, long-term outcome among bipolar-II patients has not been extensively studied. Both Angst (1986a) and Endicott and co-workers (1985) noted a more chronic course in bipolar-II than in bipolar-I patients. This increased chronicity may not primarily reflect affective symptoms per se but rather the presence of other psychiatric problems, such as alcoholism and antisocial personality, between episodes. In the NIMH collaborative 5-year follow-up study, however, Coryell and colleagues (1989b) found outcome roughly comparable in bipolar-II and bipolar-I patients, although bipolar-II patients were somewhat more likely to relapse into depression during the initial two years of follow-up (Coryell et al., 1987b).

The phenomenon of *double depression* refers to the persistence of milder depressive states (dysthymia) following recovery from an episode of major depression (Keller et al., 1983). As noted in Chapter 4, Klein and colleagues (1988) noted that, compared with other unipolar patients, those with double depression have a higher incidence of hypomanic episodes during follow-up.[30]

Suicide, a frequent outcome in manic-depressive illness, is in some respects a function of illness course. For example, the severity of attempts correlates with overall duration of ill-

ness (Roy-Byrne et al., 1988). These issues are discussed in Chapter 10. Although suicide is the single most important factor contributing to increased mortality,[31] other causes contribute as well. Indirect consequences of psychotic behavior during untreated episodes—malnutrition, exposure, and exhaustion—all compromise general health and presumably contribute to a higher mortality rate. As reviewed in Chapters 17 and 18, some of the biological dysfunctions noted in manic-depressive patients involve systems other than the brain. These dysfunctions could contribute to higher than normal mortality rates.

Early studies of mortality rates in manic-depressive illness, which did not separate bipolar from unipolar forms, claimed very substantially increased mortality; up to six times the rate expected for the same age group in a normal population (Table 6-12). More recent studies indicate a less striking but still considerable increase in mortality, averaging approximately 2.28 times the expected rates. Differences between the older and the more recent studies probably reflect improvements in psychiatric care, particularly the availability of specific treatments for the depressive and manic phases. Thus, in Derby's study (1933), 22 percent of the hospitalized manic patients died, and 40 percent of these deaths were from "exhaustion," whereas in the Iowa-500 follow-up, Tsuang and associates (1980) found a significant increase in "circulatory" death among women. Corroborating the earlier Iowa findings in a follow-up of 1,593 affective patients, Black and colleagues (1987a) found that natural death was excessive only in those patients with a concurrent medical disorder.

SUMMARY

The natural course and outcome of manic-depressive illness contribute to its definition and its differentiation from schizophrenia. For the clinician, understanding natural course can help answer a patient's questions about the most important estimate of all—the prognosis—"Will it return?" "When will it return?" Today, estimates of course must include the effects of variable treatment, both acute treatment of episodes and prophylaxis. We also must accept the reality that patients who are doing well—perhaps the majority—are unlikely to enroll themselves in

Table 6-12. Mortality Rates in Manic-Depressive Illness

Study	Subjects N	Years Observation	Deceased %	Excess Mortality[a]	Suicide % of all Deaths	Comments
Derby, 1933	4,341	20	22.5			45.3 exhaustion deaths
Slater, 1938b	138		42.8		15.3	
Langelüddeke, 1941	341	37	78.8		15.3	
Lundquist, 1945	319	6-30	37.3		14.3	21% cardiovascular deaths
Schulz, 1949	2,004		24.5		13.4	
Odegård, 1952	94 M 192 F	1-25	100 100	3.8 6.2		
Stenstedt, 1952	216	2-20	19.4		14.3	
Helgason, 1964	81	1-60	42	3.0	52	17% cardiovascular deaths
Perris & d'Elia, 1966b	57 M 63 F		25 21		7 15	BP mortality > UP mortality, but no significant differences in suicide incidences
Brattos & Haug, 1968	215	2-12	15.3	2.75	12.1	27% cerebral insult deaths, 39% cardiovascular deaths
Taschev, 1974b	70 M 52 F 21 M 17 F	post-mortem	100 100 100 100		24.3 30.8 9.5 5.9	First group were cyclothymic, second were recurrent manic. "All suicides were made in the depressive phase" (in recurrent manics, in a hypo-depressive phase post-mania)
Winokur & Tsuang, 1975b[b]	76	30-40	62		8.5	No significant differences in suicide rate compared with UP and schizophrenics

Study	N	Duration (yrs)	%	Ratio[a]		Comments
Petterson, 1977[a][b]	69 / 123	50 / up to 10	93 / 2.4	1.8	4.7 / 0	No demonstrable increased mortality; short observation time (<5 years in over half)
Tsuang, 1978[b] / Tsuang et al., 1980[b]	92	40	59	1.35	11.1	MR includes UP deaths Increased risk of circulatory deaths in females
Eastwood et al., 1982	199 M / 386 F	9.5	12.1 / 8.0	1.14 / 1.55	25 / 35	Suicides measured as "unnatural causes", also includes homicides and accidental deaths
Norton & Whalley, 1984	751	1-10	44	2.83	24	42% cardiovascular deaths; 12% cancer deaths; 64% of suicides in BP; risk of death by suicide in younger > older, by CVS in older > younger
Black et al., 1985	556 M / 875 F	10	6.8 / 4.8	1.10 / 1.36	23.7 / 38.1	Suicides measured as "unnatural causes", also includes homicides and accidental deaths
Martin et al., 1985[b]	19	6-12	11		50	Part of a larger sample of "psychiatric outpatients"
Weeke & Vaeth, 1986	843 M / 1,325 F	5-7	18.9 / 11.3	2.17 / 1.45	30.8 / 18	BP mortality > UP mortality from non-violent causes only; BP suicide and violent death < UP
Berglund & Nilsson, 1987	506 M / 700 F	14-27	43.7 / 36.4	1.29 / 1.20	20.8 / 22.4	BP < UP mortality from suicide; Excess mortality in BP from physical disorders
Black et al., 1987a	1,593	14	9.9	1.19 for natural death 7.26 for unnatural death		"Unnatural death" included suicide, homicide, accidents, war; BP < UP mortality for unnatural causes
			Weighted Average:	2.28		

[a] Ratio of observed mortality to expected mortality based on a comparison population
[b] Data are for bipolar patients only

153

follow-up studies. Even with this limitation, however, it is important that prospective follow-up studies continue. There are still considerable gaps in our knowledge, gaps that limit our ability to plan and conduct optimal maintenance treatment. For example, a better understanding of the relationships between relapses and specific environmental stresses, as they relate to individual patient characteristics, could make the psychosocial aspects of maintenance treatment more focused and deliberate.

In a sense, the contemporary data on course and outcome, derived from patients receiving average community treatment (or no treatment), represent the baseline, the bare minimum. Once the majority of clinicians have acquired the requisite knowledge and skill, patients with manic-depressive illness have every right to expect a more favorable outcome. The treatment section provides a framework.

NOTES

1. As discussed in Chapter 5 (The Psychoses—Separate or Continuous?), many patients whose symptoms, course, or outcome appear to be intermediate between schizophrenia and the affective disorders represent a challenge to the Kraepelinian dichotomy. Angst (unpublished and 1986d) has even suggested that "course should be dropped completely as a criterion for the classification of endogenous psychoses." He argues that differences in course could result from nonspecific factors and that many patients show "affective" and "schizophrenic" symptoms at different times in their life history of illness. He points out that one cannot use diagnosis to predict course unless the former has been arrived at independently of the latter.

2. Although not directly relevant to some of these studies, using the SADS-L to apply the RDC (see Chapter 5) has been found to be a reliable method for determining the age of onset for affective disorder over periods up to 6 years preceding the index episode (Prusoff et al., 1988; see also Mazure and Gershon, 1979; Bromet et al., 1986).

3. One problem with reports of the initial onset of bipolar illness among the elderly, however, is that earlier episodes are more likely to have been forgotten or misdiagnosed (Spar et al., 1979).

4. Kay, 1959; Mendlewicz, 1976; Shulman and Post, 1980; Taylor and Abrams, 1981a; Stone, 1989.

5. Perris (1968) found 83 percent with 4 or more episodes, and 43 percent with 7 or more. In a 1978 paper, Angst updated a careful longitudinal study of 95 bipolar patients who at that time had been followed for an average of 26 years (SD ± 11.9). The study included both retrospective and prospective phases, the latter involving direct patient and family contact at least every 5 years. Patients by and large did not receive prophylactic treatment, although most had individual episodes treated with medications. The number of episodes ranged from 2 to 54, with a median of 9; 84 percent had 5 or more episodes, 69 percent had 7 or more, and 42 percent had 11 or more. A naturalistic study of 51 bipolar patients who received unsystematic acute and prophylactic treatment showed that all but 2 patients had 3 or more episodes, with a median of 15 (Roy-Byrne et al., 1985a). Although this is consistent with earlier data, it is important to remember that the patient groups are not comparable, since the research setting of the Roy-Byrne study tended to select treatment-resistant patients. In a chart review study of 236 bipolar patients from the prepharmacotherapy era (between 1920 and 1950), Winokur and Kadrmas (1989) found that, during a follow-up period averaging 2.4 years, 28 percent had 1 episode, 22 percent had 2, 14 percent had 3, 11 percent had 4, 4 percent had 5, 2 percent had 6, 0.8 percent had 7, 0.4 percent had 8, and 11 percent had 9 or more.

6. Angst's Dm group is roughly analogous to the bipolar-II subgroup in DSM-III-R, although in DSM-III-R, hospitalization is not necessary for the diagnosis of either major depression or mania.

7. Kraepelin, 1921; Lange, 1928; Kielholz, 1959; Taschev, 1974; Angst, 1978, 1981b; Zis et al., unpublished; Roy-Byrne et al., 1985a.

8. Unfortunately, since the study of Keller and colleagues (1982) focused on the proportion of patients relapsing at certain times rather than on the distribution of time intervals prior to relapse, it cannot be compared with previous studies. In addition, patients at various stages of their illness were grouped together, and their outcome following the selected index was tracked, confounding the effect of illness course with relapse time when averages are presented.

9. Swift, 1907; MacDonald, 1918; Pollock, 1931; Angst and Weis, 1967; Zis et al., 1979.

10. The 1989 study of Winokur and Kadrmas, although limited by its chart review methodology, is nevertheless of interest because it is based on the prepharmacology era. The authors report that patients with a polyepisodic course (> three episodes per average follow-up of 2.4 years) were significantly more likely to have an early age of onset (below age 20) than those with one or two episodes.

11. Whether patients received prophylactic medications during some interepisode intervals is not specified in this report (Angst 1986d). In an earlier article, Angst and colleagues (1980b), apparently reporting on a portion of the same sample, attempted to determine the types of treatment pa-

tients received between episodes. In that sample, bipolar patients received pharmacotherapy during 11.3 percent of the intervals.

12. Kukopulos et al., 1980, 1983; Kuyler, 1988; Wehr et al., 1988.

13. Dunner et al., 1977b; Kukopulos et al., 1983; Alarcon, 1985; Wehr et al., 1988; Parry, 1989. However, among 10 cases of rapid cycling in mentally retarded subjects, there was no female predominance.

14. The relationship between rapid cycling and evidence of disturbed thyroid function is controversial, with three studies finding a relationship (Cho et al., 1979; Cowdry et al., 1983; Bauer and Whybrow, 1988b) and two not (Joffe et al., 1988a; Wehr et al., 1988).

15. In their 5-year follow-up of patients with an index episode of major depression treated naturalistically, Coryell and colleagues (1989b) found that those with a bipolar-II history developed hypomanic or manic-like symptoms more slowly than those with a bipolar-I history. Among the bipolar-I patients, half of those who developed such symptoms had done so by week 20, whereas among the bipolar-II patients, it took 60 weeks before half of those who would eventually develop manic or hypomanic symptoms had done so. Since most of these patients were treated with antidepressant medications, this difference may differentiate vulnerability to drug-induced mania or hypomania in bipolar-I vs bipolar-II patients, as reported by Wehr and Goodwin (1987a,b) (see Chapter 20).

16. This discrepancy might be more apparent than real if the Swift, Kraepelin, and Rennie studies counted patients with a late course chronic hospitalization who were cycling in the hospital as having one long episode.

17. Bratfos and Haug, 1968; Shobe and Brion, 1971; Morrison et al., 1973; Roy-Byrne et al., 1985a.

18. Keller and co-workers (1986a) examined a treated population prospectively and found that, after 1 year, a higher proportion of patients had recovered from pure manic than from pure depressive episodes, also implying that depressive episodes last longer than manic ones.

19. The NIMH collaborative project evaluated patients referred to university-based centers in the 1980s. It may therefore include a higher proportion of treatment-resistant patients than that for the earlier Angst or Grof patient samples.

20. Both the Grof et al. (1979) and the Coryell et al. (1989b) studies include treated episodes. Thus, the findings could reflect the fact that, for many patients with recurrent disorder, the interval between the appearance of symptoms and the beginning of treatment may be relatively constant.

21. Perris and d'Elia, 1966; Dunner et al., 1976b; Winokur et al., 1969; Carlson et al., 1974; Petterson, 1977a; Angst, 1978; Roy-Byrne et al., 1985a.

22. In the Kukopulos and associates (1980) study, the course was analyzed over an average of 18 years, the prospective phase averaging 4.5 years, the retrospective 13.4 years.

study sample (Coryell et al., 1989b), 55 percent were bipolar II and 45 percent were bipolar I, roughly comparable to Angst's sample.

24. Since some patients will be counted in more than one category (e.g., some depressive episodes can be both preceded and followed by a manic episode), the percentage will add up to more than 100 percent.

25. See, for example, Holmes and Rahe (1967) for a systematic approach to gauging this influence.

26. See reviews by Lloyd, 1980; Paykel, 1982b; Thoits, 1983; Roy et al., 1985a.

27. Clayton, 1982; Brockington et al., 1983; Angst, 1986c; Coryell et al., 1989b.

Because of the shifting boundaries between manic-depressive and schizoaffective illness in the literature, it is difficult to be precise about the impact of schizoaffective patients on average outcome results. Indeed, now that DSM-III-R has broadened the definition of mania and major depression to include psychotic patients who in other diagnostic schema would be considered schizoaffective, it could be anticipated that outcome among DSM-III-R manic-depressive patients might, on average, be less favorable than that recorded among manic-depressive patients defined somewhat more narrowly. In the literature on long-term course and outcome of schizoaffective disorders, diagnostic definitions vary. For example, in their carefully executed studies, Marneros and colleagues (1988, 1989) used DSM-III-R definitions for the various kinds of episodes recorded, but their definition of schizoaffective disorder—"the concurrent or sequential presence of schizophrenic (or mood incongruent paranoid) symptoms and melancholic or manic symptomatology"—is broader than the DSM-III-R definition and would certainly include some DSM-III-R manic-depressive patients (see Chapter 5). Other studies of outcome in schizoaffective illness also define it in such a way as to overlap with DSM-III-R manic-depressive illness (e.g., Rzewuska and Angst, 1982; Angst, 1980, 1986d). Indeed, in his 1986 study of outcome among DSM-III manic-depressive patients, Angst found that only 20 percent of those with mood-incongruent delusions had full remission, compared with 45 percent of those with mood-congruent delusions; Angst noted that he considers mood-incongruent delusions to be synonymous with schizoaffective. For a scholarly and thorough review of the schizoaffective disorders, the reader is referred to the book *Schizoaffective Psychoses,* edited by A. Marneros and M. T. Tsuang (1986).

28. Lundquist, 1945; Rennie, 1942; Bratfos and Haug, 1968; Carlson et al., 1974.

29. The question of whether manic-depressive illness ever evolves into schizophrenia and whether such an evolution could be distinguished from a diagnostic error is discussed in Chapter 5. In their often-quoted study, Piotrowski and Lewis (1950) estimated a 50 percent rate, but given their nosological concepts ("the diagnosis of manic-depressive psychosis can be made only by the elimination of schizophrenia . . . even a trace of schizophrenia is schizophrenia"), a discrepancy is understandable.

30. The greater frequency of hypomanic episodes during follow-up of patients with double depression may be due to more vigorous antidepressant treatment; this is not unlikely, given the greater severity and persistence of their depressive symptoms than in typical unipolar patients.

31. In a postmortem study of 122 bipolar patients, for example, Taschev (1974) found that 27 percent had died by suicide. Among manic patients from the Iowa 500 series, Winokur and Tsuang (1975b) reported that 8.5 percent of the deaths were suicides. Perris and d'Elia (1966) found that 11 percent of the deaths in their patients resulted from suicide, exactly the same proportion as in Tsuang's (1978) 40-year follow-up. Reviewing the literature, Guze and Robins (1970) noted that about 15 percent of all deaths in major affective disorder can be traced to suicide. See Chapter 10 for a more comprehensive review.

7

Epidemiology

Mood disorders are common and costly and thus are the subject of intense public health concern. The unanimity of opinion reflected in this concern quickly dissipates when finer distinctions are introduced, however. At the level of populations, the severe forms of manic-depressive illness—clinically among the most easily recognizable of all mental disorders—have been surprisingly difficult to characterize. Frustrated by biases, inconsistencies, and inadequacies in the psychiatric epidemiological literature in general, investigators have become increasingly more systematic and sophisticated in their methodology. Yet even the newer data are problematic. As a consequence, this chapter concentrates heavily on the methodological questions that must be considered in interpreting the epidemiological literature on bipolar illness. That literature, as we shall see, poses demanding challenges to the next generation of epidemiologists.

Ideally, epidemiological evidence can provide a measure of the magnitude of an illness, the pattern of its distribution in the population, and the aggregation of risk factors associated with it. The public health consequences of an illness are only the most obvious reason for collecting such data.[1] Epidemiological evidence is also used to link the occurrence of an illness with genetic, psychological, social, and environmental factors—correlations that can later be explored under controlled experimental conditions. In addition, epidemiological data can be used to assess the effectiveness of preventive intervention programs in the community.

Methodological problems in epidemiological studies of manic-depressive illness, the subject of the next part of this chapter, can be traced to variable diagnostic, treatment, and hospitalization practices, as well as inconsistencies in research design. There is reason to believe that most of the biases in this literature are in one direction; that is, they tend to result in underestimates of the incidence and prevalence of bipolar illness.

Methodological artifacts are not the only sources of disagreement over rates of manic-depressive illness. Some are traceable to changes and confusion in the definition of the disorder. As originally defined by Kraepelin (1921), manic-depressive illness included all forms of serious and recurrent affective illness.[2] That conception, used in most European studies, is clearly broader than the bipolar illness identified in recent American studies. Confusion arises even when bipolar illness is specified, however. Investigators tend to confine the term's use to cases that show an episodic pattern of mania and depression (bipolar-I disorder) and ignore those with a pat-

157

tern of hypomania and depression (bipolar-II). This practice contributes to the variable, often incomplete, ascertainment of manic-depressive illness.

As should be obvious from these caveats, epidemiology is not the straightforward counting operation it might appear to be. The field is mined. Traversing it requires unyielding precision in language and relentless rigor in logic. We begin the discussion with a review of types of epidemiological data and their uses. Then, as noted, in the next section we examine methodological problems that complicate the collection and interpretation of epidemiological data about manic-depressive illness. Next, we review reported rates of incidence and prevalence. Finally, we analyze demographic, cultural, and seasonal factors associated with the disorder.

Rates of illness typically are calculated from data gathered in three major types of epidemiological studies (modified from Krauthammer and Klerman, 1979). Each yields different types of data:

- In census studies, an entire population is examined during some period of time. A variation of this type of study is the community survey, which uses a carefully designed sample of the entire population. Although these studies are best suited to determining prevalence, they can be used to calculate new cases (incidence) by returning to the same sample in a second wave of interviews. Because census studies depend on field interviews to ascertain cases, they tend to yield the highest rates.
- In biographical studies, a cross-section of the population, identified retrospectively, is followed over time. Krauthammer and Klerman point out that the biographic study is well suited to determining morbid risk.
- Treatment–admission studies, which extrapolate population rates from the number of patients admitted, traditionally used hospital admission rates alone, but increasingly rates are determined from admission to both inpatient and outpatient care. Admission studies are appropriate for determining incidence and period prevalence rates, which tend to be lower than in other types of epidemiological studies. Diagnoses are, by and large, more accurate, but distortions are produced by differential avail-

ability and use of services, diagnostic and therapeutic fashions, and public attitudes.

METHODOLOGICAL CONSIDERATIONS

Many sources of variance can influence the collection and interpretation of epidemiological data. For convenience, we have conceptualized these as (1) variance in diagnostic criteria, (2) nonstandardization of data collection, (3) variance in defining a case—determining who is entered into the epidemiological system—which is primarily caused by biases in diagnosis and treatment, and (4) variance in illness rates caused by the introduction of effective treatment.

Variable Diagnostic Criteria

Diagnostic variance is perhaps the best-described source of error in psychiatric epidemiology. Acknowledged for years as a major problem, it was given particular emphasis by the United States–United Kingdom Diagnostic Project (Cooper et al., 1972). The U.S.–U.K. study showed that psychiatric patients in New York were nearly twice as likely to be diagnosed as schizophrenic and 6 times as likely to carry a label of alcoholism as those in London. Patients in London, on the other hand, were 12 times more likely to be diagnosed as manic and 5 times more likely to be diagnosed as psychotically depressed. When consistent research diagnostic criteria were applied, however, most of these differences were not sustained.[3] Psychiatrists in New York clearly had a far broader notion of schizophrenia than had their London counterparts (discussed in Chapter 5), diagnosing as schizophrenia what the British frequently labeled as depressive illness and almost always diagnosing as schizophrenia what the British diagnosed as mania.

Inconsistencies in diagnosis, which lead to disparities and errors in reported rates of illness, can be traced to several causes. First, poor reliability results from the imprecise definitions of many diagnostic terms (Boyd and Weissman, 1981). Second, criteria for what constitutes a case vary enormously, so that the threshold for diagnosis changes from one study to another (Boyd and Weissman, 1981; Turns, 1978; Wing et al., 1978). A related problem is that mild forms of affective illness, including cyclothymia, go undetected and unstudied by current epidemiological methods.[4] The often arbitrary cutoff points tend to obscure the spectrum or subtle variations of an illness. Third, problems arise in making cross-sectional diagnoses without longitudinal follow-up data to evaluate the correctness of an initial differential diagnosis (Carlson and Goodwin, 1973; Gagrat and Spiro, 1980).

Further problems in understanding the meaning of reported rates of affective illness are illustrated by the significantly different findings from two studies that used different inclusion criteria. In their study in New Haven, Connecticut, Weissman and Myers (1978) found an exceptionally high lifetime rate for all depression and mania of 28 percent, whereas Winokur (1979a) found only 8 percent in the Iowa 500 sample. In his 1980 analysis of these differences, Winokur suggests that criteria for determining a case contributed to the disparate findings. The New Haven group used the RDC, which stipulate that symptoms must have been present for a minimum of 2 weeks; the Iowa group used the Feighner criteria, which require a month of dysfunction. In addition, the New Haven group included secondary depressions in its admission criteria. It is clear that any interpretation of differences in rates must rest solidly on an understanding of the diagnostic criteria involved.

Nonstandard Data Collection

Although diagnostic systems are becoming increasingly objective and reliable, inconsistencies in diagnostic criteria still contribute to confusion in collection methods. Epidemiological investigators have gathered data through clinical interviews (with or without standardized interview schedules), rating scales, and interview schedules administered to a sample of an entire community (with clinical interviewing techniques of varying quality). Diagnostic criteria and standardized interview schedules have evolved rapidly over recent years from the Feighner criteria (Feighner et al., 1972), the Renard Diagnostic Interview (L.N. Robins et al., 1977), the RDC (Spitzer et al., 1978a), the Present State Examination (Wing et al., 1967), the Schedule for Affective Disorders and Schizophrenia (Spitzer and Endicott, 1978; Endicott and Spitzer, 1978), and the Diagnostic Interview Schedule (Robins et al., 1979).

The short duration of many manic and depressive episodes, to say nothing of mixed states, causes another problem. These short episodes, which are counted in some studies, are overlooked in others that use diagnostic instruments with long duration criteria. Short episodes also are responsible for large differences in rates of point and yearly prevalence. Gagrat and Spiro (1980) explain this difficulty and underscore the problems created by studying a phenomenon with a low baseline rate:

Point prevalent studies for a short-duration disorder with a yearly prevalence of 0.7% would require the screening of very, very large numbers. . . . Even allowing for a mean duration of the manic episode being two months, the point prevalence rate would be of the order of .2% if the yearly prevalence in the population at large was 1.0%. This means that one must screen a thousand people to find two active cases. Epidemiologic studies of several hundred thousand people at a time would be required to find the natural point prevalence in the population at large. Moreover, it is questionable whether current epidemiologic research instruments would be reliable in such studies. This perhaps explains why the definitive study, either of mania or of bipolar affective disease, has yet to be performed. (pp. 294-295)

Case Definition Inconsistencies

In treatment or hospital admission studies, traditionally the most common type of epidemiological investigation, large variances in illness rates result from the very method used to identify cases. By definition, these studies register only diagnosed cases—only those brought to professional attention—and predictably they result in overall underestimation of cases (Gagrat and Spiro, 1980). The major contributors to this problem are biases in diagnosis, treatment, and hospitalization practices that are traceable to social class, race, and cultural factors.

As Weissman and Boyd point out in their 1984 review, diagnostic bias and inconsistency are common problems. Some authors argue that upper class patients are more likely to be diagnosed manic-depressive than lower class patients, even though the illness they suffer is the same (Rosenhan, 1973; Rowitz and Levy, 1968; Walsh, 1969b). All 12 of Rosenhan's "pseudopatients" were admitted to different hospitals with the same amorphous complaint of an auditory hallucination, and 11 were diagnosed as schizophrenic. The remaining patient, the only one admitted to a private hospital, was given a diagnosis of manic-depressive psychosis, which generally has a better prognosis. Walsh (1969b) also observed the diagnostic bias in private hospitals toward the more prognostically favorable manic-depressive illness.

Manifestations of affective symptoms, which may vary with social class and subculture, constitute another possible contributor to diagnostic discrepancies and epidemiological inconsistencies. This issue is discussed more fully later in the chapter but can be demonstrated in Friedman's terse descriptions (1965) of the differential presentation of depressive symptoms in different social classes: Depressed patients in social class V, the lowest, have a tendency to "behave badly," in IV to "ache physically," in III to "defend fearfully," and in the two highest classes to be "dissatisfied with themselves." In addition, distress is expressed differently across cultures, so that different presenting symptoms may represent a common underlying syndrome. Cultural differences might, for example, alter the form or relative frequencies of disturbances of cognition, affect, and volition or might influence interpretations of levels of function (Dohrenwend and Dohrenwend, 1974).

Further confounding epidemiological evidence are the class, racial, and cultural differences in treatment and hospitalization practices.[5] These differences clearly affect the decision to hospitalize a patient, the choice of private or public hospital, the point in the illness at which the hospitalization occurs (thereby possibly influencing the chronicity of course and choice of treatment), and the reasons for hospitalization (Birtchnell, 1971; Monnelly et al., 1974; Ödegaard, 1956). Hospital admission rates also are influenced by the number of psychiatric beds available in the community, access to psychiatric treatment outside hospital, and the local community's acceptance of individuals with a history of mental hospitalization (Schou, 1968). The stigmatization of individuals with psychiatric problems varies widely from country to country and from subculture to subculture within the same country.[6] These features are discussed in detail later in the chapter.

Changing Treatment Modalities

A final source of variance in reported illness rates is the introduction of an effective method of treatment into the health care system.[7] As Krautham-

mer and Klerman (1979) note, diagnoses become more exact as treatments become more specific. Differential diagnosis of bipolar illness from schizophrenia mattered little when the only treatment modalities were the same for both disorders—hospitalization, electroconvulsive therapy, and psychotherapy. The introduction of phenothiazines almost certainly biased diagnostic practice in the direction of the overdiagnosis of schizophrenia.

To explore these issues, Baldessarini (1970) studied the 1944 to 1968 rates of affective and schizophrenic diagnoses in the Johns Hopkins' Henry Phipps Clinic. He found that, during the ascendancy of the neuroleptics, diagnoses of schizophrenia increased, and diagnoses of manic-depressive illness decreased. After lithium was introduced, however, the diagnostic trends reversed directions for first admissions and readmissions (Parker et al., 1985). Baldessarini (1970) attributed this change in diagnostic practice to "observer bias, modified by the availability of novel and effective therapies." The prelithium and postlithium frequencies of affective psychoses are shown graphically in Table 7-1. Kendell (1975), with a note of irony, echoed Baldessarini's findings: ". . .an epidemic of mania appeared to sweep through the eastern United States in the 1960s," and he too attributed this increase to the introduction of lithium.

Symonds and Williams (1981) studied a related point in their investigation of hospital admission rates for the years 1970 to 1975. They observed that, although lithium compounds had been widely used since 1968, admission rates for mania did not decrease appreciably (in fact, there

Table 7-1. Mean Frequencies[a] of Affective Psychotic Diagnoses (Manic-Depressive plus Schizoaffective) Since 1960

Period	Mean Incidence[b]	SD
1960-1965 (before lithium)	5.2	± 1.9
1966-1968 (lithium in use)	11.2	± 2.0

[a] As percentages of all discharges per year

[b] $p < .01$

Adapted from Baldessarini, 1970

was a slight increase in rates for women). They attributed this stability to changes in diagnostic practices, not to an actual increase in the illness or ineffectiveness of the lithium. The authors concluded that the very availability of an effective treatment for mania predisposed psychiatrists and general practitioners to view the illness as treatable and thus enhanced the probability that they would diagnose it. Symonds and Williams also noted that increased use of lithium for atypical conditions led some clinicians to diagnose patients as manic to "justify" the treatment. There may be additional explanations for their findings, such as the many patients with only a partial lithium response, the varying degrees of lithium compliance, and a genuine increase in recognizing manic-depressive illness that resulted from the better information that accompanied lithium's success. Malpractice concerns about suicide, as well as about neuroleptic use and tardive dyskinesia, almost certainly have affected diagnostic practices as well.

INCIDENCE, LIFETIME RISK, AND PREVALENCE RATES

Diagnostic ambiguity seriously confounds efforts to quantify the extent of bipolar manic-depressive illness in the general population. We are indebted here to the careful work of Weissman and Boyd, who reviewed the major epidemiological studies of affective illness.[8] Their identification of studies that differentiated bipolar from unipolar illness was particularly useful, as was their exclusion of studies that were diagnostically vague or that merged unipolar and bipolar disorders. For the sake of completeness, however, we include data from selected studies excluded from their review. These early studies, done before the seminal Amish and catchment area studies to be described later, provide a context in which to interpret results from the very recent, more methodologically sophisticated studies.

Selected Early Studies

The early European, British, and American studies used the term *manic-depressive illness* in the Kraepelinian sense to refer to both recurrent unipolar and bipolar illness. More recent studies, which have well-specified inclusion criteria as part of their research protocols, are preferable when fine analytical distinctions are needed.

Of all patients subsumed under the general diagnosis of manic-depressive (affective) illness, estimates of the bipolar fraction range from 15 to 35 percent, with an average of 20 percent (Krauthammer and Klerman, 1979). Asano (1967) found that 15 percent of 162 patients with a diagnosis of manic-depressive psychosis had a history of one or more manic episodes. Bratfos and Haug (1968) studied 215 patients, of whom 20 percent presented with a manic episode or had a history of one, and Perris (1966b) concluded that 19 percent of his patients with major affective illness were bipolar. These figures are significantly lower than those found in studies conducted in two Middle Eastern countries: 45 percent in Israel (Gershon and Liebowitz, 1975) and 44 percent in Iraq (Bazzoui, 1970). It is unclear whether these discrepancies represent true cross-cultural differences in rates or manifestations of illness, artifacts of diagnostic and sampling procedures, or some combination of these factors. Interestingly, Belmaker and Van Praag (1980a) dedicate their book on mania to the city of Jerusalem, in part because of its disproportionate rate of bipolar affective illness:

> . . . every other depressed patient in Jerusalem is bipolar, whereas only every fifth patient in Sweden is bipolar. . . . Jerusalem might represent a natural laboratory for the study of mania and bipolar illness . . . and the high incidence of mania in Jerusalem might somehow provide a key to understanding some of the complexities of the illness' causes.

Recent epidemiological studies of the incidence of bipolar illness are shown in Tables 7-2, 7-3, and 7-4, each of which presents incidence rates based on different information-gathering methods. Various criteria for bipolar affective illness were employed, taken from the DSM-III, ICD-8 and -9, PSE, and CATEGO (see Chapter 5 for explanation of these systems). Summary statistics show that the lifetime risk of bipolar disorder is generally less than 1 percent in industrialized nations (ranging from 0.6 to 0.9 percent, with 1.2 percent being a combination of bipolar-I and -II patients). The annual incidence of bipolar disorder is 0.009 to 0.015 percent (or 9 to 15 new cases per 100,000 per year) for men, and 0.007 to 0.03 percent (or 7 to 30 new cases per 100,000 per year) for women. Boyd and Weissman (1981)

Table 7-2. Annual First Hospitalization Rates for Bipolar Illness

Study	Site and Date	First Hospitalization %		
		Male	Female	Total
Spicer et al., 1973	England and Wales 1965 - 1966	.003	.004	.004
Leff et al., 1976	Aarhus County, Denmark 1969 - 1970	.003	.002	.003
Leff et al., 1976	Camberwell Section, London, England, 1965 - 1973	.003	.002	.003
Nielsen & Biørn-Henriksen, 1979	Samsø Island, Denmark 1957 - 1974			.006
Weeke 1984	Central Danish Registry 1970-72, 1978	.004	.004	.004

Adapted from Boyd and Weissman, 1985

found that the rates from comparable studies of nonbipolar depression are, as expected, higher. They noted that the advent of systematic diagnostic criteria has resulted in consistency across studies in rates for both bipolar and unipolar illness.

A few studies have been conducted on the incidence of mania and hypomania. Leff and colleagues (1976) compared the annual incidence (first admission rates) of mania per 100,000 in London and Aarhus, Denmark. Using the Present State Examination and a schedule of manic items drawn up by the authors, they found the same rate, 2.6, in both cities. Dickson and Kendell (1986) reported that new admissions for mania in one Scottish hospital had significantly increased between 1970 and 1981, whereas Eagles and Whalley (1985) found no significant difference in mania in age-standardized groups during roughly

the same period in all of Scotland. The various explanations for this discrepancy are well detailed by Dickson and Kendell (1986).

The range of morbid risk rates for manic illness, 0.24 to 0.77 percent (Table 7-5), is consistent with the low figures in the studies of bipolar illness reviewed by Boyd and Weissman (1981), that is, less than 1 percent. Earlier, Krauthammer and Klerman (1979) had concluded that the mania figures were consistent with rates obtained by multiplying the risk for manic-depressive illness by the bipolar fraction. They also pointed out that the figures confirm the clinical impression that mania is the rarest type of major psychosis.

Finally, although very few studies have been conducted, it is important to mention the epidemiology of the spectrum of manic states (see Chapter 4). Several authors have expressed con-

Table 7-3. Annual Incidence for Bipolar Disorder[a]

Study	Site and Date	Annual Incidence %		
		Male	Female	Total
Weeke et al., 1975	Aarhus County, Denmark 1960 - 1964	.015	.017	.016
Nielsen & Biørn-Henriksen, 1979	Samsø Island, Denmark 1957 - 1974	.014	.007	.011
Helgason, 1979	Iceland 1966 - 1973	.009	.033	.021

[a]Data are for persons 15 years of age or older seeking treatment

Adapted from Boyd and Weissman, 1985

Table 7-4. Percent Lifetime Risk of Bipolar Disorder[a]

Study	Site and Date	Lifetime Risk %
Fremming, 1951	Denmark 1951	0.61
Parsons, 1965	England 1961	0.88
James and Chapman, 1975	New Zealand 1967	0.24
Weissman and Myers, 1978	New Haven, Connecticut 1975–1976	0.6[b]
Helgason, 1979	Iceland 1957–1971	0.79
Weissman et al., 1988a	United States 1980–1984	1.2[c]

[a] Studies of manic-depressive illness are omitted if bipolar disorder is not separated from nonbipolar disorder
[b] This is the lifetime prevalence for BP I. If BP II is included, the lifetime prevalence is 1.2 percent
[c] Combination of BP I and BP II

Adapted from Boyd and Weissman, 1985

cern about the neglect of this aspect of affective illness.[9] Weissman and Myers (1978) found that bipolar-I and bipolar-II disorders each had a lifetime prevalence of 0.6 percent, which combine to 1.2 percent for all bipolar patients. Depue and colleagues (1981) studied an even wider range of the mood spectrum using the General Behavioral Inventory (see Chapter 4), a self-report instrument designed to identify individuals at high risk for bipolar illness. In looking for cyclothymic phenotypes too low in intensity to require outpatient treatment, they obtained a prevalence of true positive cases of bipolar-II, bipolar-III,[10] and dysthymic disorders of 7.8 percent. By including

Table 7-5. Percent Morbid Risk of Mania

Study	Country	Morbid Risk %
Fremming, 1951	Denmark	0.61
Helgason, 1961	Iceland	0.77
James & Chapman, 1975	New Zealand	0.24

Adapted from Krauthammer and Klerman, 1979

false-negative cases, the prevalence increased to 12 percent. It is difficult to know what to make of these preliminary findings, yet they are of interest because of their appreciation of the unstudied subtleties of the affective spectrum.

Two recent studies, which merit special attention, have greatly contributed to knowledge of the incidence and prevalence rates of manic-depressive illness, the Amish and the Epidemiologic Catchment Area studies. Both are notable for their standardized diagnostic procedures and comprehensive surveys of large samples.

The Amish Study

The Amish study of Egeland and colleagues (1983) is unusual in its assessment of the prevalence of affective disorders in a population that is culturally and genetically homogeneous. This subculture, a very conservative Protestant religious sect in Pennsylvania, offered an "unheralded opportunity to study multigenerational pedigrees with large sibships" (Egeland and Hostetter, 1983). Variables that confounded past research are not present in this population: Alcohol and drug abuse are virtually nonexistent, for example, and rarely do acts of crime or violence occur. Other obstacles had to be overcome, however. In applying specific diagnostic criteria to this group, the RDC definitions for mania and depression needed to be translated into Amish behavioral terms. Manic behaviors, to the Amish, include:

racing one's horse and carriage too hard . . . buying or using machinery or worldly items . . . excessive use of the public telephone . . . or planning vacations during the wrong season. (Egeland et al., 1983, p. 68)

The Old Order Amish, 12,500 people who live primarily in Lancaster County, Pennsylvania, keep extensive genealogical and medical records of ancestors back through 30 generations (Egeland and Hostetter, 1983). The Amish study, which spanned a 5-year period from 1976 to 1980, attempted to identify all individuals who were actively ill, thus giving incidence and period prevalence rates. As Egeland and Hostetter (1983) point out, the close interactions among the Amish prevented even mild cases of emotional disturbance from being overlooked. Once an active case was identified, medical records were abstracted and sent to a psychiatric board, which made a consensus diagnosis based on RDC criteria. If medical records did not exist, patients were directly interviewed using the SADS-L.

Reliability estimates were made on the agreement between board consensus and a separate psychiatrist's diagnosis (Hostetter et al., 1983). Kappa statistics for reliability generally were high and consistent for any major affective disorder, that is, unipolar depression, and bipolar-I disorder (0.87, 0.95, and 0.86, respectively). Only with bipolar-II disorder was the kappa coefficient much lower (0.68), suggesting a possible misrepresentation of this diagnosis among the Amish and less reliability in the diagnostic category.

During this period, 112 cases of mental illness were reported, 80 percent of which were affective disorders (71 percent major affective disorders), involving 1 percent of the Amish population (Egeland and Hostetter, 1983). A further breakdown of these rates revealed that 34 percent of the psychiatric cases were either bipolar-I or bipolar-II disorder, and 37 percent were unipolar depression. The remaining 9 percent were made up by minor depression and hypomanic disorder (8 and 1 percent, respectively). As Egeland and Hostetter (1983) point out, the rate of major affective disorder, as well as the rate of mental illness in general, appear to be below the U.S. average.

The most interesting finding is the apparent equivalence in rates of bipolar and unipolar illness. Other studies have shown a lopsided ratio. Weissman and colleagues (1988a) reported an almost 4:1 unipolar/bipolar diagnosis ratio across the United States, and some rates have shown a 10:1 ratio (Clayton, 1981). In an attempt to explain these discrepant findings, Egeland and Hostetter (1983) noted that their sample of bipolar patients would have been greatly reduced had not community reports of "highs" led to early SADS-L interviewing. Another explanation for the discrepancy is the finding by Egeland and colleagues (1983) that 79 percent of their bipolar-I patients had earlier been diagnosed as schizophrenic. Cultural factors may be partly responsible for the misdiagnosis, since earlier clinicians, unlearned in the customs of the Amish, may have viewed thought disorder, paranoia, and grandiosity as symptoms of schizophrenia rather than mania (Egeland and Hostetter, 1983; Egeland et al., 1983). Of particular note are the grandiose symptoms with marked religious overtones; religion is a central theme of the Amish. If other manic symptoms are not noted or are overlooked (as is apparent from early medical records), these symptoms could easily be seen as schizophrenic. Misdiagnosis is reviewed further in the sections on race and cross-cultural comparisons later in this chapter, and manic delusions are reviewed in Chapter 11. Assortative mating, the tendency for individuals with affective illness to marry each other (see Chapters 12 and 15), is likely to be even more prevalent in a small, inbred culture and thus may also raise the relative rate of bipolar illness. Likewise, it is probable that the most ill of the Amish stay within the community, whereas the less ill may migrate outwards.

Among bipolar and unipolar patients in the Amish study, gender was equally distributed. While this finding is consistent with others for bipolar illness, the majority of studies find a 2:1 female/male ratio in unipolar depression. The most obvious explanation for this discrepancy, according to Egeland and Hostetter (1983), is that alcoholism and sociopathy do not mask depression in Amish males as they do in males in the general population. Although the findings of this study will likely be discussed and debated for years, they provide a view of major affective disorder relatively untainted by violence, alcohol and drug abuse, and other variables that might otherwise mask their presence.

The Epidemiologic Catchment Area Program

The second noteworthy study is the Epidemiologic Catchment Area (ECA) program of the National Institute of Mental Health. It is a multicenter population survey of representative samples of five U.S. catchment area centers: New Haven, Connecticut, Baltimore, Maryland, St. Louis, Missouri, Piedmont County, North Carolina, and Los Angeles, California. ECA investigators acknowledge that the study is not wholly representative of the entire American population, but it is the most comprehensive epidemiological study of mental illness in the United States to date (Eaton et al., 1981). A brief summary of the history and purpose of the ECA follows (comprehensive reviews can be found in Regier et al., 1984; Eaton et al., 1981; Eaton and Kessler, 1985).

Background

The ECA program was intended to produce accurate, uniform, and comparable epidemiological data on mental disorders in the United States and to assess the adequacy of services to the mentally ill (Regier et al., 1984). It was built on four early and comprehensive, but smaller scale, epidemiological studies of mental illness.[11] The design required representative sampling of populations from both community and institutional settings, at two different times (wave 1 and wave 2). In wave 1, prevalence data were gathered for DSM-III diagnosable illnesses over periods of a lifetime, 6 months, 1 month, and 2 weeks. Wave 2 is a follow-up to ascertain rates of relapse and remission, as well as to determine incidence rates (better than prevalence rates in the study of etiology) (Eaton et al., 1981).[12]

The Diagnostic Interview Schedule

Nearly 20,000 persons were interviewed in the ECA by lay interviewers, who used a specially designed structured diagnostic instrument, the Diagnostic Interview Schedule (DIS), with criteria from the DSM-III, RDC, and Feighner diagnostic systems.[13] Subjects were first asked whether they had ever experienced a symptom at any time during their lives, which became the basis for ECA lifetime prevalence rates. Then they were asked whether they had experienced

the symptoms during the last 2 weeks, the last month, the last 6 months, and the last year, and this information was used to calculate 1-month, 6-month, and 1-year prevalence rates. The DIS determined the severity of a disorder in addition to its presence and duration.[14]

The DIS appears to have relatively high reliability for diagnosing major depression but considerably less reliability for manic episodes.[15] Some questions remain about its continued use and interpretation of the data it yields (see, e.g., Anthony et al., 1985). The accuracy of lifetime recall has been questioned, for example, as has the lack of comparability of diagnoses made by DIS lay interviewers with those of experienced clinicians, whose pattern recognition and access to family history are likely to produce a more accurate diagnosis. For example, Robins (1985) compared 1-month prevalence rates of depression and mania at two ECA sites (St. Louis and Baltimore) as diagnosed by psychiatrists and by lay interviewers using the DIS. He noted a curious finding. Although rates of mania and depression were not significantly different when determined by psychiatrists and lay interviewers in Baltimore, rates of both disorders were diagnosed three times more often by psychiatrists than by lay interviewers in St. Louis. This anomaly suggests that some caution should be applied to interpreting ECA data, although, on the whole, the study is methodologically superior to past attempts at estimating the prevalence and incidence of manic-depressive illness.

Findings in Affective Disorders

Results of the ECA program are summarized here and noted in many of the demographic correlate sections.

Prevalence and Demographics. Weissman and colleagues (1988a), in the most complete summary of the ECA data for affective disorders from all five sites, give the following mean cumulative prevalence rates per 100 persons for bipolar disorder (defined as a manic episode): for periods of 2 weeks, 0.7 percent; 1 month, 0.8; 6 months, 0.9; 1 year, 1.0; and lifetime 1.2. Consonant figures for major depression are 1.5, 1.6, 2.2, 2.6, and 4.4 percent, respectively.

The breakdown of these prevalence rates by sex and age by site is shown in Table 7-6. The

Table 7-6. One-Year Prevalence Rates/100 Persons of DIS/DSM-III Bipolar Disorder by Age, Sex, and ECA Site[a]

	New Haven		Baltimore		St. Louis		Piedmont		Los Angeles		Total	
	N	(%)	N	(%)	N	(%)	N	(%)	N	(%)	N	(%)
Male	2,057	(1.1)	1,279	(0.9)	1,182	(1.3)	1,505	(0.3)	1,475	(0.7)	7,498	(0.9)
Female	2,965	(1.4)	2,056	(0.9)	1,789	(1.5)	2,321	(0.8)	1,634	(0.6)	10,765	(1.1)
Sex ratio, F/M	1.3		1.0		1.2		2.7		0.9		1.2	
Age 18-44	1,655	(2.0)	1,691	(1.4)	1,696	(2.1)	1,597	(0.8)	2,084	(0.9)	8,723	(1.4)
45-64	802	(0.5)	815	(0.5)	715	(0.5)	1,055	(0.4)	646	(0.4)	4,033	(0.4)
65+	2,565	(0.1)	829	(0.0)	560	(0.4)	1174	(0.1)	379	(0.0)	5,507	(0.1)
Total	5,022	(1.3)	3,335	(0.9)	2,971	(1.4)	3,826	(0.6)	3,109	(0.6)	18,263	(1.0)

[a]Unweighted N and weighted percentages

From Weissman et al., 1988a

prevalence of bipolar illness in females is 1.2 times that of males across all five sites, but the ratio ranges from a low of 0.9 to 1 in Los Angeles to 2.7 to 1 in the Piedmont. Age data were consistent with earlier studies (see Chapter 6). The 18 to 44 age group had the highest prevalence of bipolar disorder (1.4 percent), and the 65 and over age group had the lowest (0.1 percent). Myers and colleagues (1984) and Regier and co-workers (1988), studying 6-month and 1-month prevalence rates, respectively, broke the 18 to 44 age

group down to 18 to 24 and 25 to 44 but found no differences in diagnoses of manic episode.

One-year prevalence rates for major depression by age, sex, and site (Table 7-7) are similar to those for bipolar illness. The ratio of females to males is 2.75 percent, with a range from 1.9 percent in Los Angeles to 5.0 percent in St. Louis. Rates were highest among the 18 to 44 age group (1.6 percent for males, 4.8 percent for females) and lowest among the 65 and over age group (0.4 percent for males, 1.4 percent for females).[16]

Table 7-7. One-Year Prevalence Rates/100 Persons of DIS/DSM-III Major Depression By Age, Sex, and ECA Site[a]

	New Haven		Baltimore		St. Louis		Piedmont		Los Angeles		Total	
	N	(%)	N	(%)	N	(%)	N	(%)	N	(%)	N	(%)
Men 18-44	719	(2.3)	654	(1.0)	690	(1.1)	705	(0.7)	1,023	(2.7)	3,791	(1.6)
45-64	340	(1.6)	294	(1.1)	283	(0.6)	415	(1.5)	298	(1.3)	1,630	(1.3)
65+	997	(0.8)	329	(0.3)	208	(0.1)	385	(0.1)	154	(0.7)	2,073	(0.4)
Women 18-44	936	(6.7)	1,037	(3.3)	1,006	(4.9)	892	(3.1)	1,061	(5.2)	4,932	(4.8)
45-64	462	(2.8)	520	(2.2)	433	(4.8)	640	(2.0)	348	(3.3)	2,403	(2.9)
65+	1,565	(1.8)	498	(1.5)	351	(0.6)	787	(1.2)	225	(1.2)	3,426	(1.4)
Sex ratio, F/M	2.5		2.9		5.0		2.9		1.9		2.7	

[a]Unweighted N and weighted percentages

From Weissman et al., 1988a

Aside from age and gender, several other demographic variables were studied in the ECA program, although data are not reported from all five sites (only from New Haven, Baltimore, and St. Louis). Robins and associates (1984), examining lifetime prevalence rates by race, reported no overall difference between blacks and nonblacks in diagnoses for manic or major depressive episodes, with one exception. Only at the Baltimore site was there a significantly higher lifetime prevalence of manic episodes among blacks (2.5 percent vs 0.7 percent), but blacks were oversampled there.

Mexican-Americans were sampled by the Los Angeles catchment area (Burnam et al., 1987; Karno et al., 1987). Lifetime and 6-month prevalence rates showed nonsignificant decreases in manic and major depressive episodes in Mexican-American subjects compared with non-Hispanic white subjects. These findings were stable across gender and age groups and did not differ significantly from findings at the other four ECA sites.

Rural–urban differences have also been studied. Robins and colleagues (1984) found no significant differences across three sites in lifetime prevalence rates of manic or major depressive episodes among central city areas, inner suburbs, and small town–rural areas. However, Blazer and co-workers at Duke University (1985) found that the Piedmont catchment area had significantly higher rates of major depression in urban areas than in rural areas, but no data on manic episodes were given. There were no significant differences in educational achievement (college graduate vs other) across three sites (Robins et al., 1984).

Use of Health Services. ECA investigators also examined the use of mental health services by patients with affective disorders (Shapiro et al., 1984). Thirty-one percent of respondents with DIS-diagnosed affective disorder across three sites (St. Louis, Baltimore, and New Haven) made a mental health visit over a 6-month period. No information was given about bipolar–unipolar differences or the proportion making mental health visits for another psychiatric problem (e.g., substance abuse).

Incidence. Wave-2 findings, reported by Eaton and colleagues (1989), show that, across four of the five sites,[17] the annual incidence of major depression is 1.6 percent. Within this group of depressed individuals, women outnumbered men 2:1, a ratio consistent with the findings of other studies. Age differences were also apparent: 18- to 29-year-old men showed a greater incidence than older men, the rate gradually declining through the group of men 65 and older. In women, annual incidence is greatest for the 18- to 29- and 30- to 44-year-olds and turns downward after age 45. Sex differences across age groups are similar to the overall 1:2 ratio, with the greatest difference occurring in the 45 to 64 age group, where depressed women outnumbered depressed men by 3:1.

Most of these data are presented again in the context of their relationship to other studies that investigated similar demographic correlates in affective disorders.

ASSOCIATED FEATURES

In the study of bipolar illness, epidemiology, like clinical description, serves primarily heuristic purposes. Where clinical impressions stimulate research on phenomenology and treatment, epidemiological findings point toward promising approaches to understanding pathological processes. In this and the following sections, we examine demographic and cross-cultural correlates of manic-depressive illness as well as seasonality factors. These variables are often called "risk factors," but to avoid possible causal implications, we use instead the term *associated features*.

Demographic Correlates

Several demographic correlates need to be taken into account when reviewing studies of manic-depressive illness. These include age, gender, social class, race, marital status, and urban–rural differences. Although few studies compensate for all of these factors, many of them are used for national, cross-national, and cross-cultural comparisons.

Age

As noted in Chapter 6, data on the age of onset of bipolar illness in the United States generally fit a unimodal distribution. Manic-depressive patients have a mean age of onset of 30, whereas those with major depressive disorder first become ill between the ages of 40 and 50. A significant percentage of patients experience their first manic or depressive episode before the age of 20 (see Chapter 8). According to Faris and Dunham (1939), the incidence of manic-depressive illness rises until the age of 35 and then gradually declines. Myers and associates (1984) and Weissman and colleagues (1988a) reported similar findings: Onsets of affective disorders generally are less frequent in the 65 and older age category and are highest between the ages of 18 and 44. Early studies reporting bimodal data (Angst, 1978; Zis et al., 1979) have not been well supported by later findings.

Spicer and associates (1973) found that the incidence of mania consistently increased with age and that half of the new cases occurred in those over the age of 50. Earlier, both Wertham (1929) and Roth (1955) presented data confirming the onset of mania after age 60. One explanation for this seemingly recent decrease in the age of onset is the advent of lithium (Baldessarini, 1970; Horgan, 1981). Boyd and Weissman (1985) postulated that the reason for the drop in the age of onset of mania following the advent of lithium may be an increased awareness of the diagnosis earlier in patients' histories. Despite the few studies that found a large late-onset group, it generally can be said that persons under the age of 50 are at much greater risk for a first attack than those over 50 and that those who have already had one attack have a very high risk of recurrence. In terms of episode duration, Krauthammer and Klerman (1979) point out that, with increasing age, the interval between episodes decreases and the length of episodes increases.

Although age groups are often correlated with other demographic factors, such as gender, race, and culture, no significant age differences have been found across these variables. Cross-cultural epidemiological studies have reported ages of onset similar to those of U.S populations (see Table 6-1). Gender differences also show no effect across age groups, even in the five-site ECA data (Weissman et al., 1988a).

Finally, cohort studies provide data on the changing patterns of illness at different points in history. Rice and associates (1987) found that age of onset is significantly related to risk of illness in relatives. Low birth cohorts (<25 and 26–44) had lower age of onset compared with those 45 and older. Although this difference may result from faulty memory and inadequate record keeping, among other factors, it is possible that susceptible individuals may now express their phenotype at a younger age. The cohort studies and related genetic theories are discussed in greater detail in Chapter 16.

Gender

Affective illness is generally found to be more prevalent in women than in men, but the difference is due in large part to the higher prevalence of unipolar depression in women. A sampling of studies from around the world shows that the ratio of affective illness in females/males ranges from 1.3:1 to 3:1.[18] In the ECA study, Regier and colleagues (1988a) found an approximately 2:1 female/male ratio of affective illness, ranging from 1:1 in Los Angeles to 2.7:1 in the Piedmont. When only those with manic episodes were considered (the ECA bipolar group), the ratio was equal, with an overall prevalence of 0.4 percent. Bolstering this bipolar finding was the ECA analysis by Weissman and colleagues (1988a) that showed that the rate of major depressive disorder among women at every ECA site and in every age category was greater (1.9:1) than that for men, whereas the rate of bipolar disorder was almost equal (1.2:1).

An exception to this pattern of findings was discovered in the Amish study: 58 percent of bipolar patients were male and 42 percent female, and the unipolar patients were divided almost evenly between the sexes. According to Egeland and Hostetter (1983), these seeming discrepancies may be explained by two characteristics of Amish culture. First, since alcoholism and sociopathy do not mask the expression of affective disorder among Amish men, a truer picture of the distribution of the illness is possible than in most populations. Second, female depression may not be detected because Amish women occupy the role of protective, self-sufficient household managers and, because of the dominant work ethic, may discount somatic symptoms.

Thus, although rates of major depression are higher among women than men, this is not true for manic-depressive illness, which is equally prevalent across gender.

Social Class

The suggestive relationship between manic-depressive illness and social class is not only fascinating but also important because of its relevance to studies of genetics, creativity, social systems, treatment compliance, and etiology. In this section, we review the major methodological problems in such studies, discuss the results of research to date, and briefly examine hypotheses about the relationship.

Studies of social class and manic-depressive illness have been hampered, and the interpretation of data has been made difficult, by two major types of methodological problems: diagnostic bias (and diagnostic overinclusiveness) and treatment bias. Together, these factors can contribute to incorrect and inaccurate reporting of incidence and prevalence rates of manic-depressive illness among various social classes. For example, upper and middle class people are more likely to be diagnosed as manic-depressive, whereas lower class individuals, especially among poor urban black populations, are more likely to be diagnosed as schizophrenic (often mistakenly so), and are consequently treated as such. Minorities generally are underrepresented in these studies as well. Further, criteria for social class vary across studies. Some authors have used the system of Hollingshead and Redlich (1958), others used occupation alone or parental social class, and still others used only educational achievement.

Landis and Page (1938) attributed the lack of a significant downward social drift in individuals with manic-depressive illness to aspects of the natural history of the illness: (1) it is an illness with a good prognosis and without the progressive deteriorative course[19] that would affect earning potential, (2) the onset of the illness is usually sudden, with no prolonged prepsychotic period, (3) the onset is usually after college age so that it does not seriously interfere with opportunities for higher education,[20] and (4) individuals with manic-depressive illness frequently have compensatory energy and ambition.

Two other possible sources of error include statistical artifacts—where significant results may be secondary to other social factors, such as place of residence, marital status, and so on—and sex biases. Sex bias enters in because women often do not drop in social class through illness

but retain the social class of their husbands (Ödegaard, 1956). All of these methodological problems can be found in, and across, the studies presented in Table 7-8. Although the problems are considerable—in addition to those outlined above, there are difficulties in sampling techniques, geographical inconsistencies and biases, and so on—these studies remain interesting, for their span across decades, their historical significance, and their great range across countries and cultures.

With the methodological considerations in mind, it appears that the majority of studies report an association between manic-depressive illness and one or more measures reflecting upper social class. While many studies have failed to find the association with social class, none found a significantly lower than expected rate of the illness associated with indices of upper social class (defined by educational status, occupation, economic status, or parental social class). Thus, considered in its entirety, the literature is highly suggestive of an association. Although a comprehensive review of each study is beyond the scope of this book, a brief synopsis of recent studies, which are more standardized and diagnostically sound, should provide a flavor of the findings.

Bagley (1973), in an extensive review of the literature, concluded:

The studies reviewed suggest that there is some support for the view that some types of "depression" and upper class economic position are related. This finding seems to hold in several cultures, and in different points in time in the present century. . . . The definition of depression has often been unclear in many studies, but there is some evidence that the finding may apply to "psychotic" rather than "neurotic" depression, and to the classic manic depressive psychoses in particular. (p. 331)

Bagley compared the distribution of occupational positions in the adult English population at large with those among all 1,500 patients with new episodes of affective illness over a 3-year period in England. Using a sophisticated diagnostic system for affective illnesses, he distinguished six major categories. Only in the category that we would term *bipolar illness* was there any significant difference in distribution across occupational classes. In this group of patients, members of the professional and managerial classes were significantly overrepresented.

Table 7-8. Social Class Studies of Manic-Depressive Illness

Study	Characteristics of Study	N	Results
Stern, 1913	Germany; compared male SCZ and MD admissions to psychiatric clinic in Frieburg, 1906-1912	395	MDI is more common than SCZ in business and professional men; opposite true for artisans, farmers, factory workers, and laborers
Stern-Piper, 1925	Germany; studied male admissions to Frankfurt psychiatric units, 1920-1924	300	MDI is particularly likely in professional and business classes
Luxenburger, 1933	Germany; studied occupational categories in families of patients of a psychiatric clinic serving all classes	13, 624	MDI is more frequent in highest occupational class as in general population 4 times as likely in professional classes
Faris & Dunham, 1939	U.S.; all new first admissions to 4 public mental hospitals in Illinois, and several private	734	Tendency for MDI to be more frequent in higher socioeconomic groups than SCZ
Myerson & Boyle, 1941	U.S.; 1. Studied incidence of MDI in a selected group of prominent American families	20	MDI is most common diagnosis
	2. Compared admissions to McLean (middle and upper class private) Hospital with those to Massachusetts State Hospital	1,467	<u>MDI</u> <u>SCZ</u> McLean (5 yr) 235 80 MA State (1 yr) 400 752 Private hospital admissions are disproportionately manic-depressive
Tietze et al., 1941	U.S.; first admissions for SCZ and MDI to state and private hospitals	14,712 Sch 10,416 MDI	MDI is more common in upper social classes, SCZ in lower
Clark, 1949	U.S.; sociological study of first admissions to Chicago hospitals, public and private, 1922-1934	12,168	For all diagnoses except MDI there was a marked negative correlation with class (SCZ: -0.8; alcoholism: -0.5; MDI: 0.0)
Hare, 1955	England; ecological correlations to study relationship between mental illness and social conditions in Bristol, males	1,264 (352MDI)	The observed class distribution of MDI was not significantly different from expected rates
Malzberg, 1956	U.S.; all first admissions to private and public mental hospitals in N. Y.	46,471	MDI is more prevalent at higher and middle economic levels in whites but not in blacks.
Ødegaard, 1956	Norway; all first admissions for groups, psychoses to all psychiatric hospitals, in Norway, 1926-1950	34,457	No significant variation of MDI across admission rates among social classes
Hollingshead & Redlich, 1958	U.S.; studied residents of New Haven, Connecticut entering psychiatric treatment, 1950-1951	1,451 psychotic diagnoses	"the higher the class, the larger the proportion of patients who are affective psychotics" (p. 228)
Brooke, 1959	England & Wales; first admissions to mental hospitals in England and Wales,1956	170	Higher rate of MD reaction in lowest social classes but less prominent when compared with SCZ
Parker et al., 1959	U.S.; male MD patients, North Carolina Veteran's Administration Hospital	62	Disproportionate representation (52%) middle and upper social classes; religious affiliations consistent with class differences

Continued

Table 7-8 Continued. Social Class Studies of Manic-Depressive Illness

Study	Characteristics of Study	N	Results
Jaco, 1960	U.S.; admissions to public and private mental hospitals in Texas, 1951-1952	5,649 (953 MDI)	Rate for affective, or MD disorders high among professionals and semi-professionals; more MD treated in private hospitals than public; diagnostic correlation with income = 0.89
Astrup et al., 1962	Norway; follow-up study of patients with functional psychoses	1,102 (61 MD)	Majority of MD were from middle class; upper and lower class prevalence was as expected
Sundby & Nyhus, 1963	Norway; first admission males to Oslo psychiatric wards from urban and suburban areas	2,976 (118 AD)	"The most well-to-do areas...have the highest admission rates of this disease. In other areas the distribution is fairly even." (p. 532)
Noreik & Ødegaard, 1966	Norway; follow-up study, using mental records of Norwegians with higher education; graduation dates 1916-1925	12,843	Affective psychoses overrepresented, 3 times expected rate in women; among professionals rate was 2 times that of general population
Rao, 1966	India; first admissions to state hospitals in India, 1958-1960	4,039	"Excess of MDI among patients with high prestige and high income backgrounds."
Stenbäck & Achté, 1966	Finland; first admissions of male residents to Helsinki psychiatric wards and mental hospitals	1,216 (37 AD)	Rate of AD (age corrected) was much higher in upper social class compared with lower social class
Hare, 1968	England; admissions to Bethlem Royal and Maudsley hospitals in London, 1964-1966	4,520	Marked tendency for MD patients to be from middle and upper occupational classes
Rowitz & Levy, 1968	U.S.; all patients admitted to 44 public and private institutions in 1961	10,653	MD "tend to come from more affluent areas with higher median school years completed and larger % of white collar employees."
Woodruff et al., 1968	U.S.; compared occupational and educational achievement in primary affective disorder patients and their same-sexed siblings; Feighner diagnostic criteria	100	Patients with primary affective disorder compared with siblings did not demonstrate higher or lower levels of occupational or educational achievement
Walsh, 1969b	Ireland; first admissions and re-admissions to Dublin hospitals in 1962	3,352	Diagnosis of MDI twice as likely in private hospitals compared to SCZ; SCZ 4 times more likely in Local Authority hospitals
Birtchnell, 1971	Scotland; compared male referrals to psychiatric facilities in Northeastern Scotland with random sample of males from local population; did not distinguish between affective and SCZ psychoses	2,861 pts 1,487 gen. pop.	"In no diagnostic group does the social class of parent distribution vary significantly from the age-adjusted, expected distribution for the patient sample."
Woodruff et al., 1971b	U.S.; compared BP and UP with ill and well brothers	198 (29 BP) (41 UP)	BP attained higher educational but not occupational levels than UP. Neither differed from siblings in education or occupation levels

Continued

Table 7-8 Continued. Social Class Studies of Manic-Depressive Illness

Study	Characteristics of Study	N	Results
Hare et al., 1972	England; randomized sample of patients attending London's Bethlem-Maudsley Hospital as inpatients and outpatients; all patients Protestant and born in Great Britain	109	Parental social class not significantly different as a function of diagnosis; highest in middle social class
Bagley, 1973	England; 3-year study of new episodes of illness recorded by the Camberwell Register; used sophisticated diagnostic breakdowns of affective disorders across occupations	1,500	Only significant difference was in BPs; They were significantly more likely to be professional and managerial
Monnelly et al., 1974	U.S.; all consecutive male admissions during 12-month period; compared family achievement in BPs and UPs, and in those hospitalized privately and publicly	25 BP 21 UP	Overall, no significant differences in education or socioeconomic level between UP and BP; BPs receiving private hospitalization and their brothers had higher education levels as opposed to those in public hospitals
Gershon & Liebowitz, 1975	Israel; first admissions to psychiatric hospitals from Jewish population of Jerusalem, 1969-1972; BP, UP, and neurotic depressions classified as affective disorder	833	Diagnosis of affective disorder is associated with middle and upper social classes than with lower social classes
Petterson, 1977a	Sweden; MD patients collected from cases treated at Stockholm's St. Goran's Hospital, 1961-1970; compared education, occupation, economic status of patients and their fathers with the general population	123	% MD Parent Gen Pop Social Class I 25 30 8.4 Social Class II 50 41 37.1 Social Class III 25 29 54.5 BPs overrepresented in higher social classes
Weissman & Myers, 1978	U.S.; used Research Diagnostic Criteria in a community sample study of households in New Haven, Connecticut; serial follow-up interview design	938	The rates of BPI and BPII disorders were 4.6% in social classes I and II combined; 1.0 in Class III; 0.9% in Class IV; and no cases in Class V; ($p < .05$)
Jones et al., 1981	U.S.; randomly selected black psychiatric patients admitted to acute psychiatric unit in South Bronx; retrospective diagnosis of cases	117	15% diagnosed as MD, 4 times national admission rate; concluded, as a result of social class analysis, that MDI in lower class blacks is less common than in higher class whites
Eisemann, 1986	Sweden; compared patient and parental social class in UP, BP, and controls	34 UP 22 BP	Lower social class overrepresented in UP and BP compared to general population; however, upper social class overrepresented in BPs parents' social class compared with controls
Coryell et al., 1989a	U.S.; used RDC, SADS, and Holligshead scales in patients presenting for treatment in any of 5 university hospitals (New York, Boston, Chicago, St. Louis, Iowa City)	88 BPI 64 BPII 422 Non-BPMDD	Male BPII probands particularly likely to occupy managerial or professional jobs. Female probands did not differ across occupation or education. Relatives of BPI and BPII probands had superior levels of occupational and educational achievement

MD, MDI = Manic-depressive illness, SCZ = Schizophrenia, RAD = reactive affective disorders, AD = affective disorder
MDD = major depressive disorder
Review, partially based on data in Bagley (1973)

In an extensive, well-designed study of 123 bipolar patients in Sweden, Petterson (1977a) also found a highly significant overrepresentation of bipolar patients in the upper social and educational classes. Weissman and Myers (1978), using specified research criteria for diagnosis, conducted a community sample study of residents of New Haven, Connecticut. Like Petterson, they found a strong relationship between bipolar disorder and upper social class. Another study (Gershon and Liebowitz, 1975) correlated affective illness with higher social class when affective illness was compared with all other diagnoses. Although the authors did not compare only bipolar patients, their affective study sample, drawn from the first admissions to psychiatric hospitals from the Jewish population of Jerusalem, was almost half bipolar manic-depressives.

In a series of studies, Woodruff and colleagues (1968, 1971; Monnelly et al., 1974) examined bipolar and unipolar probands as well as siblings who either had been diagnosed with an affective disorder or were well. Although they found no difference in social class (as defined by occupation and educational status) between probands and their siblings, they did note that bipolar patients had more years of education than unipolar patients, although this advantage seemingly did not translate into a higher occupational status. The most striking differences were among the siblings of probands. Specifically, brothers of bipolar patients had higher education and occupational levels than did brothers of unipolar patients. This is of interest in its similarity to a recent study conducted by Richard and associates (1988), who found that non-ill siblings of bipolar patients enjoyed a relative benefit in creativity over bipolar probands, and especially over never-ill or diagnosed controls (see Chapter 14).

Jones and associates (1981), studying black patients in New York City, found none of their manic-depressive patients to be in the upper social classes. Because their sample population was from poor, urban areas, it is clearly unrepresentative of the total population, but it highlights the similar deficiencies of earlier investigations that surveyed mostly suburban, white patients admitted to private hospitals. (A more lengthy discussion of this topic is found in the race correlates section later in this chapter.)

One last notable study is that of Eisemann (1986), who investigated the social class distribution of bipolar and unipolar patients. He found that both subgroups of patients predominated in the lowest social class (agricultural worker, blue collar worker, and unskilled workers), 77 and 88 percent, respectively. These figures are significant in comparison to the general population, where 58 percent fall in this class. Eisemann also compared the parental social class of bipolar and unipolar patients and found similar but nonsignificant results. Most recently, Coryell and colleagues (1989a) studied 442 probands with nonbipolar major depressive disorder and 152 with bipolar disorder. They found that the family backgrounds of the bipolar patients were characterized by higher socioeconomic status than those with nonbipolar depression.

Finally, as we discuss in greater detail in Chapter 14, two main types of arguments have been advanced to explain the hypothesized greater incidence of manic-depressive illness in the middle and upper social classes. First, some authors suggest that a relationship exists between certain personality and behavioral correlates of affective (primarily bipolar) illness and a rise in social position (Bagley, 1973; Myerson and Boyle, 1941). In fact, many features of hypomania, such as outgoingness, increased energy and intensified sexuality, and heightened productivity, have been linked with increased achievement and accomplishments (see Chapter 14).

The second hypothesis posits that manic-depressive illness is secondary to the stresses of being in or moving into the upper social classes. This hypothesis is implausible because it assumes that, compared with lower classes, there is a special kind of stress associated with being in the upper social classes, one capable of precipitating major psychotic episodes. Further, it ignores genetic factors and evidence suggesting that parental social class is often elevated as well. As Birtchnell (1971) has argued, any differences from parental social class (upward or downward mobility) that are observed between manic-depressive patients and the general population make such differences more likely to be etiological (or correlative) and not consequences of illness. It would be possible to hypothesize a stress-diathesis model to explain genetic aspects, but this has not been done and research findings remain less than parsimonious.

Race

The literature on race overwhelmingly focuses on comparisons between white and black patients. Studies of Asian, Hispanic, or other ethnic group patients are primarily cross-cultural and are dealt with in that section of this chapter.

Over the past century, several studies have examined racial similarities and differences in the prevalence and incidence of manic-depressive illness. Many factors, apart from the previously mentioned sources of variance, cloud the accurate determination of the these rates: inadequate sampling from different socioeconomic groups, cultural differences and consequent presenting problems (dealt with in a later section), the misdiagnosis of schizophrenia, and possible racist sentiment or racial insensitivity among early researchers. These factors must be accounted for to obtain a more complete picture of racial comparison. The effects of these confounding variables are important enough to warrant more attention before reviewing the literature.

The first problem encountered in reviewing racial comparisons regarding any diagnosis is the predominant socioeconomic class of the race being investigated. For example, sample populations of black patients (predominantly lower class) often are compared to samples of middle and upper class whites. Jones and colleagues (1981) reported that 15 percent (more than four times the national admission rate) of their sample of black psychiatric patients were DSM-III-diagnosed manic-depressive. All of these patients were from the lowest social classes,[21] which makes cross-class comparisons difficult, much less comparisons with national rates. This result is similar to that of Warheit and associates (1973), who found higher rates of manic-depressive illness among lower socioeconomic blacks than in some white populations. This factor is quite significant, especially for manic-depressive illness, since different socioeconomic levels produce different stresses, set different limitations, and establish different goals among their populations. Drug abuse in the lower social classes may also complicate accurate diagnosis (Jones et al., 1988).

Results of several studies (Cooper et al., 1972; Simon et al., 1973; Welner et al., 1973) suggest a second obscuring factor, that black manic-depressive patients may be more likely to be misdiagnosed as schizophrenic than whites. Misdiagnosis of patients with clear manic symptoms as schizophrenic has been a continual impediment in ascertaining correct incidence and prevalence rates among black populations. Mukherjee and colleagues (1983), systematically controlling for age, gender, and marital and socioeconomic status, still found that blacks (and Hispanics) were more likely to be misdiagnosed as schizophrenic than whites. Taylor and Abrams (1973b) and Bell and Mehta (1980) proposed that this misdiagnosis in blacks can result from language barriers between patients and physicians who are unfamiliar with cultural aspects of black patients' language and behavior. Misdiagnosis might account for the especially low prevalence rates of manic-depressive illness in blacks reported by Faris and Dunham (1939), Malzberg (1956), and Rowitz and Levy (1968).

Such misdiagnosis is not solely characteristic of black populations, however. Comparing records of Amish patients, a Caucasian subculture, to those of other whites reveals that a substantial portion of bipolar-I patients in that sample were originally misdiagnosed as schizophrenic (Egeland et al., 1983). Horgan (1981) likewise reported an overrepresentation of manic-depressive patients previously misdiagnosed as schizophrenic in the United Kingdom. This suggests that the misdiagnosis may result more from nonrecognition (or ignorance) of manic symptoms by physicians than from racial insensitivity.

Speculation has arisen about the presence of racism or racial insensitivity in early studies of prevalence and incidence rate differences between blacks and whites. Since manic-depressive illness was often labeled as white upper class disorder in the early part of this century (Kolb, 1968), studies that reported lower incidence rates in blacks attributed it to their "primitive" mentality (reviewed by Thomas and Sillen, 1972). One striking example is a summary statement of Lewis and Hubbard in their 1931 study that found no difference in hospital diagnoses of manic-depressive illness:

Most investigators who have studied the abnormal mental reactions of negroes (and other "uncivilized" peoples) in their more primitive state, that is, in situations where there has been a minimum of contact with the white man and his ways, concur that such reactions as manic depressive insanity . . . are exceedingly rare, if they occur at all. If this is so, perhaps it is an indication that "higher" types of psychosis require a certain type of common or racial consciousness such as is found among the higher orders of civilized peoples. (p. 815)

This racist sentiment is not evidenced in later studies, many of which reported equal or higher rates of manic-depressive illness in black patients.

Mindful of these caveats, a brief overview of the epidemiological literature considering race differences yields an unclear picture. In 1931, Pollock published the results of a 4-year survey of first-admission diagnoses of manic-depressive illness in New York State hospitals in which he found a lower rate in white compared with black patients (0.9 vs 1.53 percent). Wagner (1938) likewise reported higher annual incidence rates for manic-depressive illness in blacks than whites in both Cincinnati and New York, the latter having a higher overall rate. A later survey by Malzberg (1944) reported similar findings: 1.5 percent admission diagnoses of manic-depressive illness in whites compared with 2.0 percent in black patients. This is an interesting finding, considering that in his later study, Malzberg (1956) reported that manic-depressive illness was diagnosed 26:1 in whites compared to blacks in all New York State hospitals from 1939 to 1941.

The most replicated finding of racial differences in manic-depressive illness is a lower incidence rate among blacks. When one excludes the four earliest studies[22] because of possible bias, however, this majority is significantly diminished. Three studies published in the early 1960s (Simon, 1965; Prange and Vitols, 1962; Jaco, 1960) reported lower rates in Florida, North Carolina, and Texas, respectively. In a 10-year study of first admissions to hospitals in the northeastern United States (1969–1979), using the DSM-II diagnosis of manic-depressive illness, Marquez and co-workers (1985) replicated these findings of lower incidence among treated blacks compared with whites, an average white/black ratio of 2.4:1.

Finally, Lewis and Hubbard (1931), Faris and Dunham (1939), Helzer (1975), and Weissman and Myers (1978) found equal rates of diagnosis of manic-depressive illness in blacks and whites. Recent national epidemiological studies, such as the NIMH ECA program, with a much broader sampling population than previous studies, likewise report no significant difference in the prevalence or incidence rates of manic-depressive illness among races (Blazer et al., 1985).

Thus, despite a majority of studies reporting lower rates of manic-depressive illness in blacks than in whites, the data, because of the presence of uncontrolled factors, such as misdiagnosis, cross-class comparisons, and racial biases, yield no clear picture. It appears that no race distinction (at least between black and white patients examined) exists in the prevalence and incidence rates of manic-depressive illness.

Marital Status

Many epidemiological studies investigating marital status among patients report that manic-depressive illness is slightly more common in single and divorced persons (Boyd and Weissman, 1985). As Krauthammer and Klerman (1979) point out, however, marital status may change as a result of the disorder rather than lead to its onset. To our knowledge, no causal relationship between these two variables has as yet been established. A brief overview of some of these studies highlights this confusion. Further discussion is found in Chapter 12.

Faris and Dunham (1939) found more divorced people among those with manic-depressive illness than in the general population. However, they found no significant differences in percentages of single, married, or widowed persons. A later study by Weeke and co-workers (1975) similarly reported that manic-depressive patients were less likely to be married and more likely to be separated or divorced than the general population. In many of the latter cases, however, the illness preceded, and presumably contributed to, the divorce. This finding was consistent with that reported by Astrup and colleagues (1962). Sundby and Nyhus (1963) reported that among males in Norway, the prevalence of affective disorders was above the predicted rate among married and divorced males and below the predicted rate in single and widowed males. In studies of black and Hispanic bipolar patients (the majority of whom were also single, divorced, or separated), Jones and colleagues (1981, 1983) consistently found a strong relationship between marital disruption, marital conflict, and bipolar illness.

It is plausible that being single or divorced does, in some populations, constitute a risk for bipolar illness. However, the evidence compiled currently suggests that these states are not, by themselves, risk factors for bipolar illness. It is also plausible that stressful marriages may, under some circumstances, precipitate affective episodes.

Urban–Rural

Results of urban–rural comparisons have, for the most part, been inconclusive. Malzberg (1940) reported finding a slight increase in the incidence of manic-depressive illness in urban areas compared with rural ones, and Murphy and colleagues (1963) noted that delusions of grandeur were more associated with rural than urban life. Jaco (1960) found that major affective disorder was significantly increased in urban areas, and Tietze and colleagues (1941) demonstrated a 2:1 difference in the rates of manic-depressive illness in public hospitals in urban areas compared to rural areas. Helgason's study (1961) in Iceland yielded an opposite finding, a slight increase in manic-depressive illness among rural populations. Similarly, Sundby and Nyhus (1963) found the highest rate of affective disorders in wealthy suburban areas but also high rates in lower class downtown Oslo. Lower class suburban areas, however, had one of the lowest rates per 100,000 of affective disorders. The investigation by Weeke's group of Aarhus County (1975) produced no differences between urban and rural communities in the incidence of manic-depressive illness. In findings similar to Malzberg's results, Robins and co-workers (1984) and Canino and colleagues (1987) reported nonsignificant increases of the incidence of both manic and major depressive episodes in urban compared with rural areas at three ECA sites. Blazer and co-workers (1985), analyzing the ECA Piedmont area data only, found significantly higher rates of depression in urban than in suburban areas, but no bipolar illness comparison was made. The inconsistent results of these studies suggest that differences in prevalence rates of affective disorders may have to do with the interplay of living location, migration patterns, socioeconomic status, and environment among others, rather than simply one variable.

Prevalence Rates Among the Homeless

Homelessness is a growing problem, and mental illness in the homeless population has become a special interest of mental health professionals. The homeless population itself is very hard to define, and the prevalence of mental disorders within this community is even harder to ascertain. As Rossi and colleagues (1987) point out, estimates of the total population of homeless in the United States vary from as little as 250,000 to over 3 million people. Estimates of the prevalence of mental disorders are similarly diverse, ranging from 15 percent (Snow et al., 1986) to 90 percent (Bassuk et al., 1984). As Koegel and associates (1988) suggest, this range is too broad to be explained by regional variation, and even after limiting their definition to severe mental illness, the best estimate that the American Psychiatric Association's Task Force on the Homeless Mentally Ill could give was between 25 and 50 percent (Arce and Vergare, 1984).

Among the mental disorders that exist within this population, schizophrenia, substance abuse, personality disorders, and affective disorders are the most prevalent (Arce and Vergare, 1984). Affective disorders make up 5 to 30 percent of mental disorders found among the homeless (Table 7-9).

The most comprehensive and best standardized of these studies (Koegel et al., 1988) used the DIS to diagnose disorders among the homeless in Los Angeles. Aside from the general findings listed in Table 7-9, Koegel and colleagues reported risk ratios for mental disorders among the homeless compared with the general population of Los Angeles. Over the course of their lifetimes, these homeless individuals were 3.4 times more likely to have had any affective disorder, 17.7 times more likely to have had a manic episode, and 2.9 times more likely to have had a major depressive episode than people in the general population. Similarly, over a period of 6 months, the risk ratios were many times greater among the homeless than in the general population (6.1, 37.5, and 5.0, respectively). Only one significant difference among ethnic group was found by these investigators: Blacks were more likely to have a manic episode within a 6-month period than were Hispanics. The prevalence of sub-

Table 7-9. Prevalence of Affective Disorders Among the Homeless Mentally Ill

Study	N	AD%	UP%	BP%	Comments
Whitley, 1955	16	50			Diagnosed at admission to lodging house
Lodge Patch, 1971	122	8			
Arce et al., 1983	179	5.6	3.9	1.7	
Baasher et al., 1983	24 117			21 19	Alexandria, Egypt Cairo, Egypt
Bassuk et al., 1984	78	9	4	5	
Bassuk et al., 1986	80	10			
Fisher et al., 1986	51	16 2			Lifetime prevalence 6-month prevalence
Koegel et al., 1988	328	29.5 20.9	18.3 15.5	10.6 7.5	Lifetime prevalence 6-month prevalence
Herrman et al., 1989	382	25 12	20 7	3 1	Lifetime prevalence Current prevalence

AD = affective disorder

stance abuse also was very high among the homeless population.

Besides Koegel and colleagues (1988), two other studies of the homeless studied bipolar–unipolar differences (Arce et al., 1983; Bassuk et al., 1984). Both studies reported unipolar depression in 4 percent of their homeless, mentally ill samples, but whereas Bassuk and colleagues (1984) found a 5 percent rate of bipolar illness, Arce and co-workers found a rate of only 1.7 percent.

One must keep in mind, however, when looking at these data, that these are prevalence rates within the homeless mentally ill population and not within the general homeless population. Still, when converted to rates within the general homeless population, these disorders are more prevalent than rates in the general population.

One other note regarding prevalence rates within this population is that substance abuse can easily mask another underlying mental disorder, especially affective disorders (see Chapter 9), and therefore these already high rates may be even higher.

Cross-Cultural Findings

Few systematic studies have been done of cross-cultural differences in rates and phenomenology of manic-depressive illness. As in so many other aspects of research into affective illness, clear distinctions between unipolar and bipolar disorders are rare; and as noted earlier, other than the studies reviewed by Boyd and Weissman (1981, 1985), very little standardized research into the epidemiology of manic-depressive illness per se has been done. Exceptions include the limited number of epidemiological investigations reviewed earlier and summarized in Tables 7-2, 7-3, and 7-4, all of which were carried out in industrialized, western nations. These investigations were carried out in Denmark, Britain, the United States, and New Zealand and revealed few cross-national differences in incidence. In fact, the consistency in rates that emerged when diagnostic criteria were held constant was impressive. It is not difficult to understand why such studies are few. Methodological problems in cross-cultural research are truly formidable; requisite

Table 7-10. Influence of Culture on Development, Manifestation, and Incidence of Depression

I. Factors generating or reinforcing depression

   a. Early formative influences
- amount of physical contact, breast feeding, etc.
- time of weaning
- degree of independence training
- parental severity
- use of symbolic sanctions vs. physical punishment

   b. Culture change
- industrialization
- urbanization
- westernization
- breakdown of family traditions and other social institutions
- changes in values, ideas, and attitudes
- acculturation
- migration

   c. Social cohesion

   d. Miscellaneous
- role deprivation (lack of a meaningful role)
- rigidity of family structure
- value saturation (individuals overly imbued with values of culture)
- anomie
- minority status

II. Factors counteracting depression

   a. Rituals and beliefs
- religious and mourning rituals
- cathartic strategies (feasts, carnivals, dances)

   b. Extended family system

   c. Status provision
- for aged, postmenopausal women, adolescents

   d. Permissiveness in early childhood training

   e. Lack of inhibition of aggression

III. Factors altering manifestations or determining their choice in depression

   a. Cultural sick role
- sick role for depression may be totally denied
- depression may be acceptable only as somatization
- culturally sanctioned
- exploited

   b. Beliefs
- witchcraft, sexual or somatic complaints, guilt

IV. Factors altering observed prevalence

   a. Differences in :
- community tolerance
- availability of treatment facilities
- somatic problems
- symptom identification
- referral procedures
- assessment techniques

Adapted from Singer, 1975

funding is limited, and until recently, diagnostic criteria have been far from reliable.

It is difficult to sort out constant features of the illness from cultural manifestations and to ascertain whether observed differences (either in rates or symptomatology) are real, secondary to differences in measurement systems, artifactual to cultural differences in tolerance levels for varying types of psychopathology, or due to cultural differences in admission criteria to treatment systems. Cultural habits, languages, and religions vary across geographic regions; so too do gene pools, nutritional standards, light and temperature conditions, and degrees of population inbreeding. The combinations and permutations of psychological, sociological, environmental, and biological variance and their possible influence on psychopathology form a significant obstacle

that is not easily overcome. Moreover, virtually all of the cross-cultural research studies on affective illness have looked at depressive, rather than manic-depressive, illness. It is to these investigations that we must first turn for perspective, recognizing the limitations in extrapolating from unspecified depressive illnesses to bipolar illness.

Singer (1975) has discussed many of the factors involved in the influence of culture on the development, manifestation, and incidence of depression (Table 7-10). Although a number of these factors are less applicable to the more biologically determined bipolar illness, his review does form a good background for a discussion of cross-cultural differences in manic-depressive illness.

Societies vary in types and degrees of accommodation to psychopathology in child-rearing practices (which, in turn, influence the ability of both the culture and the individual to handle the illness), in what is defined as pathological, and in what caretaking obligations are assumed. The role of psychological and environmental stress in precipitating the first and subsequent affective episodes also is far from understood. It is quite possible that cultural influences on the development, manifestation, and handling of stress are more important than is now realized.

Earlier investigators, limited by language differences and primitive psychiatric nosologies, made general, often unqualified, observations about differences in incidence. For example, Kraepelin (1904b) observed an increased incidence of manic illness and a greater incidence of depressive illness in the inhabitants of Java and Singapore than in European subjects. Van Wulfften-Palthe (1936) and Oesterreicher (1951) noted a higher rate of depressive illness in the Chinese population in Java than in the native Javanese, although Tan (1977) has suggested that this difference may be due to the relative urbanization of the Chinese, which contributes to an increased use of mental health facilities. A more recent study by Dunner and colleagues (1984) suggests that when specific diagnostic criteria, such as DSM-III, are used, bipolar disorder in China is similar to that seen in the United States.

One rather unique population study was the Hutterite society, a group living in North America, known for supporting their members from "the cradle to the grave" (Dohrenwend and Dohrenwend, 1974). Among this population, researchers found a very high rate of manic-depressive illness and attributed it to the high degree of communal cohesiveness, with an extreme emphasis on religion and duty to society (Eaton and Weil, 1955). It may well be, however, that other issues (e.g., assortative mating and inbreeding) may be important as well.

Various other cultural investigations of prevalence rates of manic-depressive illness yield differing results. For example, in a sequel to their 1981 investigation of urban blacks, Jones and associates (1983) studied poor urban Hispanics in New York, finding that 11 percent of their sample carried a DSM-III diagnosis of manic-depressive illness, a figure more than three times the United States admission rate.

Figures slightly more consistent with overall rates of manic-depressive illness in Western countries are found in Chinese studies. Zhang and Xu (1980) reported a 2 to 3 percent prevalence of affective disorder in Chinese psychiatric admissions, and Hsia and Zhang (1980), studying almost 60,000 consecutive admissions to a Chinese psychiatric center, identified 1.2 percent of these patients as diagnosed with manic-depressive illness. Neither these nor any other large-scale study of manic-depressive illness using standardized research diagnostic criteria has as yet been undertaken in China. In the most comprehensive Chinese study to date, Shan-Ming and associates (1982), using semi-structured interviews and diagnostic criteria similar to those used in two U.S. studies (Taylor and Abrams, 1975; Feighner et al., 1972), reported an annual prevalence rate of mania of about 3 percent. Although these researchers reported their findings to be consistent with findings of Taylor and Abrams (1973b) in the United States, their figures are more than 14 times that of the period of $3\frac{1}{2}$ years at the same facility prior to this research, demonstrating the worth of standardized diagnostic criteria.

The Amish population studied by Egeland and colleagues (1983) provides yet another cultural comparison. The total number of bipolar and unipolar cases made up 71 percent of the total number of psychiatric cases diagnosed between 1976 and 1980, but this is less than 1 percent of the Amish population, which is half of the normal rate for all urban U.S. populations. Including minor depression, hypomania, and schizoaffective disorder, the rate among the Amish is still only 1.2 percent. The ratio of unipolar/bipolar cases is just greater than 1:1, markedly different from the 10:1 ratio reported by Clayton (1981) in inpatient studies. She suggests, however, that a change will be seen in these figures "as psychiatrists become more astute in recognizing mania and hypomania . . . (which are) probably more common than previously reported."

This sentiment also can be related to the problem of misdiagnosis of schizophrenia, which is seen among minority, primarily lower class, manic-depressive patients and is also prevalent among the Amish. Seventy-nine percent of the bipolar-I subjects in the Amish study had originally been diagnosed as schizophrenic. Egeland and her co-workers (1983) attribute this partially to the cultural differences, the intense religious dedication, and excessive involvement in activities of the members of this community, which physicians might not fully understand.

Perhaps the most quantified cross-cultural studies of the incidence of manic-depressive illness have been carried out in Jewish populations. Few, however, have differentiated bipolar and unipolar illness. Grewel (1967) found manic-depressive illness rates higher in Ashkenazic Jews (born in Europe or the Americas) than in Gentiles, with no differences between Sephardic Jews (born in Asia or Africa) and Gentiles. Miller (1967) found affective psychosis far less common in Sephardic Jews than in Ashkenazic Jews. Gershon and Liebowitz (1975) replicated this study, finding a twofold increase in the rate of affective psychosis in Ashkenazic over Sephardic Jews. However, Halpern (1938) and Hes (1960), in their studies of Jewish subpopulations in Palestine/Israel, did not find the incidence of affective psychosis particularly high among Jews compared to other cultures. Malzberg (1962) found that Jews in New York and Canada were significantly more likely than Gentiles to have manic-depressive psychosis, a finding Cooklin and colleagues (1983) replicated in London.

Gershon and Liebowitz (1975) determined polarity within their affectively ill population and found that 45 percent of their patients in Jerusalem had bipolar illness. They compared these findings with those of Perris (1966), showing that 19 percent of his Swedish affective patients had bipolar illness (figures consistent with those of Bratfos and Haug, 1968, and Asano, 1967). The large bipolar fraction in the Jerusalem study is comparable only to that found by Bazzoui (1970) in Iraq (44 percent).

As is evident even from this brief overview, several discrepancies exist between cultural studies. What might account for these differences? Methodological problems, differences in diagnostic criteria, and language difficulties are obvious sources of variance. So too are differences in referral procedures and community tolerances for psychopathology. Differential availability of psychiatric facilities and differences in symptom presentation, such as somatization (discussed more fully below) may be contributing factors.

The presentation of symptoms also varies from society to society. Most of the studies that looked at such differences were done in a time of unsophisticated diagnostic methods and are, therefore, hard to interpret. However, one finding remains fairly constant from early to recent studies: depressed patients in non-Western and developing societies are much more likely to manifest somatic complaints than are their industrialized counterparts. This tendency to manifest physical symptoms and complaints (analogous to masked depressions), rather than more strictly cognitive and mood dysfunctions, has been noted in African cultures,[23] in Saudi Arabia (Racy, 1980), and in Iraq (Bazzoui, 1970). In a sophisticated World Health Organization study of four developing countries—Colombia, India, the Philippines, Sudan—physical symptoms were the presenting complaint in the majority of depressed patients (Harding et al., 1980).

In a direct cross-cultural comparison of depression in Peru and the United States, Peruvians scored much higher on somatization factors (Mezzich and Raab, 1980). This was true for Colombians in another direct country-to-country comparison with the United States. In this latter study, patients in two American cities—Minneapolis and Memphis—were compared with patients in Bogotá in a double-blind antidepressant protocol. The Hamilton Rating Scale and RDC were used as assessment methods. The Colombians complained more of sexual and physical problems; the Americans scored higher on measures of agitation. French Canadians were found to be more likely than British Canadians to register somatic complaints (Murphy, 1974).

Other cultural differences in depressive symptom patterns include manifestations of guilt and suicide. Kimura (1965) noted that depressed Japanese were more likely than depressed Germans to feel guilt toward their parents, ancestors, and fellow workers. The Germans, however, felt more guilt toward their children and God. Sartorius (1973) observed more guilt in depressed Europeans, Americans, and Arabs and less guilt in Japanese, Africans, and Filipinos. Several investigators found fewer signs of guilt in depressed patients from India than in comparable populations in Britain (Kiloh and Garside, 1963; Carney et al., 1965; Teja et al., 1971). A few authors observed that guilt is rare in depressive individuals from developing countries (Singer, 1975; Sartorius and Jablensky, 1977), but this generalization, like many others, is subject to criticism.

Suicide is also rare in developing countries

(Singer, 1975), although sophisticated research into the question is even rarer. Mezzich and Raab (1980) reported higher suicide rates among Americans than Peruvians, and several researchers have reported low rates of suicidal thought and behavior in African cultures, compared to their Westernized counterparts (e.g., Lambo, 1956; A.H. Leighton et al., 1963; Binite, 1975).

Interesting studies of auxiliary symptoms have been carried out. Murphy (1974), comparing depressed British and French Canadians, found more cognitive complaints among the British Canadians. For example, the British group complained far more frequently of impaired concentration and difficulty in thinking and expressing themselves.

A few general statements about the manifestation of depressive symptoms across cultures can be made. Most recent studies have identified a core depressive syndrome in diverse geographical and cultural areas, regardless of development or socioeconomic or political status.[24] Those signs and symptoms commonly associated with depression in all places are changes in mood, disruptions in physiological functions (sleep, appetite), and changes in energy levels. Those symptoms most likely to vary in frequency and intensity across cultures are guilt, suicide, somatization, and disturbances in cognitive functioning.

This variability has several possible explanations. Increased somatization in nonindustrialized and non-Western cultures, for example Hispanic, has been attributed to stigmatization of the mentally ill by such societies, a lack of psychiatric sophistication, and an attempt to legitimize health-seeking behavior (Escobar et al., 1983). The actual extent and nature of differences in manifestations of guilt are less clear, and the methods for ascertaining guilt and differentiating it from shame have been strongly criticized (Yap, 1965). Intrapsychic phenomena, such as guilt, are more subject to interpretative error than are the more objective and easier to communicate symptoms, such as changes in appetite and sleep, or somatic complaints.

Many explanations for differences in suicidal thought and behavior have been proposed, among them that suicide is a marker for depressive and manic-depressive illness and that a lower rate of suicide in developing countries may represent a true finding, namely, that serious affective illness occurs less frequently in such cultures. However, the lower rate may be an artifact of the reporting system and simply reflect the lack of an efficient civil service or the presence of a strong social disincentive to report suicide (Wittkower and Rin, 1965).

Far less research has been carried out on cross-cultural aspects of mania and bipolar illness than of depression. Although Tan (1977) reports that mania is reported more frequently than depression in non-Western societies, there are few data to substantiate this. Studies of African societies indicate more manic symptoms and shorter affective episodes compared to reports from Western societies, and Bazzoui (1970) has reported that in Iraq paranoia and irritability are far more characteristic than elation in manic episodes.

Cultural variants of mania are cited infrequently in the literature. Matiruku, a Fijian type of periodic insanity, is interesting for both its similarities and dissimilarities to manic-depressive illness. Price and Karim (1978), who have studied Matiruku, suggest that it best corresponds to hypomania. The syndrome is characterized by a short duration (2 days to a week), frequent recurrence (often once a month), pronounced periodicity (every month, or the same time of the year), reversibility, and intensification of symptoms in the morning. Behavioral changes include increased talkativeness and psychomotor activity, elated mood, occasional violence, decreased sleep, and a sense of health, life, freshness, and being "of the wind." There are no perceived advantages of this syndrome, either to the individual or others around him, nor is there progression to a more serious mental disorder.

One of the few direct cross-cultural comparisons of mania was conducted by Leff and colleagues (1976). They compared manic patients in Aarhus, Denmark, with a group in London and found an overrepresentation of West Indian men in the London sample. This finding is similar to that of Hemsi (1967) who reported that West Indian male immigrants to London suburbs were overrepresented among manic individuals 3:1.

Leff and associates (1976) concluded that, "The native-born English manic patients were very similar to the Aarhus patients in terms of social and clinical characteristics. The immigrants in the London sample, however, showed a significantly higher proportion with manic delusions" (p. 436). There were no significant differences in delusional symptomatology between the English and Danish patients. The West Indians were, however, significantly more likely to have delusions of special abilities, of grandiose identity, and of a special mission. All in all, they were far more likely to manifest a delusion of some kind.

The authors suggest two possibilities to explain their findings. First, they hypothesize that there may be a lower threshold for developing delusions among immigrants (non-Westerners), somewhat of a restatement of their findings. They cite Brody's study (1973) of first admissions to hospitals in Rio de Janeiro, which revealed that a much higher proportion of the recent migrants than of the settled reported grandiose delusions or auditory and visual hallucinations. Leff and coworkers (1976) attribute this finding to the possible effects of less education and sophistication. Contradicting this explanation, however, is the common clinical observation of flagrant delusional systems in highly educated and sophisticated manic patients.

Their second explanation is that immigrants may show greater tolerance for disturbed behavior (short of delusions), resulting in the selective admission to hospitals of deluded patients. There may also be a selection factor among manic individuals who choose to immigrate; that is, manic patients may have extra drive, grandiosity, and initiative and may, therefore, be more apt to emigrate.

It will be interesting, as more sophisticated studies are done, to re-examine many of the periodic psychoses (such as amok) in more primitive societies to see what relation they bear to bipolar disorders. We believe that much of what has been labeled "schizophrenia" in non-Western societies will be found to be a form of manic-depressive illness.

Studies of Immigration

Another interesting correlate of epidemiological work is the concentration on the prevalence of mental disorders among immigrants. Rates of manic-depressive illness among immigrants compared to native citizens were first quantifiably studied by Roberts and Myers (1954). They reported that although the percentage of the total psychiatric patients to the general population was comparable in immigrants and natives, the incidence of affective disorders in those who immigrated to the United States was almost twice as great as among natives. This trend appeared to be more specific to immigrants from Italy (18.5 percent) and Poland and Russia (14.4 percent) than those from Ireland (9.8 percent) and northwestern Europe (9.0 percent), but all were greater than the incidence in natives (7.0 percent). Rowitz and Levy (1968) and Gershon and Liebowitz (1975) both reported that immigration (foreign-born) correlates positively and highly with manic-depressive illness, and Malzberg (1964) found an overall higher rate of manic-depressive illness among immigrants compared to natives.

Two studies specifically looked at bipolar–unipolar differences. Pope and colleagues (1983a) reported that bipolar patients and their families have a relatively high rate of immigration, similar to an earlier finding (Astrup et al., 1962). Grove and co-workers (1986) did not replicate this but instead found that the rate of immigration is significantly higher in probands with primary unipolar depression.

Eitinger (1959) points out that the higher incidence of psychoses among immigrants may be due partly to the fact that most of those surveyed (at least in earlier studies) were voluntary emigrants, that is, it was a free choice for them to leave. Westermeyer (1988) mirrored this sentiment, that aversive migration (as opposed to non-aversive migration) has been shown to correlate with an increase in, among others, depression and substance abuse. Eitinger goes on to suggest that these increased rates can be attributed to one or more of the following: (1) a higher incidence of psychosis in the native land of the refugee, (2) the premorbid personality of the refugees, and (3) the mental (and physical) stress during the interval between the uprooting and the outbreak of the disorder. It may also be that impulsivity, high energy, and risk-taking are characteristics common to both emigration and manic-depressive illness.

What accounts for these findings of increased rates of manic-depressive illness remains unclear, but the data do support a foreign–native difference. A comprehensive investigation like the Roberts and Myers (1954) study, but using

Table 7-11. Peak Incidence of Affective Episodes by Month[a]

Study	J	F	M	A	M	J	J	A	S	O	N	D
Kraines,[b] 1957			D						D			
Angst et al.,[b] 1968				AE						AE		
Perris, 1974				AE								
Zung & Green, 1974			D	D								
Eastwood & Peacocke,[c] 1976			D			D	D		D	D	D	
Milstein et al.,[b] 1976		AE	AE		AE							
Symonds & Williams,[d] 1976								M	M			
Sedivec, 1976			AE	AE	AE			AE	AE	AE		
Walter, 1977 males						M	M					
Walter, 1977 females								M	M			
Eastwood & Stiasmy,[e] 1978			D	D	D				D	D	D	
Myers & Davies, 1978 males							M	M				
Myers & Davies, 1978 females					M		M	M				
Frangos et al.,[b] 1980					M,D							
Carney et al., 1988			M				M		M			

D = depressive episode, M = manic episode, AE = affective episode, polarity unspecified

[a]For those studies in which peak seasons rather than specific months were given, we assumed equal monthly incidence as follows: Spring (March, April, May), Summer (June, July, August), Autumn (September, October, November) and Winter (December, January, February)
[b]Peak incidence by date of onset, all other studies are by first hospitalization
[c]Psychotic depression peak in spring, neurotic depression peak in autumn
[d]Females only
[e]Endogenous depression peak in spring (females only), neurotic depression peak in autumn (both sexes)

more standardized diagnostic techniques, may clarify some of the confusion surrounding this issue.

Seasonality

It is disconcerting how few studies have examined seasonal patterns of affective episodes despite its clinical and theoretical importance and despite the fact that seasonal components in depression and mania have been observed for centuries. Certain patterns emerge from an examination of those studies that have looked at seasonal patterns (Table 7-11). Two peaks are evident in seasonal incidence of affective episodes: spring (March, April, May) and autumn (September, October, November). This pattern tends to parallel the seasonal pattern for suicide which shows a large peak in the spring and a smaller one in October (see Chapter 10). The data on mania are scarcer and, therefore, less compelling, but the peak incidences occur in the summer months. Carney and colleagues (1988), who found significant seasonal variation in the prevalence of mania in Ireland (admission rates were higher in sunnier months and in months with greater average day length), suggest that this presentation of mania may result from abnormal response to light in these patients (see Chapter 19).

There are many sources of variance in the collection of seasonality data. For example, hospital admission dates, although likely to be meaningful markers for the onset of manic episodes, are unlikely to reflect the true onset of depressive episodes. In fact, hospitalizations for depressions are more likely to reflect severity or lethality of illness than time of onset. Voluntary admissions and hospital schedules (rotation of physician staff or holidays) also may affect reported seasonal patterns. Despite these methodological problems, the consistency of findings in the seasonality studies of both affective episodes and suicide (see Chapter 10) is impressive. It gains further weight from the fact that virtually all the studies were carried out after the widespread use of lithium had begun, which may have dampened the natural pattern of seasonal variability.

Far more data are available on suicide and seasonality, and dating a suicide is obviously far more accurate than dating the onset of an affective episode. We reviewed more than 20 studies of the peak monthly incidence of suicide. One of these examined data from 16 countries (Takahashi, 1964); another examined data from 4 countries (Bolander, 1972). Two did separate analyses for males and females. As shown in Figure 10-4, we counted these results separately, which resulted in over 40 data points. There is an obvious peak incidence of suicide in May across studies and a second peak in October. These findings are consistent with the peaks for affective episodes. The second suicide peak in October may reflect not only an increase in unipolar depressive episodes but also bipolar depressions following the increase in manic episodes during the summer months (i.e., it may represent suicidal postmanic depressions).

SUMMARY

Epidemiological studies of manic-depressive illness are important to its understanding, treat-

ment, and possible prevention. Methodological problems are numerous and often raise difficult pragmatic and interpretive issues. All recent studies find bipolar illness to be a relatively common disorder, affecting both sexes approximately equally. Differences in rates of manic-depressive illness across cultures, marital status, social classes, and racial groups are less clear. Finally, mania, depression, and suicide all show pronounced seasonal patterns.

NOTES

1. Strictly speaking, biometric surveys and epidemiological studies together provide a sketch of the dimensions of the problem for society and serve as the basis for public health policies that determine allocation of research and treatment resources.
2. As discussed in Chapter 3, the original Kraepelinian synthesis provided for patients who experience recurrent episodes of depression and/or mania to be grouped under manic-depressive illness. The partitioning of this concept by Leonhard, Perris, and Angst led to the view of manic-depressive illness currently accepted throughout Europe that includes bipolar and recurrent unipolar patients. The American version of the bipolar–unipolar distinction is quite different: The unipolar category has become a catchall for all serious affective illness that is not bipolar.
3. The rate of alcoholism remained higher in New York, however, and the overall rate of affective illness was higher in the London sample (44 percent) than in the New York sample (32 percent).
4. Nielsen and Biörn-Henriksen, 1979; Akiskal et al., 1977; Depue et al., 1981; Gagrat and Spiro, 1980; Helgason, 1979.
5. Birtchnell, 1971; Monnelly, 1974; Ödegaard, 1956; Walsh, 1969a.
6. Schou (1968) states that in Denmark, "It is, on the whole, no longer considered a social stigma to have been admitted to a mental hospital," but most societies cannot yet make this claim.
7. Baldessarini, 1970; Kendell, 1975; Krauthammer and Klerman, 1979; Symonds and Williams, 1981.
8. Boyd and Weissman 1981, 1985; Weissman and Boyd, 1984; Weissman et al., 1985.
9. Nielsen and Biörn-Henriksen, 1979; Akiskal et al., 1977; Depue et al., 1981; Helgason, 1979.
10. Bipolar-III disorder, discussed in Chapter 4, is defined as recurrent unipolar depression with a family history of mania or hypomania.
11. The Stirling County study (Hughes et al., 1960; D.C. Leighton et al., 1963), the Baltimore morbidity study (Pasamanick et al., 1957), the Midtown Manhattan study (Srole et al., 1962), and the

Weissman and Myers (1978) study of New Haven, Connecticut.

12. There are several advantages to the ECA program. The integration of community and institutional surveys gives a more accurate reading of the prevalence of mental illness. Its several sites offer the opportunity for cross-site replications and give access to special populations for assessing ethnicity, age, rural–urban differences in rates (Regier et al., 1984). To ensure large enough sample sizes for these subgroup comparisons, some groups were oversampled at particular sites. For example, in St. Louis and Baltimore, blacks were oversampled, whereas older populations were oversampled in both Baltimore and New Haven.

13. These three criteria all share a common heritage, that is, they provide a diagnosis from a descriptive rather than an etiological perspective.

14. Severity is defined as the degree to which the disorder limits activity, whether a physician or other professional had been consulted, or whether medication had been taken (Regier et al., 1984). The DIS has been translated into Spanish and German for use in different parts of the United States as well as in other countries.

15. The reliability and validity of the DIS lay interviews have been tested extensively (e.g., Robins et al., 1981) and challenged (e.g., Anthony et al., 1985). Questions remain about whether it can elicit enough data to diagnose specific disorders accurately. Burke (1986), in a comprehensive review, noted that test–retest and interrater reliability estimates have been the major focus of studies on the DIS, some of them pertaining to affective illness. Relevant findings of Burke's review can be summarized as follows. Test–retest reliability of the DIS has been investigated in five studies, and the results are consistently positive and high. Two that investigated reliability of a diagnosis of a manic episode (using the DIS Spanish version) produced quite different results. Burnam and colleagues (1983) reported a very low kappa coefficient (-0.03) because of a low prevalence of manic episodes, whereas Canino and associates (1987), with a slightly larger prevalence rate, reported a kappa coefficient of 0.43. Eight studies examined differences between DIS and psychiatrists' diagnoses and reported consistently high correlations across clinical samples for Major Depression. Reliability coefficients for community samples were comparable but only when Yule's Y was employed. The data for Manic Episode are very consistent with findings for Major Depression across community and clinical samples (i.e., high kappa coefficients in clinical samples and low kappas in community samples). This rather striking difference, especially with regard to Manic Episode,

may be easily explained. As Burke (1986) points out, in the community samples:

> . . . the pathology may not be so severe or so prototypic as in clinical samples, and the subjects may be harder to interview because there is no presenting complaint. . . . For these reasons, it has been suggested that findings in clinical samples may not carry over to community samples. (p. 260)

Lifetime diagnoses made by the DIS have also been shown to correlate highly with diagnoses of the SADS-L (Hesselbrock et al., 1982; Weissman, personal communication to J. Burke, 1986). This is especially true for Major Depression, but not enough data are available for Manic Episode.

16. Again, Myers and colleagues (1984) and Regier and co-workers (1988a), studying 6-month and 1-month prevalence rates, respectively, broke the 18 to 44 age group down to 18 to 24 and 25 to 44 but found no difference in diagnoses of major depression.

17. Data were not reported for the New Haven site because the longitudinal aspect of design and the questionnaire used were sufficiently different to make comparison of incidence rates very difficult (Eaton et al., 1989).

18. Pollock, 1934; Tietze et al., 1941; Malzberg, 1956; Astrup et al., 1962; Malzberg, 1964; Gershon and Liebowitz, 1975; Weissman and Myers, 1978; Canino et al., 1987; Weissman et al., 1988a; Mezzich et al., 1989. Weissman and Klerman (1977) provide an excellent of review of epidemiological studies of affective illness.

19. Although Landis and Page were writing before lithium treatment, the course of illness at that time may not have been as severe because of the sharp delineation between manic-depressive illness and schizophrenia.

20. Several studies reported finding no significant difference with respect to education level in manic-depressive patients (Jaco, 1960; Woodruff et al., 1968; Monnelly et al., 1974; Gershon and Liebowitz, 1975). Only one study looked at bipolar–unipolar differences with regard to educational achievement (Woodruff et al., 1971b). These authors reported a significantly higher education level for male bipolar patients compared with male unipolar patients.

21. This is based on Hollingshead's Two-Factor Index of Social Position (Hollingshead, 1957).

22. Babcock, 1895; O'Malley, 1914; Green, 1914; and Bevis, 1922.

23. Laubscher, 1951; Tooth, 1950; Carothers, 1953; Lambo, 1956; A.H. Leighton et al., 1963; Binite, 1975.

24. Pfeiffer, 1968; Sartorius and Jablensky, 1977; Mezzich and Raab, 1980; Escobar et al., 1983.

8

Childhood and Adolescence

Once . . . he wrote a poem.
And he called it "Chops",
Because that was the name of his dog, and
    that's what it was all about.
And the teacher gave him an "A"
And a gold star.
And his mother hung it on the kitchen door,
    and read it to all his aunts . . .

Once . . . he wrote another poem.
And he called it "Question Marked Innocence",
Because that was the name of his grief, and
    that's what it was all about.
And the professor gave him an "A"
And a strange and steady look.
And his mother never hung it on the kitchen door
    because he never let her see it . . .

Once, at 3 a.m. . . . he tried another poem . . .
And he called it absolutely nothing, because
    that's what it was all about.
And he gave himself an "A"
And a slash on each damp wrist,
And hung it on the bathroom door because he
    couldn't reach the kitchen.
        —Written by a 15-year-old boy 2 years before he committed suicide[1]

Evidence that manic-depressive illness frequently emerges in adolescence, perhaps even in childhood, has generated increasing interest in the early features of the illness. The clinical presentation of early-onset illness differs from bipolar illness with later onset, as does the patient's experience of it. Diagnosis is difficult, and bipolar illness is frequently mistaken for conduct disorder, schizophrenia, or attention deficit disorder. In this chapter, we discuss manic-depressive illness in childhood and adolescence—its diagnosis, clinical description, subjective experience, predictors of bipolarity, and studies of high-risk children. Several related areas are discussed else-

where. Nonbipolar childhood depression is covered in other books and reviews,[2] natural course and outcome are dealt with in Chapter 6, except for studies specific to prognosis in early- vs late-onset bipolar illness, and treatment issues are discussed in Chapters 21 through 27.

EARLY ONSET

Many patients experience their first episode of manic-depressive illness before the age of 20. As indicated in Table 8-1, most studies find such early onset in 20 to 30 percent of patients. Kraepelin (1921) concluded that the greatest fre-

Table 8-1. Percentage of Bipolar Patients
With Onset of Illness Prior to Age 20

Study	Patients N	Results
Kraepelin, 1921	900 BP & UP	Greatest frequency of initial attacks between ages 15 and 20; 0.4% had first attack prior to age 10
Wertham, 1929	2000 Manic	20% had first hospitalization prior to age 20
Olsen, 1961	450 BP	6.2% had onset between age 13 and 19
Perris, 1968	138 BP	40% had first treatment between age 15 and 25
Winokur et al., 1969	61 BP	34% had first symptoms prior to age 20
Loranger & Levine, 1978	200 BP	33% had first hospitalization before age 25; 20% had onset in adolescence
Zis et al., unpublished data 1981	105 BP	20% had first symptoms prior to age 20
Baron et al., 1983b	142	1st treatment or hospitalization: 28% by 24 years of age; 11% as adolescents; 2% before 15 years of age

quency of first attacks occurs between the ages of 15 and 20 years. This figure is consistent with our analysis of contemporary studies that examine their data in 5-year epochs (see Figure 6-2). Weissman and colleagues (1988c) report a greatly increased rate (14-fold) in the onset of depression before age 13 in children of probands who had an onset before age 20.

Childhood Onset

Although the occurrence of mania and depression in adolescence is well established, early childhood onset remains controversial. Kraepelin found that 0.4 percent of his patients had displayed manic features before the age of 10. Anthony and Scott (1960) reviewed the psychiatric literature from 1884 to 1954 and uncovered only 28 cases of alleged manic episodes in young children. After applying systematic diagnostic criteria (Table 8-2) to these clinical reports, Anthony and Scott dismissed all of the cases as misdiagnosed. In three cases, the age of onset was 11, or late childhood. The authors concluded that

". . . the occurrence of manic-depression in early childhood as a *clinical phenomenon* has yet to be demonstrated," and they criticized the early studies for not following their cases into adulthood to verify the existence of adult bipolar illness. They presented their own case, a child first admitted to a psychiatric hospital when 12 years of age and readmitted at ages 19, 21, and 22. Again, however, the age of onset was at the borderline between late childhood and early adolescence. Weinberg and Brumback (1976) reported several apparent cases of mania in early childhood, but Loranger and Levine (1978) argued, as Anthony and Scott did in the earlier context, that:

. . . they will have made a more convincing case for this [early childhood onset] when such children have been followed up through adolescence and adulthood and then give evidence of bipolar affective illness. (p. 1348)

Prepubertal manic-depressive illness has been reported in several additional isolated case histories,[3] including four cases of rapid-cycling beginning at age 11 or 12. In our review of contemporary studies that included 898 patients (Chapter 6, Figure 6-2), onset was under age 10 in only 3 patients, whereas it was between 10 and 14 in 24 patients (3 percent).

Although the question of early childhood onset remains open, onset in late childhood seems established although uncommon (Coll and Bland, 1979). The issue may be clarified by the ongoing developmental and high-risk studies discussed later in this chapter. Thus, Winokur and colleagues (1969) described onset prior to puberty, and Loranger and Levine (1978) concurred:

. . . as far as mania is concerned, we favor the view expressed almost ten years ago by Winokur et al.: "The data indicate that manic-depressive disease can occur in childhood and probably begin before the onset of menstruation or pubertal changes. Whether it may occur in early childhood is still open to question." (p. 1348)

Kron and colleagues (1982) argue that true bipolar illness, with its biphasic periodicity and elation, is "extremely rare" before the age of 12. No cases of mania or hypomania were found in the studies of juvenile offspring completed by four groups of investigators.[4] Another group (Akiskal et al., 1985b) found that three of ten prepubertal children exhibited hypomanic features, but that full-blown manic psychosis did not appear before

Table 8-2. Anthony-Scott Diagnostic Criteria for Prepubertal Bipolar Manic-Depressive Illness

1. Evidence of an abnormal psychiatric state at some time of the illness approximating to the classical clinical description as given by Kraepelin, Bleuler, Meyer, and others.

2. Evidence of a "positive" family history suggesting a manic-depressive "diathesis."

3. Evidence of an early tendency to a manic-depressive type of reaction as manifested in:
   a. A cyclothymic tendency with gradually increasing amplitude and length of the "oscillations"
   b. Delirious manic or depressive outbursts during pyrexial illnesses.

4. Evidence of a recurrent or periodic illness. This entails the observation of at least two episodes, separated by a period of time (gauged in months or years), and regarded as clinically similar. There should be diagnostic agreement by different clinical judges on the nature of any one episode and diagnostic agreement by different clinical judges on the identity of different episodes.

5. Evidence of a diphasic illness showing swings of pathologic dimension from states of elation to states of depression and vice versa.

6. Evidence of an endogenous illness indicating that the phases of the illness alternate with minimal reference to environmental events.

7. Evidence of a severe illness as indicated by a need for inpatient treatment, heavy sedation, and ECT.

8. Evidence of an abnormal underlying personality of an extroverted type as demonstrated by objective test procedures.

9. An absence of features that might indicate other abnormal conditions such as schizophrenia, organic states (e.g., alcohol delirium).

10. The evidence of current, not retrospective assessments

Adapted from Anthony and Scott, 1960

puberty. The findings are consistent with Carlson's view (1983) that puberty may be a requirement for the onset of mania.

The Role of Puberty

Carlson (1980), investigating the rarity of mania in childhood, studied the interaction between cognitive maturity and manic-depressive illness in a test of a hypothesis advanced by Rutter (1972), Anthony (1975a), and Lester and LaRoche (1978). According to their hypothesis, cognitive and psychodynamic maturity is necessary to sustain and express both mania and severe depression. Carlson compared 19 bipolar children who were chronologically immature (i.e., prepubertal but functioning appropriately for their age) with 21 bipolar adults who were biologically mature but functioning intellectually at a much younger age equivalent (i.e., mentally retarded bipolar).[5] Ten of the children had first episodes of mania, and the other 9 had first episodes of depression; 18 of 19 had family histories of manic-depressive illness or cyclothymia. Carlson

found that affective disturbances in bipolar children are manifested more by irritability and crying than by depressive or elated appearance. It was the older children who were more likely to appear depressed or elated. In depressed children, agitation was present as often as psychomotor retardation, which was found only in the older children. Carlson also found that affective preoccupations were absent in younger children but present in older children and in the mentally retarded bipolar adults. Carlson (1980) concluded:

There seem to be qualitative differences that increasing chronologic age superimposes. These maturational changes seem to occur in the cognitively normal around 8 or 9 years of age, and account for the more "adult-like" affective symptoms of the later latency-age child. In contrast, there is no change in symptom manifestations of [manic-depressive illness] between the moderately and mildly retarded, as one would have predicted if cognitive development alone accounted for the changes.

In summary, this review suggests that immature cognitive functioning affects the content of manic or depressive preoccupations, and possibly the patient's awareness of his mood state; it does not, however, seem to determine the presence or absence of mania and depression, nor does it explain other age-related symptom disparities between young children and adults. . . . it is further felt that other reasons must be sought to explain the relative absence of bipolar [manic-depressive illness] in childhood and its increasing incidence with biologic maturity. (pp. 287-288)

Formal diagnostic criteria for bipolar illness are the same in children, adolescents, and adults. DSM-III-R states that "Because the *essential* features of Affective Disorders . . . are the same in children and adults, there are no special categories corresponding to these disorders" (p. 27).

MANIC-DEPRESSIVE ILLNESS IN ADOLESCENCE

Diagnosis and Clinical Description

Issues in Diagnosis

Difficulty in correctly diagnosing childhood or adolescent manic-depressive illness can be traced to several sources. Although bipolar illness is a relatively frequent diagnosis, many clinicians continue to associate manic-depressive disorders with a later age of onset.[6] Many also wish to avoid psychiatric labeling during adolescence, tend to avoid probing and explicit questioning of adolescents, and fail to inquire sufficiently into the presence of depressive symptomatology (Carlson and Strober, 1979). Likewise, there is a tendency for many child psychiatrists to avoid the use of medications; consequently, they are likely to choose a diagnosis that does not require drug therapy (Bowden and Sarabia, 1980).

The fluid and often tumultuous nature of adolescence confounds the problem of accurate diagnosis. The common assumption of upheaval within this developmental period can mask severe underlying psychopathology. Likewise, the rapidity and intensity of changes in normal adolescents can obscure chaos of a frightening and dangerous level in those with manic-depressive illness. The normal heightening of denial in this age group and sense of adolescent omnipotence also affect communications to a clinician. Carlson and Strober (1979) note other complicating factors:

What, if anything, then, distinguishes the larger group of adolescent manic-depressives from their adult counterparts? Obviously, the psychosocial context in which affective symptoms unfold in adolescents is different. For instance, parents rather than spouses will complain of the profound changes in the patients; school work suffers as concentration becomes impaired; and it is the school that will call increasing withdrawal or frenzied manic behavior to parents' attention. Secondly, the phenomenological content of the teenager's ruminations and/or delusions can merge imperceptibly with such age-appropriate issues as drugs, sex, identity confusion, and struggles with parents. In this regard, factors unique to adolescence may broaden or amplify the young person's illness, coming as it does in a period of major personal, social, and biological change. (p. 516)

Adolescence also is a period marked by many first-time events; the language, contextual, and cognitive systems necessary to comprehend such events generally are primitive and still forming. The signs and symptoms of depression, hypomania, mania, and mixed states may be perceived by such developing systems as just more new, or first, events. The complexity of an adolescent's social and psychological sphere also is relevant to the likelihood of accurate recognition and diagnosis of affective illness. The very fact that an adolescent is usually deeply and complexly enmeshed with disparate social systems—peers, school, family—makes it relatively easy for one part of the system (1) to see only one side or aspect of the problem, (2) to see it in very different and often seemingly explainable ways, and (3) to assume that another part of the social system is aware of, and doing something about, the difficult situation. Further, those most likely to recognize a serious problem—friends, teachers, clergy—may not conceptualize the difficulties as medical or psychiatric, or they may feel bound by confidentiality and pledges of personal loyalty. Several studies have found that children report more psychiatric illness in themselves than their parents report.[7]

Once an adolescent is brought to the attention of a psychologist or psychiatrist, differential diagnosis can be problematic. Several categories of medical and psychiatric disorders create particular confusion (see Chapter 5 for a more comprehensive discussion). Depression often is mistaken for physical disease. Decreased energy levels and lethargy, particularly in a normally active adolescent, can cause such an error. In addition, mood is not always affected, the child may have age-specific problems in communicating moods and other subjective states, and physicians tend to think of depression and manic-depressive illness as illnesses of adulthood.[8]

Hypomania can be misdiagnosed as hyperactivity because of its psychomotor component and cognitive changes, such as distractibility and shortened attention span. Several features of hypomania can aid in differentiating it from hyperactivity: it is more episodic and is characterized by rapid mood swings, a family history positive for affective illness, and episodic hyperactivity (Bowden and Sarabia, 1980). Nieman and Delong (1987), using the Personality Inventory for Children, compared 20 children with mania with 20 children who had attention deficit disorder. The manic children showed significantly greater behavior pathology and overall maladjustment. Their psychopathology manifested itself in psychosis, depression, aggression, excitability, rapid mood swings, hostility, inappropriate affect, and a disregard for the feelings of others.

Bipolar illness in adolescents can also be confused with antisocial personality disorders. The two disorders are marked by overlapping behaviors, such as impulsivity, shoplifting, substance abuse, difficulties with the law, and aggressiveness. Factors that may be useful in differentiating adolescent affective illness from antisocial personality disorder include family history, premorbid personality, and the association, in bipolar patients, of antisocial behavior with elevated or irritable mood, the absence of a disorder of conscience, and a relative lack of peer group influence on behavior (Bowden and Sarabia, 1980). In some individuals, of course, a DSM-III-R Axis-I diagnosis of bipolar manic-depressive illness coexists with an Axis-II diagnosis of antisocial personality disorder. Here, as in most cases where Axis-I and Axis-II diagnoses are present in the same patient, differential diagnosis can be difficult. Pfeffer and Plutchik (1989), in a study of co-morbidity in child psychiatric patients, found that their patients with major depressive disorder (n = 39) were also given DSM-III diagnoses of borderline personality disorder (46 percent), specific developmental disorder (38.5 percent), conduct disorder (28 percent), adjustment disorder (23 percent), anxiety disorder (20.5 percent), and attention deficit disorder (13 percent). Only 7.6 percent of their patients were without a co-diagnosis.

Mixed states can cloud the diagnostic picture.

Most bipolar illness in young adolescents occurs as a mixed state or a rapid-cycling disorder, according to Ryan and Puig-Antich (1986), who recommend considering a diagnosis of a mixed state in depressed adolescents who are notably irritable or angry. They also point out that mixed states often are misdiagnosed as conduct disorders in adolescents who have an affective syndrome with symptoms of extreme irritability and repeated deviant behavior. Mixed states can appear spontaneously or be precipitated by drug or alcohol abuse. Detoxification must precede recognition of affective illness in alcohol abuse. Ryan and Puig-Antich warn that, because tricyclic antidepressants can aggravate mixed states, accurate differential diagnosis is essential.

The importance of alcohol and other drug abuse in the presentation, exacerbation, and treatment of manic-depressive illness is discussed in Chapters 9 and 26. Here we wish to call attention to the fact that, among preadolescent children, alcohol abuse is very closely associated with affective illness. Famularo and colleagues (1985) documented that seven of their ten cases of preadolescent alcohol abuse or dependence were bipolar or cyclothymic, and the remaining three had closely related disorders (major depression with conduct disorder, atypical psychosis, and atypical affective disorder).

Perhaps the major error in the differential diagnosis of manic-depressive illness in adolescents results from the overdiagnosis of schizophrenia. Although no large-scale epidemiological studies have been done, Weiner and Del Gaudio (1976), in a study of 1,300 adolescent patients in Monroe County, New York, found that only 1 patient was diagnosed as manic-depressive; schizophrenia was diagnosed 40 times as frequently. In a more recent study (R.A. Weller et al., 1986), the histories of 157 "severely disturbed" children were reviewed. Almost half of those diagnosed as manic had originally received a different diagnosis. Despite the fact that psychotic features are a well-established part of adolescent manic-depressive illness (Carlson and Strober, 1979; Rosen et al., 1983b), many clinicians continue to believe that thought disorder, grandiosity, and bizarre delusional and hallucinatory phenomena are pathognomonic of schizophrenia. Difficulties often arise in differentiating blunted from depressive affect, thought blocking from depressive affect and from depression-induced latency of response, and schizophrenic from depressive apathy (see Chapter 2 for further discussion). Bipolar illness in adolescents also is commonly misdiagnosed as atypical psychosis (Hsu and Starzynski, 1986). Despite these difficulties in diagnosis, many studies make it clear that adolescent-onset manic-depressive illness can be identified reliably through the use of standardized adult diagnostic criteria, such as the Feighner criteria,[9] the RDC and the Schedule for Affective Disorders and Schizophrenia (SADS),[10] and the DSM-III-R.[11]

Symptoms and Onset of Illness

A comparison of affective symptoms in manic-depressive adolescents and adults (Carlson and Strober, 1979) is summarized in Table 8-3. Carlson and Strober's analysis, which was based on a chart review of nine adolescents and studies

Table 8-3. Comparison of Patients with Various Affective Symptoms in Manic-Depressive Adolescents[a] and Adults[b]

	Adolescents %	Adults %
Depressed Phase		
Dysphoric mood	100	100
Low self-esteem	66	91
Recent poor school performance	83	91[c]
Anhedonia	50	
Fatigue		75
Insomnia		100
Anorexia	50	97
Somatic complaints		66
Suicidal ruminations	83	82
Agitation/irritability	50	75
Psychomotor retardation	83	82
Paranoid delusions	66	75
Auditory hallucinations	50	75
Confusion	66	33
First-rank symptoms		
Manic Phase		
Euphoria	89	90
Irritability	100	100
Distractibility	67	70
Grandiosity	67	100
Insomnia	78	
Hyperactivity	100	100
Hyperverbosity	89	100
Hypersexuality	78	80
Flight of ideas	56	75
Delusions	56	65
Paranoid grandiosity	44	
Auditory hallucinations	33	40
Regressed	56	45
Formal thought disorder	44	70

Missing data: symptom was not examined in that group

[a]N = 9; based on chart review

[b]The corresponding figures are summarized from Winokur et al.,1969, for the depressive phase and Carlson and Goodwin, 1973, for the manic phase

[c]Poor concentration is the corresponding adult item for comparison

Adapted from Carlson and Strober, 1979

of adult bipolar patients (Carlson and Goodwin, 1973; Winokur et al., 1969), revealed a remarkable consistency in symptom frequencies and expression between the groups. Psychotic symptoms during the depressed phase were, however, much more common in the adolescents. This is consistent with results from other investigations showing floridly psychotic symptoms in adolescent manic-depressive illness (Ballenger et al., 1982; Carlson and Strober, 1978), more non-Schneiderian delusions in bipolar-I patients with a younger age at onset (Rosenthal et al., 1980b), and a larger number of different psychotic symptoms associated with an earlier age at onset (Rosen et al., 1983b; McGlashan, 1988). The declining of psychotic symptoms with increasing age is shown diagrammatically in Figure 2-1. Psychotic symptom score and age at onset were negatively correlated, -0.40 ($p < 0.001$) (see Chapter 2). Rosen and associates (1983b) found that bipolar-I patients with an early age of onset not only have more florid psychotic symptoms but also poorer global functioning.[12]

In a study of psychotic symptoms in 58 prepubertal children with major depressive disorder (MDD), W.J. Chambers and colleagues (1982) found that auditory hallucinations were far more common and delusions far less common in their sample than in adolescents or adults studied by other investigators (Table 8-4). They concluded:

1. In prepubertal children with disorders diagnosed systematically and by RDC as MDD, about one-third report psychotic symptoms, primarily hallucinations.
2. The psychotic symptoms reported are similar in form, content, and temporal characteristics to those reported in samples of adults with the same disorder, although the patterns of frequency differ.
3. The precise psychopathologic implications of psychotic symptoms in children with MDD are uncertain, because of the immature cognitive and social development of prepubertal children. (p. 927)

Friedman and associates (1983b) studied depressive symptoms in 26 adolescent and 27 young adult inpatients who met RDC for major depressive disorder (Table 8-5). Although mania and hypomania were specifically ruled out for the current episode, it is illustrative to see the striking similarity between symptoms of depression in the two age groups, as well as the overlap, except in terms of severity, with the findings from Strober's group (Strober et al., 1981). Finally, Carlson and Kashani (1988a) reviewed the pre-

Table 8-4. Characteristics of Psychotic Symptoms in Children, Adolescents, and Adults

Sample Characteristics	Present Findings	Strober et al., 1981	Baker et al., 1971
Patients N	58	40	100
Psychotic symptoms, N(%)	28 (48)	5 (12.5)	
Age range	6-12	12-17	16-76
Mean age	9.3	15.0	45.9
Auditory hallucinations			
N (%)	28 (48)	4 (10)	9 (9)
Affective	20 (34)	4 (10)	
Nonaffective	1 (2)	0	
Themes			
Command	18 (31)	0	
Conversing	2 (3)	0	
Persecution	8 (14)	4 (10)	
Religious	3 (5)	0	
Other verbal	5 (9)	0	
Delusions			
N (%)	4 (7)	5 (12.5)	27 (27)
Depressive	3 (5)	5 (12.5)	16 (16)
Nondepressive	2 (3)	0	14 (14)
Themes			
Sin, guilt	2 (3)	5 (12.5)	
Punishment, persecution	1 (2)	5 (12.5)	
Nihilism	2 (3)	2 (5)	
Somatic themes	0	2 (5)	
Control	1 (2)	0	
Grandiosity	1 (2)	0	

From W.J. Chambers et al., 1982

sentation of depressive symptoms in different age groups: preschool, prepubertal, adolescent, and adult. Those symptoms that increase or decrease with age, show a curvilinear relationship with age, or are independent of it are shown in Table 8-6.

The mode of onset of affective disturbances in the children and younger siblings of manic-depressive patients was studied by Akiskal and colleagues (1985b). The 68 subjects were observed prospectively, within 1 year of the onset of a variety of psychopathological conditions.[13] The authors concluded that bipolar psychosis most often is preceded by depressive episodes and dysthymic–cyclothymic disorders. Consistent with other studies reported earlier, no full-blown manic psychosis occurred before puberty, al-

Table 8-5. Frequency of SADS Items of Depression in Adolescents and Young Adults
with Major Depressive Disorder

	Frequency (%)[a]		
	Current Sample		Strober et al., 1981
Item	Adolescents (N=26) (Mean age = 16.3)	Adults (N=27) (Mean age = 25.8)	Adolescents (N=40) (Mean age = 15.0)
1. Loss of interest or pleasure	100	100[c]	70[d]
2. Discouragement	96	100[c]	50[d]
3. Subjective depressions	92	100	95
4. Suicidal tendencies	92	100	70
5. Negative self-evaluation	92	93[c]	63[d]
6. Diminished concentration	92	85	70
7. Lack of energy	85	74	55[d]
8. Self-reproach	77	81[c]	55
9. Social withdrawal	73	74	78
10. Worrying	69	81[c]	43
11. Nonreactivity of mood	69	74	35[d]
12. Insomnia (any)	58	81	65
initial	62	59[c]	28[d]
middle	27	26	43
terminal	27	37	25
13. Indecisive	58	67	58
14. Loss of appetite	58	63	68
15. Irritability	58	59	38
16. Distinct quality of mood	54	74	50
17. Depressed appearance	54	67[c]	95[d]
18. Weight loss	54	59	50
19. Lack of specific concerns	54	56	58
20. Psychomotor agitation	46	37[c]	10[d]
21. Psychomotor retardation	46	37	18[d]
22. Weight gain	42	44	25
23. Increased appetite	38	26	28
24. Excessive sleep	31	48	28
25. Mood worse in evening	19	30	10
26. Mood worse in morning	15	37	35
27. Bodily concerns	15	33	30
28. Affective hallucinations	15	11	
29. Delusions (guilt, nihilism, sin, or disease)	8	15	
30. Self-pity	4[b]	33	28[d]

[a]Based on primary interviewer's rating of symptom present to at least a mild degree
[b]Chi-square yields $p < 0.05$ compared to current sample of adults
[c]Chi-square yields $p < 0.05$ compared to adolescent sample of Strober et al., 1981
[d]Chi-square yields $p < 0.05$ compared to current sample of adolescents

From Friedman et al., 1983b

though 3 of the 10 prepubertal children had hypomanic features. Mood-incongruent features were seen in 4 of the 11 manic or mixed state patients and in 2 of those having major depressive disorder. These features were present in only 1 patient's subsequent episodes, however. Of the total sample, 32 percent had not yet shown evidence of bipolarity 3 to 4 years after onset.

The following case history, taken from Akiskal and associates (1985b), illustrates the nature of symptoms and onset of illness in one manic-depressive adolescent. The change in polarity from depression to mania appears to have been triggered by tricyclic antidepressant treatment.

Table 8-6. Depressive Signs and Symptoms in Four Age Groups with Major Depression

Sign or Symptom	Preschoolers (N = 9)[a]		Prepubertal Children (N = 95)[b]		Adolescents (N = 92)[b]		Adults (N = 100)[c]		p
	N	(%)	N	(%)	N	(%)	N	(%)	
Increases with age									
Anhedonia	2	(22.2)	63	(66.3)	68	(73.9)	77	(77)	0.003
Worse in morning	0		18	(18.9)	13	(14.1)	46	(46)	0.0000
Hopelessness	0		19	(20)	43	(46.7)	56	(56)	0.0000
Psychomotor retardation	3	(33.3)	27	(28.4)	33	(35.9)	60	(60)	0.000
Definite delusions	0		4	(4.2)	4	(4.3)	16	(16)	0.003
Decreases with age									
Depressed appearance	8	(88.9)	23	(24.2)	15	(16.3)	0		0.0000
Self-esteem	6	(66.7)	60	(63.2)	53	(57.6)	38	(38)	0.002
Somatic complaints	9	(100)	55	(57.9)	45	(48.9)	29	(29)	0.0000
Any hallucinations	0		28	(22)	13	(14.1)	9	(9)	0.0005
Curvilinear relationship with age									
Fatigue	8	(88.9)	62	(65.3)	66	(71.7)	97	(97)	0.0000
Agitation	7	(77.8)	57	(60)	38	(41.3)	67	(67)	0.001
Anorexia	9	(100)	30	(31.6)	33	(35.9)	80	(80)	0.0001
Nonsignificant relationship with age									
Depressed mood	9	(100)	86	(90.5)	81	(88)	100	(100)	0.004
Poor concentration	5	(55.6)	71	(74.7)	73	(79.3)	84	(84)	0.140
Insomnia	9	(100)	57	(60)	58	(63)	71	(71)	0.054
Suicidal ideation	6	(66.7)	48	(50.5)	45	(48.9)	0		0.156
Suicide attempts	0	(0)	24	(25.3)	31	(33.7)	15	(15)	0.010

[a]From Kashani and Carlson, 1987
[b]From Ryan et al., 1987
[c]From Baker et al., 1971

From Carlson and Kashani, 1988a

A 16-year-old girl first came to psychiatric attention because she was found unconscious in a bathtub after having cut both wrists with a razor. During the previous year, she had had repeated pediatric workups because of six-week periods of listlessness, irritability, crying, anergia, oversleeping, menstrual irregularities, and lack of interest in school work and dating. Premorbidly, she had been a quiet, studious girl who got along well with friends and family. She had recently moved and changed schools due to her father's transfer, and did not seem to be adjusting well; however, even before that move, she had experienced short-lived retarded hypersomnic episodes. She was given desipramine hydrochloride, the dosage of which was gradually raised to 100 mg/day, and on the ninth day she began to exhibit decreased need for sleep, a surge of energy and creativity (ie, writing poetry), overconfidence, and rapid speech. Although the dose of medication was decreased, hypomanic symptoms increased to manic intensity, with extreme psychomotor acceleration and delusions of grandeur (ie, "I am the woman poet of all time"). She responded to treatment with lithium carbonate and, in a three-year follow-up, there have been no depressive or manic recurrences; her

menses are now regular. She is currently a fine arts major in a prestigious college. (p. 1000)

Seasonal affective disorder (see Chapters 5 and 19) has been observed in children and adolescents (N.E. Rosenthal et al., 1986a). Indeed, 33 percent of adult patients with seasonal affective disorder report that their illness began before age 19. Another 9 percent state that onset was prior to age 11 (Rosenthal et al., 1984). Although the early-onset syndrome is similar to that found in adults, the symptoms appear to be milder and less well defined.

Predictors of Bipolarity and Prognosis

One of the most important clinical issues arising from the treatment of depressed children and adolescents is the prediction of which individuals will go on to become bipolar and which will remain unipolar depressives. Strober and Carlson (1982) studied prospectively, for 3 to 4 years, 60 adolescents hospitalized for major depressive disorder. Of those 60, 20 percent became bipolar. The mean length of time elapsing between the index hospitalization and the shift in polarity was 28 weeks (standard deviation of 17 weeks, range of 10 to 76 weeks). Bipolarity was predicted by (1) *symptom cluster*—rapid symptom onset, psychomotor retardation, and mood-congruent, psychotic features, (2) *family history*—loading of affective disorder in family pedigree, family history of bipolar illness, and three-generational history (Strober et al., in press), and (3) *pharmacologically induced hypomania*. Psychoticism, as manifested by delusions and/or hallucinations, was experienced by 6 percent of adolescents who remained unipolar but by fully 75 percent of those who subsequently switched into bipolar illness. These findings are consistent with those of Akiskal and colleagues (1983b), who, in their prospective study of adolescent patients, found that psychotic symptoms and hypersomnic–retarded behavior were sensitive and highly specific precursors of switches into mania. Weissman and co-workers (1984b), in a family study of major depression, found that the prevalence of bipolar illness was nearly six times higher in relatives of delusional patients than in relatives of nondelusional patients or controls (see Chapter 11).

Strober and Carlson (1982) hypothesize that the increased incidence of psychotic symptoms in their adolescent population reflects the existence of a "continuously distributed gradient of vulnerability underlying all forms of major affective disorder, wherein bipolar illness reflects the phenotypic outcome of a more extreme or deviant point on the liability curve" (p. 554). They further assume that the age at onset is under at least partial genetic control, that early onset reflects even greater liability from the combined effects of the genetic load and adverse environment.

Although Carlson (1983) was unable to determine any particular personality patterns that seemed to predispose to bipolar manic-depressive illness, SADS intake interviews showed that unipolar patients (when depressed) were far more likely than their depressed bipolar counterparts to be rated as irritable, self-pitying, and demanding (Strober and Carlson, 1982). Issues relating to personality and manic-depressive illness are discussed more fully in Chapter 12.

Comparisons of Early- and Late-Onset Illness

It might be expected that the prognosis for individuals with adolescent-onset affective illness would be poorer than it is for those with a later age of onset, but this prediction is not supported by the data available. Studies comparing late onset (above 30) with more typical onset (under 30) found no relationship to prognosis (Winokur et al., 1969; Coryell and Norten, 1980; Taylor and Abrams, 1981a), although Taylor and Abrams did report that the early-onset patients made more errors on an aphasia screening test and had more nondominant temporoparietal errors (see Chapter 11). They suggested that early-onset illness may be a more severely expressed form of the disorder.

More to the point are comparisons of early onset with later onset. Carlson and colleagues (1977) compared 28 patients who had their first affective episode before the age of 20 with 20 patients with onset after age 45. There were no significant differences between the two groups in sex distribution, type of episode at onset, distribution of episodes, number of episodes per year, divorce rates, educational achievement, and overall functioning (school, job, family, social interactions). They concluded:

. . . having the onset of a major affective episode in adolescence determines neither the severity of the illness nor its course. . . . Although one might hypothesize that having a first episode of mania or depression in late childhood or adolescence could predispose patients to a poorer outcome by virtue of their having been afflicted at an earlier and more critical time or having had a longer duration and therefore more episodes of illness, most of our data suggest that early age of onset has little measurable impact on outcome. (p. 921)

Carlson and Strober (1979) summarized their clinical impressions about the impact of manic-depressive illness on the formative years of adolescence:

Most impressive is the degree of growth and maturity shown by most of these patients in spite of their often devastating episodes of illness. In other words, we feel that with alleviation of affective episodes and some additional therapeutic intervention (though the effect of the latter is difficult to document systematically), most adolescent manic-depressives are not hindered developmentally and during their euthymic periods remain undistinguishable from their peers who are not affectively disturbed. (p. 518)

It should be noted, however, that Strober and colleagues (1988) did find that bipolar patients with prepubertal onset were significantly less likely to respond well to lithium treatment. A long-term (15-year) follow-up study of 35 adolescent-onset patients in a private psychiatric hospital found that their outcome was as good as, if not better than, that of 31 adult-onset patients (McGlashan, 1988).

Campbell (1953), three decades earlier, described a tendency for manic-depressive children and adolescents to want to "get on with it," to try and catch up quickly for that which they had missed, and to forgo further dwelling on their problems:

Furthermore, it was also conspicuous throughout this series that the patients seemed utterly incapable of self-analysis. They were co-operative, but notably not introspective. Like adult manic-depressive patients, any attempt to arouse insight in them only seemed to bore these young patients. Speaking to them about possible dynamic factors, these patients usually responded thus: "Yes, but what I want to do is get well." (p. 201)

The following description of an adolescent depressive episode was written by a 17-year-old girl who went on to experience several further depressive and hypomanic episodes before becoming floridly manic in her 20s. This passage depicts the resilient recovery described by Carlson and Strober (1979). It also underscores the disconcerting ability of some manic-depressive adolescents to continue the illusion of normal functioning even though severely ill. Additionally, the passage illustrates many of the obscuring issues of adolescence and the effects of intense peer loyalties.

I was 17 and it was autumn—a wonderfully intense season full of life, friends, sports, desires, and controlled uncertainty about the future. And, then one day, although the days were shorter they seemed interminably longer. I awoke deeply tired, a feeling as foreign to my natural self as being bored or indifferent to life. Those were next. Then a gray, bleak preoccupation with death, dying, decaying, that everything was born but to die, best to die now and save the pain while waiting. I dragged exhausted mind and body around a local cemetery, obsessed with how long each of its inhabitants had lived before the final moment. I sat on the graves writing long, dreary, morbid poems, convinced that my brain and body were rotting, that everyone knew and no one would say. Laced into the exhaustion were periods of frenetic and horrible restlessness;

no amount of running brought relief. I started drinking vodka in my orange juice before setting off for school in the mornings and I thought often of killing myself. It was a tribute to my ability to present an image so at variance with what I felt that few noticed I was in any way different. Certainly no one in my family did. Two friends were concerned but I swore them to secrecy when they asked to talk with my parents. One teacher noticed and the parent of a friend called me aside to ask if something was wrong. I lied readily: Fine, but thank you for asking.

Anyway, it was a time in life for all of us for death, for existential readings, ennui, and giving testament to the absurd and futile nature of life. My friends were attracted to these dark edges of bleakness and despair—as it were to the small liberating doses of it standing in sharp contrast to their otherwise normal and vital lives. I was, in fact, actually on the edge. But I got well and made up for the lost months quickly, although never quite completely. My previously grim and despairing thoughts became distant and finally unimaginable.

Looking back I am amazed I survived, that I survived on my own, and that high school contained such complicated life and palpable death. I aged rapidly during those months, as one must with such loss of one's self, with such proximity to death, and such distance from shelter. (Author's files)

HIGH-RISK STUDIES

Studying children of manic-depressive parents offers the rare opportunity to follow the development of the illness prospectively over many years. Because the illness is genetic, having a manic-depressive parent confers a much greater likelihood of inheriting a vulnerability to the illness than is found in the general population. This fact makes prospective research feasible, so that future patients can be observed while they go through infancy, childhood, and adolescence and then enter adulthood. The genetic penetrance is only partial, however, and the so-called high-risk research strategy can be used to tease out relative and different contributions of genetic and environmental factors. Early, premorbid signs and symptoms of affective illness can be detected, early phases and natural course of the illness can be charted, and early diagnostic and treatment strategies can be developed. As discussed in Chapter 15, high-risk studies also provide one approach to evaluating genetically relevant markers for manic-depressive illness.[14]

Childhood psychopathology can derive from inherited vulnerability from one or both parents, contagion or modeling of abnormal mood patterns or other pathologies, or unstable and inadequate parenting. In this section, we focus on research findings—social, personality, cognitive, and diagnostic—from studies of high-risk children. Interpersonal aspects of manic-depressive illness, and parenting behavior of individuals who have bipolar illness are discussed at length in Chapter 12.

High-risk studies are, unfortunately, especially prone to methodological difficulties in conception and execution. Control of parental and family variables is a particular problem. Sources of error and variance include the heterogeneity or nonspecification of parental diagnosis (bipolar I, bipolar II, unipolar), intactness and stability of parental marriage, nature, duration, and treatment responsiveness of parental illness (potentially affecting both genetic vulnerability and the environment of the high-risk child), heritability of type, severity, and age of onset of parental illness, compensatory genetic and environmental factors, parental role of ill parent, whether father or mother, perinatal and nutritional effects if mother is the ill parent, socioeconomic status, number of other siblings, and number and influence of other affectively ill family members. The role of other types of parental psychopathology (e.g., substance abuse or personality disorders) remains virtually unexamined in bipolar high-risk studies, underscoring the need for systematic observations not only of children but of parents as well. Finally, the important and common pattern of assortative mating in individuals with affective illness (see Chapter 15) presents further issues of interpretation.

A lack of adequate comparison or control groups is another frequent problem in the high-risk literature. Ideally, in the comparison group, affective illness (especially bipolar) should be ruled out not only in the parents but also in other first- and second-degree relatives. In addition to controlling for demographic characteristics of both parents and children, it is important to control for nonspecific effects of having a chronic illness. Here, a desirable but infrequently used paradigm is to study children of parents with chronic medical illnesses.

General measurement issues obtain as well. Raters of children's behavior and those who make the diagnosis are not always blind to the diagnoses of the parents. The children often are assessed indirectly (i.e., interview with parents and teachers), interview schedules and behavior-rating scales are not standardized, seasonal factors are not taken into account, and diagnostic measures are inconsistent and range widely.

Additionally, most high-risk studies involve a very small sample size and little or no follow-up into adulthood. At a more basic conceptual level, it is rare for a study to present specific hypotheses about types of behavior and psychopathology that might be expected in high-risk children. In one exception to this common failing, Klein and colleagues (1985) predicted a disproportionate rate of cyclothymia in offspring of bipolar patients. The hypothesis, which was verified, was based on the high rate of cyclothymia in manic-depressive families, the cyclothymic nature of the patients' premorbid personality, the increased rate of bipolar illness in their families, the association of cyclothymia with an increased risk for developing bipolar illness, and cyclothymia's place on the manic-depressive spectrum.

Finally, the value of high-risk studies in characterizing the natural development of an illness is compromised by ethical imperatives. When an effective treatment is available, investigators are ethically bound to intervene with children (and parents) who appear to be going into a manic or depressive episode.

Personality and Social Findings from High-Risk Studies

Twelve studies produced findings on personality and social factors; they are summarized in Table 8-7. Certain personality characteristics, especially increased aggressiveness, appear to be associated with the high-risk children (Worland et al., 1979; Kron et al., 1982). Obsessionality, linked to bipolar illness in some studies of adults (see Chapter 12), was correlated with cyclothymia in Klein and Depue's investigation (1985). Kron and colleagues (1982) found that approximately one third (32 percent) of their high-risk children could be classified as extraverted, another one third (29 percent) as introverted, and one-fifth (19 percent) as impulsive. Affective expression, as assessed by proportionately greater color to movement response on the Rorschach, was much higher in the high-risk children than in the control group ($p < 0.005$).

Table 8-7. High-Risk Studies: Personality and Social Findings

Study	High-Risk Parents	High-Risk Children	Comparison Parents	Comparison Children	Measures	Results
O'Connell et al., 1979	4 BP I Fa 8 BP I Mo	13 M 9 F X̄ age: 11.5 range: 6-17			Clinical interview and observations, Children's Psychiatric Rating, Clinical Global Impression Scales	10 HRC had separation anxiety and denial; 12 nonsymptomatic HRC were preoccupied with health of family.
Worland et al., 1979	7 MD Fa 11 MD Mo (8 BP, 10 UP)	23 M 30 F X̄ age: 10.2 range: 6-20	13 SCZ Fa 17 SCZ Mo 9 PI Fa 10 PI Mo 38 normal	51 M 43 F X̄ age: 9.5 30 M 43 F X̄ age: 9.1 63 M 56 F X̄ age: 9.2	WISC, Rorschach, TAT, Draw-a-Person, Beery-Buktenica Developmental Form Sequence	HRC significantly more aggressive than CSCZ, CPI, & CN. TAT protocols of HRC showed negative affect, destructive coping, and negative interactions
Kuyler et al., 1980	27 BP (7 UP spouses)	27 M X̄ age: 13.7 22 F X̄ age: 13.4 range: 6-18			Structured parental interview	If both parents ill: HRC more likely to be irritable, show decline in school work, have "dyssocial" behavior with peers, are better able to plan ahead and take good care of possessions
Kron et al., 1982 & Decina et al., 1983	11 BP I 7 BP II	14 M X̄ age: 10.5 17 F X̄ age: 11.4 range: 7-14	Neg history of AD in 1st deg or BP in 2nd deg relatives	9 M X̄ age: 11.4 9 F X̄ age: 11.3 range: 9-14 Matched for sex, age, SES	Semistructured interview, Global Assessment Score, WISC-R, Motoric Lateralization Questionnaire, RDC/DSM III, Rorschach	HRC > CC (p<.05): overactivity, attractiveness, aggressiveness, HRC more likely to have more interests Personality patterns of HRC: extroverted 32% inhibited 29% impulsive: 19% Affective expression (Rorschach color > movement in response) HRC 48% CC 5% (p<.005)
Gaensbauer et al., 1984	3 BP Fa 4 BP Mo (5 UP spouses) in remission	7 M	Normal	7 M Matched for age, SES, race	Riccutti measures of affiliative behavior, Ainsworth ratings of attachment, NIMH ratings of modulation of emotional expression Tested at age 12, 15, and 18 mo	HRC show disturbance in quality of emotional attachments at 2 yr, greater avoidance/withdrawal from mothers, and generalized disturbance in regulating emotions. Severity of disturbance increases with age
Zahn-Waxler et al., 1984a	3 BP Fa 4 BP Mo in remission	7 M age 2	No history of AD	10 M 10 F Matched for age, SES, race, parental age	Structured observations in novel, neutral, affectionate, or hostile environments	HRC show heightened distress and preoccupation with conflicts and suffering of adults, difficulty with friendly social interactions and increased and inappropriate hostility

Study	Index group	Index group ages	Comparison group	Comparison ages	Measures	Findings
Zahn-Waxler et al., 1984b (same sample as above)	3 BP Fa, 4 BP Mo (5 UP spouses)	7 M, age 2	No history of AD	10 M, 10 F, Matched for age, SES, race, parental age	Object relations measures: Agent Use, Self-awareness, Object permanence, Interpersonal Scales. Tested at age 12-14, 18, 24 and 30 mo	HRC impaired in interpersonal object relations of role-taking abilities and attachment
Klein & Depue 1985 & Klein et al., 1986a	12 BP Fa, 14 BP Mo, $\bar{x}$ age: 48.5	21 M, 20 F, $\bar{x}$ age: 17.95, range: 15-21	5 Fa, 10 Mo, $\bar{x}$ age: 46.7 NonAD; 6 Fa, 8 Mo, $\bar{x}$ age: 45.1 normal	13 M, 10 F, $\bar{x}$ age: 17.96; 16 M, 10 F, $\bar{x}$ age: 17.65	Life Activities Inventory, General Behavior Inventory, DSM III	HRC not significantly different from CC on social adjustment; however, CYC offspring had poorer social adjustment than nonCYC CC (p<.001)
Pellegrini et al., 1986	16 BP I	11 M, 12 F, range: 7-18	19 normal	16 M, 17 F, range: 7-18	WISC-R, WAIS-R, Means-Ends Problem Solving Test, Locus of Control, Harter's Perceived Competence Scale, Social Network Structure and Support	Low level of perceived social support associated with psychiatric disorder in HRC and CC. Nondisordered HRC had better profile of personal resources than disordered HRC. Absence of best friend associated with AD for both groups
Hammen et al., 1987	9 BP Mo; 13 UP Mo	5 M, $\bar{x}$ age: 13.6; 7 F, $\bar{x}$ age: 13.0; 10 M, $\bar{x}$ age: 13.5; 9 F, $\bar{x}$ age: 12.3	14 PI Mo; 22 normal Mo	9 M, $\bar{x}$ age: 12.8; 9 F, $\bar{x}$ age: 12.9; 18 M, $\bar{x}$ age: 12.6; 17 F, $\bar{x}$ age: 10.6	SADS-L, Beck Depression Inventory, Children's Depression Inventory, Child Behavior Checklist, school and teacher ratings	Children of UP Mo had poorest psychological functioning (social competence, behavioral problems)
Zahn-Waxler et al., 1988 (follow-up of Zahn-Waxler et al., 1984a,b)	3 BP Fa, 4 BP Mo (5 UP spouses)	7 M, 5-6 yr		12 M, Matched for age, sex, race	Child Assessment Schedule, Achenbach Child Behavior Checklist, DSM-III	HRC had more difficulties with empathy, insight, establishment of relationships, and regulation of affect, fewer self-image problems and generated more problem-solving strategies than CC

Fa = fathers, Mo = mothers, PI = physically ill, CSCZ = children of schizophrenic parents, CPI = children of physically ill parents, CN = children of normal parents, HRC = high-risk children, CC = comparison children, AD = affective disorder, CYC = cyclothymia

Mean age reported in years

The most in-depth studies of interpersonal and social behavior in children at risk for manic-depressive illness have been conducted by Zahn-Waxler and colleagues at the NIMH.[15] Unfortunately, they are flawed by small sample size (n = 7) and an extremely high rate of unipolar affective illness in the nonbipolar spouses (5 of 7). The detailed observations and follow-up design of these investigations make them important, however. By the end of the first year and during the second year of life, these high-risk children had significant psychological problems, such as disturbed regulation of emotion, especially hostility, which increased with age. The children also had trouble with empathy and emotional attachments and were overconcerned with the suffering of adults. A 4-year follow-up investigation of the same group of children, at ages 5 and 6 (Zahn-Waxler et al., 1988), found a continuation of these earlier behavior and emotional patterns.

Problems in interpersonal relationships were also more frequently found in high-risk children with cyclothymia (Klein et al., 1986a) and affective or other psychiatric disorders (Pellegrini et al., 1986). Children who were not disordered, on the other hand, were as likely as control children to have good, even superior, relationships with others. In fact, high-risk children demonstrated assets in several of the studies: an ability to plan ahead and take good care of possessions (Kuyler et al., 1980), a greater number of interests and more involvement in hobbies and other activities (Kron et al., 1982), fewer self-image problems, an ability to generate more problem-solving strategies (Zahn-Waxler et al., 1988), and greater emotional expressiveness (Kron et al., 1982).

Cognitive Findings from High-Risk Studies

Table 8-8 summarizes cognitive studies of high-risk children. They showed no differences from control children on measures of object permanence (Zahn-Waxler et al., 1984b), developmental sequences (Zahn-Waxler et al., 1984b), or perceptual–analytic ability (Worland, 1979). Consistent with findings from cognitive studies of adult manic-depressive patients (see Chapter 11), Kestenbaum (1979) found that high-risk children performed as well as control subjects on the verbal portion of the WISC but did markedly less well on the performance subtests. Kron and colleagues (1982) reported a similar and signifi-

cant verbal performance discrepancy in their high-risk sample; the discrepancy, associated with right hemisphere impairment (see Chapter 11), was greatest in the offspring of bipolar-I parents and next greatest in bipolar-II offspring compared with controls. Of the high-risk children, the extroverted subgroup was the most likely to show this cognitive pattern. The possibility that this discrepancy might be a trait marker is discussed, along with other interpretations, in Chapter 11. Kron and colleagues further describe an overproduction of "florid fantasy" in the high-risk children.

Harvey and associates (1982) compared speech production in the offspring of bipolar, unipolar, schizophrenic, and normal individuals. They found that verbal productivity was greater in bipolar offspring than in other groups. Cohesion of speech was similar in bipolar and normal offspring and higher in these groups than in unipolar or schizophrenic offspring. A similar pattern, but in the opposite direction, held for total speech deviance and ambiguity of reference. The authors concluded:

The children of unipolars were more deviant than the children of manics and nearly as deviant as children of schizophrenics. . . . the deviant speech of these children is consistent with the results of laboratory investigations of their cognitive and attentional deficits (e.g., Winters et al., 1981) and their low social competence as judged by both teachers and peers (Emery, Weintraub, and Neale, 1982). (Harvey et al., 1982, p. 386)

Diagnostic Findings from High-Risk Studies

Diagnostic findings from the high-risk studies are presented in Table 8-9. In studies where no comparison groups were used, there was a wide range of diagnostic results. O'Connell and colleagues (1979), for example, found that 45 percent of their high-risk children had significant psychopathological symptoms, whereas LaRoche and associates (1981) found that only 6 percent of their high-risk children (mean age approximately 10 years) were disturbed enough to be referred for treatment. Fifty-five percent of the children in the study of Kuyler and colleagues (1980), who had a mean age of approximately 14, showed significant psychopathology. On the other hand, Waters and co-workers (1983b) found that 32 percent of their high-risk children met diagnostic criteria for major affective disorder; more disturbing is the fact that two of the children, both male, had committed suicide. These researchers also found that although bipolar high-risk children were equally likely to be male or female, a unipolar diagnosis was much more likely to be held by a female. Age clearly affected the rate and nature of presenting symptoms. Waters and associates (1983b) observed that no children in the age range of 6 to 15 years met the diagnostic criteria for primary affective disorder, but more than one third (37.5 percent) of those 16 years and older did. Likewise, Kuyler's group noted that of the few children who were diagnosed as having depressive disorder, all were at least 13 years old and had two ill parents. Somatic and cognitive symptoms characterized the younger children, whereas motivational symptoms were more characteristic of the older age group. McKnew and colleagues (1979) reported that 53 percent of their high-risk children were depressed at one or both of two interviews spaced at 4-month intervals, and Kestenbaum (1979) found that 38 percent of their high-risk children had depressed mood or a learning problem in conjunction with a depressed mood (38 percent). Of the 22 children interviewed by O'Connell and colleagues (1979), 8 boys and 2 girls were reported symptomatic by parents; most common were symptoms of manifest anxiety, although 3 children became overtly depressed and made suicide attempts.

For reasons discussed earlier in this section, the more meaningful rates of psychopathology in high-risk children come from studies that use comparison groups. Kron and colleagues (1982), comparing 31 high-risk children with 18 offspring from parents with no family history of affective disorder, found rates of depressive disorder of 25 percent in the high-risk group and 6 percent in the controls. More than half (52 percent) of the high-risk children received an RDC/DSM-III diagnosis of any kind, compared with 6 percent of the comparison group. Additionally, the authors speculate that of the personality subtypes in the high-risk children (see Table 8-7), the cyclothymic children are most likely to become bipolar, the inhibited most likely to become depressive, and the impulsive most likely to become sociopathic or alcoholic.

Comparably elevated rates of psychopathology were found in two other high-risk studies (Klein et al., 1985; Zahn-Waxler et al., 1988). Klein's group found a much higher rate of psychiatric disorders in the high-risk children than in the comparison children from parents who had nonaffective psychiatric problems (43 percent and 18 percent, respectively). Affective diagnoses, in particular, were far more common in the high-risk children (38 percent) than in the comparison group (5 percent). Of the high-risk children, 24 percent had cyclothymia and 27 percent bipolar disorders, whereas in the control children none had either diagnosis. There was no significant difference between the groups in the rate of nonaffective disorders. Zahn-Waxler and colleagues (1988) reported that 43 percent of their high-risk children met criteria for depression, conduct disorder, or overanxiety; none of the comparison group did.

An excellent study reported by Grigoroiu-Serbănescu and colleagues (1989) found an overall rate of psychopathology in 61 percent of their high-risk children compared with a rate of 25 percent in their control children. The high-risk children were significantly more likely to meet diagnostic criteria for nonbipolar depressive disorders, anxious disorders, attention deficit disorders with hyperactivity, and personality disorders. The severity of psychopathology in the children was significantly correlated with the severity of the illness of the bipolar parent, the presence of psychopathology in the nonbipolar parent, number of mixed and manic (but not depressive) episodes in the bipolar parent, and the age of onset of the parent's bipolar illness.

Two groups of investigators used offspring of unipolar parents as a comparison group (Conners et al., 1979; Hammen et al., 1987), and both found that the children of unipolar parents showed higher rates of psychopathology than did children of bipolar parents. This is consistent with the research on speech pathology (Harvey et al., 1982) reported earlier. Conners and associates comment that:

Unipolars may represent a vulnerable group characterized by an anxious-reactive response system, whereas bipolars become symptomatic only when some genetic variable becomes operative after adolescence. (p. 607)

Cyclothymia in adolescence was found to occur early, between 12 and 14 years of age, in three studies (Klein et al., 1985; Akiskal et al., 1985b; Depue et al., 1981). The mean age of onset in the Klein study was 12.4 years. In all cases, the hy-

Table 8-8. High-Risk Studies: Cognitive Findings

Study	High-Risk Parents	High-Risk Children	Comparison Parents	Comparison Children	Measures	Results
Kestenbaum, 1979	Not specified	13 M			Clinical report, WISC	Verbal > Performance in 6 of 9 children tested
Worland, 1979	7 MD Fa 11 MD Mo (8 BP, 10 UP)	51	13 SCZ Fa 17 SCZ Mo 48 PI normal All children between 6 and 20 yr	79 59 116	Rorschach, WISC	Perceptual-analytic ability: HRC = CPI = CN > CSCZ
Worland et al., 1979	7 MD Fa 11 MD Mo	23 M 30 F $\bar{X}$ age: 10.2 range:6-20	13 SCZ Fa 17 SCZ Mo 9 PI Fa 10 PI Mo 38 normal	51 M 43 F $\bar{X}$ age: 9.5 30 M 43 F $\bar{X}$ age: 9.1 63 M 56 F $\bar{X}$ age: 9.2	WISC, Rorschach, TAT, Draw-A-Person, Beery-Buktenica Developmental Form Sequence	No significant differences
Harvey et al., 1982	27 BP 30 UP	18 M 20 F $\bar{X}$ age: 14.2 22 M 21 F $\bar{X}$ age: 13.3 range: 7-18	16 SCZ 42 normal	12 M 11 F $\bar{X}$ age: 13.3 25 M 28 F $\bar{X}$ age: 14.2 range: 7-18	Rochester & Martin Method for Evaluation of Speech	Verbal Productivity: CBP > CN > CUP > CSCZ Cohesion of speech: CBP = CN > CUP > CSCZ Ambiguity of reference: addition of nonexistent referent: CSCZ > CUP > CBP > CN Total speech deviance: CSCZ > CUP > CBP > CN

Study	Index parents	Control criteria	HR offspring	Comparison offspring	Measures	Results
Kron et al., 1982	11 BP I 7 BP II	Neg history for AD in 1st deg or BP in 2nd deg relatives	14 M X̄ age: 10.5 17 F X̄ age: 11.4	9 M X̄ age: 11.4 9 F X̄ age: 11.3	Semi-structured interview, Global Assessment Scale, WISC-R, Motoric Lateralization Questionnaire, RDC/DSM III, Rorschach	Lefthanded: 29% HRC vs. 6% CC ($p < .05$), Verbal IQ: NC, Performance IQ: CC > HRC ($p < .05$) Verbal > Performance discrepancy $\geq$ 15 points 39% HRC vs. 11% CC ($p < .05$) BP I > BP II offspring greater in extroverted subgroup. HRC > CC: distractability, overproduction of "florid fantasy"
Waters et al., 1983b	17 BP		24 M 29 F		SADS-L, Educational & occupational history, Medical history	Educational problems: • not associated with enhanced risk to AD • significantly associated with earlier onset of disorder
Zahn-Waxler et al., 1984b	3 BP Fa 4 BP Mo (5 UP spouses)	No history of AD	7 M tested at 12-14 mo, 18, 24 & 30 mo	10 M 10 F matched for age, SES, race, parental age	Object relations measures: Agent Use Scale (Watson & Fisher), Self-Awareness (Bertenthal & Fisher) Object Permanence (Uzgiris-Hunt) Interpersonal (Ainsworth)	No significant differences

Fa = fathers, Mo = mothers, PI = physically ill, CPI = children of physically ill parents, CN = children of normal parents, CBP = children of bipolar parents, CUP = children of unipolar parents, HRC = high-risk children, CC = comparison children, AD = affective disorder CSCZ = children of schizophrenic parents, CSP = children of schizophrenic parents, CC = comparison children, AD = affective disorder

Mean age reported in years

Table 8-9. High-Risk Studies: Diagnostic and Clinical Findings

Study	High-Risk		Comparison		Measures	Results
	Parents	Children	Parents	Children		
Conners et al., 1979	9 Fa 50 Mo (16 BP, 43 UP)	63 M 63 F $\bar{x}$ age: 12 range: 1-18			Conners' Parent Questionnaire	CUP > CBP: conduct problems, anxiety, impulsivity-hyperactivity CBP vs CUP: (NS) learning problems, psychosomatic, perfectionism, antisocial, muscle tension
Kestenbaum, 1979	Not specified	13			Clinical report	Of 13 HRC: • 38% learning problems with depressed mood • 8% hyperactive with behavior problems • 38% depressed mood • 15% behavior problem
McKnew et al., 1979	14 BP or UP	14 M $\bar{x}$ age: 9.9 range: 6-15 16 F $\bar{x}$ age: 10.5 range: 5-15			Structured interviews at two 4 month intervals, Conners' Parent Questionnaire, Children's Personal Data Inventory	77% of HRC were depressed at one or both interviews, 47% at one only, 30% at both. Boys had greater correlation for depression on both interviews
O'Connell et al., 1979	4 BP I Fa 8 BP I Mo (all lithium responders)	13 M 9 F $\bar{x}$ age: 11.5 range: 6-17			Clinical interview and observations, Children's Psychiatric Rating Scale, Clinical Global Impression Scale	The 10 symptomatic HRC met DSM-II criteria for various behavior disorders, 2 for depression (3 suicide attempts), and none for manic-depression
Worland et al., 1979	7 MD Fa 11 MD Mo (8 BP, 10 UP)	23 M 30 F $\bar{x}$ age: 10.2 range: 6-20	13 SCZ Fa 17 SCZ Mo 9 PI Fa 10 PI Mo 38 normal	51 M 43 F $\bar{x}$ age: 9.5 30 M 43 F $\bar{x}$ age: 9.1 63 M 56 F $\bar{x}$ age: 9.2 range: 6-20	WISC, Rorschach, TAT, Draw-A-Person, Beery-Buktenica Developmental Form Sequence	General Psychopathology Factor: HRC & CSCZ > CPI & CN

Study	Diagnosis	Subjects	Controls	Measures	Results
Kuyler et al., 1980	27 BP	27 M X̄ age: 13.7 22 F X̄ age: 13.4 range: 6-18		Structured parental interview	55% had significant psychopathology, 37% had symptoms related to personality disorder, adjustment reactions, and AD, 8% had depressive disorder; all were at least 13 yrs old and had 2 ill parents. Children < 12 have more somatic and cognitive symptoms. Children > 12 have more motivational symptoms. Children in BP I, BP II, BP III had comparable rates of illness
Waters & Marchenko-Bouer, 1980	8 BP Fa 8 BP Mo	22 M X̄ age: 27.0 26 F X̄ age: 26.3		Cattell 16 Personality Factors Inventory	42% of daughters and 13% of the sons had primary affective disorder. 1st symptoms were 5-10 years before study. 2 sons committed suicide prior to study
Apter et al., 1981	BP and UP, % BP Fa/Mo not specified	10 M 8 F X̄ age: 14 range: 10-19 3-5 yr follow-up		Children's Psychiatric Rating Scale, Children's Affective Rating Scale	Of 12 children originally diagnosed as depressed, only 5 met the criteria at follow-up. These 5 had dysthymic disorder. 5 others met DSM-III criteria for other psychiatric diagnoses
LaRoche et al., 1981	5 BP Fa 5 BP Mo	11 M 6 F X̄ age: 10.1 range: 8-18		Conners' Patient Questionnaire, Children's Data Inventory and Symptom History, clinical interview	1 HRC had symptoms severe enough for psychiatric treatment
Kron et al., 1982	11 BP I 7 BP II	14 M X̄ age: 10.5 17 F X̄ age: 11.3 range: 7-14	9 M X̄ age: 11.4 9 F X̄ age: 11.3 Matched for sex, age, SES Neg history of AD in 1st deg or BP in 2nd deg relatives	Semistructured interview, Global Assessment Score, WISC-R, Rorschach, RDC/DSM III, Motoric Lateralization Questionnaire	52% HRC vs 6% CC had RDC/DSM-III diagnosis (25% HRC vs 6% C had depressive diagnoses) 2 of 8 depressed HRC had adult attention-deficit disorder and 2 were over-anxious. Authors speculate that of HRC subtypes (see Table 8-7) cyclothymic most likely to become BP, inhibited to become depressive, and impulsive to become sociopathic or alcoholic

Continued

Table 8-9 Continued. High-Risk Studies: Diagnostic and Clinical Findings

Study	High-Risk Parents	High-Risk Children	Comparison Parents	Comparison Children	Measures	Results
Waters et al., 1983b	17 BP	24 M 29 F all > 15 yr			SADS-L, educational occupational, and medical history	32% HRC met RDC for major affective disorder: $\quad$ M $\;$ F % BP I or BP II $\quad$ 17 $\;$ 17 % Hypomanic $\quad$ 0 $\;$ 7 % UP $\quad$ 4 $\;$ 17 2 male suicides prior to study
Akiskal et al., 1985b	67 BP	68 referred juvenile offspring or siblings $\bar{x}$ age of onset: 15.9 onset range: 6-24 3-yr prospective follow-up			Clinical interview Feighner Criteria, Mood Clinic Data Questionnaire	Manic episodes did not appear before puberty. 4/10 prepubertal (6-11 yr) had hypomanic features. 7/10 adolescents with cyclothymia became BP I or BP II. Acute depressive episodes and dysthymic-CYC disorders are most common in referred offspring and younger siblings of BP parents. 12% had psychotic depressive onset and 16% had acute manic or mixed onset
Klein et al., 1985	24 BP $\bar{x}$ age: 48.4	19 M 18 F $\bar{x}$ age: 17.9 range: 15-21	14 non-AD	13 M 9 F $\bar{x}$ age: 17.8 range: 15-21	Structured diagnostic interviews, RDC/DSM III	$\quad\quad$ HRC% $\;$ CC% $\;$ p Any disorder $\;$ 43 $\;$ 18 $\;$ .05 Affective $\;$ 38 $\;$ 5 $\;$ .005 BP $\;$ 27 $\;$ 0 $\;$ .01 CYC $\;$ 24 $\;$ 0 $\;$ .01 Nonaffective $\;$ 19 $\;$ 14 $\;$ NS Age of onset of CYC: 7-15 yr ($\bar{x}$ age : 12.4)
Hammen et al., 1987	9 BP Mo 13 UP Mo	5 M 7 F $\bar{x}$ age: 13.6 $\bar{x}$ age: 13.0 10 M 9 F $\bar{x}$ age: 13.5 9 F $\bar{x}$ age: 12.3 range: 8-16	14 Pl Mo 22 normal mothers	9 M $\bar{x}$ age: 12.8 9 F $\bar{x}$ age: 12.9 18 M 17 F $\bar{x}$ age: 12.6 $\bar{x}$ age: 10.6 range: 8-16	SADS-L, Beck Depression Inventory, Children's Depression Inventory, Child Behavior Checklist, school and teacher ratings	$\quad\quad$ CBP% $\;$ CUP% Major depression $\;$ 25 $\;$ 47 Dysthymia $\;$ 8 $\;$ 32 Most affective and behavioral problems were in CUP

Study	Parents	High-risk children	Comparison children	Measures	Findings
LaRoche et al., 1987	17 BP Mo, 4 BP Fa	25 M, 12 F, X̄ age: 16.2, range: 8-25		Feighner criteria (parents) DSM-III (children), Children's Psychiatric Rating Scale, Children's Affective Rating Scale, Achenbach Child Behavior Profile, Kovac's Self-Esteem Inventory	24% HRC had DSM-III diagnosis: 5% CYC, 3% MDD. Better marital adjustment associated with absence DSM-III diagnosis in offspring
Zahn-Waxler et al., 1988 (4 yr follow-up of Zahn-Waxler et al., 1984)	4 BP Mo, 3 BP Fa (5 UP spouses)	7 M, range: 5-6	12 M, range: 5-6	Child Assessment Schedule, Achenbach Child Behavior Checklist, DSM-III	DSM-III Diagnosis / HRC% / CC%: Depression 43 / 0; Conduct disorder 43 / 0; Overanxious 43 / 0. Severity of disturbance, as measured by multiple diagnoses and/or receiving treatment for emotional problems more common in HRC than CC ($p < .001$)
Grigoroiu-Serbanescu et al., 1989	28 BP I Mo, 19 BP I Fa	34 M, 38 F, X̄ age: 12.9, range: 10-17	61 normal; matched for sociocultural and marital status; 34 M, 38 F, X̄ age: 13.1, range: 10-17	DSM-III, Parental Attitude Scales, K-SADS-E, interviews concerning psychological and school functioning	HRC% / CC% / p: Non-BP Dep. 8 / 1 / .05; BP 1 / 0 / NS; Suicide Attempt 1 / 0 / NS; Anxious Disord. 12 / 4 / .05; ADDH 21 / 7 / .001; Personality disorders 12 / 3 / .05; Overall psycho-pathology rate 61 / 25

Fa = fathers, Mo = mothers, PI = physically ill, CSCZ = children of schizophrenic parents, CPI = children of physically ill parents, CN = children of normal parents, CBP = children of bipolar parents, CUP = children of unipolar parents, HRC = high-risk children, CC = comparison children, AD = affective disorder, CYC = cyclothymia, MDD = major depressive disorder
Mean age reported in years

pomanic and depressive episodes began within a year of one another; the average duration of a depressive episode was 2.3 days, a hypomanic episode 1.8 days. The durations of depressive and hypomanic episodes were highly correlated with one another ($r = 0.81$), and 80 percent of patients who met criteria for cyclothymia experienced more than 12 episodes a year. Akiskal and colleagues (1985b), in a 3-year prospective study of 68 referred juvenile offspring (or siblings) of adult bipolar patients, average age 15.9 years, found that no full-blown manic episodes occurred before puberty. The most common psychiatric disorders observed in the high-risk group were acute depression and dysthymic or cyclothymic disorders. Acute mania or mixed states accounted for 16 percent of onsets, and psychotic depression accounted for another 12 percent. Fully 70 percent of adolescents with cyclothymia went on to develop either bipolar-I or bipolar-II illness.

SUMMARY

Manic-depressive illness often first occurs in childhood and adolescence, making it especially important that child psychiatrists, psychologists, pediatricians, parents, and teachers be aware of early signs and symptoms. Many confounding issues of adolescence can mask, change, or make difficult to recognize symptoms of affective illness. Despite these problems, many studies have demonstrated that adolescent-onset bipolar illness can be identified reliably through the use of standardized adult diagnostic criteria. Several predictors of bipolarity have been suggested, including family history, symptom constellations, and pharmacologically induced hypomania. Prognosis does not seem to differ appreciably between early and late onset of illness groups.

Although methodologically difficult, high-risk studies represent an important paradigm for understanding manic-depressive illness. Personality and interpersonal studies suggest that aggressiveness, obsessionality, and affective expression are greater in high-risk children than in comparison groups. It is unclear the extent to which social problems exist in the non-ill siblings of psychiatrically disturbed high-risk children. Indeed, there is some evidence that interpersonal assets exist in the high-risk group in general and in the non-ill group in particular.

Cognitive patterns similar to those found in adult manic-depressive patients—that is, significant verbal performance discrepancies on the WISC, suggestive of right hemisphere impairment—were found in the high-risk children. Speech productivity and cohesion were not impaired in bipolar offspring, although unipolar offspring did have deviant performances. Rates of affective disorder, although variable, were considerably higher in children at risk. Age affected both the rate and nature of presenting symptoms.

NOTES

1. From Norwich, 1982, p. 105.
2. For excellent discussions of childhood depression, see Orvaschel et al., 1980; Kashani et al., 1981; Strober et al., 1981; Kovacs et al., 1984; Ryan and Puig-Antich, 1986; Ryan et al., 1987; Keller et al., 1988; Angold, 1988; Carlson and Kashani, 1988a; Kovacs, 1989.
3. R.E. Davis, 1979; Dvoredsky and Stewart, 1981; Poznanski et al., 1984; Sylvester et al., 1984; Reiss, 1985; Jones and Berney, 1987. The four cases of early-onset, rapid-cycling patients reported by Jones and Berney were all of low intelligence, which raises the question of concomitant organic factors. One of the children had gone through puberty, and one definitely had not, but it is not clear whether the children were prepubertal.
4. Greenhill and Shopsin, 1979; McKnew et al., 1979; O'Connell et al., 1979; Kuyler et al., 1980.
5. Her subjects were derived from case histories reported in the literature. The children had onsets earlier than 12 years of age.
6. Earlier studies indicated that 30 to 40 percent of adolescents hospitalized in a psychiatric facility had bipolar diagnoses (King and Pittman, 1969; Hudgens, 1974; Gammon et al., 1983). That figure may have dropped, however, because of the greater number of adolescents now being hospitalized with diagnoses of borderline personality disorder or substance abuse. Although not strictly comparable, unpublished biometric data from surveys done in 1986 by the Survey and Reports Branch, Division of Biometry and Applied Sciences, National Institute of Mental Health, show that the figure has dropped. The overall proportion of teenagers with a diagnosis of bipolar disorder admitted to all inpatient services in 1986 was 3.6 percent. This included state and county, private psychiatric hospitals, the psychiatric wards of general hospitals, and the inpatient service of multiservice mental health organizations. There was considerable variability in these rates from one type of institution to another, ranging from 0.5 percent in state and county hospitals to 6.5 percent in multiservice mental health organizations. The

preponderance of cases in absolute numbers was in private psychiatric and nonpublic general hospitals. Figures for affective disorders in teenagers for the same institutions ranged from 20 percent to more than 40 percent.

7. Costello and Edelbrock, 1985; Kashani et al., 1985; Lobovits and Handel, 1985; Moretti et al., 1985; Weissman et al., 1987b; Carlson and Kashani, 1988b.

8. Kasanin, 1952; Campbell, 1953; McHarg, 1954; Carlson and Strober, 1979.

9. King and Pittman, 1969; Hudgens, 1974; Carlson and Strober, 1978; Engstrom et al., 1978; Chambers et al., 1985.

10. Carlson and Strober, 1978; Friedman et al., 1983b; Gammon et al., 1983; Strober et al., 1988, 1989.

11. Hsu and Starzynski, 1986; Bashir et al., 1987; Jones and Berney, 1987; Carlson and Kashani, 1988b.

12. Of the 71 bipolar-I patients in the Rosen et al. (1983b) study, 53 had been psychotic at some time during their illness. Of those 53, 25 also met RDC for schizoaffective disorder. Findings from the study "raise the question as to whether some schizoaffective disorders defined by RDC are a form of early-onset bipolar I disorder" (p. 1524).

13. The mean age at onset was 15.9 years. Onset of affective illness in 24 patients was major depressive disorder; in 8 it was mania, and in 3 it was a mixed state. Of the remainder, 12 first presented with dysthymia, 10 with cyclothymia, and 11 with polydrug abuse.

14. The broader question of the use of biologically based diagnostic tests of affective disorders in children has been reviewed by Casat and Powell (1988).

15. Gaensbauer et al., 1984; Zahn-Waxler et al., 1984a,b,c; Zahn-Waxler et al., 1988.

9

Alcohol and Drug Abuse in Manic-Depressive Illness

I became insane, with long intervals of horrible sanity. During these fits of absolute unconsciousness, I drank—God only knows how often or how much. As a matter of course, my enemies referred the insanity to the drink, rather than the drink to the insanity.   —Edgar Allan Poe, 1848

Referring the insanity to the drink, rather than the drink to the insanity, remains a difficult problem in the differential diagnosis and treatment of affective illness, alcoholism, and substance abuse disorders. Relationships between alcohol and drug abuse and affective illness have been postulated for more than 2,000 years. Plato (cited in Ackerknecht, 1959) referred to alcoholism as a demonstrable cause of mania; Soranus (c. 100 AD, cited in Zilboorg, 1941) echoed the sentiment that alcoholic excess frequently caused mania and assailed those who prescribed it as treatment for mania. Aretaeus (c. 90 AD, cited in Whitwell, 1936) suggested that mania may be produced by excess of wine or opiates but concluded that the resulting states cannot properly be termed mania, just temporary deliria. Early in this century, Kraepelin (1921) summarized his findings of alcoholism in manic-depressive illness as follows:

Alcoholism occurs among male patients in about a quarter of the cases, but is to be regarded as the consequence of debaucheries committed in excitement, not as a cause. (p. 178)

The differing views about whether alcoholism precedes or follows manic-depressive illness persist today, but there is a growing appreciation of the importance of comorbidity or dual diagnosis. Investigators approach the problem from both di-

rections, many of them particularly concerned about its development in the young.

Why and to what extent manic-depressive patients self-administer mood-altering drugs are not entirely clear. The problem has not been studied as extensively in bipolar patients as it has in unipolar patients. In this chapter, we review what is known about relevant diagnostic and methodological problems: the rates of bipolar illness in substance abusers, as well as the rates of substance abuse in bipolar patients, and the hypothesized relationships among manic-depressive illness, alcoholism, and drug abuse, including genetic factors, phase of illness, seasonal influences, masking of symptoms, self-medication theories, precipitation of episodes, and modification of course through the impact of pathophysiological mechanisms, such as kindling.

METHODOLOGICAL AND DIAGNOSTIC ISSUES

Several general methodological problems are associated with the study of alcohol and drug abuse in manic-depressive patients. We consider these first and then turn to specific diagnostic issues.

First, it is often difficult to obtain accurate histories of alcohol and drug abuse from patients. Compounding this problem is the tendency for clinicians to skirt this general line of inquiry. Second, patients vary tremendously in the development and expression of both manic-depressive illness and substance abuse. Third, many studies do not adequately differentiate substance abuse from the more serious and persistent disorder of true dependence. Fourth, the lack of control groups makes interpretation of research findings difficult; for example, data indicate a coexistence of alcoholism with depression, but it is not always clear that the alcoholism rate is significantly different from that in the general population (Morrison, 1974). Fifth, because manic-depressive illness has a low baseline rate, relationship to alcoholism and drug abuse is not easy to demonstrate.

Inconsistency and unreliability of diagnostic criteria are particular problems when investigators attempt to diagnose and study several, generally quite separate, disorders and to determine which is primary and which is secondary. Schuckit (1986) has summarized several major sources of diagnostic confusion related to alcohol: (1) alcohol can cause depressive symptoms in anyone, (2) signs of temporary serious depression can follow prolonged drinking, (3) drinking can escalate during primary affective episodes in some patients, especially during mania, (4) depressive symptoms and alcohol problems occur in other psychiatric disorders, and (5) a proportion of manic-depressive patients have independent alcoholism. As Dilsaver (1987) points out, the symptomatic overlap between substance abuse and affective disorders is considerable, since both involve disturbance of mood and affect. Teasing them apart presents a challenge for the clinician. Psychopathological changes in mood and behavior secondary to drug and alcohol intoxication have been well documented.[1] More specifically, the dysphoric mood, depression, withdrawn behavior, and anxiety caused by chronic alcohol use have been reviewed by many authors,[2] as have the hostility, depression, and emotional withdrawal precipitated by heroin and morphine abuse,[3] and the profound changes in mood, energy, and thought brought about by cocaine.[4]

Boyd and colleagues (1983) point out that variability in diagnostic criteria has major effects on the estimates of comorbidity with major depression. Recent studies more often use standardized criteria, such as the DSM-III, DSM-III-R, and

RDC, however. Table 9-1 presents DSM-III-R criteria for psychoactive substance dependence and abuse. It should be noted that the criteria for abuse are far less stringent than those for dependence and, more important, quite inclusive in their nature. Drinking patterns secondary to affective episodes often will meet these criteria.[5]

Age almost certainly plays an important role in this issue. A recent study indicates that patients who began abusing alcohol before the age of 20 were more likely to exhibit hostility and physical violence. They also were three times more likely than older-onset alcoholics to be depressed and four times more likely to have attempted suicide (Buydens-Branchey et al., 1989).

Diagnostic subtypes of bipolar illness also present different problems in the study of alcohol and substance abuse. The common assumption that substance abuse among bipolar-I patients is largely state dependent has been challenged by the recent data from the Epidemiological Catchment Area program showing a predominance of substance dependence over abuse alone. Bipolar-II patients are more likely to show chronic abuse patterns (Himmelhoch et al., 1976a), which are likely to worsen the course of their illness. Ascertaining whether the abuse is primary or secondary in bipolar-II patients is also problematic.

Differentiating symptoms secondary to an underlying psychiatric disorder from those secondary to substance abuse problems can be difficult (a general review of overlapping symptoms and pathophysiologies of substance abuse and affective disorder can be found in Dilsaver, 1987, and a review of the specific problems in adolescents can be found in Bukstein et al., 1989). Affective, cognitive, and psychotic symptoms can result from alcohol and from a wide variety of classes of drugs, such as amphetamine, cocaine, and hallucinogens. Likewise, alcohol and other drugs can both mask and precipitate affective symptoms. The onset of psychotic illness also can be precipitated through drug intake.[6] Kraepelin observed many years ago that manic attacks occasionally begin with delirium tremens. More recently, LSD- and PCP-induced manic attacks have been observed in biologically vulnerable individuals. These issues are discussed further later in this chapter.

The importance of a detailed chronology of the onset of symptoms (i.e., did difficulties with sub-

Table 9-1. DSM-III-R Criteria for Psychoactive Substance Dependence
and Psychoactive Substance Abuse

There are many problems with the DSM–III distinction between substance abuse and dependence: problems using social and occupational consequences to define abuse, inadequacy of tolerance or withdrawal as a required criterion for dependence, and inconsistencies in the relationship of abuse to dependence for various substances. In DSM–III–R the definition of dependence is broadened to define a syndrome of clinically significant behaviors, cognitions, and other symptoms that indicate loss of control of substance use and continued use of the substance despite adverse consequences. Most cases of DSM–III abuse are subsumed under the DSM–III–R category of dependence. The DSM–III–R category of abuse is a residual category for cases in which the disturbance does not meet the criteria for dependence, yet there is a maladaptive pattern of use.

In DSM–III–R the same general criteria for dependence, index of symptoms, and criteria for abuse are used for all of the categories of psychoactive substances.

Criteria for Psychoactive Substance Dependence
A. At least three of the following:
  1. substance often taken in larger amounts and over a longer period of time than the person intended
  2. persistent desire or one or more unsuccessful efforts to cut down or control substance use
  3. a great deal of time spent in activities necessary to get the substance (e.g., theft), taking the substance, or recovering from its effects
  4. frequent intoxication or withdrawal symptoms when expected to fulfill major role obligations at work, school, or home (e.g., does not go to work because hung over, goes to school or work "high," intoxicated while taking care of his or her children), or when substance use is physically hazardous (e.g., drives intoxicated)
  5. important social, occupational, or recreational activities given up or reduced because of substance use
  6. continued substance use despite knowledge of having a persistent or recurrent social, psychological or physical problem that is caused or exacerbated by the use of the substance (e.g., keeps using heroin despite family arguments about it, cocaine-induced depression, or having an ulcer made worse by drinking)
  7. marked tolerance: need for markedly increased amounts of the substance (i.e., at least a 50% increase) in order to achieve intoxication or desired effect, or markedly diminished effect with continued use of the same amount
  Note: The following items may not apply to cannabis, hallucinogens, or phencyclidine (PCP):
  8. characteristic withdrawal symptoms (see specific withdrawal syndromes under Psychoactive Substance-induced Organic Mental Disorders)
  9. substance often taken to relieve or avoid withdrawal symptoms

B. Some symptoms of the disturbance have persisted for at least one month, or have occurred repeatedly over a longer period of time.

Continued

Table 9-1 Continued. DSM-III-R Criteria for Psychoactive Substance Dependence
and Psychoactive Substance Abuse

Criteria for Severity of Psychoactive Substance Dependence:
Mild: Few, if any, symptoms in excess of those required to make the diagnosis, and the
symptoms result in no more than mild impairment in occupational functioning or in usual
social activities or relationships with others.
Moderate: Symptoms or functional impairment between "mild" and "severe"
Severe: Many symptoms in excess of those required to make the diagnosis, and the symptoms
markedly interfere with occupational functioning or with usual social activities or relationships
with others.
In Partial Remission: During the past six months, some use of the substance and some
symptoms of dependence.
In Full Remission: During the past six months, either no use of the substance, or use of the
substance and no symptoms of dependence.

Criteria for Psychoactive Substance Abuse
A. A maladaptive pattern of psychoactive substance use indicated by at least one of the following:
1. continued use despite knowledge of having a persistent or recurrent social, occupational,
psychological, or physical problem that is caused or exacerbated by use of the psychoactive
substance
2. recurrent use in situations in which use is physically hazardous (e.g., driving while
intoxicated)

B. Some symptoms of the disturbance have persisted for at least one month, or have occurred
repeatedly over a longer period of time.

C. Never met the criteria for Psychoactive Substance Dependence for this substance.

stance abuse predate affective symptoms, or vice versa?), severity of presenting symptoms, and family history can aid in a differential diagnosis (Hesselbrock et al., 1985; Schuckit, 1986). Further discussion of possible concurrent diagnosis of affective illness and substance abuse, along with the relevant treatment approaches, is presented in Chapter 26.

RATES OF ALCOHOL AND DRUG ABUSE IN MANIC-DEPRESSIVE ILLNESS

As with many of the topics discussed in this book, the association among alcohol abuse, drug abuse, and affective illness has been far more thoroughly studied for unipolar depression than it has for bipolar illness.[7] We concentrate on issues concerning bipolar patients.

Alcohol Abuse and Alcoholism
The lack of consistency in the use of diagnostic criteria has led to widely disparate estimates of

the rates of depression in alcoholism, ranging from 3 to 98 percent, depending on whether clinical scales or more formal diagnostic criteria were used (Keeler et al., 1979; Himmelhoch et al., 1983). The estimates of the prevalence of affective disorders in primary alcoholics range from 12 to 57 percent when affective disorders are defined by formal diagnostic criteria but are as high as 98 percent when rating scales are used (Berndt and Murray, 1986).

Rates of alcohol abuse and alcoholism in patients with manic-depressive illness are summarized in Table 9-2. Comparison figures for the general population (which focus on alcoholism) are presented in Table 9-3. The general rate of alcohol abuse and alcoholism in manic-depressive individuals, summarized across an admittedly widely varying range of estimates in a highly variable group of methodologies, is about 35 percent. In the general population, males tend to have a higher rate of drinking problems and females tend to have higher rates of affective dis-

Table 9-2. Rates of Alcohol Abuse or Alcoholism in Patients with Manic-Depressive Illness

Study	Observations/Comments
Kraepelin, 1921	25% rate of alcoholism in males with manic-depressive illness
Cassidy et al., 1957	21% of males, 2% of females became alcoholics; BP–UP differences not specified
Parker et al., 1960	33% of manic-depressive patients were alcoholic
Mayfield & Coleman, 1968	At least 20% of affectively ill patients drank to excess
Freed, 1969	65% of bipolar patients, manic phase, abused alcohol
Schuckit et al., 1969	27% of alcoholic patients had affective disorder predating their drinking problem
Mendlewicz et al., 1972a	45% of bipolar patients were alcoholic
Morrison, 1974	44% of BP patients reported periods of some alcohol problems
Reich et al., 1974	Approximately 50% of manic-depressive patients drank to excess
Dunner et al., 1979a	19% of male and 0% of female BPIs had drinking problems
Hensel et al., 1979	21% of male and 12% of female BPIIs had drinking problems
Lewis et al., 1982	3% of patients with MDD had secondary alcoholism; 15% of "all other depressives" (including BPs) had secondary alcoholism
O'Sullivan et al., 1983	11% of primary affective disorder patients were alcoholics
Mirin et al., 1984a	Among patients with affective illness, 30% to 40% abused alcohol
Estroff et al., 1985	75% of BP manic and 60% of BP depressed patients abused alcohol
Hasin et al., 1985	24% of patients with MDD or BP showed evidence of clinically significant levels of alcohol abuse. BP-UP differences were not significant
Bernadt & Murray, 1986	25% of BP depressed and 20% of BP manic patients abused alcohol
Louks & Smith, 1988	53% of their sample of homeless people with major affective disorders abused alcohol
Miller et al., 1989	18% of BP patients abused alcohol
Regier et al., 1990	Lifetime prevalence of alcohol abuse or dependence among BPI patients was 46% (ECA study). The rate for alcohol abuse only is 15%

MDD = major depressive disorder

orders, particularly depression. From a diagnostic point of view, only one group examined differences in bipolar-I and bipolar-II patients (Hensel et al., 1979; Dunner et al., 1979a) and found that bipolar-II women (12 percent) were much more likely to drink to excess than their bipolar-I counterparts (0 percent), whereas among the men, bipolar-I and bipolar-II patients were equally likely to have drinking problems (19 percent and 21 percent, respectively). Bedi and Halikas (1985) reported higher rates of alcoholism in their female affective patients (43 percent) than in their male patients (29 percent) but made no bipolar–unipolar comparison. The Epidemiologic Catchment Area (ECA) data for alcohol abuse and dependence in patients with affective illness show

Table 9-3. Rates of Alcohol Abuse or Alcoholism in the General Population

Study	Total Population %	Males %	Females %	Comments
Winokur & Tsuang, 1978	3.5			Current rate of definite or probable alcoholism
	7.6			Morbid risk
Weissman & Myers, 1980	2.6			Current rate of alcoholism
	6.7			Lifetime rate
Robins et al., 1984	11.5	19.1	4.8	New Haven ECA data, alcohol abuse & dependence, lifetime prevalence
	13.7	24.9	4.2	Baltimore
	15.7	28.9	4.3	St. Louis
Schuckit, 1986		8-10	3-5	Review of literature, meet criteria for alcoholism
Regier et al., 1988	13.3			Lifetime rate
	4.0			6-month rate
	2.8	5.0	0.9	1-month current rate
				Data from 5 ECA sites

a strikingly high lifetime prevalence rate (Table 9-4) of 21 percent in unipolar patients and 46 percent in bipolar patients (Regier et al., 1990). Three other studies (Freed, 1969; Morrison, 1974; Estroff et al., 1985) show that when bipolar patients were specifically queried, they reported consonant rates of alcohol abuse, 60 to 75 percent.[8] These estimates are significantly higher than earlier estimates of alcoholism in the general population, which were 6 to 7 percent for morbid or lifetime risks (Winokur and Tsuang, 1978; Weissman and Myers, 1980). The ECA study of

Table 9-4. ECA Lifetime Prevalence Rates for Substance Abuse among Persons with Affective Disorders

	BP I %	Major Depression %
Alcohol abuse or dependence	46	17
Abuse only	15	5
Dependence	31	12
Drug abuse or dependence	41	18
Abuse only	13	7
Dependence	28	11
Any substance abuse or dependence	61	27

Data from Regier et al., 1990 Based on DSM-III diagnoses

alcoholism and psychiatric comorbidity (Helzer and Pryzbeck, 1988) found that mania was strongly associated with alcoholism (odds ratio = 6.2) but that major depression (odds ratio = 1.7) was not.

Rates of affective illness in alcoholics are shown in Table 9-5. The rates of primary affective disorder range from 6 to 46 percent, and the rates of secondary affective disorder range from 24 to 41 percent with a weighted average of 33 percent. One problem with trying to interpret these findings is that no distinction was made in these studies between bipolar and unipolar illness, dysthymia, or cyclothymia. Despite diagnostic differences between these studies, it may be said that they show a significantly higher rate of affective disorder among alcoholics compared with the general population.

The data from the six studies that specifically examined the rates of bipolar illness in a population of alcoholics are displayed in the far right column of Table 9-5. Except for the study by Ross and colleagues, the rates of bipolar illness (6 to 9 percent) are several times what one would expect in the general population, approximately 1 to 3 percent (Weissman and Myers, 1980).

In summary, many studies using a wide variety of diagnostic criteria and patient populations and conducted over a period of more than 50 years are quite consistent in finding elevated rates of alco-

Table 9-5. Percent of Affective Illness in Patients with Alcohol Abuse or Alcoholism

Study	N	SA	MDD	BP/MDP
Tillotson & Fleming 1937	120			6
Amark, 1951	407			9
Sherfey, 1955	161			7
Winokur et al., 1970	173	41		
Cadoret & Winokur, 1974	171	41		
Weissman & Myers, 1980	34		44	6
O'Sullivan et al., 1983	194	24		
Schuckit, 1983	577	30		
Bowen et al., 1984	48		46	8
Dackis & Gold, 1984	70		7[a]	
Bedi & Halikas, 1985	421	33		
Schuckit, 1986	Review of literature		20-30% of alcoholics met criteria for a secondary affective disorder	
Ross et al., 1988	511[b]		24	2

SA = secondary affective disorder, MDD = major depressive disorder, MDP = manic-depressive psychosis

[a]Current depressive illness at time of admission for alcoholism
[b]Sample included substance abusers as well as those with alcohol problems (87% of sample)

hol abuse and dependence in manic-depressive patients and a significantly increased percentage of bipolar patients among populations of alcoholics and alcohol abusers.

Drug Abuse

The data on concurrent rates of manic-depressive illness and drug abuse are much less extensive and consistent than those on alcohol abuse. Much of the work in this field has been done by Weiss, Mirin, and colleagues in Boston and Rounsaville and colleagues at Yale. To avoid confusion between depressants and stimulants, we discuss cocaine, opiates, and other drugs separately. As depicted in Table 9-6, the rate of bipolar illness (including cyclothymia) among drug abusers is somewhat less than unipolar illness in some studies but equivalent or greater in others. The recent findings from the ECA, based on an extremely large sample size, show that the drug abuse rate in bipolar-I patients is far higher than in unipolar patients (18 percent and 41 percent, respectively).

Cocaine

The rate of bipolar illness among cocaine abusers is, as it is with alcohol abusers, several times higher than in the general population (Table 9-7). The majority of bipolar patients in Weiss and

Table 9-6. Percent of Affective Illness in Drug Abusers

Study	N	UP	BP	CYC
Cocaine				
Mirin & Weiss,[a] 1986	36	31	22	
Weiss & Mirin,[b] 1986	30	30	7	16
Weiss & et al., 1988	149	9	5	11
Nunes et al., 1989	30	13[c]	30	17[d]
Opiates				
Mirin et al., 1984a	91	18	3	
	33[e]	18[e]	6[e]	
Kosten & Rounsaville, 1986	533	24[c]	5[f]	
Weiss et al., 1988	293	12	3	3

CYC = cyclothymia

[a]6 of these 36 patients abused amphetamines
[b]Chronic cocaine abusers
[c]Major Depresssive Disorder
[d]Subset of 30% listed under BP
[e]CNS depressant abusers
[f]Includes BPI and BPII; increases to 11.6% if those with hypomanic disorder are included

Mirin's study (1986) reported using cocaine more often when manic than when depressed. This is consistent with the findings of Estroff and associates (1985), who observed that 58 percent of their manic bipolar patients abused cocaine compared with 30 percent of their depressed bipolar patients (Table 9-8). However, Miller and associates (1989) reported a much lower rate (10 percent) of cocaine abuse among their manic patients. Weiss and colleagues (1986) found that the overall rate of affective illness was higher in chronic cocaine abusers than any other type of drug abusers, especially opiate and other depressant abusers. Later expanding on this, Weiss and associates (1988)

Table 9-7. Rates of Drug Abuse in the General Population

Study	Total Population %	M %	F %	Comments
Robins et al., 1984	5.8	6.5	5.1	New Haven ECA data[a]
	5.6	7.1	4.4	Baltimore ECA data[a]
	5.5	7.4	3.8	St. Louis ECA data[a]
Regier et al., 1988	5.9[a]			Combined ECA data, from five sites[a]
	2.0[b]			
	1.3[c]	1.8	0.7	

[a]Drug abuse or dependence, lifetime prevalence
[b]Drug abuse or dependence, 6-month rate
[c]Drug abuse or dependence, 1-month current rate

Table 9-8. Percentage of Drug Abuse in Bipolar Patients

Abused Drug	Manic (N=12)	Depressed (N=10)	A/M (N=14)
Cocaine	58	30	28
Heroin	25	20	28
Marijuana	66	50	71
LSD	33	30	28
PCP	25	0	7

A/M = atypical/mixed

Data from Estroff et al., 1985

reported that, although bipolar illness was more prevalent among cocaine abusers than among opiate and depressant abusers, rates of unipolar depression were more evenly distributed across the drug abuse categories. As Weiss and colleagues (1986) point out, the large number of bipolar and cyclothymic patients among cocaine abusers is consistent with Silberman and colleagues' finding (1981) that amphetamine produces euphoria more often in depressed bipolar patients than in unipolar patients. It is unclear whether this implies that bipolar symptoms are secondary to the drug abuse or whether there are other features of bipolar illness (e.g., nature of depressive symptoms, presence of mixed states, desire to reinduce or accelerate elevated mood and energy states) that lead to greater cocaine abuse.

Opiates and CNS Depressants

The most quantitative analysis of affective illness in opiate and CNS-depressant abusers is that of Kosten and Rounsaville (1986). They studied 533 opiate and depressant abusers; 24 percent of the total were diagnosed with major depressive disorder, and 5.4 percent were either bipolar I or II (Table 9-6). Mirin and co-workers (1984a) found similar rates of unipolar depression among opiate addicts but a doubled rate of bipolar illness among CNS-depressant abusers in comparison. Mirin and colleagues (1984a) also reported that almost three times more female than male opiate addicts were diagnosed as bipolar (10.8 vs 3.7 percent). This rate of bipolar illness is substantially higher than that found in the general population.

Only two studies examined drug abuse in bipo-

lar patients. Estroff and colleagues (1985) reported that 25 percent of their manic patients abused heroin compared with 20 percent of depressed bipolar patients. These findings cannot be generalized, however, because of the small sample size. Miller and associates (1989), studying a larger sample, reported that only 5 percent of their manic patients abused opiates.

Overall, the rates of bipolar illness, although not as dramatically high as in cocaine abusers, are nevertheless greater than those found in the general population. Most opiate addicts with affective illness suffer from major depression. Determining the sequence of comorbidity of affective illness and drug abuse presents the same methodological problems as it does in alcoholism and alcohol abuse. The ECA data show that comorbidity is more likely (1.3 times) to start with affective disorder than the other way around.

Marijuana, LSD, and PCP

No specific study has been undertaken to ascertain the rate of affective illness in marijuana users. Several studies have reported on the affective features associated with marijuana use. Harding and Knight (1973) found four patients whose marijuana use increased concurrent with the onset of hypomanic or manic symptoms. The authors suggest that the patients' mania already existed and that the marijuana use was symptomatic of the illness. Rottanburg and colleagues (1982) reported that their marijuana-using manic-depressive patients had more hypomanic symptoms and agitation and less flattening of affect than did psychotic (primarily schizophrenic) controls. After detoxification, the marijuana-using patients' psychotic symptoms decreased much more than those of the controls, suggesting a possible cannabis-induced psychosis with hypomanic features.

Rates of manic-depressive illness have likewise been scarcely studied in LSD and PCP users. Only one study (Bowers, 1977) examined LSD-induced psychoses. The author postulated that:

It may be that a group of patients who develop extended psychoses following psychotomimetic drug use have an organismic vulnerability to developing acute psychoses with affective features . . . by virtue of genetic loading for manic-depressive illness. (p. 835)

Table 9-9. Alcohol Intake and Phase of Bipolar Illness

Study	Depressed Phase			Manic Phase		
	Increase	Decrease %	No change	Increase	Decrease %	No change
Minski, 1938	100	0	0	29	0	71
Mayfield & Coleman, 1968	26	43	31	83	0	17
Winokur et al., 1969	27	0	73	42	0	47
Reich et al., 1974	3	0	97[a]	50	0	50[a]
Hensel et al.,[b] 1979	21	22	57	14	7	79
Bernadt & Murray, 1986	38	25	36	20	23	57

[a]No information given as to decrease or no change
[b]Depressed phase approximated, excluding unipolar patients

Finally, as Table 9-8 shows, Estroff and colleagues (1985) reported higher rates of marijuana abuse among manic than depressed bipolar patients (66 vs 50 percent). A similar trend was seen for PCP (25 vs 0 percent) but not for LSD (33 vs 30 percent). The sample size here is small, however, and another study of marijuana use in a larger sample of manic patients found a rate of only 8 percent (Miller et al., 1989). On the other hand, the ECA findings (Table 9-4) do suggest that the comorbidity of bipolar-I illness with either drug or alcohol abuse is indeed very high (61 percent).

RELATIONSHIPS AMONG MANIC-DEPRESSIVE ILLNESS, ALCOHOLISM, AND DRUG ABUSE

Of the many possible complex relationships among manic-depressive illness and alcohol and drug abuse, only a few have been translated into specific hypotheses. We focus here on those that link substance abuse disorders with the bipolar subgroup. They are based on our own formulations and those of Harding and Knight (1973), Himmelhoch and his colleagues (1976a, 1979), Ballenger and Post (1978), and Meyer and Hesselbrock (1984).

Phase of Illness

Alcohol Abuse and Dependence

Although it is perhaps more intuitive to link increased alcohol use with the depressed phase of manic-depressive illness, evidence suggests that increased alcohol consumption more frequently is associated with hypomania, mania, and the mixed or transitional states. Indeed, bipolar patients who increase alcohol consumption generally do so during the manic phase (Zisook and Schuckit, 1987). Table 9-9 summarizes six studies of alcohol intake and phase of illness. Mayfield and Coleman (1968) reported that patients were far more likely to increase their drinking when manic than when depressed, a finding replicated by Reich and colleagues (1974). Winokur and associates (1969) found a similar but less striking increase in drinking during mania over that in depression. Bernadt and Murray (1986), on the other hand, found that more bipolar patients drank when depressed than when manic, a finding similar to Minski's study (1938), in which all patients increased their drinking when depressed but only about one third increased their drinking when manic. Hensel and co-workers (1979) reported that twice as many patients increased as decreased their alcohol intake during mania. This was much more so than during the depressed phase.

One conclusion reached by Reich and colleagues (1974) was that chronic excessive drinking predominated in the manic phase, whereas periodic excessive drinking predominated during depression. The majority of their patients hospitalized for depression stated that they more frequently drank when manic. Attempting to explain a similar finding, Pitts and Winokur (1966) suggested that, in mania, excess alcohol use occurs in conjunction "with other evidences of euphoria, overactivity and poor judgement" (p. 37).

Whereas alcohol use increases during mania, some investigators report a profound decrease during depression (with the few noted exceptions). Mayfield (cited in Liskow et al., 1982) elaborates on this point:

A decrease in drinking, which appears quite rare in mania, is common in depression, and it is not unheard of for an excessive drinker to cease drinking during a depressive episode. (p. 145)

Alcohol, to a point, does seem to provide some relief for the irritability, restlessness, and agitation associated with mania. In this sense, it is understandable why its use increases more during mania.

Men are more likely than women (54 percent vs 35 percent) to increase their drinking when manic, according to Winokur and colleagues (1969). These same investigators found that, for those who increased their alcohol intake (expressed in ounces of 80 proof whiskey), the amount of alcohol consumed during mania is also greater for men (10 to 37 ounces per day) than for women (6 to 17 ounces). This finding is consistent with Cassidy and associates' observation (1957) that men (79 percent) were more likely than women (48 percent) to increase their drinking when affectively ill. The polarity of the phase of illness, however, was not specified in their study. Gender differences were not pronounced in drinking behavior while depressed (Winokur et al., 1969). The average amount of alcohol consumed during bipolar depression, by those who drank, was 16 ounces per day.

Only one study systematically compared drinking behavior during unipolar and bipolar depressive episodes (Bernadt and Murray, 1986).

These authors found that bipolar depressed patients (38 percent) were much more likely than unipolar depressed patients (15 percent) to increase their drinking. Twice as many unipolar as bipolar (68 percent vs 36 percent) patients reported no change in their alcohol consumption when depressed. The tendency for manic-depressive individuals in this study to drink more heavily when depressed may reflect increased agitation and perturbation associated with coexisting transitional or mixed states, discussed below. This finding would be consistent with Pauleikhoff's observation (1953) that those patients who drank when depressed were more likely to exhibit features of agitation and "inner tensions."[9]

Finally, Winokur and co-workers (1969) found that the percentage of patients increasing their alcohol consumption was more similar during mixed and manic states (43 and 42 percent, respectively) than during bipolar depression (27 percent). None of their patients reported decreasing the use of alcohol when in a mixed state; 57 percent reported no change. Himmelhoch and associates (1976a) later noted that the major differentiating feature between mixed- and nonmixed-state bipolar patients was rates of alcohol and drug abuse. The mixed-state patients were twice as likely to abuse these substances.

Drug Abuse and Dependence

The incidence of manic-depressive illness in individuals heavily using cocaine and other stimulants is, as the rates presented previously indicate, very high. Clinical researchers studying the role of cocaine in the affective disorders have emphasized cocaine's selective ability to alleviate potential symptoms and mood states across all phases of the illness.

Although there are no quantitative studies of cocaine use as a function of phase of illness, clinical research suggests that bipolar patients do use cocaine when depressed but are more likely to use it during hypomania and mania, in a pattern similar to alcohol use. For example, in one study (Weiss and Mirin, 1986), five of seven bipolar and cyclothymic patients reported that they used cocaine more often when manic than when depressed. The reasons for cocaine's use during these elevated phases were not only to alleviate associated dysphoria but also to bring about, sustain, or heighten the euphoric states often associated with hypomania and mania (Weiss and Mirin, 1986). These mood-altering uses of cocaine are described by several investigators.

The use of cocaine in hypomanic states has been described by Khantzian (1985) ". . . to *augment* a hyperactive, restless lifestyle" (p. 1263) and by Gawin and Kleber (1986), who describe the use of cocaine by cyclothymic individuals:

Cocaine use did not precipitate manic episodes, and it was initially well controlled. . . . Cocaine use early on reestablished hypomanic functioning during dysthymic cycles. However, cocaine use eventually was extended to continuously regulate mood state. When these subjects began to perceive that cocaine use was harmful, they successfully refrained from cocaine during dysthymic phases. Paradoxically, 80% described that when mood state improved toward hypomania, judgment of the seriousness of cocaine-related problems deteriorated, and cocaine use recurred. (pp. 110-111)

The use of cocaine for control of both depressed and elated phases of manic-depressive illness was described in some detail by Weiss and Mirin (1984):

We were impressed by the perceived utility of [cocaine] in the regulation of both dysphoric and elated mood. Typically, depressed patients reported symptom relief at moderate doses but also noted the need to gradually increase the dose or the frequency of drug administration. . . . Bipolar and cyclothymic patients hospitalized for chronic cocaine use reported that they used the drug most frequently to enhance endogenously elevated mood in the manic phases of their illness. (pp. 49-50)

A recent clinical report of two patients with seasonal fluctuations in cocaine abuse or craving suggests a link with the dysphoric features of seasonal affective disorder (Satel and Gawin, 1989).

Genetic Factors

Alcohol Abuse

Manic-depressive illness may be a risk factor for substance abuse through common genetic factors. Family studies of the link between alcoholism and affective disorder are, by their nature, complex. Pertinent conceptual and methodological issues have been reviewed by Cloninger and associates (1979) and D. Goodwin and colleagues (1979). Genetic theories and data positing an underlying biological relationship

among alcoholism, depressive illness, and manic-depressive illness (e.g., Winokur et al., 1971; Behar and Winokur, 1979), reviewed in Chapter 15, have generally shown that the alcoholism in the absence of affective disorder is not in the genetic spectrum of bipolar manic-depressive illness. Many studies have demonstrated no significant increase in the rates of alcoholism in relatives of patients with bipolar or unipolar major depressive disorders.[10] Several studies have, however, reported significantly increased rates of alcoholism in relatives of affectively ill patients compared with controls.[11] Price and Nelson (1986), having determined a significantly higher morbid risk of alcoholism in the relatives of unipolar patients with nonmelancholic features (16.1 percent) than in those with melancholic features (4.6 percent), further demonstrated a higher morbid risk in melancholic patients without delusions (6.7 percent) than in those with delusions (2.2 percent). They concluded that their unipolar nonmelancholic patients were equivalent to Winokur's depressive-spectrum disease and emphasized the importance of diagnostic subtyping. In other studies of affective subtyping, Dunner and colleagues (1979a) found that most alcoholism in relatives of male bipolar-I patients may be genetically unrelated to the affective disorders, but they earlier found that bipolar-II families showed a higher rate of alcoholism (Dunner et al., 1976d). Studying the concomitant incidence of alcoholism and manic-depressive illness in the Jewish population (among whom rates of manic-depressive illness are unusually high), Malzberg (1960) noted a far lower incidence of alcoholism in manic-depressive patients compared to the general population. Malzberg suggested that the two illnesses are transmitted separately by genetic or environmental factors or both. Findings indicate that the rates of alcoholism in first-degree relatives of bipolar manic-depressive patients are not different from those of control families (see Chapter 15). Rosenthal and Wehr (1987) found that 34 percent of 220 patients with seasonal affective disorder had at least one first-degree relative with a history of alcohol abuse.

The data, although limited, are more consistent for studies of rates of affective disorders in the first-degree relatives of alcoholics. Winokur and associates (1970) reported an increase in rates; however, other researchers have been unable to

Table 9-10. Usage Trends and Affective Disorders in Cocaine Abusers

	1980-1982			1982-1986		
	Number at Risk	N	%	Number at Risk	N	%
Cocaine Abusers[a]		154	19.5		288	41.3
Affective Disorder[b]	30	15	50	119	25	21
Affective Disorder in female first-degree relatives[c]	58	18	31	227	26	11.5
Affective Disorder in male first-degree relatives[c]	56	8	14.3	227	5	2.2

[a]Total percentage of cocaine abusers in treatment facility
[b]$p < .01$
[c]$p < .001$

Adapted from Weiss et al., 1988

replicate this finding.[12] Winokur and co-workers (1970) did state that the affective disorder usually seen in both patients and relatives of alcoholics is not bipolar illness. Separating male from female relatives of alcoholics, the results show a higher rate of affective disorders among female first-degree relatives, as is true for the population in general (Schuckit et al., 1969; Winokur et al., 1970, 1971). The difference is even greater for female relatives of female alcoholics. Mirin and colleagues (1984b) concluded that:

. . . being alcoholic did not increase the probability that one would have a relative with affective disorder. Conversely, having affective disorder did not increase the probability that the patient would have one or more alcoholic relatives. (p. 100)

Similarly, Zisook and Schuckit (1987) concluded that the best explanation for the coappearance of alcoholism and affective illness is that, although both are genetically distinct, the presence of one or both in family members of alcoholics adversely affects their illness in an additive way.

Drug Abuse

The genetic data linking drug abuse to manic-depressive illness are much less systematic than those for alcoholism and have been studied mainly in cocaine and some opiate abusers. Weiss and colleagues (1986) reported that 19 percent of their patients who abused cocaine and 7.5 percent of those who abused opiates had a first-degree relative with an affective disorder. In a more recent inquiry (Weiss et al., 1988), although the rates of

affective disorder in relatives of opiate abusers remained constant, the rate of affective disorder in relatives of cocaine abusers dropped to 10 percent (Table 9-10).

Only two studies distinguished bipolar and unipolar illness among first-degree relatives of cocaine abusers. Mirin and co-workers (1984b) reported that rates of bipolar illness and unipolar depression in first-degree relatives were higher than those found in the general population. Gershon and colleagues (1988) reported nonsignificant increased risks for bipolar and unipolar disorders in relatives of patients who abused drugs. Combining the bipolar and unipolar disorders in Gershon's study denoted a significantly higher risk.

It is possible that there is some predisposition for affective illness among drug abusers. However, not enough quantitative evidence has been gathered to make an accurate assessment.

Self-Medication Hypothesis

Manic-depressive illness also may be a risk factor for substance abuse through self-medication that occurs to alleviate affective symptoms. As Khantzian (1985) points out:

The drugs that addicts select are not chosen randomly. Their drug of choice is the result of interaction between the psychopharmacologic action of the drug and the dominant feelings with which they struggle. (p. 1259)

The theory of self-medication by substance abuse of affective illness has been suggested in many ways for many hundreds of years. Many of the hypotheses emerged from early psychoanalytic theorizing about use of drugs and alcohol by patients to defend against aggression and depression, and from this grew a more conceptual and well-defined hypothesis.[13]

In 1884, Freud recognized that cocaine, with its mood-elevating properties, could be used as a potent antidepressant. As Khantzian (1985) noted, "Cocaine has its appeal because of its ability to relieve distress associated with depression, hypomania, and hyperactivity" (p. 1259) and that addicts experienced improved self-esteem when using cocaine. This latter notion closely followed the findings of Milkman and Frosch (1973):

. . . that heroin addicts preferred the calming and dampening effects of opiates and seemed to use them to shore up tenuous defenses and reinforce a tendency toward withdrawal and isolation, while amphetamine addicts used the stimulating action of amphetamines to support an inflated sense of self-worth and a defensive style involving active confrontation with their environment. (Khantzian, 1985, p. 1260)

Self-medication in depressed patients has been nicely described by McLellan and colleagues (1985):

. . . [depressed, self-medicating patients] often appear to be suffering from more lethargic, retarded, anergic symptoms (especially loss of interest in previously stimulating events) . . . It may be that the sedative drugs are preferred by patients with more agitated forms of depression, while the stimulant drugs are selected for their energizing qualities by patients with retarded forms of depression. (p. 152)

Contrary to theories positing a use of stimulants to counter depressive states, most patients report using cocaine primarily when hypomanic or manic to enhance or induce euphoric moods associated with those states. Weiss and colleagues (1988), for example, reported that the majority of their bipolar and cyclothymic patients abusing cocaine claimed that they were not self-medicating depression but rather lengthening and intensifying euphoric effects of hypomania. These same authors had noted earlier (Weiss and Mirin, 1984) that the bipolar and cyclothymic cocaine abusers' manic phase was characterized by euphoria whereas:

. . . substance abusers who experienced dysphoria during mania or hypomania seemed to prefer to "self-treat" their symptoms with opiates or other central nervous system depressants (including alcohol). (p. 50)

This notion of self-treatment of dysphoric feelings by opiates echoes similar results from Rounsaville's group (1982) and Castaneda and colleagues (1989) and, in part, those of Khantzian (1974) and Wurmser (1974), who suggested that use of opiates was a mechanism for combating the "psychologically disorganizing effects of overwhelming rage" (p. 358) (Weiss and Mirin, 1987). Evidence suggests, however, that alcohol and such drugs as heroin and PCP also may produce increased symptoms of dysphoria, irritability, and anxiety.

Why then do bipolar patients continue to abuse cocaine, for example, after they have switched mood states or alleviated the painful state from which they were trying to escape? Weiss and colleagues (1986) suggest that low to moderate doses of cocaine may make affectively ill patients feel better (as Post et al., 1974b, found in depressed patients) by relieving anxious, agitated feelings, and this effect promotes further drug use. Once chronic, other factors assume importance in maintaining drug-taking behavior, and a chronic addiction often results (Castaneda et al., 1989). This also may be true for opiate and alcohol abuse in manic and depressed patients who continue to drink or abuse drugs despite the realization of the substances' adverse effects on mood (Weiss and Mirin, 1987).

Self-medication of affective illness by alcohol has been postulated but is not as well founded as self-treatment with cocaine and opiates. Reich and colleagues (1974) and many other clinicians observed that increased alcohol consumption appears to be self-medicating, an attempt to slow down, relax, and take the edge off the dysphoria. These authors hypothesized that excessive alcohol use was a sign of more severe mania and that it was used to control the manic symptoms, especially those of sleep disturbance and hyperactivity. Weiss and Mirin (1987) suggest that, in addition to self-medication, the increased use of drugs and alcohol during manic episodes could be attributed to impulsiveness, recklessness, and poor judgment. Liskow and associates (1982) suggested that "Drinking may simply be another manifestation of mania—manics tend to do more of everything" (p. 145) and point out that "the self-medication hypothesis relating alcoholism to affective disorder appears to be simplistic if not entirely erroneous" (p. 146).

Finally, recalling that patients with mixed states tend to be twice as likely as other patients to abuse drugs and alcohol, Himmelhoch and associates (1976a) point out that the switch phase can be dysphoric and uncomfortable and substance abuse may be used as a treatment for this dysphoria.

Attention has been give to the self-medication hypothesis in substance abuse among affectively ill patients. However, it will likely be debated for some time before the issue is resolved. The recent ECA findings, discussed earlier, show a greatly increased rate of major depression preceding substance abuse rather than substance abuse preceding depression. Although this has not been shown in bipolar illness, it may reflect some of the self-medication hypothesis for major depression.

Precipitation of Illness

The underlying manic-depressive illness/psychosis may be precipitated by alcohol or drug abuse; for example, the first manic episode in a biologically vulnerable individual may be triggered by hallucinogen or amphetamine use. Potential and observed interactions between those who are predisposed, their substance abuse patterns, and the onset of psychotic or severe depressive episodes have been described by many clinicians and investigators.

The most demonstrable drug-precipitated manic-depressive psychoses are those resulting from hallucinogenic drugs, such as LSD and PCP. The psychotic symptoms associated with the use of these drugs have been well documented by several authors.[14]

Amphetamine abuse, also recognized as a precipitant of psychosis, was noted by Ellinwood and Petrie (1979) as being indistinguishable from paranoid schizophrenia. Many of the presenting symptoms (e.g., delusions of persecution and grandeur and visual and auditory hallucinations), however, often are present in manic psychoses as well. Although no studies have specifically focused on cocaine-precipitated manic-depressive illness, it seems logical that cocaine abuse by vulnerable individuals could precipitate manic-depressive illness. This possibility is especially likely given the evidence from animal studies that cocaine is a very potent inducer of a process analogous to kindling in the CNS (sensitization) (Post et al., 1984e). The role of kindling–sensitization

processes in the pathophysiology of manic-depressive illness is discussed in Chapter 16.

Marijuana has been seen as a precipitant producing psychoses similar to those induced by other hallucinogens (Bowers and Freedman, 1975; Weller et al., 1988). Rottanburg and colleagues (1982) noted that, after detoxification, symptoms of a seemingly cannabis-induced psychosis decreased in several patients, revealing hypomanic and agitated symptoms. Hekimian and Gershon (1968) and Keup (1970) also noted that several of their manic-depressive patients became psychotic after marijuana use.

Alcohol abuse as a precipitant of affective episodes has not been well studied, despite the numerous reports of coexisting alcoholism and affective illness. As noted earlier, Kraepelin (1921) had observed that mania was occasionally precipitated by delirium tremens. Morrison (1974) concluded:

. . . when alcoholism and manic-depressive illness do occur together, no conclusions as to temporal relationship can be drawn: one is as likely as the other to have had the earlier onset. (p. 1133)

Ballenger and Post (1978a) hypothesized that repeated alcohol abuse can produce a kindling-like impact on the CNS (see Chapter 16).

Although many of the psychoses noted here have been attributed to schizophrenia rather than manic-depressive illness, the symptoms often are typical of both, as noted among marijuana users (Harding and Knight, 1973). Pope (1979) remarked that patients who develop psychotic symptoms as a result of drug use may have latent schizophrenia or manic-depressive illness:

The latter diagnosis seems particularly plausible in that it might explain both the drug abuse and the psychosis: the patient may abuse stimulants during the depressed phase, only to be hospitalized subsequently with a manic phase triggered or exaggerated by drug abuse. (p. 1341)

Lending further support to the notion that many of these psychotic reactions may in fact be manic-depressive illness is the strong evidence that many schizophrenics are misdiagnosed manic-depressives.

It has been postulated that individuals with drug-precipitated psychoses have an earlier age of onset than those with psychoses that are not induced by drugs (Breakey et al., 1974; Erard et al., 1980). This has not been well studied in manic-depressive illness, but could provide a possible diagnostic aid if proven accurate.

Masking of Symptoms

The use of alcohol and other drugs may mask or partially mask the symptoms of mania and depression; that is, manic-depressive illness may manifest itself as alcoholism, marijuana abuse, or other types of substance abuse. The emergence of affective illness after detoxification can be seen easily in Tables 9-2, 9-5, and 9-6.

Much of the literature comprising this area concerns the masking of affective illness by the use of alcohol. Masking presents a very complex problem for the clinician, since it confounds diagnosis (Freed, 1970). As Arieti (1978) points out, "A considerable number of depressed people hide their depressions by making immoderate use of alcohol, and are therefore considered alcoholic" (p. 67). These patients' underlying affective symptoms are then discovered during periods of no alcohol use.

Noting alcohol's complicating effects on manic-depressive illness, Campbell (1953) remarked that cases of the illness "including repeated psychotic episodes, are obscured for years by the more conspicuous effects of alcohol" (p. 281). Indeed, Morrison (1974) reported that the mean duration of current illness before admission was substantially higher in alcoholic bipolar patients (203 days) than in nonalcoholic bipolar patients (37 days), suggesting that this may be due to a masking of affective symptoms by alcohol.

The literature on masking of manic-depressive illness by drug abuse is scarce. The potent effects of such drugs as marijuana, cocaine, heroin, LSD, and PCP leave little doubt, however, that manic-depressive symptoms could easily be masked by drug abuse. Harding and Knight (1973), for example, noted that in their four hypomanic and manic patients, marijuana use was symptomatic of their illness. All presented in a hypomanic state, and all reported having used marijuana for several years before hospitalization. Marijuana use may have masked their affective illness.

Modification of Course

Alcoholism and drug abuse may modify the course and expression of manic-depressive ill-

ness; they may especially worsen the course and prognosis of those who have mixed states or who are rapid cyclers (Himmelhoch et al., 1976a; Himmelhoch, 1979).

The switch process, described in detail by Bunney and associates (1972a,b,c), and its precipitating factors are still not totally understood. While alcohol and drug abuse have not been thoroughly studied in the switch process, the data available are fairly consistent and in need of further replication. The earliest reporting of substance abuse in rapid-cycling patients was by Mayfield and Coleman (1968), who observed that "Several cyclic patients had onset of increased drinking at the transition from depression to mania" (p. 472). The authors offered several explanations for this finding: (1) that drinking was a successful attempt to alleviate depression, (2) that depression precipitated the manic swing, or (3) that drinking was an early expression of a manic swing. Following this, several authors reported that alcohol and drug abuse was significantly higher in mixed or cycling manic-depressive patients (Winokur et al., 1969; Himmelhoch et al., 1976a; Himmelhoch and Garfinkel, 1986). Himmelhoch and associates (1976) comment that ". . . drug abuse (particularly alcohol and sedatives) alters the clinical presentation of manic-depression swings, and that the impact of oversedation or withdrawal or both on a 'pure' affective state is to make it dysphoric and mixed" (p. 1065). Excessive polysubstance, cocaine, and amphetamine abuse in bipolar manic patients may indicate, according to Estroff and colleagues (1985), "that the drug abuse either causes or exacerbates manic symptoms" (p. 39). It is not clear whether alcohol and drug abuse directly modify the course of manic-depressive illness by inducing a switch, but it is evident that their use is elevated during the switch process.

There may be a common underlying process between manic-depressive illness and the substance abuse disorders that has not yet been identified. Mayfield (1985) expanded on this point in discussing the relationship between affective illness and alcoholism:

The relationship is not simply one mediated by the manifest mood disturbance and the easily observable psychopharmacological effects of alcohol. These apparent causal links may indeed be irrelevant or frankly misleading clues to the causal mechanism. (p. 80)

SUMMARY

Alcohol and drug abuse are common in patients with manic-depressive illness. Likewise, patients with affective illness (unipolar and bipolar) constitute a significant proportion of the total alcohol- and drug-abusing population. The correct identification of these patients is an important social and clinical concern.

Many methodological problems make it difficult to understand fully the sequencing of comorbidity (i.e., whether affective illness precedes or follows the alcohol or drug abuse problem), although recent data on major depression from the ECA study provide impressive support for the hypothesis that comorbidity is more likely to start with depression than the other way around.

Increased drug and alcohol abuse in manic-depressive patients has been related to changes in mood states, genetic factors, and self-medication of affective symptoms (both to diminish painful or unpleasant states and to induce, sustain, or exacerbate hypomanic states). Alcohol and drug abuse also mask the symptoms of manic-depressive illness and modify its course, complicating both diagnosis and treatment.

It is important for clinicians to detect substance abuse in manic-depressive patients because it is a particularly strong predictor of lethality in suicide, especially in males. Alcohol and illicit drugs diminish impulse control, impair judgment, and worsen the course of affective illness. These substances often are used as an attempt by the patient to lessen the severe anxiety and panic associated with suicidal depression. The combination greatly increases the risk of suicide. Therefore, it is clear that recognition and treatment of a substance abuse must be a priority.

NOTES

1. For example, Stein, 1964; Schildkraut, 1965; Duarte-Escalante and Ellinwood, 1972; Baldessarini, 1975; Castellani et al., 1985.
2. Mendelson and Mello, 1966; Mayfield and Allen, 1967; Freed, 1970; Nathan et al., 1970; Davis, 1971; Winokur, 1983.
3. Wikler, 1952; Griffith et al., 1968; Haertzen and Hooks, 1969; Babor et al., 1979.
4. Post et al., 1974b; Post and Kopanda, 1976; Siegel, 1977.
5. In DSM-III, the criteria for substance abuse were more stringent, and it was these criteria that were used in the ECA study (see Table 9-4), the largest population-based assessment of comorbidity to date. It appears that DSM-IV will return to the more demanding criteria.
6. Safer (1987) found that more than 70 percent of a sample of young adult chronically mentally ill (schizoaffective and bipolar disorder) were under the influence of an abused substance just before one or more of their psychiatric hospital admissions.
7. For good reviews of alcohol and drug abuse in unipolar depressive illness, see Cloninger et al., 1979; Woodruff et al., 1979; Dackis et al., 1986; Schuckit, 1986.
8. A more detailed discussion of alcohol abuse in mania and depression is presented in the phase of illness section.
9. Another hypothesized difference between bipolar and unipolar illness and alcoholism is the connection between bipolar illness and type II alcoholism. Type I alcoholism generally has its onset after age 25, frequently involves psychological dependence as well as guilt and fear about dependence, and infrequently involves fighting and arrests. Type II alcoholism, on the other hand, generally has its onset before age 25, is frequently associated with fighting and arrests and spontaneous alcohol seeking, but less frequently involves psychological dependence or guilt and fear about dependence. Thus, when alcoholism is present with unipolar illness, it is often associated with anxiety as is typical in the type I alcoholic. When alcoholism is comorbid with bipolar illness, it usually has an early age of onset and is characterized by impulsive and aggressive behavior. In these respects, type II alcoholism and bipolar illness are very similar.
10. For example, Gershon and Liebowitz, 1975; James and Chapman, 1975; Morrison, 1975; Dunner et al., 1976d; Gershon et al., 1982a; Lewis et al., 1982.
11. For example, Slater, 1938b; Pitts and Winokur, 1966; Winokur et al., 1969; Helzer and Winokur, 1974; Dunner et al., 1976d; Andreasen and Winokur, 1979; Hensel et al., 1979.
12. James and Chapman, 1975; E. Robins et al., 1977; D. Goodwin et al., 1979; Schuckit, 1983, 1985; Mirin et al., 1984b.
13. Glover, 1932; Rado, 1933; Lettieri et al., 1980; Khantzian, 1985; Weiss and Mirin, 1987; Pervin, 1988; Castaneda et al., 1989.
14. El-Guebaly, 1975; Horowitz, 1975; Bowers, 1977; Erard et al., 1980; and Weller et al., 1988.

10

Suicide

The patients, therefore, often try to starve themselves, to hang themselves, to cut
their arteries; they beg that they may be burned, buried alive, driven out into the
woods and there allowed to die. . . . One of my patients struck his neck so often
on the edge of a chisel fixed on the ground that all the soft parts were cut through
to the vertebrae. p. 25   —Emil Kraepelin, 1921

Patients with depressive and manic-depressive
illnesses are far more likely to commit suicide
than individuals in any other psychiatric or medical risk group. The mortality rate for untreated
manic-depressive patients is higher than it is for
most types of heart disease and many types of
cancer. Yet this lethality often is underemphasized, a tendency that may be traceable to the
erroneous but widespread belief that suicide is
volitional.

Suicidal thinking and behavior in both bipolar
and unipolar major depressive disorders have
been underscored in DSM-III-R, which gives a
specific diagnostic criterion for suicidal potential:

Recurrent thoughts of death (not just fear of dying),
recurrent suicidal ideation without a specific plan, or a
suicide attempt or a specific plan for committing suicide. (p. 272)

On the other hand, the general suicide literature,
despite its staggering size, offers relatively little
guidance for the management of suicidal patients.
The guidance that is available is often more speculative than empirical, and it is not particularly
relevant to the study and prevention of suicide in
manic-depressive illness. The lack of research in
this area is particularly surprising given the well-
documented and extensive overlap among suicide, suicide attempts, and affective disorders.
Even fewer articles or books deal specifically

with the clinical problems or predictors of suicidal behavior in bipolar patients, especially the
unique pharmacological and psychological issues
raised by this group.

In this chapter, we discuss several basic prem-
ises. First, suicide in untreated, inadequately
treated, or treatment-resistant bipolar patients is
far too common and often can be avoided. Second, although relatively little scientific literature
deals specifically with the clinical management
of suicidal bipolar patients, enough is known
from the combination of recent biological studies, a formidable psychopharmacology literature,
and extensive clinical knowledge of manic-
depressive illness to justify reviewing the field
and making specific clinical suggestions (see
Chapter 27). The literature on suicidal behavior
in unipolar patients is, cited for the sake of comparison or to supplement that on self-destructive
behavior in bipolar patients.

RATES OF SUICIDE IN MANIC-DEPRESSIVE
ILLNESS

General Issues

Determining suicide rates under any conditions is
difficult, but doing so for manic-depressive patients presents problems idiosyncratic to the ill-

227

ness. Completed suicides are relatively easier to determine than suicidal thoughts and behavior, which form a complicated, frequently unrecognized spectrum from ideation through threats, attempted suicide, and completed suicide. The relationship of these manifestations of suicidal potential to actual behavior has not been well studied, certainly not in bipolar patients. But the discrepancy between those who attempt suicide and those who actually commit suicide is far less important in manic-depressive patients—an exceptionally high risk group—than it is in other populations.

Interpreting suicide rates presents its own difficulties. They generally reflect prelithium realities, for example, and as a result they probably yield a more realistic picture of the untreated natural course of the illness than is now available. However, these data are compromised by the unsophisticated diagnostic and sampling techniques used for their collection. Ethical considerations now preclude a clinical trial comparing medicated with unmedicated bipolar or recurrent unipolar patients to evaluate the impact of pharmacological treatment on suicide rates.

Changes in suicide rates also are difficult to decipher. Diagnostic criteria vary across time and from one year to the next, and treatments change, both for the illness itself and for the medical consequences of attempted suicide. For example, Brown (1979) found no systematic studies on the impact of improved treatments for self-poisoning and their efficacy on overall suicide rates. However, he also noted that British suicide rates had declined because traditional methods of suicide had become less lethal—barbiturates were replaced by benzodiazepines for many patients, and the carbon monoxide content of domestic gas was reduced in Great Britain, where, in 1961, almost 50 percent of suicide deaths were caused by carbon monoxide poisoning.

Methodological problems confound interpretation. Diagnostic criteria often are unclear, and bipolar and unipolar distinctions only recently became standard in the literature. Particularly critical is the enormous variance across studies in follow-up periods, which results in variable periods of risk. Most studies are done with hospitalized patients as subjects, a practice that skews the data toward the more severely ill. Many of these and other methodological problems are similar to issues raised throughout this book and will

not be elaborated here. (Methodological issues bearing on outcome measures are discussed in Chapter 6.)

Rates of Suicide

Although many early researchers noted the strikingly high rate of suicide in patients with manic-depressive illness, Guze and Robins (1970) were the first to review and document systematically the extent of suicide risk. They reviewed 14 follow-up studies, two population surveys, and one family study (Table 10-1). Guze and Robins found that in every study at least 12 percent of all deaths among manic-depressive patients were the result of suicide (like most of the early studies, both unipolar and bipolar patients were included). In nine studies, 12 to 19 percent of deaths were due to suicides, and in eight studies the suicide rate ranged from 35 to 60 percent. They concluded that by the time all the patients had died, about 15 percent would have committed suicide, at least 30 times what one would find in the general population.

Findings from our more recent review of 30 studies of completed suicide in manic-depressive patients (Table 10-1) do not differ significantly from those of Guze and Robins. We found a range, 9 to 60 percent, of manic-depressive deaths secondary to suicide, with a mean of 19 percent. In 13 of the 30 studies, or about one half, the figure was in the 10 to 30 percent range. One fifth of the studies concluded that at least half of their manic-depressive patients had died because of suicide. The question of whether risk of suicide is different among subgroups of major affective disorder is discussed later in the chapter.

From a different perspective, Robins and co-workers (1959b) found that 46 percent of individuals who committed suicide had manic-depressive illness. Barraclough (1972) estimated that 64 percent of the suicides in his sample had a primary affective disorder, and 60 percent of the suicides in the sample studied by Helgason (1979) had an affective disorder. Hagnell and associates (1981), in a survey of 3,563 residents of Lundby, Sweden, found a 78-fold increase in risk for suicide among patients with depressive disorder (bipolar and unipolar combined) when compared with those with no psychiatric disorder. Weeke (1979) found many more suicides than expected in the general population, an increase observed in both men and women (Figure 10-1).

Table 10-1. Rates of Suicide in Manic-Depressive Illness

Study	Patient & Study Characteristics	Subjects N	Deaths due to Suicide unless Otherwise Specified %
Bond & Braceland, 1937	MDI	204	38
Slater, 1938b	MDI	138	15
Langelüddecke, 1941	MDI	341	15
Lundquist, 1945	MDI	319	14
Ziskind et al., 1945	MDI	109	60
Huston & Locher, 1948a	MDI	80	60
Huston & Locher, 1948b	MDI	93	36
Schulz, 1949	MDI	2,004	13
Fremming, 1951	MDI	45	50
Stenstedt, 1952	MDI	216	14
Watts, 1956	MDI	368	19
Hastings, 1958	MDI	238	35
Astrup et al., 1959	MDI	256	17
Seager, 1959	MDI	206	54
Helgason, 1964	MDI	103	51
Pitts & Winokur, 1964	Study of causes of death in first-degree relatives with affective disorders (index relatives depressed)	56	16
Perris & d'Elia, 1966	BP (F = 81, M = 57)	138	23
Bratfos & Haug, 1968	MDI	207	12

Continued

Table 10-1 Continued. Rates of Suicide in Manic-Depressive Illness

Barraclough, 1972	Postmortem study of consecutive suicides	100	64
Tashev, 1974	Postmortem study of BP patients	122	27
James & Chapman, 1975	BP patients (46) & first-degree relatives (52) with affective illness	98	46
Winokur & Tsuang, 1975b Tsuang, 1978	30-40 year follow-up study of mortality in schizophrenics (SCZ), manics (M), depressives (D) and surgical controls (S/C)	SCZ = 170 M = 76 D = 182 S/C = 109	10.1 8.5-11.1 9.3-10.6 0.0
Dunner et al., 1976d	BP, follow-up 1-9 years post-index hospitalization	90	9 (BPI, 5.9%; BPII, 18.2%)
Helgason, 1979	Manic-depressive psychoses in cohort of all Icelanders born 1895-1897 and alive in 1910		60% of probands who committed suicide had affective disorder (majority had manic-depressive psychosis)
Weeke, 1979	MDI (M = 2,840; F = 5,296)	8,136	Suicide risk in males: 11/1,000/year, in females: 5/1,000/year
Hagnell et al., 1981	Epidemiological survey	3,563	78-fold increase in risk associated with depressive disorders over those in population with no psychiatric diagnosis
Egeland & Sussex, 1985	Biographical survey of all suicides between 1880 and 1980 among the Old Order Amish	26 suicides	92% of the suicides were committed by those diagnosed with major affective disorder; clustered in 4 primary pedigrees, suggesting the role of inheritance in suicide
Black et al., 1987a	Risk of suicide in UP and BP as compared to general population	586 BP 1,007 UP	17 in BP, 30 in UP
Angst, 1988	26 year follow-up of psychiatric admissions	215 BP 173 UP	15 in BP, 20 in UP
	Total N = 9,389[a]		**Weighted Mean = 18.9%**

MDI = manic-depressive illness. In these studies the bipolar-unipolar distinction was not made, so it must be assumed that both subgroups were included. The traditional European designation of MDI is limited to those with a prior course; i.e., it would include bipolar and recurrent unipolar.

[a]Excluding Helgason, 1979; Weeke, 1979; Hagnell et al., 1981

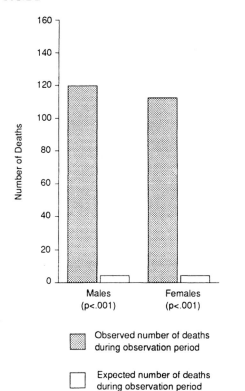

Figure 10-1. Expected vs. observed deaths in manic-depressive patients (from Weeke, 1979).

Rates of Attempted Suicide

Studies of attempted suicide in bipolar patients (Table 10-2) show that 25 to 50 percent attempted suicide at least once. Combining data for both sexes results in an attempted suicide rate ranging from 20 to 56 percent. Women, however, appear far more likely than men to attempt suicide, showing both a higher minimum and maximum rate, 15 and 48 percent, respectively. The attempted suicide rate for men was consistently lower, ranging from 4 to 27 percent. Johnson and Hunt (1979), the only investigators to specify the severity of suicide attempts, classified 90 percent of them as serious enough to warrant hospitalization.

Sex Differences in Attempted and Completed Suicide

In the general population, women attempt suicide two to three times more often than men, but men actually commit suicide two to three times more often than women. Table 10-3 shows sex differences in rates for manic-depressive individuals.

Like the general female population, manic-depressive women more often attempt suicide, but unlike the general population, there is not a clear predominance of males among manic-depressives who actually commit suicide. Three of the seven studies actually note a female predominance for completed suicides among manic-depressive patients. Roy-Byrne and colleagues (1988a), in their study of 67 bipolar and 20 unipolar patients, note that violent attempts and completed suicide were equally common in men and women. Linkowski and colleagues (1985a) found that a family history of suicide (mainly violent) greatly increased the frequency of violent suicidal behavior in both depressed males and females.

Evidence of sex differences among suicide attempters may be marred by reporting biases when patients are asked about past suicidal behavior. Bipolar women may more readily admit attempts, whereas men may be more prone to the suicidal equivalents—such as extreme risk-taking, car accidents, and substance abuse—that are less often explored in surveys.

The course of the illness may affect men and women differently (the impact of course in general is discussed later). Johnson and Hunt (1979) found that more men (42 percent) than women (17 percent) attempted suicide at the onset of manic-depressive illness, but this sex difference later dissipated. Attempts by women were more evenly distributed across time. Although all women's attempts occurred within approximately 15 years of onset, those by men were more extremely, and bimodally, distributed. Thus, 60 percent of the men who attempted suicide did so within 2 years of the onset of the illness; the other 40 percent attempted suicide after 23 years or more.

These sex differences may be accounted for by various explanations. Women may accommodate to mood swings, through adaptation to mood changes secondary to the menstrual cycle, for example. Cultural and sexual differences in adaptation to catastrophe or acute stress may also be responsible.

Rates of Other Suicidal Behavior

Little is known about the prevalence of other suicidal behavior, such as suicidal ideation or threat, in manic-depressive illness. The experiences, thoughts, severity, and persistence of suicidal

Table 10-2. Rates of Suicide Attempts in Manic-Depressive Illness

Study	Patient & Study Characteristics	Subjects N	BP Suicide Attempts %	Comments
Kraepelin, 1921	MDI	995		
Astrup et al., 1959	MDI	96		
Perris & d'Elia, 1966	BP psychoses (F = 81, M = 57)	138	26	37% female, 11% male
Winokur et al., 1969	BP (F = 35, M = 26)	61	25	40% female 4% male, $p < .005$
Woodruff et al., 1971a	Primary affective disorders (BP = 19, UP = 139)	158	32	14% of UPs attempted suicide
Dunner et al., 1976d	BP	90	38 BP I 56 BP II	
Johnson & Hunt, 1979	BP patients and first-degree relatives (F = 19, M = 31)	50	20	26% female, 16% male; 90% required hospitalization
Stallone et al., 1980	BP I, BP II	72 BP I 53 BP II	33 BP I 45 BP II	49% female, 29% male
Roy, 1983	Psychiatric inpatients with (S-P) and without (S-N) family history of suicide	243 S-P (incl. 58 BP, 32 UP) 5,602 S-N	38	Suicide attempts: 48.6% of S-P 21.8% of S-N 40.6% of UP
Goldring & Fieve 1984	Primary affective disorders	Incl: 24 BP I 6 BP II 7 UP	55 BP I 60 BP II	17% of UPs attempted suicide
Linkowski et al., 1985a	Major depressive illness	244 BP 269 UP	26	37% of UPs attempted suicide; a family history of suicide strongly increased chances the attempt would be violent
Kupfer et al., 1988a	Major depression	27 BP II 188 UP	48 BP II	24% of UPs attempted suicide. Significant BPII/UP differences ($p < .01$)
Mitterauer et al., 1988	MDI with family history of MDI, with and without family history of suicide	342 S-P 80 S-N		25% in S-P group made attempts, 11% in S-N group; S-N group had more delusions

Continued

Table 10-2 Continued. Rates of Suicide Attempts in Manic-Depressive Illness

Roy-Byrne et al., 1988	Major affective disorder	67 BP 20 UP	58	65% female, 42% male with violence equally common; 50% of UPs attempt suicide
Regier et al., 1988b	Epidemiological survey, lifetime prevalence rates	Over 20,000	24	18% for UP, 17% for dysthymia, 1% for those with no life-time history of mental disorder

S-P = suicide-positive family history, S-N = suicide-negative family history
MDI = Manic-depressive illness. In these studies the bipolar-unipolar distinction was not made, so it must be assumed that both subgroups were included. The traditional European designation of MDI is limited to those with a prior course, i.e., it would include bipolar and recurrent unipolar.

feelings remain largely unexamined, although there have been a few attempts to determine the frequency of suicidal ideation. Winokur and co-workers (1969) found that 82 percent of their depressed bipolar patients, during their depressive phase, had suicidal ruminations. Carlson and Strober (1979) found essentially the same rate of suicidal ruminations in their chart review of nine bipolar adolescents (83 percent) as in the adult bipolar group (82 percent).[1] Among a bipolar sample studied by Johnson and Hunt (1979), 16 percent had contemplated or threatened suicide in addition to the 20 percent who had actually attempted it. Stallone and colleagues (1980) found approximately the same rates of suicide attempts and suicidal ideation in their study of 125 bipolar patients. A positive family history of suicidal behavior was twice as prevalent among attempters and contemplators as in a nonsuicidal group. They concluded that "attempters and contemplators were a good deal more similar to one another than either was to the nonsuicidals" (p. 386).

Table 10-3. Sex Differences in Rates of Suicide and Attempted Suicide in Manic-Depressive Illness

Study	M > F	M = F	F > M
Completed Suicide			
Ahlstrom, 1942[a]	X		
Dahlgren, 1944[a]			X
Stenstedt, 1952[a]	X		
Ringel, 1953[a]			X
Ettlinger, 1964[a]			X
Weeke, 1979[a]	X		
Hegnell et al., 1981[a]	X		
Egeland & Sussex, 1985[a]	X		
Attempted Suicide			
Kraepelin, 1921[a]		X	
Astrup et al., 1959			X
Perris & d'Elia, 1966			X
Winokur et al., 1969			X
Woodruff et al., 1971a	X		
Johnson & Hunt., 1979			X
Stallone et al., 1980			X
Goldring & Fieve, 1984			X
Linkowski et al., 1985a			X
Mitterauer et al., 1988		X	
Roy-Byrne et al., 1988			X

[a]Bipolar-unipolar distinction not made

Bipolar–Unipolar Differences

Table 10-4 displays the eight studies that have compared rates of suicide attempts or suicides in unipolar and bipolar patients. Typical of this literature is the study of Black and colleagues (1988b), who followed a large group of patients with major depression (n = 1,593) for 1 to 14 years. They found no bipolar–unipolar differences in suicide rates, although the total number of suicides was small during these relatively brief and variable follow-up periods. As Table 10-4 shows, when weighted means are compared, bipolar patients and unipolar patients do not differ significantly in the rates at which they attempt or commit suicide.

In a study of risk factors among adolescents who had died from suicide, Brent and co-workers

Table 10-4. Rates of Attempted and Completed Suicide in Unipolar and Bipolar Illness

Study	Suicide Attempts				Suicides			
	UP		BP		UP		BP	
	N	(%)	N	(%)	N	(%)	N	(%)
Woodruff et al., 1971a	139	(14)	19	(32)				
Roy, 1983	32	(41)	58	(38)				
Goldring & Fieve, 1984	7	(17)	35	(43)				
Linkowski et al., 1985a	269	(37)	244	(26)				
Black et al., 1987a					1,007	(3)	586	(3)
Angst, 1988					173	(12)	215	(7)
Kupfer et al., 1988a	188	(24)	27[a]	(48)				
Roy-Byrne et al., 1988	20	(50)	67	(58)				
Weighted means	**655**	**(28)**	**450**	**(35)**	**1,180**	**(4)**	**801**	**(4)**

N refers to the total number of patients in the study; rates of attempted or completed suicides are in parentheses

[a]Bipolar II only

(1988) found that 22 percent were bipolar, and half as many were unipolar. Among the high-risk attempters (n = 54), only 5 percent were bipolar. The presence of four risk factors accounted for 82 percent of the suicides: bipolar diagnosis, substance abuse comorbidity, lack of prior treatment, and availability of firearms. Of these, bipolar diagnosis contributed the most to the prediction.

According to Himmelhoch (1987), suicidal unipolar depressed patients show greater anxiety and agitation than bipolar patients. Bipolar depressions become suicidal later in the course of the episode, and lethality intensifies with recurrence.

In their study of the premorbid personality of psychiatric patients, Angst and Clayton (1986) found that bipolar patients did not differ significantly from matched controls but did have a significantly lower aggression score than the unipolar group. In the National Institute of Mental Health (NIMH) collaborative study on the psy-

chobiology of depression (Fawcett et al., 1987), diagnostic subgroups did not differentiate patients who committed suicide from those who did not, but mood cycling during the index episode did ($p < 0.002$). The authors of the study concluded that a bipolar or schizoaffective diagnosis is implied by this cycling, the only subtype of affective illness associated with a suicidal outcome. The association was particularly strong in men. Although the suicides of bipolar patients were not analyzed separately in this prospective study, in the absence of other data, these findings are sufficiently compelling to serve as a guide to clinical practice. A retrospective analysis of patients with unipolar depression while on the census at the New York State Psychiatric Institute between 1955 and 1980 showed an unusually high rate of delusions among those who committed suicide (Roose et al., 1983). Again, bipolar patients were not considered in this study, but the findings are at least suggestive of symptom patterns associated with high risk of suicide. Black and colleagues (1987b) found no increased suicide risk among affectively ill patients who were psychotic, however.

Other Diagnostic Correlates

Delineating diagnostic subgroups with increased incidence of suicide is one of the first steps toward identifying individual bipolar patients at particularly high risk. Dunner and co-workers (1976d) found that bipolar-I patients, those with histories of severe depressive and manic episodes, had lower rates of suicide and attempted suicide than bipolar-II patients. Stallone and colleagues (1980), using the same diagnostic system in 125 bipolar patients, found the same higher rates in the bipolar-II subgroup. Angst and colleagues (1980a), using their own, similar system for designating subgroups (see Chapter 4), found no patient suicides in the 43 Dm (BP II) patients, but 3 in the 36 MD (comparable to bipolar I) patients. This finding conflicts with the findings of the previous two studies, but the sample sizes were small, and problems inherent to retrospective diagnoses confound the results.[2] The Angst group did find that morbid risk of suicide in the first-degree relatives of his patients followed a pattern that was similar to the earlier findings: the risk was higher in the Dm group (bipolar II) than in the MD group (bipolar I) and lowest in the Md group (predominance of manic symptomatology with little or no history of depression). Although not formal diagnostic subgroups, mixed and delusional states (discussed in greater detail later) are also associated with greater vulnerability to suicide.

In summary, the separation of bipolar patients into subgroups may increase the ability of clinical researchers to predict suicide. It should be emphasized, however, that, along with a history of suicidal attempt, the diagnosis of bipolar manic-depressive illness itself remains the best predictor of suicide.

CLINICAL DESCRIPTION AND CORRELATES

Phenomenology

My life felt so cluttered and obstructed that I could hardly breathe. I inhabited a closed, concentrated world, airless and without exits. I doubt if any of this was noticeable socially: I was simply more tense, more nervous than usual, and I drank more. But underneath I was going a bit mad. I had entered the closed world of suicide, and my life was being lived for me by forces I couldn't control. (p. 259)—A. Alvarez, 1973

The subjective reports of patients who attempt or commit suicide are particularly helpful in understanding this otherwise inexplicable phenomenon and provide insight into the thoughts and motivation of individual patients. In addition, they are an important, if neglected, source of hypotheses for clinical and basic researchers. Patients' descriptions of diurnal or other cyclic patterns of suicidal mood and activity, subjective reports of feelings of violence or agitation, and patterns of acute perturbations or diminution of such feelings convey the cognitive content and patterns of suicidal ideation. All are of potential value to both the researcher and the clinician. Good subjective descriptions can aid in identifying high-risk groups, culling out more specific pharmacological treatments for different subgroups of manic-depressive patients (e.g., those with violent vs nonviolent thoughts and feelings), adding correlative subjective data to more objective measures, and developing an increasingly sophisticated diagnostic system through a more refined understanding and differentiation of patients' experiences.

Alvarez (1973), in his book on suicide, *The Savage God,* vividly portrayed the despair, violence, and highly individualistic motives involved in suicide. In citing Cesare Pavese, the Italian writer who committed suicide and who wrote that "no one ever lacks a good reason for suicide," Alvarez reminds us of the limits of knowing the mind of any suicidal individual. Without accepting a nihilistic notion of such limits, it remains important to recognize the ultimate inaccessibility of many complex, idiosyncratic motivations:

It goes without saying that external misery has relatively little to do with suicide. . . . Suicide often seems to the outsider a supremely motiveless perversity, performed, as Montesquieu complained, "most unaccountably . . . in the very bosom of happiness," and for reasons which seem trivial or even imperceptible. . . . At best they assuage the guilt of the survivors, soothe the tidy-minded and encourage the sociologists in their endless search for convincing categories and theories. The real motives . . . belong to the internal world, devious, contradictory, labyrinthine, and mostly out of sight. (Alvarez, 1973, pp. 95, 97)

Feelings of isolation and pain characterize the remarks of many suicidal manic-depressive patients. One of our patients who was in a hospital on continual suicide watch wrote:

I have prayed to God to kill me—isn't there some pill they can give me to take my life? I put my neck across the back of a chair and tried to put weight on it. I'm a failure. I've lived my whole life and accomplished nothing, I just want to die. I dread to wake up in the morning and face another day of emptiness. I'm tired of feeling as though I'm standing in the foyer of mankind and can't go in.

This sense of "standing in the foyer" is described by many seriously depressed and suicidal patients. Alvarez (1973) wrote of such an abyss:

A suicidal depression is a kind of spiritual winter, frozen, sterile, unmoving. The richer, softer and more delectable nature becomes, the deeper that internal winter seems, and the wider and more intolerable the abyss which separates the inner world from the outer. Thus suicide becomes a natural reaction to an unnatural condition. Perhaps this is why, for the depressed, Christmas is so hard to bear. In theory it is an oasis of warmth and light in an unforgiving season, like a lighted window in a storm. For those who have to stay outside, it accentuates, like spring, the disjunction between public warmth and festivity, and cold, private despair. (pp. 79-80)

The cumulative effects of manic-depressive illness and their influence on the decision to commit suicide were reflected in Virginia Woolf's suicide letter to her husband:

Dearest, I feel certain I am going mad again. I feel we can't go through another of those terrible times. And I shan't recover this time. . . . So I am doing what seems the best thing to do. . . . I don't think two people could have been happier until this terrible disease came. I can't fight any longer. (Bell, 1972, p. 266)

Many of the feelings described earlier—despair, isolation, violence, hopelessness—are expressed in the following passage written by one of our patients, a woman with manic-depressive illness. She, too, described the tremendous havoc wrought in relationships. Before writing this she had been suicidal for several months, experiencing intermittent exacerbations characterized by a mixed manic and depressive state and clearly perceived as extremely painful. The episode described here was an acute and particularly serious one, which led to a nearly lethal suicide attempt:

I remember that in a rage I pulled the bathroom lamp off the wall and felt the violence go through me but not yet out of me. "For Christ's sake," he said, rushing in—and then stopping very quietly. Jesus, I must be crazy, I can see it in his eyes: a dreadful mix of concern, terror, irritation, resignation, and why me, Lord? "Are you hurt?" Turning my head with its fast scanning eyes I see in the mirror blood running down my arms, collecting into the tight ribbing of my beautiful, erotic negligee, only an hour ago used in violence of an altogether different and wonderful kind. "I can't help it. I can't help it," I chant to myself but I can't say it; the words won't come out and the thoughts are going by far too fast. I bang my head over and over against the door, God make it stop, I can't stand it, I know I'm insane again. . . . He really *is* concerned I think, but within ten minutes he too is screaming, and his eyes have a wilder look from contagious madness, from the lightning adrenaline between the two of us. "I can't leave you like this" but I say a few truly awful things and then go for his throat in a more literal way and he does leave me, provoked beyond endurance and unable to see the devastation and despair inside. I can't convey it and he can't see it, there's nothing that can be done. I can't think, I can't calm this murderous cauldron, my grand ideas of an hour ago seem absurd and pathetic, my life is in ruins and—worse still—ruinous; my body is uninhabitable. It is raging and weeping and full of destruction and wild energy gone amok. In the mirror I see a creature I don't know or like but must live and share my mind with.

I understand why Jekyll killed himself before Hyde had taken over completely. I took a massive overdose of lithium with no regrets.

Suicidal feelings are difficult for patients to express because they are often embarrassed by such impulses and lack the appropriate language to articulate such feelings. Psychotic thinking, cognitive slowing, and psychomotor retardation further impair description of painful and incomprehensible emotions and thoughts. Some common themes about suicide do emerge from the writings and remarks of manic-depressive patients: the impact of severe depression, the devastating cumulative effects of the illness on the patient and on his or her relationships with others, and the almost intolerable subjective experience of mixed states and feelings of violence. Anger, either nonspecific or directed toward another, feelings of isolation, a sense of hopelessness and lack of control over feelings and thoughts, and a conviction that the current emotional state is endless also contribute to suicidal thought and feeling.

Treatment History

Several investigators have examined the amount and timing of contact with physicians by those who have committed suicide, but the greater part of this literature does not differentiate bipolar from unipolar patients. Robins and colleagues (1959b) found that 73 percent of the manic-depressive patients[3] in their sample of 134 suicides had received medical care in the year before the suicide, and 53 percent had received it within 1 month. Likewise, within a year before their deaths, 15 percent had been hospitalized in a psychiatric facility, and 11 percent had been hospitalized in a medical facility with symptoms of a psychiatric illness. Among Barraclough's sample (1970) of depressed patients who committed suicide, 70 percent had been in touch with a physician within 30 days of their death, and nearly 50 percent had seen their doctors during the preceding week. Of the 49 suicides in Murphy's study (1975a,b), 71 percent had been seen by a physician within 6 months of death. To our knowledge, only one study examined these issues specifically among bipolar patients. James and Chapman (1975) found that 50 percent of the bipolar patients and their first-degree affectively ill relatives who committed suicide had been seen by a psychiatrist in the 3 months before their death. Thus, although a very high percentage of patients who killed themselves had recently seen a physician (often a psychiatrist), it is unclear what conclusions can be drawn from such data. Patients may present themselves for medical problems seemingly unrelated to manic-depressive illness. It would be important to know the baseline rates of physician contact for a comparable group of individuals from the general population.

Most studies imply that physicians should have been more sophisticated in the diagnosis and appropriate treatment of such patients. Though this is true in many cases, patients often are depressed intermittently or prefer not to reveal the time, nature, and extent of their psychological distress. It is within this context that the specific nature of the physician–patient contacts and the treatments prescribed before suicide take on critical meaning.

Retrospective analyses of physicians' treatment regimens for patients who subsequently killed themselves have been carried out by several researchers.[4] Barraclough and co-workers (1974) found that barbiturates, phenothiazines, and minor tranquilizers were overprescribed in depressed patients who went on to commit suicide. They also concluded that in half of the patients treated with antidepressants, the medication had failed, and in the other half, the medica-

tion had not been given a fair trial (56 percent) or the wrong antidepressant, for example, a monoamine oxidase inhibitor instead of a tricyclic, was given (44 percent). In any event, in only one case was a tricyclic accompanied by some improvement before death, leading to the inevitable question of why alternative treatments or hospitalization had not been recommended. Lithium, not yet in widespread use at the time of the study, was given to only one manic-depressive patient. A small but significant proportion of patients who committed suicide (6 percent) did so early in the course of electroconvulsive therapy. The same proportion (6 percent) refused to take their medication. Black and colleagues (1988c) compared mortality risk in 1,076 patients with affective disorders (160 bipolar) to matched controls from the general population. The patients were divided into four treatment groups, including electroconvulsive therapy, adequate antidepressants, inadequate antidepressants, and no treatment. Although, as expected, the risk for suicide was higher in the patient groups, the mode of therapy had little influence on subsequent mortality, including suicide.

Murphy (1975a,b) found that general physicians tended to underdiagnose depression and to miss histories of suicidal behaviors (e.g., 71 percent of the patients had threatened or attempted suicide, but only 39 percent of the physicians knew of such episodes). An alarming 50 percent of the patients who died from a medication overdose obtained the lethal dose in a single prescription.

Most authors[5] have concurred in several conclusions: (1) most people who committed suicide were seen by physicians not long before their deaths, (2) few were adequately diagnosed or treated for their affective illness, (3) tranquilizers were overprescribed, (4) prejudice, outdated information, or obstructive legislation kept many practitioners from using electroconvulsive therapy, (5) tricyclics frequently were prescribed in inadequate doses and without proper monitoring, and (6) outpatient follow-up and posthospitalization aftercare services were inconsistent and often poor.

Effect of Lithium on Suicide Rate

One of the more interesting questions in preventive medicine today is the impact of lithium on suicide rates. There are no current and systematic data available, although a well-documented answer may be possible within the next 10 years. Until then, we must rely on preliminary speculations and clinical observations.

Barraclough (1972) hypothesized that because there was a high rate of suicide in affective disorders and because lithium was very effective in treating such disorders, the drug might well be expected to decrease the suicide rate. He studied the records of 100 suicides in West Sussex and Portsmouth and found that 64 could be diagnosed as having primary affective disorders (11 percent had been treated by a psychiatrist for mania). Forty-four of these had a history of a previous affective illness and 21 met the criteria of Coppen's group for recurrent affective disorder:

. . . a clear history of affective disorders and . . . at least one affective illness per year for 3 years, or three affective illnesses in the previous 2 years, or two illnesses during the previous year. The affective illnesses could be either manic or depressive or both. (Coppen et al., 1971b, p. 275)

Such criteria would tend to underestimate the incidence of recurrent affective illness. On the basis of these figures, Barraclough estimated that had lithium been used, there would have been at least a 21 percent reduction in suicides. Although Barraclough probably underestimated the number of individuals in the sample who had recurrent affective illness, given that 44 out of 64 had histories of prior episodes, he also almost certainly overestimated the lithium response rate and the extent of compliance (apparently assuming total response and complete compliance).

In a study by Page and colleagues (1987) involving a mixed group of 65 bipolar patients and 35 recurrent unipolar patients followed on lithium maintenance, 6 patients committed suicide. All were bipolar.

Kay and Petterson (1977) noted that in their follow-up of a group of treated bipolar patients, presumably at high risk for suicide, there were no suicides. They concluded that this was probably due to either a relatively short follow-up period or to the prophylactic effects of lithium. Yet another contributing factor may have been the highly specialized and competent medical care available at a clinic treating only affective disorders.

Weeke (1979) hypothesized that suicide was related to whether individuals were taking lithium at the time of their suicide. He found that of 222 individuals who had committed suicide, 10 percent were on lithium at the time of their deaths, 8 percent had been on lithium at a previous time, and 82 percent had never been on lithium. He concluded:

Together with the information that 40% of the suicides during the observation period occurred within the first six months after first admission . . . [it appears] that most suicides occur before lithium-therapy has been considered. There are, however, no control figures for the use of lithium in the surviving manic-depressive patients at the same point of time after the first admission. (p. 298)

It is also possible that lithium had been considered but rejected by some patients who had not yet been through enough episodes to accept the reality of the illness or, for some other reason, refused to take lithium.

A related and important issue, discussed further in Chapter 23, is the determination of the number of episodes necessary to warrant maintenance lithium. If suicides occur relatively early in the illness but lithium is not recommended unless a sufficient number of episodes elapse, the risk of suicide might be unnecessarily high. Clayton (1981) pointed out that some studies (Akiskal et al., 1978a; Petterson, 1977a) indicated a lower suicide risk in bipolar patients than was found in earlier investigations (Guze and Robins, 1970; Tsuang, 1978). Such lower risk might be attributable to a shorter follow-up period or to the effects of lithium. Prien and colleagues (1973a,b), in a related study of the efficacy of lithium, found that the only two suicides in their samples were the two patients on placebo rather than on lithium.

Additional data come from the clinical observations of Fieve (personal communication) and of Akiskal (personal communication), both at specialized clinics for affective disorders. Four suicides were reported in their combined clinical populations of more than 9,000 patients receiving lithium treatment. Schou and Weeke (1988), in a retrospective analysis of the treatment received by 92 manic-depressive patients who had committed suicide, found that 70 percent had taken their own lives despite having the best medical and prophylactic treatment available. The other 30 percent of suicides might have been prevented by more attention to risk factors, such as previous attempts, but Schou and Weeke caution that the study's methodological limitations make their conclusions tentative. In the same article, they reviewed three other studies of suicidal behavior during prophylactic lithium treatment of manic-depressive illness (Poole et al., 1978; Hanus and Zapletalek, 1984; Causemann and Müller-Oerlinghausen 1988). Poole's group followed 100 manic-depressive patients 5 years before and 5 years after they began lithium prophylaxis and found that 7 patients made more suicide attempts after being maintained on lithium, and 14 patients made fewer. Hanus and Zapletalek followed 95 manic-depressive patients over the same periods of time and found that 25 patients made suicide attempts before they took lithium, whereas 4 did so while taking lithium (chi-square = 13.3, $p <$ 0.001). The 78 patients in Causemann and Müller-Oerlinghausen's study had all made at least one suicide attempt and had taken lithium for at least a year. Over a period averaging 7.9 years, a mean of 1.17 suicide attempts were made per patient before lithium was started and 0.18 per patient (11 attempts and 3 suicides) during prophylactic treatment.

Very little systematic follow-up on suicide has been done in these or other specialty clinics to our knowledge. Further, the variety of highly specialized pharmacological and psychological treatments available at these clinics confounds any interpretations based on lithium as the sole reason for decreased suicide rates. However, it is impressive that within these clinics, treating a referral-based sample of particularly difficult, predominantly bipolar population of manic-depressive patients (including, presumably, a disproportionately high proportion of lithium noncompliers and nonresponders), there should be so few suicides among so many patients. The significantly low suicide rate in such a high-risk population is only suggestive but extremely promising.

Suicide and the Course of Illness

Little is known about the relationship between suicide and the course of manic-depressive illness. We are interested here in the amount of elapsed time from the onset of the illness or the episode to the suicide or suicide attempt. Evidence suggesting an increased risk of suicide early in the first episode of affective illness is fairly consistent (see, e.g., Guze and Robins, 1970). Tsuang and Woolson (1977) found that an in-

creased risk for suicide in patients with manias and depressions was largely limited to the first decade following first admissions, and Weeke (1979) determined that 40 percent of suicides occurred within the first 6 months after first admission and more than 50 percent occurred within the first year. Roy-Byrne and colleagues (1988a), studying 67 bipolar and 20 unipolar patients, found that none of the patients, regardless of polarity or history of suicidal behavior, differed in prior course of illness. Initial suicide attempts occurred early in the course of the illness. However, the severity of the worst attempt was positively correlated with the duration of the illness. Himmelhoch (1987) has suggested that suicide may be simultaneously psychologically and neuronally kindled. That is, in addition to the biological aspects of kindling, patients also become increasingly less tolerant with each new episode of depression and so increase their risk of suicide as the duration of the illness increases. These findings underscore the importance of early recognition, accurate diagnosis, and aggressive treatment and the need for continuous reappraisal of suicidal risk (see Chapter 27).

Johnson and Hunt (1979) were among the first to study the timing of suicide attempts in bipolar patients. All of the suicide attempts were classified as serious, and 90 percent of them warranted hospitalization. The authors found that 30 percent of the suicide attempts occurred at the onset of the illness or during the first episode of depression. The median lag was 5.5 years, indicating that the risk was greatest early in the course of illness. Their data (Figure 10-2) show that half of the serious suicide attempts occurred within 5 years of the onset of illness, yet the range (0 to 27 years) is striking. The sample size in the Johnson and Hunt study is small, but the increased risk period early in the illness is consistent with findings by Guze and Robins (1970), Tsuang and Woolson (1977), and Weeke (1979).

Few studies have considered the issue of episode length and suicide. Robins and colleagues (1959b) found that 57 percent of episodes had lasted less than 6 months and 87 percent less than 12 months at the time of death. Barraclough and co-workers (1974), in their study of endogenously depressed patients, found 50 percent and 67 percent, respectively. It is difficult to interpret these data, since they are simply consistent with

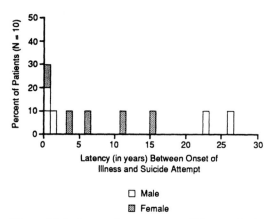

Figure 10-2. Latency between onset of illness and suicide attempts in bipolar patients (adapted from Johnson and Hunt, 1979).

what is known about the natural length of affective episodes and do not give any specific insight into patterns of suicide within episodes.

Clinical State Preceding Suicide and Attempted Suicide

Communication of Suicidal Intent

Patients who commit suicide generally communicate their intentions to others. Since little is known about communication patterns specific to bipolar patients, we must again draw on the general suicide literature and data obtained from depressed patients. Shneidman (1975) and others have estimated that 80 percent of people who commit suicide had communicated their intent to kill themselves. Dorpat and Ripley (1961), after studying the records of 114 consecutive suicides, found that 83 percent had indicated suicidal intent in some manner, usually directly.

In their study of 134 consecutive suicides (approximately half of whom had bipolar or unipolar illness), Robins and co-workers (1959a) found that 68 percent of the manic-depressive patients had communicated their suicidal ideas, most frequently through a direct and specific statement of the intent to commit suicide. They also observed that (1) men and women did not differ significantly in their frequency of suicidal communication, (2) expression of suicidal ideas was diverse, even for an individual, and (3) communications were repeated and expressed to a number of different persons. The authors further noted that, "In the vast majority of instances the relatives and friends did not regard these communications as efforts to manipulate the environment by playing on the emotions of the hearers." Of the entire sample, 86 percent expressed suicidal ideas for the first time or had shown a recent intensification of these ideas. Suicidal potential most frequently was expressed to spouses and other relatives (60 percent and 51 percent, respectively), then to friends (35 percent), and to physicians (18 percent). Robins and colleagues (1959b) observed:

> If we had found that suicide was an impulsive, unpremeditated act without rather well defined clinical limits, then the problem of its prevention would present insurmountable difficulties using presently available clinical criteria. The high rate of communication of suicidal ideas indicates that in the majority of instances it is a premeditated act of which the person gives ample warning. (p. 897)

Fawcett and colleagues (1990), in a study of 955 affectively ill patients (bipolar and unipolar), found a high rate of suicidal ideation, which was not, however, a good predictor of completed suicide. Because Fawcett and colleagues were conducting a prospective study, they may have been listening for communications of suicide intent that were indirect or made to others. On the other hand, in a retrospective study, such as that completed by Robins, investigators are looking for any clue to suicide in the individual's communications. This discrepancy underscores the importance of gathering information from all available sources.

When Barraclough and colleagues (1974) studied warnings of suicide in 64 endogenously depressed patients, they found that 30 percent of those who killed themselves had left a trail of "unequivocal threats, not enlightened hindsight." The many subtle meanings of suicidal communication were summarized by the authors:

> Talk indicating thoughts of suicide [is] sometimes a statement of fact; or coercive; or may imply mental conflict between the wish to die and the wish to live; or may indeed be a real supplication. (p. 367)

Clinical State

Robins and colleagues (1959b), in their study of 134 suicides, found that no one had committed suicide in the manic phase; all were depressed at the time of death. Mixed states were not specified and, by their nature, are far more difficult to elicit by history or postmortem questioning of family members and friends. Winokur and co-workers (1969) found no suicide attempts during mania, although suicidal ideation occurred during 7 percent of manic episodes. They did find suicidal thoughts or attempts in 13 percent of depressive episodes following mania and a strikingly high rate of suicide threats and attempts in mixed states (43 percent). Suicidal thoughts or behavior during these mixed states was reported only in women. Kotin and Goodwin (1972) also described the coexistence of suicidal behavior and mixed states, as did Kraepelin (1921) in his original clinical monograph.

To Jameison (1936), the mixed state was the most dangerous clinical phase of illness for suicide risk. In his study of 100 suicides (half with manic-depressive psychosis), he noted that the combination of depressive symptoms, mental alertness, and tense, apprehensive, and restless behavior was particularly lethal. Mixed states may represent a critical combination or potentiation of depressive affects and cognition, with a particularly dysphoric state, heightened energy level, and increased impulsivity. The following clinical account of mixed states in manic-depressive illness is apt:

Finally there are the patients with mixed manic-depressive states. The majority of these show the usual depression, numerous self-accusations, ideas of guilt and punishment and a varying degree of hypochondriasis. At the same time there is a mental alertness, associated with tense, apprehensive and restless behavior. The retardation of thought and action that paralyzes the acting out of the wish for death in the average depressed patient is entirely absent in these persons. They are, therefore, the most dangerous types of patients with mental disease, so far as suicide is concerned. The records of the fifteen patients in the group emphasize this strikingly. Three of these patients committed suicide twenty-four hours after leaving the hospital, two within forty-eight hours, another within a week and still another within two weeks. The patient who was longest outside the hospital lived two months, and the average period for this group was fifteen days! (Jameison, 1936, p. 4)

Schweizer and colleagues (1988) describe two patients who committed suicide while switching into depression from a hypomanic state. They emphasize the importance of rapidly cycling mood as a suicide risk factor.

Other behavioral clues to suicide have been examined. Insomnia and excessive concern about sleep disturbances have been noted as correlates of increased potential for suicide,[6] as has the presence of pervasive hopelessness (Beck et al., 1975; Reich and Kelly, 1976). Concomitant substance abuse has been noted to increase the risk of suicide, particularly in the young (Murphy, 1988).

Roose and colleagues (1983) found that delusional depressed inpatients were five times more likely to commit suicide than nondelusional ones, and delusional males were particularly vulnerable. Their sample comprised unipolar patients only, but their findings may well be relevant to bipolar patients because recurrent unipolar depression and bipolar illness have many phenomenological and clinical similarities, including the fact that both types of patients frequently are delusional. Roose and colleagues hypothesized that the coexistence of depressive suicidal thoughts with a delusional process may transform suicidal ideation into a suicidal act. Black and colleagues (1988b), in a study of 1,593 affectively ill patients, found no increased risk of suicide among the 27.8 percent of the patients who were psychotic at the time of their index hospitalization. Likewise, Coryell and Tsuang (1982) and Frangos and colleagues (1983) did not find an increased risk of suicide in delusional depression.

Severe depression, not surprisingly, correlates with increased lethality (Jameison and Wall, 1933; Barraclough et al., 1974; Weeke, 1979). Weeke found that at the time of death, 58 percent of patients were in a constant or worsening depressive state. Of particular interest, however, is the fact that fully 30 percent of the patients were classified as "depressive state, recovering," a finding consistent with that of Jameison and Wall (1933), who found a sudden improvement in depression in many of their patients immediately before suicide.

Keith-Spiegel and Spiegel (1967) compared the clinically rated affective states of 61 psychiatric patients immediately preceding their suicides with those of 51 matched control patients of comparable age and diagnoses who had not committed suicide or who had no history of a suicidal attempt. Those who killed themselves had histories of more frequent and severe depressions and more suicide attempts, threats, and suicidal ideation. Especially noteworthy, however, is that, just before death, those who committed suicide were assessed by their clinicians to be calmer and in better spirits than were members of the control group. An apparently unwarranted mood shift had been observed in those who killed themselves. Several hypotheses might account for the latter, counterintuitive, observation. The improvement might reflect calmness once a decision to die has been made—a resolution of ambivalence. It may represent a genuine calm before the storm brought about by biological changes or a transition from one phase of the illness into another (e.g., depression into hypomania, mania, or a mixed state). It may also reflect genuine clinical improvement, with a concomitant level of frustration when symptoms recur. In some instances, a previously indecisive and lethargic patient becomes able to make lethal decisions and is energized to act on them. Finally, improvement may be a deliberate deception of physicians, hospital staff, and family in order to carry out a suicide plan. Weeke (1979), who studied clinicians' evaluations of suicide risk in patients who later killed themselves, found that 13 percent of the patients had been assessed as "seriously suicidal," 58 percent assessed as "suicide possible, not likely," and 28 percent as "suicide quite unexpected."

Problems in assessing clinical improvement were pointed out in 1936 by Jameison:

> It is only when the depression is lifting, often some weeks before the morbid and self-accusatory ideas have disappeared, that the possibility of suicide is less remote. Unfortunately, at this time a tendency to project the inner distress on the environment leads to complaints and pleadings, so that relatives, noting the improvement, agree with the patient that the hospital restrictions are prolonging the illness. The patient is then removed at a time when he is potentially more suicidal than at any time before. (p. 4)

Fawcett and co-workers (1988), in their prospective study of 955 bipolar and unipolar patients, found that risk factors among the 14 who committed suicide within 1 year of assessment were anhedonia, severe psychic anxiety, moderate alcohol abuse, and panic attacks. The abuse of alcohol in addition to another drug is a significant risk factor, especially in males. Another 13 killed themselves in the next 4 years. These late suicides, those completed after the first year, were most associated with severe hopelessness, somatic anxiety, suicidal ideation, and a history of suicide attempts. The findings of Fawcett and

colleagues underscore the importance of assessing patients in terms of acute vs long-term suicide risk.

Like Fawcett and colleagues, others have noted an association between alcohol abuse and suicide. Barraclough and colleagues (1974) found that as the number of suicide attempts increased, so did the chances that the attempter was alcoholic. In a study of 204 suicides, Rich and associates (1988) found substance use disorders and affective disorders to be the most frequent diagnoses for men and women. In a total of 342 completed suicides (Robins et al., 1959b; Dorpat and Ripley, 1960 Barraclough et al., 1974), 48 percent had an affective disorder, and 23 percent were alcoholic, the two most common diagnoses in the sample. Morrison (1975) found that bipolar patients who were also alcoholic had a higher rate of suicide in their family histories than bipolar patients without alcoholism. Runeson (1989), in a study of suicide in adolescents and young adults, found that co-existing substance abuse occurred in 47 percent of the suicides. Depressive disorders were diagnosed in 64 percent of those who committed suicide (major depressive disorder = 41 percent).

The connection between suicide and substance abuse may be attributable to increased impulsivity or aggressiveness. As discussed in Chapter 17, low levels of 5-hydroxyindoleacetic acid (5-HIAA), the principal serotonin metabolite, are correlated with aggression and impulsivity, and it has been shown that patients with the most violent and impulsive suicide attempts have low 5-HIAA levels. It is of interest that Rosenthal and colleagues (1980a) found significantly lower levels of 5-HIAA among depressed patients with a family history of alcoholism compared with those with a negative family history. Low 5-HIAA levels also have been found in alcoholics after recovery (Ballenger et al., 1979). Therefore, not only do substance abusers have impaired judgment and decreased inhibition from the drugs themselves, they may also carry a biological risk for suicide.

The relationship between suicide and aggressiveness, violence, anger, impulsivity, and irritability goes beyond an association with substance abuse. Such features have been associated with self-destruction for many years (Jameison and Wall, 1933; Reich and Kelly, 1976; Myers and Neal, 1978). Analogous to the concept of perturbation developed by Shneidman (1975), this association is important to both a theoretical understanding of manic-depressive illness and its effective clinical management. Exacerbations of dysphoric states, often accompanied by increased energy and activity that are commonly of a wired or dysphoric type, may well signify a mixed state in a sizable subsample of patients. Not surprisingly, predicting a relatively infrequent behavior, such as suicide attempts, in the midst of subtle and fluctuating mood states is difficult. Nonetheless, it is particularly important to identify these patients rapidly and to treat them both aggressively and specifically.

In summary, a review of the clinical studies of suicide leads to several conclusions: (1) suicidal intent is often communicated beforehand; (2) disrupted sleep often occurs before suicide, with, perhaps, disproportionate concern over the disruption; (3) a high suicide rate is found in mixed states; (4) suicide often follows an improvement (or seeming improvement) in mood after a severe depression, and 5) there is an association between suicide and increased aggressiveness and impulsivity.

Genetic factors in suicide and their relationship to the genetics of manic-depressive illness are discussed in Chapter 15, and possible biological correlates of suicide in manic-depressive illness are reviewed in Chapter 17.

Seasonality
May is a pious fraud of the almanac,
A ghastly parody of real Spring
Shaped of snow and breathed with eastern wind.
    — James Russell Lowell, *Under the Willows*

As noted in Chapter 7, seasonality affects the timing of manic and depressive affective episodes. Far more data are available on suicide and seasonality, however, and dating a suicide is obviously far more accurate than dating the onset of an affective episode. We reviewed more than 20 studies of the peak monthly incidence of suicide. One of these examined data from 16 countries (Takahashi, 1964), another examined data from four countries (Bolander, 1972), and two did separate analyses for males and females. As shown in Figure 10-3, we counted these results separately, which resulted in over 40 data points. There is a striking peak incidence of suicide in

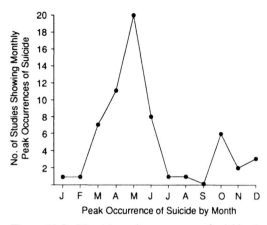

Figure 10-3. Monthly peak occurrences of suicide: A review of studies. The several studies that have appeared since this figure was constructed continue to show the main peak in the spring and a smaller peak in the fall (e.g., see Näyhä, 1982; Egeland and Sussex, 1985; Souêtre et al., 1987).

(Based on a review of 61 studies.)

May across studies and a second, much smaller peak in October. These findings are consistent with the peak hospitalization rates for affective episodes. The second suicide peak in October may reflect an increase not only in unipolar depressive episodes but also in bipolar depressions following the increase in manic episodes during the summer months (i.e., it may represent suicidal postmanic depressions). In a review of the world's literature on seasonal incidence of suicide, Aschoff (1981a) observed environmental factors that may play a role in the increased risk of suicide at certain times of the year. He found that seasonal variation in suicide rates was greatest in the least industrialized nations and declined with more industrialization during the past century. Some aspects of industrialization (e.g., artificial light, central heating) may insulate patients from environmental risk factors for affective episodes. Seasonal variation was greatest in the temperate latitudes, not in the north with its extremes of light and temperature. Seasonal variation also was most correlated with hours of clear sunshine (not day length per se). This observation, which implicates brightness and duration of light (rather than its timing) in the seasonal occurrence of depression, is consistent with conclusions about the properties of phototherapy in seasonal affective disorder. There are not enough data to draw any meaningful conclusions about latitudinal differences in seasonal incidences of affective illness. Two studies have been carried out in the southern hemisphere, both in Australia (Takahashi, 1964; Parker and Walter, 1982). In both, suicide seasonality was consistent with the pattern seen in the northern hemisphere—that is, peaks in the spring, although women in the Parker and Walter study in New South Wales showed two peak suicidal periods (in May and November) rather than one. Unfortunately, there are no seasonality statistics specific to bipolar patients.

Sex differences in seasonal patterns of suicide in Italy were examined by Micciolo and colleagues (1989). They found that cyclical fluctuations in the number of suicides occurred in both sexes but that there was only one significant peak per year for men and two for women. The most significant peak for both men and women was in May; women had a subsidiary peak in October and November.

NOTES

1. Fewer unipolar depressed adolescents (61 percent) reported such thinking.
2. Consistent with the general female predominance among attempters discussed earlier, Goldring and Fieve (1984) found the highest frequency of suicide attempts among bipolar-II females, 67 percent compared to 50 percent among bipolar-II males, and 55 percent among bipolar-I patients of both sexes.
3. The patients were not classified as bipolar or unipolar, but all were depressed at the time of suicide.
4. Barraclough et al., 1974; Murphy, 1975a,b; Avery and Winokur, 1976; Myers and Neal, 1978; Ottosson, 1979.
5. Barraclough et al., 1974; Murphy, 1975a,b; Avery and Winokur, 1976; Myers and Neal, 1978; Ottosson, 1979.
6. Jameison and Wall, 1933; Slater and Roth, 1969; Barraclough et al., 1974; Motto, 1975.

PART THREE

PSYCHOLOGICAL STUDIES

Temperament also enters fully into the system of illusions and shuts us in a prison of glass which we cannot see. There is an optical illusion about every person we meet. In truth they are all creatures of given temperament, which will appear in a given character, whose boundaries they will never pass; but we look at them, they seem alive, and we presume there is impulse in them. In the moment it seems impulse; in the year, in the lifetime, it turns out to be a certain uniform tune which the revolving barrel of the music-box must play. . . . the individual texture holds its dominion, if not to bias the moral judgments, yet to fix the measure of activity and of enjoyment.
                                                                          —Ralph Waldo Emerson[1]

Despite its indisputable biological roots, manic-depressive illness—as experienced by patients and as expressed to the world—is exquisitely psychological. It manifests itself as temperament and as fluctuations around that temperament. It reveals itself in thoughts, perceptions, language, behavior, and intellect. And it displays itself in interactions with family members, friends, colleagues, and society. "The individual texture," as Emerson wrote, does indeed "hold its dominion."

This section of the book presents psychological perspectives on manic-depressive illness. First, in Chapter 11, we consider studies of formal thought disorder, perception, and cognition. We discuss similarities and dissimilarities in the nature and extent of thought disorders found in manic, depressed, and schizophrenic patients, and we compare them to the thought patterns of normal individuals. Speech patterns are similarly examined. In the second part of Chapter 11, we discuss hallucinations and delusions in mania and depression and then examine what we know about psychotic depression in bipolar and unipolar illness. Cognitive functioning in manic-depressive illness forms the chapter's final section. There we review the available literature on intellectual and neuropsychological assessment completed during mania, depression, and normal states—that is, the findings from studies of cognitive and psychomotor speed, general intellectual functioning, associational patterns, memory and learning, and lateralization. Substantial limitations of methodology make it difficult to interpret many of the findings, yet the consistency of results in some areas (e.g., lateralization) is both gratifying and indicative of promising areas for future research. It is clear that deeper understanding of thought and behavior will, in part, derive from the important methods developed by neuropsychologists. Their work will, in turn, be greatly enhanced by use of brain-imaging techniques.

In Chapter 12, we review descriptive and systematic investigations of personality and interpersonal behavior focusing on bipolar manic-depressive illness. We examine studies of personality that were performed with patients when they were manic, depressed, or normal and then compare personality functioning in remitted bipolar patients and normal individuals. Studies comparing bipolar and unipolar

1. Ralph Waldo Emerson: "Experience." In: *Essays, Second Series*, 1844. Reprinted in Penguin Books, Middlesex, 1982. p. 290.

patients, when ill and well, also are reviewed. Investigations of patients' perceptions of themselves across different affective states, coexisting personality disorders, and the effects of lithium on personality complete the first half of Chapter 12.

In the second half of that chapter, we look at the interpersonal lives of patients who have manic-depressive illness: their marriages and families, friendships, sexual relationships, and their functioning as parents. Lithium usually profoundly alters the nature of these relationships, and such changes also are discussed.

Chapter 13 is concerned with matters of measurement, in particular the rating scales developed to assess mania and depression. We discuss the advantages and disadvantages of observer-rating and self-rating scales, as well as those of specific scales. We explore here, as we have in many chapters, the insufficiency of studying mania and depression as separate and opposite states and reemphasize the importance of measures that attempt to assess mixed or rapidly fluctuating psychological and behavioral phenomena.

Manic-depressive illness is perhaps unique in the coexistence of beneficial qualities with destructive ones. It is these qualities that are discussed in Chapter 14. An association between "madness" and artistic creativity has long been a part of the history of ideas. Here we develop the biographical and scientific basis for one important aspect of that relationship. Cognitive, behavioral, and emotional characteristics of manic-depressive illness are similar to many attributes intrinsic to the creative process. We discuss their nature, potentially enhancing capacities, and liabilities. Recent systematic studies of the relationship between mood disorders and creativity also are presented. We have allocated an entire chapter to the topic of manic-depressive illness, creativity, and leadership because it is an interesting and important subject in its own right. We also believe, however, that the theoretical, clinical, social, and ethical implications of the issues discussed in Chapter 14 are exceedingly important and need to be considered.

Because of the clearly biological underpinnings of manic-depressive illness, the psychology of the disorder has been relatively less emphasized. Fortunately, in recent years, this has begun to change, and we are optimistic that in time the perspectives and methods of psychology will provide many more answers than now exist. Effective treatment of manic-depressive illness is predicated on an understanding of its psychological as well as biological aspects.

11

Thought Disorder, Perception, and Cognition

I roll on like a ball, with this exception, that contrary to the usual laws of motion I
have no friction to contend with in my mind, and of course have some difficulty in
stopping myself when there is nothing else to stop me. . . . I am almost sick and
giddy with the quantity of things in my head—trains of thought beginning and
branching to infinity, crossing each other, and all tempting and wanting to be
worked out.
—John Ruskin[1]

Disorders of thinking are central to manic-depressive illness. Changes in the rate, quality, and fluency of thought and speech, alterations in associational patterns and logical processes, and impairments in learning and memory are as fundamental to depression and mania as are changes in mood and behavior. The clinical importance of these changes is underscored by their inclusion and emphasis in all diagnostic and evaluation systems (see Chapters 2 and 5). This chapter reviews formal thought disorder and communication and perceptual and intellectual deficits in manic-depressive illness. It is not intended to be a comprehensive discussion of the complex concepts and research on memory, attention, learning, or cognitive disturbances, nor is it meant to be a critical examination of measurement techniques or their reliabilities and validities. Although our focus is on bipolar manic-depressive illness, in some areas (such as studies of formal thought disorder) the dearth of specific bipolar data requires that we broaden our focus to include recurrent unipolar illness as well. Also, the bipolar–unipolar distinction is not specified in much of the literature. Additional topics of relevance to changes in thinking associated with manic-depressive illness are covered elsewhere in this book. The clinical description and frequencies of cognitive and perceptual symptoms (e.g., dis-

tractibility, impaired concentration, confusion, racing thoughts, psychomotor slowing, subjective complaints of memory deficits, delusions and hallucinations) are presented in Chapter 2, relevant diagnostic criteria and differential diagnostic criteria in Chapter 5, laterality studies other than neuropsychological ones (electrophysiological approaches, dichotic listening, handedness studies, event-related potentials) in Chapter 18, intellectually enhancing aspects of hypomania in Chapter 14, and cognitive effects of lithium in Chapter 23.

Methodological problems are varied and vast in the study of thought disorders and intellectual deficits in manic-depressive illness. There are few theoretical models that attempt to tie together existing findings and to guide future research. Data from high-risk populations are virtually nonexistent, and there are few longitudinal studies of thought disorder and cognitive deficits carried out before, during, and after affective episodes. Normative data from the general population are inadequate, and there is a dearth of data from meaningful comparison samples, such as family members who are free of the illness and—other than schizophrenic patients—other psychiatric diagnostic groups. Gender differences are rarely discussed, and age and IQ seldom are controlled for. As noted, there are essentially no studies of formal thought disorder in bipolar depression.

Few studies of disorders of thinking in manic-depressive illness have controlled for specific illness variables, such as number of previous affective episodes and their polarities, elapsed time since first and most recent episodes, phase of illness during assessment period, including the rapidity and severity of fluctuating mood states, number and nature of subclinical affective episodes, diurnal, seasonal, and premenstrual fluctuations and their effects on mood and cognition at the time of assessment, patterning, or sequencing, of episodes, severity of mood cyclicity and of episodes (both manic and depressive), presence or absence of psychotic features, suicidal potential (and possible neurological sequelae from previous suicide attempts), impulsivity, duration of episodes, and chronicity.

Treatment variables are likewise seldom controlled for in a systematic way—for example, current and past use of neuroleptics and lithium, treatment with electroconvulsive therapy, current medication levels, combined use of medications, degree of treatment response, and possible confounding influences of long-term hospitalization (e.g., inadequate nutrition and lack of social interaction or intellectual stimulation). Other methodological problems occur with the assessment process itself. Mania, especially, creates difficulties in accurate measurement because of distractibility, poor cooperation, impaired attention span, and irritability. Many studies of cognition and perception in psychiatric patients were conducted before the development or common use of standardized diagnostic criteria, and even in most recent research, subtypes of bipolar illness—bipolar I, II, and cyclothymia—are rarely specified. Controlling for even such basics as level of intelligence is compounded by the obvious overlapping nature of several variables in both neuropsychological and intelligence assessment. The specificity of neurological deficits is generally limited and highly variable across neuropsychological measurement techniques. Likewise, even if a deficit is specified, it may occur across a wide variety of psychiatric and neurological conditions.

The first section of this chapter reviews the literature on thought and communication disorders in manic-depressive illness, the second section reviews hallucinations and delusions, and the third discusses cognitive deficits. There is, of course, tremendous overlap in these areas—overlap that is biological, anatomical, attentional, perceptual, and clinical—and distinctions between the areas are occasionally arbitrary.

THOUGHT DISORDER AND COMMUNICATION

[Robert Lowell's] whole conversation became very fragmentary and disconnected. I used to think of it as a great knot which would twist and twist and twist and then a sentence would come out of it, pushed by a sort of strange breathy impulsion, and it was always in a totally unexpected direction.—Keith Botsford [2]

Definitions and Assessment

There is no single or comprehensive definition of formal thought disorder. Instead, thought disorder has been used as a general phrase to describe problems in the ability to attend, abstract, conceptualize, express, or continue coherent thought. At one time more generally described—"Kraepelin thought of the patient's thought and speech as a train which kept derailing, Bleuler's image was that of a torn and poorly mended fabric" (Andreasen, 1984)—specific deficits in thought and language are now defined by specific measures of those deficits (e.g., the Thought Disorder Index, or the Scale for the Assessment of Thought, Language and Communication). This increased specificity allows disentanglement, at least in part, of thought from language or speech disorders. Although difficult, this distinction is important, since it is possible to have thought disorder without language disorder, and vice versa (Holzman et al., 1985). Much of thought is nonverbal, and individuals often say one thing while thinking another (Andreasen et al., 1985). We use here, as a working definition of thought disorder, that provided by Solovay and colleagues (1987): Thought disorder ". . . is not intended to denote a unitary dimension or process; rather, it refers to any disruption, deficit, or slippage in various aspects of thinking, such as concentration, attention, reasoning, or abstraction" (p. 13).

Certain psychotic features of mania and bipolar depression—delusions and hallucinations—are relevant but not central to the concept of thought disorder. They have been described in Chapter 2 and are discussed later in this chapter. The specificity of thought disorder to the major psychoses—mania and schizophrenia—represents an important conceptual issue and is a major focus of the first part of this chapter. Holzman and his colleagues (1985) have asked the question:

Is thought disorder a non-specific accompaniment of psychotic behavior, whatever the etiology of that psychosis, just as fever is nonspecific for a variety of systemic conditions; or is there a set of specific disorders of thinking that accompanies specific psychotic conditions? (p. 228)

To answer these and other questions, several methods have evolved for the study of thought and communication disorders in schizophrenia and affective disorders. These methods have been described and reviewed by Harvey (1983) as (1) clinical (the examination of speech patterns on the basis of clinical interactions, e.g., in the manner of Kraepelin and Bleuler), (2) laboratory (the study of underlying cognitive processes that result in or contribute to disordered speech), and (3) natural language studies (the examination of speech samples, from a variety of sources, in an attempt to "identify the discourse processes that lead to the problems listeners have in understanding the speech of psychotics" [p. 368]). Several specific measures have been developed, three of which, summarized below, form the basis of most of the research relevant to the study of thought disorder in manic-depressive illness. Taken together, these three measures can provide a reasonably comprehensive assessment of formal thought disorder.

Holzman and his colleagues, using verbal protocols (most typically verbatim responses to the Rorschach test), developed the Thought Disorder Index. Based on earlier indices (Rapaport et al., 1968; Watkins and Stauffacher, 1952), the Thought Disorder Index comprises 23 different categories of thinking disturbances, evaluated at four levels of severity (Johnston and Holzman, 1979; Shenton et al., 1987; Solovay et al., 1987). These categories and examples of them are outlined in Table 11-1.

Andreasen has characterized different language behaviors that she considers to be subtypes of thought disorder and has developed them into a measure of thought disorder, the Scale for the Assessment of Thought, Language and Communication (Andreasen, 1979a,b). Definitions of

these types of thought disorders are given in Table 11-2. Some subtypes occur frequently in psychotic speech (e.g., poverty of content of speech, pressure of speech, tangentiality, derailment, loss of goal, and perseveration), whereas others are relatively uncommon and, correspondingly, less useful (e.g., clanging, blocking, echolalia, neologisms, and word approximations).

Finally, Harrow and colleagues[3] have used a battery of measures taken from the WAIS (Social Comprehension subtest), the Goldstein-Scheerer Object-Sorting Test, and the Gorham Proverbs Test to assess bizarre and idiosyncratic thinking and behavior, as well as conceptual style. Detailed discussions of the development, reliability, and validity of their test battery are reported elsewhere.[4]

Thought Disorder in Mania and Schizophrenia

Virtually all studies of formal thought disorder in mania and schizophrenia, the results of which are summarized in Table 11-3, find comparably high levels in both diagnostic groups.[5] In fact, although Resnick and Oltmanns (1984) reported more thought disorder in schizophrenics, Harrow and associates (1982) found a trend toward greater levels in manic patients.[6] There is, therefore, no indication that thought disorder per se is in any way specific to schizophrenia. This is consistent with the evidence for the strong presence in mania, as well as in schizophrenia, of psychotic features, such as hallucinations and delusions (see Chapter 2). Qualitative comparisons between manic and schizophrenic thought disorder are less consistent, although increased pressure of speech appears more characteristic of mania,[7] as does increased derailment, loss of goal, and tangentiality (Andreasen, 1984; Simpson and Davis, 1985). Poverty of speech, and other negative symptoms, have been reported by Andreasen (1984) to be more characteristic of schizophrenic thought, although Ragin and Oltmanns (1987), using the same scale, did not confirm this. Studies of differences between manic and schizophrenic patients on measures of idiosyncratic and/or bizarre thinking report mixed conclusions, with some authors finding higher levels in manics (Andreasen and Powers, 1975; Harrow et al., 1982) but others reporting higher levels in schizophrenics (Simpson and Davis, 1985; Shen-

Table 11-1. Thought Disorder Index Categories and Levels of Severity with Selected Examples

0.25 Level

1. Inappropriate distance
    A. Loss or increase of distance: "I'm afraid of what else it could be...It scares me to think of what else it could be"
    B. Excessive qualification
    C. Concreteness: "Some kind of fancy military jet flying up the card"
    D. Overspecificity: "A four-legged lamb"
    E. Syncretistic response (on Wechsler Adult Intelligence Scale: How are wood and alcohol alike?): "They both have atoms"
2. Flippant response: "I see another vagina; I guess I'm a sex maniac...ah, that's getting written down? Uh-oh, they'll tell the police on me"
3. Vagueness: "Nothing but two figures on each side. I don't know what kind of figures. They don't look like animals or people. They just looked like two smears"
4. Peculiar verbalizations and responses
    A. Peculiar expression: "A reverse reflection"
    B. Stilted, inappropriate expression: "It's a piece of animation"
    C. Idiosyncratic word usage: "He's all *clowned* up in some kind of suit"
5. Word-finding difficulty
6. Clangs
7. Perseverations
8. Incongruous combinations
    A. Composite response: "It looks like a mastodon wearing shoes"
    B. Arbitrary form-color responses: "An orange pelvic bone," "green fire"
    C. Inappropriate activity response: "A beetle crying"

0.50 Level

9. Relationship verbalization (an allusion back to an earlier one): "That being the mandibles in the very first picture"
10. Idiosyncratic symbolism: "The red...shows action"
11. Queer responses
    A. Queer expressions: "Inward type of photograph of a flower's reproductive cells"
    B. Queer imagery: "Idealized fire"
    C. Queer word usage: "Pestals on a flower"
12. Confusion: "Some people smoking matches and burning cigarettes"
13. Looseness: "Because it's black, dark, darkness, lovemaking"
14. Fabulized combinations, impossible or bizarre: "Two crows with afros and they're pushing two hearts together"
15. Playful confabulation: "An evil witch doing a square dance...She had her dress like this and she was do-si-do-ing"
16. Fragmentation

0.75 Level

17. Fluidity: "The head of a rocket or the head of a bear or the head of a bird...looked like something was becoming something else"
18. Absurd responses: "This is sticking out there. Remember that's the-uh-cure there. It's our cure, it's called"
19. Confabulations
    A. Details in one area generalized to a larger area
    B. Extreme elaboration: "The light bulb is — I think it's man-made. And the pink is down here and it gives energy for the light bulb...and the vapors from the pink...cause the green and the orange to...be there..."
20. Autistic logic: "I see something rather like an appendix. Looked to me totally useless, so then I thought of the appendix"

Continued

Table 11-1 Continued. Thought Disorder Index Categories and Levels of Severity
with Selected Examples

1.00 Level
21. Contamination: "This is definitely a man...a man butterfly, a butterfly with a man's face — could
    be a dark cloud that's dark because it swallows up all...uh...the dark particles — man
    butterfly...it could be a cloudlike man-butterfly"
22. Incoherence: "A duck...their disarrangement. They follow out together, they follow one another.
    The two toes together, meeting one another. They jacked up in back, like spinal cord being
    broken"
23. Neologisms: "That's tavro or neoglyphics"

From Solovay et al., 1987

ton et al., 1987). Simpson and Davis (1985) made the useful distinction that manics appear to be more disordered in *thought structure,* whereas schizophrenics appear to be more disordered in *thought content.* Jampala and colleagues (1989) argue that manic patients with formal thought disorder may "have a more severe rather than a different condition than manic patients without formal thought disorder. The fact that more manic patients with formal thought disorder had a first-degree relative with affective illness supports this interpretation" (p. 462).

Qualitative differences in thought disorder between mania and schizophrenia are more distinct in the use of combinatory thinking, the "tendency to merge percepts, ideas, or images in an incongruous fashion" (Shenton et al., 1987). In a study of 20 manics, 43 schizophrenics, and 22 normal subjects, Solovay and colleagues (1987), using the Thought Disorder Index, found no significant difference in the quantity of thought disorder in manics and schizophrenics. Manic thought disorder was, however, "extravagantly combinatory, usually with humor, flippancy, and playfulness." Schizophrenic thought disorder, on the other hand, was "disorganized, confused, and idealistically fluid, with many peculiar words and phrases." The same authors elaborated further on these differences:

. . . manic thought disorder manifests itself as ideas loosely strung together and extravagantly combined and elaborated. . . . appearance of irrelevant intrusions into social discourse that may at times appear inappropriately flippant and playful. . . . Schizophrenic thought disorder, on the other hand, seems devoid of the playful, compulsively elaborative, and ideationally loose constructions of the manic patients. Characteristic of the schizophrenic patients in this study were fluid thinking, interpenetrations of one idea

by another, unstable verbal referents, and fragmented and elliptical communications. (pp. 19-20)

These differences are portrayed graphically in Figure 11-1, which shows standardized Thought Disorder Index scores (on factors derived from a principal components analysis) for 12 schizoaffective (manic) and 10 schizoaffective (depressed) patients, as well as for the manic, schizophrenic, and normal subjects discussed earlier (Shenton et al., 1987). Of note, on the one "manic" factor (combinatory thinking), schizoaffective manics were most similar to the manic group, but on the five "schizophrenic" factors (idiosyncratic thinking, autistic thinking, fluid thinking, absurdity, and confusion), they performed more like the schizophrenics. The schizoaffective depressed patients more strongly resembled the normal subjects. Andreasen (1984) found that her schizoaffective patients were midway in thought disorder between the manics and schizophrenics. Jampala and associates (1989) observed a greatly increased rate of flight of ideas in their manic patients (72 percent) compared with schizophrenic patients (10 percent). Interestingly, in a study of conceptual style in writers, manics, and schizophrenics, Andreasen and Powers (1975) concluded:

Creative writers resemble patients suffering from bipolar affective disorder, manic phase, in their conceptual style more than they resemble schizophrenics. That is, they tend to show considerable overinclusive thinking, based on both the quantity of objects that they sort [on the Goldstein-Scheerer Object Sorting Test] and their conceptual overinclusiveness. Both writers and manics tend to sort in large groups, change dimensions while in the process of sorting, arbitrarily change starting points, or use vague distantly related concepts as categorizing principles. (p. 72)

Table 11-2. Types of Thought Disorders: Definitions

Poverty of Speech (Poverty of Thought, Laconic Speech). Restriction in the **amount** of spontaneous speech, so that replies to questions tend to be brief, concrete, and unelaborated. Unprompted additional information is rarely provided.

Poverty of Content of Speech (Poverty of Thought, Empty Speech, Alogia, Verbigeration, Negative Formal Thought Disorder). Although replies are long enough so that speech is adequate in amount, it conveys little information. Language tends to be vague, often overabstract or overconcrete, repetitive, and stereotyped.

Pressure of Speech. An increase in the amount of spontaneous speech as compared with what is considered ordinary or socially customary. The patient talks rapidly and is difficult to interrupt. Speech tends to be loud and emphatic.

Distractible Speech. During the course of a discussion or interview, the patient repeatedly stops talking in the middle of a sentence or idea and changes the subject in response to a nearby stimulus.

Tangentiality. Replying to a question in an oblique, tangential, or even irrelevant manner. The reply may be related to the question in some distant way. Or the reply may be unrelated and seem totally irrelevant.

Derailment (Loose Associations, Flight of Ideas). A pattern of spontaneous speech in which the ideas slip off the track onto another one that is clearly but obliquely related, or onto one that is completely unrelated.

Incoherence (Word Salad, Jargon Aphasia). A pattern of speech that is essentially incomprehensible at times. It differs from derailment in that the abnormality occurs at the level of the sentence, within which words or phrases are joined incoherently. The abnormality in derailment involves unclear or confusing connections between larger units, such as sentences or ideas.

Illogicality. A pattern of speech in which conclusions are reached that do not follow logically.

Clanging. A pattern of speech in which sounds rather than meaningful relationships appear to govern word choice, so that the intelligibility of the speech is impaired and redundant words are introduced.

Neologisms. New word formations. A neologism is defined here as a new word or phrase whose derivation cannot be understood.

Word Approximations (Paraphrasia, Metonyms). Old words that are used in a new and unconventional way, or new words that are developed by conventional rules of word formation.

Circumstantiality. A pattern of speech that is very indirect and delayed in reaching its goal idea.

Loss of Goal. Failure to follow a chain of thought through to its natural conclusion. This is usually manifested in speech that begins with a particular subject, wanders away from the subject, and never returns to it.

Perseveration. Persistent repetition of words, ideas, or subjects so that, once a patient begins a particular subject or uses a particular word, he continually returns to it in the process of speaking.

Continued

Table 11-2 Continued. Types of Thought Disorders: Definitions

Echolalia. A pattern of speech in which the patient echoes words or phrases of the interviewer.

Blocking. Interruption of a train of speech before a thought or idea has been completed. Blocking should only be judged to be present if a person voluntarily describes losing his thought or if on questioning by the interviewer he indicates that that was his reason for pausing.

Stilted Speech. Speech that has an excessively stilted or formal quality. It may seem rather quaint or outdated, or may appear pompous, distant, or overpolite.

Self-Reference. A disorder in which the patient repeatedly refers the subject under discussion back to himself when someone else is talking and also refers apparently neutral subjects to himself when he himself is talking.

Paraphasia, Phonemic. Recognizable mispronunciation of a word because sounds or syllables have slipped out of sequence.

Paraphasia, Semantic. Substitution of an inappropriate word during an effort to say something specific.

Adapted from Andreasen, 1979a

Clearly, although the conceptual style of these writers may be similar to that of manic patients, the research does not imply that they suffered from thought disorders. This conceptual style is well illustrated by John Custance (1952), a manic-depressive writer who, during one of his psychiatric hospitalizations, described the nature of his manic (and depressive) patterns of mental associations:

As I sit here, looking out of the window of the ward, I see flocks of seagulls who have been driven inland by the extreme cold. The mere sight of these seagulls sets up immediately and virtually simultaneously in my mind the following trains of thoughts:—

1. A pond called Seagull's Spring near my home.

2. Mermaids, i.e. Sea girls, sirens, Lorelei, Mother Seager's syrup, syrup of figs, the blasted fig-tree in the Gospels, Professor Joad who could not accept Jesus as the supremely perfect Man owing to particular incident. Here the chain stops as I cannot remember the exact title of Joad's book, which was a confession of the failure of his agnosticism.

3. The Mental Hospital where I spent nearly a year during my worst attack of suicidal depression. The weather that winter was also very cold, and quantities of seagulls came into the courts of the hospital. At that time I was suffering from the delusion that I was a supremely evil person who had sold his soul to Satan, and the gulls terrified me for two reasons: firstly because I thought of myself as a sort of super-gull who had been gulled into selling his soul; and secondly because I thought I was responsible for all the death and

evil in the world and that the spirits of all the lost seamen since the world began were in those gulls calling for vengeance on me.

It is interesting to note that both in manic and in depressive periods of sufficient intensity animistic conceptions of this kind impel themselves forcibly upon me; I cannot avoid seeing spirits in everything.

4. Gulls equals girls, lovely girls, lovelies, filmstars, countless stars on the infinite wastes of space, query: is space really infinite? According to Einstein it is not. . . (pp. 33–34)

In summary, although the overall amount of thought disorder does not differentiate manic from schizophrenic patients, qualitative differences do exist. Manic patients are far more likely than schizophrenics to exhibit pressured speech, grandiosity, flight of ideas, combinatory and overinclusive thinking, and a strong affective component to thought that is characterized by humor, playfulness, and flippancy. The causal relationships between affect, psychomotor acceleration, and the often strikingly different manifestations of the underlying thought disorders in mania and schizophrenia remain unclear.

Thought Disorder in Depression

Very little research has specifically considered the issue of thought disorder in bipolar depression (psychotic features, such as delusions and hallucinations, are discussed subsequently and in

Table 11-3. Thought Pathology in Mania and Schizophrenia: Similarities and Differences

Study	Thought Disorder Measure	Similarities	Differences
Breakey & Goodell, 1972	Bannister Grid Test	Same frequency of thought disorder	
Andreasen & Powers, 1975	Goldstein-Scheerer Object Sorting Test		**Manics:** ↑ behavioral overinclusion, ↑ conceptual overinclusion, ↑ idiosyncratic thinking **Schizophrenics:** ↑ underinclusiveness
Grossman et al., 1981	Gorham Proverbs Test, Goldstein - Scheerer Object Sorting Test, Social Comprehension(WAIS)	Similar in overall level of severity, course of disturbance, and loose association of ideas; intermingling of inappropriate personal ideas or concerns into responses to neutral stimuli; gaps in communication of ideas, odd outlooks, and other manifestations of bizarre thinking	**Manics:** ↑ behavioral activity and responsivity, ↓ response time on word association test, ↓ deficits in behavioral activity or impoverished activity, ↑ grandiose ideas
Harrow et al., 1982	Gorham Proverbs Test, Goldstein - Scheerer Object Sorting Test, Social Comprehension(WAIS)		**Manics:** may be more thought disordered than schizophrenics, "although the results are not conclusive"; ↑ bizarre - idiosyncratic thinking
Andreasen, 1984	Thought, Language and Communication Scale	Similar in number of abnormalities	**Manics:** more positive thought disorder; ↑ tangentiality, ↑ derailment, ↑ incoherence, ↑ illogicality, ↑ pressure of speech **Schizophrenics:** more negative thought disorder; ↑ poverty of speech, ↑ poverty of content **Schizoaffectives:** thought disorder is midway between manics and schizophrenics
Resnick & Oltmanns, 1984	Global ratings of thought disorder		**Manics:** less overall thought disorder; ↑ pressure of speech

Study	Measure		Findings
Simpson & Davis, 1985	Thought, Language and Communication Scale; Brief Psychiatric Rating Scale		**Manics:** more disordered thought structure; ↑loss of goal, ↑tangentiality, ↑derailment, ↑circumstantiality, ↑illogicality, ↑pressure of speech, ↑incoherence. **Schizophrenics:** more disordered thought content; ↑hallucinatory statements, ↑hallucinatory behavior, ↑unusual thought content
Ragin & Oltmanns, 1987	Thought, Language and Communication Scale	Similar levels of poverty of speech, derailment, loss of goal	**Manics:** ↑pressure of speech
Shenton et al., 1987	Thought Disorder Index	High level of thought disorder in both manics and schizophrenics	**Manics:** ↑combinatory thinking. **Schizophrenics:** overall higher level of thought disorder; ↑idiosyncratic and autistic thinking, ↑absurdity, ↑confusion. **Schizoaffectives:** thinking disorders more similar to schizophrenics than manics
Solovay et al., 1987	Thought Disorder Index	Equal amount of thought disorder	**Manics:** Thought disorder "extravagantly combinative, usually with humor, flippancy and playfulness". **Schizophrenics:** "disorganized, confused, and ideationally fluid, with many peculiar words and phrases"
Jampala et al., 1989	Authors' measures of thought disorder		**Manics:** ↑flight of ideas. **Schizophrenics:** ↑nonsequiturs, ↑tangentiality, ↑drivelling, ↑neologisms, ↑private use of words, ↑paraphasias

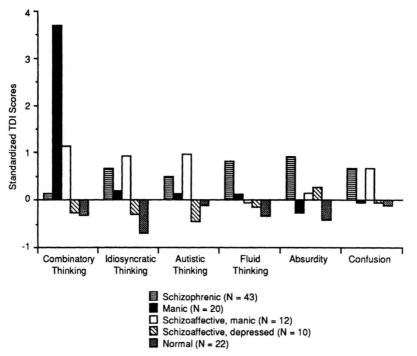

Legend:
- Schizophrenic (N = 43)
- Manic (N = 20)
- Schizoaffective, manic (N = 12)
- Schizoaffective, depressed (N = 10)
- Normal (N = 22)

Figure 11-1. Standardized Thought Disorder Index scores on factors derived from principal components analysis for five groups of subjects (adapted from Shenton et al., 1987).

Chapter 2); much of the review here necessarily focuses on unipolar as well as bipolar depression. McPherson and co-workers (1973), in an early study, found no significant differences between normal subjects and patients with recurrent depression in their performance on the Bannister-Fransella Grid Test of Thought Disorders and no bipolar–unipolar differences. Using a thought disorder scale similar to that developed by Cancro

(1969) and Phillips (1953), Ianzito and colleagues (1974) compared 47 unipolar hospitalized depressed and 34 schizophrenic patients. Tables 11-4 and 11-5 show the rates of formal thought disorder and disturbed content of thought in their patient populations. The authors concluded that (1) moderate-to-severe formal thought disorder was present in approximately 20 percent of the depressed patients, (2) moderate-

Table 11-4. Formal Thought Disorder in 47 Hospitalized Unipolar Depressed and 34 Schizophrenic Patients

Severities of Thought Disorder	Characteristics	Depressives % (N = 47)	Schizophrenics % (N = 34)
None	No formal thought disorder detected	68	38
Mild	Circumstantiality; vagueness	13	6
Moderate	Paralogical or unrelated responses; tangentiality; flight of ideas	15	35
Severe	Neologisms; echolalia; perseveration; clang associations; word salad	4	21

Adapted from Ianzito et al., 1974

Table 11-5. Disturbed Content of Thought in 47 Hospitalized Unipolar Depressed Patients

Severity	Characteristics	% (N = 47)
None	No content disorder detected	15
Mild	Phobias; obsessions; compulsions; ideas of reference; thoughts of guilt or worthlessness; repetitive thoughts	40
Moderate	Depersonalization; derealization; thought interference, control, insertion; withdrawal, or broadcasting; audible thoughts; feeling that mind can be read	22
Severe	Hallucinations; structured or systematized delusions, not including suicidal ideation	23

Adapted from Ianzito et al., 1974

to-severe content disorder was present in almost one half (45 percent) of the unipolar patients, (3) depressed patients reported more, but exhibited less, observable impairment in thinking, and (4) formal thought disorder predicted a more severe episode of depression (Ianzito et al., 1974).

The frequencies of thought disorder in manic, depressed, and normal subjects (as measured by the Scale for the Assessment of Thought, Language and Communication) have been analyzed by two principal studies, and the results are given in Table 11-6. Manic patients were more likely

Table 11-6. Frequency of Thought Disorder in Manic, Depressed, and Normal Subjects

Type of Thought Disorder[a]	Manics[b] % (N = 32)	Depressives[b] % (N = 36)	Normals[c] % (N = 94)
Poverty of speech	6	22	5
Poverty of content of speech	19	17	1
Pressure of speech	72	6 (2)[d]	6
Distractible speech	31	0	3
Tangentiality	34	25 (5)[d]	2
Derailment	56	14	32
Incoherence	16	0	0
Illogicality	25	0	0
Clanging	9	0 (0)[d]	0
Neologisms	3	0 (1)[d]	0
Word approximation	3	0	2
Circumstantiality	25	31 (21)[d]	6
Loss of goal	44	17	18
Perseveration	34	6 (2)[d]	8
Echolalia	3	0 (2)[d]	0
Blocking	3	6	1
Stilted speech	6	3	1
Self reference	22	11	1
Global rating	88	53	6

[a]Assessed by Thought, Language and Communication Scale
[b]Data from Andreasen, 1979a
[c]Data from Andreasen, 1984
[d]Data from Ianzito et al., 1974, (N=47)

than the depressives to exhibit pressured speech, distractibility, derailment, illogicality, loss of goal, perseveration, and overall global rating of thought disorder. Depressive patients, on the other hand, were more likely than the manic patients to demonstrate poverty of speech. There were no differences between manic and depressed patients on ratings of poverty of content of speech, tangentiality, clanging, neologisms, word approximations, circumstantiality, echolalia, blocking, or stilted speech. When compared with normal subjects, depressed patients displayed greater poverty and content of speech, as well as increased tangentiality, circumstantiality, and self-reference. Normal subjects were more likely than depressed patients to exhibit derailment. Andreasen (1979a,b, 1984) found less evidence of thought disorder in her depressed patients than in schizophrenic patients, perhaps reflecting differences in illness severity, assessment techniques, and diagnostic criteria (bipolar–unipolar differences were not specified).

Follow-up Studies of Thought Disorder

A few studies have followed the course of manic thought disorder over time. Andreasen (1984) observed that most manic patients, unlike schizophrenic ones, demonstrated a reversible thought disorder. Other than a continuing pressure of speech, they showed nearly complete recovery over time. Schizoaffective patients, to a lesser extent than the manic patients, also recovered. Ragin and Oltmanns (1987), on the other hand, found that manic patients displayed moderate levels of derailment and loss of goal at initial testing and, unlike other thought-disordered subjects, did not show significant decreases in either of these at follow-up. The most extensive longitudinal studies of manic thought disorder have been conducted by Harrow and colleagues (Harrow et al., 1982, 1986; Grossman et al., 1986). Using a battery of cognitive tests designed to assess bizarre-idiosyncratic thinking (Goldstein-Scheerer Object Sorting Test, Gorham Proverbs Test, and the WAIS subtest measuring social comprehension), the investigators tested manic thought disorder in the acute phase (Harrow et al., 1982), 1 year after hospitalization (Harrow et al., 1986), and 2 to 4 years after hospitalization (Grossman et al., 1986). Initial levels of manic thought pathology and changes over time were

compared with those obtained from schizophrenics, nonpsychotic psychiatric patients, and normal subjects. These findings are summarized in Figure 11-2 and further by the authors:

In the *acute phase:* (1) manic patients were extremely thought disordered; 94 percent demonstrated some definite evidence of abnormal thinking, and 73 percent of hospitalized manic patients showed severe levels of bizarre-idiosyncratic thinking, (2) there were no significant differences in levels of thought disorder between medicated and unmedicated manic patients, and (3) manic patients were at least as thought disordered as, if not more than, schizophrenics (Harrow et al., 1986).

In the *short-term follow-up phase* (7 weeks): (1) manic thought disorder in medicated patients improved, although some patients continued to show severe thought disorder, and (2) manic patients did not show a more rapid reduction in thought pathology than did the schizophrenics (Harrow et al., 1982).

One year after hospital discharge: (1) a "surprisingly large number" of manic patients showed relatively severe bizarre-idiosyncratic thinking or positive thought disorder (Figure 11-2). An example of such thinking is provided by Harrow and colleagues (1986) from one manic patient's response to the proverb "Don't cast pearls before swine":

If you be on a mission—and I watched this on TV myself—if you're on a mission at Lake Michigan, covering something, and a fish come and bite you, bite you on the gill, if you got the will power, the guts, the determination, you got to keep on going, keep on trucking. (p. 783)

(2) There was a significant reduction in severity of thought pathology for both manic and schizophrenic patients at follow-up, and (3) there was a trend for greater reduction in manic patients (from 73 percent to 27 percent rated as severe or very severe) when compared with schizophrenics (from 50 percent to 27 percent) (Harrow et al., 1986).

Two to four year follow-up data revealed that (1) 30 percent of manic patients had severe or very severe thought disorder, and another 30 percent had definite signs of abnormal thinking, (2) of the 14 formerly hospitalized manic patients who showed severe or very severe thought disorder, only 4 were rehospitalized at the time of the

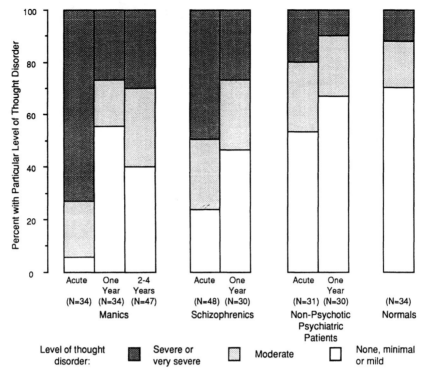

Figure 11-2. Composite level of thought disorder during and after hospitalization in manic, schizophrenic, and nonpsychotic psychiatric patients, and normals (adapted from Harrow et al., 1982, 1986; Grossman et al., 1986).

follow-up assessment, (3) positive thought disorder was associated with manic behavior, that is, those patients who showed more manic behaviors had more severe thought disorder (Table 11-7), (4) there was a significant correlation between thought disorder and psychosis (Table 11-7), but psychotic symptoms alone did not account for all of the variance associated with thought disorder at follow-up, and (5) manic patients with more than one previous hospitalization, or with a more chronic manic course, had significantly more thought disorder than patients with only one or no previous hospitalizations (Grossman et al., 1986).

Table 11-7. Relationship of Manic Behavior and Psychosis to Thought Disorder in 47 Formerly Hospitalized Manic Patients at 2-4 Years Follow-up

	No or Mild Thought Disorder % (N = 19)	Signs of Abnormal Thought Disorder % (N = 14)	Severe or Very Severe Thought Disorder % (N = 14)
Ratings of manic behavior			
None	58	71	29
Equivocal	42	7	36
Definite	0	21	36
Ratings of psychosis			
None	74	29	43
Equivocal	26	36	29
Definite	0	36	29

From Grossman et al., 1986

These results from Harrow's group are indicative of the fact that manic thought disorder can prevail long past an acute episode, a point that suggests caution in accepting assumptions of a relatively benign course of illness or of return to normality for all patients with manic-depressive illness. The findings must be leavened, however, by certain methodological constraints, especially by one relevant to recent research investigations. Manic-depressive patients seen and treated in university teaching hospitals, in the current era, represent a disproportionately ill and treatment-refractory group. Bipolar patients with a more typical (i.e., salutary) course are now treated, for the most part, by the general psychiatric community. Those patients less responsive to standard medical interventions are more frequently referred to research centers for evaluation and treatment. Further confounding interpretation of the findings are possible medication effects and seasonal biases (e.g., annual assessments, if completed 1 year, 2 years, or 4 years after an acute episode, may increase the likelihood of testing during a periodic recurrence rather than a remission). The continuance of significant thought pathology in many manic patients is of both clinical and theoretical relevance and is an important area for further research. There is, unfortunately, no comparable follow-up research on thought disorder in bipolar depression.

Speech Patterns

Comparison of Speech Patterns in Mania and Schizophrenia

Investigators have been unable to find consistent and significant differences in linguistic patterns between manic and schizophrenic patients (Kagan and Oltmanns, 1981; Harvey, 1983; Ragin and Oltmanns, 1987). Calev and colleagues (1989) found no significant differences in word fluency between manic patients who were matched on age with stable bipolar patients. Hoffman and colleagues (1986), however, found that total speech deviance and utterance length were greater in manic than in schizophrenic patients; the authors concluded that "manic speech difficulties were due to shifts from one discourse structure to another, while schizophrenic speech difficulties reflected a basic deficiency in elaborating any discourse structure" (p. 836). In a

related study, Fraser and associates (1986) found that schizophrenics have less syntactically complex speech than do manics. These structural differences in language are schematized in Figure 11-3 and illustrated in the following speech segment (along with the investigators' comments) taken from one of their manic patients:

[Speaker responding to a question about the things he likes to do] I like playing pool a lot, that's one of my releases, that I play pool a lot. Oh what else? Bartend, bartend on the side, it's kind of fun to, if you're a bartender you can, you can see how people reacted, amounts of alcohol and different guys around, different chicks around, and different situations, if it's snowing outside, if it's cold outside, the weather conditions, all types of different types of environments and types of different types of people you'll usually find in a bar . . .

[Authors' commentary] Here the speaker begins talking about things he likes to do, including bartending, which offers him interesting experiences that include different situations or environments. One set of different environments includes references to the weather, which indeed can induce environmental variability, but which has no obvious relationship to bar-based situations and environments. This progression from bar to variable environments to the weather corresponds to a break in transitivity in the statement hierarchy that induces an experience of incoherence for the listener. If the speaker ended here, this hierarchical deviance would suggest that the patient demonstrates a basic deficiency in elaborating complex discourse structures. However the speaker continues with the following statements.

You know the ones that are really, uh, fuddy duddies they might come in for one glass of wine and then leave, you know, as a social thing, then you've got the wallow-away drunks that—young kids that don't know where the hell they are going, and they just want to get drunk and impress chicks—chicks don't like that, then you have the ones that are suave and debonair. They come in as the macho man. Yes the bar's a very interesting place. It's a very, I think it's a really, well, it's not a complete representative cross-section of, of, society, but it's close enough as far as the younger generation goes.

[Authors' commentary] Thus, the speaker successfully elaborates on the "bar society" topic, and by so doing demonstrates the ability to complete a complex discourse hierarchy. (Hoffman et al., 1986, p. 835)

Hoffman and colleagues (1986) speculate that the shift from one discourse structure to another is related to the manic patient's increased distractibility and general level of overactivation, both of which involve both verbal and nonverbal behavior.

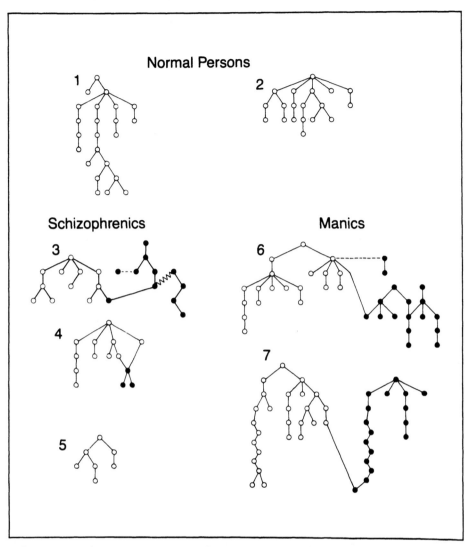

Figure 11-3. Sample of discourse structures taken from three groups. Nodes correspond to statements generated by text. Linkages are formed from dependency relations. Substructures identified by open circles correspond to largest subtree embedded in segment. Jagged line indicates nontransitive dependency; broken lines represent nondependent associations. Upward branching nodes can be seen to receive more than one chain of superordinate statements. Two manics have larger subtrees compared with three schizophrenics. 1, 2, and 5 are well-formed trees (from Hoffman et al., 1986).

Comparison of Speech Patterns in Mania and Depression

Predictability of verbal communication has been studied through close analysis, a measure of the ability of normal judges to guess words deleted from transcripts of speech samples. Using this technique, Ragin and Oltmanns (1983) found that depressed speech was the most predictable, schizophrenic the least, and manic speech was somewhere in between. Andreasen and Pfohl (1976) analyzed the frequency of syntactical elements in speech samples taken from 16 manic and 15 depressed patients. These results are summarized in Table 11-8 and by the authors:

The analysis of syntactical elements was particularly useful in distinguishing between the two groups. . . . depressive speech tends to be more vague, qualified, and personalized, while manic speech is more colorful and concrete. . . . depressed patients tend to qualify more, to talk more in terms of a "state of being," and to talk more both about themselves and other people.

Table 11-8. Frequency of Syntactical Elements in Manic and Depressed Patients[a]

Manic = Depressed	Manic > Depressed	Depressed > Manic
• Lexical diversity (number of words, number of different words) • Syntactical complexity	• Colorfulness • Action verbs • Adjectives • Concreteness • Words reflecting power and achievement	• Vagueness • Qualifying adverbs • First person pronouns • Overstatement

[a]N = 16 manic patients, N = 15 depressed patients

Adapted from data in Andreasen and Pfohl, 1976

Manics, on the other hand, tend to talk more about things than about people, to discuss them in terms of action, and to use more adjectives to describe them. (p. 1366)

HALLUCINATIONS AND DELUSIONS

. . . I saw the stars rushing at each other—and thought the lamps of London were gliding through the night into a World Collision. . . . Nothing was more notable to me through the illness than the general exaltation of the nerves of sight and hearing, and their power of making colour and sound harmonious as well as intense—with alternation of faintness and horror of course. But I learned so much about the nature of Phantasy and Phantasm—it would have been totally inconceivable to me without seeing, how the unreal and real could be mixed. —John Ruskin[8]

Delusions and hallucinations are common and important features of manic-depressive illness but neither necessary nor specific to its diagnosis. We discussed in earlier chapters the incidence of psychotic features in mania and bipolar depression, methodological problems associated with their assessment, the nature of their clinical presentation, and patients' subjective accounts of delusional and hallucinatory experiences (see Chapter 2), the relationship between psychotic features and diagnosis (see Chapters 4, 5, and 8), and their correlation with age, severity, and outcome (see Chapters 2 and 8). Here, after a brief summary of the incidence data presented in Chapter 2, we focus on the nature and content of bipolar hallucinations and delusions, as well as the relationship between the psychotic features of unipolar depressive illness and those that occur in bipolar manic-depressive illness.

Hallucinations

In the night, not long after we had gone to bed, Robert got up and wrote down a melody which, he said, the angels had sung to him. Then he lay down again and talked deliriously the whole night, staring at the ceiling all the time. When morning came, the angels transformed themselves into devils and sang horrible music, telling him he was a sinner and that they were going to cast him into hell. He became hysterical, screaming in agony that they were pouncing on him like tigers and hyaenas, and seizing him in their claws. The doctors who came only just managed to control him. —Clara Schumann[9]

Hallucinations, the perceptions of sensory impressions without the existence of external physical stimuli, represent a fascinating, not uncommon, and yet relatively unstudied part of the clinical phenomenology of affective illness. They occupy a portion of the continuum of dream state–illusory–hallucinatory phenomena that ranges from distortions and misperceptions, on the one hand, to the total conjuring of fully developed images on the other. These illusions and hallucinations can vary on a wide variety of aspects, such as their extent (frequency and duration), location, constancy, intensity, effect on overt behavior, affect produced, content, and causal attributions (Lowe, 1973). Despite these complexities, hallucinations are most commonly presented in the psychiatric research literature as simply present or absent in a given sensory modality (e.g., auditory or visual).

Hallucinations occur less frequently than delusions in both the manic and depressed phases of bipolar illness. The lifetime history data presented in Chapter 2 suggest that at least half of all patients report a history of delusions, but only about a fifth report the experience of hallucinating while depressed or manic. Auditory hallucinations, averaged across the data-based studies, are more common than visual ones.

Kraepelin (1921) observed that in mania the perception of external impressions was "invariably encroached upon" and that defective perceptions often were related to "extraordinary distractibility of attention." He described not only the blurring of illusions, hypnagogic phenomena, and hallucinations but also their overlap with mood and thinking in manic-depressive illness:

> Isolated Hallucinations are observed frequently and in the most different states, although they do not very often appear conspicuously in the foreground. It is generally a case of illusionary occurrences, the appearance of which is favoured by the incompleteness and slightness of perception, but especially by the lively emotions peculiar to the disease. The substance of the illusions therefore is invariably in close connection with the trains of thought and the moods of the patients. (p.8)

Auditory hallucinations frequently appear only in the night-time, or at least much more then. They seem, as a rule, not to possess complete sensory distinctness. They are voices "as in a dream" . . . . Their origin is relatively seldom referred to the external world. . . . Much more frequently the hallucinations have their seat in the patient's own body. (p.11)

In an early study, Bowman and Raymond (1931–1932b) compared hallucinations in 1,009 patients with manic-depressive psychoses, 1,408 with schizophrenia, and 496 with general paresis. They found a general tendency for more women than men to have a history of hallucinations (especially of a visual nature), and that women with "seclusive personalities" were at particularly high risk for auditory and visual hallucinations. The authors found no significant relationship between the presence of hallucinations and religion, age at admission, or level of intelligence. They did observe a close relationship between the clinical nature of the hallucinations in manic-depressive illness and those present in patients with general paresis. This latter finding is consistent with Lowe's conclusion (1973) that manic-depressive hallucinations resemble more those of the organic psychoses than those of schizophrenia or paranoia. (This similarity to organic psychosis (toxic vs defect) is also discussed in Chapters 5 and 18.)

Winokur and colleagues (1969) noted that manic hallucinations tended to be brief, grandiose, often part of a delusional idea, usually religious ("the face of God," "Heaven in all its glory"), and frequently in the form of a command from God. Manic and depressive hallucinations shared in common a fragmented and fleeting quality and usually occurred in the most severely disturbed patients. The authors also stressed the theoretical importance of a severity profile in manic-depressive illness, after noting that hallucinations—the least common of symptoms—were also the first symptoms to disappear during recovery from a manic episode, followed in turn by delusions, flight of ideas, push of speech, and distractibility (a general pattern later confirmed by Carlson and Goodwin, 1973; see Chapters 2 and 4):

> If symptoms that are present in fewest of the patients tend to disappear first, then we may think of them as being manifestations of severity of the illness occurring at its apex. Conversely, the symptoms that are most frequently present may be considered as the clinical core of the illness. The order of disappearance of symptoms might also say something about possible underlying neural mechanisms and enable correlation between biologic and psychologic phenomena. Finally, psychopathologic mechanisms might be uncovered if some symptoms are necessary to the appearance of others, the *basic* symptoms tending to disappear last. (Winokur et al., 1969, p. 77)

D. Goodwin and colleagues (1971) in St. Louis, although finding hallucinations of generally limited use in differential diagnosis, did draw several conclusions about the nature of affective hallucinations in their study of 28 patients (7 bipolar) with affective illness: (1) the modality of hallucinations (e.g., auditory or visual) was not consistent from one affective episode to another, (2) patients with affective illness were far more likely than those with schizophrenia to hallucinate only when no other person was there, (3) color was usually normal, (4) hallucinated people were usually of normal size and appearance, (5) the hallucinations were intermittent, (6) they were often in several sensory modalities, and (7) accusatory voices were not specific to affective illness—indeed, they were more common in schizophrenia.

Lowe (1973), in a particularly intensive and interesting investigation of hallucinations, studied 22 manic-depressive patients. He found, in comparing these patients with others who had organic, paranoid, or schizophrenic psychoses, that manic-depressive patients reported mainly auditory and visual hallucinations, that these were less frequent and briefer than hallucinations occurring in other neuropsychiatric conditions, that, in retrospect, the hallucinations were believed by patients to be "less real" but were also perceived to be less controllable, that women were more likely to report rarer types of hallucinations, and, finally, that the hallucinations were always considered by the patients to be experienced only by themselves. As mentioned earlier, Lowe concluded that manic-depressive hallucinations were more similar in nature to those reported by the patients with organic psychoses than by those with schizophrenia or paranoia.

Lerner (1980), who also investigated qualitative differences between the psychotic experiences of mania and schizophrenia, concluded that mania was more characterized by enhanced sensory awareness and ecstatic or beatific experiences. Manic hallucinations tended to be more of the visual type, strikingly vivid and associated with bright, colorful sensations, and often coupled with intensely pleasurable or ecstatic feelings (similar to psychedelic experiences). Silberman and colleagues (1985) compared histories of transient sensory phenomena in 44 euthymic affective patients (34 bipolar), 37 complex partial seizure patients, and 30 hypertensive controls. Affective and epileptic patients were similar in their reports of sensory changes, including visual and auditory hallucinations, and altered perceptual intensities. Epileptic patients, however, were far more likely to have experienced epigastric, vestibular, and gustatory hallucinations.

In summary, hallucinations occur less frequently than delusions in both the manic and depressed phases of bipolar illness. Hallucinatory phenomena appear to represent the extreme end of the symptomatic picture, being nonexistent in milder forms of depression and mania and most pronounced in the gravest, most delirious states. Hallucinations during mania are frequently ecstatic and religious in nature, brief and fleeting in duration, and inconstant in their modality of expression. They appear qualitatively, at least in a few studies, to be more similar to organic than schizophrenic psychoses. Gender differences in the experience of hallucinatory phenomena are unclear.

Delusions in Manic-Depressive Illness

But there are cases . . . in which the patient perceives justly; associates naturally, judges correctly, but reasons erroneously, that is, draws false conclusions from just prepositions [sic]. Sometimes he discovers the reverse of this state of mind, by drawing just conclusions from erroneous perceptions, associations and judgments. Thus, when he fancies himself to be a king,

he errs in all the ways that have been mentioned. But observe his conduct: he covers himself with a blanket which he calls a robe, he puts a mat upon his head which he calls a crown, struts with a majestic step, and demands the homage due to royalty from all around him.—Benjamin Rush[10]

Delusions are common in manic-depressive illness, occurring in approximately one half (48 percent) of manic episodes and in 33 to 56 percent of severe bipolar depressive episodes (see Chapter 2). In mania, grandiose (47 percent) and persecutory/paranoid (28 percent) delusions are relatively frequent; delusions of passivity (15 percent) are less common. Delusions, like hallucinations, vary widely in their severity, fixedness, content, and effect on overt behavior. The degree to which they are contingent on fluctuating affect also varies. Kendler and co-workers (1983), emphasizing the dimensional aspects of delusional experiences, defined five as especially central:

1. *Conviction*—the degree to which the patient is convinced of the reality of the delusional beliefs. . . .
2. *Extension*—the degree to which the delusional belief involves various areas of the patient's life. . . .
3. *Bizarreness*—the degree to which the delusional belief departs from culturally determined consensual reality. . . .
4. *Disorganization*—the degree to which the delusional beliefs are internally consistent, logical, and systematized. . . .
5. *Pressure*—the degree to which the patient is preoccupied and concerned with the expressed delusional belief. (pp. 466-467)

Kendler and colleagues, like Winokur and associates (1969) in their discussion of the sequencing of hallucinations, have stressed the potential implications of the temporal course of psychotic decompensation:

. . . individual dimensions of delusional experience often change independently of one another during the course of a psychotic episode. An investigation of the pattern of change in dimensions of delusional experience during psychotic decompensation or resolution might provide insights into the nature of the psychotic process. (p. 468)

Further discussion of definitional and measurement aspects of delusions are covered elsewhere.[11]

Manic delusions are usually grandiose and expansive in nature, often religious, and not infrequently paranoid. They generally can be differentiated from schizophrenic delusions by their tendency to be wish-fulfilling in nature and more oriented toward communion rather than segregation (Lerner, 1980); also:

> The delusions that are seen in schizophrenia usually last for months or years and are often primary in that they do not explain a real or disordered perception. They fulfill the definition of a delusion as a fixed, false belief. In mania the delusions are quite different. They are often evanescent, appearing or disappearing during the course of a day, or even during an interview. They also vary with the patient's total state, being more frequent when he is more active; and his flights of ideas become more pronounced and fading as he becomes more quiet. Frequently they are extensions of the patient's grandiosity.
>
> At times the patient can be talked out of his delusion, and at other times he gives the impression that he is only being playful rather than really being deluded. In our group the delusions were often secondary to the patient's exalted affect. This was especially true of those patients who felt their mood could be described only as a religious experience.
>
> The most subtle and earliest distortions of reality are manifest in the frequent extravagance and grandiose self-image expressed by the patients. (Winokur et al., 1969, p. 70)

Kraepelin (1921) also emphasized the changing nature of manic delusions (especially when contrasted to those expressed during the depressive phase, which he thought were for the most part "uniformly adhered to"): manic delusions "change frequently, emerge as creations of the moment and again disappear." Kraepelin noted that manic delusions "move very frequently on religious territory," tending to be grandiose, and that the "patients often narrate all sorts of journeys and adventures, secret experiences." He also observed that the same delusional ideas often appeared again in subsequent attacks. Winokur and colleagues (1969), like Kraepelin, described delusions of mania as being "not well systematized and, apart from grandiose optimism, tend not to be acted upon" (p. 72). The fact that manic patients seldom act on their delusions (a point perhaps worth disputing) was attributed by the authors to the brief duration of the delusions and the patient's "inability to make any sort of concerted action" (p. 72). Both manic and depressive delusions, which occur primarily in the most disturbed patients, tend to be appropriate to the patient's mood and not to be systematized (Winokur et al., 1969). The same investigators found that religious themes were the most common manic delusions in both men and women. Political themes were more common in men than

Table 11-9. Themes of Manic Delusions

	Males % (N = 37)[a]	Females % (N = 63)[a]
Religious	27.0	30.1
Political	18.9	3.2
Sexual	13.5	9.5
Wealth	5.4	7.9

[a]Number of manic episodes

Adapted from Winokur et al., 1969

women, and sexual and financial themes were about equally common (Table 11-9).

Depressive delusions tend to focus on fixed ideas of guilt and sinfulness, poverty, hypochondriacal and somatic concerns, and feelings of persecution.[12] Kraepelin, in his discussion of hypochondriacal tendencies and somatic delusions, described the "delusional interpretation of harmless sensations" so common in depressive states and contrasted them to manic perceptions:

> This heightened sensitivity for the processes in their own bodies is in vivid contrast with the lowering of central excitability in manic states. We observe here a very striking lack of sensibility towards heat and cold, hunger and thirst, pain and injury. (p. 13)

Winokur and colleagues also examined the nature of delusions during mixed states and found, not surprisingly, that the type of delusion fluctuated with the patient's mood. Although depressive delusions were more frequent, manic-like delusions (nondepressed, grandiose, all religious) also occurred. Himmelhoch (1979) emphasized the importance of manic delusions in differentiating unipolar agitated depression from mixed states:

> The clue to recognizing it [a mixed state] is the presence of distinct maniacal coloration of the psychotic material in the midst of all the severe depressive symptomatology . . . [for example] . . . grandiose, radiant, beatific religious delusions . . . out of tune with the patient's misery. (p 453)

In summary, delusions are common in the manic, depressed, and mixed phases of bipolar illness. Manic delusions generally are expansive, grandiose, and often religious. They differ from schizophrenic delusions in being less fixed, more fleeting, and more communal in nature. Depressive delusions tend to focus on guilt, poverty, somatic, and persecutory concerns.

Table 11-10. Psychotic Symptoms in Bipolar and Unipolar Patients

Study	N	% with Delusions and/or Hallucinations		Comments
		BP	UP	
Beigel & Murphy, 1971b	25 BP 25 UP	12	36	Depressed phase; matched for age, sex, level of depression
Guze et al., 1975	19 BP 139 UP	53	17	Phase unclear
Winokur, 1975	15 BP 216 UP	60	57	Depressed phase
Brockington et al., 1982a	32 BP 122 UP	13	37	UP > BP: ideas of reference; auditory hallucinations
Winokur, 1984	122 BP 203 UP	64	56	BP > UP: auditory and visual hallucinations
Endicott et al., 1985	178 BP 204 UP	27	14	Lifetime history of a psychotic depressive episode (i.e., with delusions and/or hallucinations)
Andreasen, 1988 (and personal communication)	177 BP (93 I, 84 II) 422 UP			BP I > BP II > UP for delusions, no significant differences for hallucinations
Black & Nasrallah, 1989	628 BP 763 UP	21 BPD 58 BPM	11	BPM > BPD, UP for hallucinations and delusions. Hallucinations: 9% BPD, 14% BPM; Delusions: 12% BPD, 44% BPM (overlap not specified)

BPD = bipolar depressed, BPM = bipolar manic

Psychotic Depression in Bipolar and Unipolar Illness

Psychotic symptoms probably occur more often in bipolar depressed patients than in unipolar depression, as shown by the rates summarized in Table 11-10. Although some studies fail to show a higher rate of delusions or hallucinations in bipolar depression,[13] others do (e.g., Guze et al., 1975), and the more recent and better designed studies (Endicott et al., 1985; Andreasen, 1988 and personal communication, 1988) support the conclusion that psychotic features are more common in bipolar depression. Corroborating evidence comes from the Coryell and associates (1985) study of psychotic symptoms in relatives of affectively ill probands with lifetime diagnoses of major depression. Both delusions and hallucinations were most frequent in the bipolar-I relatives and least frequent in the nonbipolar major depressive group.

Clinical, demographic, and course differences in delusional and nondelusional (unipolar) depression are summarized in Table 11-11. There are no consistent demographic differences (gender, age of onset) between the two groups, nor are there consistent significant clinical differences in sleep disturbance, loss of appetite, or decreased libido. Course and outcome variables are similarly inconclusive in their relationship to the presence or absence of delusions in unipolar depressed patients. The most significant clinical difference between the groups is on psychomotor agitation–retardation. Delusional patients demonstrated greater agitation in several studies (Charney and Nelson, 1981; Frances et al., 1981; Frangos et al., 1983), whereas in others, delusions were more strongly associated with psychomotor retardation and depressive stupor (Glassman and Roose, 1981; Frangos et al., 1983). This apparent discrepancy is not, however, inconsistent with clinically observed fluctuations in activation patterns, nor is it incompatible with the coexistence of psychomotor agitation and psychomotor retardation in severely depressed patients:

Although seemingly contradictory, it is important to note that the presence of retardation does not preclude the concurrent presence of agitation: for example, we have observed delusional patients who walk slowly, speaking in a halting monotone, while wringing their hands and reporting a sense of internal restlessness. (Roose and Glassman, 1988, p. 79)

There is a strong tendency for the presence or absence of psychotic symptoms to be consistent across episodes. Charney and Nelson (1981) found that 95 percent of their delusional patients had had prior delusional episodes, whereas only 8 percent of their nondelusional patients had experienced prior delusional episodes. Among patients whose index admission was psychotic, 89 percent of all previous episodes were psychotic as well. Helms and Smith (1983) reported that 92 percent of their psychotic depressives with recurrent illness experienced another admission for psychotic depression, and Lykouras and colleagues (1985) found that 92 percent of their delusional depressives had had previous episodes with delusional ideation compared with 36 percent of their nonpsychotic depressives. Nelson and associates (1984) observed:

It would appear that the presence of delusions during an index episode of depression may be not merely an indicator of severity of that episode, but additionally a distinct stable trait which would be expressed in the biologically vulnerable individual during prior and subsequent episodes. (p. 298)

Aronson and co-workers (1988), studying bipolar as well as unipolar delusional depressives, also found a consistency of psychotic expression across episodes as well as a marked rate of relapse. They remarked that "psychoticism may

Table 11-11. Clinical Correlates[a] of (Unipolar) Delusional Depression

Study	N	Psychomotor Agitation	Psychomotor Retardation	Sleep Disturbance	Appetite Changes	Age at First Episode	# Previous Episodes	Family History of Affec. Ill.	Suicide	Gender
Charney & Nelson 1981	54D 66ND	↑	↓	NS	NS	NS	NS			
Frances et al., 1981	30P 34NP	↑	NS	↑		NS	NS	NS		
Glassman & Roose, 1981	21D 42ND	↓[b]	↑	NS	NS		↓			
Coryell & Tsuang, 1982	115D 97ND							NS		
Frangos et al., 1983	145P 119NP	↑	↑[c]			NS	NS	NS	NS[d]	NS
Roose et al., 1983	14S 28DC							↑		
Nelson et al., 1984	13D 12ND							↑		NS
Black et al., 1988b	183P 824NP								NS	

NS = no significant difference, D = delusional patients, ND = nondelusional patients, P = psychotic patients, NP = nonpsychotic patients, S = suicides, DC = depressed control patients

[a]Based on comparisons between delusional and nondelusional patients
[b]Authors point out that psychomotor retardation does not preclude presence of agitation
[c]Depressive stupor
[d]Suicide attempts

represent an independent variable that may be associated with either unipolar or bipolar illness." This issue of psychoticism breeding true is discussed in Chapter 15, as are family history studies of bipolar and unipolar delusion depression. Additional reviews of clinical correlates of unipolar delusional depression are covered elsewhere.[14]

COGNITIVE FUNCTIONING

My thoughts are like loose dry sand, which the closer it is grasped slips the sooner away. . . . I lose every other sentence through the inevitable wanderings of my mind, and experience, as I have these two years, the same shattered mode of thinking on every subject and on all occasions. If I seem to write with more connexion, it is only because the gaps do not appear. —William Cowper[15]

Mania and depression unquestionably affect the ability to think, concentrate, formulate ideas, reason, and remember. Less clear are the nature and extent of such changes, as well as their specificity to affective illness, their etiology, or their existence before the onset of affective symptoms. The degree of progression, chronicity, and reversibility of cognitive impairment in treated or untreated manic-depressive illness is, likewise, inadequately understood. Many of the conceptual and methodological problems specific to studying intellectual functioning in patients with depression or mania have been discussed in the introduction to this chapter and are reviewed extensively elsewhere.[16] Problems of particular significance arise when attempting to distinguish between general factors that might account for intellectual impairment across psychiatric, psychological, or medical conditions—e.g., distractibility, attention, fatigue, or motivation—and those specific to bipolar depression and mania—e.g., lateralization differences.

We present first a brief review of the literature on cognitive and psychomotor speed in manic-depressive illness and then cover neuropsychological findings: general intellectual functioning, learning, memory, and associational processing, and finally, results from lateralization studies conducted on bipolar patients. Excellent reviews of cognitive deficits in unipolar depressive disorders have been written by, among others, Miller (1975) and Weingartner and Silberman (1984).

Thought Association Patterns

Early clinical researchers described many changes in the associational patterns that oc-

curred during depression and mania. Kraepelin (1921) observed that rhymes and sound associations increased during mania. His own work and that of Isserlin led him to conclude that association response time was much longer during depression and shorter during mania; also:

. . . whereas in mania the associations according to external relations, especially after linguistic practice, are greatly in excess, they decrease greatly in the depressed patients in favour of associations dependent on content. As a further expression of this displacement the almost complete disappearance of pure clang associations may be taken, which play such a large part in mania. In the same way digression which is so characteristic of the distractibility of manic patients is completely absent in depression, and lastly also the repetition of the stimulus word, which is frequent in manic patients and is probably caused mostly by inattention. (p. 17)

Murphy (1923), in an early study, also found that rhymes and sound associations increased during the manic states. Later, Henry and colleagues (1971) studied associational patterns and found that during mania, the number of statistically common responses decreased by 35 percent and the idiosyncratic responses increased threefold. The change in word association patterns was directly proportional to the severity of manic symptoms. In a related study, Pons and associates (1985) found that bipolar patients had fewer repetitions of common responses than controls and concluded that, since these findings did not appear to be affected by mood state, "aberrancies in associational processes may be a trait characteristic of persons with bipolar affective disorder." Calev and colleagues (1989) found no significant differences in word fluency between manic patients who were matched on age with stable bipolar patients. Hoffman (1987), who has developed computer simulations of neural information processing, suggests that increased randomness may be the underlying cause of the neurocognitive processes central to the active manic states:

The model predicts that mania is due to increased randomness of state adjustments of individual neurons, which destabilizes memories. It should be stressed that the manic behavior of this model is due not to increased activation (ie, firing rate) of the neurons in the system but to increased randomness; increased firing rate per se would only cause the system to run its programs at a faster rate.

The randomness model of manic cognition suggests that accessibility of memories is markedly enhanced due to jumps from one memory to another, though the stable generation of the correct nearest gestalt based on input information is impaired. This may account for the grandiose self-assessments of manics. Their minds might in fact be extraordinarily capable of accessing large numbers of gestalts. The price they pay, however, is a devastating instability of their mental constructions. (p. 187)

Related work on the randomness of underlying biological processes by Mandell and colleagues (1984) is discussed in Chapter 20, and further discussions of associational processes can be found earlier in this chapter, as well as in Chapter 14.

Cognitive and Psychomotor Speed

Subjective complaints of slowed mental processes are common in depression. For example, as we reviewed in Chapter 2, fully 91 percent of depressed patients report diminished speed of thought. Clinical data also show a high incidence of psychomotor retardation in depression. Winokur and colleagues (1969) found that 76 percent, and Carlson and Strober (1979) 83 percent, of bipolar depressed patients displayed psychomotor retardation. Even though there is some evidence that depressed patients tend to underestimate their performance on motor speed tests and overestimate their degree of retardation, there is no doubt that slowed thinking and movement are central to the depressive state (Morgan, 1967; Colbert and Harrow, 1967; Miller, 1975). Indeed, Widlöcher (1983) has stated that "cognitive slowing seems a constant dimension of depression and, probably, its core." Mania and hypomania, on the other hand, are more characterized by an acceleration in thought, speech, and psychomotor activity. Three components of cognitive and psychomotor speed—reaction time, speech, and psychomotor activity—are reviewed briefly here. For more extensive reviews, the reader is referred to Miller (1975), Greden and Carroll (1981), Widlöcher (1983), and Sackeim and Steif (1988).

Reaction Time

Virtually all studies of reaction time have been carried out during the depressed rather than the hypomanic or manic phases of bipolar illness. Most studies have failed to specify diagnostic subtypes, possible existence of mixed states (which can involve both increases and decreases in psychomotor speed and activity), number of prior episodes, gender, age, and medication status. There is, however, an impressive consistency in finding that depressed patients show slower reaction times than do normals.[17] Pfeiffer and Maltzman (1976), in contrast, did not find significant state-dependent differences in warned reaction times, and Gill and Horne (1974) found no significant differences between normals and depressives on reaction time tasks. Manic-depressive and "endogenously depressed" unipolar patients have been found to have significantly faster reaction times than chronic schizophrenics (Huston and Senf, 1952; Hall and Stride, 1954).

Slowed reaction time is not specific to depression and is probably more likely to reflect severity of illness. There is, however, some evidence that reaction time performance deteriorates more quickly in depressed than in normal individuals and that the last reaction time in a series is slower than the first. Several explanations have been offered for these findings: (1) depressives may have an increased susceptibility to fatigue, (2) may be lacking in sustained motivation, (3) may be unable to maintain concentration, and (4) may be lacking in physiological preparedness to react (Miller, 1975). There is some evidence that distraction (from external stimuli) can to some extent break up psychomotor retardation in manic-depressives (Foulds, 1952). Clinical improvement in depression has been shown by several investigators to correlate with an increase in response speed and a decrease in psychomotor retardation.[18] Although depressed patients clearly show cognitive slowing, just what the slowness reflects and where in the processing it occurs remain unclear.

The few studies that have examined manic and hypomanic response patterns found more premature responses in mania (Hemsley and Philips, 1975). They also found that manic illness did not seem to affect speed functions very significantly and, in fact, that at certain speeds manic patients were better able than depressed ones to solve problems (Blackburn, 1975). In another study (Pfeiffer and Maltzman, 1976), hypomanic patients were faster than euthymic patients on warned reaction time tasks.

Speech

Clinical studies reviewed in Chapter 2 are consistent in reporting rapid and pressured speech as one of the most characteristic features of mania, occurring in 98 percent of patients, averaged across studies (see Table 2-4). Changes in rate of speech in mania and depression were discussed earlier in this chapter in the review of thought disorder. Specific studies of the psychomotor component of speech show that depressed patients exhibit slowed speech, with a low rate of total speech rate and a high rate of silence (Pope et al., 1970) and long pause times (Szabadi et al., 1976; Greden et al., 1979, 1981; Greden and Carroll, 1980). One study found a diurnal variation in rate of speech, with greater slowing in the morning (Greden et al., 1979). Studies of rate of speech in mania have demonstrated a greater number of words spoken per minute (Lorenz and Cobb, 1952), faster spontaneous talking and longer spontaneous sentences (Hutt and Coxon, 1965), and an increase in the amount of speech as patients switch into mania (Stoddard et al., 1977).

Psychomotor Activity

In general, studies of psychomotor activity are consistent in showing a decrease during depression.[19] (Descriptive studies of psychomotor activity are discussed in Chapter 2 and circadian aspects in Chapter 19.) Bipolar depressed patients tend to exhibit more retardation, and unipolar depressed patients tend to exhibit relatively more activity.[20] An increase in nighttime psychomotor activity was related in one study to the development of psychotic features (Weiss et al., 1974).

Learning and Memory

Generalized Level of Cognitive Impairment

The most generalized and consistent finding about cognitive impairment in affective illness is that it increases with increasing levels of severity of depression.[21] Fewer studies have examined the relationship between severity of cognitive impairment and levels of mania; Henry and colleagues (1971), however, found that impairment in serial learning performance occurred in direct proportion to increasing levels of mania. Although many factors confound the interpretation of findings (e.g., severity of depression, male to female ratios, and medications), several studies have found that bipolar patients show greater cognitive impairment when depressed than do unipolar patients. Wolfe and associates (1987) found this to be so on verbal recall and fluency tasks, and Savard and co-workers (1980) and Rubinow and colleagues (1984b) demonstrated the point on concept formation and problem solving tasks. Wolfe and colleagues (1987) were especially impressed by the debilitating extent of memory problems in their bipolar depressed patients:

A particularly important finding from this study is that the performance of bipolar depressed patients may quantitatively resemble the memory dysfunction found in neurologic patients [Huntington's] with damage to certain basal ganglia structures (i.e., the caudate nuclei) on tasks of verbal learning and verbal fluency. (p. 90)

Henry and associates (1971, 1973), on the other hand, found more memory impairment in unipolar patients, although they speculated that it may reflect the greater severity of their depression. Brand and Jolles (1987) found no significant differences between bipolar and unipolar patients, although there was a trend for the unipolar patients to have greater cognitive difficulties.

Short-Term Memory and Attentional Deficits

Short-term memory usually is assessed by testing recall after a short delay (most often less than 10 seconds). In this paradigm, patients are tested for the number of items they can recognize or recall immediately after presentation (average range of 5 to 9 in normal subjects). Results of short-term memory assessment in depressed patients are equivocal. Several investigators have found minimal, if any, impairment during depression,[22] whereas others have reported short-term memory problems (Breslow et al., 1980; Steif et al., 1986a). Even where such differences do exist, the general consensus in the literature is that the impairment is secondary to attentional dysfunction rather than the capacity for short-term memory storage (Sackeim and Steif, 1988).

The inability to attend and concentrate are part and parcel of the memory and learning problems that occur during affective illness. Kraepelin (1921) noted this in his depressed patients:

. . . facility of attention is distinctly disordered. The patients are not able to turn their attention easily and quickly to any impressions or ideas. They are not able either to pay attention, or to turn away of themselves from ideas which emerge in their own minds or which are suggested to them from without. This lack of freedom of attention certainly displays innumerable gradations. (p. 7)

Poor concentration and distractibility are among the most common symptoms of both manic and depressed states. Our reviews of the clinical studies (see Chapter 2) found that 71 percent of manic patients reported impaired concentration and distractibility (see Table 2-2), and 91 percent of depressed patients reported impaired concentration (see Table 2-5). Attention and concentration deficits have been observed in depressed patients tested on a wide variety of experimental tasks (e.g., Caudrey et al., 1980; Raskin et al., 1982; Frith et al., 1983). Although detailed discussion is beyond the scope of this chapter, the specific mediational processes that might account for cognitive impairment during affective illness are reviewed extensively by Sackeim and Steif (1988). These problems include, in addition to attention, level of effort, levels of processing, storage vs retrieval, and mood congruence. Depressed patients, for example, have been shown to have shallow encoding of information, but when external coding is provided (i.e., words are categorized), the depressed patients are able to perform at a better level (Weingartner et al., 1981a). Sackeim and Steif (1988) conclude, on the basis of these findings, that:

. . . when exposed to new material, depressed patients are less likely to link information to preexisting knowledge and thereby impose the organization that facilitates learning and memory. (p. 277)

Level of effort, the ability to recall stimuli, and severity of depression appear to correlate substantially with one another (R.M. Cohen et al., 1982; Roy-Byrne et al., 1986; Calev et al., 1989; Golinkoff and Sweeney, 1989), further compounding the difficulties of assessing memory impairment in affectively ill patients. Only one study (Koh and Wolpert, 1983) examined bipolar–unipolar differences and found none.

Long-Term Memory

Several studies of depressed patients have found a decrease in the ability to acquire new information without a reduction in the ability to retain it (Cronholm and Ottosson, 1961; Sternberg and Jarvik, 1976; Steif et al., 1986b), and some investigators have concluded that little or no impairment exists (Whitehead, 1973; Gass and Rus

sell, 1986). Differences in findings may result from differences in methods of assessment, since several researchers have noted that the memory and learning deficits in depression are more apparent for unstructured rather than structured material.[23] One implication of this research is that clinicians should, whenever possible, structure material for their depressed patients.

Both unipolar and bipolar patients show evidence of impaired verbal learning (Calev and Erwin, 1985; Wolfe et al., 1987), which has been most commonly interpreted as reflecting an inability to transfer information from short-term to long-term storage (Henry et al., 1971, 1973; Sackeim and Steif, 1988). The degree to which these learning deficits represent only state-dependent changes or reflect more underlying trait characteristics remains unclear and is discussed further in studies of lateralization.

Mood Congruence and State Dependence

Mood state affects the content of recalled material. Mood congruence has been defined by Blaney (1986) as assuming:

. . . that some material, by virtue of its affectively valenced content, is more likely to be stored and/or recalled when one is in a particular mood; concordance between mood at exposure and mood at recall is not required or relevant. (p. 229)

The consistency of research findings is stronger for mood congruence than for state-dependent recall (where stored material is recalled better when the mood of recollection is the same as the mood of storage). For detailed discussion of the mood–congruence literature, the reader is referred to several substantive reviews.[24] Most studies have found that depressed patients are better able to recall words with depressive content; nondepressed subjects show the opposite tendency (H. Davis, 1979a,b; Kuiper and Derry, 1982; Bower, 1983). Depressed patients also are more likely to recall negative experiences,[25] and to underestimate success (Blaney, 1986). Failure tasks are also recalled more often by depressed than nondepressed subjects. Conversely, success tasks are recalled more frequently by nondepressed subjects (Blaney, 1986).

State-dependent learning has been observed in drug and alcohol studies in both humans and animals (Reus et al., 1979). Weingartner and colleagues (1977) found that patients who cycled between manic and normal states were better able to recall material (verbal associations) during similar rather than disparate moods; that is, they were better able, when manic, to recall material generated during mania. Likewise, when normal, they were better able to recall material generated when normal. They concluded:

The findings presented here suggest that mood state determines not only how we encode events but also how we search memory or how we decide what are the relevant, meaningful features of an event. (p. 283)

General Intellectual Functioning

Tests of general intelligence, such as the Wechsler Adult Intelligence Scale (WAIS), show an inconsistent pattern in patients with manic-depressive illness. This pattern is in rather marked contrast to the relative evenness of results shown in neuropsychological test batteries. Early studies of intelligence, conducted before lithium or other effective treatments were in use, reported general intellectual impairment in manic-depressive patients (Wittman, 1933; Rapaport, 1946; Shapiro and Nelson, 1955); these studies concluded, however, that the cognitive deterioration was reversible, not progressive in nature. Davidson (1939) reported that clinical improvement was paralleled by increased performance on the Stanford-Binet test. Conversely, those patients whose clinical profile worsened also worsened on their intelligence testing.

Mason (1956) found that patients with manic-depressive illness performed better than the general population norms on the Army General Classification Test, the only psychiatric group to do so. Overall and colleagues (1978) concluded that WAIS performance suffered less with moderate hypomania than with other types of psychopathology, and Donnelly and colleagues (1982) found that hypomania was related to increased intellectual functioning. Beneficial cognitive features associated with manic-depressive illness are discussed at length in Chapter 14.

Knowledge of premorbid intellectual level in affectively ill patients and family members is scarce, and interpretation of pre- and post-illness functioning data is correspondingly difficult. As Miller (1975) pointed out with respect to studies of depressed patients, "No study has made the direct comparison of the depressives' premorbid IQs with their IQs during the depressive episode." Further complicating the issue are findings that although manic-depressive patients and their families show evidence of above-average creative, professional, and educational attainment (see Chapters 7 and 14):

. . . comparisons of unipolar and bipolar patients in the depressed phase of illness have not revealed IQ differences (e.g., Donnelly et al., 1982) or different levels of neuropsychological impairment (Abrams and Taylor, 1980). This indirectly leads to the possibility that compared with premorbid functioning, during the depressed phase of illness there may be greater intellectual deterioration in bipolar than unipolar patients. (Sackeim and Steif, 1988, p. 278)

Intellectual functioning in acutely depressed and remitted patients has been reviewed by Miller (1975) and Sackeim and Steif (1988). Studies show fairly consistently that patients in remission perform better than when they are ill. Although not surprising, this finding is still open to question. Along with others, Sackeim and Steif argue that practice effects may account for at least some of the difference because, in the usual paradigm, patients are tested first when ill and then when euthymic.

Recent studies of intellectual functioning in manic-depressive illness are summarized in Table 11-12. (Neuropsychological profiles, a more sensitive gauge of possible underlying cognitive differences between affectively ill and normal populations, are discussed later in this chapter.) In comparing affectively ill patients with those suffering from schizophrenia and organic brain disease, Abrams and colleagues (1981) found that manic and depressed patients performed comparably; both groups obtained higher WAIS scores than their comparison groups. Donnelly and co-workers (1982), as reported earlier, found no significant group differences on full-scale WAIS performance between unipolar and bipolar patients. Hypomania was related to some increase in intellectual functioning. Kerry and associates (1983) found a normal distribution of full-scale IQ in a sample of manic-depressive patients and concluded that there was no evidence of cognitive deterioration. On the other hand, Clark and colleagues (1985) found that affectively ill patients did significantly less well than controls on measures of IQ and abstract reasoning and that recurrent unipolar depressives and bipolar-II patients showed the least intellectual impairment.

Table 11-12. General Intellectual Functioning in Manic-Depressive Illness

Study	Patients N	Measures	Results
Abrams et al., 1981	43 manic 9 depressives 17 SCZ 8 OBD	WAIS	Verbal, Performance, & Full scale IQ: M = D > SCZ = OBD
Donnelly et al., 1982	56 BP 40 UP	WAIS	Full scale IQ: no significant group differences. BP > UP: block design; object assembly. Hypomania related to ↑ intellectual functioning
Kerry et al., 1983	27 MD	WAIS; Verbal Paired Associate Learning Test; Memory for Designs; Names and Events Memory Scale	Full scale IQ: normal distribution. No WAIS subtest pattern. No evidence for cognitive deterioration
Clark et al., 1985	954 affectives 98 SES matched controls	Shipley Institute of Living Scale	Affective patients vs. controls: ↓ IQ ($p<.001$), ↓ abstraction ($p<.001$) Recurrent UP and BP II depressives showed the least intellectual impairment. Cognitive symptoms of depression not predictive of intellectual impairment

SCZ = schizophrenic, OBD = organic brain disease, MD = manic-depressive, SES = social economic status

Interestingly, intellectual functioning could not be predicted by cognitive symptoms of depression (e.g., impaired memory and concentration).

In summary, it is not possible on the basis of intelligence testing alone to state whether the changes seen in the intellectual functioning of affectively ill patients reflect an underlying deficit or difference because at least some of them may be due to methodological problems, such as practice or medication effects. Nor is it possible to ascertain the degree of post-illness decline without good measurements of pre-illness levels of ability. The possibility that manic-depressive patients may start with greater than average cognitive abilities makes especially difficult any conclusions along these lines.

Neuropsychological Functioning

Neuropsychological studies of patients with affective illness, summarized in Table 11-13, show a surprising degree of consistency in their findings. Patients with depressive and manic-depressive illness, as a group, typically demonstrate deficits in right hemisphere or nondominant hemisphere functioning, long associated with problems in perception, spatial relations, integra-

tion of holistic figures, and complex nonverbal tasks (right hemispheric functions are well reviewed by Walsh, 1987). Fragmented thinking and a general inability to integrate thoughts or relate elements in a complex pattern also are associated with right hemisphere cortical damage (Daniels et al., 1988). The patterns of findings across individual studies presented in Table 11-13 are consistent with, and to some extent overlap, the similar conclusions reached in several reviews.[26] The specificity to right hemispheric impairment is most consistent in depressed patients (Sackeim and Steif, 1988), with indication that functioning improves after effective treatment (electroconvulsive therapy or antidepressants) or during remission (Staton et al., 1981; Fromm-Auch, 1982; Fromm and Schopflocher, 1984). The extent to which hemispheric deficits and differences are state or trait dependent, primary or derivative, relatively more pronounced in bipolar or unipolar illness, or in manic or depressive states, remains unclear. For example, children of bipolar probands, who are by virtue of that fact at high risk for developing manic-depressive illness, show significant discrepancies between their verbal and performance scores on

Table 11-13. Neuropsychological Profiles in Affective Illness

Study	Patients N	Measures	Treatment Status	Findings	Presumptive Lateralization
Gilliland et al., 1943	32 manic 87 SCZ 92 paretic	WAIS	NR	Verbal > Performance (affectives)	Right hemisphere impairment[a]
Waldfogel & Guy, 1951	16 manic 21 BP dep 21 reactive dep	WAIS	NR	Verbal > Performance	Right hemisphere impairment
Friedman, 1964	55 dep (BP, agitated, & involutional)	WAIS	Tested before start of treatment	↓ Digit symbol in dep	Right hemisphere impairment
Brown, 1967	7 manic 42 SCZ 21 dep psychoses 20 psychoneurotic	WAIS	NR	Verbal = Performance in affectives; Verbal > Performance among SCZ	Unclear
Donnelly et al., 1972	13 BP & UP 13 TLE	Halstead-Reitan	Drug-free 2 - 4 wks	69% of affectives and 54% of TLE patients performed as mildly-severely brain damaged	Unclear. No results given for subtests
Taylor et al., 1975	24 BP & UP 9 SCZ	Reitan Trail-Making Tests and Aphasia Screening Test	Most patients on neuroleptics	SCZ had more abnormal perfor-mance on Global Aphasia Screen Test (both dom and nondom hemisphere functioning)	Unclear
Kronfol et al., 1978	18 dep	Temporal Orien-tation; right and left hemisphere tests; Self Rating Depression Scale	NR	Nondom hemisphere functions more abnormal than dom	
Flor-Henry & Yeudall, 1979	29 BP 31 UP 54 SCZ	25 neuropsy-chological variables	1/2 of patients med-free	"Cerebral disorganization" greater in mania than depression	Depressed & manic states associated with nondom dysfunction: more pronounced in mania

274

Study	Groups	Test	Medication	Verbal > Performance	Right hemisphere impairment
Kestenbaum, 1979	13 HRC	WISC	NR		Right hemisphere impairment
Taylor et al., 1979	83 manic 22 dep 22 SCZ 99 C	Aphasia Screening Test	More SCZ drug-free than affectives at testing	Affective vs controls: ↑ total errors ($p < .0001$) ↑ dom parietal errors ($p < .025$) ↑ nondom parietal errors ($p < .0001$) Affective vs schizophrenics: ↓ total errors ($p < .05$) ↓ dom temporal/temporoparietal errors ($p < .0025$) Similar distribution of frontal, dom and nondom parietal errors	Dom and non-parietal impairment Nondom > dom impairment
Donnelly et al., 1980	35 BP 29 UP 49 NC	Halstead-Reitan Category Test	Drug free at least 1 wk	Depressed groups had significantly more errors than controls No significant BP-UP differences BP vs NC ($p < .007$), UP vs NC ($p < .07$)	Right hemisphere impairment
Savard et al., 1980	15 BP dep 11 UP dep 14 C	Halstead-Reitan Category Test	Variety of medications	% scoring in abnormal range: BPs: 87 UPs: 64 C: 36 BP vs C ($p < .001$) Older BPs had more errors than younger, remained in abnormal range even at remission and demonstrated more impairment than both SCZ and CNS cortical damage group	Right hemisphere impairment
Abrams et al., 1981	43 manic 9 endogenous dep 17 SCZ 8 OBD	WAIS	Psychotropic drugs withheld during study	Digit symbol D > M	Relative right hemisphere impairment in mania
Taylor & Abrams, 1981a	80 BP onset < 30 yr 54 BP onset > 30 yr	Aphasia Screening Test	NR	Early onset made more AST errors than late	Non-dom temporo-parietal impairment
Decina et al., 1983	31 HRC	WISC-R	NR	Verbal > Performance (≥15 points): HRC: 39% deficit Normals: 11% deficit BPI children > BPII children on verbal-performance discrepancy	Right hemisphere impairment

Continued

Table 11-13 Continued. Neuropsychological Profiles in Affective Illness

Study	Patients N	Measures	Treatment Status	Findings	Presumptive Lateralization
Flor-Henry, 1983	25 manic 28 psychotic dep 28 SCZ 24 neurotic dep	Wisconsin Card Sort, Memory for Designs, WAIS, Halstead-Reitan	NR	Psychotic dep: impaired right frontal and bilateral temporal lobe function relative to left frontal area. Manics: maximal dysfunction of the frontal areas relative to the temporo-parietal regions. Gender differences: greater lateralized dysfunction shown by manic males (dom > nondom) and psychotically dep females (nondom > dom)	Nondom hemisphere impairment in manic-depressives
Silberman et al., 1983	7 BP dep 6 UP dep 13 NC	Levene method for examining hypothesis testing in discrimination learning	All but 2, med-free	Dep: abstract and logical reasoning deficits; performed less well than NC on discrimination learning tasks. Errors: inability to reduce the set of possible solutions, and perseveration on discontinued hypotheses	Right hemisphere impairment (comparable to patients with right temporal-lobectomy)
Taylor & Abrams, 1983	30 manic 67 dep 62 SCZ	Aphasia Screening Test, Halstead-Reitan, Luria Nebraska	NR	Moderate to severe cognitive impairment: 45% of affectives 75% of SCZ	Nondominant hemisphere impairment
Deptula & Yozawitz, 1984	8 BP 20 UP 15 NC	Verbal and visual list learning tasks	NR	Recall asymmetry consistent with right hemisphere impairment, but without recognition asymmetry	Right hemisphere impairment
Brumback, 1985	61 dep children 36 C	WISC	NR	Verbal > Performance dep: 34% deficit C: 14% deficit	Right hemisphere impairment
Robertson & Taylor, 1985	18 BP (incl 2 UP manics) 6 UP 6 reactive dep 41 NC (all male prisoners)	WAIS, verbal fluency, visual attention & visual recognition tests	NR, but addicts excluded	BPs superior on verbal tasks: similarities & vocabulary subtests BPs inferior on visual/holistic tasks: embedded letter and broken figure subtests	Right hemisphere impairment
Dalby & Williams, 1986	15 BP manic 30 SCZ 28 alcoholic 21 C	WAIS-R, Wechsler Memory Scale	Some on antipsychotics	BPs: Verbal > Performance (only group to show this discrepancy)	Right hemisphere impairment

Study	Sample	Tests	Treatment status	Results	Interpretation
Sapin et al., 1987	20 BP euthymic 20 C	Face recognition tasks, WAIS: Block Design, Digit Span, Benton Visual Retention Test, Street Gestalt Completion Test	Drug-free 2 wk	No significant differences between BP and C in tasks for right or left hemisphere impairment. However, BPs relied on individual facial features for recognition whereas NCs synthesized multiple elements. On task requiring holistic synthesis of multiple stimulus elements (Gestalt) BPs made significantly more errors than NCs ($p < .00001$)	Right hemisphere impairment
Gruzelier et al., 1988	21 psychotics: (9 manic, 12 dep) 36 SCZ 29 C	Recurring Digit and Block-Span Memory Test, Spatial and Non-spatial Learning Tests, Verbal Fluency Tests	12 drug-free, NR for others	Affectives > SCZ > C: right-sided impairment SCZ > affectives > C: left-sided impairment Affectives: spatial deficits > nonspatial; depressives impaired on digit span SCZ: Active syndrome (grandiose & religious delusions, excitement, cognitive acceleration, overactivity) associated with right hemisphere impairment & integrity of left hemisphere. Withdrawn syndrome (blunted affect, poverty of speech & social withdrawal) associated with left hemisphere impairment	Right hemisphere impairment, left temporohippo-campal dysfunction implicated during depressive states
Wade et al., 1988	10 manic 30 SCZ	WAIS; Wechsler Memory Scale Subtests, Modified Wisconsin Card Sort; Shipley Abstraction Index; Verbal Fluency	NR	Only the degree of frontal-lobe dysfunction reliably discriminated SCZ from BPs; did not differ on dom & nondom hemisphere measures	Moderate bilateral cerebral dysfunction

NR = treatment status not reported, SCZ = schizophrenic, TLE = temporal lobe epileptics, HRC = high-risk children (parental history BP), C = control, NC = normal control, OBD = organic brain disease

[a]See text for evidence that a significant discrepancy between verbal and performance scores on the WAIS, where V > P, is suggestive of right hemisphere impairment.

the WAIS-R (Kestenbaum, 1979; Decina et al., 1983). This discrepancy, reflected in verbal scores that are higher than performance scores, also is found in depressed children (Brumback, 1985) and is consistent with an extensive psychometric literature that demonstrates a similar WAIS profile associated with right hemisphere damage caused by localized lesions.[27] Although there are substantive issues in the interpretation of such verbal performance discrepancies (Matarazzo, 1972), there is consistency within the high-risk studies discussed, within the WAIS studies of adults with affective illness (e.g., the early studies of Gilliland and colleagues, 1943 and Waldfogel and Guy, 1951, as well as the more recent work of Robertson and Taylor, 1985), and across the age groups. Robertson and Taylor (1985), in discussing their specific findings, also summarize the major findings in this area:

> The general picture presented by the MD group is that of men with intact, indeed superior, verbal reasoning ability and inadequate, inferior functioning on two spatially biased subtests of the visual recognition test.
>
> The consistent relationship found between spatial/holistic functioning and affective illness lends further support to the view expressed by Flor-Henry and others that disorders of mood are associated with impairment of right hemisphere functioning. A specific impairment of spatial/holistic functions was not found either in schizophrenic subgroups which were studied . . . or in the "normal" group of men. (pp. 306–309)

Sackeim and Steif (1988), in their review of the lateralization findings for mania, depression, and schizophrenia, concluded: (1) Overall impairment is greater in mania than in depression. It remains unclear whether deficits are bilateral or involve, as in depression, primarily right hemisphere dysfunction. (2) There is greater left hemisphere impairment (reflecting deficits of changes in verbal, symbolic, logical, or expressive capacities) in schizophrenia than in mania (Taylor et al., 1979, 1981; Taylor and Abrams, 1983). (3) Mania exacts a greater toll on left hemispheric functioning than does depression (Flor-Henry, 1983), consistent with other findings that euphoric mood states may affect left hemisphere functioning (Sackeim et al., 1982).

The consistency of right or nondominant hemispheric impairment in affective illness is quite apparent in the studies summarized in Table 11-13. The particular deficits in spatial learning and memory are portrayed in graphic manner in

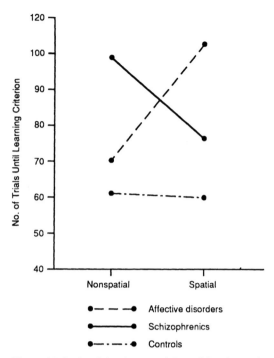

Figure 11-4. Spatial and nonspatial conditional associate learning performance (from Gruzelier et al., 1988).

Figure 11-4 (Gruzelier et al., 1988). Further evidence of an affectively linked right hemisphere deficit comes from a study by Post and colleagues (R.M. Post, personal communication, 1989), who compared 75 patients with affective illness, 56 of whom (three fourths) were bipolar, with 34 controls on an 80-item questionnaire designed to assess subjective evaluations of facility with language and music, logical–sequential vs emotional–spatial processing, and other areas thought to reflect hemispheric laterality. The only items that revealed significant differences between the groups were those assessing perceived difficulty with spatial relations: good at reading maps ($p = 0.0001$), good sense of direction ($p = 0.0045$), good sense of geography ($p = 0.0052$), trouble with street directions ($p = 0.001$), and easily lost in a strange city ($p = 0.0001$). These differences were found only in women with affective illness except for map reading, where the male patients with affective illness were also significantly more likely ($p = 0.03$) to report having difficulty. The gender-by-diagnosis interaction is clear and underscores the importance of analyzing results along this dimension. These results may tie in with another recent study that linked sex hormones to task performance, finding that spatial ability in women was significantly influenced by their menstrual cycle.[28]

The relationship between the observed neuropsychological deficits in manic-depressive illness and independent studies of neuroanatomical and neurochemical correlates is discussed in Chapter 18. As for the neuropsychological measures, there remains an enormous need for sufficiently subtle assessment procedures. When developed, particularly when used in conjunction with imaging techniques in prospective paradigms (e.g., Parks et al., 1988), such procedures should allow more solidly based interpretations to be made. Future studies of lateralization must additionally include not only more specialized attention to the cognitive processes involved in manic and mixed, as well as depressed, states but also lateralization of hallucinations, delusions, and thought disorders in bipolar patients.

SUMMARY

Thought and perception are profoundly changed in manic-depressive illness. Although there are few quantitative differences in formal thought disorder between manic and schizophrenic patients, qualitative differences do exist. Manic patients are far more likely than schizophrenics to exhibit pressured speech, flight of ideas, grandiosity, and combinatory and overinclusive thinking. In many manic patients the thought disorder continues long after the acute episode has subsided. The nature and extent of thought disorder in depression are less clear, and distinctions between bipolar and unipolar are often not considered.

Speech patterns in manic patients tend to be characterized by greater total speech, greater complexity of speech, and multiple shifts from one discourse structure to another than is demonstrated by schizophrenic patients. Compared with depressed speech, that of manic patients generally is less predictable, more colorful, more concrete, and more oriented toward action.

Hallucinations are less common than delusions in both mania and depression. When they do exist, they are associated with more severe illness. Manic hallucinations are characterized by their ecstatic and religious nature and tend to be fleeting in duration. They are qualitatively more similar to organic than schizophrenic psychoses. De-

lusions are common in mania, depression, and mixed states. Manic delusions are generally expansive, religious, grandiose, communal, and relatively less fixed than schizophrenic delusions. Depressive delusions are most frequently characterized by themes of poverty, guilt, persecution, and somatic concerns.

Recent studies indicate a greater rate of psychotic features in bipolar than in unipolar depression, but the data are as yet inconclusive. Although there are few consistent clinical or demographic differences between delusional and nondelusional unipolar depression, there is a strong tendency for the presence or absence of psychotic symptoms to be consistent across episodes.

Several general conclusions can be made about cognitive functioning in manic-depressive illness. Psychomotor speed, reaction time, and speech all are slowed in depression, and the opposite obtains for manic states. Methodological problems prevent meaningful conclusions being drawn about results of general intelligence testing in bipolar patients. Associations responses are increased during mania. Poor concentration, distractibility, and deficits in learning are characteristic of both depression and mania. One of the most consistent findings in the neuropsychological literature is right hemispheric or nondominant hemispheric impairment in affective illness. The extent to which this reflects a state or trait condition is unclear.

NOTES

1. Cited by John Rosenberg in *The Darkening Glass,* p. 151.
2. K. Botsford, cited by Ian Hamilton in *Robert Lowell,* 1982, p. 301.
3. Harrow et al., 1972a,b, 1982, 1983, 1986; Harrow and Prosen, 1978; Harrow and Quinlan, 1977.
4. Harrow et al., 1972a,b, 1986; Himmelhoch et al., 1973; Adler and Harrow, 1974; Harrow and Quinlan, 1977; Grossman et al., 1981.
5. Breakey and Goodell, 1972; Grossman et al., 1981; Andreasen, 1984; Shenton et al., 1987; Solovay et al., 1987.
6. The discrepancy between the results of these two groups may be due, in part, to differences in the assessment of thought disorder. Resnick and Oltmanns used a global rating, whereas Harrow and associates used specific tests.
7. Andreasen, 1984; Resnick and Oltmanns, 1984;

Simpson and Davis, 1985; Ragin and Oltmanns, 1987.

8. Cited by Joan Abse in *John Ruskin: The Passionate Moralist,* 1980, p.302.

9. From the diary of Clara Schumann, 1854; cited in R. Taylor's *Robert Schumann: His Life and Work.* London: Granada, 1982, p. 314.

10. From Rush, 1812, pp 151–152.

11. Jaspers, 1913; Strauss, 1969; Mullen, 1979; Kendler et al., 1983; Garety, 1985.

12. Kraepelin, 1921; Bowman and Raymond, 1931–1932a; Schneider, 1959; Beck, 1967; Winokur et al., 1969.

13. Beigel and Murphy, 1971; Winokur, 1975, 1984; Brockington et al., 1982.

14. Charney and Nelson, 1981; Frances et al., 1981; Glassman and Roose, 1981; Coryell and Tsuang, 1982; Nelson et al., 1984; Spiker et al., 1985; Roose and Glassman, 1988.

15. From a letter written in 1796 (Cowper, edited by W Benham, 1884. pp. 310–311).

16. Chapman and Chapman, 1973; Miller, 1975; Kupfer and Rush, 1983; Buchwald and Neale, 1984; Weingartner and Silberman, 1984; Johnson and Magaro, 1987; Walsh, 1987; Sackeim and Steif, 1988.

17. Franz, 1906; Wells and Kelley, 1920; Lundholm, 1922; Brower and Oppenheim, 1951; Huston and Senf, 1952; Hall and Stride, 1954; Payne and Hewlitt, 1960; Friedman, 1964; Martin and Rees, 1966; Mayo, 1966; Court, 1968; Hemsley and Philips, 1975; Bruder et al., 1980.

18. Fischer, 1949; Hall and Stride, 1954; Pichot et al.,

19. Post et al., 1977; Wehr et al., 1980, 1982; Wolff et al., 1985.

20. Kotin and Goodwin, 1972; Kupfer et al., 1974; Weiss et al., 1974; Blackburn, 1975; Dunner et al., 1976a.

21. Cronholm and Ottosson, 1961; Henry et al., 1973; Miller, 1975; Sternberg and Jarvik, 1976; Strömgren, 1977; Frith et al., 1983; Silberman et al., 1983; Mormont, 1984; Pettinati and Rosenberg, 1984; Warren and Groome, 1984.

22. Davis and Unruh, 1980; Henry et al., 1973; Koh and Wolpert, 1983; Gass and Russell, 1986.

23. Weingartner et al., 1981a; R. M. Cohen et al., 1982; Weingartner and Silberman, 1984; Sackeim and Steif, 1988.

24. Bower et al., 1981; Bower and Cohen, 1982; Bower, 1983; Ingram, 1984; Blaney, 1986; Johnson and Magaro, 1987; Sackeim and Steif, 1988.

25. Lloyd and Lishman, 1975; Teasdale and Fogarty, 1979; Clark and Teasdale, 1982; Fogarty and Hemsley, 1983; Slife et al., 1984.

26. Flor-Henry and Yeudall, 1979; Flor-Henry, 1983; Flor-Henry and Gruzelier, 1983; Leventhal and Tomarken, 1986; Sackeim and Steif, 1988.

27. Reitan, 1955; Lansdell, 1962; Blackenmore et al., 1966; Satz, 1966; Satz et al., 1967; Zimmerman et al., 1970; Simpson and Vega, 1971; Matarazzo, 1972.

28. Reported in Research News, "Sex and Violence in Neuroscience," *Science* 242:1509, 1988.

12

Personality and Interpersonal Behavior

PERSONALITY AND MANIC-DEPRESSIVE ILLNESS

He [Robert Schumann] could be extremely lively and excited, and again quite introverted, sunk in revery and apathetic, gruff, and peevish. Then again, when he woke from his dream world, he could be a perfectly fascinating heart-winner, full of the most devoted amiability.   —Franz Brendel[1]

That the individual is a system of patterned uniqueness is a fact. That science likes universals and not particulars is also a fact. Yet personality itself is a universal phenomenon though it is found only in individual forms. Since it is a universal phenomenon science must study it; but it cannot study it correctly unless it looks into the individuality of the patterning!   —Gordon Allport[2]

The subtlety and complexity of the relationship between biology and psychology are nowhere more apparent than in the study of personality and manic-depressive illness. It is daunting to try to disentangle personality characteristics from a psychologically expressed, yet constitutionally based illness. Temperament is enmeshed with perceptions, expectations, and ways of interacting with others, and mild or devastating affective illness has compounding effects on personality structure. Individual personalities are unique by most common definitions, making their assessment difficult and subject to intense controversy. The shading of normal into pathological patterns is the subject of long-standing social and academic debate. Despite a tradition in psychology of sophisticated theory and measurement in the field of personality studies, the relationship between affective illness and personality is only partially delineated.

In this chapter, we first briefly review the major psychological theories of personality and their associated methods of measurement. Our focus is on personality studies in bipolar manic-depressive illness, a focus that involves a review of direct bipolar–unipolar personality comparisons.

The study of personality and affective illness can aid in understanding the relationship between temperamental factors and personality, delineating the role of mood in personality development and expression, generating theories about the plasticity of personality, and describing the relationships between clinical states and personality traits. It can also contribute to developing more subtle and accurate differential diagnostic techniques (especially between personality disorders and manic-depressive illness; see Chapters 4 and 5), clarifying the impact of personality structure on the clinical presentation of symptoms, and identifying personality predictors of treatment responsiveness and compliance.[3]

Conceptual Issues

Personality, Character, and Temperament
Defining words and concepts, such as personality, character, and temperament, is difficult but

necessary. In common usage, personality generally refers to the unique aspects of an individual,
especially those most distinctive or likely to be
noticed by others in social interactions. Allport
(1961) wrote simply that personality is "what a
person 'really is,'" (p. 35) his or her most typical
and deeply characteristic features. Psychological
definitions of personality are as many as the theorists writing. Hall and Lindzey (1970) summarized them succinctly as focusing on one or more
of the following facets: "the individual's social
stimulus value; the integrative or organizational
function of personality; an individual's general
adjustment; the unique or individual aspects of
behavior; and the essence of man" (p. 8). Hall and
Lindzey, like most personality researchers, end
by defining personality empirically—namely,
personality is that which is measured by tools of
assessment used within a particular conceptual
framework. This pragmatic definition underlies
our discussions of personality and affective disorder.

Character has been defined as "personality
evaluated"— that aspect of an individual bearing
a moral stamp. Allport (1961) has observed that
whereas *personality* derives from the Latin word
for "mask," *character* derives from the Greek for
"engraving," "the mark of a man—his pattern of
traits or his life-style" (p. 31). Character is less
frequently used in the United States as a concept
than it is in Europe, although the terms often are
used interchangeably.

Temperament has always been viewed as having a more constitutional, genetic, and biological
basis than has either personality or character.
Hippocrates and Galen, for example, based their
theories of temperament on the four humors of the
body. The relationship of personality to temperament is, of course, of considerable theoretical and
clinical interest in personality and mood disorders. Allport (1961) described temperament as a
"class of 'raw material' from which personality is
fashioned" and wrote that temperament was:

. . . the "internal weather" in which personality
evolves. The more anchored a disposition is in native
constitutional soil the more likely it is to be spoken of
as temperament. . . .
    Temperament refers to the characteristic phenomena
of an individual's emotional nature, including his susceptibility to emotional stimulation, his customary
strength and speed of response, the quality of his prevailing mood, and all peculiarities of fluctuation and
intensity in mood, these phenomena being regarded as

dependent upon constitutional make-up, and therefore
largely hereditary in nature. (pp. 33-34)

Except where otherwise indicated, our discussion of personality and temperament will assume,
in addition to our earlier operational definition, a
broad definition of personality, one encompassing temperamental endowment as well as learned
or acquired components of behavior, attitudes,
and values.

Conceptual Differences in Theories of Personality

This chapter focuses on empirical studies of personality, emphasizing results from psychometric
investigations. However, many different assumptions underlie major theories of personality,
and some theories lend themselves more readily
to empirical research than others.[4] Of particular
importance in any discussion of personality and
affective illness are assumptions about the stability of personality structure over time and circumstance and the relative importance of genetic
factors in determining behavior.

Relationship of Personality to Affective Disorders

Klerman (1973), Hirschfeld and Klerman (1979),
and Akiskal and colleagues (1983a) have outlined
the complicated relationship and interactions between personality and affective illness. From
their work and that of others, four major interactional hypotheses have been formulated:

1. *Personality as predispositional to affective illness.* This hypothesis assumes that personality patterns precede and, therefore, predispose an individual to develop affective
   illness. This view, fundamental to psychoanalytical thought and writing, also is reflected to
   varying degrees in the writings of cognitive
   and behavioral psychologists.
2. *Personality as an expression of affective illness.* Personality patterns are viewed as manifestations of mild to moderate forms of the
   underlying affective illness. The individual's
   temperament is assumed to be intricately
   bound up with the genetic predisposition to
   mania and depression. This view, integral to
   the work of Kraepelin and Kretschmer, is
   shared, in part, by most of the modern researchers who posit a continuum of affective
   states.

3. *Personality as a modifier of affective illness.*
Chodoff (1972), Klerman (1973), and Von Zerssen (1977) have emphasized the role of personality in determining the clinical presentation of affective symptom patterns (especially in obsessive, dependent, or hysterical personality types), response to psychotherapy and medication, and adherence to prescribed treatment regimens. They also view personality as an important determinant of the nature and extent of interpersonal relationships. These, in turn, can affect both precipitating events and the likelihood of emotional support during affective episodes. The ability to handle the enormous stress and complications of affective illness is assumed to be strongly affected by premorbid personality and character structure.

4. *Personality as altered by affective illness.* In this frame of reference, personality is assumed to be altered by the experience of affective illness. Changes in self-esteem, social interaction patterns, ability to sustain meaningful relationships and employment, and frequent fluctuations in moods, energy, perceptions, and thinking are all thought to cause and reflect short-term or long-term personality changes that can be reversible or irreversible. The obvious importance and impact on personality of such illness variables as frequency, duration, severity, and nature of episodes have not been well studied.

Methodological Issues

In addition to the conceptual issues raised previously, many specific methodological problems are intrinsic to the study of personality and manic-depressive illness. Most central is the problem of *trait and state,* or disentangling manifestations of illness from the more stable and lasting structures of personality. Specific problems include the substantial difficulty of separating the current clinical state from measured personality traits. Assessing the effects of medications on personality (independent of their effects on the underlying affective illness), sorting through the personality effects of previous manic and depressive episodes, and delineating the effects of subclinical episodes on personality are also problems.

Fundamental issues of measurement and philosophy emerge when the pivotal question is posed: What aspects of personality are being studied when assessing the successfully treated manic-depressive—true premorbid ones or affectively changed and attenuated ones? To what extent is personality a function of medication level or a function of the cumulative effects of disease? These issues are discussed in a later section.

Another set of problems concerns issues of *diagnostic and illness heterogeneity.* Heterogeneity is well recognized in the unipolar depressive disorders (in symptom patterns, etiology, severity, episodic patterning, and frequency). Although bipolar illness is more homogeneous, it too can be confusingly varied. Few investigations of personality distinguish between bipolar I and bipolar II, and fewer still consider other issues related to the wide spectrum of bipolarity, such as the stage or severity of depressive and manic illness at the time of testing, the ratio of manic to depressive episodes, the age of illness onset, the frequency and nature of mixed states, the duration and patterning of episodes, and the characteristic nature of the manic episodes (euphoric and expansive, e.g., rather than paranoid and destructive). All of these variables are likely to have both long-term and short-term effects on the expression of personality.

Other variables generally not controlled for in personality studies of affective illness include seasonal factors of importance to studies done both during remission and illness, the competence and sophistication of clinical care, including such common problems as prescribing wrong drug dosages or the incorrect medication, and selection factors intrinsic to the nature of remission studies, that is, a selection bias favoring healthier, more normal manic-depressive patients.

Measurement and design also are problematic. Until recently, comparison groups were inadequate. Early studies compared manic-depressive with schizophrenic patients; more recent ones have used unipolar depressed patients. Studies of subjects from the general population as controls, although a clear improvement, too often have not controlled for important demographic variables, such as age, intelligence, socioeconomic status, and sex. Standard problems of measurement, such as the reliability and validity of the psychometric tests used, are well reviewed elsewhere.[5]

Several study designs have been used to investigate personality and manic-depressive illness, including studies of patients across different mood states. In addition, comparisons have been made between affectively ill bipolar and unipolar patients, remitted bipolar and unipolar patients, and remitted bipolar patients and members of the general population. These design strategies are more fully discussed in later sections.

Personality Assessment

Many types of assessment techniques have been developed to measure both the universals and particulars of personality, including detailed studies of single individuals through their writings, video and audio recordings of speech and behavior, and open-ended questionnaires. Self-ratings and ob server ratings of personality traits, values, attitudes, and behaviors have been used extensively, as have social psychological measures of group affiliations, status, and perceived roles. Projective tests, such as the Rorschach, Sentence Completion Test, and the Thematic Apperception Test, also have been used to study personality in general and patients with mood disorders in particular.

Most extensively developed and used, especially in investigations of unipolar and bipolar affective illness, are assessment techniques rooted in the psychometric tradition that emphasizes measurement of individual and group differences. These include tests developed to measure a single or a few traits (e.g., the Eysenck Personality Inventory[6]) or multidimensional scales to measure several or many traits, such as the Minnesota Multiphasic Personality Inventory (MMPI), the Guilford-Zimmerman Temperament Scale (GZTS), the California Psychological Inventory (CPI), the 16 Personality Factor Inventory (16PF), or the Comrey Personality Scales (CPS). Most of our discussion will focus on studies using the various psychometric techniques.

Descriptive Studies

Clinical Typologies

As reviewed in Chapter 2, clinical investigators in the early part of this century assumed that personality structure in manic-depressive illness reflected the underlying disease process.[7]

Psychoanalytic Perspectives

Psychoanalytic theorists considered two major issues in their writings on manic-depressive illness: the etiology of mania and depression and the un derlying personality structure of patients with bipolar illness. Most psychoanalysts primarily discussed the origins and nature of depression rather than mania. Their formulations on this subject are well known and are not presented here. Instead, we briefly outline psychoanalytic concepts of mania and the manic-depressive personality. Although neither time nor research has supported the psychoanalytic perspective on bipolar affective illness, it is historically important, especially in the United States, because it deeply influenced generations of psychiatrists, psychologists, and social workers.

From a psychoanalytic perspective, mania can best be understood as a defense against underlying depressive affect. This fundamental concept has been stated in different ways by many authors.[8] Although interesting, the psychoanalytic perspectives suffer from the usual difficulties of interpreting open-ended, clinical observations: They are retrospective, interpretative, and speculative. Comparison groups are lacking, and there are few, if any, ways of subjecting the theory to test. Finally, as Kotin and Goodwin concluded in 1972 from their data-based studies of mania:

Our data suggest that if mania is a defense against depression, it is often an inadequate defense, since depressive symptoms remain prominent during the manic phase. (p. 684)

The manic-depressive personality was viewed by the psychoanalysts as narcissistic (Freud, 1917; Fenichel, 1945), masochistic (Gerö, 1936; Jacobson, 1953; Garma, 1968), extraverted (Dooley, 1921; Stone, 1978; Wilson, 1951; Arieti, 1959), and highly conventional (Arieti, 1959; Cohen et al., 1954; Gibson et al., 1959; Smith, 1960). Rado (1928) discussed at length the belief that manic-depressive individuals have an "obsessive need for the approval of others."[9]

Alexander (1948) described the manic-depressive personality as warm, outgoing, and practical, a person who prefers the concrete to the abstract. Not surprisingly, he noted a tendency for the emotions to rule reason. English (1949) characterized the manic-depressive person as perfectionist, egocentric, logical, wise, talented, afraid to hate (except when manic), and rigid. Dooley (1921), Wilson (1951), and Cohen and colleagues (1954) highlighted somewhat different constellations of traits and the problems they pose for the therapist and others.[10]

PERSONALITY STUDIES DURING OR ACROSS AFFECTIVE EPISODES

Bipolar–Unipolar Differences During Depression

Donnelly and colleagues examined numerous bipolar–unipolar personality differences during acute depression. In their first study, Donnelly and Murphy (1973) compared 30 bipolar patients with 29 unipolar patients on the MMPI, Barron's Ego Strength Scale, Edward's Social Desirability Scale, and Gough's Social Status Scale. Bipolar patients were significantly less depressed and introverted and scored significantly higher on the ego-strength, social-desirability, and social-status scales. Scores on the MMPI depression scale and the social desirability scale were highly correlated in the bipolar ($r = -0.65$) but not the unipolar ($r = 0.07$) groups. The authors concluded that the tendency of the bipolar patients to endorse socially desirable items, rather than real differences between the groups, accounted for the greater degree of psychopathology reported by depressed unipolar patients.

Donnelly and colleagues (1975) also looked at Rorschach differences in drug-free, hospitalized bipolar and unipolar patients. The perceptual approach of their unipolar patients was at a "higher development level of differentiation and integration" than was the more "global approach" of the bipolar patients. The relative lack of attention to formal detail on the inkblots, coupled with the more amorphous percepts in the bipolar protocols, seemed to indicate less neurotic involvement, anxiety, and depressive content in the bipolar group. Based on Rorschach's original assumption of an association between color-reactive percepts and impulsive emotional discharge and on the finding that the bipolar patients had responded and referred to primary colors more frequently than had the unipolar patients, Donnelly and associates (1975) concluded:

The results of the present study suggest that the color-reactive response style of the bipolar group underscores the potential for manic (impulsive) behavior in the midst of a depressive episode. These data support biologic and pharmacologic evidence that mania and depression, although representative of "opposite" poles on a continuum, cannot be considered "opposite" states in all instances. It should also be noted that the unipolar-bipolar differential represents a dimension and not a dichotomy. (p. 1131)

Finally, Donnelly and co-workers (1978b) compared 29 acutely depressed hospitalized bipolar patients with 21 acutely depressed hospitalized unipolar patients on the IPAT Anxiety Scale. Bipolar patients showed significantly less covert and overt anxiety than unipolar patients, but their scores were still higher than normal.

In summary, bipolar and unipolar patients, when acutely depressed, showed several significant differences in personality functioning. Bipolar patients showed a greater social desirability response set, less neuroticism, less impulse control, and less anxiety than unipolar patients. These differences are summarized in Table 12-1.

Comparisons of Mania with Depression

Studies contrasting personality functioning during depressive and manic[11] or hypomanic states often—and not surprisingly—reveal dramatic differences. These differences have been examined, for the most part, through projective techniques such as the Rorschach, the Thematic Apperception Test (TAT), the Semantic Differential, and paintings or drawings obtained during art therapy sessions.

Consider, for example, the responses of a 25-year-old male patient to the blank card from the TAT when he was asked to construct a story about what is happening on the card. This third-generation manic-depressive patient, who had been repeatedly hospitalized for both manic and depressive episodes, responded during both types of episodes. His manic response is characterized by loose associations, paranoid overtones, overt thought disorder, and dysphoria:

It's really clear, except for some spots. There are lots of germs, that's why I'm not holding it close to my face. It would look better with some color. There is an absence of all color except there are bits of color. I identified with the hero, afraid of germs. Color of lithium. Shapes of butterflies. Lots of symmetry, counterparts. Candy-colored bullshit. I feel like I'm being held involuntarily in a fog, don't see much blue. Don't see any flowers. A guy sees a bunch of black guys and weirdos, he follows the man and they find a civilization, walking like robots until they find it. They escape, find a lot of secrets about the trap. They have a run-in with the police, find a guy who looks like God who is arrested for having sex with his wife, who should have been having a test-tube baby. There is a lot of electrocardiac shock in the fog, a lot of homosexuals

Table 12-1. Bipolar – Unipolar Personality Differences During Acute Depressive Episodes

Study	Psychological Measure	Higher Mean Score
Donnelly & Murphy, 1973	MMPI	
	Depression	UP
	Social Introversion	UP
	Barron's Ego Strength Scale	BP
	Edward's Social Desirability Scale	BP
	Gough's Social Status Scale	BP
Blackburn, 1974	Hostility and Direction of Hostility Questionnaire	
	Intropunitiveness	BP=UP
	Extrapunitiveness	UP
Donnelly & Murphy, 1974	MMPI	
	Mania	BP
	Psychasthenia	UP
Donnelly et al., 1975	Rorschach	
	Primary color responses	BP
	Frequency of color responses	BP
Donnelly et al., 1978b	IPAT Anxiety Scale	
	Overt anxiety	UP
	Covert anxiety	UP

and green and gray people who travelled through fog into an insane asylum. They emerged out into the world and found the sun for the first time in a hundred years.

The depressed response to the same blank card is characterized by relative brevity, self-doubt, a well-formed and original story, lack of thought disorder, and a depressive ending:

"The Fog." I don't get it. Anything. This is the view to a flier pilot in World War I as he's been assigned to go over Heidelberg, Germany, and shot from his plane. He's in the middle of a cloud seeing nothing but whiteness and fear. Fears he won't be successful and in fact he wasn't successful. He was shot down a little less than one hour after he began his mission. End of story.

Owen and Nurcombe (1970) reported on the different profiles shown on the Semantic Differential Test by a 14- year-old girl when hypomanic and when depressed. The test was administered once during hypomania and twice during depression. The two profiles obtained during depression were identical. Figure 12-1 shows the comparison of manic and depressive profiles. There was a greater variability in the portrayal of others during mania than during depression; conversely the portrayal of the self was less variable when manic than when depressed. In addition, the self was portrayed more positively and others more negatively during mania than during depression.

In 1970 Wadeson and Bunney carried out the first systematic, blind study of spontaneous art productions in manic-depressive illness. Nineteen pictures were obtained from one rapid-cycling patient, a woman who alternated every 24 hours between mania and depression. The seven independent judges rated each picture as manic or depressed and distinguished between the two states at a statistically significant level. The patient's depressive drawings centered on prisons, cages, tombs, and coffins, whereas manic themes were characterized by the images of bursting out. Depressive symbols tended to be concentrically organized forms within forms, and manic symbols often were spirals with much motion.

Wadeson and Bunney also found that manic drawings were more likely to be vivid, full of motion and bold lines, busy, confused, and characterized by anger, sensuousness, wildness, and ebullience. Depressed drawings were pale, tentative, static, tight, and characterized by listlessness, hopelessness, emptiness, less affect, and a sense of being trapped or enclosed.

Rorschach findings consistently demonstrate that manic patients show more color, whole, and texture responses than do depressed patients.[12] This is usually interpreted as reflecting a greater degree of affect, especially outwardly expressed

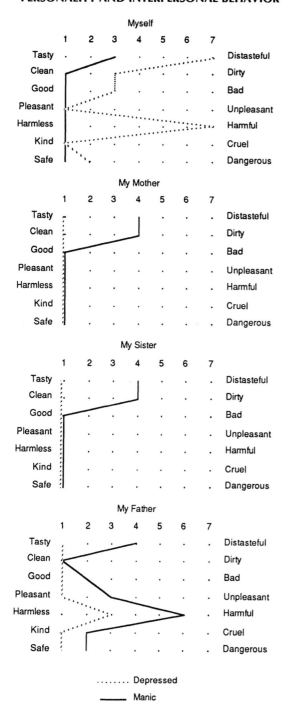

Figure 12-1. Personal constructs on the semantic differential in a 14-year-old girl when depressed and when manic (from Owen and Nurcombe, 1970).

affect, during the manic phase. Differences in human movement responses are less consistently shown between depressed and manic patients.

A number of studies have revealed that artistic productions during mania and depression generally are quite different. Major differences in expression are summarized in Table 12-2. Colors used during mania tend to be brighter, warmer, and more vivid than the somber, darker tones used during depression. The content of manic art is often sexual and full of joie de vivre, whereas depressive art usually reflects a poverty of ideas and decaying, fearful, hopeless imagery. The greater impulsiveness and overall production of art work during mania has been contrasted with the sparser, more sterile productions of depressed patients.

Although these manic and depressive differences have been reported in almost all studies of art production in affectively ill patients, Wadeson and Carpenter (1976), in a large study of 104 affectively ill and 62 schizophrenic patients, found considerable variability within diagnostic groups and overlap between groups. They did not find, for example, that manic drawings differentiated out as a group, although they did find significant age differences. The younger unipolar and bipolar patients demonstrated "more colorful, more full, more formed, and more developed" drawings (p. 337) than did the older affective psychotic patients.

Comparisons of Mania and Bipolar Depression with the Remitted State

Mania and Remitted State. In 1974, Blackburn found that actively manic patients scored significantly higher than those in a recovered group on extrapunitive but not intropunitive measures from the Hostility and Direction of Hostility Questionnaire. Their response pattern appeared to be state-dependent; it reverted to normal levels as the manic symptomatology cleared. Manic patients, according to Blackburn, are the only diagnostic group (other than "selected paranoids") to show a predominance of extrapunitiveness over intropunitiveness and the only group in which the level of extrapunitiveness changes significantly with recovery. Levels of intropunitiveness, on the other hand, tend to fluctuate with illness and across diagnoses.

Price and O'Kearney (1982), studying 30 bipo-

Table 12-2. Artistic Expression During Mania and Depression

	Mania	Depression
Color	Vivid, hot, sharply contrasting (Zimmerman and Garfinckle, 1942); wild (Reitman, 1950); highly colored, without the time to use a variety of colors (Dax, 1953); vivid (Plokker, 1965); bright, warm, optimistic (Enâchescu, 1971); color did not differentiate manics as a diagnostic group (Wadeson & Carpenter, 1976)	Somber (Reitman, 1950); somber, usually black with upper portion darkest (Dax, 1953); dark colors, upper portion of picture generally darker than lower, lightening of palette as depression begins to clear (Plokker, 1965); dark, dirty, cold, somber (Enâchescu, 1971); bipolar more colorful than unipolar (Wadeson & Carpenter, 1976)
Content	Sexual, setting sun, orifices (Zimmerman & Garfinckle, 1942); often obscene (Dax, 1953); flowers, landscapes, sunrises, fires, waterfalls, animals, people, dance scenes (Enâchescu, 1971)	Poverty of ideas (Reitman, 1950); immobile figures with sunken heads, signs of death, starless nights rather than days, trees broken off, no flowers (Dax, 1953); representations of delusions (sin, poverty, hypochondriasis), torture, suicide (Plokker, 1965); mourning scenes, physical or moral disaster, abandonment, physical decompensation (Enâchescu, 1971)
Affect	Positive, assured (Zimmerman and Garfinckle, 1942); excitement (Reitman, 1950); careless (Dax, 1953); euphoric (Enâchescu, 1971)	Useless, depressive, cold, gloomy (Enâchescu, 1971)
Form and Activity	Extreme agitation, productive, fluid composition, swirl-like forms (Zimmerman and Garfinckle, 1942); restless, disordered, incoherent lines (Reitman, 1950); rapidly produced, lacking in restraint (Dax, 1953); deterioration in composition (Plokker, 1965); rapid and expansive, far more productive than in depressed phase; lines are rash, thick, and crossed (Enâchescu, 1971)	Bareness and lack of detail (Dax, 1953); rarely engaged in artistic activity (Plokker, 1965); less creative activity (Enâchescu, 1971)

lar patients, found, as had Blackburn, that scores on the Hostility and Direction of Hostility Questionnaire were significantly higher during hypomania than on recovery; especially changed were the extrapunitive aspects of hostility. This reflected the tendency for patients, when hypomanic, to be more critical of others and to have a higher level of paranoid hostility. In addition, individuals differed markedly in patterns and degree of hostility during the hypomanic episodes.

Bipolar Depression and Remitted State. Several studies have examined changes in personality profiles between depressed and recovered bipolar patients (Table 12-3). Scores on the neuroticism scale of the Maudsley Personality Inventory (MPI) decreased from depression to recovery in all three studies using the MPI (Perris, 1971; Liebowitz et al., 1979; Hirschfeld et al., 1983).

Extraversion scores, in contrast, increased at recovery in the first and third study and were unchanged in the second. Blackburn (1974) found that intropunitiveness scores significantly decreased on recovery from depression ($p < 0.01$) but that extrapunitiveness scores remained the same.

Donnelly and colleagues (1976) compared MMPI profiles on admission and at recovery in bipolar depressed patients (Figure 12-2). The t-scores for the depression, paranoia, and schizophrenia scales decreased with recovery but remained above 60 at remission for both the psychopathic deviate (Pd) and mania (Ma) scales. The authors interpreted the relatively normal profile of bipolar depressed patients as reflecting either less psychopathology in the bipolar group or "successful denial of conflict by activity or by other-directed behavior often attributed to manic-

Table 12-3. Test-Retest Personality Differences in Depressed and Recovered Bipolar Patients

Study	Psychological Test	Direction of Change on Recovery
Perris, 1971[a]	Maudsley Personality Inventory	↑ Extraversion (E), ↑ E/N ratio, ↓ Neuroticism (N)
Blackburn, 1974	Hostility and Direction of Hostility Questionnaire	↓ Intropunitiveness, [NS]Extrapunitiveness
Donnelly et al., 1976	MMPI[b]	↓ Depression (scale 2),↓ Paranoia (scale 6), ↓ Schizophrenia (scale 8)
Liebowitz et al., 1979[a,c]	Maudsley Personality Inventory	↓ Neuroticism, ↓ Extraversion
Hirschfeld et al., 1983[a]	Items from GZTS, Interpersonal Dependency Inventory, Lazare-Klerman-Armor Personality Inventory, Maudsley Personality Inventory, MMPI (2 subscales)	↓ Neuroticism, ↓ Interpersonal Dependency, ↑ Emotional Strength, ↑ Extraversion, [NS]Rigidity, [NS]Level of activity, [NS]Obsessionality, [NS]Impulsivity

[a] Bipolar and unipolar patients combined
[b] Scales 4 (Psychopathic Deviate) and 9 (Mania) both remained at t-scores above 60
[c] Patients euthymic at index, depressed at follow-up

depressive patients" (p. 236). This interpretation is problematic, however, because the protocols of patients with t-scores above 80 on the F scale, a measure of validity, were eliminated from the sample. The authors interpreted the continuity of elevated Pd and Ma scores from depression to recovery as a phase-independent lack of impulse control. This is consistent with the findings of Hirschfeld and co-workers (1983), who found, in their combined sample of bipolar and unipolar

Figure 12-2. Comparison of admission and remission profiles in bipolar depressed patients (adapted from Donnelly et al., 1976).

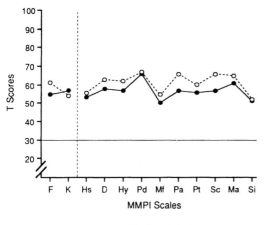

patients, that impulsivity scores were unchanged from depression to remission. Hirschfeld and colleagues also found no state-dependent changes in measures of rigidity, obsessionality, restraint, reflectiveness, demandingness, and dominance. They also found no state-dependent changes in level of activity, a surprising finding that may reflect similar psychomotor activity patterns during depression in both unipolar and bipolar patients (canceling out their usual differences). They did find, however, that patients, when recovered from their depressions, scored lower on measures of emotional lability, neuroticism, passivity, hypersensitivity, and interpersonal dependency while scoring higher on measures of emotional strength, resiliency, and extraversion. For a subgroup of patients who had not recovered from depression at the time of follow-up, scores on the personality tests did not change, giving credence to the authors' interpretation that "the changes recorded for the recovered patients reflect the influence of the depressed state" (p. 698).

Mania, Bipolar Depression, and Remitted State. A few studies have looked at personality profiles across all three major affective states: mania, depression, and euthymia. Lumry and colleagues (1982) administered the MMPI to 22

bipolar-I patients. All had family histories of severe psychiatric disorder and personal histories of
multiple affective episodes, and all but 1 were
stabilized on lithium. The MMPI profiles obtained from 12 patients when manic or hypomanic and from 10 depressed patients (5 patients
overlapped the manic/hypomanic group) were
classic manic and depressive profiles. The mean
profile for the 12 euthymic patients was entirely
within normal limits. The mean MMPI profiles
obtained during hypomania or mania and depression are shown graphically in Figure 12-3. The
authors concluded that the normal profile pattern
obtained during euthymia in most of their
lithium-stabilized patients indicated "complete
restitution of normality."

In a 1982 study of 10 manic and 20 depressive
patients, Ashworth and co-workers used the repertory grid to assess state-related changes in self-
esteem. Grids obtained from the depressed patients were characterized by low self-esteem and
those from the manic group by high self-esteem.
Most of the original patient sample (16 depressive
and 9 manic patients) were then retested on recovery (Ashworth et al., 1985). Self-esteem appeared to be clearly state dependent. It markedly
increased in the recovered depressed patients and
decreased in the recovered manic ones. The recovered groups did not differ significantly from
one another or from the nonpsychiatric control
group.

Figure 12-3. Mean MMPI profiles of bipolar probands during a hypomanic/manic phase ($n = 12$) and
during a depressive phase ($n = 10$); 5 cases overlap
(adapted from Lumry et al., 1982).

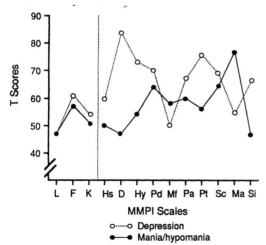

Perceptions of Self Across Affective States

Widely discrepant views of the self emerge during mania, depression, and normal functioning.
Indeed, these differences in self-perception have
been incorporated into the DSM-III-R diagnostic
criteria for both mania and depression ("inflated
self-esteem or grandiosity" and "feelings of
worthlessness or excessive or inappropriate
guilt," respectively). Platman and co-workers
(1969), in an attempt to study alternating views of
the self in depression and mania, administered the
Emotions Profile Index weekly to 11 bipolar patients. This psychological measure was designed
to assess eight primary emotions: fear, anger, acceptance, rejection, surprise, exploration, joy,
and deprivation. Twelve staff members were
asked to give their conceptions of mania and depression. This collective profile was then compared with profiles actually produced by patients
while manic or depressed. The staff's and patients' conceptions of depression were strikingly
similar on all eight dimensions. For both groups,
depression was characterized by decreases in sociability, interest in new experiences, and feelings of acceptance, as well as by increases in
feelings of deprivation, aggression, and rejection
of others. Mania, on the other hand, was perceived in very different ways by staff and patients, with seven of eight mean scores showing
differences at the $p < 0.01$ level. Patients while
manic saw themselves as sociable, trusting, moderately impulsive, and cautious and not at all
stubborn or aggressive. Staff members, however,
saw them as only moderately sociable, somewhat
distrustful, extremely impulsive and aggressive,
quite rejecting of others, and completely incau-
tious and unafraid. Response patterns from patients were far more variable than those from staff
members, suggesting a more stereotypic view
from the latter group.

Patients were asked, when normal, to recall
their previous manic and depressive episodes.
Their recalled depressive profile was similar to
that produced while actually depressed, and both
resembled the staff-generated depressive profile.
By contrast, profiles of recalled manic episodes
did not resemble those actually obtained during
mania. The patients' recall of mania was far more
highly correlated with staff perceptions of mania
($r = 0.95$) than with their own ratings produced
while manic ($r = 0.35$). The authors concluded:

These facts imply that the self-critical judgmental process is severely impaired in the manic state but not in the depressed state. This is consistent with the well-known fact that manic patients do not usually admit to any illness, or that they deny the maladaptive nature of their behavior. This is also why it is difficult to detect the presence of manic states by means of self-description type inventories; these usually show that the manic patient is normal.

One interesting theoretical question posed by these findings is whether the manic patient is deliberately misrepresenting his feelings and behavior, or whether he is simply unable to discriminate the specific feelings and behaviors which are judged by an outside observer as pathognomonic of mania. (Platman et al., 1969, p. 213)

In a subsequent study, Plutchik and colleagues (1970a) asked 14 euthymic bipolar patients, 16 staff members, and 52 college students to complete the Plutchik Emotions Profile Index as if describing their normal self, ideal self, and least-liked self. All three groups viewed their ideal self as a person who is "unusually sociable, friendly, accepting and trusting, unaggressive, not at all depressed or sad, moderately cautious, but usually interested in having new experiences" (p. 402). The three groups also agreed on their least-liked self: an individual with "almost no social involvements, does not trust or like other people; is extremely aggressive, hostile, rejecting; severely depressed and gloomy; not cautious or anxious; and not at all interested in having new experiences" (p. 402). The authors pointed out the striking similarities between the clinical description of depression given by patients and staff in the earlier study and the profile of the least-liked self obtained in the current investigation. They also note:

The changes that occur in the manic state, however, are like neither the ideal self nor the worst self. Instead, there is a unique constellation of traits characterized by moderate sociability, extremely high impulsivity,

Figure 12-4. Perceptions of self as a function of affective state (from Jamison et al., unpublished data).

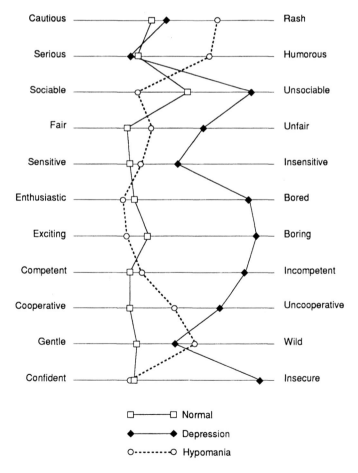

moderate aggression, and low anxiety. This profile is not a simple mirror-image of the depression profile. As the patient describes himself, the depression profile is much more socially undesirable than the manic one. (Plutchik et al., 1970a, pp. 404-405)

Jamison and colleagues (unpublished data) examined self-perceptions across affective states in 69 euthymic bipolar patients, using the Semantic Differential, a combination of associational and scaling procedures. Patients were tested with 22 pairs of opposite adjectives (e.g., good–bad, strong–weak, complex–simple) shown as the polar ends of a 7-point continuum. Patients indicated their perceptions of themselves when manic, hypomanic, depressed, and normal by marking the most descriptive point between each polar pair. Analyses of variance, with repeated measures of sex and phase, were performed on the adjective pairs. The phase of illness affected all pairs except masculinity–femininity, indicating that changes in self-perception across the affective states of bipolar illness were consistent and widespread (Figure 12-4).

Newman-Keuls comparisons, conducted to identify significant differences between each two phases, revealed a number of consistent patterns, particularly for the adjective pairs reflecting a positive–negative, or valuative, dimension. On all of these dimensions self-perceptions in the depressed phase were significantly more negative than in the other phases ($p < 0.01$ on all dimensions). More interesting, on all except two dimensions (exciting–boring and active–passive), the ratings for the hypomanic phases did not significantly differ from the ratings for the euthymic phase. Compared with men, women rated themselves overall as less active and as more "cold" and "boring" during the depressed phase, and more "exciting" and "warm" during the manic phase. Women also perceived themselves as overall more changeable than did the men ($p < 0.02$).

Men's and women's perceptions of their masculinity–femininity in various phases of illness are presented in Figure 12-5. Women felt less feminine and men less masculine in the depressed phase than in the euthymic phase; the opposite was true for the hypomanic and manic phases. In other words, depression had a neuterizing effect and hypomania or mania had a polarizing or enhancing effect on sexual identity.

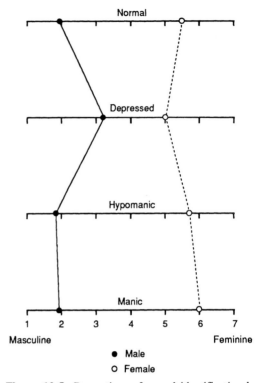

Figure 12-5. Perceptions of sexual identification by affective state: Sex differences (from Jamison et al., unpublished data). Affective state × sex; ANOVA F = 16.2; $p < .001$.

Throughout their bipolar cycles, patients underwent not only mood swings but also substantial changes in their perception of self, self-esteem, energy expenditure, interpersonal conduct, and sexual identity. The study revealed that, as expected, bipolar patients had high self-esteem in the hypomanic phase and low self-esteem in the depressive phase. Of more interest, self-esteem in the euthymic state did not substantially differ from that in the hypomanic phases. That is, bipolar patients generally held themselves in high regard; their apparently low self-esteem during the depressive phase was encapsulated, without long-term adverse effects. Interpersonal conduct was perceived by patients to be less socially desirable in the hypomanic phase than during euthymia. Such findings are especially revealing in light of the common conception that bipolar patients are outgoing and socially engaging during their highs, suggesting that patients may have some insight into the one-sidedness of their social engagement in the manic and hypomanic phases.

PERSONALITY STUDIES DURING REMISSION

Comparisons of Remitted Bipolar Patients with Normal Groups

Two major dimensions of personality—extraversion and neuroticism—have been compared in remitted bipolar patients and normal groups. The findings from studies of these two dimensions, and of several others less often investigated, are summarized in Tables 12-4 and 12-5.

Extraversion–Introversion

The primary psychological measure of extraversion used in affective illness research has been the Maudsley Personality Inventory (MPI) (later known as the Eysenck Personality Inventory). Extraversion is characterized by a "dual nature": impulsivity (typi-

cal item: "Are you inclined to be quick and sure in your actions?") and, sociability (typical item: "Would you be very unhappy if you were prevented from making numerous social contacts?"). In normal populations, impulsivity and sociability correlate 0.5, producing a second-order factor of extraversion. Introversion can be further subdivided into social introversion (characteristic of people who prefer not to have much social contact with others) and neurotic introversion (characteristic of people who are afraid to have contact with others and are basically unsure of themselves and their interpersonal competence) (Eysenck, 1956).

The authors of the Maudsley/Eysenck Personality Inventories (MPI/EPI) (Eysenck, 1959; Eysenck and Eysenck, 1963a,b) described a typical extravert as one who is:

. . . sociable, likes parties, has many friends, needs to have people to talk to . . . craves excitement, takes

Table 12-4. Neuroticism in Remitted Bipolar Patients and Normal Groups

Study	Patients N	Psychological Measure	Neuroticism Greater In
Frey, 1977	45 BP ND	AUPI (based on Maudsley Personality Inventory)	NS
Hirschfeld & Klerman, 1979	24 BP PN	Maudsley Personality Inventory	NS
Liebowitz et al., 1979	71 BP[a] 13 C	Maudsley Personality Inventory	NS
Bech et al., 1980	23 BP PN	Eysenck Personality Inventory	NS
Ashworth et al., 1982	9 BP NC	Repertory grid: Self-Esteem	NS
Matussek & Feil, 1983	19 BP 44 NC	Autodestructive-Neurotic Tendencies	BP
Winters & Neale, 1985	16 BP 16 NC	Self-Report Inventory: Self-Esteem	NS
Hirschfeld, 1985	31 BP (F) ND	Maudsley Personality Inventory	NS
Hirschfeld et al., 1986	45 BP (F) 463 NIR	Maudsley Personality Inventory Guilford-Zimmerman Temperament Survey (Emotional Stability)	BP BP
Jamison et al., unpublished	35 BP PN	Eysenck Personality Inventory	NS

ND = normative data, PN = published norms, C = control, NC = normal control, F = female, NIR = never-ill relatives

[a]Patients instructed to report what they are like when well

Table 12-5. Extraversion-Introversion in Remitted Bipolar Patients and Normal Groups

Study	Patients N	Psychological Measure	Extraversion Greater In
Frey, 1977	45 BP ND	AUPI (based on Maudsley Personality Inventory)	NS
Hirschfeld & Klerman, 1979	24 BP PN	Maudsley Personality Inventory	NS
Liebowitz et al., 1979	71 BP[a] 13 C	Maudsley Personality Inventory	NS
Bech et al., 1980	23 BP PN	Eysenck Personality Inventory	NS
Hirschfeld, 1985	31 BP (F) ND	Maudsley Personality Inventory	ND, PN or C
Popescu et al., 1985	45 BP PN	Cattell 16 Personality Factor Inventory	BP
Hirschfeld et al., 1986	30 BP (F) 15 BP (M) 463 NIR	Maudsley Personality Inventory	NIR (F) NS (M)
Jamison et al., unpublished	35 BP PN	Eysenck Personality Inventory	NS

ND = normative data, PN = published norms, C = control, F = female, M = male, NIR = never-ill relative

[a]Patients instructed to report what they are like when well

chances . . . is generally an impulsive individual . . . easy going, optimistic . . . prefers to keep moving and doing things . . . and to lose his temper quickly.

A typical introvert, on the other hand, is a:

. . . quiet, retiring sort of person, introspective, fond of books rather than people . . . reserved and distant except to intimate friends . . .tends to plan ahead . . . distrusts the impulse of the moment . . . does not like excitement . . . likes a well-ordered mode of life . . . keeps his feelings under close control . . . does not lose his temper easily . . . [is] reliable, somewhat pessimistic.

The extraversion–introversion scale of the MPI/EPI, unlike the neuroticism scale, is relatively impervious to the effects of mood or clinical state. In six studies comparing extraversion in remitted bipolar patients and normal individuals, five found no significant differences between the two groups.[13] Two studies found remitted bipolar patients to be less extraverted than published norms or never-ill relatives (Hirschfeld, 1985; Hirschfeld et al., 1986). One study reported that remitted bipolar patients were more extraverted than a normal population (Popescu et al., 1985).

Neuroticism

The neuroticism scale of the MPI/EPI is more likely to reflect changes in clinical state than is the extraversion scale. Several authors have shown that neuroticism scores decrease following recovery in patients with endogenous depression (Crookes and Hutt, 1963; Coppen and Metcalfe, 1965; Ingham, 1966). In normal populations, extraversion and neuroticism are independent factors, but in psychiatric patients, the correlation between the two measures is usually quite high.[14]

Eysenck and Eysenck (1963a,b) defined neuroticism as "a largely inherited lability of the autonomic nervous system" and as a general measure of emotionality. Its principal components include mood swings, inferiority, poor emotional adjustment, lack of social responsibility, suspiciousness, lack of persistence, social shyness and hypochondriasis, and lack of relaxed composure. Moodiness, which has the single highest loading on the neuroticism factor, is illustrated by positive answers to the following sample items: "Do you sometimes feel happy, sometimes depressed, without any apparent reason?" "Are you inclined to be moody?" and "Do you have frequent ups and downs in mood, either with or without apparent cause?"

Of seven studies comparing neuroticism scores on the MPI/EPI, none found significant differences between remitted bipolar patients and normal populations, and one found lower neuroticism in non-ill relatives of bipolar patients than in the patient group.[15] Matussek and Feil (1983), however, reported that remitted bipolar patients were more likely than normal medical patients to show "autodestructive-neurotic" tendencies.

In summary, there are few significant differences between remitted bipolar patients and normal individuals on the two most frequently assessed personality dimensions, extraversion–introversion and neuroticism. Studies using other psychological measures have found similar results.[16]

Lepkifker and colleagues (1988) found that self-assessment of life satisfaction and adjustment in 50 lithium-treated, euthymic bipolar patients revealed no significant differences between the manic-depressive group and 50 healthy controls. Both of these groups, however, scored significantly higher levels of adjustment and satisfaction than did a control group of 50 patients with personality disorders. Likewise, both the bipolar patients and healthy controls rated their current life satisfaction as higher than at 5 years previously. Again, the reverse was true for the patients with personality disorders.

MacVane and colleagues (1978) found no significant differences in their study of remitted bipolar patients and normal controls on a variety of other psychological measures (Social Desirability Scale, Internal and Powerful Others Locus of Control Scales, Personal Orientation Inventory, Embedded Figures Test, Brief Psychiatric Rating Scale). They concluded:

> Mood swings do not appear to be associated with major persistent psychological deficits in persons with this disorder, nor leave them begging for approval from "normal" society or feeling totally bereft of power and control over their lives. These findings also attest to the resiliency of the human personality. (p. 1354)

Von Zerssen (1977, 1982) has strongly emphasized the difficulties of interpreting data from heterogeneous bipolar samples and the necessity for separating out patients who are exclusively or primarily manic from those with more typically manic-depressive symptomatologies and natural histories. In his view, the lack of differences between personality traits in bipolar patients and normal subjects can be at least partially explained by sample heterogeneity.

Comparisons of Remitted Bipolar Patients with Remitted Unipolar Patients

Extraversion and neuroticism are the major dimensions on which remitted bipolar and unipolar patients have been compared. Results from studies of these and other factors are summarized in Tables 12-6 and 12-7.

Extraversion–Introversion

In five studies of extraversion using the MPI/EPI,[17] and two using the extraversion factor from the Cattell 16 Personality Factor Questionnaire (Murray and Blackburn, 1974; Popescu et al., 1985), remitted bipolar patients scored higher on extraversion than did remitted unipolar patients. Two studies (Bech et al., 1980; Hirschfeld, 1985) found no significant differences between the two groups. Hirschfeld and colleagues (1986) found no significant differences in women, but they did find that bipolar men scored higher on extraversion measures than did unipolar men.

Three studies of dominance, a closely related personality factor, found that bipolar patients were more dominant than unipolar patients (Strandman, 1978; Abou-Saleh and Coppen, 1984; Popescu et al., 1985).

Neuroticism

Seven studies revealed no bipolar–unipolar differences on neuroticism scores obtained during remission.[18] Six studies reported that unipolar patients scored higher in the direction of neuroticism, low self-esteem, or emotional instability, and two studies (Abou-Saleh and Coppen, 1984; Popescu et al., 1985) revealed bipolar patients to be more neurotic than unipolar patients.

Summary

Most studies have shown remitted bipolar patients to be more extraverted than remitted unipolar patients. Differences in neuroticism, if they

Table 12-6. Extraversion-Introversion and Dominance in Remitted Bipolar and Unipolar Patients

Study	Patients N	Psychological Measure	Extraversion/ Dominance Greater In
Murray & Blackburn, 1974	18 BP 18 UP	Cattell 16 Personality Factor Inventory	BP
Frey, 1977	45 BP 65 UP	AUPI Questionnaire (based on Maudsley Personality Inventory)	BP
Strandman, 1978	16 BP 26 UP	Cesarec-Marke Personality Inventory	BP
Liebowitz et al., 1979	71[a] & 46[b] BP 21[a] & 73[b] UP	Wish to dominate/lead others Maudsley Personality Inventory	BP BP
Hirschfeld & Klerman, 1979	24 BP 73 UP	Maudsley Personality Inventory	BP
Bech et al., 1980	25 BP 13[c] UP	Eysenck Personality Inventory	NS
Abou-Saleh & Coppen, 1984	86 BP 149 UP	Eysenck Personality Inventory Foulds Personality Deviance Scale Dominance	BP BP
Hirschfeld, 1985	31[d] BP 55[d] UP	Maudsley Personality Inventory	NS
Popescu et al., 1985	45 BP 69 UP	Cattell 16 Personality Factor Inventory Extroversion Dominance	BP BP
Hirschfeld et al., 1986	45 BP 78 UP	Extraversion-Introversion Cluster[e]	BP (M) NS (F)
Jamison et al., unpublished	35 BP 26 UP	Eysenck Personality Inventory	BP

M = male, F = female

[a] Patients instructed to report what they are like when well
[b] Degree of remission unclear; "manifest symptoms had largely abated"
[c] ≥ 3 episodes
[d] All female
[e] Derived from the Maudsley Personality Inventory, Guilford-Zimmerman Temperament Survey, Thoughtfulness and Restraint Scales, and MMPI

exist at all, are far less compelling. Other studies using different scales show similar results.[19] Donnelly and colleagues (1976) concluded that most bipolar–unipolar differences on the MMPI are limited to the acute depressive phase, except for impulsivity, which appears independent of phase and highly characteristic of ill or remitted bipolar patients. This finding is consistent with the increased extraversion scores among remitted bipolar patients, since one of the two primary components of extraversion is impulsivity.

Most personality researchers have concluded that the personality profiles of remitted bipolar patients are more normal than those of remitted unipolar patients,[20] although some authors report few or insignificant differences between the two groups (Liebowitz et al., 1979; Bech et al., 1980; Hirschfeld, 1985). Inconsistencies in findings derive in part from heterogeneity within populations (due to differing diagnostic criteria), types and degrees of illness (as well as degree of recurrence within unipolar patients), inconsistent criteria for "remission," and inclusion or exclusion of patients with "double depressions."

Table 12-7. Neuroticism and Emotional Instability in Remitted Bipolar and Unipolar Patients

Study	Patients N	Psychological Measure	Neuroticism/ Emotional Instability Greater In
Perris, 1966e	50 BP 50[a] UP	Marke-Nyman Temperament Survey (Stability)	UP
Perris, 1971	25 BP 55[a] UP	Maudsley Personality Inventory (Neuroticism)	NS[b]
Murray & Blackburn, 1974	18 BP 18 UP	Cattell 16 Personality Factor Inventory (Emotional Stability)	UP
Frey, 1977	45 BP 65 UP	AUPI (based on Maudsley Personality Inventory)	NS
Hirschfeld & Klerman, 1979	46[c] BP 73[c] UP	Maudsley Personality Inventory	UP
Liebowitz et al., 1979	71[d] BP 21[d] UP	Maudsley Personality Inventory	UP
Bech et al., 1980	23 BP 13[a] UP	Eysenck Personality Inventory	NS
Matussek & Feil, 1983	19 BP 95 UP	Neurotic Personality Structure	NS
Abou-Saleh & Coppen, 1984	86 BP 149 UP	Marke-Nyman Temperament Survey (Solidity)	BP
Hirschfeld, 1985	31[e] BP 55[e] UP	Maudsley Personality Inventory	NS
Popescu et al., 1985	45 BP 69 UP	Cattell 16 Personality Factor Inventory (Emotional Stability) Marke-Nyman Temperament Survey: Solidity Stability	UP BP BP
Winters & Neale, 1985	16 BP 16 UP	Self-Report Inventory: Self-esteem	UP
Hirschfeld et al., 1986	45 BP 78 UP	Maudsley Personality Inventory Guilford-Zimmerman Temperament Survey (Emotional Stability)	NS NS
Jamison et al., unpublished	35 BP 26 UP	Eysenck Personality Inventory	NS

[a] ≥ 3 episodes
[b] UP > BP at discharge but not at follow-up
[c] Degree of remission unclear; "manifest symptoms had largely abated"
[d] Patients instructed to report what they are like when well
[e] All females

PERSONALITY DISORDERS AND MANIC-DEPRESSIVE ILLNESS

It may be said, simply, that severe emotional upsets ordinarily tend to subside, but that mild emotional states, when often provoked or long maintained, tend to persist, as it were, autonomously. Hence the paradox that a gross blatant psychosis may do less damage in the long run than some meagre neurotic incubus: a dramatic attack of mania or melancholia, with delusions, wasting, hallucinations, wild excitement and other alarms, may have far less effect on the course of a man's life than some deceptively mild affective illness which goes on so long that it becomes inveterate. The former comes as a catastrophe, and when it has passed the patient takes up his life again . . . while with the latter he may never get rid of his burden. (p. 998)   —Aubrey Lewis, 1936

Only in recent years has the complicated relationship between manic-depressive illness and personality disorders been approached systematically. Clearly, personality disorders may precede, coexist with, or be secondary to affective illness. They may also represent untreated, or inadequately treated, affective illness. Akiskal and colleagues, for example, have emphasized that overlapping symptom patterns make it difficult to differentiate bipolar illness and borderline personality (Akiskal, 1984; Akiskal et al., 1985a,c).

A few studies have examined the coexistence of bipolar and personality disorders (Table 12-8). In all but one of the largest and best-controlled studies, the rate of coexistent bipolar illness and personality disorder was relatively low, 4 to 12 percent. However, Charney and colleagues (1981a) found a rate of 23 percent. It is difficult to interpret the results from other studies because of their very small sample sizes (Friedman et al., 1983a; Val et al., 1983). Prevalence rates of personality disorders in affectively ill patients are difficult to compare with such rates in the general population because information on the latter is exceedingly limited. Charney and co-workers (1981a) did compare rates of personality disorders in bipolar and unipolar patients, however, and found that personality disorders were significantly ($p < 0.001$) more common in unipolar nonmelancholic depressed patients (61 percent) than in melancholic unipolar (14 percent) or depressed bipolar patients (23 percent).

McGlashan (1986) compared 33 bipolar patients who did not have Axis-II diagnoses with 33 bipolar patients who did. He found that bipolar patients with personality disorders had more chaotic interpersonal relationships, more anger, greater social isolation, and less rapport than those without. Long-term (15-year) outcome did not differ between the two groups, except for greater alcohol abuse in the bipolar patients with Axis-II diagnoses.

Effects of Lithium on Personality

Evidence for a strong effect of lithium on personality functioning comes from several sources: studies of lithium effects on normal subjects, prima facie evidence derived from both clinical and systematic observation of lithium's profound effect on behavior, mood, and personality in affectively ill patients, and comparisons of personality studies completed in the prelithium era with those completed after lithium treatment became widespread. The latter studies, as discussed earlier, indicate that personality differences between bipolar patients and other groups pale considerably, and often entirely, once lithium is used effectively.

We return, then, to a series of interesting philosophical and treatment issues. Does lithium make the personality of a manic-depressive individual revert to pre-illness levels, or does it decrease variability in mood and personality functioning beyond those levels? Does lithium create an abnormally stable personality and mood system? To what extent is personality in lithium-treated patients a function of blood level? Does a patient who is inadequately treated or only partially responsive to lithium show premorbid personality or subsyndromal disease? How does lithium's in-

Table 12-8. Prevalence Rates of Personality Disorders
in Patients with Bipolar Affective Disorders

Study	N	Type of Personality Disorder	%
Charney et al., 1981a	30	Any personality disorder	23
Gaviria et al., 1982	88	Borderline	12
Baxter et al., 1984	26	Borderline	4
Boyd et al., 1984	46	Antisocial	4

Two studies, with a combined total of 7 BP patients, reported that all patients met criteria for borderline personality disorder (Friedman et al., 1983a; Val et al., 1983)

Based on data in Docherty et al., 1986

fluence on personality affect medication compliance?

Several authors have examined the effects of lithium on personality function in normal subjects. Schou (1968) was the first to describe systematically the cognitive, behavioral, and personality effects of lithium in normal people. At relatively low blood levels, lithium had minimal effects on personality functioning in medical student volunteers. In three researchers taking lithium at higher levels, however, effects were more pronounced. They noted occasional hypersensitivity but also decreased responsivity to their environment, an increased indifference and malaise, greater passivity, and cognitive changes (discussed further in Chapters 14 and 23). Judd and colleagues (1977a), studying lithium effects on normal male volunteers, found that, in addition to reporting a mood-lowering effect, their subjects reported less inclination and desire to "deal with the demands of the environment." Normal men studied by Kropf and Müller-Oerlinghausen (1979) showed, while on lithium, decreased social involvement, activity, and concentration, as well as increased boredom and lethargy. When White and colleagues (1979) administered the Profile of Mood States (POMS) to 10 normal volunteers treated with lithium, the subjects reported a reduced sense of well-being and fewer social interactions. They also complained of fatigue, anxiety, lack of initiative, and decreased efficiency. In an indirect measure of lithium's ability to attenuate emotional responsiveness, Belmaker and colleagues (1979) found that, on lithium, neither normal subjects nor patients experienced the predicted increased heart rate generally caused by participating in cognitive tasks. Both of these studies, although important, were relatively short-term trials (1 to 3 weeks and 2 weeks, respectively), and there is some indication that longer periods of time on lithium result in at least partial accommodation to some of these side effects.

The most clear-cut influences of lithium on bipolar personality were summarized earlier in the reviews of personality studies done on euthymic, lithium-stabilized patients. Additionally, a few studies have examined personality and mood stabilization over time in lithium-treated, affectively ill patients. Bonetti and colleagues (1977) administered the Eysenck Personality Inventory and the Marke-Nyman Temperament Scale to 33 recurrent (minimally three episodes) unipolar and 28 bipolar patients at the end of their index episode and at least 3 months later. They found that personality changes were more pronounced in the bipolar patients, especially on measures of sociability, initiative, and impulsiveness. Neuroticism scores decreased most dramatically within the unipolar group (test–retest differences, $p < 0.001$). The authors speculated that lithium both reduced symptoms and altered habitual patterns of personality, such as high activity levels and impulsiveness in bipolar patients and anxious–neurotic traits in unipolar patients.

In an interesting and important study of the relationship between lithium dose and personality change, Kropf and Müller-Oerlinghausen (1985) conducted a double-blind study of lithium dose reduction (20 percent) in 14 long-term, lithium-treated patients (5 unipolar, 9 bipolar), all of whom were euthymic when tested. Eleven patients (3 unipolar, 8 bipolar), maintained at their regular lithium levels, acted as controls. The patients on higher levels of lithium tended to be less active, less obsessive, and less elated. Specifically, those on lower levels of lithium scored higher on Von Zerssen's measures of initiative and assertiveness ($p < 0.05$) and of social resonance (social acceptance and assertiveness), transparency (social openness and sensitivity), and social potency (sociability and "ability for devotion"). However, a significant proportion (29 percent) of the patients in the experimental group became affectively ill at a reduced lithium level.

Mood stability in lithium-treated patients, although not a direct measure of personality, clearly is related to personality functioning. Folstein and colleagues (1982) administered the Visual Analogue Mood Scale (VAMS) for 30 days to 65 euthymic manic-depressive patients on chronic lithium therapy and to 36 nonpatient control subjects. The mean mood ratings for the two groups were similar; the patients, however, reported significantly less mood variability. The authors attributed this unusual degree of mood stability to the effects of lithium treatment and suggested that euthymic patients may view this change as an undesirable aspect of lithium therapy. DePaulo and colleagues (1983) administered the VAMS to 17 euthymic bipolar patients and to 21 nonpatient controls. They found, like Folstein and co-workers, that the mean mood ratings were similar in the two groups and that the patients' moods were less variable than those of the controls. Three manic-depressive patients were studied separately, during and after lithium treatment. Two became manic and the third, who remained euthymic while off lithium, showed markedly increased variability in daily mood ratings. The authors were uncertain whether these results reflected baseline differences in reporting between affectively ill patients and normal controls, lithium's therapeutic effect, or a medication side effect.

Personality Predictors of Lithium Response

Personality variables do not consistently predict response to lithium therapy. Studies using the MMPI, the most commonly used personality instrument, as well as four studies using other psychological measures, are summarized in Table 12-9. No MMPI scale was predictive in more than two studies, and the one scale specifically derived to predict lithium response (Donnelly et al., 1978a) was not predictive in three subsequent investigations (Burdick and Holmes, 1980; Garvey et al., 1983; Campbell and Kimball, 1984). Findings from other psychological tests have been inconclusive or not replicated. The personality factors most predictive of lithium response are psychasthenia and the related quality of obsessiveness.[21] The psychasthenia scale from the MMPI, reflecting Pierre Janet's original concept, includes items designed to assess obsessive and compulsive reactions, indecisiveness, preoccupied and fearful thinking, perfectionism, insecurity, and guilt feelings.

It is difficult to interpret specific findings or, indeed, a lack of findings. Lithium compliance was not adequately controlled in any of the stud-

Table 12-9. Personality Predictors of Lithium Response

Study	Psychological Test	Correlates of Lithium Response
Steinbrook & Chapman, 1970	MMPI	Acquiescence Scale
House & Martin, 1975	MMPI	↑ depression ↑ psychasthenia
Anath et al., 1979	MMPI	↑ hypochondriasis ↓ psychopathic deviance ↓ paranoia ↑ psychasthenia ↓ mania ↑ social introversion
Kerry & Orme, 1979	Middlesex Hospital Questionnaire	↑ obsessiveness
Abou-Saleh, 1983	Foulds Personality Deviance Scale	↑ dominance ↓ deviant personality
	Eysenck Personality Inventory	↑ psychoticism: male responders ↑ EPI lie scale ↑ neuroticism: female nonresponders
Smigan, 1985	Karolinska Hospital Personality Inventory	↑ psychasthenia ↑ muscular tension
Abou-Saleh & Coppen, 1986	Fould's Personality Deviance Scale	↓ intropunitiveness
	Eysenck Personality Inventory	↓ neuroticism ↑ extraversion
	Crown-Crisp Experiential Index	↓ anxiety ↓ depression ↓ hysteria

ies, and it is unclear whether compliance or true responsiveness to lithium was being predicted. Further, in virtually all studies, the affective state at the time of personality testing was variable, as were the diagnostic inclusion criteria and measures of treatment success. Finally, as Lane (1985) has pointed out:

. . . these studies have investigated the relationship of a temporally unstable predictor (MMPI data obtained during acute episodes) to a temporally unstable criterion (short-term response to lithium), so that failure to replicate is unremarkable. (p. 1388)

INTERPERSONAL BEHAVIOR IN MANIC-DEPRESSIVE ILLNESS

No one has the slightest idea of what I've been through with Cal [Robert Lowell]. In 4½ years, counting this present breakup, he has had four collapses! Three manic, and one depression. These things take time to come and long after he is out of the hospital there is a period which can only be called "nursing." The long, difficult pull back—which does not show always to others. I knew the possibility of this when I married him, and I have always felt that the joy of his "normal" periods, the lovely time we had, all I've learned from him, the immeasurable things I've derived from our marriage made up for the bad periods. I consider it all a gain of the most precious kind. But he has torn down this time everything we've built up . . . how difficult these break-ups are for both of us.
—Elizabeth Hardwick[22]

Moods are by nature compelling, contagious, and profoundly interpersonal. Mood disorders alter the perceptions and behaviors not only of those who have them but also of those who are related or closely associated. Manic-depressive illness—marked as it is by extraordinary and confusing fluctuations in mood, personality, thinking, and behavior—inevitably has powerful and often painful effects on relationships. Violence, poor judgment, and indiscreet financial and sexual behavior are almost always destructive and embarrassing to spouses, children, family members, and friends. Trust is not easily restored in the wake of mania, nor are goodwill and love always regenerated after months of severe, depleting, and unremitting depression. In this section, we review the issues and studies concerned with patients who have manic-depressive illness and their relationships with other people.

Overview of Interpersonal Behavior: Psychoanalytic Perspectives

Psychoanalysts, with rare exceptions, have regarded the interpersonal lives of manic-depressive patients as unstable and chaotic, narcissistically based, bereft of empathic regard for the rights of others, too dependent or independent, singularly rigid, and full of rage. These conclusions are not surprising given that they have been based substantially on experiences with patients in the prepharmacotherapy era. Understandably, such perceptions led most psychoanalysts to be wary and reluctant to treat these patients. Since the psychoanalytic relationship with manic-depressive patients was seen as superficial and distant, countertransference was the subject of considerable discussion and writing about such patients (see Chapter 24). Most psychoanalytic writers were primarily interested in the origins of the illness and the personality structure of manic-depressive patients, but we present here a brief review of their observations and interpretations of interpersonal behavior.

Abraham (1911, 1924), one of the earliest writers to formulate psychodynamic principles in manic-depressive illness, described the patients' abnormal character development and inability to maintain good relationships. These features, he speculated, were coupled with an ongoing sense of impending loss of objects, which produce a "rageful" stance toward these objects and their inability to "gratify narcissistic demands." Freud (1917), for the most part, concurred: "Manic-depressives show simultaneously the tendency to too-strong fixations to their love-object and to a quick withdrawal of object cathexis. Object choice is on a narcissistic basis." Lewis (1931), after psychoanalyzing four manic-depressive patients, summarized his observations:

The conscious strong attachment to the parents with more or less unconscious love and hate ambivalencies, which do not mature and differentiate. . . . and make for infantile modes of reaction in society and particularly in married life. . . . The capacity for love and hate is very highly developed, with the sadistic components often more openly expressed during the elated phases and more deeply repressed in the depressed, pessimistic, accusatory and "sense of guilt" periods. (p. 771)

The attitude of manic-depressive individuals toward others was described by Blalock (1936) as "a selfish one serving in its several aspects the narcissistic needs of the patient" (p. 342). Equally critical in his views, Fenichel (1945) regarded manic-depressive patients as "love addicts," narcissistic, and incapable of love. To English

(1949), the manic-depressive person was egocentric, incapable of relating warmly to others, rigid, afraid to hate except when manic, and powerfully influenced by the intensity of feelings:

> The manic-depressive is afraid of extremes of emotion, of great love, or of hostility, and yet these are the very things he may show in his illness. One patient . . . said, "To live is like opening all my pores on a cold day and subjecting myself to a catastrophe." The manic-depressive therefore has a defect in catching the feelings of others. He ignores what others feel and want as long as he can. Thus in trying to avoid being hurt he avoids the strengthening influence of friendship. (p. 131)

Fromm-Reichmann (1949), in a similar vein, described a "lack of subtlety," a "lack of any close interpersonal relatedness," and a tendency to exaggerate the intensity of their interactions with other people. While describing manic-depressive individuals as manifesting a "particular kind of narcissistic dependency on their love objects," Jacobson (1953) provided a perspective remarkably at variance with the earlier psychoanalytic writers:

> We are also surprised to see that as long as they are not sick, they may be delightful companions or marital partners, a feature that Bleuler mentioned especially. In their sexual life they may show a full . . . response, and emotionally, in contradistinction to schizoid persons, a touching warmth and unusual, affectionate clinging to people they like . . . (they) are potentially able to function extraordinarily well. (p. 66)

Cohen and colleagues (1954), however, commented on what they viewed as the illusion of normal relationships in manic-depressive patients:

> The appearance of closeness is provided by the hypomanic's liveliness, talkativeness, wittiness, and social aggressiveness. Actually, there is little or no communicative exchange between the hypomanic and any one of his so-called friends. . . .
> The concept of reciprocity is missing; the needs of the other for similar experiences are not recognized. (p. 119)

Finally, Gibson and colleagues (1959) stressed the dependent nature of the manic-depressive person—the difficulties in dealing with feelings of envy and competition and the "common use of denial as a defense, there being a notable lack of subtlety, and of awareness of their own or the feelings of others in their interpersonal relations" (p. 1102). (The views of more recent psychoanalytic writers are presented in later sections on bipolar marriages and families.)

Mania: Clinical Observations

The complex, subtle, enraging, and potentially infuriating aspects of manic interpersonal behavior were observed by most of the early clinical investigators (see Chapter 2). Hypomanic behavior, especially, was noted for its powerful and confusing influence on others. The positive, engaging, and often charismatic aspects of many individuals with manic-depressive illness are discussed extensively in Chapter 14. Kraepelin (1921) wrote of the skill of hypomanic patients in manipulating fellow patients:

> It is just the peculiar mixture of sense and maniacal activity, frequently also an extensive experience of institutions, which makes them extremely ingenious in finding out means to satisfy their numerous desires, to deceive their surroundings, to procure for themselves all kinds of advantages, to secure the property of others for themselves. They usually soon domineer completely over their fellow-patients, use them for profit, report about them to the physician in technical terms, act as guardian to them, and hold them in check. (p. 61)

Gibson (1963) described the manic-depressive person as "extraordinarily perceptive on an unconscious level, . . . "skillful" . . . in evoking and utilizing feelings, especially guilt, in the other person. . . . manipulative, exploitative" (p. 93). The observations of Kraepelin and of Gibson are quite consistent with the more recent work of Janowsky and colleagues (1970, 1974), who assessed the interactional style of acutely manic patients with tape recordings of psychotherapy sessions (both group and individual), physician and social worker notes, observations of milieu therapy, and nurses' behavioral descriptions and ratings of patients. Janowsky's group (1970) observed five basic types of interpersonal activity in their acutely manic patients:

> Type 1. Manipulation of the self-esteem of others: sensitivity to issues of self-esteem in others, with the increasing or lowering of another's self-esteem as a way of exerting interpersonal leverage.
> Type 2. Perceptiveness of vulnerability and conflict: the ability to sense, reveal, and exploit areas of covert sensitivity in others.
> Type 3. Projection of responsibility: the ability to shift responsibility in such a way that others become responsible for the manic's actions.
> Type 4. Progressive limit testing: the phenomenon

whereby the manic extends the limits imposed on him, "upping the ante."

Type 5. Alienating family members: the process by which the manic distances himself from his family. (p. 253)

The manic person's interpersonal maneuvers are, according to these authors, "simultaneously cementing and distancing." Their study, although perhaps presuming too much conscious control and manipulation on the part of the patient, is one of the few clinical reports to describe in perceptive detail the interpersonal behavior of manic patients. We quote, as an example, from their work on the manic patient's perceptiveness to vulnerability and conflict:

Intimately related to the manic's ability to appeal to the self-esteem systems of others is his extraordinary perceptiveness. In interpersonal encounters, the manic possesses a highly refined talent for sensing an individual's vulnerability or a group's area of conflict, and exploiting this in a manipulative fashion. This sensitivity may be utilized in dealing directly with a given individual or in focusing on areas of conflict between others. In either case, the manic patient is able to make covert conflicts overt, causing the person or group with whom he is dealing to feel discomfort. . . .

What he says cannot be dismissed as untrue or unreal, for the areas attacked truly do exist and, indeed, are areas of vulnerability. (p. 254)

Mania: Interpersonal Studies

Here we briefly review the findings of data-based studies of mania (summarized in Chapter 2) that are relevant to its interpersonal aspects. Mood changes during mania clearly affect both manic individuals and those around them. Prominent changes in mood include euphoria, reported in 71 percent of all patients studied, as well as the considerably more disruptive and distressing symptoms of irritability (80 percent) and depression (72 percent) (see Chapter 2 for sources of data). Affective lability, confusing and disturbing to most family members and friends, has been reported in 70 percent of manic patients. Financial extravagance and irregularities, sources of anxiety and friction in most relationships of manic-depressive individuals, are present in a substantial majority of episodes. Additionally, Akiskal and colleagues (1977) reported repeated buying sprees, financial extravagances, or financial disasters in 75 percent of their cyclothymic patients. (Changes in sexual behavior during mania, another source of turmoil and conflict, are discussed

later in this chapter.) Violence and assault, of clear concern to relatives and acquaintances, occur in most manic episodes (46 to 75 percent).

Fluctuations in levels of sociability almost define manic-depressive illness. Energetic seeking-out of other people and uninhibited social behavior are common features of mania. Winokur and colleagues described this in their 1969 monograph:

A most characteristic sight when the patient is brought to the hospital is a frightened and exhausted family, which has frequently been awake for 1 or more nights being lectured to by a bright-eyed and excited patient. (p. 63)

Murphy and Beigel (1974), in their study of 30 bipolar patients, found two distinctive behavioral characteristics of mania: noticeably increased psychomotor activity and, of relevance here, a need for increased interpersonal contact ("people-seeking"). Akiskal and associates (1977) reported that half of their cyclothymic patients alternated periods of uninhibited people-seeking with periods of introverted self-absorption.

Janowsky and colleagues (1974), in an attempt to quantify their earlier clinical descriptions of the interpersonal aspects of mania, had nurses rate features of manic behavior (including testing limits, projecting responsibility, being sensitive to others' vulnerabilities, flattering others, and angering others) in nine schizophrenic, ten schizoaffective, and ten manic patients. Their study had several methodological problems, including the choice of comparison groups and the highly questionable assumption of scoring purely schizophrenic and purely manic symptoms as two ends of a continuum. In addition, diagnostic criteria were unclear, especially for manic, excited type and agitated schizophrenia. Further, a nonpsychiatric control group was lacking, and it was uncertain that nurses were blind to patient diagnosis. Despite these limitations, the study is conceptually important. Janowsky and associates found, not surprisingly, that manic patients obtained a higher average score on the Manic Interpersonal Interaction Scale (MIIS) than did schizophrenic and schizoaffective patients. In addition, there was a high positive correlation between the Bunney-Hamburg global mania score and the MIIS score ($r = .84$): In the five manic patients evaluated longitudinally, MIIS scores dramatically diminished as remission occurred (regardless of whether the remission occurred spontaneously or after pharmacotherapy). The authors concluded:

What may be unique in the acutely manic patient is the fact that he appears to have changes in his style of interpersonal interactions that fluctuate dramatically with the phases of the psychotic illness. This may be theoretically important, since styles of interpersonal relating are usually thought to be long-term and continuing characteristics of behavior, in contrast to symptoms, which can fluctuate over brief intervals. Thus, our observations suggest that the acute manic disorder has a widespread effect on personality, affecting not only drive and subsequent defenses but also those aspects of ego structure that govern an individual's personality style. (Janowsky et al., 1974, p. 253)

Depression: Interpersonal Studies

The social context clearly shapes the features, severity, and consequences of depression. Although not considered a definitive symptom of depression, impaired relationships with other people are almost universal. They have been explored in several lines of research conducted primarily on unipolar depressed patients.

An extensive longitudinal study of neurotically depressed women revealed that impaired social adjustment persisted even when depressive symptoms had diminished (Paykel and Weissman, 1973; Bothwell and Weissman, 1977). For these women, the most enduring difficulties in social relationships were marital problems and general interpersonal friction. Social impairment has also been observed when depressed people interact with relative strangers. Youngren and Lewinsohn (1980), for example, showed that depressed people differ significantly from psychiatric and nonpsychiatric controls on a variety of interactional measures of nonverbal behavior and social skill, as well as on self-reported discomfort in social situations.

Communication deficits in depression have been studied by several investigators and well reviewed by Miller (1975). Hinchliffe and colleagues (1971) reported that depressed individuals, when compared with controls, showed lower rates of speech, more negators such as "not" and "never," and more personal references. Depressed subjects also spoke more slowly than controls but did not exhibit more or longer pauses. Libet and Lewinsohn (1973), in a study of college students, found that depressed students spoke more slowly and had lower rates of verbal behavior than did nondepressed students. They also exhibited fewer positive interpersonal reactions and had a longer latency of response time. Ekman and Friesen (1974) found that depressed persons showed few hand motions that were illustrative (i.e., furthered communication) but many that were not, such as scratching and rubbing. With clinical improvement, the number of the facilitating communications increased, and the number of nonfacilitating ones decreased. Andreasen (1982b) reported that depressed patients showed an unchanging facial expression, decreased spontaneous movements, paucity of expressive gestures, slowed speech, poor eye contact, affective flattening, and a lack of vocal inflections. Communication deficits are further discussed in Chapter 11.

The symptomatology of depression appears to contribute to patients' interpersonal difficulties. For example, irritability is common in bipolar depression. Winokur and co-workers (1969) observed it in 76 percent of their patients. Depressed men and women report diminished enjoyment of formerly gratifying activities, including relationships, and often withdraw from both personal and social contacts. Akiskal's group (1977) found "introverted self-absorption" in half of their cyclothymic patients, and Winokur and colleagues (1969) reported that all their bipolar depressed patients were socially withdrawn.

Friends and family may be frustrated by the exaggerated dependence of the depressed patients, especially when they seem unable to relieve his or her despondency. Moreover, the depressed person may be particularly sensitive to perceived rejection or criticism, and minor or even nonexistent slights are exaggerated or inaccurately interpreted. All of these common symptoms of depression can thwart the best intentions and efforts of friends and family members.

Interpersonal tension may be further intensified by the depressed individual's marked guilt and feelings of worthlessness and self-blame for real or perceived negative social encounters. Coyne and colleagues (1987), in a study of 42 adults living with a depressed individual (who was hospitalized or in outpatient treatment), found that the most burdensome symptoms were the patients' lack of interest in social life, fatigue, feelings of hopelessness, and worrying.

Depressed people frustrate themselves and others and depress those around them. Coyne (1976), in a study of 45 normal subjects conversing with depressed patients, nondepressed patients, or normal controls, found that subjects were significantly more depressed and rejecting after interacting with depressed patients than they were after being with nondepressed patients or normal controls. The patient's depressed mood had a greater effect than their hostility, even though depressed patients were significantly more hostile than the other groups. Coyne suggested that depressed patients' unusual willingness to discuss "intensely personal matters" contributed to inducing a depressed mood in others. Coyne noted that his results were consistent with the overall finding of Weissman and Paykel (1974) that the "social consequences of the illness may themselves be stressful and tend to perpetuate the condition" (p. 216).

Hammen and Peters (1977), in a study based on written descriptions of depressed individuals, found that subjects evaluated depressed men more negatively than they did depressed women. The same investigators examined telephone interactions between same-sex and opposite-sex pairs. In each pair, one person enacted a depressed or nondepressed role (Hammen and Peters, 1978). They found that depressed people were more strongly rejected than nondepressed people, especially by individuals of the opposite sex. Interacting with depressed people made listeners significantly more depressed than did interacting with nondepressed persons, and the listeners attributed significantly more feminine traits to depressed than nondepressed individuals regardless of gender.

Hammen and Peters (1977, 1978) also found that depressed people were viewed as undesirable potential friends or lovers and were seen as impaired in various social roles. Depression elicited more rejection than did anxiety or unemotional and detached reactions to stress, suggesting that, beyond emotional dysfunction, something unique to depression results in others' negative judgments.

Rejection of depressed individuals also has been demonstrated by Boswell and Murray (1981), Gotlib and Robinson (1982), and Strack and Coyne (1983). In a recent review of the psychological literature, Gurtman (1986) concluded that rejection of depressed persons is a robust finding and consistent across studies and methodologies.

The depressed person, therefore, already burdened by a paralyzing sense of futility, helplessness, and self-deprecation, must also face the likelihood of provoking or eliciting negative social encounters. It seems clear that for patients with persistent episodes of depression, a self-perpetuating cycle of upset and frustration in interpersonal situations may be established.

Marriage and Manic-Depressive Illness

I am tired of papering over the cracks and pretending to friends and relatives that life is wonderful. It is the nearest and dearest who come in for the bulk of the barrage. . . .

It is the Jekyll and Hyde syndrome. I never know which is going to walk in through the door, and the unpredictability is most unnerving. It is like living on a knife-edge. You can never relax or take anything for granted and any thought of lapsing into "placid serenity" is completely out of the question. —Anonymous[23]

Marriage and Unipolar Depression

The disruptive influence of mood disorders on marriage has been more assumed than measured. The research literature on this important aspect of life is sparse, although the volume has increased in recent years. Marriages involving unipolar depression have received more study than those involving bipolar illness. Because of their relevance to the discussion of bipolar marriages, these unipolar studies are briefly reviewed here.

In an early study of life events and depressive illness, Paykel and colleagues (1969) found that the most frequent event reported by depressed women was an increase in the rate of arguments with their spouses. Weissman and Paykel (1974) characterized the marriages of depressed women as fraught with friction, inadequate communication, dependency, overt hostility, resentment and guilt, poor sexual relationships, and a lack of affection. McLean and co-workers (1973), who observed marital communication patterns, noted that when spouses of depressed patients gave what they viewed as "constructive criticism," their spouses saw it as hostile behavior. In a study of 45 divorced unipolar depressives, Briscoe and Smith (1973) concluded:

. . . depressions associated with divorce, unlike the depressions of bereavement . . . can be the result or cause (or both) of the marital turmoil. (p. 817)

Hinchliffe and associates (1975) used the Revealed Difference Questionnaire to compare communication patterns in 10 depressed inpatients and their spouses with 11 surgical controls and their spouses. They tested patients during hospitalization and during recovery 3 to 12 months later. When depressed, patients' communication styles were characterized by high levels of tension, negative expression, self-preoccupation, and diminished nonverbal communication patterns. There were ". . . major differences in both verbal and non-verbal modes of communication between hospital psychiatric patients and their spouses and the hospital surgical patients and their spouses" (p. 170). Over time, however, as patients recovered from their depression, their communication patterns became more like those of controls. Interestingly, although there were no significant sex differences during hospitalization, the long-term course for men and women was quite different. In male but not female patients, negative expression decreased significantly from hospitalization to recovery.

Arkowitz and colleagues (1979), using the Marital Interaction Coding System, coded videotapes of couples discussing a topic on which they disagreed. The researchers concluded that husbands of depressed women reported more hostility after the discussion than did husbands of nondepressed psychiatric or normal control women. They also found that depressed women and their husbands had significantly lower rates of positive nonverbal behavior and that "husbands of depressed women were feeling hostile, attempting to hide this, but leaking it nonverbally."

Merikangas and co-workers (1979), studying interactions between nine depressed inpatients and their husbands, found that spouses influenced the patients significantly less at the last of six treatment sessions than at the first. These researchers attributed their findings to a redistribution of power within the relationship, reflecting a more equal balance.

Hautzinger and colleagues (1982) investigated communication patterns in 26 couples with equally severe marital problems, 13 of whom had a spouse with unipolar depression. Eight 40-minute conversations were recorded over a 3- to 4-week period. The depressive couples showed "uneven, negative and asymmetrical communication" in contrast to the nondepressive couples, who were "positive, supportive and reciprocal." The depressed patients tended to speak negatively of themselves and positively of their spouses, while their nondepressed spouses "rarely spoke of their somatic and psychological well-being . . . evaluated their relationship and partner less positively . . . and offered their partner more help, but in an ambivalent way" (p. 312).

Finally, Kahn and colleagues (1985) used the Impact Message Inventory to compare laboratory-based discussions in depressed patients and their spouses and in normal control couples. They found that, after the discussion, couples with a depressed member were more angry and sad than were the normal controls and more likely to view one another as hostile, mistrusting, competitive, and inhibited. They were less likely than the controls to find one another agreeable, nurturant, or affiliative, and the evaluations by both spouses were equally negative.

Marriage and Bipolar Illness

The marriages of untreated, inadequately treated, or treatment-nonresponsive manic-depressive patients tend to be turbulent, fluctuating, and uncertain. An excellent overall clinical description is given by Janowsky and colleagues (1970):

Diametrically opposed styles of marital relating, occurring during depressed or manic phases respectively, seem intolerable to the spouse. The depressive phase is usually viewed by the spouse as an illness over which the patient has little control. Here, spouses offer significant physical care and emotional support. The patient, during the depressive phase, often expresses much guilt and self-blame and sometimes speaks of the spouse in laudatory and absolving terms. . . .

In contrast, the attitude of the spouse undergoes a marked change when the patient is manic. The manic phase is perceived as a willful, spiteful act. Lip service only is given to seeing the mania as an illness. There is always an underlying feeling that the manic can control his actions, and does not do so out of maliciousness, selfishness, and lack of consideration. This impression is fostered by the fact that the manic often has periods of seeming reasonableness. . . .

Related to the issue of the spouse feeling betrayed and experiencing diminished self-esteem is the problem of marital infidelity. Often, manic patients speak of divorce, make sexual advances to other people, become engaged in affairs. . . .

In all these situations, the spouses felt trapped in what they perceived as an impossible situation. They felt caught in a whirlwind of activity, personally threatened, powerless to enforce limits . . . Their moods and feelings were intimately related to the disease state of the sick partner. (p. 259)

Ablon and colleagues (1975) conducted a psychodynamic study of eight couples in which one spouse was manic-depressive (bipolar I). (Seven of the patients were men, and five were on lithium.) The couples, married 12 to 34 years, were all in conjoint group therapy, during which several themes emerged: threat and fear of recurring mania, hostility between spouses, massive denial, symbiosis and dependence, and the weak or absent father. Consistent with other authors, these noted how differently patients and spouses perceived mania: ". . . the patient viewed mania as an overwhelming force . . . [but] mania was seen by the spouse as an expression of the patient's true feelings, under his control and for which he was responsible" (p. 857). The observations of Ablon's group, based on years of intensive psychotherapeutic experience with affectively ill patients, are clinically important. However, their findings are difficult to interpret. There was no comparison group (presumably, several of the themes mentioned would be common to most marriages), men were disproportionately represented in the patient group, and it is unclear how dependent these observations were on the clinical state of the patients (or, indeed, their spouses). Finally, the efficacy or duration of lithium treatment in these patients was not specified.

Hoover and Fitzgerald (1981) compared marital interactions in 42 manic-depressive and depressive inpatients and their spouses, with 30 normal couples from the community. Using the 67-item Conflict in Marriage Scale (designed to measure resolution of conflicts, ways of dealing with anger, and content of disputes), they found that the couples with an affectively ill spouse scored higher on expressed conflict than did the community controls ($p < 0.001$). Within the affectively ill group, couples with a bipolar-I member expressed more conflict than those with a unipolar member, who, in turn, scored higher on this factor than those with a bipolar-II member. Hoover and Fitzgerald also found patients to be more sensitive to their spouses' marital dissension and proposed several possible explanations:

It may be that conflict with an ill partner is more difficult to acknowledge and express.

Another possibility is that the spouses of manic-depressive patients derive some personality reinforcement, a tested sense of ability or moral fulfillment, from caring for a recurrently sick partner. Or perhaps some spouses need to be a trifle oblivious and not too sensitive to remain with a manic-depressive patient through the years.
Finally, there remains the possibility that, in a complementary sense, mercurial persons seek out cheerful, denying persons to marry whereas stolid maintainers of the peace search for more spontaneous, mood-varying types. (p. 67)

Relevant to these findings are those of Hooley and colleagues (1987), who found that spouses of patients with florid, positive symptoms (auditory or visual hallucinations, grandiosity, agitation, speech disorganization, delusions, elated mood, silliness, or inappropriate affect, appearance, or behavior) reported significantly higher levels of marital satisfaction than spouses of patients with negative symptom patterns (social isolation, depression, lack of emotion, or routine or leisure time impairment). The authors attribute this difference to the fact that the more bizarre and flagrant positive symptoms, unlike the negative ones, are perceived by the spouse as being caused by an illness and thus beyond the patient's volition. Although seemingly contradictory to the observations that mania is perceived as being within the patient's control (Janowsky et al., 1970; Ablon et al., 1975), it is most likely that only the less severe and nonpsychotic forms of mania are seen as volitional or as the patient's "true feelings." Likewise, the marital satisfaction ratings may simply reflect a stronger association between positive symptoms and overall long-term interpersonal adjustment.[24] Mayo (1979), studying 12 manic-depressive patients, also found them to be most "anti-spouse" when hypomanic or mildly to moderately depressed. When severely depressed, they tended to be overtly accepting of their spouses. Both patients and spouses were most loving toward one another when their moods were normal.

Targum and associates (1981) administered the Family Attitudes Questionnaire to 19 bipolar patients and their well spouses to determine their attitudes and beliefs about the etiology, familial risk, and long-term burden of manic-depressive illness, as well as their attitudes toward marriage and childbearing. The long-term burdens of the illness included financial difficulties, home and child neglect, marital problems, loss of status and prestige, constant tension, and fears of recurrence of acute illness. These researchers concluded that the "bipolar patient, compared with his or her spouse, more often minimizes the burden of affective illness, denies the heritable/familial nature of affective illness." When asked whether they would have married their spouses if they had known more about manic-depressive illness, 5 percent of the bipolar patients and 53 percent of their spouses said they would not have ($p <$ 0.01). Similarly, when asked whether they would have had children, 5 percent of the bipolar patients but fully 47 percent of their spouses said they would not have ($p < 0.01$).

Both patients and spouses perceived violent behavior as the most troubling characteristic of mania. Patients also were especially worried by their poor judgment during mania. Spouses were particularly concerned by impulsive spending, overtalkativeness, and decreased need for sleep. Both groups saw suicide threats and attempts as the most troubling aspect of depression, and patients were also bothered by the hopelessness and poor concentration accompanying depression, whereas spouses were disturbed by the lowered self-esteem and withdrawal from others. Overall, the most troublesome long-term social problems resulting from manic-depressive illness were financial difficulties, unemployment, marital problems, recurrences of illness leading to rehospitalization, and social withdrawal due to depression. The authors concluded:

> Well spouses who have coped with affective illness for many years perceived bipolar illness as a profound burden that had seriously disrupted their lives. . . .
> The regrets of the well spouse are a most striking feature of this study . . . Whereas affective episodes may not be directly associated with major persistent psychological deficits, the damaging effects of these episodes may still yield psychological and economic consequences, particularly for the spouse. The spouse is the person who bears the brunt of manic episodes. . . . In depression, the spouse is the most frequent target of demands and hostility, and often feels inordinate responsibility for the mood state of the patient. (Targum et al., 1981, p. 568)

Targum and colleagues were the first to examine and compare systematically the attitudes of manic-depressive patients and their spouses and to highlight spousal distress. But, as in other studies noted in this chapter, several methodological

problems make such findings difficult to interpret. Most significantly, there was no comparison group. In addition, differences in response sets almost certainly occurred between spouses and patients. For patients, relationship problems may well pale into relative insignificance compared with the traumatic nature of experiencing mania and depression, and denial may be more of a necessity to patients for both emotional and physical survival. Further, the authors did not examine possible assets in the marriages in these couples. Patients and spouses had been married an average of 22 years at the time of the study. It would be interesting to know why so many marriages lasted as long as they did. Did psychopathology alone bind patient and spouse together? Were there any offsetting advantages to these marriages, or, as in most relationships, was there a complex combination of ill and good? Other research design problems include the tremendous variability in the lengths of marriages within the sample (1 to 45 years), nonspecification of the role of lithium in the marriages, and the lack of clarity in defining a "well" spouse. In addition, given the long duration of these marriages, it is difficult to know how much of the mental conflict is attributable to patterns of interaction established before the regular use of lithium.

Frank and colleagues (1981), in a study of 16 couples, one of whom in each couple had remitted bipolar illness, corrected for the most problematic of the difficulties in the studies just described by comparing the bipolar couples with 16 nonpatient couples (matched for age and other demographic variables). They found no significant differences between the two groups of couples in overall marital satisfaction, sexual satisfaction, methods of handling disagreements (except that more nonpatients reported sulking during disagreements), or in their perceptions of courtship and the first year of marriage. In striking contrast to the earlier described study, Frank and colleagues found that individuals in both groups were equally likely to assert that if they had their life to live over, they would "marry the same person," "marry a different person," or "not marry at all." They concluded that:

> Our findings point to the value of nonclinical comparison groups for clinical populations. An evaluation of the marriages of bipolar patient-well spouse couples

done in isolation could lead to the conclusion that these are relatively troubled, unsatisfactory relationships; however, when viewed in comparison with a nonpatient population, we are reminded that even normal marriages suffer from economic problems, serious illness in children, multiple moves from city to city, etc. (Frank et al., 1981, p. 767)

The fact that all of the patients in their study were treated and in remission is, no doubt, also an essential variable in their findings.

Comparison of Marriages of Bipolar and Unipolar Patients

There are many clinical differences between bipolar and unipolar patients that might be expected to contribute to substantial differences in their marriages. Janowsky and associates (1970), in one of the few comparative studies of marriage in both patient groups, concluded:

The discussion of separation in the marriages of manic patients occurred so frequently as to be a diagnostic differentiator between patients with manic-depressive psychosis and those with unipolar depressive illness. Significantly, none of the spouses had known the manic patients during a manic episode prior to marriage. (p. 258)

Brodie and Leff (1971), who reviewed the case records of 30 bipolar and 30 unipolar patients matched by age and sex, found a highly significant difference ($p < 0.01$) in the divorce rates for the two groups: 57 percent in bipolar and 8 percent in unipolar patients. They, like many others, emphasized the singularly damaging effect of mania:

These findings suggest the probable incompatibility of manic symptoms with stable marriage. We found, for example, that divorce occurred only after a manic attack and never before a bipolar patient had experienced at least one period of mania. (p. 1089)

On the other hand, Ruestow and co-workers (1978) found no bipolar–unipolar differences among wives on the marital adjustment scale but found that among the husbands it was actually the unipolar patients who reported a poorer marital adjustment. The bipolar patients were stabilized on lithium, an obviously important factor to be discussed separately.

Coryell and colleagues (1985), in a study of depression in relatives of affectively ill probands, found the highest rates of separation or divorce (in those ever married) in the bipolar-II group (33 percent), followed by the bipolar-I group (21 percent) and the nonbipolar depression (17 percent) group. The rates were significantly different between the nonbipolar and bipolar-II groups ($p < 0.01$). These findings parallel those reported for the probands themselves (see Chapter 2).

Jamison and colleagues (unpublished data) compared bipolar and unipolar patients' perceptions about the disruptiveness of depression to the marital relationship. Unlike mania, which they saw as exceedingly disruptive to the overall family system (see discussion to follow), depression, as reported by most of the bipolar (55 percent) and unipolar (64 percent) patients, caused relatively little marital disruption. The two groups did not differ significantly in overall ratings. It is important to note, however, that these were the patients' perceptions not those of their spouses.

Lithium Treatment and Marriage

Clinical experience suggests that lithium has a very stabilizing effect on manic-depressive marriages because it partially or totally eliminates both highly volatile and disruptive manic episodes and frightening and depleting depressive ones. These benefits appear to be corroborated by the few marital studies of adequately treated bipolar patients,[25] although these results were not found in the study by Targum and co-workers.

Demers and Davis (1971) administered the Marital Partner Attribute Test to 14 married manic-depressive patients and their spouses. Lithium produced a highly significant decrease in spouses' negative ratings of the patients but no significant change in patients' ratings of their spouses. In fact, 13 of 14 manic-depressive patients (93 percent) were rated by their spouses as improved and as having significantly fewer undesirable attributes ($p < 0.01$) after lithium treatment. Spouses particularly noted decreases in nervousness, bizarre, threatening, and violent behavior, withdrawn or demanding behavior, guilt, sadness, and undue exaggeration of abilities. But they also reported missing the enthusiasm and heightened sexuality associated with hypomanic phases:

Hypomanic joviality, enthusiasm, and spontaneity are often regarded as social pluses; and manic-depressives and their spouses complain about the loss of these valued attributes. When pressed to discuss the sexual compatibility of the marriage, frequently they will say it is worse since lithium treatment started, as the lithium-treated spouse has less libidinal strivings. (p. 352)

Although 77 percent of the spouses rated the marriage as considerably improved, only 43 percent of the manic-depressive patients expressed this opinion. Patients may be more sensitive to the loss of positive experiences associated with bipolar illness, whereas their spouses may be more aware of lithium's beneficial effects. Such a possibility would be consistent with the discrepancies in perceptions reported by Targum and colleagues (1981). These results again underscore the importance of sophisticated clinical management and subtle titration of lithium to the lowest possible level consistent with efficacy.

O'Connell and Mayo (1981) studied the effects of lithium treatment on 12 manic-depressive patients and their families. They found that lithium increased the direct care of the children by both patients and spouses, significantly alleviated marital friction, and resulted in increased cooperative planning, communication, and trust.

Holinger and Wolpert (1979) found that the majority (59 percent) of their 56 manic-depressive patients showed improvement in their relationships with spouses, families, or friends as a result of being on lithium. Slightly over one third (39 percent) showed no change. The primary changes observed by the authors were decreases in impulsivity, fragility, and erratic behavior; confidence in relationships increased. The bipolar patients were far more likely than the lithium-treated unipolar patients to demonstrate a change in interpersonal behavior (59 percent and 11 percent, respectively). In a study by Lepkifker and colleagues (1988), psychiatrists' ratings of marital relationships and other interpersonal relationships were significantly higher for the 50 bipolar and 50 unipolar patients (all of whom were euthymic and lithium-treated) than they were for 50 psychiatric controls with personality disorders. There were no significant bipolar–unipolar differences.

Finally, Ruestow and co-workers (1978), in the study reported earlier, suggested that bipolar manic-depressive patients, especially men, could have good marriages if stabilized by lithium. While emphasizing the importance of adjunctive use of marital therapy, they also suggested "that patients be treated with appropriate medication . . . prior to the initiation of marital therapy and that the need for intensive marital therapy be reassessed after the patient's illness has been stabilized."

Sexual Behavior in Manic-Depressive Illness

Again judging from my own experience, the sexual symptoms of the manic state seem to be the most powerful and important of all. . . . The normal inhibitions disappear, and sexual activity, instead of being placed, as in our Western Christian civilization, in opposition to religion, becomes associated with it. This release of the underlying sexual tension . . . seems to me to be the primary and governing factor of all the ecstasies and many other experiences of the manic state. —John Custance, 1952

Changes in sexual desire, thought, and behavior during depression and mania were observed centuries ago. Aretaeus of Cappadocia (150 AD), for example, observed that "a period of lewdness and shamelessness exists with the highest type of [manic] delirium" (Jelliffe, 1931, p. 20). In our century, Kraepelin (1921), Bleuler (1924), Campbell (1953), and Mayer-Gross and colleagues (1955) also have described heightened sexuality during mania and decreased sexuality during depression (see Chapter 2).

Fluctuations in sexual drive are sufficiently important in manic-depressive illness to warrant inclusion as diagnostic criteria in the DSM-III ("sexual indiscretions" for manic episodes, and "decrease in sexual interest or drive" for depressive episodes). Items pertaining to sexual behavior are on most self- and observer-rating instruments for both mania and depression (see Chapter 13). Beigel and colleagues (1971), for example, required nurses to judge 26 items most characteristic of manic behavior, thought, and affect. Of those items, the two pertaining to sex ("Talks about sex" and "Is sexually preoccupied") had high concordance with independent ratings on both a psychiatrists' global mania scale and a nurses' manic-symptom checklist.

The actual data on changes in sexual behavior and thinking during different phases of manic-depressive illness are relatively limited. Quantified observational data are presented in Chapter 2 and can be summarized here. Hypersexuality was observed or reported in 57 percent of manic patients (averaged across seven studies, with a range of values from 25 to 80 percent), and actual nudity or sexual exposure was reported in 29 percent (averaged across three studies, with a range of values from 23 to 33 percent). Akiskal and colleagues (1977) reported that 40 percent of their cyclothymic patients had "episodic or unexplained promiscuity or extramarital affairs." Allison and Wilson (1960) studied the sexual behavior of 24 manic patients using data based on physician observations and on historical information from patients and their relatives. They found no relationship between sexual display during mania and age, religion, duration of illness, previous episodes, or social class. Women were far more sexually provocative and seductive than the men (58 percent and 0 percent, respectively) on a 5-point rating scale. However, men and women were equally likely to have both increased "libidinal drives" and increased frequency of sexual relations. In a total of 78 percent of the patients, the frequency of sexual intercourse substantially increased while manic.

Winokur and colleagues (1969) found that 65 percent of manic episodes were characterized by increased sexuality. In one third (32 percent), it was of a socially approved type, that is, within the marriage or a long-lasting relationship. In 10 percent of the Winokur group's patients, the increased sexuality was in thought or discussion only, and in 11 percent increased sexuality was manifested in socially disapproved behavior. In this last group, patients were homosexually or heterosexually promiscuous or both; in all cases the hypersexuality was clearly associated with being ill. Like those studied by Allison and Wilson (1960), the women (18 percent) in the study by Winokur and co-workers were more likely to have increased sexual contacts (noncoital) than the men (3 percent), but men and women were equally likely to have an increased frequency of intercourse (35 percent and 30 percent, respectively).

Spalt (1975) studied lifetime sexual behavior in 42 patients with unipolar depression, 19 with bipolar illness, 56 with secondary affective illness, and 38 with nonaffective illness. Extramarital sexual experiences were more frequent among bipolar patients (29 percent had more than 10 experiences) than among unipolar patients (12 percent). Bipolar patients (21 percent) also were more likely than unipolar patients (10 percent) to have had more than 10 sexual partners during a lifetime. These figures almost certainly reflect many other behavioral differences between the two groups, including hypersexuality and differences in sexual drive during normal periods, as well as differences in levels of gregariousness, sociability, and interpersonal turmoil.

Jamison and colleagues (1980) studied changes attributed to affective illness in 35 bipolar and 26 unipolar patients. Twice as many women (41 percent) as men (20 percent) reported that sexual intensity was "very much increased" during hypomania; 40 percent of the men and 18 percent of the women stated that sexual intensity during hypomania was "somewhat increased." Women rated increased sexual intensity as the most important or enjoyable change they experienced during hypomania.[26] Bipolar patients were significantly more likely than unipolar patients ($p < 0.01$) to feel that increased sexual intensity was a lasting characteristic attributable to their mood disorders.

Manic-depressive illness also can be associated with decreased sexual drive. For example, Winokur and associates (1969) reported that 63 percent of patients with mixed manic-depressive psychosis reported decreased sexual interest. Indeed, approximately three fourths of bipolar depressed patients experience a loss of sexual interest, 73 percent reported by Winokur and co-workers (1969) and 77 percent by Casper and associates (1985).

Sexual responsiveness can also be dampened in patients taking lithium.[27] Sheard (1971, 1975) and Lion (1975) attributed this to a common effect on aggressive and sexual behaviors, both often occurring together in manic-depressive patients. Lorimy and colleagues (1977) reported that half of their patients on prophylactic lithium experienced troublesome side effects affecting their sexual activities, including decreases in sexual intensity, frequency of sexual drive, and frequency of sexual intercourse. However, patients reported that once intercourse began, there was no decrement in enjoyment or orgasmic ability.

It is unclear what accounts for these lithium-induced changes. Among the possible explanations are lithium-induced hypothyroidism, decreased frequency or intensity of hypomanic episodes, or the direct effect of lithium on the central nervous system mechanisms underlying sexual drive and behavior. Yet another possible reason for these changes is vacillation in interpersonal relationships brought about by lithium, with secondary manifestations in the sexual domain.

Manic-Depressive Illness and the Family

The issue here is not that the family finds that home life [is] made unpleasant by the sick person. . . . The issue is that meaningful existence is threatened. (p. 374) —Erving Goffman, 1969

The families of manic-depressive patients and their environments deserve research and clinical attention because they may influence the development and course of illness and they may serve as predictors of treatment compliance and outcome. Further, studying families gives clinicians an empathetic understanding of what they and the patients themselves experience. Until recently, despite much speculation, very little was known about the family's role in this disorder. Most studies were retrospective, entirely descriptive, and done without comparison groups. Few investigators examined families in the light of lithium's stabilizing effects.

Here we review the studies that have been done, including those based on psychodynamic formulations, those focusing on patients' perceptions about how their illness affects the rest of the family, recent studies of communication factors and their value in predicting the long-term course of bipolar illness, and finally interaction patterns of manic-depressive parents and their children.

Psychodynamic Formulations

Psychoanalytical studies of manic-depressive families have tended to emphasize the role of rigid conformity within the family system (Finley and Wilson, 1951; Wilson, 1951; Cohen et al., 1954). Such writers speculated that the combination of a domineering parent and unrealistically high expectations led to a "walled-in existence" and pervasively deep hostility later manifested as depression and mania.

Cohen and associates (1954), in their classic study of 12 families of manic-depressive patients, stressed conformity and aspiration as key issues differentiating these from normal families:

In every case, the patient's family had felt the social difference keenly and had reacted to it with intense concern and with an effort, first, to improve its acceptability in the community by fitting in with "what the neighbors think" and, second, to improve its social prestige by raising the economic level of the family, or by winning some position of honor or accomplishment. In both these patterns of striving for a better social position, the children of the family played important roles; they were expected to conform to a high standard of good behavior, the standard being based largely on the parents' concept of what the neighbors expected. . . .

In a number of cases, the child who was later to develop a manic-depressive psychosis was selected as the chief carrier of the burden of winning prestige for the family. (p. 114)

The lack of systematic comparison to normal families or to other psychiatrically ill families makes it difficult to generalize from these observations.

Davenport and associates (1979) looked more comprehensively at the structure of six families in which at least one member had been manic-depressive—for three generations in the case of four families and for two generations in the other two. Although an interesting clinical report, like the study by Cohen and co-workers it suffers from several methodological problems, especially a lack of a comparison group and small sample size. Further, the role of lithium is not clearly specified, the study is interpretative rather than observational, and state–trait issues are largely ignored. The observations of Davenport and co-workers are important, however, and the study remains unique in the population and problems examined.

Essentially, these researchers found several recurrent themes among patients and family members: fears related to the heritable aspects of the disease, concerns with absence and loss, problems with multiple parenting, and issues with "domineering, depressed and withholding mothers." Several of their conclusions overlap with those of Cohen and co-workers (1954), but many observations were unique to them. They concluded that manic-depressive families avoided affect and used denial to manage hostility and anxiety. Davenport and colleagues (1979) observed that family members had unrealistic standards of conformity and self-expectations and found it hard to initiate and sustain intimacy apart from the family. Parents appeared to displace their low self-esteem onto their children. According to these investigators, ". . . all efforts for change were resisted" and "a capacity for awareness and expression of needs, as well as a pattern of resolution, also appears lacking or poorly developed." "Spouses and children almost uniformly prefer the affected parent to be depressed rather than manic" (pp. 29-30).

Communication Patterns

The relative disruptiveness of mania and depression to the family lives of 35 bipolar patients was examined by Jamison and colleagues (unpublished data). Mania was seen as much more disruptive to families by the men (47 percent) than by the women (18 percent). Conversely, 40 percent of men and 54 percent of women reported that their depressions were more disruptive to family life. The majority of men (53 percent) saw their mania as the illness phase causing most concern to others; for most women (64 percent), the most negative effects were attributed to depression. Some of these sex differences may stem from the fact that the women patients were predominantly bipolar II, not bipolar I. Both sexes, but especially men, felt that depression was much more likely than mania to promote family closeness or unity.

Mayo and co-workers (1979), in their study of manic-depressive families, investigated the communication patterns between spouses and their effects on children:

The relationship between the spouses proved critical to childrearing patterns. The balance between mutuality/isolation in the husband-wife relationship was strained by the birth of successive children. Many of the spouses of patients tended to view manic or depressive episodes as willful abdications of responsibility or as manifestations of weakness of character and self-indulgence that had to be met with a firm display of power and control. The unspoken but forcefully communicated dictum to the child that mommy (or daddy) is "sick" through some fault of his or her own thrust the child on the horns of the dilemma: the "sick" parent was lovable but irresponsible, while the well parent was responsible but also to be feared. Thus a pattern was set in which caretaking roles were vague, loyalties were tenuous, and affection and approval were dependent on degree of health and responsibility. (p. 1538)

Miklowitz and co-workers (1988), in a study of 23 bipolar manic-depressive patients and their families, tried to determine the extent to which negative family communication factors, such as those measured by expressed emotion (EE, parental emotional attitude toward the patient) and affective style (AS, emotional–verbal interaction with the patient), predict the longitudinal course of bipolar illness.

The present findings suggest that the affective climate of the family to which a recently manic bipolar patient returns following hospitalization is predictive of his or her subsequent course of illness and subsequent functioning. Our findings are consistent with those reported by Vaughn and colleagues and Doane et al., who found that negative family attitudes (EE) and interactional behaviors (AS) are important predictors of the short-term course of schizophrenic illness.

These two measures of the intrafamilial affective climate were unrelated to each other in our sample and were most powerful as conjoint predictors of outcome. Interestingly, EE and AS were interactive rather than additive predictors of patient outcome: If either indicator of a high level of family stress was present, relapse was highly likely (15/16, or 94%), whereas only those patients from families rated low on both family factors had a low relapse rate (1/6 or 17%). (p. 229)

Although this investigation did not control for the mood and diagnostic status of family members, which are critical in a genetically based illness, it is an important contribution to the literature because of its systematic nature and longitudinal perspective.

Gibson (1959) followed up on the earlier Chestnut Lodge studies (Cohen et al., 1954) by comparing family backgrounds and early life experiences in 27 manic-depressive and 17 schizophrenic patients. He found that manic-depressive families were more characterized by accentuated concerns for social approval and prestige, often coexisting in a background of intense envy and competitiveness. It is unclear how much this pattern represents psychopathology and how much it simply reflects a family situation where, unlike that of schizophrenia, competition and achievement are more realistic expectations of life.

Manic-Depressive Illness and Parenting

In this section, we focus on general parental factors that might influence the development of children of manic-depressive parents. Clearly, it is not always easy to separate genetic factors, manifested in childhood or adolescent expressions of affective illness, from true effects of the psychological and social impact of bipolar parenting. Given the lack of complete penetrance, the combination of both environmental and genetic influences is not only the most probable but also the most conceptually interesting likelihood. High-risk studies of bipolar offspring—early symptoms, natural course, predictors, and so on—are discussed in Chapter 8; family and other genetic studies are covered in Chapter 15.

In addition to the pivotal issue of attribution of causality—that is, the relative influences of the psychological environment and genetic predisposition—many methodological problems exist: lack of prospective design, short follow-up periods, lack of appropriate comparison groups, small sample sizes (the Radke-Yarrow studies, which comprise a significant proportion of the relevant research literature, are based on seven children), lack of ascertainment of degree of parental impairment (and degree of responsiveness to treatment), alternative sources of emotional support (e.g., from well siblings, other members of the immediate or extended family, friends, nonfamily member adults), personal resources (e.g., intelligence, emotional resilience, or other temperamental variables), and a surprising lack of control for assortative mating (in the NIMH studies, five of the seven spouses who had manic-depressive illness were themselves diagnosed as having unipolar major depressive disorder). Adoption studies would be useful in sorting out at least some of the etiological issues of manic-depressive parental influence on childhood development.

Additional problems remain. Eisenbruch (1983) emphasized the diagnostic nonspecificity of emotional turmoil in families and highlighted the importance of the child's developmental level in terms of parental impact. He also pointed out the necessity for precise definition of the phenomena to which the child is ostensibly responding; for example, extended separation from the parent or ongoing depression in the parent.

The difficulties experienced by depressed women in fulfilling their maternal roles has been researched extensively by Weissman and colleagues.[28] In comparing 35 unipolar depressed and 27 normal mothers, Weissman found that mothers, during an acute depressive episode, were less involved with their children, had impaired communication and increased friction, guilt, and resentment, were overprotective, more rejecting, irritable, and distant (Weissman et al., 1972; Weissman and Paykel, 1974). The depressed women also reported greater degrees of discord with their children than with their friends, colleagues, or other members of their family. Increased hostility by depressed mothers toward their children has been observed by several investigators (Fabian and Donohue, 1956; Rutter, 1966; Weissman and Paykel, 1974).

Many areas of childrearing are affected by maternal depression: degree and type of involvement in the school, family and social lives of children, neglect of physical care and lessened involvement in play activities, lack of time and emotional resources to adequately deal with the needs of children, often leading to children discussing their problems with others, or not at all, and maternal self-preoccupation (Weissman, 1979).

Few empirical studies exist on parental deficits specific to manic-depressive parents, although several authors have made clinical observations and speculations. Anthony (1975b), for example, describes the emotional environment created by a manic-depressive parent:

. . . cycles of omnipotence and impotence, of high and low self-esteem, of surplus and depleted energy, of adequate and defective reality testing, and of optimism and pessimism, and, above all, the surprising variations in mood. (p. 288)

Anthony suggests that, under these circumstances, children of manic-depressive parents suffer from inconsistency in their emotional upbringing, problems of identification with the ill parent, and the tendency to become "magic helpers," that is, to try and exert unrealistic levels of influence over their parent's chaotic world.

Zahn-Waxler and colleagues (1984) hypothesize that problems in parent–child bonding occur in manic-depressive families because of the lack of parental consistency and stability, as well as the existence of emotional extremes in sadness, excitability, irritability, and other manifestations of "disregulation of affect." The same authors, in their follow-up study of seven children of bipolar parents (Zahn-Waxler et al., 1988), characterized the families as disorganized, unpredictable, and "alienated." Davenport and colleagues (1984), in a study of the same families, found that mothers in the index families, when compared with those in normal control families, were less attentive to their children's health needs, were more overprotective, less organized, and less active with their children, were more unhappy and tense, demonstrated greater negative affect toward their children, and were less consistent in their behavior. Again, however, interpretation of these findings is difficult because of the extremely small sample size and high rate of psychiatric illness in the parent who was not manic-depressive.

Patterns of attachment in 2- and 3-year-olds were studied by Radke-Yarrow and colleagues (1985) in 99 children of 14 bipolar depressed mothers, 42 unipolar depressed mothers, 12 mothers with minor depression, and 37 with no history of affective disorder. Children of normal mothers showed more than twice the level of security of attachment than children of mothers with bipolar depression. Assortative mating was relatively frequent in the couples, and the authors concluded that:

In families in which mothers were depressed, depression in the father did not increase the likelihood of anxious attachment between mother and child. However, if mothers with a major affective disorder were without a husband in the household, risk of an insecure mother-child attachment was significantly increased. (p. 884)

Perris and colleagues (1985) found that Italian bipolar and unipolar patients in remission perceived both their fathers and mothers as demonstrating significantly less emotional warmth than did a comparison group of 200 healthy controls. No significant differences were found on measures of rejection and overprotection. The same results did not obtain for a group of Swedish bipolar patients, although the unipolar patients again reported a significantly lower degree of perceived parental emotional warmth (Perris et al., 1986). Joyce (1984b) found no significant differences between manic-depressive and general practice patients on a retrospective measure of the care and protection experienced with each parent during the first 16 years of the patients' lives.

Divorce or separation of the biological parents has been associated in several studies with an increased risk of affective illness or other significant psychopathology in children of manic-depressive parents (Kuyler et al., 1980; Lavori et al., 1988), as has a lack of marital adjustment in the well parent, especially the father (LaRoche et al., 1985, 1987). Older current age of the parent, duration of illness, and younger age of exposure to parental illness were also correlated with less favorable outcome in high-risk children. Sex, social class, number of hospitalizations, age of illness onset, and marital adjustment score in the mother were not so correlated (LaRoche et al., 1985). The authors stress the role of the father in providing important support if the mother is affectively ill.

SUMMARY

The relationship between affective illness and personality is a complicated one. Methodological problems make the determination of what is illness and what is temperament even more difficult. Several general conclusions can be made, however.

During acute depression, bipolar patients show less neuroticism, less anxiety, greater social desirability response set, but less impulse control than do unipolar patients. During remission, bipolar patients do not differ from unipolar patients on measures of neuroticism but score higher on tests of extraversion.

In studies of manic-depressive illness, measures of neuroticism, self-esteem, and introversion are more consistently state dependent than are measures of impulsivity, rigidity, obsessionality, and reflectiveness. When bipolar patients in remission are compared with normal control groups, there are no significant differences on most personality variables, including neuroticism and extraversion. Personality profiles of remitted bipolar patients are, for the most part, more normal than those of remitted unipolar patients.

Consistent with these observations is the finding that personality disorders, or Axis-II diagnoses, are relatively less prevalent in patients who have manic-depressive illness.

Lithium, in addition to its direct effect on personality through ameliorating the underlying affective illness, has at least subtle effects on personality in both normal and manic-depressive subjects. These include increased passivity, decreased social involvement and activity, decreased initiative and impulsivity, and increased mood stability. The dearth of normative data, especially data on the long-term use of lithium, renders these findings tentative, however. Personality predictors of lithium responsivity also remain inconclusive.

Interpersonal aspects of both mania and depression are pervasive, usually profound. Fluctuating levels of sociability, impulsivity, dependency, hostility, and sexuality are part and parcel of manic-depressive illness. Marriages and families are strongly affected and can, in turn, affect the course and outcome of the illness. Lithium and other treatments have radically changed the nature of these relationships.

NOTES

1. Cited in Schauffler, 1945
2. From Allport, 1961, p. 9.
3. For general reviews of these and related issues, see Von Zerssen (1977, 1982) and Hirschfeld and Klerman (1979).
4. These differences have been well summarized by Hall and Lindzey (1970): the relative importance of the uniqueness of the individual (the idiographic–nomothetic controversy), whether or not man should be viewed as possessing purposive or teleological qualities, the importance of group membership, the relative importance of conscious and unconscious determinants of behavior, the number of motivational concepts, the importance of the principles of reward and association, the relative emphasis on stable structures or the process of change in personality, the functional independence of personality structure at any particular point in time, the relative importance of genetic factors in determining behavior, and the relative importance of early developmental experiences.
5. Eysenck, 1959, 1970; Guilford, 1959a; Eysenck and Eysenck, 1971; Cattell, 1973; Von Zerssen, 1982.
6. Earlier known as the Maudsley Personality Inventory.
7. Thus, Kraepelin (1921), like Reiss (1910) before him, delineated four fundamental types of temperament: *depressive, manic, irritable*, and *cyclothymic*. Kretschmer (1936) stressed the overlap among these personality types in the prepsychotic, *cycloid personality* of manic-depressive patients: ". . . they form layers or patterns in individual cases, arranged in the most varied combinations." Campbell (1953), too, described a cycloid personality, which could occur in one of three forms—*hypomanic, depressive*, and *cyclothymic*—"with innumerable gradations and mixtures between the three." He, like Kraepelin, regarded all of these personality types as ". . . part of the same disease process, and that any one of these may change into any other." Leonhard (1957), who separated major affective illness into unipolar and bipolar types, also regarded many personality patterns in manic-depressive patients as subclinical, or "diluted," forms of the primary illness itself. Mayer-Gross and colleagues (1955) derived personality topologies similar to those of Kraepelin, Kretschmer, and Campbell: *cyclothymic* (sociable, good-hearted, kind, and easygoing), *hyperthymic* (elated, humorous, lively, and hot-tempered), and *hypothymic* (quiet, calm, serious, and gentle). Rowe and Daggett (1954) and Von Zerssen (1977) summarized premorbid personality traits of manic and depressed patients, which are quite consistent with the earlier clinical topologies.

8. Dooley (1921) wrote:
   The behavior found in the manic attack, in which the patient throws himself with almost equal vim into every possible avenue of expression, is in itself a defense reaction. By thus taking the offensive he keeps himself safe from the approach of the painful thought or feeling which is usually a realization of some failure or degradation, or fundamental inferiority of his own. When he is depressed his defense is no longer possible and he is weighed down by the pain of the acknowledged defect. (p. 167)

   More specifically, Schwartz (1961) described the dynamic purpose for hyperactive behavior and grandiose thought:
   The hypermotility in mania may have a twofold purpose. First, it may serve as a method for distracting attention from the perception of deprivation; second, it is a diffuse and multidirectional effort to obtain pleasure, in which some realistic basis for the denial of deprivation may be grasped. . . . Grandiosity is a defense by denial against emptiness, however . . . may even represent, additionally, an intellectual attempt at a further regression, in the service of the ego, to the stage of omnipotence. (p. 244)

   Grotstein (1986) has described the manic mechanism of denial in terms of power and self-regulation:
   The psychical state which is set up to regulate this primal state of powerlessness is that of a fraudulent state of power, including that of a severe superego and/or compulsive and/or hypomanic defenses which seek to create an artificial "floor" over a "floorless" psyche.

9. This concept was explained in a different way by Arieti (1959):
   The receptiveness to others and willingness to introject the others determines, at this early age, some aspects of the personality of the patient. He tends to become an "extrovert"; at the same time he tends to become a conformist, willing to accept what he is given by his surroundings (not only in material things but also in terms of habits and values). (p. 431)

10. Dooley (1921):
    The personality of the manic depressive individual also presents an obstacle. Those who manifest frequent manic attacks are likely to be headstrong, self-sufficient, know-it-all types of persons who will not take suggestions or yield to direction. They are "doers" and managers, and will get the upper hand of the analyst and everyone else around them if given the opportunity. . . . (p. 39)
    The manic-depressive character is extroverted, he tries always to relate himself to his environment, he minimizes the subjective element and makes use of every object in the range of his senses. (p. 166)

    Wilson (1951) further discussed the therapist's problems in treating the manic-depressive patient:
    From the psychiatrist's point of view he is uninteresting because he is hard to get at. He is friendly and superficially cooperative, but soon personality investigation ceases because the patient refuses to be self-analytical. When the patient is depressed or manic his illness seems to explain his unapproachableness, and when he is well he will have nothing to do with you except in a very superficial way. This impenetrable shell is characteristic of persons with this illness and sets them

apart from those having other forms of depression. (p. 362)

Cohen and colleagues (1954) described the manic-depressive personality as dependent, even during states of normal functioning:

> We see, then, in the adult cyclothymic, a person who is apparently well adjusted between attacks, although he may show minor mood swings or be chronically overactive or chronically mildly depressed. He is conventionally well-behaved and frequently successful, and he is hardworking and conscientious; indeed, at times his overconscientiousness and scrupulousness lead to his being called obsessional. He is typically involved in one or more relationships of extreme dependence, in which, however, he does not show the obsessional's typical need to control the other person for the sake of power, but instead seeks to control the other person in the sense of swallowing him up. His inner feeling, when he allows himself to notice it, is one of emptiness and need. He is extremely stereotyped in his attitudes and opinions, tending to take over the opinions of the person in his environment whom he regards as an important authority. Again this contrasts with the outward conformity but subtle rebellion of the obsessional. It should be emphasized that the dependency feelings are largely out of awareness in states of well-being and also in the manic phase; in fact, these people frequently take pride in being independent. (p. 120)

11. Indeed, one can question whether projective tests during mania can really reflect anything about personality, given the impact of the psychoses on cognition and perception, as described in Chapter 11.
12. Levy and Beck, 1934; Rorschach, 1942; Schmidt and Fonda, 1954; Spielberger et al., 1966.
13. Frey, 1977; Hirschfeld and Klerman, 1979; Liebowitz et al., 1979; Bech et al., 1980; Jamison et al., unpublished data.
14. Jensen, 1958; Sigal et al., 1958; McGuire et al., 1963; Levinson and Meyer, 1965; Ingham, 1966.
15. Frey, 1977; Hirschfeld and Klerman, 1979; Liebowitz et al., 1979; Bech et al., 1980; Hirschfeld, 1985; Hirschfeld et al., 1986; Jamison et al., unpublished data.
16. Other personality studies using various psychological measures also have looked at bipolar patients and normal groups. They include Becker, 1960; Becker and Altrocchi, 1968; Hofmann, 1973; Marsella and Murray, 1975; MacVane et al., 1978; Hirschfeld and Klerman, 1979; Lumry et al., 1982; Matussek and Feil, 1983; Mandel et al., 1984; Winters and Neale, 1985; and Hirschfeld, 1985.
17. Frey, 1977; Hirschfeld and Klerman, 1979; Liebowitz et al., 1979; Abou-Saleh and Coppen, 1984; Jamison et al., unpublished data.
18. Perris, 1971; Frey, 1977; Bech et al., 1980; Matussek and Feil, 1983; Hirschfeld, 1985; Hirschfeld et al., 1986; Jamison et al., unpublished data.
19. Other personality studies using a variety of psychological scales comparing remitted bipolar and unipolar patients include Perris, 1966c,e; Hoffman, 1973; Blackburn, 1974; Donnelly et al., 1976; Strandman, 1978.
20. Perris, 1966; Donnelly and Murphy, 1973, 1974; Strandman, 1978; Hirschfeld and Klerman, 1979; Von Zerssen, 1982.
21. House and Martin, 1975; Anath et al., 1979; Kerry and Orme, 1979; Smigan, 1985.
22. Cited in Hamilton 1982, p. 214.
23. Published in *The Times* (London), January 24, 1986.
24. Ludwig and Ables (1974) studied the interactions of a 45-year-old bipolar man and his 38-year-old wife over 33 weeks over which the patient experienced one episode each of depression, mania, and hypomania and two normal periods. Both patient and spouse made daily ratings of the patient's moods and of one another's positive and negative attributes. The authors concluded:

> . . . it appears as though the mood swings of the patient and spouse are concurrent—namely, the spouse becomes upset when the patient experiences any major mood shifts, either a high or low, and feels more tender and cheerful during his normalthymic periods. Second, the findings corroborate the notion that it is mania that is the most disruptive of the marital relationship. Not only is the spouse upset during this time, but in contrast to the depressed state, the patient comes to view her in far more negative terms, thereby introducing more overt friction into the relationship. (p. 417)

25. Demers and Davis, 1971; Ruestow et al., 1978; Frank et al., 1981; O'Connell and Mayo, 1981.
26. Stoddard and co-workers (1977) studied eight affective episodes in a 39-year-old rapid-cycling woman. They collected systematic behavioral data twice a day and observed that she became sexually provocative during mania. Conversely, a significant predictor of her switch into depression was a decrease in sexual preoccupation ($p < 0.05$).
27. In addition to references in this paragraph, see Demers and Davis (1971).
28. Weissman et al., 1971, 1972; Weissman and Klerman, 1973; Weissman and Paykel, 1974.

13

Assessment of Manic and Depressive States

INTRODUCTION

Standardized measures of mania and depression, by minimizing differences in the way that clinicians record their observations, provide a common language and standard for a wide variety of observers in very different settings. Such measures are used in determining the severity of illness, assessing and predicting treatment response, making differential diagnoses and delineating illness subtypes, and ascertaining the incidence of different types of affective states. Quantitative rating scales can be especially important in longitudinal studies (e.g., to describe the natural course of the illness and the individual depressive and manic episodes), identifying the progression and resolution of symptom patterns, studying euthymic states in bipolar patients, and correlating manic and depressive states with other aspects of behavior, cognition, personality, and biochemistry.

Several general types of measurements have evolved to classify and quantify change in affective states. The major categories, delineated by Von Zerssen and Cording (1978), are: observer ratings, usually made by clinicians, self-ratings, made by patients, analyses of behavior (including linguistic analyses of speech or written produc-

tions), and objective measurements, either of spontaneous activities (physical activity) or of reactions within a standardized situation (objective psychometric tests). This chapter necessarily is limited to an overview of self-rating and observer rating scales constructed to measure manic, depressive, and cyclothymic states; analyses of behavior and various objective measurements are discussed in Chapters 11 and 12.[1] Measurement issues specific to particular topics are covered in the relevant chapters. For example, measurement of childhood and adolescent conditions is discussed in Chapter 8, diagnostic assessment is covered in Chapter 5, and measures of personality are covered in Chapter 12. Only those rating scales that are generic and have been most widely used or replicated are presented here.[2]

Methodological Issues

Several factors can interfere with accurate measurement of depressive or manic states. The problem of defining clinical populations and diagnostic criteria clearly affects the range, distribution, and interpretation of rating scale data. Factors that can confound the interpretation of measurement include seasonal, diurnal, menstrual, and other cyclic variations. As discussed in detail later, mixed states also confound the utility of bipolar scales—those constructed on the assumption that mania and depression are, in all respects, opposite states. The specificity of scales also can be problematic, since it has been demonstrated that depressed patients, although distinguishable from normal populations on most scales, may not be readily distinguished from other clinical populations, such as general medical patients, schizophrenics, or other psychiatric patients (Mendels et al., 1972b; Murphy et al., 1982b). Additionally, Snaith (1981) criticized the proliferation of rating scales, lack of follow-through with the requisite reliability and validity studies, and the often seemingly arbitrary use of particular rating scales.

The importance of recognizing relative strengths and weaknesses in different types of measurement has been emphasized by Raskin and Crook (1976) and by Murphy and colleagues (1982b). For example, rating scales completed by nursing staff often are the most sensitive in detecting specific behavior and drug side effects, whereas mood effects are usually most effectively portrayed through self-ratings completed by patients. Meaningful measurement often requires the use of more than one type of rating scale.

Other problems in assessing manic-depressive illness include a lack of focus on those aspects of depression that are most specific to bipolar illness (see Chapter 3),[3] and a lack of consistency in training criteria and the level of clinical experience required for raters. The advantages and disadvantages of the two major methods for measuring manic and depressive states—self-rating and observer rating—are presented in the following sections.

Self-Rating of Affective States

There are obvious advantages in using self-ratings by affectively ill patients. First, as Murphy and colleagues (1982b) point out, patients are in a unique position to provide information about their feelings and moods—key symptoms in any assessment of mood disorders. The value of self-ratings was confirmed by Raskin and associates (1970), who found that a mood scale completed by patients was one of the best measures of significant treatment effects. The patient is also, for the most part, free of the theoretical biases affecting the development and use of observer ratings and

"has access to the totality of his experience, rather than only a subset of behavior that the observer views" (Murphy et al., 1982b). For example, when Zealley and Aitken (1969) analyzed independent recordings made by patients and nursing staff, they concluded:

. . . the patient's gradual swing from depression, through normality to hypomania may be discerned by the nurse only after several days' delay, resulting in a "phase shift" between the patient and nurse analogue score curves. A second tendency in other patients was for the nurse to be patently unaware of the patient's feeling state day by day, indicated by a clustering of nurse's line scores around the centre point.

In both these situations, it is clear that the patient was the better guide to his affective state than the nurse. Since psychiatric treatment is largely directed towards symptom relief, due weight should be given to the validity and immediacy of the patient's record. (p. 995)

Figure 13-1, reproduced from their report, illustrates the lag between a patient's self-rating and a nurse's ratings of the patient. There are several

Figure 13-1. Visual Analogue Scale scores obtained from nursing staff and from patient with manic-depressive illness (adapted from Zealley and Aitken, 1969).

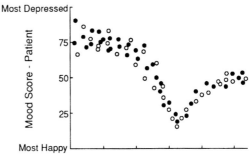

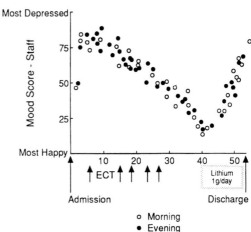

practical advantages in using patient self-report measures: They require relatively little professional time and expense, can be rapidly completed, and can be used as repeated measures (Hamilton, 1976; Murphy et al., 1982b).

Self-ratings have obvious disadvantages, however. Patients must be literate, cooperative, not too depressed or too manic, and able to concentrate (Hamilton, 1976; Murphy et al., 1982b; Snaith, 1981). Other difficulties derive from patients' idiosyncratic interpretations of the language of rating scales, their highly variable degrees of insight, and the scales' inability to clearly differentiate between symptoms (e.g., mood and energy changes) when they occur simultaneously (Pinard and Tetreault, 1974; Snaith, 1981). Finally, there is some evidence that severely depressed patients tend to underestimate the severity of their psychopathology (Paykel and Prusoff, 1973; Donovan and O'Leary, 1976). Prusoff and colleagues (1972a) assessed 200 depressed patients with semistructured clinical interviews and self-reports. They found that self-report ratings, although useful in measuring the presence or absence of symptoms, were not a reliable index of their severity. Self-report and clinically obtained measures were far more highly correlated at follow-up than during the acute episode. In a related report, Prusoff and co-workers (1972b) examined the nature of the discrepancy in scores derived from self-ratings and clinical ratings. They found that patients who rated symptoms higher than clinicians did tended to be younger, less severely depressed, and more hysterical. Conversely, those who minimized their symptoms tended to be older, more severely depressed, and obsessive. In another study, however, Rush and colleagues (1986b) gave self-administered and clinician-administered versions of the Inventory for Depressive Symptomatology to a mixed group of unipolar and bipolar depressed patients and they found that total scores for the two samples were nearly identical and suggest that "self-reported symptom severity may be fairly reliable when each item has clear anchors and items are unconfounded" (p.78).

Observer Rating of Affective States

In a summary of the advantages of observer ratings, Hamilton (1976) included the observer's ability to:

. . . evaluate the intensity of any one symptom by comparing it against the background of experience which he has . . . penetrate the mask which the patient holds up, whether deliberately or unintentionally . . . rate and assess certain manifestations of illness which the patient would find impossible or extremely difficult to do. For example, . . . loss of insight, . . . mild retardation, . . . hypochondriasis and delusions. An observer can rate all grades of severity of an illness, . . . whereas a patient can be too ill to complete a questionnaire. (p. 158)

The drawbacks of observer ratings, implicit in the earlier discussion of the advantages of self-ratings, were discussed at length by both Lorr (1974) and Bech (1981). Lorr noted that variability in the degree of the patient's disturbance from one interview to another affects both self-ratings and observer ratings. Furthermore, observers may differ in efficiency and manner in relating to the patient, and rating scales may be ambiguously worded or require too much inference. Bech (1981) stressed sources of variance in observer rating, including the differences that occur because information is not gathered from the same sources, in the observers' perceptions when the same phenomena are observed differently by different observers, and in the terminology used when the same phenomena are observed but the results are couched in different terminologies. Variable mood of the observer affects ratings of some items (Bunney and Hamburg, 1963), especially anger and anxiety ratings, which can be distorted if the observer projects his own feeling state onto the patient.

ASSESSMENT OF MANIC STATES

Self-Rating Scales

Self-rating scales are, for obvious reasons, rarely used to measure manic states. Poor judgment, uncooperativeness, cognitive impairment, distractibility, and denial combine to make meaningful measurement essentially impossible. Platman and co-workers (1969), in a study reported in Chapter 12, found a very low correlation (0.35) between self-ratings made by patients during manic episodes and ratings made by staff. After recovery, however, the patients' recall of mania was highly correlated (0.95) with staff perceptions. Murphy and colleagues (1982b) concluded that "some ability to discriminate subjective states, at least on the MMPI hypomania scale, is maintained during mania" (p. 375). However, the MMPI (Minnesota Multiphasic Personality Inventory; Hathaway and McKinley, 1951) is a measure of personality, not a rating scale.

If there is a use for self-rating scales in mania, it is clearly for the less severe, or hypomanic, end of the severity continuum. One such scale is the M-D Scale, developed by Plutchik and associates (1970b). Its 16 items, demonstrated to discriminate hypomania from normality, use a yes/no format. Sample items include: "I have boundless energy," "Lately I feel like breaking things," and "I've been telephoning a lot of friends recently."

There is little reliability or validity information available.

Observer Rating Scales

Manic State (Beigel) Scale

One of the first systematic observer rating scales to be developed for the measurement of mania was constructed at the National Institute of Mental Health (Beigel et al., 1971; Murphy et al., 1974b). The scale is made up of 26 items, rated from 0 to 5 on both frequency and intensity dimensions. It was designed to be used by a trained research nursing staff (Table 13-1). The 11

Table 13-1. Manic-State Rating Scale

Part A - Frequency (How much of the time?)	The Patient	Part B - Intensity (How intense is it?)
0 to 5		0 to 5
_____	1. Looks depressed	_____
_____	*2. Is talking	_____
_____	*3. Moves from one place to another	_____
_____	4. Makes threats	_____
_____	*5. Has poor judgment	_____
_____	6. Dresses inappropriately	_____
_____	7. Looks happy and cheerful	_____
_____	8. Seeks out others	_____
_____	*9. Is distractible	_____
_____	10. Has grandiose ideas	_____
_____	*11. Is irritable	_____
_____	12. Is combative or destructive	_____
_____	13. Is delusional	_____
_____	14. Verbalizes depressive feelings	_____
_____	*15. Is active	_____
_____	*16. Is argumentative	_____
_____	17. Talks about sex	_____
_____	*18. Is angry	_____
_____	19. Is careless about dress and grooming	_____
_____	*20. Has diminished impulse control	_____
_____	21. Verbalizes feelings of well-being	_____
_____	22. Is suspicious	_____
_____	23. Makes unrealistic plans	_____
_____	*24. Demands contact with others	_____
_____	25. Is sexually preoccupied	_____
_____	*26. Jumps from one subject to another	_____

* = core feature of mania

Adapted from Beigel et al., 1971

starred items were found to be core features of mania—elements present in all patients and most characteristic of manic severity. Reliability and validity data are good, and the evidence suggests that the scale can be easily taught to new nursing staff. On the other hand, the Manic State Scale has been criticized as being too extensive to be practical. It is also thought to have inadequately defined items and scale steps, to require too much time to complete, and to exclude certain core features of mania, such as sleep changes (Petterson et al., 1973; Tyrer and Shopsin, 1982).

Petterson Scale

Attempting to develop a shorter but still reliable rating scale for mania, Petterson and colleagues (1973) devised a seven-item mania scale, using a 5-point severity system. The behavior assessed includes motor activity, pressure of speech, flight of ideas, noisiness, aggressiveness, orientation, and elevated mood. As with the other scales that measure only mania, the Petterson Scale is flawed both theoretically and empirically by not assessing mixed states (simultaneously existing manic and depressed states). Although the Petterson Scale rates fewer symptoms of mania than the Beigel Scale does, its measures of severity are far more precisely defined, and because of its relative brevity, it can be readministered easily to obtain serial ratings. The interrater reliability is good, but several salient aspects of mania, such as sleep and work disturbances, are not assessed. Validity measures have not been presented.

Mania (Young) Rating Scale

Young and colleagues (1978) sought a mania rating scale broader than the Petterson Scale but "shorter and more explicit in its rating of item severity" than the Beigel Scale. To this end, they devised an 11-item measure, using a 5-point scale of severity, modeled on the Hamilton Depression Rating Scale. They based their choice of items on published descriptions of the core symptoms of mania—those cutting across the entire spectrum of illness severity. Ratings are based on subjective reports by patients and on behavioral observations by the clinician made during the interview. Items assessed during the 15- to 30-minute interview include elevated mood, increased mo-

tor activity (energy), sexual interest, sleep changes, irritability, speech (rate and amount), language–thought disorder, disruptive and aggressive behavior, appearance, and insight. The authors report that the scale is a reliable, valid, and sensitive measure of mania. Unfortunately, however, it has not yet been widely used by others or extensively compared with other scales.

Bech-Rafaelsen Mania Scale

The main purpose of the Bech-Rafaelsen Scale, according to its authors, is to "cover relevant items of the whole affective spectrum of manic-melancholic states" by using it in conjunction with the Hamilton Depression Scale (Bech et al., 1979a). There are 11 items, rated on a 5-point scale, with highly specific ratings of severity; for example, a score of 1 on the sleep item represents a reduction of sleep by 25 percent, and a score of 2 represents a reduction by 50 percent. To control for diurnal variation in mood and behavior, the investigators specified that the 15- to 30-minute interview should always take place at a fixed hour. The scale items are motor activity, verbal activity, flight of thoughts, voice/noise level, hostility/destructiveness, mood (feelings of well-being), self-esteem, contact with others, sleep changes, sexual interest, and work activities. Data demonstrating the scale's adequate interrater reliability and a high degree of item homogeneity are presented in the article by Bech's group (1986).

Manic Diagnostic and Severity Scale

Secunda and colleagues (1985), in the National Institute of Mental Health Collaborative Study of Depression, aggregated items from physician- and nurse-rated instruments to create the Manic Diagnostic Severity Scale (MADS). The two subscales taken from physician-rated scales—the SADS-C Scale 17 (Spitzer and Endicott, 1978) and the Global Severity Scale (Katz and Itil, 1974)—correspond, respectively, to the elation–grandiose index and the paranoid–destructive indices proposed by Beigel and Murphy (1971a). Two factors derived from the nurse-rated Affective Disorder Rating Scale (Murphy et al., 1982a) also draw on items designed to measure these two major subtypes of manic symptoms. The MADS subtests measure elevated mood, sleep and energy changes, grandiosity, guardedness, anger, disturbances in insight and judgment, negativism, restlessness, impulsivity, and distractibility. Detailed reliability and validity data have not yet been published.

Two other rating scales for mania have been published. The Modified Manic State Rating Scale (Blackburn et al., 1977; Loudon et al., 1977) comprises 28 items and uses a 6-point rating scale. Information is derived from interviews and data from nursing staff and case notes. The authors found good validity when using a global rating scale as an independent measure. Further, the scale was highly reliable when used in a structured interview by several independent raters. As its name implies, the scale is based largely on the earlier Manic State Scale developed by Beigel and Murphy. The 17-item Shopsin-Gershon Social Behavior Checklist, designed for both inpatients and outpatients, uses a 5-point measure of severity (Shopsin, 1979). The checklist is unusual in containing several quite specific behavioral changes characteristic of mania (e.g., litigious behavior, excessive spending and use of telephones, wanting to divorce spouse). Unfortunately, no reliability or validity data have been presented.

Williams and colleagues (1987) developed a Hypomania Interview Guide for Seasonal Affective Disorder that is based on the Hypomania Rating Scale (Rosenthal and Wehr, unpublished), the Criteria for a Hyperthymic Period (Depue, 1987), and the Structured Clinical Interview for DSM-III (Spitzer et al., 1984). Designed to supplement the related depression scales designed by this group (discussed later in this chapter), this scale is still in the preliminary stages of development.

Several general rating scales measure features of mania even though they were not developed specifically for that purpose. These scales include the Inpatient Multidimensional Psychiatric Scale, Brief Psychiatric Rating Scale, and the Clinical Global Inventory. The Differential Diagnostic Scales, Bellevue Differential Inventory, and Schedule for Affective Disorders and Schizophrenia, devised for differentiating mania from schizophrenia and not directly relevant to the measurement of mania per se, are not reviewed here.

ASSESSMENT OF DEPRESSIVE STATES

Self-Rating Scales

Beck Depression Inventory

The Beck Depression Inventory (BDI) is the most widely used self-rating scale of depression. Developed by Beck and colleagues (1961), the scale consists of 21 items, each containing a series of statements with content ranging in severity from not depressive to severely depressive. Patients select the items that correspond most to their current clinical states. The items include assessments of mood, guilt, irritability, social withdrawal, indecisiveness, fatigability, sleep and appetite disorders, and loss of libido. The following sample item concerning suicidal ideation illustrates the range of severity assessed:

0. I don't have any thoughts of harming myself
1. I have thoughts of harming myself but I would not carry them out
2a. I feel I would be better off dead
2b. I feel my family would be better off if I were dead
3a. I have definite plans about committing suicide
3b. I would kill myself if I could

The BDI emphasizes the mood and cognitive features of depression, but it provides little assessment of the more somatic symptoms. For example, there are no items assessing hypersomnia, diurnal variations, psychomotor agitation or retardation, or weight gain. Although sleep and appetite are covered, only the loss of each is scored, making the items unsuitable for many depressed bipolar patients. The BDI correlates reasonably well with global ratings of depression made by physicians (0.62, Metcalfe and Goldman, 1965) and with the Hamilton Depression Scale (0.68–0.75, Bailey and Coppen, 1976; Schwab et al., 1967), the D scale from the MMPI, and the Zung Depression Scale (Beck and Beamesderfer, 1974; Bech et al., 1975), although these correlational studies have focused on nonbipolar patients.

Zung Self-Rating Depression Scale

The Zung Self-Rating Depression Scale, a 20-item scale, with a 4-point scale of severity, measures somatic, psychological, and mood aspects of depression. It is a modified version of the earlier Zung Depression Scale (Zung, 1965, 1974). To an item such as, "I have trouble sleeping through the night," the patient is expected to indicate which of the following responses is most appropriate: "None or a little of the time," "Some of the time," "Good part of the time," or "Most or all of the time." Note that a graded response applies only to frequency, not to the extent of sleep loss. Further, the scale does not rate hypersomnia, a frequent symptom among patients with bipolar depression.

The Zung Scale, which does not correlate highly with the Hamilton Depression Scale (Murphy et al., 1982b), has been criticized on the grounds that depressed patients find it hard to judge the degree and frequency of their symptoms, and endogenous symptoms are underrepresented (Rush et al., 1986b). Hamilton (1988) also reports that a major shortcoming of the Zung Scale is that it is relatively insensitive to clinical improvement following treatment (Rickels et al., 1968; Feighner et al., 1984).

Carroll Rating Scale

The Carroll Rating Scale was developed to closely parallel in item content the observer-scored Hamilton Depression Scale (Carroll et al., 1981; Feinberg et al., 1981a; Smouse et al., 1981). The inventory consists of 17 general item groupings, with either five or three statements representing varying degrees of endorsement of the items. These 52 items are presented in random order in a yes/no format. Sample items are: "It must be obvious that I am disturbed and agitated," "Dying is the best solution for me," and "I wake up before my usual time in the morning." The scale's developers report good concurrent validity (based on comparisons with the Hamilton Depression Scale and BDI), acceptable face validity, and reliability. They concluded that their scale may be a good alternative to the BDI (Carroll et al., 1981). Both the Carroll and Beck scales provide information not available from an observer rating scale such as the Hamilton (HRS):

[Both] . . . had access to a subjective dimension of depression that could not be predicted from HRS scores. The complementary uses of self ratings and observer ratings are evident from these results. (Carroll et al., 1981, p. 194)

The Carroll Rating Scale, although similar in structure and content to the Hamilton, is less time-consuming and expensive to administer. Initial reports indicate that the Carroll may, in fact, be a good alternative (Smouse et al., 1981;

Tandon et al., 1986). Among its disadvantages are its unequal weighting of items and its failure to represent certain types of endogenous symptomatology (Rush et al., 1986b). Correlations with other depression scales suggest that it is as sensitive to bipolar as it is to unipolar depression.

Inventory for Depressive Symptomatology

The most recent addition to self-report measures of depression, the Inventory for Depressive Symptomatology (IDS-SR), was devised by Rush and colleagues (1986b). The scale comprises 28 items, rated 0 to 3, measuring four basic dimensions of depression: vegetative symptoms (e.g., psychomotor changes, libido, weight and appetite, sleep), cognitive symptoms (e.g., suicidal ideation, self-esteem), anxiety symptoms (e.g., panic and phobia, somatic reactions), and endogenous symptoms (e.g., quality of mood and anhedonia, diurnal variation). Although little information is available on reliability and validity, the inventory holds considerable promise because of its comprehensiveness and specificity of item content. Two items, one measuring sleep disturbance and the other measuring quality of mood, illustrate its specificity:

4. Sleeping too much:
   0 I sleep no longer than 7–8 hours/night, without napping during the day
   1 I sleep no longer than 10 hours in a 24-hour period, including naps
   2 I sleep no longer than 12 hours in a 24-hour period, including naps
   3 I sleep longer than 12 hours in a 24-hour period, including naps
10. Quality of mood:
   0 Mood (internal feelings) that I experience is very much a normal mood
   1 My mood is sad, but this sadness is pretty much like the sad mood I would feel if someone close to me died or left
   2 My mood is sad. But this sadness has a rather different quality to it than the sadness I would feel if someone close to me died or left
   3 My mood is sad. This sadness is different from the type of sadness associated with grief or loss.

Other self-rating scales of depression that are not as widely used as those discussed include the Center for Epidemiologic Studies Depression scale (CES-D, Weissman et al., 1977), the Inventory to Diagnose Depression (Zimmerman et al., 1986), and the Wakefield Self-Assessment Depression Inventory (Snaith et al., 1971, 1976).[4] The Visual Analogue Scale (Hayes and Patterson, 1921; Zealley and Aitken, 1969), a global rather than symptom-specific scale, is used to measure both manic and depressive states and, therefore, is discussed in the section on combined measurement instruments.

Observer Rating Scales

Hamilton Depression Scale

The Hamilton Depression Scale remains the most widely used observer-rated measure of depression. It was developed by Hamilton (1960) to measure the severity and changes over time in the clinical state of depressed patients. Although not developed as a diagnostic tool, it has been used with success in making retrospective diagnoses from chart reviews (Thase et al., 1983). It also has been used to evaluate treatment response, correlate depression severity with biological parameters, and evaluate depression subtypes. It is focused much more on somatic and behavioral symptoms than on mood and cognitive symptoms. In its most commonly administered form, the Hamilton is a 17-item scale (9 items on a 5-point scale and 8 items on a 3-point scale, with a score range from 0 to 4 for 9 items, 0 to 2 for the 8 others) measuring mood, guilt, suicidal ideation, sleep disorders, changes in work and interests, psychomotor agitation and retardation, anxiety, somatic symptoms, hypochondriasis, loss of insight, and loss of weight.

Interobserver reliability is good, although various factor analyses have extracted inconsistent numbers and types of factors.[5] The high reliability, ease of administration, and emphasis on somatic symptoms have been cited as reasons for the enormous popularity of the Hamilton (Murphy et al., 1982b). Critics of the Hamilton believe that somatic symptoms are disproportionately represented, that the differential weighting of symptoms is arbitrary, and that anchor points are ambiguous. Furthermore, certain symptoms, such as hypersomnia, increases in weight and appetite, and changes in quality of mood, are not assessed (Bech, 1981; Rush et al., 1986b). This last point may be an especially important limitation in the assessment of bipolar depression.

Recently, the Structured Interview Guide for the Hamilton Depression Rating Scale (SIGH-D) was developed to standardize the administration of the scale. Preliminary findings suggest that the use of the SIGH-D results in increased reliability (Williams, 1988). Another new structured interview guide for the Hamilton was specifically designed to assess seasonal affective disorder.

Bech-Rafaelsen Melancholia Rating Scale

The Bech-Rafaelsen Melancholia Rating Scale, developed to combine the Hamilton and the Cronholm-Ottosson Depression Scales, comprises 11 items rated in five degrees of severity (Bech et al., 1979a; Bech and Rafaelsen, 1980; Rafaelsen et al., 1980). Items are decreased motor activity, decreased verbal activity, intellectual and emotional retardation, psychic anxiety, suicidal impulses, lowered mood, self- depreciation, sleep disturbances, tiredness and pains, and decreased motivation and productivity with work and interests. The interview is designed to be completed within 15 to 30 minutes and, to control for possible diurnal variation, to be administered at approximately the same time of day. Guidelines for ratings are highly specific, for example:

Retardation (intellectual)
0 Normal intellectual activity
1 The patient has to make an effort to concentrate on his work
2 Even with a major effort it is difficult for the patient to concentrate or make decisions. Less initiative than usual. The patient easily experiences "brain fatigue"
3 Marked difficulties with concentration, initiative and decision-making. For example, can hardly read a newspaper or watch television. Score 3 as long as the retardation has not clearly influenced the interview
4 When the patient during the interview has shown marked difficulties in following normal conversation

The interobserver reliability of the Bech-Rafaelsen Melancholia Scale has been found to be as high as that of the Hamilton Depression Scale (Rafaelsen et al., 1980) and the item–total score correlations are adequate (Bech and Rafaelsen, 1980; Rafaelsen et al., 1980).

Montgomery and Åsberg Depression Rating Scale

Yet another observer rating scale of depression is that of Montgomery and Åsberg (1979), developed to measure changes in depression secondary to antidepressant treatment. Easily administered by clinicians, the scale's ten items measure the major components of clinical depression: apparent sadness, reported sadness, inner tension, reduced sleep, reduced appetite, concentration difficulties, lassitude, inability to feel, pessimistic thoughts, and suicidal thoughts. Items are rated on a 7-point scale (0–6), with illustrative anchor points given for ratings of 0, 2, 4, and 6. For example, ratings for the item measuring "pessimistic thoughts" are:

Pessimistic Thoughts
Representing thoughts of guilt, inferiority, self-reproach, sinfulness, remorse and ruin
0　No pessimistic thoughts
1
2　Fluctuating ideas of a failure, self-reproach or self-depreciation
3
4　Persistent self-accusations, or definite but still rational ideas of guilt or sin. Increasingly pessimistic about the future
5
6　Delusions of ruin, remorse or unredeemable sin. Self-accusations which are absurd and unshakable

The Montgomery and Åsberg Depression Scale exhibits construct validity and concurrent validity relative to the Hamilton Depression Scale (Davidson et al., 1986). Further, it is easily and relatively quickly administered, has well-defined items, and provides for equal weighting of symptoms (Rush et al., 1986b). On the other hand, its unidirectional rating of sleep change (i.e., decreased sleep) may be a disadvantage when it comes to rating bipolar patients.

Additional major observer rating scales for depression include the Cronholm-Ottosson Depression Scale (Cronholm and Ottosson, 1960), the Inpatient Multidimensional Psychiatric Scale (Lorr, 1974), Physicians' Global Assessment Scale (Carney et al., 1965; Endicott et al., 1976), and the clinician-rated Inventory for Depressive Symptomatology (Rush et al., 1986b) and the Newcastle Rating Scales (Roth et al., 1985), which have been of special interest in biological studies because of their sensitivity to endogenous or melancholic items. As one might expect from the symptomatic differences reviewed in Chapter 3, bipolar and unipolar depressed patients show different patterns of response to some of the same standard rating instruments (Paykel and Prusoff, 1973). In light of this, it is unfortunate that there are no systematic studies of the differential sensitivity of rating scales to bipolar depression. To our knowledge, the only scale that has been designed specifically with bipolar patients in mind is the Affective Disorders Rating Scale (Murphy et al., 1982b), to be described.

COMPARISON OF SCALES FOR MANIA AND DEPRESSION

There are many ways of comparing rating scales; here we focus primarily on differences in item content.[6] Content profiles of the items in observer rating measures of mania and self- and observer rating measures of depression are presented in Figures 13-2 through 13-5. The classification of items is, of necessity, occasionally arbitrary. For example, symptoms of mood and cognition often overlap (hopelessness and pessimism), as do symptoms of behavior and activity level. Working within these and other constraints, we can draw up item-content profiles—that is, the items in each scale that are designed to assess a particular feature of depression or mania. Figure 13-2 illustrates relative weightings in observer rating measures of mania for mood, cognition, sleep, psychomotor activity, speech, and behavior. Figure 13-3 portrays content profiles for more specific types of manic behavior—aggression and hostility, hypersexuality, impaired judgment, seeking out others, impulsivity, and appearance. Mood items represent approximately 15 percent of the total number of observer-rated mania items. Most emphasis is placed on euphoric and expansive mood, although all but two scales (Petterson and Bech-Rafaelsen) also include items measuring dysphoric, angry, irritable, or negativistic mood.

Despite the frequency of depression during mania (see Chapter 2), only one scale (Manic State Scale) assesses this. The proportion of cognitive items is high on all scales, especially the Manic Diagnostic and Severity Scale and the Petterson Scale. Sleep disorder symptoms, although integral to the diagnosis and pathophysiology of mania, are the least represented of symptoms on the rating scales. Indeed, two scales do not inquire at all into sleep changes. Psychomotor activity and speech symptoms are measured by all of the mania scales. Behavior changes, like cognitive symptoms, are widely represented, especially by Beigel and Murphy's Manic State Scale.

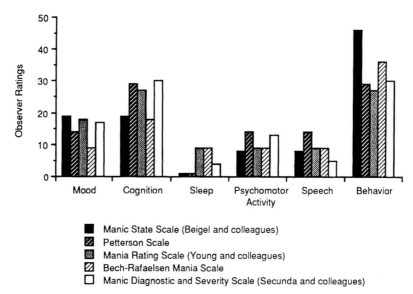

Figure 13-2. Relative weighting of item content: Observer rating measures of mania.

The breakdown of behavior symptoms, shown in Figure 13-3, shows that the most consistently and widely represented symptoms are aggression and hostility, followed by hypersexuality and seeking out others. Impaired judgment, impulsivity, and appearance are less consistently assessed.

The use of a particular rating scale for mania is determined not only on the basis of the item con-

tents but also the nature of the patient population and the training of the raters administering the scale. Thus, the Manic Rating Scale and the Bech-Rafaelsen Mania Scale are more appropriate for less severely ill patients and they require a less experienced rating staff. The Manic State Rating Scale is more comprehensive but also requires sophisticated nurse raters. If patients are

Figure 13-3. Relative weighting of item content for behavior items: Observer rating measures of mania.

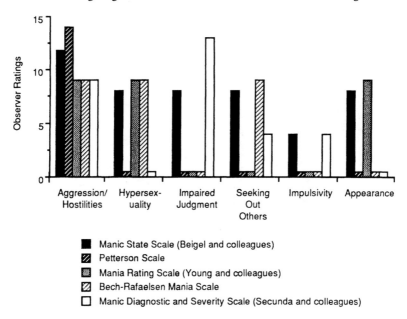

only hypomanic rather than manic, additional useful subjective information may be obtained by using self-rating forms.

The relative weighting of item contents in self-rating measures of depression is shown in Figure 13-4 and in observer rating measures in Figure 13-5. Mood and cognitive symptoms are the most represented of symptom groups in both types of measures. The Beck Depression Inventory is particularly weighted toward cognitive items, and the Montgomery and Åsberg Depression Rating Scale is particularly weighted toward both mood and cognition. Somatic and sleep symptoms are most strongly represented on the Hamilton Depression Scale and on its self-rating parallel, the Carroll Rating Scale. There are no other major differences in relative weightings of item contents. Behavior items are not substantially represented on either self-rating or observer rating inventories, except for work activities and interests which together comprise 7 percent of the total self-rating and 6 percent of the total observer rating items (of the latter, all were on the Hamilton Depression Scale). As in the assessment of mania, the choice of instruments to assess depression depends on the type of patients being evaluated, the level of interviewer training involved, and the nature of the clinical or research issue being addressed. It is often useful to combine a self-rating with an observer rating measure.

COMBINED ASSESSMENT OF MANIC AND DEPRESSIVE STATES

A single rating scale that measures depression and mania along one continuum creates both theoretical and practical difficulties, since it implies that depression and mania are opposite states—an assumption that is clearly contrary to what is known about the nature and expression of manic-depressive illness, as documented extensively in Chapter 2. Monopolar scales (e.g., Bech, 1981) also generally preclude the measurement of mixed and transition states, rapid-cycling states, and diurnal or other cyclic variations in mood, behavior, and activity. Individual measures of depression and mania can be used together[7] to alleviate these problems, or other combined measures, such as those discussed here, can be used.

Visual Analogue Scale

The Visual Analogue Scale (VAS) (Hayes and Patterson, 1921; Zealley and Aitken, 1969), in its most commonly administered form, comprises a 100-mm line anchored at either end with opposite descriptors (e.g., "worst I have ever felt" and "best I have ever felt"). The patient is asked to place a mark or line across the point on the scale that best characterizes his or her mental state. Ratings are made frequently, typically once or

Figure 13-4. Relative weighting of item content: Self-rating measures of depression.

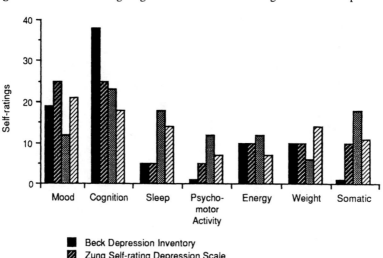

Beck Depression Inventory
Zung Self-rating Depression Scale
Carroll Rating Scale
Inventory for Depressive Symptomatology (Rush and colleagues)

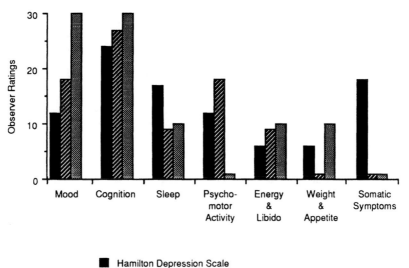

Figure 13-5. Relative weighting of item content: Observer-rating measures of depression.

twice a day, a characteristic that makes the VAS especially appropriate for longitudinal studies of mood and treatment effects. Further advantages include the rapidity of assessment, economic feasibility, involvement of patients in their research and treatment protocols, relative lack of cultural and educational bias, and good reliability and validity (Zealley and Aitken, 1969; Folstein and Luria, 1973; Luria, 1975). The simplicity of the test makes it ideal for depressed patients who are very ill or indecisive. Moderately high correlations exist between the Visual Analogue Scale and the Zung and Hamilton Depression Scales and global ratings by psychiatrists (Folstein and Luria, 1973; Luria, 1975). Correlations with clinical judgment tend to decrease after acute treatment (Zealley and Aitken, 1969). The VAS is not sensitive at lower levels of depression and other types of psychopathology. However, the most important limitation of these scales is that they are global measures not designed to assess specific psychopathological states or symptoms.

Affective Disorder Rating Scale

The Affective Disorder Rating Scale (ADRS, Murphy et al., 1982b) comprises 34 specific assessing mania and depression, using a 6-point scale for frequency and intensity of the behavior and global ratings (on a 15-point scale) of mania,

depression, psychosis, anxiety, and anger. For the global ratings, specific guidelines for assigning scores are provided. For example, in the mild range (within normal limits), scores of 2 or 3 on the mania scale reflect "especially talkative, active, enthusiastic, gregarious or boisterous behavior," and, at the extreme end of the scale, scores of 13 to 15 reflect "nearly continuous manic activity and other symptoms, with uncontrolled, impulsive behavior requiring close supervision and often seclusion for the majority of the day."

Interrater reliability for the global depression rating from the ADRS is reasonably good ($r = 0.77$) although it is somewhat lower for the cluster of individual depression items (Murphy et al., 1982b).

Since the ADRS was designed with the bipolar patient in mind, it is of interest to compare it with other, more generic scales. The depression cluster correlates modestly with the Hamilton Depression Scale ($r = 0.56$), the Beck Depression Inventory ($r = 0.55$), and the POMS-D ($r = 0.56$) but not with the Zung ($r = 0.33$).

The ADRS mania cluster shows relatively high correlations with other measures, such as the IMPS Excitement and Grandiose/Expansiveness subscales ($r = 0.69$ and 0.62, respectively), but less so with the relevant POMS subscales ($r = 0.50$ and 0.45) (Murphy et al., 1982b). Murphy's group reports similar correlations between the ADRS global mania rating and these other scales.

AMDP System

The Association for Methodology and Documentation in Psychiatry (AMDP, originally AMP) was a group of Australian, Swiss, and German psychiatrists interested in establishing valid, reliable psychopathology measures for use in clinical psychopharmacology trials and in European multicenter collaborative research investigations. Their extremely rich clinical assessment system currently is being evaluated as a basis for the major European diagnostic system. Thirteen major categories of psychopathological symptoms have been developed (Guy and Ban, 1982): Intellectual Deficit, Disorders of Consciousness, Disturbances of Orientation, Disturbances of Attention and Memory, Formal Disorders of Thought, Phobias and Compulsions, Delusions, Disorders of Perception, Disorders of Ego, Disturbances of Affect, Disorders of Drive and Psychomotility, Circadian Disturbances, and Other Disturbances. Each of these broad categories comprises several specific descriptive individual items. The detailed quality of the AMDP system can be seen in a few illustrations of individual symptom items (from Disturbances of Affect), with their brief descriptions:

Inner Restlessness: Complaints or feelings of psychic unrest. The patient complains spontaneously—or in answer to questions—that he is stirred by and suffers from agitation and tension. Do not include Item 83 ("Motor Restlessness") here. Inner restlessness is fre-

quently associated with depressive, fearful, hopeless, and despondent feelings and with manic states, delusional mood, and delusional states with various content. (p. 73)

Affective Lability. Rapid changes in affect. Increases in affective variability in which an affect persists for only a very short period and shows many ups and downs. Take into consideration native temperament or cultural tradition. (p. 74)

The AMDP system is especially useful in assessing mixed and cycling affective states, and the richness of its phenomenological description is unique. It has been used successfully in collaborating research centers, with good reliability and validity.[8]

Comprehensive Psychopathological Rating Scale

The Comprehensive Psychopathological Rating Scale (CPRS) was developed in 1971 by the Swedish Medical Research Council to measure treatment effects (Åsberg et al., 1978). Four scale steps, with detailed descriptions for each, are allocated for each item. The scale, designed to be used by all trained mental health workers, can assess both reported and observed behaviors. Items include elevated and sad mood states, indecision, lassitude, fatigability, concentration difficulties, reduced or increased sexual interest, ideas of grandeur, and ecstatic experiences.

Reliability studies in depressed patients in the United Kingdom (Montgomery et al., 1978a) and in cross-cultural populations of Swedish and British depressed patients (Montgomery et al.,

Table 13-2. Sample Items from the General Behavior Inventory

Question Content	Extreme Polar Descriptors
Stimulus seeking/excitement (Receptivity toward and stimulation by the world)	Passionately absorbed in the world's excitement; my sensations and feelings incredibly intensified; I seek out novel stimulation Life is too much trouble; sick of everything
Flight of ideas/thought retardation (Thought processes)	Brilliant penetrating ideas emerging spontaneously and with great rapidity My mind is cold, dead; nothing moves
Decisiveness/doubt	Supremely confident in my judgment and strength of mind; I can instantly see problems which confuse others and solve them Utterly immobile, frozen by doubts; nothing is certain or solid for me

From Depue et al., 1981

1978b) indicate that the CPRS is "highly reliable and highly sensitive . . . easily communicable" (Perris, 1979, p. 413).

General Behavior Inventory

The General Behavior Inventory (GBI) was developed to identify individuals at high risk for developing manic-depressive illness, particularly adolescents and young adults (Depue et al., 1981). Five dimensions of bipolarity were defined as characterizing manic-depressive illness: its core behaviors and symptoms, their intensity, frequency, and duration, and rapid shifts of mood and behavior. Sample question contents (taken from a longitudinal mood-rating study), with their extreme polar descriptors, are presented in Table 13-2. Each item is rated on a 4-point frequency scale.

The GBI, uniquely designed to measure subsyndromal variants of manic-depressive illness (see Chapter 4), has been validated in an initial series of studies through interview-derived diagnoses, interviews with college roommates, family histories of affective illness, clinical characteristics, and longitudinal mood-rating investigations (Depue et al., 1981). Recently the GBI has been further validated in a study of the offspring of bipolar-I patients (Klein et al., 1986b).

SUMMARY

Many rating scales exist for the assessment of mood, behavior, and cognitive changes that take place during mania and depression. Except for the Affective Disorder Rating Scale designed by Murphy and colleagues, none of the depression rating instruments has been designed with the bipolar patient in mind. This oversight can lead to mistaken assessments of bipolar patients. For example, hypersomnia can result in a lower score on many depression scales. Another problem is that few measures exist for the simultaneous assessment of manic and depressive symptoms. Self-rating and observer rating forms both have strengths and liabilities, and the comprehensive assessment of manic-depressive states often requires the use of more than one type of measure.

Each scale used in the measurement of mania and depression has a different profile of item content reflecting different degrees of emphasis on somatic, cognitive, and behavioral components of the illness.

NOTES

1. For theoretical considerations of measurement, including detailed discussions of scale construction, reliability, and validity, the reader is referred to several excellent reviews (Guilford, 1954; Carroll et al., 1973; M. Hamilton, 1976, 1982; Bech, 1981; Boyle, 1985). Structured interview schedules and diagnostic measures are covered elsewhere (see Chapter 5), as are issues of classification and specific diagnostic techniques, such as factor analysis (Lorr, 1974; Andreasen and Grove, 1982; Feinberg and Carroll, 1983). Detailed discussions of global rating measures can be found in other reviews; they include the Brief Psychiatric Rating Scale (Overall and Gorham, 1962; Overall, 1974), symptom checklists, such as the Hopkins Symptom Check List and Symptom Check List—58 items (Derogatis et al., 1974), and the Inventory of Psychic and Somatic Complaints (Raskin et al., 1967, 1969, 1970; Raskin and Crook, 1976), adjective checklists, such as the Depression Adjective Checklists (Lubin, 1965; Zuckerman and Lubin, 1967) and the Profile of Mood States (McNair et al., 1971), social adjustment rating scales (Weissman and Paykel, 1974), or behavioral and linguistic analyses (Emrich and Eilert, 1978; Polsky and McGuire, 1979).
2. Good reviews of other measures may be found in Murphy and colleagues (1982b) and Bech (1981).
3. For example, hypersomnia, the more typical sleep disturbance among bipolar depressed patients, may not register as an indicator of depression on scales that focus on the "typical" symptom of insomnia.
4. General reviews of self-rating measures of depression can be found in McNair (1974) and Raskin and Crook (1976).
5. Hamilton, 1960, 1967; Baumann, 1976; Cleary and Guy, 1977.
6. Detailed comparisons of reliability, validity, and intercorrelations can be found elsewhere (e.g., Murphy et al., 1982b; Feinberg et al., 1981a; Schaefer et al., 1985).
7. For example, the Bech-Rafaelsen Mania and Depression Scales or the Manchester Nurse Rating Scales (Brierly et al., 1988).
8. Baumann and Angst, 1975; Helmchen, 1975, 1985; Woggon, 1979; Woggon and Dittrich, 1979; Baumann, 1985.

14

Manic-Depressive Illness, Creativity, and Leadership

Schumann's greatness lies on the one hand in his wealth of emotion, on the other in the depth of his spiritual experience and his striking originality. . . . With the shadow of his insanity already hanging over him, this inspired poet of human suffering seemed incapable of finding moments of tranquility.　—Tchaikovsky, 1872[1]

. . . had he been a stable and equable man, he could never have inspired the nation. In 1940, when all the odds were against Britain, a leader of sober judgement might well have concluded that we were finished. (pp. 4-5)
—Anthony Storr, *Churchill: The Man*

INTRODUCTION

For the many centuries that man has observed man, extremes in mood have been linked with extremes in the human experience: madness, creativity, despair, ecstasy, inspiration, romanticism, charisma, and destructiveness. Extreme mood swings, when removed from the sphere of poets and historians and placed in the more modern, analytical clinics of psychologists and psychiatrists, lose their association, however tumultuous, with growth, sensuality, creativity, and other positive attributes, becoming instead representations of psychopathology. This is, in many ways, understandable. Clinicians are called on to treat symptoms, not to mystify them, and clinical objectivity is essential to avoid the risks of overlooking or minimizing a patient's pain and suicide potential. For these and many other reasons, a psychopathological approach to mood disorders has resulted in a psychiatric literature generally slighting the positive aspects of affective illness, especially manic-depressive illness and its variants. In this chapter we examine several areas of human accomplishment that have been linked, both anecdotally and systematically, with mood disorders.

Brief History of an Association

Robert Browning's 19th century description of the poet's soul and its close relationship to divine inspiration—"Visibly through his garden walketh God"—is similar, in a Victorian way, to those from thousands of years earlier. The notion of an intimate relationship among the gods, madness, and creators is described in pre-Grecian myths, most dramatically in the Dionysian struggles between violence and creation or madness and reason. These worship rituals symbolized the ancient belief that self-knowledge emerged through violence and destruction and that the god Dionysus, himself inflicted with madness by Hera, "afflicted human beings with madness and violence, becoming the god of fertility, the principle of creation in nature" (Feder, 1980, p. 43). Restoration of sanity, renewed vitality, and creative inspiration followed such blood feasts, which often involved the dismemberment of animals or humans. Interestingly, these rituals, characterized by ecstatic worship, wild dances, and violent death, were cyclic in nature and tied to the seasons, representing the common themes of death and rebirth. We see later how the seasonal and regenerational themes also represent additional ties between the nature of manic-depressive illness and creativity.

By the time of Plato and Socrates, common lore held that priests and poets communicated with the gods through their demons, or "geniuses." These demons were the basis for the idea of divine madness, and inspiration was thought obtainable only during particular states of mind, such as loss of consciousness, affliction with illness, or under states of "possession" (Becker, 1978). Aristotle wrote:

Why is it that all men who are outstanding in philosophy, poetry or the arts are melancholic, and some to such an extent that they are infected by the diseases arising from black bile . . . ? For Heracles seems to have been of this character. . . . The same is true of Ajax and Bellerophontes. . . . In later times also there have been Empedocles, Plato, Socrates and many other well-known men. The same is true of most of those who have handled poetry. (pp. 55–157)

Becker, in *The Mad Genius Controversy,* (1978) describes the Middle Ages as relatively indifferent to extraordinarily endowed individuals and the Renaissance as displaying renewed interest in the relationship among extreme talent, melancholy, and madness. During that era, an important distinction was made between sane melancholics of high achievement and individuals whose insanity prevented them from using their ability. The 18th century witnessed a sharp change in attitude; balance and rational thought were seen as the primary components of genius. This comparatively brief period, which associated moderation with genius, was completely reversed by the 19th century Romantics, who once again emphasized the more spontaneous, inspired, and possessed-by-the-muses qualities of genius. William Wordsworth, in his poem about Thomas Chatterton, the brilliant, 18th century poet who committed suicide at the age of 17, described the fate of poets as:

By our own spirits are we deified;
We Poets in our youth begin in gladness;
But thereof comes in the end despondency and
  madness.

Lord Byron, the personification of moody intensity among the Romantic poets, wrote of his brooding roots in Canto the Third, from "Childe Harold's Pilgrimage":

Yet must I think less wildly:—I *have* thought
  Too long and darkly, till my brain became,

In its own eddy boiling and o'erwrought,
A whirling gulf of phantasy and flame:
And thus, untaught in youth my heart to tame,
My springs of life were poisoned.

In the same year that Lord Byron published "Childe Harold's Pilgrimage," Benjamin Rush, signer of the U.S. Constitution and Professor of Medicine at the University of Pennsylvania in the early 19th century, recorded his observations about the relationship between milder manic and creative states:

From a part of the brain preternaturally elevated, but not diseased, the mind sometimes discovers not only unusual strength and acuteness, but certain talents it never exhibited before. . . . Talents for eloquence, poetry, music and painting, and uncommon ingenuity in several of the mechanical arts, are often involved in this state of madness. . . . The disease which thus evolves these new and wonderful talents and operations of the mind may be compared to an earthquake, which, by convulsing the upper strata of our globe, throws upon its surface precious and splendid fossils, the existence of which was unknown to the proprietors of the soil in which they were buried. (1812, pp. 153–154)

An ironic exception to the 19th century writers who emphasized deep, mysterious, and overwhelming forces giving rise to genius was the essayist Charles Lamb, himself hospitalized for what would now be called manic-depressive illness, and constant companion to a sister intermittently insane with manic-depressive psychosis. In *The Sanity of True Genius,* he argued for a balance of faculties, much as the 18th century writers had done:

So far from the position holding true, that great wit (or genius, in our modern way of speaking), has a necessary alliance with insanity, the greatest wits, on the contrary, will ever be found in the sanest writers. It is impossible for the mind to conceive a mad Shakespeare. The greatness of wit, by which the poetic talent is here chiefly to be understood, manifests itself in the admirable balance of all faculties. Madness is the disproportionate straining or excess of any one of them. . . . The ground of the mistake is, that men, finding in the raptures of the higher poetry a condition of exaltation, to which they have no parallel in their own experience, besides the spurious resemblance of it in dreams and fevers, impute a state of dreaminess and fever to the poet. But the true poet dreams being awake. He is not possessed by his subject, but has dominion over it. (pp. 212–213)

The late 19th and early 20th centuries saw a moderation of earlier views, partly due to the inevitable swing from any extreme—in this case that of the Romantics—and partly due to the subduing influences of academic psychology and psychiatry. Scholars, such as William James, and clinical researchers, such as Emil Kraepelin, emphasized positive features associated with certain kinds of madness, or "psychopathy," and speculated as to how these features combine with other talents in some instances to produce an extraordinarily creative or accomplished person. Also accented, however, were the debilitating extremes of mental illness—psychosis or morbid depressions, for example—rather than the milder hypomanias and more reflective, philosophical melancholias. These scholars underscored the need for sustained attention, discipline, and balance in the truly accomplished individual. This more moderate view has characterized most 20th century thinking about the relationship between psychopathology and genius. Madness, inspiration, and psychopathology have been relegated to roles of far less importance.

William James, like his brother Henry, was subject to profound, debilitating depressions and wrote about the potentially valuable combinations of temperament with talent:

... the psychopathic temperament [by which James meant "border-line insanity, insane temperament, loss of mental balance"], whatever be the intellect with which it finds itself paired, often brings with it ardor and excitability of character.... His conceptions tend to pass immediately into belief and action ... when a superior intellect and a psychopathic temperament coalesce—as in the endless permutations and combinations of human faculty, they are bound to coalesce often enough—in the same individual, we have the best possible condition for the kind of effective genius that gets into the biographical dictionaries. Such men do not remain mere critics and understanders with their intellect. Their ideas possess them, they inflict them, for better or worse, upon their companions or their age. (James, 1902, pp. 23–24)

Kraepelin, the premier authority on manic-depressive illness, was acutely aware of the severe psychopathology of the untreated disorder. He described it extensively but wrote of its positive aspects:

The volitional excitement which accompanies the disease may under certain circumstances set free powers which otherwise are constrained by all kinds of inhibition. Artistic activity namely may, by the untroubled surrender to momentary fancies or moods, and especially poetical activity by the facilitation of linguistic expression, experience a certain furtherance. (Kraepelin, 1921, p. 17)

Myerson and Boyle, writing from Boston's McLean Hospital in the 1940s, reiterated the position of William James with specific reference to manic-depressive illness. In discussing affective psychosis in socially prominent families, they concluded:

It does not necessarily follow that the individuals who appear in these records were great because they had mental disease, although that proposition might be maintained with considerable cogency and relevance. It may be that the situation is more aptly expressed as follows. The manic drive in its controlled form and phase is of value *only* if joined to ability. A feebleminded person of hypomanic temperament would simply be one who carried on more activity at a feebleminded level, and this is true also of mediocrity, so the bulk of manic-depressive temperaments are of no special value to the world, and certainly not of distinguished value. If, however, the hypomanic temperament is joined to high ability, an independent characteristic, then the combination may well be more effective than the union of high ability with normal temperament and drive might be. The indefatigability, the pitch of enthusiasm, the geniality and warmth which one so often sees in the hypomanic state may well be a fortunate combination and socially and historically valuable. (p. 20)

More recently, the writer Arthur Koestler (1964) and psychoanalysts Storr (1972) and Arieti (1976), whom we discuss in greater detail later, have argued for some link between psychopathology and creative work—primarily in terms of special access to primitive thought and feelings shared in common by the psychotic and creative processes. All, however, stress the need for an intact mind in creative endeavor, while minimizing an important clinical reality of manic-depressive illness—that periods of psychosis or otherwise debilitating mood states often are interspersed with periods of strong functioning.

General Methodological Issues

In this section, we examine hypothesized relationships between manic-depressive illness and accomplishment. After considering the reasons why a strong connection might be expected to exist, we examine existing evidence for such a link among manic-depressive illness, creativity, and leadership. First, we present a brief overview of methodological problems, the most striking of which is the overwhelming amount of apocryphal speculation and the lack of systematic work on the subject. Quantitative sources of data are rare. To find studies of "inspiration," ecstasy, or the elated states, one must turn to theology, music, and literature, not to psychiatry or psychology or other sciences. Likewise, to find studies linking "madness," mood disorders, and creativity, one must turn, almost entirely, to biographical and autobiographical writings. Biographical works are, of course, irreplaceable, deeply instructive sources of information about moods, their extremes, and their effects on individuals and the societies in which they lived and worked. There are only a few systematic studies[2] of creativity and affective illness using modern diagnostic and interview techniques. None exists in the field of political, military, or religious leadership.

What, then, are some of the major problems in doing research into the relationship between manic-depressive illness and accomplishment? First, any historical perspective necessarily dictates that a recounting of highly accomplished affectively ill individuals will be only a partial listing—illustrative, but by no means definitive. Always, in the analysis of individual lives, problems arise. For example, it is fairly easy to identify major 20th century American poets who were manic-depressive, but it is all but impossible to determine what proportion of the total pool of great poets they represent. How many great 19th century composers, military leaders, or novelists were there? Although there are some relevant data available for 20th century writers and artists (Andreasen and Canter, 1974; Andreasen, 1987a; Jamison, 1989), no other comparison data exist. Still, in looking at accomplishment within the fields of arts and leadership, certain general conclusions can be drawn, and, in many instances, of course, the individuals under study are sufficiently important to be interesting in their own right.

Retrospective or posthumous diagnostic studies always present special methodological problems. Historical context and prevailing social customs to some extent determine which behavior is noticed and commented on. Likewise, more detailed information exists for some individuals than for others (e.g., those more in the public eye, those existing in more modern and communicated times, those writing more about themselves, both directly and indirectly). Storr has put it well:

. . . the more we know about anyone, the easier it becomes to discern neurotic traits, mood disorders and other aspects of character which, when emphatically present, we call neurotic. The famous and successful are usually less able to conceal whatever vagaries of character they may possess because biographers or Ph.D students will not let them rest in peace. (Storr, unpublished manuscript)

Definitional and diagnostic problems also come about from differences in "language, latitudes, and lifestyles." Almost by definition, the idea of using formal psychiatric diagnostic criteria in the arts has been an anathema. Biological psychiatrists have displayed little or no interest in studying mood disorders in artists, writers, or leaders; and, certainly, those in the arts and leadership fields have been less than interested in seeing, or being seen, through a biological or diagnostic grid. Those in the best position to link the two worlds, that is, students of creativity, have not done so. By focusing on the relationship between creativity and "schizophrenia" (often misdiagnosed manic-depressive ill....ss) or diffuse notions of psychopathology, these researchers have left unexamined the specific role of mood disorders in creative work.

Further complicating matters, certain lifestyles provide "cover" for deviant and bizarre behavior. The arts have long given latitude for extremes in behavior and mood; indeed, Becker (1978) observed that the Romantic artists used the notion of mad genius to "provide recognition of special status and the freedom from conventional restraints that attended it":

The aura of "mania" endowed the genius with a mystical and inexplicable quality that served to differentiate him from the typical man, the bourgeois, the philistine, and, quite importantly, the "mere" man of talent; it established him as the modern heir of the ancient Greek poet and seer and, like his classical counterpart, enabled him to claim some of the powers and privileges granted to the "divinely possessed" and "inspired." (pp. 127–128)

Burton wrote in the 17th century that "All poets are mad," a view shared by many since. Such a view, however appealing and whatever its accuracy, tends to lead to both overdiagnosis of psychopathology, because of diagnostic over-inclusiveness, and to underdiagnosis, because of an assumption that within artistic circles madness is somehow normal. This latter point is well illustrated in Ian Hamilton's biography of the poet

Robert Lowell. The following passage describes the reactions of others to one of Lowell's many escalations into mania:

. . . Lowell had announced to all his Cincinnati acquaintances that he was determined to remarry, and had persuaded them to stand with him on the side of passion. Some members of the faculty found him excitable and talkative during this period, but since the talk was always brilliant and very often flattering to them, they could see no reason to think of Lowell as "ill"; indeed, he was behaving just as some of them hoped a famous poet would behave. They undertook to protect this unique flame against any dampening intrusions from New York. Thus, when Hardwick became convinced that Lowell was indeed sick—over a period of two weeks his telephone calls to New York became more and more confused, lengthy and abusive—she ran up against a wall of kindly meant hostility from Lowell's campus allies. Her version of Lowell was not theirs, even when they were discussing the same symptoms; what to her was "mad" was to them another mark of Lowell's genius. (1982, p. 208)

The tendency for highly accomplished individuals, almost by definition, to be highly productive and energetic, results in yet another type of diagnostic bias—an inclination to underdiagnose manic aspects of affective illness. Biographical studies indicate that writers, artists, and leaders often describe in great detail their periods of "melancholy" but that other features of their lives—more clinically describable as hypomania or even overt psychosis—are subsumed under "normal functioning," "creative inspiration," the "artistic temperament," "intense creative episodes," "eccentricity," and "chaotic lifestyle." Thus, many individuals with clear histories of profound or debilitating depressions are labeled as depressive rather than manic-depressive in temperament despite their episodic histories of extremely high levels of energy, enthusiasm, productivity, and irritability (often with accompanying lapses in financial, social, and sexual judgment). Paradoxically, the more chronically hypomanic the individual, the more noticeable and relatively pathological the depression will appear. Retrospective studies lend themselves to diagnostic errors of the opposite type. That is, some researchers have tended to overdiagnose manic-depressive illness because they observe patterns of behavior common to both hypomania and normal accomplishment (e.g., enthusiasm, high energy, and the ability to function with little

sleep) and then label as manic-depressive anyone displaying any of these symptoms.

HYPOTHESIZED RELATIONSHIPS BETWEEN MANIC-DEPRESSIVE ILLNESS AND ACCOMPLISHMENT

. . . how weirdly our lives have often gone the same way. Let's say we are brothers, have gone the same journey and know far more about each other than we have ever said or will say. There's a strange fact about the poets of roughly our age. . . . It's this, that to write we seem to have to go at it with such single-minded intensity that we are always on the point of drowning. I've seen this so many times, and year after year with students, that I feel it's something almost unavoidable, some flaw in the motor.   —Robert Lowell, letter to Theodore Roethke, 1963[3]

Both Lowell and Roethke won the Pulitzer Prize for their poetry (Lowell twice), and both were hospitalized repeatedly for manic breaks. They, with many other of the leading poets of their generation, seem to have been quite singularly hit by manic-depressive illness, Lowell's "flaw in the motor." The question we address here is the extent to which this "flaw" and "single-minded intensity" made possible their creative work, uniquely colored it, hindered it, or was independent of it.

In hypothesizing possible relationships between manic-depressive illness and accomplishment, several general areas need to be explored: characteristics of the illness (e.g., acute and long-term effects or the recurrent, cyclic nature of the illness), experiences derived from having manic-depressive illness, and the relative importance of different aspects of the illness in various types of accomplishment.

Characteristics of the Illness

Profound changes in mood, cognition, person ality, sleep, energy, and behavior can occur during all phases of manic-depressive illness. Even during normal states, many individuals experience subtle and not so subtle fluctuations in the intensity of their perceptions and feelings. All of these changes have potentially important effects on personality and level of functioning, but perhaps most relevant to our discussion of creativity and leadership are those changes occurring during the milder manic states. Table 14-1 presents the DSM-III criteria for hypomania; even the

Table 14-1. DSM-III Criteria for Hypomania[a]

Mood
Elevated, expansive

Psychomotor
More energy than usual
Physical restlessness

Speech
More talkative than usual

Sleep
Decreased need for sleep

Cognitive
Inflated self-esteem
Sharpened and unusually creative thinking
Overoptimism or exaggeration of past
    achievement

Behavior
Increased productivity, often with unusual and
    self-imposed working hours
Uninhibited people-seeking
Hypersexuality
Inappropriate laughing, joking, punning
Excessive involvements in pleasurable activities
    with lack of concern for painful consequences,
    e.g., buying sprees, foolish business invest-
    ments, reckless driving

[a]These criteria were included in the DSM-III criteria for
cyclothymia

most casual review gives prima facie evidence for a possible connection between hypomania and accomplishment. There is some truth in the easy, glib question often arising in clinical teaching situations: Who would not want an illness that numbers among its symptoms elevated and expansive mood, inflated self-esteem, more energy than usual, decreased need for sleep, hypersexuality, and—most germane to our argument here—"sharpened and unusually creative thinking," and "increased productivity?" In looking at some of these changes, especially in mood and cognition, we need to first turn to the pivotal issue of inspiration.

In the chapter's introduction we discussed associations—ancient and modern—among creativity, divine inspiration, and "madness." This special access to a power beyond what is ordinarily available to an individual or his society has extended across many different kinds of inspirations: warlike, druidic, mystical, poetic, insane, and divine. Attributions once made to the

gods or the muses (Gerard Manley Hopkins's "sweet fire the sire of muse," Emerson's "all poetry is first written in the heavens") have been transformed into the 20th century's rather more prosaic constructions of "primary process," "prelogical thought," and "bisociative thinking." Arieti, a leading psychoanalytic writer on creativity, has described the creative process in the following way:

Primary process mechanisms reappear in the creative process also, in strange, intricate combinations with secondary process mechanisms and in syntheses that, although unpredictable, are nevertheless susceptible of psychological interpretation. It is from approximate matching with secondary process mechanisms that these primitive forms of cognition, generally confined to abnormal conditions or to unconscious processes, become innovating powers. . . . I have proposed the expression *tertiary process* to designate this special combination of primary and secondary mechanisms. . . . Instead of rejecting the primitive (or whatever is archaic, obsolete, or off the beaten path), the creative mind integrates it with normal logical processes in what seems a "magic" synthesis from which the new, the unexpected, and the desirable emerge. (1976, pp. 12–13)

What Arieti said in the technical language of his field, Koestler said earlier in somewhat more literary terms. What is compelling is the similarity between their conceptualizations and how relevant are their hypotheses for relating mood disorders to creative or "inspired" thinking. Koestler (1964) wrote:

We have seen that the creative act always involves a regression to earlier, more primitive levels in the mental hierarchy, while other processes continue simultaneously on the rational surface—a condition that reminds one of a skin-diver with a breathing-tube. (Needless to say, the exercise has its dangers: skin divers are prone to fall victims to the "rapture of the deep" and tear their breathing-tubes off—the *reculer sans sauter* of William Blake and so many others. A less fatal professional disease is the Bends, a punishment for attempting to live on two different levels at once.) The capacity to regress, more or less at will, to the games of the underground, without losing contact with the surface, seems to be the essence of the poetic, and of any other form of creativity. "God guard me from those thoughts men think/In the mind alone./He that sings a lasting song/Thinks in a marrow bone" (Yeats). (pp. 316–317)

From virtually all perspectives—early Greek philosopher to 20th century specialist—there is agreement that artistic creativity and inspiration involve, indeed require, a dipping into untapped irrational sources while maintaining ongoing contact with realities of "life at the surface." The degree to which individuals can, or desire to, "summon up the depths" is one of the more fascinating of individual differences. Within the group of highly creative and accomplished individuals, most function essentially within the rational world, without losing access to the "underground." Others, the subject of this chapter, although privy to their unconscious streams and to a tumultuous emotional depth, somehow seem to be incapable of so steadily integrating deeper irrational sources with more logical processes. Individuals also vary enormously in their capacity to tolerate extremes of emotions and to live on close terms with darker forces. Yeats describes this in his essay "A Remonstrance with Scotsmen for Having Soured the Dispositions of Their Ghosts and Faeries":

You have discovered the faeries to be pagan and wicked. You would like to have them all up before the magistrate. In Ireland warlike mortals have gone amongst them, and helped them in their battles, and they in turn have taught men great skill with herbs, and permitted some few to hear their tunes. Carolan slept upon a faery rath. Ever after their tunes ran in his head, and made him the great musician he was. . . . You—you will make no terms with the spirits of fire and earth and air and water. You have made the Darkness your enemy. We—we exchange civilities with the world beyond. (William Butler Yeats, 1893, pp. 106–107)

No one yet understands what gives some people access to this "world beyond" or why—once in contact with such worlds—some should be so rich and vital, and some so uninspired. Most individuals describe their mood states during moments of greatest creative insight or inspiration as elated, expansive, and occasionally ecstatic. Although it is unclear whether these mood changes precede or follow creative thought, there is some evidence that the expansiveness of thought and the grandiosity of both mood and thought—common features in mild hypomania—can result in an increased fluency and frequency of ideas highly conducive to creative achievement (see Chapter 11). The similarities between intense creative episodes and hypomania are discussed in more detail elsewhere (Jamison, 1989), but it should be mentioned here that in successful artists and writers, very powerful mood and sleep

changes often occur just before periods of intense creative activity. This period of elated and expansive mood is described by many individuals as their time of inspiration: a time of faster and more fluid thinking, new ideas and connections in thoughts. This fluency in thought, common to hypomania and creative activity, was reported by Kraepelin in his citation of the experimental work of Isserlin:

Isserlin has specially investigated the duration of ideas in manic patients. He found that their associations show heightened distractibility in the tendency to "diffusiveness," to spinning out the circle of ideas stimulated and jumping off to others, a phenomenon which in high degree is peculiar to mania. (1921, p. 15)

The increase in speed of thoughts—ranging from a very mild quickening, to a flight of ideas, to complete psychotic incoherence—may exert its influence on creative production in several ways. Speed per se, that is, the quantity of thoughts and associations, may be enhanced. Also significant, however, may be the effect of increased quantity on the qualitative aspects of thought; that is, the sheer volume of thought might produce unique ideas and associations.

Guilford's systematic psychological studies (1957) into the nature of creativity concluded that several components comprise creative thinking (many of which relate directly to cognitive changes that take place during mild manias as well). *Fluency of thinking* is operationally defined by Guilford in several related concepts, each with tests to measure it:

1. Word fluency: the ability to produce words, each containing a specified letter or combination of letters
2. Associational fluency: the production of as many synonyms as possible for a given word in a limited amount of time
3. Expressional fluency: the production and rapid juxtaposition of phrases or sentences
4. Ideational fluency: the ability to produce ideas to fulfill certain requirements in a limited amount of time

In addition to fluency of thinking (characterized by the components outlined), Guilford developed two other important concepts in creativity: *Spontaneous flexibility*, the ability and disposition to produce a great variety of ideas, with freedom to switch from category to category, and *adaptive flexibility,* the ability to come up with unusual types of solutions (relative to the frequency of response occurrences in the general population). Guilford (1959b) also concluded, as did Hudson in his later work (1966), that creative individuals were far more characterized by "divergent" thinking ("a type of thinking in which considerable searching about is done and a number of answers will do") than by "convergent" thinking ("thinking toward one right answer").

In all of these facets of creative thought the elements of fluency and flexibility of cognitive processing are emphasized. Clearly, the mere quickening and opening up of thought in an otherwise unimaginative person will not result in creative achievement. If a creative person's cognitive processes are hastened and loosened by hypomania, however, a qualitatively different result might well emerge. A more systematic review of cognitive changes occurring during different types and stages of affective illness is presented in Chapter 11. Hyperacusis, the heightening of senses—of sight, hearing, touch, and smell—so often experienced during manic states, also may foster creativity. Richards (1981), in an excellent review of the relationship between creativity and psychopathology, explores cognitive and other features of pathological states that might benefit the creative process.

Characteristics of a noncognitive nature also link manic-depressive illness and accomplishment. The ability to function well on a few hours of sleep and to work at a high energy level, an integral part of most hypomanic states, is important to accomplishment. In her studies of outstanding artists and scientists, for example, Anne Roe (1946, 1951, 1952) found one trait that stood out in these individuals: the willingness to work hard and to work long hours. Finally, the importance of great depth or display of emotion to those in the creative or leadership fields cannot be overstated. Slater (1979) describes these aspects of temperament in composers:

In terms of temperament, these men depart from the average of mankind in having a greater capacity for feeling, for emotional reaction. Not only do they react to the environment in a more powerfully emotional way than most men, they also contain an excessive number of personalities of the cyclothymic kind, subject to biological swings of mood. In addition, the personality is more than normally energetic, vigorous,

even aggressive and combative. Despite their liability to a level of intensity of emotional reaction that the normal personality would be unable to tolerate, they are little liable to neurotic illness. (p. 102)

Haile portrays the role of mood swings and emotional depths in Martin Luther:

Such radical oscillation in mood was a most characteristic feature of Martin Luther's genius. He was very much the victim of his momentary emotional state, over which he had little control. . . . But this is not to say he was a naive creature of his moods. Martin Luther's entire greatness arose from his ability to draw knowingly upon depths of his unconscious being, placing emotional powers at the disposal of an astute intellect. . . . He was also long accustomed to drawing on his emotions for his songs, for some of his best writings, for the power of his passionate prayers. Emotionality was probably also the driving force in his penetrating thought about God and man. (pp. 745–747)

Cyclic and Contrasting Nature of the Illness

Poetry turns all things to loveliness; it exalts the beauty of that which is most beautiful, and it adds beauty to that which is most deformed; it marries exultation and horror, grief and pleasure, eternity and change; it subdues to union under its light yoke, all irreconcilable things . . . its secret alchemy turns to potable gold the poisonous waters which flow from death through life; it strips the veil of familiarity from the world . . .   —Percy Bysshe Shelley[4]

Throughout this book, we stress the recurrent, cyclic nature of manic-depressive illness—its natural history, pathophysiology, subjective experience, and treatment. Integrally tied to this conception and of particular consequence here is the significance of contrasting, recurrent mood states. Cyclic patterns are common to both mood disorders and the nature of creative work. The ebbing and flowing character of inspiration, described so often, bears a striking resemblance to changes from the vitality to nonvitality of different seasons, death and rebirth, and the antithetical qualities of the bipolar mood states. Indeed, preliminary evidence (Jamison, 1989) suggests that seasonal patterns not only exist in moods but in creative productivity as well. Such patterns, discussed in greater detail in a later section of this chapter, resemble those changes reported by many authors in seasonal patterns of mania and depression (see Chapter 19) and by Rosenthal and colleagues (1984) in their study of seasonal affective disorders. Patients studied by Rosenthal's group, for example, during the fall and winter months reported depressed mood and a decrease in physical activity, but an increase in activity and mood during the summer months. In many ways, the depressive phase seems analogous to hibernation or a metabolic slowdown. These seasonal patterns of mood and creativity provide, in addition to a continuing exposure to contrasting states, an opportunity for the incubation of ideas. William James described this aspect of creativity as the "subconscious maturing processes in results of which we suddenly grow conscious," and Koestler (1964) provides many instances of ideas needing to "brew" before coming to fruition.

Finally, the contrasting natures of the elated and depressive state provide a rich variety of experiences and sensations from which to create. The use of intense, opposite mood states was most pronounced, of course, in the romantic poets and composers. Schumann, for example, created two contrasting characters who alternated throughout portions of his compositions: Florestan, impassioned, headstrong, with a "head so full of ideas that I cannot actually form any of them," and Eusebius, an introspective, reflective, lyrical dreamer. In his preface to the "Davidbündlertänze" (a piano work illustrating the contrasting sides of his nature, with abrupt alterations of mood between tempestuous activity and introspection), Schumann wrote that "Joy and sorrow are inseparable all through life." The intense awareness of such joys and sorrows and the powerful contrasts between the extremes in mood and in vitality are potential benefits to creativity taken from the depths and heights of the emotional experiences associated with manic-depressive illness. William James portrayed the unique perspective of the "sad heart" and "sick soul" in this remarkable description of contrasts:

. . . mankind is in a position similar to that of a set of people living on a frozen lake, surrounded by cliffs over which there is no escape, yet knowing that little by little the ice is melting, and the inevitable day drawing near when the last film of it will disappear, and to be drowned ignominiously will be the human creature's portion. The merrier the skating, the warmer and more sparkling the sun by day, and the ruddier the bonfires at night, the more poignant the sadness with which one must take in the total situation. (1902, pp. 141–142)

Experiences Derived from Having Manic-Depressive Illness

. . . I do strongly feel that among the greatest pieces of luck for high achievement is ordeal. Certain great artists can make out without it, Titian and others, but mostly you need ordeal. My idea is this: The artist is extremely lucky who is presented with the worst possible ordeal which will not actually kill him. At that point, he's in business. Beethoven's deafness, Goya's deafness, Milton's blindness, that kind of thing. And I think that what happens in my poetic work in the future work will probably largely depend not on my sitting calmly on my ass as I think, "Hmm, hmm, a long poem again? Hmm," but on being knocked in the face, and thrown flat, and given cancer, and all kinds of other things short of senile dementia. At that point, I'm out, but short of that, I don't know. I hope to be nearly crucified.   —John Berryman[5]

Berryman, a contemporary of Robert Lowell and Theodore Roethke, was, like them, a winner of the Pulitzer Prize for poetry and a manic-depressive. At the end of a full but highly painful and tumultuous life, he committed suicide (as his father had before him). His remarks about the role of ordeal in the creative process suggest Nietzsche's belief that "One must harbor chaos within oneself to give birth to a dancing star." Koestler discussed the central importance to creativity of the archetypal Night Journey where, under the effect of some overwhelming experience, the hero suffers a crisis that involves the deepest foundations of his being: "he embarks on the Night Journey, is suddenly transferred to the Tragic Plane—from which he emerges purified, enriched by new insight, regenerated on a higher level of integration" (Koestler, 1964). This is, of course, a variation on the ancient theme of insight through suffering, of "having good of all one's pain," and the monomythic hero (Campbell, 1949).

The dive or journey underground often provides an increased range and intensity of experience to those in a position to inspire—through the arts, leadership, religion, whatever. Poetic, religious, and philosophical insights are perhaps the major beneficiaries of ruminative, depressive, terrifying, or ecstatic experiences. Profound depression or the suffering of psychosis can, and often does, fundamentally change the expectations and beliefs about the nature and length of life, God, and other people. Many writers have described the impact of their long periods of depression, how they have dealt with them, and how they have used them in their work.

Anne Sexton, a contemporary of Lowell, Roethke, and Berryman, was yet another Pulitzer Prize winner in poetry and a manic-depressive. After many hospitalizations for both mania and depression, she, like Berryman, committed suicide. She described the importance of using pain in her work:

> I, myself, alternate between hiding behind my own hands, protecting myself anyway possible, and this other, this seeing ouching other. I guess I mean that creative people must not avoid the pain that they get dealt. . . . Hurt must be examined like a plague. (Sexton and Ames, 1977, p. 105)

Robert Lowell, who wrote about depression that "I don't think it is a visitation of the angels but dust in the blood," also wrote:

> Depression's no gift from the Muse. At worst, I do nothing. But often I've written, and wrote one whole book—*For the Union Dead*—about witheredness. . . . Most of the best poems, the most personal, are gathered crumbs from the lost cake. I had better moods, but the book is lemony, soured and dry, the drought I had touched with my own hands. That, too, may be poetry—on sufferance. (Giroux, 1987, p. 287)

Both Lowell and Sexton wrote of their heightened psychological sensitivity and vulnerability in graphic and quite similar physical metaphors: "seeing too much and feeling it/with one skin-layer missing" (Lowell) and ". . . even illusion breaks its filament wings/on the raw skin of all I wouldn't know" (Sexton).

The importance and possible limitations of fluctuating moods, ever-changing perceptions, and a responsive temperament were crucial issues to Ralph Waldo Emerson, who wrote extensively of his own moods, which were often beyond his control or prediction:

Life is a train of moods like a string of beads, and as we pass through them they prove to be many-colored lenses which paint the world their own hue, and each shows only what lies in its focus. . . . Temperament is the iron wire on which the beads are strung. Of what use is fortune or talent to a cold and defective nature? . . . Of what use is genius if the organ is too convex or too concave and cannot find a focal distance within the actual horizon of human life? Of what use, if the brain is too cold or too hot, and the man does not care enough for results to stimulate him to experiment, and hold him up in it? or if the web is too finely woven, too irritable by pleasure and pain, so that life stagnates from too much reception without due outlet? (Emerson, 1982, pp. 288–289)

Learning through intense and deep emotional experiences, and using that learning to add meaning and depth to creative work, is probably the most widely accepted and written about aspect of the relationship between mood disorders and accomplishment. The influence of pain's dominion fills novels, biographies and autobiographies, sermons, and canvases; there is no shortage of portrayals. We end this section with one biographer's comment about Martin Luther:

> If the whole purpose of theology was to comfort the troubled in heart, "to raise one conscience up out of despair," then the taste of sorrow was the indispensable qualification for a sincere theologian. Here Luther agrees with his biographers insofar as he does feel himself eminently well qualified by the many sharp assaults the devil has directed against him. Theologians, he taught, draw both training and practice from human suffering. Unlike the physician, the theologian must *undergo* an affliction before he can comfort it. . . . He could not count himself one of the simple folk able to accept God unquestioningly. "I did not come to my theology of a sudden, but had to brood ever more deeply. My trials brought me to it, for we do not learn anything except by experience." (Haile, 1980, p. 304)

Relative Importance of Different Aspects of the Illness to Different Types of Accomplishment

I was born to go to war, and give battle to sects and devils. That is why my books are stormy and warlike. I have to root out the stumps and clumps, hack away the thorns and brambles. I am the great feller of forests, who must clear the land and level it.   —Martin Luther, 1534[6]

I cannot see that there is anything remarkable about composing a symphony in a month. Handel wrote a complete oratorio in that time.   —Robert Schumann, 1850[7]

Changes brought about by manic-depressive illness—during hypomania, mania, depression, and normal states—produce different advantages and disadvantages in various fields of creative work and other types of accomplishment. Although there are no systematic data, a review of current sources strongly suggests that the actual prevalence of manic-depressive illness is distributed unequally across professions; for example, poets appear to have an unusually high rate, scientists a much lower one. To a poet, the cognitive, energy, mood, and experiential advantages of the elated and depressive states may outweigh the disruptions, chaos, turmoil, and inconsistent productivity that would be insurmountable to most scientists. Pragmatic issues of education and job requirement also probably affect the rates of manic-depressive illness in various occupations. Composers and poets, while increasingly likely to obtain graduate levels of education or professional training, do not absolutely require it. On the other hand, medical and graduate schools—particularly highly structured programs, such as those for medicine and law—tend to select students who, by and large, have demonstrated an ability to conform to strict requirements for consistently high levels of performance over long periods of time. This may well exclude many individuals at risk or those with an actual history of manic-depressive illness, since they are more likely to show greater variability in their performance across seasons and years.

The risk period for a first manic or depressive episode overlaps considerably with the period of advanced education, eliminating some manic-depressive individuals from being selected. Further selection bias exists in the decisions made about those individuals who have actually had an affective episode, especially a manic one, while in training. The consequences of a psychotic break (personally and professionally) are far different for those in medical school, law school, or a military academy than they are for those writing poetry or composing music.

Even within the field of literary accomplishment, differences in the characteristics of manic-depressive illness are likely to produce relative gains and losses to various types of writers. Poets may benefit much more from mood and cognitive changes than do novelists, for example, because the language and rhythms of poetry are more akin to primitive thought processes and psychosis and because the nature of sustained work is probably different in poetry and fiction.

Certain aspects of manic-depressive illness probably are important and helpful in other fields of accomplishment as well. It is likely that mood changes (elevated and expansive mood, inflated self-esteem, increased enthusiasm, increased emotional intensity, and infectious mood) might be equally, if differently, important to those who create and to those who lead. This is probably true as well for increased energy levels and a decreased need for sleep. However, on a very general level, it is likely that cognitive changes (sharpened and unusually creative thinking, flight of ideas, hyperacusis, delusions, and hallucinations) are more useful to those in arts and sciences than they are to those in positions of political and military leadership. Conversely, interpersonal changes brought about by hypomania (enhanced liveliness, uninhibited people-seeking, interpersonal charm, the ability to find vulnerable spots in others and to make use of them, increased perceptiveness at the subconscious or unconscious level, and increased social ease) are probably more likely to benefit those in the leadership rather than in the arts and sciences.

MANIC-DEPRESSIVE ILLNESS AND CREATIVITY

A work of art is a corner of creation seen through a temperament.   —Emile Zola[8]

. . . there is personal anguish everywhere. We can't dodge it, and shouldn't worry that we are uniquely marked and fretted and must somehow keep even-tempered, amused, and in control. John B[erryman] in his mad way keeps talking about something evil stalking us poets. That's a bad way to talk, but there's some truth in it.   —Robert Lowell[9]

Biographical Studies

In this section, we present a few of those individuals who have distinguished themselves in two fields of the creative arts—literature and music—and who also had manic-depressive illness (or severe cyclothymia). Although within the visual arts there have been numerous seriously depressed individuals (e.g., Romney and Michelangelo), psychotics (among others, Benvenuto Cellini, who had ecstatic visions and visual hallucinations), and many suicides (Modigliani, van Gogh, Jackson Pollock, René Crevel, and Mark Rothko), we stress here only the literary arts, with a brief discussion of composers. Affectively ill writers and composers provide special insight into mood disorders because of their ability to describe their experiences through words, sounds, and images. Yeats has described literature as "being wrought about a mood, or a community of moods"; perhaps it is not surprising that it is in literature that we find such a seemingly disproportionate rate of affective illness. Poetry, in particular, seems well served by the extremes of mood disorders:

The sign of the poet, then, is that by passion he enters into life more than other men. That is his gift—the power to live. . . [Poets] have been singularly creatures of passion. They lived before they sang. Emotion is the condition of their existence; passion is the element of their being; and, moreover, the intensifying power of such a state of passion must also be remembered, for emotion of itself naturally heightens all the faculties, and genius burns the brighter in its own flames. (George Edward Woodberry, in Wilkinson, 1925, p. 13)

Our focus here is on several English language poets, especially 18th and 19th century British poets and 20th century American poets. For all of its reputation as the age of reason, the 18th century, in fact, produced a remarkable number of psychotic or intensely disturbed poets. The affective component—melancholic, grandiose, ecstatically religious, visionary—is striking.

Christopher Smart (1722–1771) was hospitalized for insanity many times throughout his life. His first break occurred just after completing his degree at Cambridge. His behavior became increasingly bizarre, and he was found praying ceaselessly in highly public parts of London. His religious mania, which led to his hospitalizations, also contributed to poetry filled with exaltation, ecstasy, and a sense of divine mission. Much of his poetry was, like that of William Blake, highly imagistic and was regarded as unique among the lyrical poems of the 18th century. Smart won the Seatonian Prize for sacred poetry five times and is represented in virtually all anthologies of English verse. In this excerpt from "A Song to David," (1763) Smart's ecstatic imagery is obvious:

> Glorious the sun in mid-career;
> Glorious th' assembled fires appear;
> Glorious the comet's train:
> Glorious the trumpet and alarm;
> Glorious th' almighty stretched-out arm;
> Glorious th' enraptured main . . .

William Collins (1721–1759), who also suffered from manic-depressive illness, began writing poetry while very young, continued during his degree work at Oxford, had his first complete breakdown when 29, and died insane at the age of 38. Although he wrote very little (fewer than 1,500 lines of poetry), his work marked an original departure from contemporary poetic conventions. Like Smart, he is represented in all major anthologies of English poetry.

William Cowper (1731–1800) suffered many periods of severe depression before his first manic break at the age of 32. He suffered repeated mental breakdowns and suicide attempts over the course of his lifetime and used these experiences (psychosis, terrors, hallucinations, despair) to portray metaphorically many of the difficulties and conflicts of ordinary life. His writing is often credited with giving English poetry a new direction, quite distinct from the highly intellectualized poetry of Pope and other contemporaries

of Cowper. In these verses, from "The Shrubbery, Written in a Time of Affliction," Cowper reveals the effects of depression on the ability to sense and feel:

> This glassy stream, that spreading pine,
> Those alders quiv'ring to the breeze,
> Might sooth a soul less hurt than mine,
> And please, if anything could please.
> But fix'd unalterable care
> Foregoes not what she feels within,
> Shows the same sadness ev'ry where,
> And slights the season and the scene.

Robert Fergusson (1750–1774), the Scots poet, was even younger than Collins when he died. Insane, he died at the age of 24 after a bout of religious mania. He was the most notable of the Scots poets before Robert Burns, and some scholars speculate that had he lived long enough, he might well have surpassed Burns (Stapleton, 1983).

Thomas Chatterton (1752–1770), one of the most influential English poets (especially on the 19th century Romantics), committed suicide at the age of 17. He left behind a small but highly powerful collection of poems, most of which were written in the context of an imaginary world of his creation. From a psychiatric perspective, however, one of the most interesting things Chatterton ever wrote was his will, composed just before he killed himself. It is, at times, acerbically witty and includes a 54-line introductory poem, instructions for a grandiose memorial monument to be erected in his honor (with six tablets inscribed variously with heraldry, old English characters, and Roman lettering), and a long series of instructions, railings, and commentaries to friends and enemies alike. A few illustrative excerpts follow:

This is the last will and testament of me Thomas Chatterton, of the city of Bristol; being sound in body, or it is the fault of my last surgeon: the soundness of my mind, the coroner and jury are to be the judges of, desiring them to take notice, that the most perfect masters of human nature in Bristol distinguish me by the title of Mad Genius; therefore, if I do a mad action, it is conformable to every action of my life, which all savour'd of insanity . . .

Item. I give all my vigour and fire of youth to Mr. George Catcott, being sensible he is most in need of it . . .

Item. I give and bequeath to Mr. Matthew Mease a mourning ring, with this motto, "Alas, poor Chatterton!" provided he pays for it himself . . . (Dix, 1837, pp. 237–242)

The last 18th century poet we consider is *William Blake* (1757–1827), the great visionary, mystic, poet, painter, and engraver. There is much controversy about Blake's "madness"—its nature, and, indeed, its existence. However, virtually all Blake biographers discuss it at some length. Most of his contemporaries thought him mad, but many of his close friends and acquaintances attributed his strange behavior to the eccentricities of genius. Two other well-known poets who knew Blake described him in the following ways:

You perhaps smile at *my* calling another Poet, *a Mystic;* but verily I am in the very mire of commonplace common-place compared with Mr. Blake. (Coleridge, 1957, p. 132)

Much as he is to be admired, he was at that time so evidently insane that the predominant feeling in conversing with him, or even looking at him, could only be sorrow and compassion . . . you perceived that nothing but madness had prevented him from being the sublimest painter of this or any other country. You could not have delighted in him—his madness was too evident, too fearful. It gave his eyes an expression such as you would expect to see in one who was possessed. (Robert Southey in Wilson, 1971, pp. 268–269)

Blake was renowned for his ceaseless energy, his ecstatic states, and, most strikingly, his frequent and extraordinary visions and visitations. He often was observed conversing with people from centuries past and tirelessly drawing or painting the strange and mystical visions that would appear before him. From the time he was a young child and first saw the forehead of God against his window and the trees full of angels with bright wings, Blake moved in and out of a visionary world. His moods fluctuated from despair to exultation, and it is perhaps not surprising that one of his greatest works should be called "The Marriage of Heaven and Hell." In the margin of a book Blake was reading on insanity, he wrote: "Cowper came to me and said . . . You retain health and yet are as mad as any of us," and in his poem "Mad Song," he wrote:

> Lo! to the vault
>   Of pavèd heaven,
> With sorrow fraught,
>   My notes are driven;
> They strike the ear of Night,
>   Make weep the eyes of Day;
> They make mad the roaring winds,
>   And with tempests play.

The diagnostic issues surrounding Blake's psychological idiosyncrasies are less clear than for the other poets we have discussed, although manic-depressive illness would appear to be consistent with what is known about his fluctuating, alternating, and grandiose mood states in conjunction with his pronounced visual and perceptual changes.

It is interesting to note that of the six major 18th century poets we have discussed, five of them are represented in the *New Oxford Book of English Verse: 1250–1950*. This is one quarter of the 18th century poets represented, a remarkably high rate of manic-depressive illness. It should be emphasized that this is a very low estimate of the total bipolar percentage in this total group of poets, for the rest of the 21 subjects have not yet been systematically reviewed.

The large number of psychotic or severely disturbed poets in the 18th century is particularly striking in an era designated as "The Age of Reason." The 19th century, however, well known for its excesses of moods and intensity of expression, produced many poets living up to the century's reputation. Several poets were clearly either manic-depressive or extremely cyclothymic, including John Clare, Edgar Allan Poe, Lord Byron, Alfred Lord Tennyson, and Percy Bysshe Shelley. Probably cyclothymic, but certainly subject to at least severe depressive illness, were Samuel Taylor Coleridge, Dante Gabriel Rossetti, and Gerard Manley Hopkins.

Of these, only *John Clare* (1793–1864) was actually hospitalized for insanity. His first psychotic break occurred when he was 40 years old, recurred within the year, and then frequently after that. His insanity was characterized by, among other things, visual hallucinations, grandiose delusions, restlessness, and walking exceedingly long distances (e.g., he once walked virtually nonstop for 3 days). His depressive side is expressed in many of his poems, including this excerpt from "I Am":

> I am—yet what I am, none cares or knows;
>   My friends forsake me like a memory lost:—
> I am the self-consumer of my woes;—
>   They rise and vanish in oblivion's host,
> Like shadows in love's frenzied stifled throes:—
> And yet I am, and live—like vapours tost

Percy Bysshe Shelley (1792–1822) has been characterized as someone who "left disorder wherever he trod" (Stapleton, 1983). Like his friend Byron, Shelley had a family history of insanity (Holmes, 1974). Even as a young boy, he was notorious for his temper and moods. One of his fellow students, Sir John Rennie, described him in the following way (quoted in Untermeyer, 1959):

The least circumstance that thwarted him produced the most violent paroxysms of rage; and when irritated by other boys, he would take up anything or even any little boy near him, to throw at his tormentors. His imagination was always roving upon something romantic and extraordinary, such as spirits, fairies, fighting, volcanoes, etc., and he not infrequently astonished his schoolfellows by blowing up the boundary palings of the playground with gunpowder. (pp. 419–420)

At Eton he was known as "Mad Shelley," where he continued his reputation for being highly strung, reckless, and of nervous temperament. He was expelled from Oxford for professing atheism and, by the age of 20, was taking laudanum to calm his nerves. His financial behavior was extravagant and characterized by reckless borrowing. After a short, very unconventional, and tumultuous life, Shelley died in a drowning accident at the age of 30.

Lord Byron (1788–1824), like his friend Shelley, led a wild and chaotic life, marked by profound mood swings and behavior radically unlike that which was socially acceptable. Enâchescu (1971) described Byron as having manic-depressive psychosis; at the very least, he was certainly an extreme cyclothymic. Byron's paternal grandfather was known for his violent temper. His granduncle, whom he succeeded in the title, was known as the "Mad Lord Byron." His father, called "Mad Jack Byron," was described as completely dissolute and financially extravagant, and he probably committed suicide. His maternal grandfather was melancholic and committed suicide, another first-degree relative on his mother's side attempted suicide, and his mother was known for her "frequent fits of uncontrollable fury" and unpredictable changes in mood. Not surprisingly, with this family history, Byron described a continual fear of going mad and referred frequently to the "curse of the Byrons."

Lord Byron was subject to wild changes in mood, melancholia, hallucinations, remarkable financial extravagance (by the age of 21, he owed £12,000), and what can only be described as extraordinary eccentricity (e.g., maintaining a large menagerie, which started with keeping a bear in his rooms at Cambridge). Shelley regarded Byron as "mad as a hatter," and Lady Byron left him after a year of marriage because "Lord Byron was under the influence of insanity." No doubt, some of Byron's odd behavior was deliberate, "Byronic," and theatrical, but intense moodiness was a constant throughout most of his life. Leicester Stanhope, Byron's friend and companion, wrote:

The mind of Byron was like a volcano, full of fire and wealth, sometimes calm, often dazzling and playful, but ever threatening. It ran swift as the lightning from one subject to another, and occasionally burst forth in passionate throes of intellect nearly allied to madness. A striking example of this sort of eruption I shall mention. Lord Byron's apartments were immediately over mine at Missolonghi. In the dead of night I was frequently startled from my sleep by the thunders of his lordship's voice, either raging with anger or roaring with laughter, and arousing friends, servants, and, indeed, all the inmates of the dwelling from their repose.

Samuel Taylor Coleridge (1772–1834), best known in his personal life for his addiction to opium, suffered throughout his life from extreme, intermittent depressions. He was also a heavy drinker, impulsive, erratically productive and—like Shelley and Byron—financially dissolute. He was inclined to great rage and, on occasion, seriously considered suicide. His description of depression, "viper thoughts, that coil around my mind," is graphic in this excerpt from "Dejection: An Ode":

A grief without a pang, void, dark, and drear,
A stifled, drowsy, unimpassioned grief,
Which finds no natural outlet, no relief,
In word, or sigh, or tear—

Edgar Allan Poe (1809–1849), noted for the morbid quality of both his poetry and prose and considered "insanely depressed," was known for his extreme morbidity of thought, his pronounced restlessness and paranoia, and his heavy financial debts and even heavier drinking. He attempted suicide at least once and died at the age of 41, a death brought on in part by his alcoholism. Of the relationship between genius and madness, he wrote:

I am come of a race noted for vigor of fancy and ardor of passion. Men have called me mad; but the question is not yet settled, whether madness is or is not the loftiest intelligence—whether much that is glorious—whether all that is profound—does not spring from disease of thought—from *moods* of mind exalted at the expense of the general intellect. (1980, p. 243)

Dante Gabriel Rossetti (1828–1882) also suffered from deep depressions, delusional at times. He abused narcotics and engaged in many rather bizarre behaviors (e.g., he housed an extensive menagerie in expectation that his dead wife might be reincarnated as an animal).

The last 19th century poet to be considered here is *Gerard Manley Hopkins* (1844–1889), who once said, "My fits of sadness resemble madness." He experienced several debilitating periods of depression. This excerpt is taken from one of his "Dark Sonnets" (which he described as having been "written in blood"):

No worst, there is none. Pitched past pitch of grief,
More pangs will, schooled at forepangs, wilder wring.
Comforter, where, where is your comforting?. . .
O the mind, mind has mountains; cliffs of fall
Frightful, sheer, no-man-fathomed. Hold them cheap
May who ne'er hung there.

That excerpt stands in marked depressive contrast to another, taken from the earlier ecstatic religious poem "The Windhover: To Christ Our Lord":

I caught this morning morning's minion, kingdom of daylight's dauphin, dapple-dawn-drawn Fal-
   con, in his riding
   Of the rolling level underneath him steady air, and
      striding
High there, how he rung upon the rein of a wimpling
   wing
In his ecstasy!. . .

The 20th century has proved no exception to the apparently high rate of affective illness—especially manic-depressive illness—in poets. A remarkable number of outstanding American poets born in the first 35 years of this century have been hospitalized and treated for manic and major depressive episodes. Table 14-2 shows a partial listing of this group of poets. A complete biographical review of all major American poets born during this period has not been completed. *Ezra Pound* (1885–1972), an extremely influential poet during this era but born before it, also has been thought by at least some to have had manic-depressive illness (Kapp, 1968).

All of the poets listed in Table 14-2 are represented in *The New Oxford Book of American Verse*. A total of 36 American poets born in this century are in the Oxford anthology. Thus, more than a fifth exhibit well-documented histories of manic-depressive illness severe enough to have warranted at least one hospitalization. Again, this is a very low estimate of the total rate of bipolar illness, since Table 14-2 is based on a review of biographical materials for these eight poets only, not for the others. Assuming a general population rate of 1 or 2 percent for bipolar affective illness, this very conservative estimate of the illness in poets signifies a striking increase in what would be expected. It should also be noted that a frighteningly high percentage of these top poets (five of eight, or 62 percent) committed suicide and that the mean age at death was 48 years (ranging from 31 to 60 years).

Although among writers, poets appear the most likely to suffer from manic-depressive illness, many novelists, playwrights, and others have as well. Those with extreme cyclothymia or psychotic forms of the disease include: Honoré de Balzac, Ernest Hemingway, Charles Lamb, John Stuart Mill, F. Scott Fitzgerald, Herman Melville, Ralph Waldo Emerson, Virginia Woolf, John Ruskin, William Inge, Johann Wolfgang von Goethe, William Saroyan, Cesare Pavese, and Eugene O'Neill. Dostoyevski and Tolstoy certainly suffered at least from severe, recurrent depressions. *Balzac* (1799-1850), for example, had an early sense of destiny, worked with a formidable level of energy and drive, was intermittently suicidal and omnipotent, and was notorious for his extraordinary spending and incurring of debt (Maugham, 1954; Storr, 1972).

Goethe (1749–1832), too, has been described as cyclothymic (Eissler, 1967; Enâchescu, 1971). Most are familiar with the despairing and suicidal aspects of Goethe's work, personified by *Werther*, but Eissler presents the other side of Goethe's personality:

But what is it to be said when, at the age of 42, a poet, author, government administrator suddenly—literally from one moment to the next—conceives the idea that the greatest physicist of his times (Newton had been dead for 64 years when the idea struck Goethe) was utterly wrong in his demonstration that white light consists of the colors of the spectrum, and from then on spends years going through the whole literature on light, finally writing a manuscript on the subject which it would take almost 2,500 pages to print? (p. 40)

Table 14-2. Partial Listing of Major 20th Century American Poets, Born Between 1895 and 1935, with Documented Histories of Manic-Depressive Illness

Poet	Pulitzer Prize in Poetry	Treated for Major Depressive Illness	Treated for Mania	Committed Suicide
Hart Crane (1899 - 1932)		X	X	X
Theodore Roethke (1908 - 1963)	X	X	X	
Delmore Schwartz (1913 - 1966)		X	X	
John Berryman (1914 - 1972)	X	X	X	X
Randall Jarrell (1914 - 1965)		X	X	X
Robert Lowell (1917 - 1977)	X	X	X	
Anne Sexton (1928 - 1974)	X	X	X	X
Sylvia Plath[a] (1932 - 1963)	X	X		X

[a]Plath, although not treated for mania, was probably bipolar II

John Ruskin (1819–1900), 19th century writer, critic, and social reformer—acknowledged by Clement Attlee to be the spiritual founder of the British Labour Party and by Gandhi to have been responsible for much of his early thought about social justice (Joseph, 1969)—was overtly psychotic for most of the last 10 years of his life and intermittently long before that. Although Joseph (1969) diagnoses Ruskin as a schizophrenic, this is at variance with available evidence and with virtually all other literary and psychiatric biographies, which consider him as having manic-depressive psychosis (e.g., Bragman, 1935; Wilenski, 1933). Ruskin's own description of his problems (1900) is quite consistent with manic-depressive illness.

Our final literary example is perhaps one of the best-known manic-depressive authors, *Virginia Woolf*. Her husband, Leonard Woolf, described the relationship of her illness to her literary creativity:

. . . I referred to the ancient belief that genius is near allied to madness. I am quite sure that Virginia's genius was closely connected with what manifested itself as mental instability and insanity. The creative imagination in her novels, her ability to 'leave the ground' in conversation, and the voluble delusions of the breakdowns all came from the same place in her mind—she 'stumbled after her own voice' and followed 'the voices that fly ahead'. And that in itself was the crux of her life, the tragedy of genius. (Woolf, 1964, p. 80)

She herself wrote:

As an experience, madness is terrific I can assure you, and not to be sniffed at; and in its lava I still find most of the things I write about. It shoots out of one everything shaped, final, not in mere driblets, as sanity does. (Woolf, 1978, p. 180)

Caramagno (in press) has discussed Woolf's manic-depressive illness in detail.

Several great composers have also suffered from manic-depressive psychosis or extreme cyclothymia (Jamison and Winter, 1988).

Robert Schumann (1810–1856) came from a family filled with affective illness. Both his mother and father were clinically depressed, two first-degree relatives committed suicide, and one son spent more than 30 years in an asylum (Slater and Meyer, 1959; Taylor, 1982; Ostwald, 1983). Schumann himself suffered from episodic depressions and manias most of his adult life. He made at least two suicide attempts and died, in 1856, in an insane asylum. Figure 14-1 presents Schumann's works by year and opus number (adapted from Slater and Meyer, 1959). The quantitative relationship between his mood state and his creative output is quite striking; when most depressed he produced least, and when hypomanic he produced at a remarkable level. The relationship of mood to the quality of production is unclear, although both the quality and the quantity of his work, as well as his mental health, deteriorated in the final years of his life. A few years before he died, Schumann wrote:

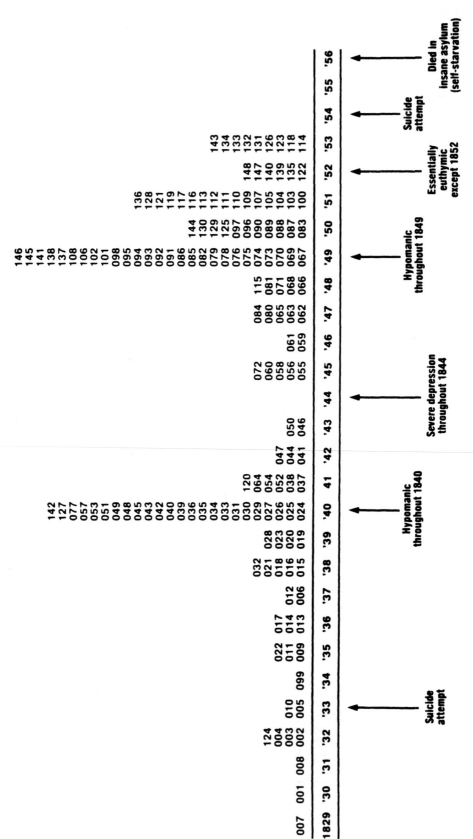

Figure 14-1. Schumann's works by year and opus number (adapted from Slater and Meyer, 1959).

. . . Lately I was looking for information about Düsseldorf in an old geography book, and there I found mentioned as noteworthy: "three convents and a lunatic asylum." To the first I have no objection if it must be so; but it was disagreeable to me to read the last . . . I am obliged to avoid carefully all melancholy impressions of the kind. And if we musicians live so often, as you know we do, on sunny heights, the sadness of reality cuts all the deeper when it lies naked before our eyes. (Niecks, 1925, p. 25)

Hugo Wolf (1860–1903) was another composer with pronounced periods of marked productivity and others of virtually no creative activity at all (Hecaen, 1934; Slater and Meyer, 1960). During periods of depression, Wolf was suicidal, filled with self-contempt, and unable even to write a letter. When hypomanic, he was described by others as warm, infectiously good-humored, charismatic, joyous, full of energy, and irritable. One friend wrote: "Who has not seen Hugo Wolf rejoice does not know what rejoicing is." Wolf entered an asylum when he was 37 years old and was able to leave it for only a few months in 1898. He again became psychotic and attempted suicide. He returned to the asylum and died there at the age of 43. Although he suffered from general paresis as well, his tempestuous mood swings predated his exposure to syphilis. Like Schumann, Hugo Wolf wrote painfully well about his moods. In 1891, he wrote:

As you know, the spring of my creative work has been practically dried up for several years. What this appalling realization means to me is quite indescribable. Since then I have led, truly, the existence of a frog and not even that of a living one, but that of a galvanic frog. To be sure, I appear at times merry and in good heart, talk, too, before others quite reasonably, and it looks as if I felt, too, God knows how well within my skin; yet the soul maintains its deathly sleep and the heart bleeds from a thousand wounds. (Walker, 1968, p. 361)

Two years later, he described himself as "leading the existence of an oyster" and wrote:

What I suffer from this continuous idleness I am quite unable to describe. I would like most to hang myself on the nearest branch of the cherry-trees standing now in full bloom. This wonderful spring with its secret life and movement troubles me unspeakably. These eternal blue skies, lasting for weeks, this continuous sprouting and budding in nature, these coaxing breezes impregnated with spring sunlight and fragrance of flowers . . . make me frantic. Everywhere this bewildering urge for life, fruitfulness, creation—and only I, although like the humblest grass of the fields one of God's creatures, may not take part in this festival of resurrection, at any rate not except as a spectator with grief and envy. (Walker, 1968, p. 322)

Other cyclothymic or manic-depressive composers include Gioacchino Rossini, Hector Berlioz, Anton Bruckner, Peter Tchaikovsky, Orlando de Lassus, Alexander Scriabin, Gustav Mahler, and Sergey Rachmaninoff. George Frideric Handel probably suffered from cyclothymia (Slater and Meyer, 1960; Storr, 1972; Young, 1975; Keynes, 1980), but the unavailability of detailed autobiographical and biographical information makes conclusive diagnosis problematic (Frosch, 1987, 1989).

Systematic Studies

There have been few systematic studies into the relationship between psychopathology and artistic creativity. Two early investigations, those of Ellis (1904) and Jura (1949), were sufficiently flawed by problems in both inclusionary and diagnostic criteria that their results are essentially meaningless.

Andreasen and her colleagues undertook the first scientific inquiries into the relationship between creativity and psychopathology in general and affective disorders in particular (Andreasen and Canter, 1974; Andreasen and Powers, 1975; Andreasen, 1987a). Andreasen's studies, using structured interviews, systematic diagnostic criteria (RDC), and matched control groups, represented marked methodological advances over prior, anecdotally based research. The size of their sample of writers was relatively small ($n = 30$), and the subjects were at varying levels of creative accomplishment (all were participants in the University of Iowa Writer's workshop, but some were nationally acclaimed writers and others were graduate students or teaching fellows not at the level of national or international recognition). Andreasen notes that because she studied only writers, her results cannot be generalized to other groups of creative individuals, such as philosophers, scientists, or musicians. Although this is true, and writers might be disproportionately likely to have affective disorders, the homogeneity of the sample is certainly valuable in its own right.

The results of the Iowa research are summarized in Table 14-3. Clearly, the writers had an extraordinarily high rate of affective illness and

Table 14-3. Lifetime Prevalence of Mental Illness in Writers and Control Subjects

RDC Diagnosis	Writers (N=30) %	Controls (N=30) %	p
Any affective disorder	80	30	.001
Any bipolar disorder	43	10	.01
Bipolar I	13	0	NS
Bipolar II	30	10	NS
Major depression	37	17	NS
Schizophrenia	0	0	NS
Alcoholism	30	7	.05
Drug abuse	7	7	NS
Suicide	7	0	NS

Adapted from Andreasen, 1987a

alcoholism. Fully 80 percent of the study sample met criteria for a major affective disorder. In contrast, 30 percent of the control sample (individuals outside the arts who were matched for age, education, and sex) met the same criteria ($p < 0.001$). Although this is a much lower figure, it should be noted that it still represents a rate much greater than that expected for the general population (5 to 8 percent). It is unclear whether this represents an overrepresentation of affective illness in the sample or the diagnostic criteria were overly inclusive for both the creative and control groups. Almost one half (43 percent) of the cre-

ative sample met the diagnostic criteria for bipolar-I or bipolar-II disorder.

The authors also investigated the family histories of the writers and the controls. Consistent with the higher rate of affective illness in the writers, their findings showed that affective illness in primary relatives, summarized in Table 14-4, was much higher for the writers than for the controls ($p < 0.001$). The overall prevalence for any type of psychiatric disorder was also much higher in the writers (42 percent) than in the controls (8 percent). Additionally, first-degree relatives of writers had a higher incidence of creativity (20 percent) than did relatives of the controls (8 percent).[10] These findings led Andreasen to suggest a familial association between creativity and affective disorders, an association consistent with findings of other researchers as well (Karlsson, 1970; McNeil, 1971; Richards, 1981).

Using a very different research design to study the relationship of creativity and psychopathology, Richards and colleagues at Harvard (1988) investigated broadly defined creativity in a sample of patients and their relatives. They hypothesized that a genetic vulnerability to manic-depressive illness is accompanied by a predisposition to creativity, which, according to this hypothesis, is more prominent among close relatives of manic-depressive patients than among the patients themselves. Such a compensatory advantage would be roughly analogous to the resistance to malaria found among unaffected carriers of the gene for

Table 14-4. Mental Illness in First-Degree Relatives of 30 Writers and 30 Control Subjects

Family History RDC Diagnosis	All Relatives			Parents			Siblings		
	Of Writers (N=116) %	Of Controls (N=121) %	p	Of Writers (N=60) %	Of Controls (N=60) %	p	Of Writers (N=56) %	Of Controls (N=121) %	p
Any affective disorder	18	2	.001	7	2	.001	20	3	.01
Bipolar disorder	3	0	.056	2	0	NS	5	0	NS
Major depression	15	2	.01	5	2	.05	14	3	.05
Alcoholism	7	6	NS	8	7	NS	5	5	NS
Suicide	3	0	NS	3	0	NS	2	0	NS
Any illness	42	8	.0001	42	8	.00003	43	8	.001

Adapted from Andreasen, 1987a

sickle-cell anemia. To test their hypothesis, Richards and her associates selected 17 manic-depressive and 16 cyclothymic patients and 11 normal first-degree relatives of such patients, using criteria that would ensure inclusion of a spectrum of disorders, and compared them with 15 normal control subjects and 18 controls with a psychiatric diagnosis but with no personal or family history of major affective disorder, cyclothymia, schizoaffective disorder, schizophrenia, or suicide. Unlike other studies in the field, which limit the definition of creativity to significant, socially recognized accomplishment in the arts or sciences, these investigators attempted to measure the disposition toward originality manifested in a wide range of everyday endeavors. They administered the Lifetime Creativity Scales, a previously validated instrument that assesses the quality and quantity of creative involvement in both work and leisure activities (see Table 14-5 for examples).

Richards and colleagues found significantly higher combined creativity scores among the manic-depressive and cyclothymic patients and their normal first-degree relatives than in control subjects (Figure 14-2). The normal index relatives showed suggestively higher creativity than did the manic-depressive patients, and the cyclothymic patients were close to the normal relatives. Modifying their original hypothesis, the authors concluded:

Overall peak creativity may be enhanced, on the average, in subjects showing milder and, perhaps, subclinical expressions of potential bipolar liability (i.e., the cyclothymes and normal first-degree relatives) compared either with individuals who carry no bipolar liability (control subjects) or individuals with more severe manifestations of bipolar liability (manic-depressives). . . . There may be a positive compensatory advantage . . . to genes associated with greater liability for bipolar disorder. The possibility that normal relatives of manic-depressives and cyclothymes have heightened creativity may have been overlooked because of a medical-model orientation that focused on

---

Table 14-5. Abbreviated Examples of Subjects at Three Rating Levels of Peak Vocational Creativity

Example 1	Example 2
No significant creativity	
Mixed and carried mortar for local brick layer for 20 years, then inherited a large income-paying trust fund and retired to a passive life on a country estate	Washed store windows for 3 years under foreman's supervision, spent 5 years on assembly lines in two factories, and, for the past 11 years, has done routine quality-control tasks in a brewery
Moderate peak creativity	
Longtime owner and manager of a small dairy farm who, after 10 years of producing cheese and other dairy products, expanded and began marketing through a local distributor	Optician who spent 4 years selling optical items, then acquired a small optical shop, and now grinds lenses to prescription while managing the retailing of standard optical products
High peak creativity	
Former avant garde dancer and choreographer who developed and directed a variety of unusual productions for several dance companies, but, postwar, has worked solely as a hotel clerk	Entrepreneur who advanced from chemist's apprentice to independent researcher of new products before starting a major paint manufacturing company, and whose operation surreptitiously manufactured and smuggled explosives for the Danish Resistance during World War II

Note. The primary distinction between avocational and vocational activities is whether the activity was financially compensated. The following points are pertinent to both avocational and vocational measures: (a) peak creativity is based only on the level of the most creative major enterprise, (b) appreciation of others' creativity is not credited on these scales, and (c) social recognition is not required as a criterion for higher creativity. Examples have been altered to protect subjects' confidentiality

From Richards et al., 1988

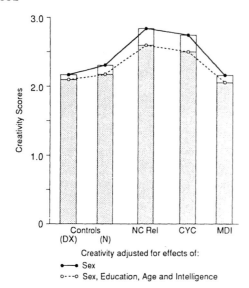

Figure 14-2. Mean creativity in selected diagnostic groups. Mean overall peak creativity scores for controls with a diagnosis (DX), normal controls (NL), normal first-degree biological relatives of cyclothymes and manic-depressives (NL REL), cyclothymes (CYCLO), and manic-depressives (MDI) (from Richards et al., 1988).

dysfunction rather than positive characteristics of individuals. Such a compensatory advantage among the relatives of a disorder affecting at least 1% of the population could affect a relatively large group of people. (p. 287)

Somewhat related but very preliminary research (DeLong and Aldershof, 1983) found an unusually high incidence of special abilities (e.g., outstanding artistic or mathematical talent, hyperlexia, and so forth) in a sample of children with manic-depressive illness.

Jamison (1989), in a study of outstanding British writers and artists, not only examined rates of treatment for affective illness within these groups but also looked at seasonal patterns of moods and productivity, the nature of intense creative episodes and the similarities between such episodes and hypomania, and the perceived role of very intense moods in the writers' or artists' work.[11] Subjects were chosen for the study on the basis of having won at least one of several specified top prizes or awards in their fields. Thus, all painters and sculptors were either Royal Academicians or Associates of the Royal Academy.[12]

Among the major criterion prizes used in the selection of poets were the Queen's Gold Medal[13] and the Cholmondeley Award. Nine of the 18 poets in the study sample were already represented in *The Oxford Book of Twentieth Century English Verse*. Six of the eight playwrights had won the New York Drama Critics Award and/or the Evening Standard Drama Award (the London critics' award); several had won both or had won one of these awards more than once.[14] Three of the five biographers had won the James Tait Black Memorial Prize, one of Britain's most prestigious literary awards.[15] The literary awards won by the novelists were distributed over a relatively larger number of prizes, but the level of prestige and associated excellence was comparable to the other groups of writers.

The artists and writers were asked whether they had ever received treatment and the nature of that treatment for a mood disorder. The results are shown in Figure 14-3. It can be seen that a very high percentage of the total sample (38 percent) had been treated for an affective illness. Three fourths of those treated had been given antidepressants or lithium, or they had been hospitalized. Poets were most likely to have received medication for depression (33 percent) and were the only ones to have received medical intervention (hospitalization, electroconvulsive therapy, lithium) for mania (17 percent). Thus, one half of the poets had been treated with drugs or hospitalized for mood disorders. This rate is strikingly high when compared with (U.S.) lifetime prevalence estimates of 1.2 percent for bipolar and 4.4 percent for unipolar major depressive disorders (Weissman et al., 1988a). The rate is even higher when one considers the fact that the proportion of those so seriously ill as to actually require treatment is much lower, perhaps one third to one half the rates reported in prevalence studies using diagnostic criteria only (Andreasen and Canter, 1974; Robins et al., 1984). A further underestimate of the total rate of affective illness in the study sample derives from its being comprised largely of British males, a group less likely than most to seek out and receive treatment. The playwrights had the highest total rate of treatment for mood disorders (63 percent), but a very high percentage (38 percent) had been treated with psychotherapy alone. It is unclear whether this was due to a difference in illness severity or in treatment preference. Visual artists and biographers

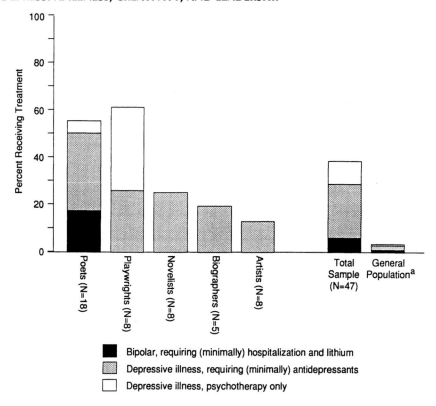

Figure 14-3. Rates of treatment for affective illness in a sample of British writers and artists (Jamison, 1989).

[a]The percentages for the general population are based on Epidemiological Catchment Area data. They indicate that less than one third of those individuals with bipolar or unipolar disorder receive treatment in any 6-month period.

had relatively lower rates of treatment (13 percent and 20 percent, respectively); all treatment was with antidepressants.

Although, with the exception of the poets, the subjects reported being treated for depression, not mania or hypomania, the design of the study did not allow systematic inquiry into hypomanic or manic episodes. However, as Figure 14-4 shows, about one third of the writers and artists reported histories of severe mood swings, and one fourth reported histories of extended elated mood states. The novelists and poets most frequently reported elated mood states, whereas the playwrights and artists were the most likely to report severe mood swings. Biographers reported no history of severe mood swings or elated states, an interesting finding, since of the five groups, they are the least likely to be associated with "creative fire" and thus provide a natural comparison group (i.e., a group highly proficient in writing abilities but perhaps less outstandingly creative by the nature of their work).

One of the major purposes of the British study was to look at the similarities and dissimilarities between periods of intense creative activity and hypomania. Hypothesized similarities were based on the episodic nature of both, the overlapping nature of the behavioral, mood, and cognitive changes associated with both, and a possible link between the duration and frequencies of the two types of experiences. Almost all of the subjects (89 percent) reported having experienced intense, creative episodes (100 percent of the poets, novelists, and artists, 88 percent of the playwrights and, consistent with results reported earlier, only 20 percent of the biographers). The modal duration of these episodes was 2 weeks (35 percent); 55 percent of the episodes lasted 1 to 4 weeks, 20 percent lasted 1 to 24 hours, and 25 percent continued for longer than 1 month. The

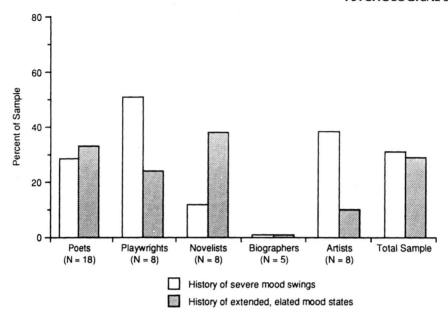

Figure 14-4. History of severe mood swings and extended elated states in a sample of British writers and artists (based on data in Jamison, 1989).

episodes were characterized by increases in enthusiasm, energy, self-confidence, speed of mental associations, fluency of thoughts, mood, and sense of well-being (Figure 14-5). Mood and cognitive changes showed the greatest degree of overlap with the episodes characterized as "intense creativity" (what would be more clinically characterized as hypomania). Approximately half of the subjects described a decreased need for sleep and increased sensory awareness, but several of the more behavioral changes typically associated with hypomania (hypersexuality, increased talkativeness, and spending of money) were reported by only a minority of subjects.

When asked open-ended questions about changes before these intense creative episodes, 89 percent reported less need for sleep. Coincident with the timing of the switch process in manic-depressive illness, 28 percent spontaneously reported waking abruptly at 3 or 4 AM and being unable to return to sleep. Fifty percent of the subjects reported a sharp increase in mood just before the beginning of an intensely creative period; for example, "I have a fever to write, and throw myself energetically into new projects," "excited, anticipatory, energetic," "more optimistic," "elated," "uplifted," "euphoric," and

"ecstatic." Dysphoria preceded creativity in 28 percent of the subjects: "more anxious," "near suicide," "increased irritability and tension," "fearfulness, general mood of distress and slight paranoia," and "irritable, antisocial." Finally, 22 percent reported mixed mood changes and psychomotor restlessness: "mixture of elation together with some gloominess, feeling of isolation, sexual pressure, fast emotional responses," "restlessness," "low ebb bordering on despair often precedes good phase when work will flow almost as though one is a medium, rather than an originator," "restless, dissatisfied." When asked specifically about the importance of very intense feelings and moods in their work, almost 90 percent stated that such moods and feelings were either integral and necessary (60 percent) or very important (30 percent). More poets than any other group regarded these intense moods as integral and necessary to what they did and how they did it.

Yet another area linking some aspects of creativity to affective illness is seasonal patterns of mood and productivity. Subjects were asked to rate their moods and productivity over the preceding 36 months. Figures 14-6 and 14-7 show mood and productivity curves for the study sample

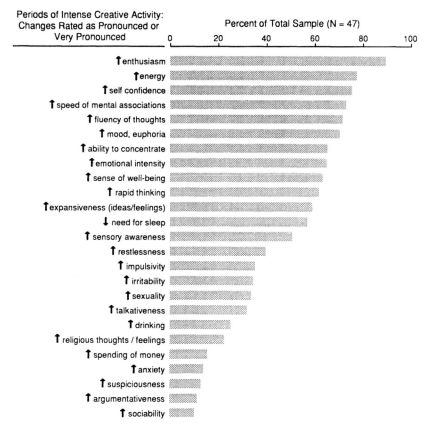

Figure 14-5. Periods of intense creativity in a sample of British writers and artists (from Jamison, 1989).

Figure 14-6. Mean mood and productivity ratings (36 months) in British writers and artists with a history of treatment for affective illness ($n = 15$) (from Jamison, 1989).

Figure 14-7. Mean mood and productivity ratings (36 months) in British writers and artists with no history of treatment for affective illness ($n = 32$) (from Jamison, 1989).

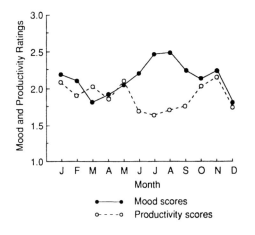

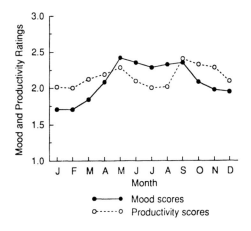

(broken down into those writers and artists with a history of treatment for an affective illness vs those with no history). Very different seasonal patterns emerged. Those with a history of treatment demonstrate inversely related curves for summer productivity and moods, whereas those in the group with no history of treatment show mood and productivity curves more directly covarying. In the treatment group, the peaks for productivity precede and follow the mood peak by 3 to 4 months. Several hypotheses can be raised to explain these differences. First, elevated productivity associated with elevated mood is less likely to lead to treatment-seeking behavior than low productivity associated with high, or any other, mood. Second, the elevated mood of the treatment group probably reflects more true hypomania (i.e., more dysphoria, greater distractibility, increased stimulus and people-seeking), which might well lead to less productivity in the acute phase. Andreasen (1980) found this in several of the writers in her study:

> Some of their periods of hypomania were clearly counterproductive. The increased energy that they experienced could not be focused and controlled so that it could be expressed creatively, and so that energy was dissipated in social or personal outlets. (p. 381)

In the no-treatment group, the periods of increased mood and productivity may represent a milder form of hypomania, with cognitive and mood changes only. These milder forms of hypomania or intensified normal functioning may result in simultaneous peaks for mood and productivity. In the treatment group, the execution of work may precede and lag behind the mood component.

One of the artists in the British study described the complicated relationship among moods, talent, and genius. It serves here as a summary statement:

> People can be talented, hardworking and masters of their craft—but it takes a kink in someone's personality to make them like a genius. This "kink" can be a bitter childhood or just a demon of frustrated energies that if not channelled into work becomes self-destructive. Mood, upbringing, or whatever passion chases talent out of someone, is irrelevant, because if someone has genius they don't need moods to heighten their work; it pours out of them. Only very talented people need madness to make themselves more special. Mozart was a genius. I am not as I rely on my moods to make my work special.

MANIC-DEPRESSIVE ILLNESS AND LEADERSHIP

Political and Military Leadership

I used to say of him [Napoleon] that his presence on the field made the difference of forty thousand men. —Arthur Wellesley, 1st Duke of Wellington[16]

. . . there is much evidence for his [Oliver Cromwell's] manic phases. "He was of a sanguine complexion . . . naturally of such a vivacity, hilarity and alacrity as another man is when he hath drunk a cup too much." . . . "I am very often judged for one that goes too fast. . . ." Cromwell admitted to the Army Council. "It is the property of men that are as I am, to be full of apprehensions that dangers are not so real as imaginary; to be always making haste, and more sometimes than good speed." (pp. 193–194) —Christopher Hill, 1970

Inspiration is as important to powerful leadership as it is to creativity in the arts. Unlike the arts, however, no systematic investigations have been done into the relationship between leadership and manic-depressive illness. Likewise, very few biographical studies exist that attempt to examine political or military leaders from this perspective. Nevertheless, hypomanic states share many characteristics with certain types of impassioned authority: high-energy level, enthusiasm, intensity of emotion, persuasion by mood, charisma, and contagion of spirit, gregariousness and extraversion, increased belief in one's self and one's ideas (including grandiosity), "grasping beyond the common grasp," optimism, hyperacusis, heightened alertness and observational abilities, risk-taking (including both impetuousness and courage), unpredictable and subtle changes in mood, eye movements, pacing, and speech, impatience and shortened attention span, and mercurial temperament. The ability to inspire—through words, actions, or traditions—is especially important in leadership. Here Napoleon, Alexander the Great, and Lord Nelson are examples of those set apart by their ability to arouse mood, enthusiasm, and energy in their followers. The Celtic languages have many names for their heroes, including *Nia* (ardor, passion) and *Niab* (vivacity and energy). All the Celtic words for hero express notions of fury, ardor, and speed: "the hero is thus conceived as the ardent one, as one who overflows with energy and life" (Sjoestedt, 1982). Many heroes and great leaders have been characterized by their excesses in rage, energy, and pride—for example, Alexander the Great or the great mythic Irish hero Cú Chulain, who was overcome by violent ecstasy and whose ardor could "heat three vats of water." Interestingly, early Irish writers noted that Cú Chulain, like so many heroes and leaders, also could go for long periods of time without sleep, an obvious asset, especially to military leaders.

An early sense of destiny, often having a grandiose quality to it, is not uncommon in great leaders. Thus, Oliver Cromwell had an early "fancy" that he should be "the greatest man in the kingdom," Napoleon and Mussolini that they had over them a "star of destiny," and Lord Nelson that he saw "suspended before him a radiant orb ever urging him onwards" (Bradford, 1979). Bluemel (1948) has written of the extremes:

. . . ill-balanced men of history who have been directed by a star of destiny, an inner voice, or a guiding light . . . Still others have displayed delusions of grandeur in their political aspirations and wars of conquest. (p. 12)

Bluemel (1948) goes on to describe the nature and role of hypomania and extraversion in some leaders:

The extrovert is regarded as capable and energetic. Actually he is a man of manic make-up. He abounds in psychomotor activity; he is often intolerant and unyielding . . . given to impulsive action, and if the action brings success he will appear gifted in foresight and decision. In any event he is a colorful figure. . . . The extrovert is vociferous because he is full of energy and at the same time full of strong purpose and burning conviction . . . the outcry attracts other extroverts and soon there assembles a group of dominant men who unite in a common cause. (pp. 14–15)

One final, common characteristic of both leadership and hypomania is decisiveness. Belloc (1934) discussed the relationship of Cromwell's temperament to his ability to lead by saying, "That intensity of nervous structure is allied to the rapidity of his decisions in the field, to the clarity of his vision and is the main source of his drive" (p. 55). Clearly, this decisiveness can be vital in a military situation but potentially disastrous in a political one. Thus, Lord Nelson's incisive and brilliant strategy at Trafalgar made the critical difference in the British naval war against the French, and his well-known remarks before the Battle of the Nile ("Before this time to-morrow I shall have gained a peerage, or Westminster Abbey") are appropriate, in most instances, to the spirit of a commanding officer. It is less clear that

some of the traits we have been discussing—impetuousness, extreme decisiveness, grandiosity, and unbridled enthusiasm—are as desirable in political leaders, especially leaders in peacetime. It is here that the issue of impaired leaders is more likely to arise, partly because of the different natures of leadership and partly because of the necessary limits of authority on military officers. Walter Bagehot described the differing requirements for leaders in "common times" and times of crisis:

The great qualities, the imperious will, the rapid energy, the eager nature fit for great crisis are not required—are impediments—in common times. A Lord Liverpool is better in everyday politics than a Chatham—a Louis Philippe far better than a Napoleon. (1867, p. 84)

We next turn to individual examples of cyclothymic or manic-depressive leaders from the 17th, 18th, 19th, and 20th centuries. As in the earlier section, these examples are meant to be illustrative, not definitive. Compared with eminent poets and others in the arts, there have been relatively few overtly psychotic political and military leaders. Most of those reported here were cyclothymic, often in a pronounced manner, but presumably the need for more sustained functioning in the public eye and the societal consequences of severely impaired judgment make psychotic forms of manic-depressive illness less likely in positions of top military and political leadership.

Oliver Cromwell (1599–1658), commander-in-chief and Lord Protector of England, suffered from severe mood swings most of his adult life. He has been described by biographers as manic-depressive (Hill, 1970), "constitutionally hypomanic" or cyclothymic (Belloc, 1934; Henry, 1975), or as having periodic "manic rages" (Fraser, 1973). In 1628, Cromwell went to a well-known London physician, who diagnosed him at the time as being *valde melancholicus,* extremely melancholic. From time to time, Cromwell felt he was dying and experienced grandiose revelations and morbid obsessions. Fraser described Cromwell's rage in the act of dismissing Parliament:

Soon the rage was full upon him, beyond anyone's control: he was talking in what Whitelocke called "a furious manner," and what by Ludlow's account must have been something almost demented, for he continued to speak "with so much passion and discomposure of mind as if he had been distracted . . .", walking up and down the House like a madman, kicking the ground with his feet and shouting. His language in itself showed the extremes almost of paranoia . . . (pp. 419–420)

As Fraser (1973) describes the rest of Cromwell's behavior that day—the rage, lack of judgment, and rhythmic-taunting quality to Cromwell's remarks about Sir Henry Vane—it is highly characteristic of manic behavior:

At last Peter Wentworth, grandson of the Parliamentary leader of Queen Elizabeth's day, had the guts to protest against Cromwell's language of abuse, all the more horrible because it was coming from the man they had all "so highly trusted and obliged." This was the last straw to Cromwell's balance. "Come, come," he riposted savagely, "I will put an end to your prating. You are no Parliament. I say you are no Parliament. I will put an end to your sitting." Then he called to Thomas Harrison who was sitting on the other side of the House and shouted: "Call them in" or words to that effect. In rushed five or six files of musketeers from Cromwell's own regiment of foot under Lieutenant-Colonel Worsley, making altogether between twenty and thirty soldiers. Cromwell pointed at the Speaker. "Fetch him down," he said grimly. Harrison, as told to Ludlow, remonstrated briefly with Cromwell—"the work is very great and dangerous." But there was no gainsaying Oliver Cromwell at this point. Harrison duly pulled the Speaker down by his gown. Seeing the musketeers, it was Vane who called out: "This is not honest, yea it is against morality and common honesty." Cromwell turned on him like a snake and cried out in a loud voice: "O Sir Henry Vane, Sir Henry Vane, the Lord deliver me from Sir Henry Vane." (p. 420)

Alexander Hamilton (1755–1804), first Secretary of the Treasury, was characterized by President John Adams for his power beyond that: "All sovereignty then existing in the nation was in the hands of Alexander Hamilton. I was as President a mere cipher" (Syrett, 1960). Hamilton, unlike most of his successful 18th century American contemporaries, arrived in New York from the West Indies as an illegitimate orphan, without money, at the age of 16. His family background was riddled with chaos and emotional turmoil. His mother was jailed for sexual indiscretions and adultery and she was divorced. Hamilton's cousin on his mother's side committed suicide, and Hamilton's eldest son died in a duel in which he refused to fire. One of Hamilton's daughters died insane. Hamilton himself suffered episodically

from extreme paranoid periods, hypersexuality, financial speculation and consequent indebtedness, a rapid and fiery temper, extreme mood swings, and inordinate energy. His writing productivity increased markedly in the summer months. Like his son a few years before him, Hamilton died in a duel. Before the duel, he stated "I have resolved . . . to reserve and throw away my first fire, and I have thoughts even of reserving my second fire" (Syrett, 1960, pp. 278–280). He did, by most eyewitness accounts, hold his fire and was killed by Aaron Burr.

Napoléon Bonaparte (1769–1821) went through well-defined depressive phases characterized by dark despair:

Always alone, though in the midst of men, I go back home that I may give myself up to my lonely dreams and to the waves of my melancholy. Whither now, do my thoughts bend? Toward death. (Bluemel, 1948, p. 94)

More characteristically, his prevailing mood was that of hypomania, euphoria, optimism, and dynamic energy (Bluemel, 1948). He, like Cromwell and others, had an early sense of destiny, that "deeds await me of which the present generation has no inkling." Although Napoleon's mood swings were not so extreme as to be incapacitating, they clearly affected, largely in a positive way, his ability to lead.

Abraham Lincoln's (1809–1865) severe, incapacitating, and occasionally suicidal depressions have been well described (Randall, 1945; Hudgens, 1973). Although popularized as a "mild bipolar manic-depressive" by Fieve (1975b), the evidence for hypomania is far less clear-cut than for his serious depressions. It is interesting that Lincoln's primary military counterpart in the South, *Robert E. Lee* (1807-1870), also suffered intermittent depressions, albeit of less severity, throughout his life. One of Lee's biographers (Connelly, 1977) wrote:

He seemed to believe that death would be a welcome release from the world. . . . Sometimes Lee's comments on the pleasant release revealed an almost suicidal tendency. . . . Early biographers always lauded his serenity and self-possession. Actually Lee's mood of depression became a central part of his behavior. . . . [He] was convinced that his star had been ill-destined. (p. 192)

Lee's family background is suggestive of bipolar manic-depressive illness, although Lee himself seems to have been of more depressive and stable temperament. However, his father, an important military and political leader in his own right, had a far more chaotic life. *Henry Lee* (1756–1818), also known as "Light Horse Harry" Lee, was a brilliant cavalry commander in the Revolutionary War, a member of the Virginia legislature and Continental Congress, Governor of Virginia, and a member of the United States House of Representatives. A close friend and confidant of fellow Virginian George Washington, it was he who eulogized Washington as "First in war, first in peace, and first in the hearts of his countrymen." After the Revolutionary War was over, Lee's behavior and personality changed:

[he started] . . . a wild mania for speculation. His every scheme was grandiose, and his profits ran to millions in his mind. He plunged deeply, and always unprofitably. . . . Desperate in his grief, and conscious at last that he had made the wrong decision when he had left the army, Lee now wanted to return to a military life. If he could not wear again the uniform of his own country there was an alternative, to which Lee turned in the wildest of all his dreams. He was head of an American state, but he would resign, go to France and get a commission in the army of the revolutionaries! But before setting out for Paris he decided to take counsel with Washington. Washington, of course, warned him to stay away. . . . For a time Henry Lee seemed to be stabilized. . . . His old passion for wild speculation returned . . . he was arrested . . . and was confined to jail. (Freeman, 1961, pp. 5–6)

Henry Lee became involved in a group opposing the War of 1812 and eventually had to leave the country, greatly in debt and dishonor.

Three 20th century leaders also bear mentioning: Theodore Roosevelt, Winston Churchill, and Benito Mussolini. The hypomanic lifestyle of *Theodore Roosevelt* (1858–1919) has been detailed by biographer Pringle (1931). As President of the United States and as adventurer, Roosevelt lived at an extraordinarily high level of energy and was frequently grandiose, elated, restless, overtalkative, and inordinately enthusiastic. He functioned on very few hours of sleep and wrote, administered, or explored ceaselessly. It is estimated that he wrote more than 150,000 letters in his lifetime and a phenomenal number of books, ranging in topics from *The Naval War of 1812* to *Hunting the Grizzly*. Although he, on occasion, became mildly depressed, Roosevelt could best be described as chronically hypomanic.

Winston Churchill (1874–1965), on the other hand, was more cyclothymic in nature, alternating between quite severe periods of depression and periods of high energy, elevated mood, increased irritability, tremendous drive, impetuousness, and—at times—questionable judgment. Storr (1968, 1988), in a psychological study of Churchill, wrote:

All those who worked with Churchill paid tribute to the enormous fertility of his new ideas, the inexhaustible stream of invention which poured from him, both when he was Home Secretary, and later when he was Prime Minister and director of the war effort. All those who worked with him also agreed that he needed the most severe restraint put upon him, and that many of his ideas, if they had been put into practice, would have been utterly disastrous. (1988, pp. 14–15)

The melancholic side of Churchill's mood swings was recorded by his physician, Lord Moran (1966):

August 14 1944
The P.M. was in a speculative mood today. "When I was young," he ruminated, "for two or three years the light faded out of the picture. I did my work. I sat in the House of Commons, but black depression settled on me. It helped me to talk to Clemmie about it. I don't like standing near the edge of a platform when an express train is passing through. I like to stand right back and if possible to get a pillar between me and the train. I don't like to stand by the side of a ship and look down into the water. A second's action would end everything. A few drops of desperation. (p. 167)

The long-standing familial side of Churchill's cyclothymic temperament has been documented by many, including Churchill himself. In describing his direct ancestor, the great English military commander and first Duke of Marlborough, Churchill wrote:

No one can read the whole mass of the letters which Marlborough either wrote, dictated or signed personally without being astounded at the mental and physical energy which it attests. . . . After twelve or fourteen hours in the saddle on the long reconnaissances often under cannon-fire; after endless inspections of troops in camp and garrison; after ceaseless calculations about food and supplies, and all the anxieties of direct command in war, Marlborough would reach his tent and conduct the foreign policy of England, decide the main issues of its Cabinet, and of party politics at home. (Rowse, 1969, pp. 249–250)

Lord Randolph, Winston Churchill's father, was Secretary of State for India, Chancellor of the Exchequer, and Leader of the House of Commons. Rowse, who described the first Duke of Marlborough as "an artist by temperament in his ups and downs" (Rowse, 1969, p. 244), described Lord Randolph as follows:

. . . he had the defect of the artistic temperament, what we in our day of psychological jargon diagnose as the manic-depressive alteration—tremendous high spirits and racing energy on the upward bound, depression and discouragement on the down. This rhythm is present in a more or less marked degree with all persons of creative capacity, particularly in the arts. (Cited in Storr, 1968, p. 7)

Benito Mussolini (1883–1945) is the final 20th century leader we present. Like Theodore Roosevelt, Mussolini is well described as a chronic hypomanic. From a young age, he was grandiose in his aspirations: he "wished to make a mark on his era, like a lion with its claw." His grandiosity remained with him throughout his life. After an assassination attempt, for example, he remarked that "The bullets pass, Mussolini remains." His behavior and mood were characterized by euphoria, ideas of grandeur, pressure of activity, irritability and intolerance, and paranoia (Bluemel, 1948). His restlessness was legendary; like P.T. Barnum, he believed that "rest is found only in action." In the ultimate description of grandiosity, Bluemel (1948) wrote, ". . . at one time Mussolini divided his energies between seven ministerial posts; he was at the same time Premier, Minister of War, Air, Marine, Foreign Affairs, Corporations, and the Interior" (pp. 75–76).

Religious Leadership

Even more, perhaps than other kinds of genius, religious leaders have been subject to abnormal psychical visitations. Invariably they have been creatures of exalted emotional sensibility. Often they have led a discordant inner life, and had melancholy during a part of their career. They have known no measure, been liable to obsessions and fixed ideas; and frequently they have fallen into trances, heard voices, seen visions . . . moreover, these pathological features in their career have helped to give them their religious authority and influence. (pp. 6–7) —William James, 1902

William James thought and wrote extensively about the relationship between moods and temperament and an individual's capacity to experience the full range of religious thought and feeling. He was particularly interested in the experience of ecstatic states, which he thought to be important in the lives of great religious innovators and leaders (the "pattern setters," those for

whom "religion exists not as a dull habit, but as an acute fever"). His belief that "Man's extremity is God's opportunity" was particularly based on observations of the similarities between extremes of mood states and acute religious experiences (e.g., conversions, mystical experiences, religious exaltation). These similarities have been observed for centuries. Maudsley wrote in 1886:

In the Hebrew and Greek languages, the same words were used to denote the ravings of insanity and the often equally unintelligible ravings of the diviner or revealer of divine things . . . it was the impressive spectacle of the singular spontaneity and brilliant flow of ideas exhibited by a mind in the inflamed state of activity which is often the prelude of actual delirium or mania; when there is an upsurging into consciousness of the latent possessions of experience, and the person enchanted with this revelation of unsuspected wealth exults in a rapid succession of ideas, a vividness of memory, a freshness of feeling, a fertility of associations and combinations of ideas, and a facility of expression that seem to him almost miraculous . . . (pp. 220–224)

Laski (1961), bringing it into more modern times, commented:

. . . in a BBC television discussion, *Sainthood and Sanity*, broadcast on June 5, 1957, one speaker assumed that the states discussed were caused by God, another by manic-depression, a third by schizophrenia, while the fourth said the power concerned was the collective unconscious which inspires poets and saints but goes sour in mental patients. (p. 168)

What are the elements common to manic-depressive illness and religious inspiration and leadership? General aspects linking affective states and leadership were discussed in the previous section. Many, if not most, of them are applicable to religious authority as well. Probably more important in religious movements than in military or political ones, however, is the active use of ecstatic and psychotic states. Sir Alister Hardy (1979) has systematically studied the nature of religious experiences and found that auditory and visual hallucinations are not at all uncommon, but especially pervasive are ecstatic experiences: a sense of joy, extreme well-being, inspiration, exaltation, and a new and heightened sensory awareness. Arieti (1976), emphasizing the nonschizophrenic nature of mystical experiences, maintains that they tend to strengthen or enhance rather than lead to disintegration. No doubt many mystical experiences are, as Arieti conceptualizes them, autohypnotic phenomena, but in this passage they could as easily be descriptions of mania:

. . . the individual who experiences them has a marked rise in self-esteem and a sense of his being or becoming a worthwhile and very active person. He has been given a mission or a special insight, and from now on must be on the move doing something important. (Arieti, 1976, p. 251)

William James (1902), in delineating the primary characteristics of mystical and conversion experiences, outlines many features that a psychopathologist would more likely label as bipolar affective illness: hyperacusis, ecstasy, hallucinatory phenomena, knowledge "perceived as full of importance and significance," a loss of all worry, a "passion of willingness," a sense of well-being, altered perceptions, and a "sense of perceiving truths not known before." James stresses again and again his belief that the ability to experience religious or any other kind of ecstasy is exactly that—an ability, a gift, an aspect of temperament:

We shall see how infinitely passionate a thing religion at its highest flights can be. Like love, like wrath, like hope, ambition, jealousy, like every other instinctive eagerness and impulse, it adds to life an enchantment which is not rationally or logically deductible from anything else. This enchantment . . . is either there or not there for us, and there are persons who can no more become possessed by it than they can fall in love with a given woman by mere word of command. (James, 1902, pp. 47–48)

We have discussed some of the characteristics that intense religious episodes share with manic-depressive illness. Turning to the opposite perspective, we find several characteristics of manic-depressive illness that are religious in nature. The DSM-III-R, of course, formally recognizes the role of delusions and hallucinations in both psychotic depressions and manias. Particularly relevant for our discussion here are the defining characteristics of the mood-congruent psychotic features of mania: "delusions or hallucinations whose content is entirely consistent with themes of inflated worth, power, knowledge, identity or special relationship to a deity or famous person." Winokur and associates (1969), in their monograph on manic-depressive illness, noted that delusions were present in 48 percent of the manic episodes they observed and that the content of 29 percent of these delusions was religious in nature

(see Chapter 11). Auditory hallucinations were present in 21 percent of manic episodes, and visual hallucinations in 9 percent. The hallucinations were characterized by being "brief, usually grandiose, usually religious." Finally, the most common cognitive theme during mania was religion, expressed by 32 percent of the patients. The high rate of religious themes in manic delusions, hallucinations, and cognitive content may simply reflect unconscious or learned material. On the other hand, it may reflect the inability of ordinary language and perceptual frameworks to express ecstatic, grandiose, and transcendent experiences in anything other than the expansive and mystical language of religion. Jonathan Edwards (1703–1758), the great theologian of American Puritanism, wrote:

Those gracious influences which are the effects of the Spirit of God are altogether supernatural. . . . They are what no improvement, or composition of natural qualifications or principles will ever produce; because they not only differ from what is natural, and from everything that natural men experience in degree and circumstances, but also in kind, and are of a nature far more excellent . . . there are new perceptions and sensations entirely different in their nature and kind from anything experienced . . . entirely different from anything which a natural man can possess, or of which he can form any proper notion. (cited in James, 1902, pp. 228–229)

Biographer Ian Hamilton (1982) quotes a draft from Robert Lowell's *Life Studies* that gives a sense of one of Lowell's religious manias (he, like John Berryman, converted from the Episcopal to the Catholic Church):

Seven years ago I had an attack of pathological enthusiasm. The night before I was locked up I ran about the streets of Bloomington Indiana crying out against devils and homosexuals. I believed I could stop cars and paralyze their forces by merely standing in the middle of the highway with my arms outspread. . . . Bloomington stood for Joyce's hero and Christian regeneration. Indiana stood for the evil, unexorcised, aboriginal Indians. I suspected I was a reincarnation of the Holy Ghost, and had become homicidally hallucinated. To have known the glory, violence and banality of such an experience is corrupting. (p. 157)

Experiencing and drawing on religious ecstasy have been integral to the work of many poets as well as religious leaders—the visionary and exalted works of Gerard Manley Hopkins, John Donne, William Blake, Christopher Smart, and

William Cowper, for example. Cowper wrote to this point:

A terrible sagacity informs
The poet's heart; he looks to distant storms;
He hears the thunder ere the tempest lowers!
And, arm'd with strength surpassing human powers,
Seizes events as yet unknown to man,
And darts his soul into the dawning plan.
Hence, in a Roman mouth, the graceful name
Of prophet and of poet was the same;
Hence British poets, too, the priesthood shared,
And every hallowed Druid was a bard.

There have been many mystics who may well have suffered from manic-depressive illness—for example, St. Theresa, St. Francis, St. John—but here we present very briefly a few individuals who were religious leaders per se. As before, our list is meant to be illustrative, not definitive. As mentioned, *Martin Luther* (1483–1546), the leader of the Reformation and the founder of the Protestant church, experienced periods of deep, psychotic, occasionally suicidal melancholy. At other times, he went through periods of inde-fatigability and exaltation, during which he had visions ("quite palpable visions of an almost stroboscopic oscillation between Christ and the devil," Haile, 1980). He also had periods of ex-treme rage and righteous tirades, when he took on the Pope, the King of England (Henry VIII), and virtually every other secular and religious head of Europe. His profound depressions are well docu-mented by himself and by his biographers. Haile (1980) describes them in the following way:

Sorrow had been his own familiar companion since boyhood. The man did not distinguish his acute spell of depression in 1527 (often diagnosed as his first heart attack) as being different in kind from earlier attacks of anxiety, but his extreme moodiness had become more pronounced afterward. As early as 1530, he announced to his congregation he would never preach to them again, and did spurn his church for several Sundays. Such spells became more frequent as the years passed. One bout, he said, followed another without teaching a thing. Looking back over his long Wittenberg career, he sighed,

> I have preached here for twenty-four years, walking the street to church so often it would be no wonder if I had worn out the soles of my feet as well as my shoes on its cobblestones. I have done what I was able—and I am satisfied. The letters I have sent would alone build a house, had I but saved them. They bear witness to my labors. Yet nothing has so exhausted me as sorrow, especially at night. (p. 301)

The 17th century gave witness to two impor-tant religious leaders, one Protestant and the other Jewish, whose religious convictions and ability to inspire change were at least partially derived from their affective states: George Fox and Sabbatai Sevi. *George Fox* (1624–1691), founder of the Society of Friends, or Quakers, is cited by William James (1902) as an example of a man who was profound and influential despite his ex-treme psychotic episodes:

The Quaker religion which he founded is something which is impossible to overpraise. In a day of shams, it was a religion of veracity rooted in spiritual inward-ness, and a return to something more like the original gospel truth than men had ever known in England. So far as our Christian sects today are evolving into liber-ality, they are simply reverting in essence to the posi-tion which Fox and the early Quakers so long ago assumed. . . . His Journal abounds in entries of this sort:—

> As I was walking with several friends, I lifted up my head, and saw three steeple-house spires, and they struck at my life. I asked them what place that was? They said, Lichfield. Immediately the word of the Lord came to me, that I must go thither. . . . Then was I commanded by the Lord to pull off my shoes. I stood still, for it was winter: but the word of the Lord was like a fire in me. So I put off my shoes, and left them with the shepherds; and the poor shep-herds trembled, and were astonished. Then I walked on about a mile, and as soon as I was got within the city, the word of the Lord came to me again, saying: Cry, "Wo to the bloody city of Lichfield!" So I went up and down the streets, crying with a loud voice, Wo to the bloody city of Lichfield! And no one laid hands on me. As I went thus crying through the streets, there seemed to me to be a channel of blood running down the streets, and the market-place ap-peared like a pool of blood. (p. 7)

Sabbatai Sevi (1626–1676) was recognized as the Messiah by a large proportion of the 17th century Jewish community of Europe, the Middle East, and North Africa (Ostow, 1980; Scholem, 1973). His behavior was classically manic-depressive in nature, alternating between days of anguish and ecstasy, "illumination" and "hiding the fire." Scholem (1973) writes: "Many times when he stood in the height of heaven, he fell again into the depth of the great abyss where the serpents tempted him." His "frenzied ecstasy" was used by Nathan of Gaza, a scholar and proph-et, to lead a new messianic movement.

One final example is *Emmanual Swedenborg* (1688–1772), a Swedish scientist, philosopher, and religious writer. When Swedenborg was in his mid-50s he had a vision in which he thought himself to be the Messiah, heard a voice saying, "I am God, the Lord, the Creator and Redeemer of the World. I have chosen thee to unfold the spiritual sense of the Holy Scriptures. I will Myself dictate to thee what thou shalt write." According to Nisbit (1900), Swedenborg conversed with the inhabitants of all the planets except Uranus and Neptune (which were not yet discovered) and thought he could discern witches. Maudsley (1886) described the controversy and impact of Swedenborg's initial and consequent hallucinations on his religious followers, as well as on dissenters:

> The visitation was the forerunner of an attack of acute mania—so overwhelming the pressure of supernatural influx upon the mental equilibrium of the natural man—which lasted for a few weeks; on recovery from which he was what he remained for the rest of his life—either, as his disciples think, a holy seer endowed with the faculty of conversing with spirits and angels in heaven and hell, and in whom the Lord Jesus Christ made His second coming for the institution of a new Church, described in the Revelation under the figure of the New Jerusalem; or, as those who are not disciples think, an interesting and harmless monomaniac, who, among many foolish sayings, said many wise and good things, attesting the wreck of a mind of large original endowment, intellectual and moral. Such the momentous difference of opinion possible, in age esteeming itself the most enlightened age of the world, between two human beings of equal capacity and understanding, each as eager as the other to know the truth and believe it! (pp. 241–242)

IMPORTANCE OF STUDYING POSITIVE ASPECTS OF MANIC-DEPRESSIVE ILLNESS

Although it certainly is possible to exaggerate or romanticize the positive aspects of mood disorders, we should be careful not to disregard these beneficial features or deal with them in only a perfunctory way. Understanding the assets that accompany manic-depressive illness, the characteristics of the illness tying it to the arts, leadership, and society at large, is as important to a thorough understanding of the illness as knowledge of its natural history, pathophysiology, and psychopathology. Three principal areas of consideration are relevant to the study of positive features in mood disorders: theoretical, clinical, and social–ethical.

Theoretical Considerations

Positive aspects of the affective disorders, including associations with accomplishment, are, of course, interesting in their own right. At first glance, the notion of advantage gained from an otherwise catastrophic illness may seem counterintuitive, yet both history and clinical experience affirm the reality of this paradox. Most clinical research understandably has focused on the depressive spectrum and given relatively little emphasis to the manic continuum. There has been next to no study of the spectrum of elated states most relevant to our discussion here. Of the many still unexamined aspects of manic-depressive illness that could profitably be studied, its positive features are particularly germane. There is little research into subtle oscillations in perception, mood, behavior, and cognition—along with corresponding biological changes—across the elated or hyperarousal states. Quantitative and qualitative changes between the milder hypomanias and manias also require more study. And we need to learn to differentiate functioning in normals—those with decreased need for sleep, coupled with high energy, productivity, and mood—from individuals with type A personalities, chronic hypomania, cyclothymia, or manic-depressive illness (see Chapter 4).

The existence of elated states also provides opportunity for cognitive psychologists to study a long-existing theoretical question: Does cognition precede or follow mood change? The current body of literature is based on studies of depression and, because of psychological assumptions about etiology, tends to assume that cognitive changes precede—indeed cause or facilitate—depressive affect. Similarly, many creative individuals and students of creativity assume that inspiration, creative ideas, and fluency of thinking precede euphoric affect. That is, many believe that the creative act creates euphoria, not that heightened mood facilitates the increased flow of thoughts and ideas. Notwithstanding these assumptions, evidence reported earlier in this chapter (Jamison, 1989) indicates that in a sizable proportion of highly creative writers and artists, mood changes precede cognitive and behavioral changes, and that intense creative episodes are, in many instances, indistinguishable from hypomania.

Yet another important theoretical issue, with enormous practical ramifications, centers on the addictive qualities of the elated or euphoric states. Such altered states of consciousness and mood can be highly potent reinforcers during euthymic or depressed periods, creating in some patients a potentially strong variable reinforcement schedule with both appreciable benefits and risks. This phenomenon is roughly analogous to drug self-administration, in which a highly pleasurable and often immediate state can be obtained. Thus, for some patients the positive aspects of the illness may be similar to stimulant addiction.

Clinical experience suggests that patients may attempt to induce mania by discontinuing lithium not just at times when they are depressed but also when they have to face problematic decisions and life events. Because the negative consequences are delayed, it is not always clear to the patient that the costs outweigh the benefits. The clinical implications of the positive aspects of mood disorders are discussed in the next section and in Chapters 24 and 25. Here it is important to mention that the addictive or addictive-like qualities of the elated states raise fascinating issues about the possible self-induction of these mood states (by sleep deprivation or psychological means), the relevance of this phenomenon to kindling models, and, of course, the use of cocaine and other stimulants to self-medicate or to induce euphoric and high-energy states. The extremely high rate of affective illness in serious cocaine abuse (Mirin et al., 1984a) may reflect not only self-medication per se but also an attempt to recapture a known previously experienced mood state, a reality that makes manic-depressive individuals perhaps uniquely vulnerable to cocaine addiction on both psychological and biological grounds (see Chapter 9).

Clinical Considerations

The existence of positive features in manic-depressive illness affects the willingness of some individuals to seek and comply with treatment. Many highly accomplished individuals in the arts, politics, the military, and business are reluctant to seek treatment for their mood disorders because of the stigma and consequences attached to the treatment of mental illness. Further, some view their serious mood problems as part of the human condition, the price one pays for being "too sensitive," for having an artistic temperament, or leading an artistic lifestyle. Indeed, in many such individuals, emotional turmoil is seen as essential to their identity as performing or creative artists. Additionally, many writers and leaders are concerned that psychiatric treatment will erode or compromise their ability to create or lead.

An increased emphasis on the potentially productive side of mood disorders may lead to a lessening of stigma and to an increased public awareness of the treatments available. An appreciation by the clinician of the "up" side of the illness can forge a stronger therapeutic bond as well as increase patients' self-respect. Strict adherence to an often arbitrary distinction between psychopathology, on the one hand, and a chaotic, tumultuous, and artistic lifestyle, on the other, can lead to unnecessary suffering and even suicide. Ironically, these seldom considered issues in affective illness give rise to one of the few instances in clinical practice where the talented and wealthy in society often receive relatively inferior medical care.

Writers and artists frequently express concern about the effects of psychiatric treatment on their ability to create and produce; these concerns are especially pronounced when it comes to taking medication. Some of this mistrust no doubt reflects unfounded preconceptions, fears of altering long-established work patterns and rituals, or simple resistance to treatment. In some instances, however, these concerns are grounded in reality. A review of the literature on lithium treatment reveals alarmingly little research on the effects of the drug on productivity and creativity or the effects of missing highs on creative individuals' ability to work or willingness to stay on lithium. What little is known can be summarized here. (Cognitive effects of lithium are discussed in Chapter 23, and those lithium side effects most implicated in noncompliance are reviewed in Chapter 25.)

Even the early lithium researchers were well aware of problems created by lithium's effects on certain useful or enjoyable qualities of the illness (e.g., decreasing or eliminating the highs of hypomania, decreasing sexuality and energy levels), as well as by the untoward side effects of lithium (possible cognitive slowing and memory impairment). Schou (1968) described the subjective effects of lithium in three "normal" subjects (medical researchers). This description has relevance, if limited applicability, to other individuals who are dependent on mind and senses for their work:

> The subjective experience was primarily one of indifference and slight general malaise. This led to a certain passivity. . . . The subjective feeling of having been altered by the treatment was disproportionately strong in relation to objective behavioral changes. The subjects could engage in discussions and social activities but found it difficult to comprehend and integrate more than a few elements of a situation. Intellectual initiative was diminished and there was a feeling of lowered ability to concentrate and memorize; but thought processes were unaffected, and the subjects could think logically and produce ideas. (p. 78)

It should be noted that Schou's study involved a relatively short-term trial of lithium, and there is some indication that patients partially accommodate to lithium's cognitive effects. Many patients, of course, experience no significant cognitive side effects, and with those that do, the risks of no treatment must always be weighed against the disadvantages of lithium. The more subtle uses of lithium are discussed in Chapter 25 and later in this chapter.

Early researchers also noted that many patients on lithium reported that life was more flat and colorless and that they had less enthusiasm and energy (Schou et al., 1970a); that they felt less creative and productive (Polatin and Fieve, 1971), and that they missed their hypomanic periods (Fitzgerald, 1972; Kerry, 1978; Van Putten, 1975). Patients report missing their highs as an important reason for stopping lithium against medical advice (Jamison et al., 1979). They also report feeling less creative while on lithium. Memory problems are among the most significant side effects cited in noncompliance (see Chapter 25).

What then is actually known about the effect of lithium on productivity and creativity? In 1971, Polatin and Fieve described their clinical experience of using lithium in creative individuals:

> In the creative individual who does his best work in the course of a hypomanic period, the complaint regarding the continued use of lithium carbonate is that it acts as a "brake." These patients report that lithium carbonate inhibits creativity so that the individual is unable to express himself, drive is diminished, and

there is no incentive. These patients also indicate that when they are depressed, the symptoms are so demoralizing and so uncomfortable that they welcome the "mild high" when the depression disappears and prefer to settle for a cyclothymic life of highs and lows rather than an apathetic middle-of-the-road mood state achieved through the use of lithium carbonate.

> Their argument is that if lithium carbonate prevents the high and may possibly prevent the "low," they prefer not to take lithium carbonate, since never to have a high as a result of the drug seems equivalent to being deprived of an "addictive-like" pleasurable and productive state. Some of these patients are terrified of having a low again, but insist on taking their chances without lithium carbonate therapy, knowing that sooner or later they will be compensated by the high, even if they do go into a low state. (p. 864)

No controlled studies of lithium's effects on productivity have been done, but Marshall and co-workers (1970) and Schou (1979a) studied a total of 30 artists, writers, and businessmen taking lithium. Their findings are summarized in Table 14-6. More than three quarters (77 percent) of the patients reported no change or an increase in their productivity while on lithium. Approximately one quarter reported a decrease. In 17 percent, the lithium was seen as leading to problems sufficient to warrant refusal to take it. It is not known how accurately these figures reflect artists and writers at the upper end of creative accomplishment. Most of these subjects, although earning their living by their creative work, were not in the top rung of artists. Schou (1979a) pointed out that lithium might affect inspiration, the ability to execute, or both and saw the following as contributing factors in a creative individual's response to lithium: the severity of illness, the type of illness, the artist's habits of using manic periods of inspiration, and individual sensitivity to the pharmacological action of lithium.

Two studies of particular relevance for artistic creativity conflict in their results. Judd and colleagues (1977b) found no effects of short-term lithium treatment on creativity in normal subjects. A study using bipolar patients as their own controls, however, found substantial detrimental effects of lithium on associational processing (Shaw et al., 1986). Differences in results may be due in part to the fact that lithium's effect on cognition is probably quite different in manic-depressive patients and normal controls (Pons et al., 1985). Individual differences in clinical state, serum lithium levels, sensitivity to cognitive side

Table 14-6. Productivity on Lithium

	Marshall et al., 1970	Schou, 1979a	Combined N	%
Subjects				
N	6	24	30	
Occupation	Artists & Businessmen	Artist & Writers		
Productivity on Lithium				
Increased	5	12	17	57
No Change	0	6	6	20
Decreased	1	6	7	23
Refused to Continue Lithium Treatment	1	4	5	17

effects, and the severity, frequency, and type of affective illness also clearly affect the degree to which an individual will experience impairment in intellectual functioning, creativity, and productivity. Artists, writers, and many others who rely on their initiative, intellect, emotional intensity, and energy for their life's work underscore the need for a re-examination of this problem.

Artists and writers represent a group at high risk for affective illness and should be assessed and counseled accordingly. Ideal treatment requires a sensitive understanding of the possible benefits of mood disorders to creativity and also the severe liabilities of untreated depression and mania, including the risk of suicide. It also requires the clinician to be aware of available medications and their side effects that might be potentially damaging to the creative process. Physicians must minimize, whenever possible, drug (especially lithium) levels. And the clinician must recognize and make sophisticated use of seasonal patterns in moods and productivity—through self-charting of moods with a Visual Analogue Scale, for example (Jamison, 1989).

Social and Ethical Considerations

Yet another reason for studying the positive aspects of manic-depressive illness should be touched on. Genetic research is progressing to the stage that ethical issues arise about amniocentesis and abortion, as well as the identification and treatment of individuals at high risk for developing manic-depressive illness. It becomes particularly important under these circumstances to have at least some broad notion of the costs and benefits of making decisions such as abortion—not

only for potential parents and the unborn child but also for society at large. The implications of losing societal variance in such basic characteristics as drive, energy, risk-taking, and personality have not yet been examined in any systematic way. Ironically, these issues were considered, to some extent, in the 1930s; in one study, carried out in Germany, the advisability of sterilization of manic-depressive individuals was examined. Luxenburger (1933) found manic-depressive illness far overrepresented in the higher occupational classes (see review of social-class literature in Chapter 7) and recommended against sterilization of these patients, "especially if the patient does not have siblings who could transmit the positive aspects of the genetic heritage." Myerson and Boyle (1941), in their study of manic-depressive psychosis in socially prominent American families, concluded:

Perhaps the words of Bumke need to be taken into account before we embark too whole-heartedly on any sterilization program, "If we could extinguish the sufferers from manic-depressive psychosis from the world, we would at the same time deprive ourselves of an immeasurable amount of the accomplished and good, of color and warmth, of spirit and freshness. Finally only dried up bureaucrats and schizophrenics would be left. Here I must say that I would rather accept into the bargain the diseased manic-depressives than to give up the healthy individuals of the same heredity cycle." (p. 20)

SUMMARY

There is strong scientific and biographical evidence linking mood disorders to artistic creativity. Biographies of eminent poets, composers, and artists attest to the prevalence of extremes of mood in creative individuals. Systematic studies are increasingly documenting the link. It should be emphasized, however, that many creative writers, artists, and musicians have no significant psychopathology. Conversely, most individuals with manic-depressive illness are not unusually creative.

We have considered the issue of the reliability— indeed, the advisability—of making a historical diagnosis of manic-depressive illness. This concern is important and valid. Labeling as manic-depressive anyone who is unusually creative, accomplished, energetic, intense, moody, or eccentric both diminishes the notion of individuality within the arts and trivializes a very serious, often lethal illness. We have been careful to base our biographical work on what is known clinically and scientifically about manic-depressive illness.

That the illness and its related temperaments are associated with creativity seems clear. The clinical, ethical, and social implications of this association are less so.

We have tried to convey that manic-depressive illness and depression are destructive, painful, sometimes fatal, and yet fascinating and important illnesses. In the great majority of instances, the effective treatments now available will not hinder creative ability. Indeed, treatment almost always results in longer periods of sustained productivity. One of our concerns, however, remains the study, public discussion, and development of treatments that will minimize side effects of currently available medications.

Perhaps some suffering must always accompany great artistic achievement. Certainly, depth and intensity of human feeling must be a part of creation in the arts. But modern medicine now allows relief of the extremes of despair, turmoil, and psychosis. It allows choices not previously available. Most of the writers, artists, and leaders discussed in this chapter had no choices.

NOTES

1. Cited in Taylor, 1982, p. 332.
2. Andreasen and Canter, 1974; Andreasen, 1987a; Richards et al., 1988; Jamison, 1989.
3. Cited in I. Hamilton, 1982, p. 337.
4. From *A Defence of Poetry,* first published in 1821, reproduced in BR McElderry, Jr, ed: *Shelley's Critical Prose.* Lincoln: University of Nebraska Press, 1967, p. 32.
5. From a *Paris Review* interview, cited in G Plimpton, ed: *Writers at Work: The Paris Review Interviews,* 1976, p. 322.
6. From Erikson, 1962, p. 161.
7. From Taylor, 1982, p. 285.
8. Cited in van Gogh, 1958, p. x.
9. Cited in I. Hamilton, 1982, p. 351.
10. Creativity and mental illness were much more overlapping in the relatives of the writers than in the relatives of the controls.
11. The 47 subjects in the study were either British citizens (87 percent) or citizens of the British Commonwealth or the Republic of Ireland (13 percent). Most were men (87 percent) and Christian (Protestant, 77 percent; Catholic, 15 percent; no affiliation or agnostic, 8 percent). The mean age of the sample was 53.2 years. There were no significant differences in demographic characteristics among the subgroups—poets, playwrights, novelists, biographers, and artists—except that the poets were disproportionately Protestant (94 percent) and the novelists disproportionately Catholic or agnostic (50 percent).
12. This honor was established by King George III in 1768 and held at any given time by only 75 British painters, sculptors, engravers, and architects. Previous recipients include J.M.W. Turner, Sir Joshua Reynolds, Thomas Gainsborough, and John Constable.
13. Previous recipients include W.H. Auden, Siegfried Sassoon, John Betjeman, Robert Graves, and Ted Hughes.
14. Previous recipients of these drama awards include Eugene O'Neill, T.S. Eliot, John Osborne, Noel Coward, Tennessee Williams, and Edward Albee.
15. Previous recipients include D.H. Lawrence, Robert Graves, Evelyn Waugh, Graham Greene, and John Le Carré.
16. From PHS Stanhope: *Notes of Conversations with the Duke of Wellington.* November 2, 1831.

PART FOUR

PATHOPHYSIOLOGY

Men ought to know that from nothing else but the brain come joys, delights, laughter and sports, and sorrows, griefs, despondency, and lamentations. . . . And by the same organ we become mad.   — Hippocrates

Except during the middle ages and again in the first half of the 20th century, prevailing opinion among medical authorities over the millennia has rested on the assumption that the origins of manic-depressive illness would be traced to pathology of the body, not the soul or mind. Many doctors, beginning with the Hippocratic writers, identified the brain as the organ of interest. Even Freud thought as much, at least before he departed from his neurological orientation to formulate his theories on melancholia. Medical scientists have now begun to realize their age-old ambition of fathoming how disturbances in brain function might be translated into impalpable, intangible thought or emotion. Biological studies comprise by far the largest literature on manic-depressive illness generated in recent history.

The next six chapters examine the evidence that has accumulated about the pathophysiology of manic-depressive illness. Provocative and promising as that literature is, it nevertheless must be examined with caution. It is easy to forget that the modern study of pathophysiology is still a relatively new undertaking, as given to excess and wrong turns as any callow youth. Before previewing the chapters that follow, we offer some cautionary observations to aid in interpreting the output of this young science.

CLINICAL DEFINITIONS AND DISTINCTIONS

Discussions of pathophysiology can be needlessly opaque unless the nature of the topic under discussion is clear. Without summarizing material covered in Chapters 3 through 6, we briefly recall that the original concept of manic-depressive illness was of a recurrent major affective disorder encompassing patients with and without mania. When Leonhard formulated his bipolar–monopolar distinction, he was subdividing patients who had a recurrent affective disorder. Since the concept of depression was more broad in the American literature, however, Leonhard's distinction sowed some confusion, and *unipolar disorder* came to mean any depression that was not bipolar. The resulting heterogeneity of the unipolar category has been reinforced by DSM-III-R, which does not require a prior episode to make a diagnosis of major depression. This use of the term *unipolar* must be kept in mind in reading the literature.

Recurrent forms of unipolar illness may have more in common with bipolar illness than with other unipolar depression. Although bipolar and recurrent unipolar illness appear to represent separate sub-groups of manic-depressive illness, they probably exist on a continuum, with many intermediate forms. The boundaries dividing manic-depressive illness from normal states and from other psychiatric illnesses, principally schizophrenia, are indistinct as well. These relationships are also consistent with a spectrum concept.

The bipolar category itself should include patients with a history of hypomania (bipolar II). Because hypomania often escapes clinical notice, bipolar-II disorders are underdiagnosed. When patients with hypomania are included in the bipolar category, the bipolar fraction of all those with major affective disorders rises to about one third.

METHODS AND CONCEPTS

Many conceptual and methodological issues are common to the entire biological literature on manic-depressive illness. One troublesome problem is that most biological studies of affective illness do not include separate analyses of data on bipolar and unipolar patients. When they do, the unipolar group is usually heterogeneous. Groups seldom are matched for the frequency of recurrent episodes, and, indeed, this parameter is almost never reported. Reported bipolar–unipolar differences are reviewed in each of the succeeding chapters; see especially Chapter 17.

Emerging evidence suggests that a bipolar patient is more likely than a unipolar patient to show greater variability on some biological measures from one sampling to the next. This *intra*individual variability is another confounding factor in interpreting research evidence. It may reflect greater instability in certain systems or the existence of more variable symptom combinations in the bipolar groups (e.g., mixed states). For these reasons, the phase of the illness can be an important source of variance.

Illness specificity is a central issue in all biological research in psychiatry, and manic-depressive illness is no exception. Is a given biological finding specific to manic-depressive illness, or may it also be found in other major psychiatric illnesses, such as schizophrenia? Can it differentiate a manic-depressive patient from one with a medical condition, such as poststroke depression or mania? Is the finding associated with the full syndrome of depression or mania or only with an individual symptom or symptom cluster? Is the biological finding normally distributed in the patient population, or does it seem to be found only in one or more subgroups? How does the variance of a biological measure in a group of manic-depressive patients relate to normal variance? Does the distribution in a comparison population shed light on the role of the biological factor in manic-depressive patients? These questions must be kept in mind when reviewing individual biological findings in the subsequent chapters.

Cyclicity is perhaps the most distinguishing clinical feature of the entity under discussion. Recurrence has rarely been studied as a variable in its own right, independent of polarity. Indeed, the bulk of the biological data are cross-sectional, as are the major hypotheses. However, in the chapters that follow, especially the synthesis of the evidence in Chapter 20, we emphasize hypotheses and models that take cyclicity into account. Do different frequencies of cycling suggest different biological processes? For example, do rapid-cycling patients and nonrapid-cycling patients have the same illness? As we shall see, only scattered biological data can be brought to bear on this question. Further, in discussing pharmacological models, we focus on putative mechanisms through which drugs can alter manic-depressive cycles.

Bunney and colleagues have applied the term *switch process* to designate the behavioral and biological events associated with the often dramatic change from depression into mania. As described in Chapter 2, the switch frequently occurs over the course of a few hours, usually during the night or early morning hours. No analogous process exists in any other psychiatric illness, except perhaps periodic catatonia and cycloid psychosis, which are probably variants of manic-depressive illness. Because of this unusual feature, detailed biological study of the switch process (as outlined in Chapter 17) offers a very real possibility of getting closer to the core pathophysiology of bipolar illness. The practical advantages are considerable as well. In regularly cycling patients, the timing of a switch can be predicted with reasonable accuracy, allowing the investigator to initiate intensive biological measures in anticipation of the event. Biological comparisons of two dramatically different states within the same patients can then be accomplished over a relatively short time. As we shall see, studies that track sequences of switches have shown that many *biological* correlates seem to follow a sine wave—that is, they rise and fall gradually over many days. *Behavioral* states, by contrast, frequently follow a square wave, with sudden shifts from depression into mania and back. (The switch from mania to depression is generally more gradual than the reverse.) If the sudden behavioral change could be demonstrably linked to—that is, driven by—the slower biological change, a threshold model would be supported. Not all manic-depressive patients experience sudden switches, of course. It is possible that in these cases, the slower onset and remission of episodes could be the stretched-out expression of a single rapid process, which, at some other phases of the illness, could be expressed as a rapid behavioral switch.

The fact that manic-depressive illness typically involves periods of remission provides investigators with the opportunity to separate state from trait. A principal focus of trait or well-state studies is genetic. In searching for a genetic marker, investigators hope to identify individuals most at risk for the illness, so that preventive measures could be taken before it becomes clinically manifest. In research on already diagnosed bipolar patients, a biological finding that (1) is present when the patient is well, (2) is independent of the particular state of the illness, and (3) differentiates manic-depressive patients from normals and from those with other illnesses is a possible marker of the genetic vulnerability. State-dependent changes, on the other hand, are of limited use, since the active state of the illness is required to bring out the biological change. At best, the absence of a given state-dependent abnormality in some ill members of a pedigree can rule it out as a primary transmitted factor in the illness. State-independent findings often are interpreted too glibly as reflecting vulnerability or predisposition, however. As we shall see, the biological factors identified as "predisposing" are, in fact, usually derived from studies of recovered patients. To date, the only markers that offer the promise of fulfilling the principal requirements of an illness marker—that it segregate with the illness in pedigrees—are the chromosomal markers. This important area is detailed in Chapter 15.

PREVIEW

The most clearly established biological fact about manic-depressive illness is that it involves a genetically transmitted vulnerability, and, therefore, the section begins with that topic. In the only guest-written chapter in this book, Elliot S. Gershon reviews the genetic–epidemiological evidence derived from twin, adoption, and family studies, which remain the most clinically useful proof of genetic transmission of the illness. Since these studies do not provide much information about transmission, investigators turn to pedigree and segregation analyses of how the illness is distributed in families of patients rather than in the population. Even more precise information can be gathered from molecular–genetic techniques. Dr. Gershon's chapter explains what can be learned from each method and evaluates the evidence for manic-depressive illness and, insofar as possible, recurrent unipolar illness.

Chapter 16, on biochemical models, is a short chapter that sets the stage for the review of biochemical and pharmacological studies in Chapter 17. It reviews the attempts at modeling depression and mania in animals and traces the evolution of the biochemical hypotheses that have so dominated the literature in the last quarter-century. Embedded in the discussion are descriptions of the brain systems that have been the focus of most of the research.

Chapter 17 covers the massive biochemical literature. It reviews the evidence for the amine hypotheses and interactions between neurotransmitter systems. Neuroendocrine abnormalities, the subject of investigation for more than a century, are reviewed next, followed by the closely related study of neuropeptides. Another pair of related areas, electrolytes and membrane transport systems, are covered next. Miscellaneous biochemical substances are reviewed, followed by discussion of studies of phasic change. Chapter 17 closes by returning to the clinical reality of the illness. Here we re-examine the evidence, not system by system but from the perspective of what it tells us about longitudinal phasic changes (the biology of cyclicity) and the interaction of state and trait. We close with a critical summary of what we know and do not know about the clinical meaning of this vast collection of data. It is sobering.

Chapter 18 deals with three different fields of investigation that share the distinction of being somewhat outside the mainstream of studies in the pathophysiology of manic-depressive illness. Although it has generally been considered counterintuitive to posit a fixed neuroanatomical lesion underlying an illness that undergoes phasic changes (including full recovery), it is also widely acknowledged that the brain is not a soup. The basic relationship between function and structure applies not only to neurotransmitter and synaptic structure but also to the macrostructure of brain organization. The advent of brain-imaging strategies is another argument for carefully examining the existing data on neuroanatomical correlates of the illness. Traditionally, the field of electrophysiology has focused on schizophrenia. Nevertheless, interesting leads have emerged from studies of manic-depressive illness. Laterality and evoked-response patterns, for example, are being evaluated for specificity and state dependency. The immunological and viral studies being done in this area are exciting, even tantalizing, but remain unproven.

Sleep disturbances accompanying affective illness are among its most troublesome symptoms, and for that reason sleep has long been of clinical research interest. In Chapter 19 we place sleep squarely in the context of other circadian rhythms and examine the link between sleep disturbances in the illness and the evidence for a more fundamental disturbance in the regulation of bodily rhythms in general. These obvious rhythmic disruptions of manic-depressive illness, an inherently cyclic disorder, have surprisingly only been explored systematically in the last two decades despite centuries-old observations of seasonal and diurnal patterns of symptoms and mood. In Chapter 19, novel hypotheses are offered to link circadian rhythm disturbances with other aspects of pathophysiology, such as neurotransmitter disturbances.

The closing chapter of the section is somewhat ambitiously intended as a synthesis. In fact, any full synthesis at this juncture would be forced and fanciful at best, given our imposing ignorance, an ignorance that we carefully document in the first section of Chapter 20. Nevertheless, in the process of our extensive and, we hope, critical review of the pathophysiology literature, some novel linkages between disparate areas of inquiry have occurred to us. We offer them in Chapter 20 in the hope of stimulating further discussion and providing some points of focus for further research.

15

Genetics

ELLIOT S. GERSHON, M.D.*

The capacity to blunder slightly is the real marvel of DNA. Without this special attribute, we would still be anaerobic bacteria and there would be no music.

—Lewis Thomas[1]

A generation ago, few mental health professionals believed that inherited vulnerabilities could be central to the development of psychiatric illness. Fearing that discovery of a genetic diathesis might cast a stigma on patients and lead to therapeutic nihilism, many clinical observers found social and developmental reasons to explain the inescapable fact that mental illness runs in families. Gradually, the genetic evidence became too compelling to ignore. Recent advances in the molecular genetics of several neuropsychiatric diseases, particularly the discovery of chromosomal linkage markers for manic-depressive illness in several pedigrees, appear to reaffirm the older evidence. If, as expected, more widespread linkage markers are found, better understanding of pathophysiological mechanisms should follow.

Along with its theoretical importance, knowledge of genetics has practical relevance, and the new discoveries could result in new diagnostic tests and improved treatment methods. Clinicians now use family histories to help diagnose an illness correctly and to manage psychotropic medications properly. They also need a familiarity with the most up-to-date evidence to answer the questions of an increasingly sophisticated population of patients, relatives, spouses, and prospective spouses requesting genetic counseling.

At present, the most clinically useful evidence for genetic transmission continues to be the traditional genetic–epidemiological findings from twin, family, and adoption studies. In addition to demonstrating genetic transmission, the genetic–epidemiological data also suggest the degree to which illness in the population is familial, and they help specify diagnoses that aggregate together. The role of age, sex, and other demographic and sociocultural variables can also be clarified from this evidence. Genetic–epidemiological studies of diagnosis do not, however, allow one to identify the mode of genetic transmission in bipolar illness. Neither they nor pedigree studies illuminate other important genetic issues: Is there biological heterogeneity? What is the pathophysiological inherited process in an illness? Where on the gene map is the disease locus (or loci)? What are the gene defects? To answer these questions, pathophysiological and genetic linkage studies are needed.

This chapter examines the several lines of evidence that establish the fact of genetic vulnerability in manic-depressive illness, clarify its

*Clinical Neurogenetics Branch, Intramural Research Program, National Institute of Mental Health, Bethesda, Maryland 20892.

This chapter includes material originally published in Nurnberger and Gershon, 1984, and in Gershon et al., 1987a.

mode of transmission, and suggest clues to its pathophysiology. It also covers genetic counseling in bipolar illness and its likely evolution as linkage markers and pathophysiological tests become more widely applicable. The focus here is on bipolar forms of illness, but we consider the central question of the genetic relationship between bipolar and unipolar subgroups, particularly recurrent unipolar illness. A common genetic diathesis for both bipolar and unipolar disorders would suggest that the correct conceptual model for these illnesses is the spectrum, or continuum, model. Different genotypes, on the other hand, would argue for a categorical model of discrete and independent affective disorders defined by clinical diagnosis (see Chapters 3 and 4).

Another set of questions we consider in this chapter concerns the mode of genetic transmission and what exactly is transmitted. Are manic-depressive disorders, particularly the bipolar forms, inherited through an X chromosome or an autosomal single major gene? Is there genetic linkage to the short arm of chromosome 11, the human leukocyte antigen (HLA) region on chromosome 6, or to the color blindness glucose-6-phosphate dehydrogenase region of the X chromosome? Are these disorders genetically or biologically heterogeneous? Are there linkage markers or biological risk factors identifying genetic vulnerability? Many of the special terms used in genetics are given in an Appendix at the end of this chapter.

A HISTORICAL PERSPECTIVE

The origins of modern genetic hypotheses about human behavior lie with Darwin and Galton, who developed their formulations in ignorance of the findings of their contemporary, Gregor Mendel (Freeman, 1983). Their model of inheritance was one of biometric correlations, similar to that of the intuitive quantitative models of selection used by the animal or plant breeder. The modern counterpart of the Darwinian or Galtonian formulations is found in statistical regression analyses of familial correlations, such as the multifactorial model, where numerous genetic and environmental events contribute additively to a measured outcome, but no single component can be identified or contributes preponderantly. The Mendelian model, by contrast, stipulates that events do

not occur in the absence of a specific causative genotype, a conception that leads to specific and testable predictions on the nature of the gene responsible. Vogel and Motulsky (1986; Vogel, 1987), who first called attention to the historical persistence of the two models, argue that as a scientific paradigm, Mendel's model proved superior. It generated a strikingly productive body of scientific theory and findings. When Mendel developed his model, the gene was an inferred construct that has since become an observable reality, with an identifiable location, a discernible coding of its information, and a specifiable product or other biological role.

Statistical regression methods—such as twin, family, and adoption studies, which do not incorporate identifiable single-locus events—have classically been invoked to account for numerous diseases in which the inheritance is complex. The proportions of ill and well relatives do not fit Mendelian ratios in these diseases (e.g., hypertension), so that single-gene inheritance is not directly implied. Multifactorial correlational models that have been applied to qualitative traits, such as psychiatric disorders, assume that an underlying variable is inherited, and affected persons have passed a threshold value on the implicit variable.[2] In this era of rapid advances in molecular genetics, however, such explanations have acquired a biological dead-end quality, even when they satisfactorily predict observed prevalences. Specific biological components—such as a gene, its sequence, and its function—cannot be identified by multifactorial interpretations. These models also have failed to exclude single-locus inheritance in such disorders as diabetes mellitus (Worden et al., 1976; Rotter and Rimoin, 1978). The distinction between multifactorial and single-locus inheritance, formerly of little interest outside of mathematical genetics, has become crucial to scientific progress in understanding many common diseases with complex inheritance, among them the major psychiatric disorders.

The possibility remains that statistical regression methods may explain some phenomena better than single genetic-loci models. In the past two decades, powerful mathematical models that incorporate single-gene effects as well as other risk factors have been developed to analyze familial events.[3] Model-free methods have been developed to study inheritance of putative illness-causing biological traits. With these methods, a characteristic is shown to be inherited by concordance in twin or family studies and then demonstrated to be more likely found in individuals who are ill or at risk for the illness than in controls.[4] These methods have uncovered possible genetic links between illness and biological phenomena, such as the muscarinic sensitivity in vulnerability to affective disorders (Sitaram et al., 1987) to be discussed subsequently.

The Galtonian approach dominated behavioral genetics until recently. Apart from the limitations of these analyses, there are historical and ideological obstacles to accepting this approach. Galton's ideas became the ideological basis of a racist eugenics movement, in which Galton himself participated (Freeman, 1983). The combination of unsavory associations with this late 19th century movement and intangible observations has led to a polemical dispute on the role of genes in human behavior that has extended to the present (Gould, 1981; Lewontin et al., 1984).

Despite these arguments, for the past few decades, prevailing scientific opinion has assumed that mental disorders are multifactorial in their transmission—that is, they result from the cumulative effect of an inherited vulnerability and numerous hypothesized developmental, social, cultural, environmental events (Gottesman and Shields, 1982). The acceptance of a genetic component is historically related to the published findings in the mid-1960s of Heston (1966) and of Kety, Rosenthal, Wender, Schulsinger, and their colleagues (Kety et al., 1975; Rosenthal and Kety, 1968), who demonstrated that schizophrenia and related disorders are found in excess in the biological relatives of adopted schizophrenics. Since the adoptions had occurred early in infancy, the findings strongly implied that the transmission was genetic, although prenatal and perinatal events might still be considered as causes. Combined with 50 years of evidence from twin and family studies pointing to the same conclusion in schizophrenia and in the major affective disorders, the adoption study findings persuaded most observers that genetics was one among many factors that could predispose a person to certain emotional disorders. But resistance to the idea that genes can produce unwanted behavior continued, along with fear that if such

knowledge were discovered it would lead to abuses and oppression (Culliton, 1975; Gershon, 1983a).

The recent demonstrations, through linkage marker studies of pedigrees, of single-major locus inheritance in manic-depressive illness, if replicated, must change this perspective radically. As described subsequently, a linkage demonstration provides strong evidence that a single, identifiable genetic event can profoundly influence complex human behavior.[5] Identifying single-locus events and elucidating their genetic and biological mechanisms have become the foremost challenges of genetic research in psychiatry. The less tangible question about relative contribution of heredity in the major psychiatric disorders is, for now, of secondary interest.

A CLINICAL PERSPECTIVE

Research on twins provided the initial genetic evidence on human behavior and on psychiatric disorders. A century ago, Galton suggested that twins could be studied as a natural experiment on the nature–nurture issue. Whereas all twins reared together share roughly the same environment, only identical (monozygotic) twin pairs have genes that are identical by descent; fraternal (dizygotic) twin pairs share only half their genes, just as other siblings do. Galton suggested that hereditary factors are probably involved when identical twin pairs are more likely to have a trait in common (concordance) than are fraternal twin pairs. Conversely, environmental factors probably determine traits equally likely to be shared by both identical and fraternal twin pairs.

Twin studies consistently show that identical twins are far more concordant for affective disorder than are fraternal twins. This evidence strongly supports a predominantly genetic contribution to vulnerability. Twin studies also demonstrate at least partial genetic overlap between bipolar and unipolar disorders, since identical twin pairs concordant for affective illness are not always concordant for type of disorder: one twin might have bipolar illness and the other unipolar.

Another clinical design, the adoption study, sorts genetic from postnatal environmental factors by studying the biological relatives of patients who have been adopted. Genetic transmission is implied if a high percentage of the biological relatives have the same illness as the patient does, although this design does not rule out prenatal environmental factors. Bipolar illness has been studied in one adoption study, which is described below.

Ascertaining whether a disease runs in families is a third clinical approach to recognizing genetic transmission. Genetic involvement is suggested by the concentration of an illness in a relatively limited number of families in a population. Although necessary, such clustering is not a sufficient condition of genetic transmission, since numerous familial characteristics are not genetic. Manic-depressive illness, clearly familial in this epidemiological sense, has been the subject of perhaps the best epidemiological–genetic study in psychiatry. A wealth of data has been collected on the prevalence of different diagnoses in the population at large and in the relatives of patients. Diagnostic criteria, differential mortality, and other factors have also been examined for their role in observed familial prevalences.

Advances in genetics and neuroscience may soon make it practical to use inherited pathophysiological defects or genetic linkage markers to identify vulnerable individuals. The prediction that the entire human genome could be mapped, so that linkage markers can be used to locate any single-locus disease gene, seemed fantastic when it was first made at the end of the 1970s. But it is now 95 percent mapped, and a complete map may be expected shortly (Donis-Keller et al., 1987). In the foreseeable future, single gene transmission might well be identifiable in a given proportion of manic-depressive patients. Genetic heterogeneity also might soon be resolved with the use of markers (Goldin et al., 1981, 1984).

Some forms of bipolar or recurrent unipolar disorder may be transmitted by multifactorial inheritance or other more complex means than single-locus inheritance. These types of complex transmission may not be understood until the inherited pathophysiological vulnerability (or vulnerabilities) can be identified. Genetic approaches to pathophysiology may require a major shift in clinical research strategies. In the classic model that predominated in the first half of the 20th century, particularly in the United States, psychiatric illness was thought to result from stress in an otherwise normal person. Unstated in this model is the assumption that the population is

genetically homogeneous in its vulnerability to such illness. The model has led to clinical research strategies of comparing the ill to the well state in patients with episodic disorders, since in the well state, they are assumed to be essentially equivalent to normal controls. Similarly, the clinical and biological effects of psychotropic drugs have been extrapolated from the drugs' universal effects on brain metabolism in experimental animals (the pharmacological bridge) rather than from their differential effects on genetic variants.

The perspective implied by the concept of genetic vulnerability is that people who become ill have a continuous, underlying constitutional vulnerability, which is present even when they are well. The etiological importance of any specific biological factor can be tested by observing whether it is genetically transmitted in families along with the illness instead of independently of it. Euthymic manic-depressive patients, their offspring, and siblings at risk are of interest because they serve as a control for observations made during illness. They also become the object of study because, even in the well state, their vulnerability for the illness should be detectable when properly compared with normal controls.

GENETIC EPIDEMIOLOGY

Twin Studies

Epidemiological–genetic diagnostic evidence comes from adoption studies, twin studies, and family studies. Over the course of 50 years, numerous studies have shown that the concordance rate between identical twins is higher than that in fraternal twins, a body of evidence that strongly argues for heritability. Price (1968) reviewed 12 cases of affective illness in one twin who was raised apart from his or her monozygotic (identical) co-twin. In that series, eight pairs (67 percent) were concordant—that is, both twins had an affective illness. This rate is quite similar to those found in monozygotic (MZ) twins raised together. One must note, however, the lack of systematic sampling for twins raised apart.

Bertelsen and colleagues (1977; Bertelsen, 1979) reported on a study using the Danish Twin Register (Hauge et al., 1968), which includes all same-sex twins born between 1870 and 1920. Questionnaires were sent to twins (or if deceased, to their relatives), and if necessary, this mailing was followed by personal interviews, thus establishing very complete information. Zygosity was checked either serologically or anthropometrically (through photographs or observed resemblances, if both were not alive). Among twin pairs in which one or both had manic-depressive illness (by Kraepelinian criteria), the concordance for the 55 MZ pairs was 0.67, whereas for the 52 dizygotic (DZ) pairs, it was only 0.20. These figures are in close agreement with the data previously summarized. Concordance for MZ twin pairs was higher for pairs in which one had bipolar illness (0.79) than for pairs in which one had unipolar illness (0.54). For DZ twin pairs, concordance rates were similar for the two disorders (0.24 for bipolar and 0.19 for unipolar illness). These data suggest that both the bipolar and unipolar forms of illness are heritable.

Concordance relates to severity of illness in this way: If one MZ twin had bipolar-I illness, 80 percent of the identical twins were also ill. In bipolar-II illness, concordance was 78 percent. When the index case had unipolar illness with three or more episodes of depression, the concordance rate for the MZ co-twin was 59 percent, whereas identical unipolar twins with fewer than three episodes had a concordance rate of only 33 percent. The unipolar data may in part reflect the fact that the population with fewer episodes may not yet have passed through the age of risk.

Further analysis of the concordant pairs for polarity reveals 11 pairs in which both had unipolar illness, 14 in which both were bipolar and 7 in which one was unipolar and the other was bipolar. These findings suggest some genetic specificity for polarity but also reveal that unipolar and bipolar illness can be associated with the same genetic makeup. These data most clearly demonstrate the inherent ambiguity in biological comparisons of bipolar and unipolar patients. At the very least, in a substantial proportion of unipolar patients, the genetic and biological vulnerability is the same as that of bipolar patients. The same conclusion can be drawn from family study data and mathematical models of observed distribution of diagnoses in families.

The question of what causes some patients to display mania or hypomania while others never do is crucial. But it cannot be assumed that unipolar patients lack this capacity, and that they should, therefore, be clearly distinguished, even on this key characteristic, from bipolar patients.

Adoption Studies

Adoption data can demonstrate that inheritance (or prenatal or perinatal events) are sufficient to predispose a person to a familial illness, as opposed to later familial environmental events. The correct comparison is between biological relatives of affected adoptees and biological relatives of control adoptees. Comparisons of adoptive with biological relatives reveal little because of the careful screening that is traditional in adoption placements (Clerget-Darpoux et al., 1986). Demonstrating that preadoption events are significant is quite important, but it is worth noting that adoption studies contribute nothing to understanding the specific genetic issues raised in the introduction (e.g., mode of transmission or mapping of genes related to illness).

In Denmark, the suicide rate among the biological relatives of 71 adoptees with affective disorder was found to be disproportionately high: 15 of 381, or 3.9 percent, compared with the rate among adoptive relatives of those probands, 1 of 168, or 0.6 percent. It was also much higher than the rate among the biological or adoptive relatives of control adoptees: 1 of 353, or 0.3 percent, and 1 of 166, or 0.6 percent, respectively (Schulsinger et al., 1979; Kety, 1979; Wender et al., 1986). The difference in suicide rates between biological relatives of patients with affective disorders and the biological relatives of controls is significant. It is not clear from the published tables whether this entity is diagnostically independent of affective disorders.

Wender and colleagues (1986) include the following in affective disorders: bipolar and unipolar disorders, neurotic depression (equivalent to RDC minor depression), and *affect reaction,* a Danish diagnostic term applied to individuals who manifest histrionic or panicky behavior or make an impulsive suicidal attempt in response to an identifiable event, usually rejection. The authors include bipolar, unipolar, and uncertain (polarity) major mood disorders as one subgroup and neurotic depression and affective reaction as another. Together, the two subgroups are called *broad affective spectrum,* and apparently the first subgroup is called *hard affective spectrum.* There were 71 relatives of bipolar probands and 132 relatives of unipolar probands, with 4.2 percent and 5.3 percent hard affective spectrum diagnoses, respectively, vs 2.3 percent among 313 controls (not significant; even combining relatives of unipolar and bipolar probands, $p = 0.08$). These rates are lower than published rates in family studies elsewhere, which may reflect the exclusive reliance on medical records, without direct interview and family history information.

Mendlewicz and Rainer (1977) found affective disorder (including depressive spectrum disorder) in 31 percent of the biological parents of 29 bipolar adoptee probands,[6] compared with only 12 percent of the adoptive parents. The morbid risk in biological parents is comparable to the risk these investigators found in parents of nonadopted bipolar patients (26 percent) and higher than biological or adoptive parents of normal adoptees (2 percent and 9 percent, respectively). In 1983, Von Knorring and co-workers reported on an adoption study from Sweden that included 56 probands with affective disorder and matched adopted and nonadopted controls. The proband diagnoses (following Perris' classification system) were: 5 with bipolar or cycloid disorder (similar to schizoaffective), 11 with unipolar and other psychotic depression, and 40 with nonpsychotic depression. Probands and relatives were diagnosed through records of the Swedish health insurance system, with additional records requested from "psychiatric hospitals and clinics throughout Sweden." The investigators found no concordance of psychopathology between biological parents and adoptees, with the possible exception of more affective disorder in biological mothers of female adoptees with affective disorder. (After correcting for the number of statistical tests, the result is of borderline significance.)

The Swedish study should not be seen as a failure to replicate the Danish adoption study. Suicide, the key outcome variable in the Danish study, could have been entirely missed in the Swedish study. Untreated psychiatric disorders and disorders treated privately or under nonpsychiatric guise could have been missed, since subjects were not examined. For example, none of 8 biological parents of adoptees with bipolar or cycloid disorder and only 1 of 18 parents of adoptees with psychotic depression showed any affective disorder. Even though this rate is similar to that found among the parents of control adoptees in this study, it is far less than the rate observed in any family study in which relatives are examined directly. Nonetheless, this study does cast some doubt on the genetic transmissibility of nonbipolar major depression because of the number of nonbipolar cases.

If we consider the entire adoption literature in bipolar illness, there are 5 bipolar probands in the adoption study by Von Knorring and associates, 10 in the study by Wender and colleagues, and 29 in the Mendlewicz and Rainer study. The positive results of Mendlewicz and Rainer do not have the advantage of sampling through population registers. The results of the other two studies are inconclusive. We would conclude that the adoption data do not provide a broad base of supportive data on the hypothesis that these disorders are transmitted before the age of adoption. The major support from epidemiological studies for genetic transmission of bipolar and unipolar affective disorders is to be found in the twin studies.

Family Studies

By *family studies* we mean case-controlled studies of illness in relatives of patients or normal controls. The key questions that can be answered by morbid risk estimates from family studies include the following: Is bipolar illness transmitted independently of unipolar (and other forms of affective disorder)? Do specific genetic models fit the familial segregation of illness? Independent transmission is assessed by studying cross-prevalences (defined as the prevalence of one illness in relatives of patients with a second illness). If two illnesses are independent, the cross-prevalences are the same as the prevalence of the illnesses in the population at large. If they are not, either or both of the cross-prevalences may be higher.

Unipolar and Bipolar Disorders in Relatives of Bipolar Patients

In the many family studies performed since the 1960s, estimates of morbid risk for relatives of patients and the general population have ranged widely. These inconsistencies, reviewed elsewhere (Gershon, 1983b), are present in more recent studies as well (Table 15-1). To a significant

Table 15-1. Affective Illness in First-Degree Relatives

	Relatives at Risk N Age-Corrected	Morbid Risk %		
		SA	BP	UP
BP Probands				
Taylor et al., 1980	600		4.8	4.2
Baron et al., 1982	135	1.5	14.5	16.3
Gershon et al., 1982a	598	1.2	8.0	14.9
Coryell et al., 1984	389		7.0	22.4
Fieve et al., 1984	1,309		2.9	8.4
Tsuang et al., 1985	608		3.9	9.1
Angst, 1986b	1,441	2.9	5.6	6.2
Rice et al., 1987b	838[a]		10.6	24.3
UP Probands				
Taylor et al., 1980	121		4.1	8.3
Baron et al., 1981b	475		3.1	16.1
Baron et al., 1982	144	4.6	2.2	17.7
Gershon et al., 1982a	138	0.7	2.9	16.6
Coryell et al., 1984	572		2.8	29.4
Fieve et al., 1984	265		1.5	8.7
Weissman et al., 1984a	656	0.3	2.7	17.0
Tsuang et al., 1985	1,366		2.2	11.0
Angst, 1986b	1,300	1.2	1.7	6.4
Rice et al., 1987b	1,176[a]	0.5	5.4	28.6
Normal Probands				
Gershon et al., 1982a	217	0.5	0.5	5.8
Weissman et al., 1984a	442	0.2	1.8	5.6
Tsuang et al., 1985	1,140		0.2	4.8

SA = Schizoaffective

[a]Interviewed only

degree, they can be attributed to differences in diagnostic definitions and procedures for gathering clinical information. Good diagnostic reliability can now be routinely attained by using recently developed family study procedures and criteria. Collaborative studies can also establish good reliability between centers and find similar prevalences in relatives, as evidenced by the findings in the collaborating studies by Gershon's group (1982a) and Weissman's group (1984a) and in the NIMH epidemiological catchment area study (Robins et al., 1984) (see Chapter 7).

Generalizations that are consistent across studies include: (1) affective disorders are familial, since the rate in relatives of patients is consistently about two to three times the rate in relatives of appropriately chosen case controls, (2) the most frequent affective disorder in relatives of bipolar patients is not bipolar illness but unipolar illness; bipolar illness is next most frequent, and

(3) among relatives of unipolar patients, there is a tendency, not always significant, for bipolar disorder to appear more frequently than it does among controls. Consistent with our earlier discussion of the twin data, these findings imply at least a partial overlap in the transmitted vulnerability to the two major forms of affective disorder.

Cohort Effect

People born in the decades starting approximately in 1940 have a higher lifetime prevalence of affective disorders than people born earlier. This so-called cohort effect has been seen in epidemiological studies and in studies of families of affective patients.[7] Surprisingly, it holds true for mania as well as for depression.[8]

In our own data, the age at onset for bipolar and schizoaffective disorders has become earlier, and the total lifetime prevalence appears likely to be much higher in the cohorts born since 1940 (Gershon et al., 1982a, 1987b) (Figure 15-1). This finding cannot be due to genetic change over such a short period nor to selective effects on reproductive fitness. It must reflect, then, a cultural influence—in the broadest sense of culture as a global environmental and biological setting—on the rate of affective illness. Whatever the cause, it interacts with familial vulnerability, since the rate remains elevated in relatives of patients.

Subgroup Differences Within Bipolar Disorder

Are there genetic differences between clinically defined subdivisions of manic-depressive illness? As discussed previously, twin studies demonstrate at least a partial overlap in vulnerability for unipolar and bipolar illness. Subgroup differences within the bipolar spectrum may also exist. Bipolar-II disorder, defined as patients with major depression who have had hypomania but not mania (Dunner et al., 1976c), is particularly difficult to diagnose reliably in family studies (Gershon and Guroff, 1984). Bipolar-II patients tend to have more bipolar-II and unipolar relatives and fewer bipolar-I relatives than do bipolar-I patients (Table 15-2). This suggests that bipolar-II illness is genetically somewhere between bipolar-I and unipolar illness, as in the multiple-threshold models for affective disorders discussed subsequently.

The suggestion that more recurrent forms of unipolar disorder may be genetically linked to bipolar disorder raises the important question of whether the tendency toward recurrence involves an independent genetic contribution. Angst and colleagues (1980a) found no significant differences in morbid risk in relatives of patients with 1 to 5, 6 to 10, or more than 10 episodes. Gershon's group (1982a) also found no morbid risk differences in their comparison of patients who had 10 or more episodes with patients who, during the 10 or more years since their affective disorders began, had fewer than 10 episodes.

An extreme form of recurrence, rapid-cycling bipolar disorder, has been defined as occurring when a patient has at least four manic and/or depressive episodes per year. Nurnberger and colleagues (1988b) did not find differences in morbid risk to relatives of rapid-cycling patients compared with other bipolar patients. They also did not find significant concordance of rapid cycling among bipolar patients who are related to each other. This implies that the specific vulnerability to rapid cycling (given a vulnerability to bipolar disorder) is not inherited.

Early-Onset and Late-Onset Bipolar Illness

Most studies have shown increased morbid risk of affective disorder in relatives of probands whose illness began relatively early in life (see review in Gershon et al., 1976). Taylor and Abrams

Figure 15-1. Bipolar and schizoaffective illness in relatives pooled into pre-1940 and post-1940 cohorts (Gershon et al., 1982b, 1987b). Life table analysis of cumulative probability of developing bipolar or schizoaffective (acute) disorder by a given age in relatives of bipolar patients studied by Gershon et al. (1982). The higher rate in later born cohorts of relatives is generalizable to the population as a whole.

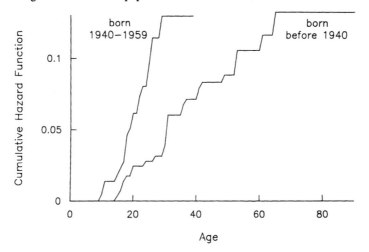

Table 15-2. Comparison of Affective Disorders in Relatives
of Bipolar-I and Bipolar-II Patients

	N	Prevalence in Relatives %			
		SA	BPI	BPII	UP
BPI Probands					
Gershon et al., 1982a	441	1.1	4.5	4.1	14.0
Fieve et al., 1984	760		3.6	1.5	6.4[a]
Coryell et al., 1984	278		2.9	2.5	22.7
Angst, 1986b	657	3.6	5.0	0.9	5.5
BPII Probands					
Gershon et al., 1982a	157	0.6	2.6	4.5	17.3
Fieve et al., 1984	549		0.7	4.2	11.1[a]
Coryell et al., 1984	111		0.9	9.8	21.4
Angst, 1986b	276	1.3	4.0	0.7	8.0

SA = Schizoaffective
[a]Includes "UP other"

Update of Gershon et al., 1987a

(1981a) divided 134 bipolar probands into 80 with early onset (starting before the age of 29) and 54 with late onset (starting at 30 or after) on the basis of the beginning of the first definite episode. Relatives of early-onset probands had a morbid risk of 9.6 percent for bipolar illness and 4.6 percent for unipolar illness; relatives of late-onset probands had 0.8 percent risk of bipolar illness and 3.0 percent risk of unipolar illness. Subsequent data did not confirm this finding for bipolar probands (Gershon et al., 1982a), although unipolar probands continue to show this phenomenon (Weissman et al., 1984c). Since the mean age of onset in bipolar illness is in late adolescence or early adulthood, considerably earlier than for unipolar depression, it is perhaps more appropriate to consider childhood-onset bipolar patients as the early-onset group. These patients do, indeed, have increased morbid risk in relatives, as found by Strober's group (Strober, 1984; Strober et al., 1988) and Dwyer and DeLong (1987). The interaction of the birth cohort effect with these findings has not been studied systematically.

Related Disorders in Relatives of Bipolar Patients

A clinical–genetic spectrum of bipolar disorders can be constructed by comparing prevalence of illness in relatives of patients with that in controls. Such data suggest that, in addition to unipolar illness, schizoaffective disorder and cyclo-thymic personality may be considered part of the spectrum of bipolar illness. The existence of a clinical spectrum with shared genetic factors has implications for both etiology and treatment, particularly with regard to lithium responsiveness in schizoaffective, unipolar, and cyclothymic relatives of bipolar patients (e.g., see Kupfer et al., 1975).

Schizoaffective Disorder. As discussed in Chapter 5, schizoaffective disorder presents something of a challenge to the Kraepelinian dichotomy. The identical twins of schizoaffective patients tend to have the same disorder, but the first-degree relatives have a considerable frequency of affective disorder, both unipolar and bipolar, and also small but consistent increases in schizoaffective disorder and schizophrenia, as compared with controls (Table 15-3). Does schizoaffective disorder, characterized by symptoms of both affective disorder and schizophrenia, demonstrate that there is a continuum in the major psychiatric disorders that includes both affective disorders and schizophrenia, according to the unitary model of Crow (1986)? Other findings also suggest a less than complete dichotomy between affective disorders and schizophrenia. As reviewed by Crow, the early literature repeatedly reported cases of schizophrenia in children of manic-depressives, although not in other relatives.

Two other possibilities suggest themselves: First, schizoaffective disorder, a rare condition, represents the unfortunate coexistence of two disorders in one individual. Such a possibility would explain the fact that, in relatives of schizoaffective patients, the frequency of schizophrenia is the same as in relatives of schizophrenics and the frequency of affective disorders is the same as in relatives of affective patients. The second possibility, proposed by Baron and colleagues (1982) on the basis of family study data, is that the schizoaffective group is a mixture of individuals who have either one of two separate inherited disorders, which can be clinically distinguished by using the Research Diagnostic Criteria (RDC) dichotomy of schizoaffective–schizophrenic-like (SA-S) and schizoaffective–affective-like (SA-A) (Spitzer et al., 1978a,b) (Table 15-3). Kendler and colleagues (1986), from somewhat similar results, conclude that the risk for schizophrenia is higher in relatives of SA-S, whereas the risk for bipolar illness is higher in relatives of SA-A. We note, however, that the schizoaffective group (SA-A or SA-S), when compared with appropriate controls, appears to have elevated risk in relatives for schizophrenia and also, but not significantly, for affective illness. Rice and colleagues (1987a) also found that schizophrenia but not bipolar-I disorder is elevated in relatives of patients they call schizoaffective/depressed, whereas the opposite is found in relatives of schizoaffective/bipolar patients. However, in the quite large study of Angst and associates (1979c,d), neither of these subdivisions of probands produces such separations of morbid risk in relatives. Our own data (Gershon et al., 1988) are similar to those of Angst (Table 15-3).

The reports of linkage of schizoaffective illness and bipolar illness to the color blindness region of the X chromosome (Mendlewicz et al., 1980b; Baron, 1977) would be consistent with the view of at least some schizoaffective disorder having the same genetic vulnerability as bipolar illness. We have reviewed these linkage data elsewhere and noted that, in view of our difficulty replicating the linkage, we take a cautious attitude to the reports.

In comparative studies that examine several forms of psychosis, including schizoaffective disorder, the number of relatives studied and the actual number of observed bipolar or schizophrenic relatives are small. Thus, the proposed subdivisions of schizoaffective disorder in rela-

tion to schizophrenia and bipolar illness and the conclusions based on them must be considered tentative. Numerous interpretations of the family study data (summarized in Table 15-3) are possible, but none of them unambiguously separates the affective and schizophrenic disorders. One possible perspective is based on the interpretation of our own data presented in Table 15-4 (Gershon et al., 1982a, 1988). From this perspective, a Kraepelinian-like dichotomy is only possible if it is formulated in a more complex way than is usual.

Our neo-Kraepelinian conceptualization is as follows. The two independent categories of psychiatric disorder categories are schizophrenia and bipolar illness. Unipolar disorder may be found (in excess) in relatives of either category of patient (bipolar or schizophrenic) when minimal additional genetic or environmental factors are present. Schizophrenic patients have relatives with acute or chronic psychoses, as well as psychoses complicated by (usually unipolar) affective syndromes.[9] Schizoaffective disorder may result when either schizophrenic or bipolar familial tendency is present, since even nonmanic schizoaffectives have bipolar relatives. This formulation could explain the increased prevalence of nonbipolar schizoaffective disorder in relatives of schizophrenic patients. It also implies that there is more than one form of schizoaffective disorder; one type includes patients who have familial bipolar illness and schizophrenia, another those that have only familial schizophrenia. On the crucial point of whether the clinical presentation of the patient predicts family history, this formulation is consistent with the findings of two studies (Angst, 1979c,d; Gershon et al., 1988) but not with two others (Baron et al., 1982; Kendler et al., 1986). In this formulation, the clinical presentation of the schizoaffective patient, as mainly affective or mainly schizophrenic, provides no necessary indication of his or her familial tendency. The astute clinician must empirically find, in each case, whether the treatment response is more like affective illness or more like schizophrenia. On the other hand, the family history may be a primary clue to therapeutic strategy in some cases.

We suspect that the true relationship of schizoaffective disorder to manic-depressive illness and to schizophrenia may be demonstrated best in

Table 15-3. Family Studies of Schizophrenia and Schizoaffective Disorder

Study	Relative N	SCZ C	SCZ NC	SA C	SA NC	BPI / BPII	UP
Angst et al., 1979c,d							
SA[a]	425	5.9[b]		3.3[c]		5.8[d]	
SA[e]	416	4.6[b]		2.9[c]		7.8[d]	
SA, mania	539	5.9[b]		4.1[c]		1.0	5.9
SA, no mania	336	4.2[b]		1.2[c]		1.2	5.2
Mendlewicz et al., 1980b							
SCZ		16.9[b]				8.6[d]	
SA		10.8[b]				34.6[d]	
BP		1.8[b]				39.4[d]	
UP		3.2[b]				28.5[d]	
Baron et al., 1982							
SCZ	178.7	7.9		1.7[a]	0[f]	0.6	4.5
SA[a]	73.2	4.1		0.7[a]	0[f]	0	10.9
SA[e]	64.4	0		0[a]	3.2[f]	1.6	26.5
BP	135.2	0.7		0[a]	1.5[f]	14.5	16.3
UP	143.5	0		0.8[a]	3.0[f]	2.2	17.7
Gershon et al., 1982a							
SA[e]	69	4.9	0	1.6	5.8	11.7	16.4
BP	738	0.3	0	0.1	0.6	7.2	14.9
UP	165	0	0	0	0.7	2.9	16.7
Kendler et al., 1986							
Schizophreniform	91	3.6	0	0		1.3[f]	5.8
SA	149	5.6	2.2	2.7		3.8[f]	7.3
SA[a]	75	8.2				1.4[f]	6.1
SA[e] (or other)	84	3.8				5.6[f]	9.1
Rice et al., 1987b							
SA / BP	139	0.7[g]		0.7[h]	0[i]	9.4	23.0[j]
SA depressed	72	2.8[g]		0[h]	0[i]	6.9	22.2[j]
BPI	567	1.1[g]		0.5[h]	0.2[i]	10.4	23.1[j]
BPII	271	0.4[g]		0.4[h]	0[i]	11.1	26.9[j]
MDD	1,176	0.3[g]		0.2[h]	0.3[i]	5.4	28.6[j]
Gershon et al., 1988							
SCZ	108	3.1	0	0	5.0	1.3	14.7
SA[a]	129	1.7	0.8	2.5	0	8.8	9.3
Control	380	0.6	0	0	0.6	0.3	6.7

SCZ = schizophrenia, C = chronic, NC = not chronic, SA = schizoaffective, MDD = major depressive disorder

[a]Schizoaffective (mainly schizophrenic) [e]Schizoaffective (mainly affective) [h]Schizoaffective (bipolar)
[b]All schizophrenia [f]BPI only [i]Schizoaffective (depressed)
[c]All schizoaffective [g]Schizophrenia (chronicity not [j]Major depressive disorder
[d]All affective specified)

Adapted from Gershon et al., 1988

chromosomal linkage marker studies rather than in additional family or clinical studies. Linkage investigations of multiple pedigrees have greater power than diagnostic epidemiological studies to resolve genetic heterogeneity, a concept clarified later in this chapter. It would not be surprising to learn that illness linked to chromosomal region A includes multiple and very disparate forms of psychiatric illness, including schizophrenia, bipolar, and schizoaffective disorders, whereas ill-

Table 15-4. Psychosis in Relatives of Schizophrenic,
Schizoaffective, and Bipolar Patients

Illness Associated in Relatives	SCZ	SA	BP
UP	Yes	Yes	Yes
BP	No	Yes	Yes
SCZ	Yes	Yes	No
SA	Yes	Yes	Yes

SCZ = schizophrenia, SA = schizoaffective

Adapted from Gershon et al., 1988

nesses linked to regions B and C include only affective disorders, primarily bipolar and unipolar, and clinical manifestations linked to regions D and E are schizophrenia and schizotypal and related personality disorders.

Alcoholism. Helzer and Winokur (1974) found an increase in alcoholism in relatives of male bipolar probands. However, elsewhere in the United States, Dunner and colleagues (1976d) found no greater alcoholism in families of bipolar or unipolar patients than in control families, although there was an increase in families of bipolar-II patients. Weissman and colleagues (1984b) found alcoholism not increased in relatives of unipolar patients. Morrison (1975) found no increase in alcoholism in families of bipolar patients unless the patients themselves were alcoholic. Gershon and colleagues (1982a) found no increase in alcoholism in relatives of bipolar probands compared with relatives of controls. Although bipolar illness and alcoholism are sometimes found in the same individual, alcoholism by itself (without affective disorder) does not appear to belong in the genetic spectrum of bipolar manic-depressive illness. For a review of the relationship of alcoholism to affective disorders, see Chapter 9.

Anorexia Nervosa. Cantwell and co-workers (1977) reported in a family history study of anorectic patients that an excess of affective disorder was present in relatives compared with controls. Winokur and colleagues (1980) investigated 25 anorectic women and 192 of their first-

and second-degree relatives in a family study. A group of 25 age-matched women with no history of anorexia or depression was used as the control. In the relatives of anorectic patients, 17.7 percent had unipolar illness and 4.7 percent had bipolar illness (not corrected for age). The corresponding figures for controls' relatives were 9.2 percent and 0.6 percent. The difference in total incidence of affective illness was significant ($p < 0.005$), suggesting a genetic relationship between the two disorders.

Our own data (Gershon et al., 1982b, 1984) were similar (Figure 15-2). In relatives of anorectic patients, we found a modest amount of anorexia (2 percent) and as much affective disorder as in relatives of bipolar patients (8.3 percent bipolar and 13.3 percent unipolar). In relatives of bipolar patients, however, there was very little anorexia (0.6 percent). Apparently, anorexia involves a unique familial vulnerability factor, possibly genetic, that can be superimposed on a genetic tendency to bipolar and unipolar affective disorder.

Cyclothymic Personality. Cyclothymic personality has been reviewed as a separate entity by Akiskal and colleagues (1977, 1979a). As reviewed in Chapter 4, evidence from family studies (Gershon et al., 1975, 1982a) suggests that this condition may be related to bipolar affective disorder, since it is found more frequently in the relatives of bipolar patients than in relatives of unipolar or normal persons.

Suicide. Suicide was common among the biological relatives of adoptees with affective disorder studied in Denmark (Schulsinger et al., 1979). In our own family study data on bipolar patients, the suicides in the proband's generation and later generations largely occurred in people with symptoms of antecedent affective disorder (by history from relatives and medical records). But in the earlier generations (the proband's parents, aunts, uncles, grandparents), there were 15 suicides (out of about 1,000 individuals); 13 of these occurred in people with no known antecedent psychiatric disorder. This probably reflects cognitive or cultural differences between generations rather than the existence of nonpsychiatric suicide as a separate entity in the affective spectrum. A parallel increase in suicide and in bipolar and

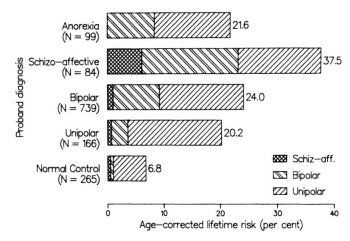

Figure 15-2. Affective disorders in parents, siblings, and adult offspring of probands. Note that bipolar disorder is more prevalent in relatives of probands than in relatives of controls, but the difference in relatives of unipolar probands is not statistically significant (from Gershon et al., 1987a).

unipolar affective disorders, which remain concentrated in families, is reviewed in the previous discussion of the cohort effect.

Childhood Depression. Depression and other psychiatric disorders of childhood have been noted repeatedly in many offspring of patients with affective disorder. These observations have understandably led to a consensus that having an affectively ill parent is associated with increased childhood psychiatric vulnerability, which may represent an antecedent of adult affective disorder (Beardslee et al., 1983; Cytryn et al., 1984). However, remarkably few observations come from controlled studies of the offspring of affectively ill parents compared with a selected group of normal parents on standardized diagnostic interviews and criteria. In their comprehensive review, Beardslee's group (1983) comments on the "need for cross-sectional studies, with adequate control groups" in studies of offspring of depressed parents.

For childhood depression, appropriate sampling can be done in two ways: from the "top down," meaning study of children ascertained through depressed patients, and from the "bottom up," where adult relatives of children with depression are studied.

Only small samples of children have been reported from the "top down." Decina and colleagues (1983) reported on 31 children (ages 7-14) of bipolar patients compared with 18 con-trol children. Eight children of patients had major or minor affective disorder, compared with only one control child with any formal psychiatric diagnosis (not specified). Gershon and colleagues (1985a) studied a similar sample of 29 children of bipolar patients and 37 children of normal controls, ages 6 to 17. There were no differences in major or minor affective diagnoses between the patient and control groups, but there was an increase of nonspecific diagnoses in the patient group. Ten percent of the patients' children and 14 percent of the controls' children had at least one episode of major depression, as diagnosed by DSM-III. Weissman and colleagues (1988c) reported on 220 offspring of patients with major depression and normal controls. They found that prepubertal depression was uncommon, and rates in patient and control offspring were similar. However, after age 12, onset was earlier and rates of depression were higher in children of patients, with female preponderance. Welner and Rice (1988) reported increased depression in 60 school-aged children of depressed parents as compared with controls.

An alternate sampling strategy is to examine adult relatives of children known to suffer from major depression. Puig-Antich and colleagues (1989) studied children, aged 6 to 12 years, who met RDC criteria for Major Depressive Disorder, endogenous type. Using family history obtained in most cases from one adult informant, they estimated significantly higher morbid risks for major depression in adult relatives of these patients than in relatives of controls. Strober and associates (1988), comparing families of bipolar adolescents with schizophrenic adolescents, found higher rates of major affective disorder in the adult relatives of the bipolar adolescents and higher rates of schizophrenia in the adult relatives of the schizophrenic patients. In a previous study of adolescents admitted for affective illness, Strober (1984) found a higher rate of affective disorder and alcoholism in adult relatives of these patients than in published rates in relatives of normals.

Taken together, these studies can be interpreted to suggest that the most severely depressed children and adolescents referred for treatment to psychiatric facilities appear to be familially related to adult affective disorders but that such cases are not found with great statistical frequency among the children of adult affectively ill patients. That is, these hospitalized children represent a rare disorder, found mainly in children from heavily loaded families. The existence of such children, who meet the stringent adult criteria for major depression, suggests that age of onset of the adult form of major depression may well extend down into the prepubertal period (Puig-Antich et al., 1989). Table 15-5 summarizes the familial relationships between bipolar illness and related disorders.

Summary of Clinical Findings Associated with Familial Illness. Unipolar disorder is common, and its clinical features are continuous with non-pathological bereavement and other life experiences. Several clinically observable findings associated with familial depression, which in all probability identify cases more likely to be inherited, include early onset, multiple depressive episodes, and severe impairment or incapacitation in the patient's occupational role performance.

Bland and colleagues (1986) found increased morbid risk in unipolar patients with more than one episode than in those with one episode. Gershon and associates (1986) similarly noted that sporadic depressions, those found in relatives of medically ill controls, are more likely to be limited to single episodes. In the same study, familial cases more frequently had occupational impairment or incapacitation.

In bipolar illness, only those rare cases with very early onset (in childhood or early adolescence) are associated with increased morbid risk in relatives (Strober et al., 1988).

SINGLE-GENE INHERITANCE

Methods for Detecting Single-Gene Inheritance

Pedigree and Segregation Analyses of Clinical Diagnosis

In contrast to genetic–epidemiological studies that examine prevalences of diagnoses in populations, pedigree and segregation analyses are used to determine the parameters of genetic transmission from the distribution of diagnoses in relatives.

Single-Locus Models. Elston and Stewart (1971) developed a general model for single-locus inheritance that allows estimation of the maximum likelihood that a particular (set of) pedigree(s) would be found under each of the different types of transmission subsumed in the model, namely, recessive, codominant, or dominant. A comparison of likelihoods of each transmission mode, as calculated in a given data set, provides a powerful way of ruling out possible transmission modes. This model is applicable to multigenerational families, variable age of onset, and different conditions of pedigree ascertainment (Elston, 1973; Elston and Yelverton, 1975; Elston and Sobel, 1979).

Goldin and co-workers (1981, 1984) have tested the power of the Elston model and a similar one by Lalouel and Morton (Lalouel and Morton, 1981; Lalouel et al., 1983) to detect single-locus

---

Table 15-5. Bipolar Diagnostic Spectrum

Diagnoses increased in relatives of bipolar patients

    Bipolar (I and II)
    Unipolar
    Cyclothymic
    Schizoaffective
    Suicide

Bipolar illness increased in relatives of these patients

    Anorexic
    Bulimic

---

autosomal transmission in simulated pedigrees, with and without a linked marker. Under certain parameter values, when there is incomplete penetrance or phenocopies (illness in persons not genetically predisposed), the power of these models to detect single-gene transmission is reduced. Genetic heterogeneity would have the same effect as phenocopies in greatly reducing the power of a segregation analysis. This is the great weakness in segregation analysis compared with systematic genomic mapping through linkage studies. Even when segregation models fail to detect single-locus inheritance in a broadly defined sample of patients with an illness, this mode of inheritance may still be present in several genetically independent subgroups.

Tsuang and colleagues (1985) applied similar models to the transmission of affective disorders, including unipolar and bipolar forms, in the families of unipolar probands. Their findings could be used to reject both dominant and recessive hypotheses but not a nongenetic hypothesis. In similar analyses of data on the families of bipolar and unipolar probands,[10] Goldin and associates (1983) also were able to reject all single-locus genetic hypotheses, even when the diagnostic classification scheme was varied. Similar results have been obtained for bipolar families (Goldin et al., 1983; Bucher and Elston, 1981). A possible single-locus effect on disease transmission in bipolar families was noted by Rice and co-workers (1987b), but because some of the estimates of transmission parameters were outside their theoretical ranges, the results were internally inconsistent.

X chromosome, single-locus transmission in bipolar illness was suggested in an early family study (Winokur et al., 1969) but has not been supported in later analyses (Goldin and Gershon, 1983).

Chromosomal Linkage: Genetic Mapping of Markers to Illness

For chromosomes that are paired, two genes on two separate chromosomes are inherited together (do not recombine) in half the gametes (sperm or egg cells) produced by an individual. This is also true for genes on the same chromosome that are separated from each other by a large genetic distance because of crossover (recombination) of

segments between paired chromosomes during gamete production (Figure 15-3). Recombination occurs between one and a few times per chromosome, depending on the size of the chromosome and other factors. For genes that are close together on the same chromosome, the observed frequency of recombination between them will be much less than one half. Such genes are said to be *linked*. The recombination frequency can be used as a definition of the genetic map distance between two genes (e.g., as contrasted with the physical distance in DNA basepairs).

Demonstration of linkage of a gene (or an illness) to a known gene is a powerful method of demonstrating that a gene exists and locating (mapping) it. The known gene is referred to as a *marker*. For a disease whose genetic nature and mode of inheritance are uncertain, linkage may prove the only way to demonstrate that a gene for the disease exists.[11]

The major impetus to linkage studies in psychiatric illness came from the successful mapping of the Huntington's disease locus by Gusella and colleagues (1983) and, more recently, from the nearly complete mapping of the human genome. These breakthroughs were made possible by the vast increase in linkage markers found through recombinant DNA technology and the perceived opportunity they offered for disease mapping (Botstein et al., 1980).

Linkage is a classic genetic strategy that is distinct from genetic vulnerability marker (risk factor) strategies. An important difference between a linkage marker and a risk factor marker is that linkage necessarily occurs in relation to a single genetic locus, whereas a risk factor may also be polygenically determined or result from complex interactions among several loci.

A second difference between the two strategies is that the risk factor is necessarily associated (across families) with the physiological process that causes the disease, whereas in linkage equilibrium, the marker is not.[12] Within families, however, any allele occupying the marker locus will be found consistently in the ill relatives.

The role of single major loci in the inheritance of the major psychiatric disorders is solvable by currently executable linkage methods, as discussed in the next section. It appears important to settle this issue. If one or more replicable single-

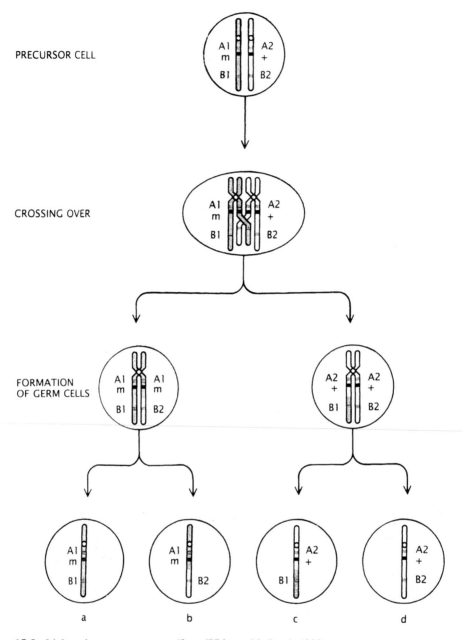

Figure 15-3. Linkage between two genes (from White and Lalouel, 1988).
Recombination fraction: Proportion of children in which two parental genes do not both appear
Two genes on two different chromosomes: Recombination = 50%
Two genes on same chromosome: Recombination = 0 to 50%
Linked genes: On same chromosome. Recombination < 50%.
Genetic distance is measured by recombination fraction; genes are close if recombination fraction is small

locus forms of bipolar illness were found, persons at high risk could be identified early and, if they requested genetic counseling, appropriate information offered to them. Finding single-locus forms would also offer important clues to the gene defect associated with the illness and perhaps crucial in causing it. If no single locus can be linked to illness, investigative attention would be forced to turn to multifactorial etiologies and inherited risk factors.

Applications of Molecular Genetics in Linkage Mapping Research

Gene mapping using molecular genetics has proven itself particularly effective in demonstrating the existence and pinpointing the location of single genes in such diseases as Alzheimer's disease. Like the psychiatric disorders, Alzheimer's disease is etiologically heterogeneous, and an actual gene defect for it is quite unknown. The many gene-mapping reports that continue to appear in the psychiatric literature make use of the basic concepts described in this section.

Two general approaches are used in molecular genetics to demonstrate a relationship between a neuropsychiatric illness and a particular gene. The first is to determine if a defect in a gene or its expression is specific to illness. The key problem is to choose the right gene, based on a pathophysiological hypothesis. The end point is to demonstrate that a defect in a particular gene or its expression is specific to patients.

The second approach is gene mapping. Polymorphisms (variants) of a marker gene are used to study whether the marker gene is linked to a specific illness susceptibility gene in pedigrees. Because a gene is inherited as part of a chromosome region millions of basepairs in length, an identified polymorphism traced through a pedigree serves as a marker for the entire region. If linkage is not found in an appropriately sized and correctly sampled series of pedigrees, it is very unlikely that there is even a proportion of cases with a major susceptibility gene in the studied region. Of course, one cannot completely rule out the existence of a very rare event on statistical grounds, but the proportion of cases that could exist and still be undetected in a series can be estimated. In a large enough series, this proportion can be very small.

The power of linkage methods in human genetics has been appreciated for decades. However, until recently, the number of available marker loci that could be used was limited, and thus the probability of detecting linkage was small (Elston and Lange, 1975). Twenty years ago, only five confirmed autosomal linkages in humans had been done (Levitan and Montagu, 1971), and only about 30 known polymorphisms were available for use as potential linkage markers to disease (blood groups, enzyme, and protein–electrophoretic variants). The proportion of the human gene map that can be studied by 30 markers is small (roughly 20 percent).

The scientific development that made linkage studies of the entire human genome possible was the demonstration of polymorphisms of DNA sequences, restriction fragment length polymorphisms (RFLPs), by Kan and Dozy in 1978. The term RFLP refers to variations in the DNA sequence by which restriction enzymes recognize where to cut DNA. Events that cause a site not to be recognized, such as a mutation at a single nucleotide, produce a recognizable polymorphism. Following the first demonstration, it was quickly appreciated that a very large number of RFLPs might be discovered.

Botstein and colleagues (1980), summarizing the power of the linkage method using RFLPs, noted that 150 evenly spaced markers would cover the genome so that no disease locus could be more than a 10 percent recombination distance from a marker locus. They predicted that because of the new availability of RFLPs, enough loci would be available in the foreseeable future to ensure a complete map. It now appears that nearly the entire genome has been mapped with RFLPs (Donis-Keller et al., 1987; Frézal and Klinger, 1987), and thus it is realistic to consider screening the entire genome for loci causing susceptibility to psychiatric disorders. With a complete gene map—that is, with a marker for every chromosomal fragment—the presence or absence of single-gene transmission can be definitively detected or ruled out.

Other major developments in linkage include more advanced analytical methods: the use of multipoint mapping (Lathrop et al., 1984; Lander and Botstein, 1986) and statistical methods with improved power for resolution of heterogeneity. Multipoint mapping uses two marker loci with a known distance between them; if inheritance of the disease is inconsistent with the inheritance of both marker loci in the persons in the pedigree, existence of a disease locus anywhere between the two loci is very unlikely. The efficiency of exclusion over the interval is greater than if one considered each marker separately, as had been done previously.

Detecting genetic heterogeneity and analyzing the proportion of cases that might be linked in large series of data have become very important in bipolar illness, schizophrenia, Alzheimer's disease, and other illnesses where initial reports of linkage to a specific locus have been followed by nonconfirmations. When linkage to a particular region has been reported in one or a few pedigrees, it is always possible to interpret a subsequent negative finding as a demonstration of heterogeneity (Hodgkinson et al., 1987). Such an interpretation is only a speculation; it does not rule out the possibility that the initial report is not reproducible.

To resolve the dilemma presented by nonreplications of linkage, large series of pedigrees are needed. In such a series, the proportion linked can be estimated directly.[13] A very large investigative effort would be required, at many centers, to systematically map the entire human genome in a large enough series of small to moderate sized pedigrees to identify the more frequent linkages in bipolar illness.

We also can anticipate that linkage methods more efficient than Southern blot RFLPs may become available. In their 1988 review, Landegren and colleagues discuss recent developments that may lead to more automated, rapid, and less expensive DNA characterization for marker and diagnostic purposes. These include new methods for analysis of nucleic acid sequences, such as allele-specific oligonucleotide hybridization, and scanning methods for detection of base substitutions, such as analysis of RNA/DNA duplexes formed to a standard RNA strand.

In the pursuit of a valid linkage marker, can we determine a priori which markers to study in which illness? One approach is not to attempt to do so but to use the nearly complete human gene map, leaving no region unexplored. A second approach is to capitalize on cytogenetic events found in rare cases of bipolar illness and to look for linkage markers in the region of chromosomal abnormality. This strategy has been successfully employed in identifying linkage markers in schizophrenia (Sherrington et al., 1988). Finally, one may consider genes of interest because of pharmacological or pathophysiological considerations, such as genes involved in neurotransmission and neuroreceptors, and attempt to locate linkage to illness in the vicinity of these genes.

Reverse Genetics

As Kidd (1987) has noted, psychiatric disorders are prime candidates for reverse genetics—learning the nature of the defect by first identifying the gene. In disorders where physiological defect implicating a particular gene is unknown, reverse genetics presents a particularly difficult challenge. For example, the Huntington's disease gene was located through linkage studies, but at the time of this writing (1989), it is not known which of the genes in the linked region is the defective gene.

The task for reverse genetics can be approached in two general ways: (1) ruling out specific genes by observing crossovers between the gene and the illness in linked pedigrees, and (2) finding a gene defect that is associated with illness across pedigrees. Each approach has its difficulties. As one gets closer to the disease gene, the frequency of crossovers decreases. To be satisfied that this frequency is effectively zero and not 0.001, thousands of meioses in linked pedigrees would need to be observed. For this reason, Bodmer (1986) recommends association across pedigrees or across unrelated ill individuals as the preferable research strategy.

It is not immediately apparent why the molecular geneticist cannot simply find out which gene is consistently inherited with illness within a single linked pedigree. Each ill person in a pedigree inherits all the genes in a chromosomal segment, one of which is the illness gene. The only exceptions occur as a result of crossovers. If the recombination fraction is 2 percent, no crossover occurs in 98 percent of meioses. In 10 generations, the probability of no crossover occurring would be 82 percent. That is, over a 2 million basepair region (containing up to 100 genes), the same genes have all been inherited from the distant ill ancestor. Each crossover event that does occur within the linkage region will rule out some candidate genes. But since the probability of crossover is low, and since a well person is never an unambiguous crossover, hundreds of ill people in a single pedigree are needed to narrow down the list of candidate genes meaningfully. Such a pedigree is yet to be found in manic-depressive illness.

Results of Linkage Mapping Studies

X Chromosome Markers

The hypothesis that manic-depressive illness is transmitted through a gene on the X chromosome was first proposed by Rosanoff and associates (1935) over 50 years ago. Two decades ago, Winokur and colleagues (1969) reported the first evidence for X linkage using genetic marker data as well as family study results. In their family study data, the morbid risk for female first-degree relatives of bipolar probands was greater than that for male first-degree relatives, and male to male transmission was not apparent. Both findings were suggestive of a dominant X-linked disease. They also presented data on two bipolar pedigrees in which color blindness (CB) segregated with affective disorder. Since this publication, numerous reports concerning possible X linkage in manic-depressive illness have been published. Mendlewicz and Fleiss (1974) reported close linkage of protan (CBP) and deutan (CBD) color blindness to 17 bipolar pedigrees, and linkage to the CB loci in 14 unipolar pedigrees was excluded. They also reported that loose linkage [recombination fraction (theta) of 19 percent] of the Xg blood group to bipolar disease was present in 23 pedigrees. The large genetic distance between these two X chromosome markers makes these two findings inconsistent, however. Subsequently, reports of additional manic-depressive pedigrees, consistent with linkage to CB or to glucose-6-phosphate dehydrogenase (G6PD) deficiency (another X chromosome marker located 3 centimorgans from CBD and CBP), appeared in the literature over the next 10 years.[14] Evidence of clear male to male transmission in some bipolar pedigrees and family studies,[15] together with a report of five pedigrees in which color blindness was not linked to bipolar disease (Gershon et al., 1979), leads to the conclusion that bipolar disease is genetically heterogeneous (Baron 1977; Risch and Baron, 1982) and that only a fraction of bipolar pedigrees could be linked to these Xq28 markers, that is, markers of the terminal fragment (28) of the long arm (q) of the X chromosome.

After reanalyzing published pedigree and family studies, Risch and Baron (1982) estimated that the fraction of bipolar pedigrees having an Xq28-linked disease is 40 to 90 percent of those without male to male transmission. Subsequently, they re-examined family study data and estimated that 33 percent of all bipolar patients may have Xq28-linked disease (Risch et al., 1986). These estimates have important implications for the classification and diagnosis of affective illness because they suggest that an X-linked form of the disease is relatively common. The estimates imply that Xq28 linkage should be detectable in any large series of pedigrees selected for absence of male to male transmission.

A more recent study confirmed that manic-depressive illness is linked to markers of the q28 region of the X chromosome, including CBP, CBD, and G6PD deficiency (Baron et al., 1987). In that study, a series of five Jewish-Israeli pedigrees, the lod score to the Xq28 markers was very significant. On inspection, it appeared that four Sephardic pedigrees were linked and the one Ashkenazi family was not. Considering only the four Sephardic families, under a hypothesis of linkage heterogeneity, the maximum lod score was 9.17 at a recombination fraction (theta) of zero.

Baron and colleagues (1987) suggested that Xq28-linked affective disorder may be particularly common among non-Ashkenazi Jews. However, a review of the positive reports suggests that Xq28 linkage has been reported in other ethnic groups. Mendlewicz and colleagues (1987) described linkage to affective disorder among nine northern European families, using a factor IX DNA polymorphism that is located approximately 35 centimorgans from the color blindness locus. It is not clear if the factor IX finding is consistent with the color blindness finding because of the large chromosomal distance between the two loci. DelZompo and colleagues (1984) reported possible G6PD/color blindness linkage to affective disorder in two Sardinian pedigrees. There have been several reports of CB linkage to affective disorder in 17 American pedigrees (Winokur et al., 1969; Mendlewicz and Fleiss, 1974; Baron, 1977), none of which has been identified as Sephardic. Risch and Baron (1982) estimated the proportion of linkage to the color blindness region of the X chromosome (Xq28) in bipolar pedigrees without male to male transmission at 64 percent.

Fourteen American bipolar pedigrees (four of which are Ashkenazi Jewish) that do not show male to male transmission of major affective disorder have been reported by one group (Gershon et al., 1979; Berrettini et al., in press). Using a highly polymorphic DNA locus in this region (Xq28), DXS52 (situated within 3 centimorgans of the CB loci), linkage to these Xq28 markers could be rejected. In simulation studies, this size series has a 90 percent power to detect linkage (at a recombination fraction of 1 percent) if only 50 percent were linked (Goldin and Gershon, 1983). The apparent epidemiological discrepancy between these findings and those reporting linkage is unresolved at present.

The conflicting reports might be interpreted as providing evidence of genetic heterogeneity in affective disorder. However, the pedigree data from Gershon's group do not support this. If an *uncommon* form of bipolar illness is linked to Xq28 markers in the United States, the hypothesis that genetic heterogeneity explains the contrasting results can best be tested in a very large pedigree series, with power to detect linkage and heterogeneity when only a small fraction (e.g., 10 percent) of the sample is actually linked to the Xq28 markers.

Autosomal Linkage Markers

Chromosome 11. Genetic investigators use very large pedigrees in linkage studies because they assume that, even in an illness that is generally heterogeneous, any given pedigree will be genetically homogeneous. This assumption is questionable for a common disease in a large population, where persons marrying into the pedigree may bring in different forms of illness, especially in view of assortative mating. In an isolated population, homogeneity might be considered more likely, at least within a pedigree. The Amish population studied by Egeland is an isolate in which several large pedigrees segregating for affective illness have been identified. In one pedigree, Egeland and associates (1987b) found autosomal dominant transmission and linkage of bipolar and unipolar illness to the insulin-*ras* oncogene region of the short arm of chromosome 11. Detera-Wadleigh and colleagues (1987) found this linkage not to be present in three smaller Maryland

pedigrees, and Hodgkinson and colleagues (1987) also failed to find this linkage in three Icelandic pedigrees. As in the X linkage findings, these failures to replicate are of concern. If they are due to genetic heterogeneity, then the Amish form of manic-depressive illness apparently is genetically uncommon in the other populations studied. If the finding is valid but peculiar to the Amish or to this Amish pedigree, it can be confirmed (or refuted) by the genotypes of a series of new individuals in the pedigree who develop illness.

Most recently, in a follow-up study of the original Amish pedigree (Kelsoe et al. 1989), the linkage between manic-depressive illness and chromosome 11 markers was no longer found. Using the same RFLPs applied to the same loci as in the original study, Kelsoe and colleagues analyzed the core pedigree, extensions of that pedigree, new genotypic information on 10 individuals whose genotypes had been incomplete, and new data on two individuals who had had an onset of affective illness since the original study. Analysis of the new information combined with the original data failed to replicate the linkage of affective illness to the Harvey-*ras*-1 or the insulin loci on chromosome 11 that was shown in the study by Egeland and colleagues (1987b). This follow-up result appears to explain the discrepancies in studies to date.

Human Leukocyte Antigen. HLA associations with unipolar and bipolar affective illness have lacked statistical significance, the various positive reports are not consistent with each other, and later reports do not support the presence of any association, as reviewed elsewhere (Goldin and Gershon, 1983). Within pedigrees, genetic heterogeneity of illness can be expected to be minimal or absent. Linkage of HLA to affective illness in bipolar families could be definitively ruled out in the data of Targum and associates (1979b). Smeraldi and colleagues (1978), who applied the identical by descent method to HLA types in sibling pairs where both had affective illness, noted increased concordance, a finding that suggests a possible linkage. Turner and King (1981) analyzed five pedigrees for linkage to HLA and proposed that bipolar illness is a heterogeneous condition, with 10 to 30 percent not linked to HLA and most of the rest linked to HLA on chromosome 6. Their assignment of diagnoses is confusing, their description suggesting that the diagnoses may have been based on family history rather than solely on clinical features.

Weitkamp and colleagues (1981) concluded that a major susceptibility gene for unipolar depression is located in the HLA region because of the increased sharing of common HLA types in ill pairs of siblings in 20 families, basing their conclusion on a subdivision of their sample by sibship size and number affected. Goldin and associates (1982) have argued that this criterion for dividing a sample is not theoretically sound. Their new data on 18 families, combined with 9 families previously published by Targum from the same study, did not support the hypothesis of a relationship of the HLA locus to unipolar depression (Goldin et al., 1983; Goldin and Gershon, 1983). In two separate studies, Suarez and Croughan (1982) and Suarez and Reich (1984) also did not replicate this linkage. Although heterogeneity could again be claimed as an explanation of nonreplication, it appears more parsimonious to conclude that this linkage is not generally present.

Current Status of Linkage Research

Although we see genetic linkage strategies as crucial in elucidating the genetics of manic-depressive illness, at present there is no widely accepted and consistently replicable linkage finding in the affective disorders. For the clinician, the excitement over recent discoveries must be tempered with patience. Validated linkages could be applied to clinical risk prediction. Knowledge about specific gene defects and improved understanding of the pathophysiology of the illness could also lead to improved treatment strategies.

PUTATIVE INHERITED BIOLOGICAL–PHYSIOLOGICAL RISK FACTORS

Methodology

In psychiatry and medicine, the common diseases are often ones in which the inherited pathophysiological mechanism is unknown and the specific genes involved are not identified. Risk factor investigative strategies are unlikely to be robust under such conditions (Gershon and Goldin, 1986; Goldin et al., 1986). By *robustness,* we mean the ability of an investigative strategy to detect or reject a putative genetic marker correctly under various conditions, such as population stratification, secondary effects of illness or treatment on a marker, biological heterogeneity of the clinical syndrome, and complex biology of the syndrome when only one component is measured.

Population stratification exists when the inherited trait studied is more frequent in one subgroup of a population than another. Sickle cell anemia, for example, is more frequent in black people; if our knowledge of this disorder were comparable to our knowledge of manic-depressive illness, it is easy to imagine a serious hypothesis that inherited anemias are heterogeneous, with the inheritance of skin pigment related to the inheritance of anemia in some cases.

If a particular marker is valid for only one of the several forms of an illness, biological heterogeneity within a clinical syndrome can obscure it. It is readily apparent that the rarer the form of illness for which a marker is valid, the more difficult it will be to detect.

In an illness with a complex biology, several risk factors must be present simultaneously for illness to occur. This is not the same as heterogeneity, in which each of several risk factors, in the absence of other factors, can lead to illness. In complex biology, many people, including relatives of known patients with a valid marker, can have the marker without being ill. Thus, the marker might not be detected as a risk factor. Two major investigative strategies aid in dealing with these issues, segregating markers in pedigrees and comparing patients by family history.

Risk Factor Segregation in Pedigrees

Rieder and Gershon (1978) designed a research strategy for identifying risk factors that tests the degree of cosegregation of the risk factor and illness within pedigrees. This strategy is designed to be sensitive to causes of false-positive or false-negative conclusions. *Cosegregate* as used here means that the prevalence of illness is higher among relatives who manifest the marker (risk factor) than among relatives who do not. This is not the precise meaning of segregation in genetics, which refers to distribution in pedigrees of single-gene locus characteristics, but it is generally analogous to single-locus segregation and can be applied to multifactorial and other complex modes of inheritance.[16]

Family History Comparisons

Family history comparisons usually are made between the frequency of a marker in patients who have ill relatives with that of patients who do not. Such a separation is inherently imprecise, even if all family members are examined directly. For many modes of genetic transmission, particularly with the small family sizes commonly encountered, a substantial proportion of cases of inherited disease will occur with no family history, purely by chance. Only if there is also a substantial proportion of nonfamilial nongenetic cases will the patients with negative family histories include fewer genetic cases than will patients with positive family histories. However, the necessity of invoking such a "best-case" assumption is a weakness of comparisons of family history-positive vs family history-negative patients. Nonetheless, the strategy has advantages. It is, perhaps, the only way to investigate state-dependent findings, such as responses to the dexamethasone suppression test.

No one investigative strategy for vulnerability markers is robust to the conditions we have considered. By itself, the study of pedigrees, with ill and well relatives compared, is the most robust, except that it is not sensitive to false-positive conclusions based on secondary effects of illness or treatment. To rule this out, it is perhaps most appropriate to use one of the strategies that examines individuals at risk who have not developed illness. One such method is the study of offspring of known patients as they enter and pass through the age of risk.

Putative Risk Factors

Gershon and colleagues (1987a) reviewed the current status of selected putative heritable risk factors from the perspective of the Rieder and Gershon paradigm (Table 15-6). They found that the following variables did not satisfy criteria for a cosegregating risk factor according to the Rieder and Gershon paradigm: *activities of enzymes of monoamine metabolism*—plasma dopamine-β-hydroxylase (DBH), erythrocyte catechol-*o*-methyltransferase (COMT), platelet monoamine oxidase (MAO); *monoamine metabolites*—cerebrospinal fluid 5-hydroxyindole-acetic acid (CSF 5HIAA); *membrane binding and transport*—lithium-erythrocyte/plasma ratio, platelet-[^{3}H]-imipramine binding, platelet α-$_2$-adrenoceptor, lymphoblast β-adrenergic receptor, and fibroblast muscarinic receptor (where the initial findings were not replicable[17]). The general study of these biological variables in manic-depressive illness is reviewed in Chapter 17.

Platelet-Imipramine Binding

Although several investigators initially suggested that values remain low after recovery,[18] subsequent studies, which examined euthymic subjects who had been recovered for at least several months, suggest that the reduced B_{max} is a state-dependent phenomenon (Berrettini et al., 1982a; Suranyi-Cadotte et al., 1982; Langer et al., 1986a). Thus, as discussed in Chapter 17, the evidence suggests that platelet-imipramine B_{max} does not represent a vulnerability trait marker for affective disorder.

Lymphocyte β-Adrenergic Receptors

Beta-adrenergic receptors on lymphocytes have been a focus of intensive investigation in affective disorders. Numerous studies have reported either decreased binding or a reduced cAMP response to β-adrenergic agonists among acutely depressed subjects.[19] Other investigators have not been able to confirm these findings (Healy et al., 1983; Cooper et al., 1985). Unfortunately, no studies have been reported with euthymic or recovered subjects, so there are no data on the state-dependent nature of this marker.

One study by Wright and colleagues (1984) suggested that a decreased number of beta receptors on cultured lymphoblasts may be a trait marker for vulnerability to affective illness. They based their suggestion on a study in which ill probands and their ill family members had lower binding values compared with values for normal subjects and well family members. Berrettini and colleagues (1987b) were unable to confirm this finding, however. One study of cultured skin fibroblast β-receptors reported no difference between patients and controls for the cAMP response to isoproterenol (Berrettini et al., 1987a). Polymorphisms of both the β$_1$ and the β$_2$ receptor genes have been used to exclude linkage to these genes in bipolar pedigrees (Berrettini et al.,

Table 15-6. Current Status of Proposed Genetic Vulnerability Markers for Affective Illness

Finding	Criteria				Study
	Patients Differ from Controls	State Independent	Heritable	Segregates with Illness	
Enzymes of Monoamine Metabolism					
Plasma DBH	No	Yes	Yes-single locus	No	Gershon et al., 1980a
Erythrocyte COMT	No	Yes	Yes-single locus	No	Rice et al., 1984
Platelet MAO	Yes	Yes	Yes-single locus	No	
Monoamine and Amino Acid Metabolites					
CSF 5-HIAA	Yes (most studies)	Conflicting data	No	Unknown	Van Praag & DeHaan, 1979; Oxenstierna et al., 1986
Membrane Transport					
Lithium Erythrocyte Plasma Ratio	Yes (some studies)	Possibly	Yes	No (most data)	Dorus et al., 1979a, 1983; Nurnberger et al., 1983b; Shaughnessy et al., 1985
Platelet ^{3}H-Imipramine	Yes	No	Possibly	No data	Berretini et al., 1982a; Mellerup et al., 1982; Langer et al., 1986b; Suranyi-Cadotte et al., 1982; Friedl & Propping, 1984
CNS Protein Polymorphism					
Duarte Pc 1 brain protein	Yes	Presumably	Yes-single locus	No data	Comings, 1979
Neurotransmitter, Receptor, and Pharmacologic Response Studies					
Muscarinic-Cholinergic					
Early induction of REM sleep by arecoline muscarinic agonist	Yes	Yes	Possibly	Possibly	Sitaram et al., 1980, 1986, 1987; Nurnberger et al., 1983a; Jones et al., 1985
Adrenergic					
Platelet alpha$_2$ adrenoceptor	Conflicting data	No	Yes	No data	Siever et al., 1984a; Kafka et al.,1980; Propping & Friedl, 1983; Healy et al.,1983; Garcia-Sevilla et al.,1981, 1986; Wood & Coppen, 1983; Daiguji et al., 1981b
Lymphoblast Beta$_2$- Receptor	Conflicting data	Yes	Yes	Almost no data	Wright et al., 1984; Berrettini et al., 1987b

Adapted from Gershon et al., 1987a

1988), suggesting that the inheritance of bipolar disease is independent of abnormalities in the genes for beta receptors.

Cholinergic Functional Measurements

As discussed in Chapters 16 and 17, the cholinergic hypothesis in affective disorders originated in the observation of mood alterations following exposure to cholinomimetic and anticholinergic agents (Janowsky et al., 1972). With advances in the anatomical and functional knowledge of acetylcholine (ACh) in brain, clinical investigative interest focused on two central muscarinic- cholinergic functions: the initiation of rapid eye movement (REM) sleep periods and the release of the anterior pituitary hormones ACTH and β-endorphin (which share the same precursor molecule). Both functions are thought to be anatomically localized to the cholinergic neuronal groupings of the medulla, which project to the hypothalamus and thalamus (Mesulam et al., 1983a,b). Janowsky and Risch (1984) demonstrated increased sensitivity to cholinomimetic-induced β-endorphin and ACTH release in depressed patients, as compared with normal controls.[20] However, this cholinergic–neuroendocrine response has not been demonstrated to be state independent or under genetic control.

As described in Chapter 19, REM sleep initiation is physiologically under muscarinic–cholinergic control and responds as predicted to pharmacological stimulation, blockade, or alterations in receptor sensitivity. Several laboratories have demonstrated independently that patients with affective disorders, whether depressed or euthymic bipolar or unipolar, were more sensitive than normal individuals to cholinergic REM induction. Sitaram and colleagues (1980) speculated that this increased cholinergic–muscarinic receptor sensitivity is a genetic vulnerability characteristic of affective disorders, since it is state independent. The method of Rieder and Gershon (1978) was used to test the validity of the hypothesized genetic vulnerability marker. Nurnberger and colleagues (1983c) demonstrated that REM induction values were highly correlated in normal monozygotic twins, suggesting that they are under genetic control. Sitaram and colleagues further showed cosegregation of sensitivity to cholinergic REM induction and affective illness within families in which the original affectively

ill proband had increased REM induction sensitivity (Sitaram et al., 1984, 1987). Within these families, there was a significant association of increased REM sensitivity with a diagnosis of major affective disorder.

Thus, the criteria for increased REM induction sensitivity as a genetic vulnerability marker in affective disorders were satisfied in these preliminary data.[21]

Melatonin Suppression by Nighttime Light Exposure

The circadian rhythm of melatonin in humans (higher amounts at night) is suppressible by light, and bipolar patients show a state-independent supersensitivity to this effect of light, a characteristic that suggests a possible trait marker (see Chapter 19). Nurnberger and colleagues (1988a) applied a high-risk strategy to investigate this phenomenon in young people (ages 15 to 25) who had a bipolar parent but themselves had never had major psychiatric disorder. In these people, supersensitivity was present, as compared with normal controls, and the proportion of supersensitive subjects was correlated with risk. That is, persons with two parents with affective illness were more sensitive than persons with one, who in turn were more sensitive that controls (who had no ill parents). This finding is of considerable interest, with implications for a role of disordered control of this system, which has been extensively studied in animal models, in the inherited vulnerability to illness.

CLINICAL APPLICATIONS

Primary Prevention

We know of no intervention that would prevent the development of manic-depressive illness in people at risk, at least not in the traditional sense of preventing its initial occurrence. As linkage markers become validated, it may become possible to identify individuals at risk within some thoroughly studied pedigrees. This knowledge will present opportunities for research on intervention strategies, and perhaps effective preclinical interventions might be developed to prevent or ameliorate illness.

An unusual case that we saw several years ago may be a forerunner of opportunities that will arise once vulnerability is predictable in specific individuals. A 22-year-old woman, the identical twin of a bipolar patient, asked if she should take lithium. After our examination revealed no psychopathology, we decided not to prescribe lithium. However, we offered her and her husband information on signs of incipient mania or depression. Within 6 months she developed mania, which was promptly treated with inpatient hospitalization. Since that time, the patient has had a very good response to lithium prophylaxis. In retrospect, it appears we would have done well to consider her 65 percent risk (without age correction) as an identical twin of a bipolar patient. Perhaps lithium treatment was indicated when the patient first consulted us. In other classes of relatives, however, we would not feel justified instituting prophylactic lithium or anticonvulsant treatment, and we know of no other primary prevention maneuver that seems promising.

Preventing and terminating pregnancies undoubtedly have been and will continue to be considered by people who see themselves at risk. It would appear that these are extreme and perhaps pathological (perhaps depressive) responses to known risk estimates, both because of the frequency of illness in children of patients and because of the potential quality of life in patients, particularly in view of the treatability of the illness. Even in the case of a fetus with markers predictive of illness genotype (in a linked family), there is a great deal of human potential to be lost through abortion (see Chapter 14).

Secondary Prevention

Secondary prevention of an illness in a population involves reducing its morbidity by recognizing and treating cases soon after the illness develops. Here, the family concentration of severe primary affective disorder offers an important opportunity for preventive intervention. In a systematic study of first-degree relatives (parents, siblings, and offspring) and second-degree relatives (grandparents, aunts and uncles, and half-siblings) of patients with bipolar disorder, we made extensive efforts to locate and examine all relatives. This included relatives at a considerable geographic distance from the patient and those who had little knowledge of or interaction with the patient. In first-degree relatives, we found the expected high incidence of affective disorders (comparable to our previous studies), which was considerably higher than the population prevalence. One fifth of the diagnosed relatives had never been treated; such people constitute a population at very high risk for future episodes, one with excellent opportunities for intervention (Gershon and Hamovit, 1979).

It is worth remembering that two thirds of bipolar patients have a positive family history, that the thought of genetic vulnerability intrudes on these people, and that active preventive efforts in relatives, rather than stirring up concerns that are best left to rest, may contribute to a sense in the patient and the family members of gaining some mastery over the inherited risk.

Genetic Counseling

Current counseling for bipolar illness, as in many other disorders, is based on empirical risk estimates not on specific genetic knowledge of susceptibility in an individual. It is to be anticipated that this will change significantly as linkage or association markers, or biological risk factors, become clinically applicable.

Generally, affective illness starts in young adulthood. This creates different needs for genetic counseling than disorders that manifest as birth defects (Targum and Gershon, 1981). Incipient or possible future illness in a teenaged or young adult relative of a patient is the most frequent concern of persons seeking genetic counseling. The next most frequent concern, in relation to affective disorders, is whether to have children. The third type of request that has appeared recently is for analysis of genetic markers from sophisticated patients who have read of recent progress in this area.

Since the patients and their spouses do not usually consider risk for the disorder to be prohibitively high (either before or after counseling), these people usually decide to have children. Except in the case of clinically unmanageable affective disorder, which makes the parental role impossible to assume, we do not advise patients against having children. Since only 15 percent of our bipolar patients have a bipolar parent, avoiding childbearing is not necessary, even from the most hardheaded primary prevention viewpoint.

For the clinician, genetic counseling is best considered as psychotherapy. The first goal is a realistic and appropriate appreciation of the patient's own family history and of the risk to relatives. A second goal is to provide a way to cope with the anxiety and narcissistic injury caused by knowledge of genetic risk. If there are eight or more living relatives with a history of illness who will participate in a genetic linkage study, it is appropriate to refer them to a linkage research center, such as the NIMH Clinical Neurogenetics Branch, the Yale program, or any number of other new programs. This may permit a linkage marker to be demonstrated in this family, leading to more precise risk estimates in any given individual. A third goal is to make appropriate plans to respond to the risk, including early treatment for relatives beginning to show signs of mood disorder.

How can one estimate the risk to the person seeking counseling who is not affectively ill? As linkage markers and, if progress continues, vulnerability genes for affective disorders become available, there will be some persons for whom a precise estimate of risk is possible. For the others, we must use empirical risk estimates, assuming that they are halved for each degree of removal of the known ill relative from the person seeking counseling. It is extremely important, however, to take a very careful family history, preferably with sources of information other than just the person seeking counseling. Extensive multigeneration pedigrees of bipolar illness are uncovered in a distinct minority of patients. These may represent dominant inheritance or several ancestral sources of illness. In those cases, we believe the risk should be considered greater than the general risk to siblings or offspring. In estimating risk in any pedigree, it is important to rely on family studies that are contemporaneous, that occur in a population comparable to that of the person seeking counsel, and that use diagnostic criteria and procedures with which the clinician is familiar, as described previously.

The risk to offspring is of most interest in genetic counseling. We found that the age-corrected risk of bipolar or unipolar disorder to 614 adult children of patients with bipolar or unipolar major affective illness was 27 percent (Gershon et al., 1982a) when the other parent was unaffected. In 300 adult offspring of one bipolar parent (other parent not ill), the risk was 29.5 percent (13 percent bipolar I or II, 15 percent unipolar, 1 percent schizoaffective). When two parents had affective

illness, with one of them bipolar, the risk of major affective disorder was 74 percent among our 28 offspring. Winokur and colleagues (1969) reported a 50 percent risk in 31 offspring of bipolar patients where the second parent had affective illness.

In estimating the risk to offspring, the increased rate of illness in recently born generations must be taken into account. It is not clear if this increased rate will apply throughout the lifetime of people who are now younger than 30 or if it will apply at all to the current generation of young children and children born in the future. A prudent approach to risk estimation in such cases would be to expect it to be higher than the figures reported so far, as discussed previously.

A second clinical use of a known family history of a major affective disorder is to take a pharmacologically aggressive approach to a newly discovered illness, particularly a mild form of illness. For example, we would treat moderate depression in a late adolescent child of a patient with bipolar illness as if it were a major affective disorder rather than as the ubiquitous developmental crisis of late adolescence.

We must also consider the patient's spouse. A tendency for assortative mating (people with similar disorders marrying each other) has been reported repeatedly in affective disorders (Gershon et al., 1973; Negri et al., 1979). It is not known whether this increases the population genetic risk, but it does give a particular quality to many of the marriages (Ablon et al., 1975). In one study of inpatients, most bipolar patients became divorced (Brodie and Leff, 1971), which was often attributed to illness, especially to manic behavior. Occasionally, we have been confronted with blunt questions: "My fiance is a manic-depressive; should I marry him or her?" Or, "My husband or wife is a manic-depressive; should we have children?" Answering these questions requires clinical skill and compassion. This important topic is covered in Chapters 12 and 24.

Children of bipolar patients who come in for counseling in childhood and early adolescence present another vexing problem for the clinician. It is tempting to discount behavioral and emotional problems in such children to reassure parents that they have not passed on a "taint." But mania has been reported in children of 8 and 9, and suicide has greatly increased in adolescents during the past few decades. We have found several adolescent suicides in our family studies of bipolar patients. In these cases, the surviving relatives cannot remember having noticed any signs of emotional problems before the act. These possibilities must be faced realistically by the consultant. On the other hand, childhood and early adolescent depression appears to be ubiquitous and overdiagnosed. If the depression is very severe, requiring hospitalization, it may best be considered an early presentation of familial major affective disorder in such a child or adolescent. Less severe depressions, even though meeting DSM-III criteria for major depression, may not be related to the parent's bipolar disorder, but careful observation and follow-up will be needed to detect cases that will worsen.

SUMMARY

Epidemiological evidence, particularly studies of concordance in identical and fraternal twins, implies that the affective disorders are heritable. A significant proportion, at the least, of bipolar and unipolar patients share the same vulnerability. In unipolar illness, early onset and multiple episodes are more familial, but this is not generalizable to bipolar illness. Other disorders, by empirical evidence, are cotransmitted with bipolar (and to a lesser extent, unipolar) illness: schizoaffective disorder, cyclothymic personality, hypomania (without depression).

Attempts to resolve the mode of inheritance of affective illness solely through clinical observations have not been successful, perhaps because of complex inheritance and biological heterogeneity. Genetic linkage methods are particularly appropriate in resolving issues of heterogeneity when there are several independent genetic mutations, any one of which makes a substantial epidemiological contribution to vulnerability to affective disorders. However, no linkage is unequivocally established in bipolar illness at this time. The reported linkage to the color blindness region of the X chromosome is the only one that has not been refuted, but, because attempts at replication have failed, it is considered tentative. Systematic genomic mapping in multiple pedigrees with bipolar illness may be expected to establish or refute the validity of this finding and

to demonstrate, if they exist, other major single genes for this illness.

Further progress may be expected as linkages become validated through replication and as reverse genetics methods are used to go from a valid linkage marker to identification of the actual disease mutation. If this were achieved, more precise knowledge of pathophysiology and rational therapeutic strategies might follow.

For the clinician, the concerns of patients and their relatives can be dealt with through counseling that draws on empirical risk figures in the majority of cases and on linkage results in members of large pedigrees that have been investigated thoroughly.

APPENDIX: GLOSSARY OF GENETIC TERMS

Allele Alternative forms of a gene, occupying a specific site on a chromosome, which determine alternative characteristics in inheritance.

Autosome Any of the nonsex chromosomes; in the case of normal humans, there are 22 pairs.

Basepairs Pairs of complementary nucleotides forming the DNA double helix.

Centimorgan A unit of distance within a chromosome. One centimorgan is approximately the distance between two genes when there is 1 percent recombination between them. There are approximately 3,300 centimorgans in the entire human genome.

Chromosome A rodlike structure found in the cell nucleus and containing the genes. Chromosomes are composed of DNA and proteins. They can be seen with the light microscope during certain stages of cell division.

Crossover See *Recombinant (in a family)*.

DNA Deoxyribonucleic acid, the substance of heredity; a large molecule that carries the genetic information necessary for the replication of cells and for the production of proteins. DNA is composed of the sugar deoxyribose, phosphate, and the bases adenine, thymine, guanine, and cytosine.

Gene A unit of heredity; a segment of the DNA molecule containing the code for a specific protein.

Genetic mapping Determining the relative locations of different genes on chromosomes.

Genome The total genetic endowment packaged in the chromosomes. The normal human genome consists of 46 chromosomes.

Genotype The full set of genes carried by an individual, including alleles that are not expressed.

Identical by descent (IBD) The frequency with which none, one, or two alleles at a locus are inherited from the same parental chromosomes in [two] siblings. Used in linkage analysis, the observed IBD distribution is compared with the theoretically expected frequency. For example, if two ill siblings have, on the average, a greater than 50 percent identity by descent at a given locus, the implication is that the locus is linked to illness.

Linkage The association between two or more allelic genes on the same chromosome that is greater than could be expected from independent assortment. The close association of a known marker gene (e.g., ABO blood type) and the gene for an illness may be inferred from evidence that the trait and the illness are inherited together.

Locus The chromosomal location (site) occupied by a gene.

Lod score The logarithm of the odds favoring linkage in a particular set of pedigree data. If an illness is more likely to be linked to marker genotypes, the lod score is higher than if there is not linkage. (Mathematically, the lod score is the logarithm of the ratio of two probabilities.)

Marker A detectable genetic variant, such as one of the ABO blood types. Some markers are found only among the victims of certain diseases and can be used to determine the presence of these diseases.

Meiosis The process of cell division that produces germ cells (sperm or egg cells).

Molecular genetics The study of genetic mechanisms at the level of the molecules DNA and RNA and their components.

Nucleotide One of the five basic molecules that make up the informational content of DNA and RNA. In DNA, bases pair across the two chains of the double helix: adenine with thymine, and guanine with cytosine. In RNA, the single-stranded nucleic acid that (among other functions) translates DNA sequences into specific proteins, contains uracil instead of thymine.

Phenotype The entire expressed physical, biochemical, and physiological constitution of an individual, resulting from the interaction of the genetic endowment with the environment.

Polymorphism An inherited variation, such as the ABO blood groups.

Recombinant DNA A fragment of DNA that is produced in the laboratory by joining together smaller fragments from different sources. The technology for DNA manipulation has become known as recombinant DNA technology.

Recombinant (in a family) A child who does not receive *both* linked genes from a single parental chromosome.

Recombination Exchange of genetic material between two paired chromosomes during meiosis. The resultant daughter chromosome is a recombinant when it contains one segment from the first of the paired chromosomes and another from the second (see legend to Figure 15-1). The distance between two genes can be expressed as the frequency of a recombinational event occurring between them. This frequency is also known as the recombination fraction.

Recombination fraction (in pedigree analy-

sis Proportion of offspring in which two particular genes from a single parent do not *both* appear.

Restriction enzyme An enzyme that recognizes a specific base sequence (usually four to six basepairs in length) in a double-stranded DNA molecule and cuts both strands of the DNA molecule at every place where this sequence appears.

RFLP Restriction fragment length polymorphism: The presence of two or more variants in the size of DNA fragments from a specific region of DNA that has been exposed to a particular restriction enzyme. These fragments differ in length because of an inherited variation in a restriction enzyme recognition site.

Segregation analysis Mathematical analysis of distribution of a characteristic in families to determine if the distribution fits a particular model of genetic transmission (such as single gene, dominant, autosomal, with variable penetrance).

X chromosome A sex chromosome; normal human females have two X chromosomes in each cell, and normal males have one X and one Y chromosome in each cell.

X-linked Refers to any gene found on the X chromosome or traits determined by such genes. Refers also to the specific mode of inheritance of such genes.

Adapted from Pines, 1984.

NOTES

1. From "The Wonderful Mistake," (p. 28) in Thomas, 1979.
2. Falconer, 1965; Reich et al., 1982; Rice et al., 1987b; Gershon et al., 1975, 1982a.
3. Elston and Stewart, 1971; Morton and Maclean, 1974; Lalouel and Morton, 1981; Lalouel et al., 1983; Bonney, 1986.
4. Rieder and Gershon, 1978; Gershon and Goldin, 1986; DeLisi et al., 1986a; Goldin et al., 1986; Sitaram et al., 1987.
5. When there is aneuploidy, such as trisomy 21 (Down's syndrome), XO, or XYY individuals, the precise cause of the behavioral alterations can be localized to a chromosome, or chromosomal region, but not to a single genetic locus. There is, thus, not the opportunity to identify a causative gene and to infer its effects from its nucleic acid sequence.
6. The probands are the index cases whose families are studied in genetic research.
7. Solomon and Hellon, 1980; Hagnell et al., 1982; Weissman et al., 1984a; Robins et al., 1984; Angst, 1985; Klerman et al., 1985.
8. Robins et al., 1984; Angst, 1985; R.A. Price et al., 1985; Gershon et al., 1987b.
9. From other reports, it is clear that the schizotypal personality is also transmitted in these families.
10. Proband data had been collected by Gershon and colleagues (1982a).

11. The statistical test for accepting or rejecting linkage is the *lod score* (Morton, 1955), which may be understood as a likelihood ratio. The term *lod* is an acronym for logarithm (base 10) of the odds favoring linkage in a particular set of pedigree data. The *odds* are the ratio of the likelihood that the distribution of illness and of marker genotypes would be found under linkage (with a given recombination fraction) vs the likelihood of the same distribution given no linkage (i.e., with recombination fraction = 1/2). The historic statistical criterion for a lod score to accept linkage is +3 and to reject linkage is -2. Although one might equate a logarithmic score of 3 with a probability of 0.001, since 3 is the logarithm of 1,000, this is not the case, for statistical reasons. In general, one may equate a lod score of 3 with a probability of 0.05 for two genes when the investigator has no prior knowledge that they are linked. With complex modes of inheritance, such as variable penetrance and analyses for heterogeneity, additional parameters may be introduced, and the significance criterion may need to be adjusted.

12. When a population association results from linkage disequilibrium or from ascertainment through probands with the same marker allele, the linkage analysis can still be performed, with appropriate modification (Gershon and Matthysse, 1977).

13. If a series is not at all supportive of linkage, one must calculate the power of the series to detect linkage heterogeneity, which is a function of the number and configuration of the pedigrees and the genetic model (including a hypothesis on the proportion linked). A conclusion that linkage with more than a certain proportion linked is ruled out in a series of pedigrees would be inconsistent with a previous report that linkage generally is present, rather than supportive of heterogeneity. The key point is that the proportion of all cases that are linked to a given marker is a parameter to be estimated separately in each series. A comparison between two series is analogous to comparisons of means in a *t*-test.

14. Belmaker and Wyatt, 1976; Baron, 1977; Mendlewicz et al., 1979b, 1980a; Gershon et al., 1980a,b; DelZompo et al., 1984.

15. For a review, see Gershon et al., 1976.

16. The requirement of cosegregation makes the strategy robust in the presence of a population association, such as the association of increased skin pigment with sickle cell anemia, since all members of a family are part of the same population. This requirement, however, applies only to pedigrees in which both the illness and the marker are present in at least one individual. With this stipulation, genetic heterogeneity is resolved, since the subgroup of families selected will be relatively homogeneous with respect to the biology of illness if the marker is valid. Nonetheless, there may be individual relatives who are in the wrong range of values. Among well relatives, there may be some who are biologically at risk but who have not manifested illness, and among ill relatives there may be phenocopies (persons who have the illness stemming from other causes).

17. Nadi et al., 1984; Gershon et al., 1985b; Kelsoe et al., 1985; Lenox et al., 1985; Lin et al., 1986.

18. Briley et al., 1980, Paul et al., 1981b,c; Raisman et al., 1982.

19. Extein et al., 1979c; Pandey et al., 1980, 1987; Mann et al., 1985; Halper et al., 1988.

20. D. Janowsky et al., 1982; Risch et al., 1981b; 1982a,b; 1983a,b. As noted by Janowsky and Risch (1984), cholinomimetic agents cause secretion of ACTH and β-endorphin, and, conversely, the muscarinic antagonist atropine, injected in hypothalamus, inhibits ACTH release.

21. The hypothesis that increased sensitivity was related to an event at the receptor level, however, was not tested in this experimental design.

16

Biochemical Models

Attempts to comprehend the brain's role in mania and depression—a quest the ancients could undertake only in rhetorical flight—began in earnest as clinically effective mood-altering drugs began to appear in the late 1950s and early 1960s. The psychopharmacological revolution fortuitously coincided with the arrival of new techniques that were making it possible to characterize neurotransmitter function in the central nervous system. Over the next three decades, a vast literature grew from research into the biochemistry and pharmacology of affective illness. Studies were, by and large, designed to detect relative excess or deficiency associated with pathological states. This too much/too little premise was an understandable supposition, given the profound changes wrought by the new medications. As experience with the drugs refined knowledge of their actions and limitations and as research results accumulated, the implicit assumptions of the early work were refined to account for interactions among neurotransmitter systems, neuromodulators, receptors, and other components of the central nervous system. More sophisticated, if less accessible, models are now emerging.

This chapter traces the evolution of the models that guided biochemical and pharmacological studies of manic-depressive illness. It begins by describing relevant animal models. It then provides a brief historical survey of the major hypotheses that have guided biochemical and pharmacological studies. By setting this context and describing relevant brain systems, the chapter serves as an introduction to the biochemical and pharmacological evidence presented in Chapter 17.

ANIMAL MODELS

Animal models provide the basis for experimental efforts to reproduce in nonhuman species the essential features of human disorders (Suomi, 1982; McKinney, 1988). Animal models of psychiatric disorders can also be defined operationally as unusual behavioral states in animals that are specifically reversed by the same pharmacological treatments that reverse symptoms of the human disorder (Petty and Sherman, 1981). A good animal model for a human behavioral disorder ideally should be simple, reproducible, and quantifiable, with homologies to the human disorder in symptoms, postulated etiology, mediating mechanisms, and treatment responses.[1] The great strength of a good animal model lies in the practical possibilities for direct studies of brain biochemistry that may underlie aberrant behavioral states. Although several interesting animal models have been developed for the symptomatic states of anxiety and depression, the more complex human psychopathology of manic-depressive illness involving genetic predisposition and a characteristic pattern of recurrent episodes and dramatic shifts (switches) between different states has not yet been modeled satisfactorily in animals. As noted by the work group on animal models at the Dahlem conference on the origins of depression (Reite et al., 1983), "Animal model systems studied to date are notable for the absence of models relevant to bipolar disorders. . . . or periodic depression" (p. 418). In this section, we review existing models that have been proposed for depression and for mania and then highlight some new approaches that may come closer to the essential features of manic-depressive illness.

The earliest animal model of depression used pharmacological treatments, such as reserpine and tetrabenazine, to deplete central catecholamines. More recently, specific lesions, such as removal of the olfactory bulbs, have provided more relevant pharmacological models, since the behavioral effect is reversed by chronic but not acute treatment with tricyclic antidepressants (TCAs) (Jesberger and Richardson, 1985a).

Behaviorally Based Models of Depression

In the 1960s, as psychologists, pharmacologists, and psychiatrists joined forces in the expanding field of psychopharmacology, formal behavioral approaches to depression models began to develop. At the University of Wisconsin, Harry Harlow discovered that infant rhesus monkeys separated from their mothers showed a despair response analogous to some forms of human depression (Harlow and Harlow, 1962). Soon afterward, Seligman and Maier (1967) found that dogs and rats given inescapable electric shock subsequently failed to learn appropriate escape responses in a situation in which escape was possible. Both paradigms have yielded interesting, albeit limited, insights into neurochemical mechanisms mediating the depressive state (Katz, 1981, 1983). There have even been efforts to explore naturalistic animal behaviors for models

of self-destructive behavior and suicide (Crawley et al., 1985).

The Primate Separation Paradigm

In its earliest version, the primate separation paradigm consisted of rearing monkeys from birth either in total isolation, completely deprived of social contact with other animals, or in wire cages with only visual and auditory contact permitted. Animals reared in either environment for the first 6 to 12 months of life, then tested socially with other animals, spend most of their time manifesting a despair syndrome: huddled alone in a corner, rocking, clasping themselves, and refraining from play or social encounters with peers (McKinney, 1988).

Subchronic treatment with TCAs, such as imipramine, can significantly reduce components of this despair syndrome, such as huddling (Suomi et al., 1978). Certain other components of the system were reversed by other categories of drugs, including a neuroleptic, chlorpromazine, and an anxiolytic, diazepam (McKinney et al., 1973; Noble et al., 1976). In a few studies, even electroconvulsive treatments (ECT) have been shown to reverse this behavioral pathology (reviewed by McKinney, 1986). Endogenous neurochemical changes noted during the separation period include reduced cerebrospinal fluid levels of norepinephrine, a condition reversed by antidepressant treatment (Kraemer et al., 1984).

Although some of the observed behaviors are roughly analogous to major depression, the fact remains that the onset of depressive illness typically occurs in adulthood. These infant monkeys are probably displaying a response more analogous to the "anaclitic depression" observed by Spitz (1946) among newborn human infants suffering from maternal deprivation. Aware of these limitations, some investigators of primates have subsequently attempted to model depression using juvenile monkeys separated from their peer groups (Kraemer et al., 1984). Of course, one of the fundamental realities of depressive illness is that it clusters in genetically predisposed individuals. Thus, the observation of considerable individual variability in the development of despair behavior among rhesus monkeys is of special importance and has prompted cross-fostering studies, which are beginning to tease apart environmental and genetic factors in individual vulnerability to separation (Mineka and Suomi, 1978; McKinney, 1988). We return to this issue later.

A rodent version of the primate separation model would allow more extensive analysis of brain neurotransmitters and receptors and also the important study of genetic factors. However, rodents generally do not show sustained behavioral changes after social separation. A nonprimate separation model of potential relevance to adult depression is found in the work of Crawley (1984, 1985), who has identified a species of Siberian dwarf hamster that appears to form male–female mating pair bonds. When members of a pair are separated, the male dwarf hamsters explore less, interact less with other animals, and gain body weight. Imipramine and tranylcypromine, a monoamine oxidase (MAO) inhibitor, were found to reverse these changes to the same degree obtained by re-pairing with the original female.

The Learned Helplessness
Model of Depression

The learned helplessness model is based on exposing animals to uncontrollable, aversive stressors (Seligman and Maier, 1967). Variations of the original paradigm include inescapable tailshock or footshock, which is varied and random, and behavioral despair, as evidenced in a test involving swimming to exhaustion. The former produces a more naturalistic situation, whereas the latter is essentially a version of learned helplessness. Rats subjected to various forms of stress, such as shock or forced swimming, are subsequently unable to acquire and perform a simple escape task. The effect lasts up to 1 week after the inescapable stress (Weiss et al., 1984). The development of the syndrome can be prevented by benzodiazepine or TCA pretreatment and can be reversed by TCAs[2] and electroconvulsive shock but not by chlorpromazine or benzodiazepines (Porsolt et al., 1977; Kametani et al., 1983).

These models suffer from some of the same limitations as the separation models: (1) Compared with the relatively low frequency of clinical depression in the populations, the behavior is produced in a substantially larger proportion of the individual animals tested. (2) The animals

require a considerable amount of stress, and severe stress does not uniformly play a critical role in the onset of major depressive episodes. In manic-depressive illness stress may be more important to the onset of the initial episode than to subsequent episodes. (3) These syndromes generally can be rather quickly reversed by restoring the animal to a normal environment, which is certainly not the case in major depressive illness. These limitations may be best overcome with new approaches that attempt to identify individual genetic vulnerability. The specificity of neurotransmitter associations with this behavioral state is not yet clear. In one series of studies, learned helplessness is associated with depletion of norepinephrine in the locus coeruleus and is mimicked by infusing the α_2-adrenergic antagonist, piperoxane, into that nucleus (Weiss et al., 1982). In another series, the role of serotonin is emphasized. The binding of [^{3}H]-imipramine in rat cortex, a reflection of presynaptic serotonergic terminals, is decreased in association with inescapable shock, and the resultant learned helplessness can be reversed by microinjecting serotonin into the cortex (Sherman and Petty, 1984). Hypercortisolemia that resists suppression by dexamethasone, a clinical finding in some depressed patients, also can be produced in animals by the learned helplessness paradigm (Haracz et al., 1988). Critical evaluations of the learned helplessness models have been provided by Katz (1981), Hellhammer (1983), and Jesberger and Richardson (1985a, 1988). Of possible relevance to the sensitization–kindling models discussed later is the observation that chronic administration of some anticonvulsant agents can reverse at least some aspects of the syndrome produced by olfactory bulbectomy (see, e.g., Lloyd et al., 1987).

Animal Models of Mania

Robbins and Sahakian (1980) suggest four behavioral aspects of mania that should be modeled: hyperactivity, irritability, elation, and a swing or switch back to a depressed state. Most animal models of mania (drug induced, lesion induced, and behaviorally induced) focus on hyperactive behavior, for the obvious reason that it is easy to measure (Murphy, 1977).

Amphetamine and related stimulant drugs, which are thought to act primarily as dopamine agonists, increase locomotion, stereotyped sniffing, intracranial self-stimulation, aggression, and startle response in rats (Creese and Iversen, 1975). Hyperactivity also has been induced by serotonin depletion, using parachlorophenylalanine and 5,6-dihydroxytryptamine lesions (Diaz et al., 1974), and by morphine (Carroll and Sharp, 1971). Chronic lithium, α-methylparatyrosine, neuroleptics, and cholinergic agonists have been shown to reduce the hyperactivity induced by these various agents (reviewed by Murphy, 1977).

Various discrete anatomical lesions of ratbrain nuclei induce hyperactivity, including those of the septum, hippocampus, frontal cortex, globus pallidus, ventral tegmentum, and raphe nucleus. Many of these nuclei are especially rich in serotonin. The reward properties of intracranial self-stimulation in hypothalamic sites have also been suggested as a model for mania; such stimulation produces a generalized activation and arousal, including increased locomotor activity.

Taken together, these various ways of modeling mania by and large center on activating dopaminergic function to increase some forms of hyperactivity and arousal. To a lesser extent, reducing serotonergic function (and perhaps enhancing endogenous opiate systems) produces the same effect as activating dopaminergic function. Unfortunately, these induced behaviors are persistent, rather than cyclic, so that, alone, their relevance to manic-depressive illness is limited.

Toward More Relevant Animal Models

Animal behavior models of manic-depressive illness must start with the two fundamental clinical realities that define the illness: cyclicity and genetic vulnerability. The most common cyclical phenomena are the daily circadian rhythms of rest and activity that occur in most, if not all, mammalian species.

One animal behavior that appears to progress through a cycle is the extinction of a learned response to an operant reward task. After the reward is removed, runway activity in rats first increases (response invigoration or frustration), then decreases (depression), and finally recovers to baseline levels (recovery) (Klinger et al., 1974; Amsel, 1967). When put in a novel environment, rats initially become hyperactive and then rest. These two states continue to alternate regularly

with a measurable cycle frequency. Both the amplitude and the frequency of this cycle are reduced by lithium treatment (Katz, 1981). Behavioral paradigms such as these provide endogenous cyclic responses to environmental stimuli.

The growing literature on the genetic determinants of behavioral traits in animals, coupled with the availability of an increasing variety of inbred rodent strains, make genetic approaches practical. Also, both the social separation paradigm in monkeys and the learned helplessness paradigm in rats demonstrate wide, remarkably stable individual differences in response (Drugan et al., 1989). For example, only about one third of the rats treated with inescapable tailshock developed the full learned-helplessness syndrome. Among this vulnerable group, extensive stress is not required, and recovery is not spontaneous. Similarly, only about half of the juvenile monkeys separated from their peer group show the complete despair response. A genetic inbreeding strategy will be useful in maximizing aberrant behavior patterns in a large number of animals, so that particular biochemical abnormalities can be more readily identified and the tools of molecular genetics can be used to identify the genetic lesion. For example, rats bred for increased sensitivity to behavioral depression induced by a cholinergic agonist also show increased vulnerability to the helplessness syndrome associated with inescapable stress (Overstreet, 1986). Such inbred animals could serve as animal models to explore hypotheses of depression that posit increased cholinergic function.

Learned helplessness has now been modeled in human subjects, and behavioral and biochemical changes analogous to clinical depression have been reported (Breier et al., 1987). In a pilot study (Breier, 1989), seven patients with bipolar or unipolar major depression showed more pronounced behavioral and neuroendocrine responses than did normal controls.

Sensitization and Kindling

Recurrences in manic-depressive illness are not simply random. Rather they show, on the average, a pattern of increasing frequency over time (see Chapter 6). Post and collaborators (Post and Kopanda, 1976; Post et al., 1984d,e; Post and Weiss, 1989) have focused on two intriguing animal models that attempt to account for this tendency of episodes to accelerate: behavioral sensitization and electrophysiological kindling. These models are of considerable interest, even though they do not provide full homologies for other aspects of the illness.

In behavioral sensitization, animals become increasingly responsive behaviorally to repeated administration of the same dose of psychomotor stimulant (e.g., cocaine).[3] Behavior becomes more severe and onset more rapid. Prior exposure to the psychomotor stimulant will produce long-lasting alterations in this behavior (motor hyperactivity and stereotypy). Since the environmental context in which the animal originally received the drug appears to be important to its later increases in responsivity, a conditioning component may be involved. Behavioral sensitization appears to involve a dopamine substrate (e.g., its development can be blocked by haloperidol), but it can also be modified by neuropeptides, including sex hormones, enkephalins, and vasopressin.

Electrophysiological kindling refers to increased behavioral and electrophysiological responsivity, either to repeated low-level electrical stimulation of the brain or to such agents as lidocaine or cocaine (in high doses) exerting local anesthetic effects. The mechanisms underlying kindling appear to be different from those mediating behavioral sensitization. Nonetheless, some characteristics are shared, including increased responsivity based on prior exposure to the same stimulation. In kindling of the amygdala, for example, repeated once-daily stimulation for 1 second initially produces no observable behavioral or electrophysiological effects. However, upon repetition, afterdischarges increase in frequency, duration, and complexity of waveform, and eventually the animal develops a full-blown major motor seizure in response to a stimulus that was previously below the threshold. If the stimulation is repeated frequently enough, the animal will eventually develop a spontaneous seizure disorder, in which seizures occur without any exogenous stimulation. Whereas concomitant stress enhances sensitization, it inhibits kindling.

How do these two models, which are not directly analogous to the behavioral or affective disturbances of manic-depressive patients, help to clarify the mechanisms underlying the accelerating longitudinal course of the illness? In considering this question, it might be helpful to review the parallels between sensitization–kindling and manic-depressive illness:

- For each, evidence exists for the predisposing effects of both genetic factors and early environmental stress.
- Each shows threshold effects (mild alterations eventuating in full-blown episodes).
- Each can show similarity of episodes through repeated occurrences.
- With each, a maximum disturbance occurs earlier in the episode as more and more recurrences occur.
- With each, early episodes may require precipitants, whereas later ones can occur spontaneously.
- With each, repeated episodes of one phase may lead to emergence of the opposite phase.
- Younger animals appear to be more vulnerable to sensitization and kindling, suggesting a parallel to the young age of onset of bipolar disorder.

Thus, these models serve to broaden the conceptual framework for linking clinical phenomenology to neurobiological mechanisms. The average pattern of cycle acceleration over time could reflect a mixture of patients with a variety of patterns. Some might accelerate dramatically over time, whereas others do so moderately or not at all. In patients who have a dramatically shorter cycle with each episode, the form of the illness may be analogous to the pattern of increasingly rapid onset of hyperactivity and stereotypy following repeated administration of psychomotor stimulant. The role of environmental stress in enhancing behavioral sensitization may resemble its postulated role in the onset of affective episodes.

These data may help to integrate psychosocial and neurobiological perspectives. Specifically, if one postulates that a psychosocial stress can precipitate manic or depressive episodes, the sensitization and kindling models would suggest that, after a certain amount of repetition, the episodes would develop spontaneously. This chain of events fits the clinical histories of many patients with manic-depressive illness (as originally described by Kraepelin), in which clear-cut psychosocial or physical stresses are associated with the onset of early episodes, but in time the episodes become more autonomous. By the time patients are seen in treatment settings, they may indeed have an autonomous illness. As Post and Weiss (1989) have pointed out, the kindling–sensitization phenomena in animals do not yet represent precise models of human cyclic mood disorders. In addition to the respective time frames being quite different, the models imply a close similarity between stress-precipitated and chemically (drug) precipitated events, a similarity that needs to be demonstrated experimentally.

These sensitization and kindling models may turn out to have their most straightforward relevance to the long-term treatment of the illness. It is of interest that the two effective agents for prophylactic treatment of some forms of manic-depressive illness, lithium and carbamazepine, have differential effects on sensitization and kindling in animals. Lithium appears to block the behavioral sensitization accompanying cocaine-induced hyperactivity and stereotypy, but it does not prevent the development of amygdala kindling. In contrast, carbamazepine, which does not block the development of behavioral sensitization to cocaine, can inhibit amygdala-kindled seizures when administered chronically (Post et al., 1984f).

The growing clinical literature reviewed in Chapter 23 indicates that carbamazepine is effective in the prophylactic treatment of some patients who do not respond to lithium, primarily those with rapid cycles. Since such rapid cycles are predominantly associated with later phases of the illness (see Chapter 6), lithium may be effective for some patients only in the earlier phases of the illness, with carbamazepine, alone or in combination with lithium, likely to be required later. This differential clinical responsivity may relate to the greater ability of carbamazepine to inhibit kindling. Whether this drug and other anticonvulsants are as effective as lithium for the typical manic-depressive patient who would ordinarily respond to lithium is not yet established. Electroconvulsive seizures are also able to inhibit kindling (Post et al., 1984e), an effect that might be considered roughly analogous to a strong current interrupting ventricular fibrillation—that is, the defibrillator. It is interesting to consider that the three treatments with beneficial effects in both the depressed and manic phases of the illness—lithium, carbamazepine, and ECT—may share some

common mechanisms of action involving interruption of kindling and sensitization.

It is implicit in these two models that early and vigorous treatment of the first few episodes of the illness may diminish the likelihood of certain later consequences, namely, rapid or continuous cycling. In fact, if a reliable marker for the illness were available (see Chapter 15), it would be reasonable to attempt to prevent the illness altogether through treatment before the onset of even the first episode, as illustrated in Figure 16-1. If the kindling–sensitization models are relevant here, one might expect to be able to discontinue all treatment later. However, the research strategies involved in testing these hypotheses are extremely difficult, and conducting properly controlled trials could raise difficult ethical issues.

Circadian Rhythm Desynchronization

Studies of biological rhythms in animals represent another approach to modeling the inherent cyclicity of manic-depressive illness. They are reviewed extensively in Chapter 19. Briefly, the animal data indicate that periodic physiological disturbances (beat phenomena) may result from an abnormal internal phase relationship between two circadian (24-hour) rhythms if one of those rhythms had escaped from entrainment to the day–night cycle and is free-running in and out of phase with the other rhythm. These beat phenomena result from the overlapping concurrence of two events intended to occur out of phase with each other. Halberg (1968), Kripke (1978, 1983), and Wehr and Goodwin (1981, 1983a) have proposed that long-term cycles of relapse and remission in manic-depressive illness might also be generated in this way—that is, the episodes or switches into episodes could represent periodic disturbances in vulnerable individuals, disturbances analogous to beat phenomena. In a pharmacologically derived animal model, chronic antidepressant drugs have been shown to uncouple circadian oscillators in animals, an effect consistent with their propensity to shorten manic-depressive cycles in some patients (see Chapter 22).

Seasonal Rhythms

Seasonal peaks in the onset of depressive and manic episodes and in suicides prominent in classic descriptions of affective illness were ig-

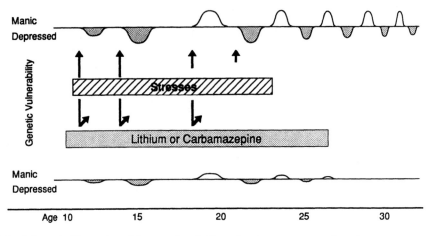

Figure 16-1. Schematic illustration of the postulated effect of early treatment on the subsequent course of bipolar disorder.

nored in modern biological formulations of the illness, only to be recently rediscovered. Contemporary systematic studies indicate that seasonal variations in light (length of the photoperiod) and probably also in temperature may be responsible for the seasonal peaks in episode onset.

The renewed clinical interest in seasonality has led to increased interest in animal models. As reviewed in Chapter 19, there are extensive animal data on seasonal behaviors and their biological substrates, much of which emphasizes the importance of the length of the photoperiod. For example, a variety of species, such as certain squirrels, abruptly enter a state of hibernation in the fall, characterized by profound physiological and endocrine changes, particularly low levels of thyrotropin-releasing hormone (TRH) in the pineal gland (Stanton et al., 1982). Microinjection of TRH into the dorsal hippocampus rapidly reverses hibernation (Stanton et al., 1981). However, the parallels between the seasonality of manic and depressive episodes and that of the animal kingdom have, at this stage, been developed only at a rudimentary level (Hallonquist and Mrosovsky, 1987).

Conclusion

If animal models are to offer promise, they must incorporate two cardinal features of manic-depressive illness: genetic vulnerability and cyclicity. The traditional models of depression and mania, although useful for illuminating important aspects of the depressed or manic state, do not adequately account for cyclicity. The models that are beginning to approach the ideal are those dealing with sensitization–kindling and circadian rhythm desynchronization and seasonal mechanisms, each of which requires considerably more elaboration. In passing, it is also worth noting that the kindling model, which predicts the clinical response to carbamazepine, has provided a clear instance in which a new psychiatric treatment received its initial impetus for a controlled trial from a hypothesis derived from animal research.[4]

EVOLUTION OF BIOCHEMICAL HYPOTHESES

The following section is organized by hypotheses for the sake of clarity. Nevertheless, most hypotheses are far from comprehensive, and most investigators have emphasized the complexity of the interrelationships between biological systems.

Amine Neurotransmitter Systems

Originally formulated in the early 1960s to explain the actions of mood-altering drugs, the amine hypotheses both stimulated and emerged in parallel with basic animal studies that were characterizing specific neuronal systems in which monoamines are the principal neurotransmitters. The cell bodies of these systems are distributed predominantly in midbrain structures making up the limbic system (Papez, 1937; MacLean,

1952), a diffuse yet highly integrated set of structures characterized by multiple feedback loops. The location of the midbrain in relation to the whole brain is illustrated in Figure 16-2, and the limbic lobe and the major interconnections of the limbic system are shown in Figure 16-3 (A and B). The limbic system is implicated in the regulation of sleep, appetite, arousal, sexual function, and emotional states such as fear and rage. It has also been shown to be involved in various self-stimulation behaviors (Kupfermann, 1985b).

Many groups of monoamine neurons, although originating from a small number of cell bodies, are distributed widely throughout the central nervous system. (For a schematic illustration of the distribution of the norepinephrine, dopamine and serotonin systems, and their interactions, see Figure 17-2, opposite page 458.) A single norepinephrine neuron projecting from the locus coeruleus to the cortex can, for example, synapse with many thousands of other nerve cells. The monoaminergic systems, by and large, do not provide the principal drive for critical life-sustaining functions. Rather, they subserve much more subtle and complex modulatory and integrative functions.

It seemed reasonable to assume that the biological substrate of a syndrome as complex as manic-depressive illness, with its interrelated cognitive, emotional, psychomotor, appetitive, and autonomic manifestations, would be found in just such systems: complex, widely distributed throughout the brain, and essentially integrative in function. Such a biological substrate would also have to be affected by drugs known to produce changes in mood or cognition. The monoamine neurotransmitter systems meet these qualifications.

The most cohesive of the early amine hypotheses was the catecholamine hypothesis (Prange, 1964; Schildkraut, 1965; Bunney and Davis, 1965), which posits that depression is associated with a functional deficiency of catecholamines

Figure 16-2. The major parts of the central nervous system and important landmarks shown in midsagittal section (from Kelly, 1985).

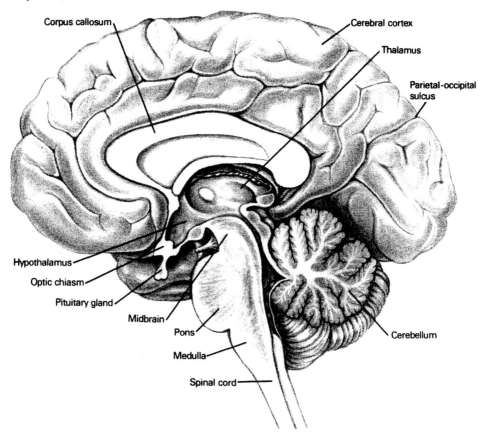

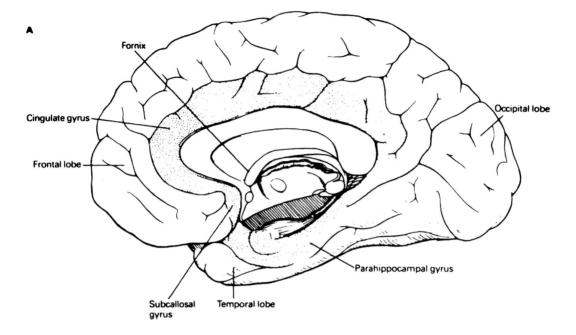

A

Fornix

Cingulate gyrus

Frontal lobe

Occipital lobe

Parahippocampal gyrus

Subcallosal gyrus

Temporal lobe

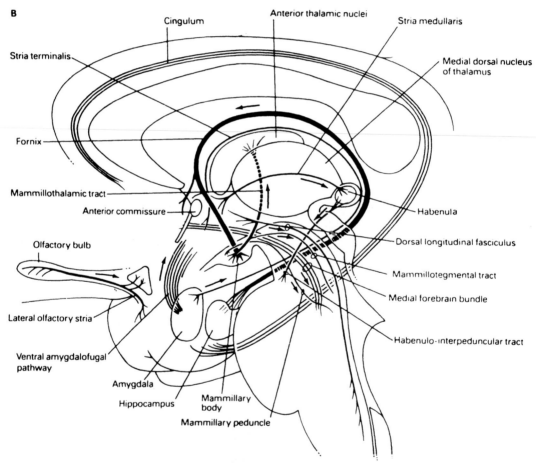

B

Cingulum

Anterior thalamic nuclei

Stria medullaris

Stria terminalis

Medial dorsal nucleus of thalamus

Fornix

Mammillothalamic tract

Anterior commissure

Habenula

Dorsal longitudinal fasciculus

Olfactory bulb

Mammillotegmental tract

Medial forebrain bundle

Lateral olfactory stria

Habenulo-interpeduncular tract

Ventral amygdalofugal pathway

Amygdala

Mammillary body

Hippocampus

Mammillary peduncle

Figure 16-3. The limbic system consists of the limbic lobe and deep-lying structures. **A.** This medial view of the brain shows the limbic lobe, which consists of primitive cortical tissue (dots) that encircles the upper brainstem. Also included in the limbic lobe are the underlying cortical structures (hippocampus and dentate gyrus). **B.** This view schematically illustrates the interconnections of deep-lying structures included as part of the limbic system. The most prominent directions of flow of neural activity are indicated by arrows, but the designated tracts typically have bidirectional activity (from Kupfermann, 1985a, adapted from Nieuwehuys et al., 1981).

and mania an excess. The neurotransmitter serotonin was hypothesized to be low in both states. The neurobiological and pharmacological bases for these hypotheses are detailed in Chapter 17.

For years, the study of drug effects in animals was limited to acute administration, despite occasional pleas by a few clinical investigators who pointed out that the therapeutic effects of these drugs in patients occurred only after chronic administration, usually for 2 weeks or more, whereas the presynaptic effects of tricyclics, MAOIs, and (in part) lithium occurred immediately (reviewed in Goodwin and Sack, 1973). Chronic administration research paradigms allowed investigators to explore drug effects that develop more slowly over time, that is, more in parallel with their clinical effects. In addition, animal behavioral models of antidepressant effects, such as the enhancement of self-stimulation behavior, have been observed more consistently using chronic drug administration paradigms.

The emphasis on chronic drug studies gave impetus to one of the most productive and exciting developments in neurobiology over the past 10 years: the discovery and characterization of neurotransmitter and drug receptors in the brain and various peripheral tissues. Receptors, which represent specific recognition sites (usually proteins) for the binding of a given neurohumoral substance, provide the selectivity by which a target tissue (or cell) responds to a biological signal. Once a neurotransmitter or hormone binds to its receptor (i.e., becomes a receptor ligand), a series of intracellular events occurs (e.g., increases in cyclic nucleotide levels and protein kinase activity, hydrolysis of phosphoinositide, PI, ion permeability changes). This results ultimately in a physiological event. Substances that produce or contribute to the activation of a receptor-mediated event are referred to as *agonists* for that receptor, whereas substances that bind to the receptor and block or interfere with its natural agonist are called *antagonists*. A given receptor is defined by its response to a series of agonists or antagonists (Nutt and Linnoila, 1988).

Since one neurotransmitter can activate more than one receptor (e.g., norepinephrine is the physiological agonist at both α- and β-adrenergic receptors) and since a given receptor can be linked or coupled to more than one second messenger system (e.g., cyclic nucleotides or PI hydroly-

sis), the possible consequences of receptor activation are quite complex, and in most cases, the neurophysiological and behavioral effects of such stimulation are unknown. Nevertheless, techniques for measuring both the number and functional activity of neurotransmitter or drug receptors are now readily available, and several have been used in studies of possible receptor alterations in manic-depressive illness.

Important to receptor techniques is the ability to distinguish nonspecific binding from true receptor activation by a neurotransmitter or drug. If the binding affinities could be shown to have a high correlation with the physiological or pharmacological effect produced, a particular recognition site could be designated as a physiologically significant receptor. Studies of chronic drug effects also can assess the biochemical consequences of receptor activation by following the generation of second messengers. Effects of chronic drug administration on presynaptic autoreceptors (which, in most instances, serve to regulate the release of transmitter) add to this increasingly complex picture. Studies of chronic effects of drugs on the firing rates of single neurons have provided a physiological confirmation of the receptor-mediated effects of these drugs.

Phasic alterations in receptor sensitivity have been hypothesized to underlie one aspect of the illness—the sudden switch from depression to mania (Bunney et al., 1972a,b,c). Given the evidence that postsynaptic receptor sensitivity tends to adapt to the level of presynaptic output of transmitter, the theory goes on to posit that the timing of this adaptation can get out of phase. Thus, a state of decreased presynaptic transmitter output would, after a while, result in an adaptive increase in the number of postsynaptic receptors (hypersensitivity). Later, if the presynaptic output were to again increase, the now greater amount of transmitter would interact with a supersensitive receptor complex, resulting in an exaggerated behavioral response, that is, mania. The reverse of this would explain the subsequent onset of depression as the excess neurotransmitter begins to down-regulate the receptor.

Neuroendocrine Systems and Neuropeptides

The hypothesis that altered endocrine function might explain or contribute to pathological mood states largely grew out of clinical observations of patients with thyroid or Cushing's disease and antedated the discovery of biogenic amine neurotransmitters. One reason that this field has evolved rapidly is the potential that neuroendocrine substances may serve as a window into the brain's neurotransmitter systems. Current explorations of pathophysiology using neuroendocrine strategies have tended to develop research tools into diagnostic tests (e.g., the dexamethasone suppression test) prematurely. But tests of this kind are most useful for research into mechanisms of illness when the illness itself remains the independent variable, an approach that allows exploration of its clinical, pharmacological, genetic, and other biological correlates independent of predetermined diagnostic boundaries.

The primary components of the neuroendocrine systems are neuropeptides, and thus the distinction between endocrine and peptide studies is somewhat artificial. New peptide neurotransmitter or neuromodulator candidates emerge with increasing frequency as methods for their isolation, characterization, and synthesis become more and more sophisticated and efficient. It is likely that we are about to experience a surge of new, as yet undreamed of peptides in the central nervous system, discoveries that will come very rapidly from application of the tools of molecular genetics (Bloom, 1987).

Electrolyte-Based and Membrane Hypotheses

Studies of total body water and electrolyte balance (principally sodium) grew out of classic observations of such state-related fluctuations in manic-depressive illness as urine volume and body weight. They also were prompted by a growing appreciation of the importance of sodium, potassium, calcium, and magnesium in nerve cell excitation, synaptic transmission, and, possibly, the mechanism of action of lithium. Although relatively prominent in the 1960s, studies in this area inexplicably died out in succeeding decades but may now be experiencing a resurgence in the emerging literature in the chemistry and biophysics of membrane function. For example, a deficiency in the membrane-bound sodium pump was initially hypothesized to explain reported excessive cellular sodium retention but later became important in its own right. Later

the lithium-sodium counterflow mechanism in the red cell was characterized, and biophysical studies revealed protein structural differences between patients and controls.

Membrane studies in manic-depressive illness occupy a special place, not only because they provide a biological handle on genetic vulnerability but also because of the vital role of membrane transport mechanisms in transmitter function at the synaptic level. Indeed, it would not be unreasonable to anticipate that all of the biological findings in manic-depressive illness ultimately may be explained on the basis of some membrane abnormality, either localized or generalized. An implicit assumption of membrane studies is that a genetically transmitted abnormality found in an available peripheral tissue, such as the red cell or platelet, will also be expressed in other tissues, including the central nervous system.

THE PHARMACOLOGICAL BRIDGE

The pharmacological bridge between biochemical pharmacology in animals and the clinical actions of drugs supported the growth of the major biochemical hypotheses of manic-depressive illness. Before negotiating our way across such a bridge in the next chapters, some caveats are in order: (1) By and large, the animal data are from genetically homogeneous normal animals, whereas the clinical data are from a small, probably genetically distinct portion of the population, probably with a specific vulnerability. (2) The fact that a clinically effective drug alters a particular neurotransmitter or receptor mechanism in a given direction does not mean that the system was involved in the pathophysiology of the illness. Strictly speaking, this caveat applies even when one can show an association between the drug-induced transmitter change in patients and clinical response, although such an association would be of considerable interest. (3) The phase during which a drug is given, whether to patients with recurrent unipolar or bipolar illness, may be critical to both the direction and intensity of effect. This factor accounts for many apparent pharmacological paradoxes, such as termination of a manic episode with a TCA. Since phase of illness is almost never specified, the major support for any bridge must rest on population studies, in which phase is presumably random, rather than on case studies.

Historically, the potential of the amine-depleting antihypertensive reserpine to induce depression was the first pharmacological bridge, one that led to formulation of the amine hypothesis. The most reasonable interpretation of reserpine's clinical effect was that it activated a preexisting vulnerability. It is not clear, however, whether a bipolar or a unipolar history confers a different degree of vulnerability to this drug or whether, continuously administered, reserpine could precipitate recurrent depressive or manic-depressive illness.[5] Reserpine's effects appear to be associated primarily with depletion of catecholamines (rather than indoleamines) because they are reversed by catecholamine and not indoleamine agonists. The relative involvement of the two catecholamines (norepinephrine and dopamine) in the behavioral effects of reserpine is not settled. Propranolol, the peripheral and centrally active β-receptor antagonist, may occasionally produce depressive episodes in standard therapeutic doses[6] and, in high doses, appears to have interesting effects on cycle length in some manic-depressive patients (see Chapter 17).

Drugs that act as stimulants in normal individuals are not generally found to be therapeutic in patients suffering from major depressive illness (Klein and Davis, 1969). Conversely, drugs that have antidepressant activity do not tend to be stimulants in normals (Oswald et al., 1972). L-Dopa, a precursor of both dopamine and norepinephrine, which at least acutely increases their output, is not an effective antidepressant. Nevertheless, it does produce some activation with increases in anger and psychosis ratings in some patients and hypomanic episodes superimposed on the depression in many bipolar patients (Goodwin et al., 1970; Murphy et al., 1971a).

Early findings on lithium were interpreted as indicating a drug-induced decrease of functional amines,[7] although the picture is now considerably more complex, giving more emphasis to the ion's effects on postsynaptic second messenger mechanisms involving cyclic nucleotides, PI, and G proteins (see Chapter 17). All neuroleptics block the action of dopamine at its postsynaptic receptor (at least in certain regions), although

they do not have uniform effects on norepinephrine. α-Methylparatyrosine, a relatively specific inhibitor of dopamine and norepinephrine synthesis, depletes the amount of transmitter available for release. Piribedil and bromocriptine are both partial dopamine receptor agonists. Both have antidepressant and possibly mania-inducing effects, although in different doses, the latter actually has antimanic effects.

The most consistent pharmacological bridge is built on the findings that direct or indirect dopamine or norepinephrine agonists can precipitate episodes of mania or hypomania in patients with manic-depressive illness.

Many of the so-called classic biochemical effects comprising one end of the pharmacological bridge are based on the ability of drugs to alter acutely the turnover of the neurotransmitter, that is, the combined rate of synthesis, release, and elimination of a particular substance. High turnover traditionally implies a higher level of function, and low turnover implies the reverse, although by itself this does not take receptor adaptation (e.g., down-regulation) into account. For the pharmacological bridge, the net action of a drug on the output of the amine system is the focus, rather than the complexities of drug effects on different components of these systems. In Chapter 17, we explore this complexity by considering the wide variety of drug effects revealed by new receptor-based and electrophysiological techniques.

Beyond the effects of a drug on the state of depression or mania are effects on the cycle length. Tricyclic antidepressants can increase the frequency of cycles in some patients. MAO inhibitors, like other antidepressants, can precipitate mania, but their long-term effect on cycles has not been studied extensively. This effect may depend on the inhibition of type-B MAO, since a selective MAO-A inhibition appears not to increase cycling. ECT apparently can both precipitate and terminate manias in bipolar patients and either increase or decrease cycle frequency depending on the phase of illness in which it is administered. Tricyclic or heterocyclic antidepressants can reverse depression, precipitate mania, and increase cycle frequency in at least a subgroup of bipolar patients. MAOIs can reverse depression, precipitate mania, and, in the case of the MAO type-A inhibitors, decrease cycle frequency, although the nonspecific (mixed A and B) MAOIs may, like TCAs, increase cycle frequency. Lithium can reverse mania, reverse depression, and decrease cycle frequency. Carbamazepine, less extensively evaluated biochemically than the others, also may have at least three classes of action. It is partially antidepressant, certainly antimanic, and anticycling. Finally, there are a growing number of antidepressants termed *second generation* and *third generation* or *heterocyclic* (because of different cyclic structures than the tricyclics); these have not been used long enough to assess whether they affect cycle frequency. Some, especially those that are primarily serotonin uptake inhibitors, may be less likely than standard antidepressants to precipitate mania. The various drug effects reviewed are illustrated in Figure 16-4.

This largely historical introduction to the phar-macological bridge has focused on the mono-amines. In Chapter 17, we broaden the focus to include proposed associations between the illness and important nonmonoamine substances, such as the widely distributed inhibitory neurotransmitter γ-aminobutyric acid.

SUMMARY

By tracing some of the theoretical and historical developments in the biology of manic-depressive illness, this chapter serves as an introduction to the chapters that follow. Its emphasis on biochemical–pharmacological aspects reflects the development of contemporary interest in this subject. Historically, the proposed linkages between the monoamine neurotransmitters and key symptoms of depressed and manic states have been a central force in modern biological psychiatry. Although the monoamine systems remain im-

Figure 16-4. Classification of drug effects on manic-depressive illness.

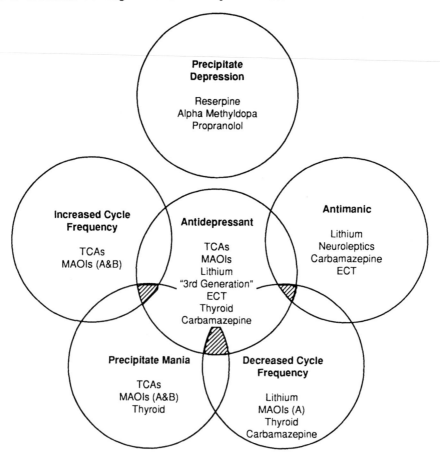

portant, our present challenge is to integrate what we know of them with emerging discoveries of a wide range of new neuromodulatory systems. In considering this integration, we should be aware that the existing biological theories, whether derived from formal animal models or from the pharmacological bridge, do not give adequate consideration to two fundamental clinical realities of manic-depressive illness: genetic vulnerability and recurrent episodes.

We return to the more daunting challenge of integrating neurotransmitter and neuroendocrine findings with other perspectives as varied as circadian rhythms, physiology, and neuroanatomy in Chapter 20.

NOTES

1. Murphy, 1977; Crawley, 1984, 1985; Willner, 1984.
2. Triiodothyronine, which can potentiate the antidepressant effects of tricyclic drugs (see Chapter 22) can also potentiate the antidepressant reversal of learned helplessness in rats (Brochet et al., 1987).
3. The analogy between cocaine-induced behavioral changes and mania is discussed in Chapter 9.
4. In the last few years, animal rights activists have intensified their attacks on the use of animals in biomedical research. This movement is a reflection of various beliefs, but at present appears to be dominated by individuals who believe that animals have the same fundamental rights that society has traditionally reserved for human beings. Its activities play into the public's misunderstanding of science, and already it has had a chilling effect on investigators using animals in disease-related research. Those whose research depends on the use of animals now must function in a climate of fear, an understandable response to the activists' destruction of facilities and direct threats against scientists. Together with the escalating cost of research animals and other factors, the movement has seriously undermined the basic research that is the foundation for clinical science. This trend is evident in the sharp reduction in literature citations to animal models of depression or mania. In the National Library of Medicine's Medline file for 1988 and 1989, no published reports of primate research were cited in this important field of inquiry. By contrast, in the early 1980s, eight to ten publications appeared each year.
5. Methyldopa, believed to act by stimulating presynaptic receptors that inhibit norepinephrine release in the central nervous system, also can precipitate depression.
6. Whether, as in the case of reserpine, the ability of propranolol to induce depression is confined to vulnerable individuals (as reflected in a personal or family history of affective illness) has not been studied.
7. The term *functional*, although somewhat imprecise, has been used to signify the level of amine in the synapse and, therefore, available to activate its postsynaptic receptor.

17

Biochemical and Pharmacological Studies

This chapter chronicles the search for the biochemical substances implicated in the etiology or pathophysiology of manic-depressive illness. Insofar as possible, the mechanisms through which neurotransmitters, neuromodulators, hormones, peptides, and other substances exert their effects are explored. The chapter follows roughly the same trail as the research.

The first studies reviewed are those that test the various forms of the amine hypothesis. Among the oldest of the biochemical hypotheses, the amine hypotheses have generated vast amounts of data since they were first formulated in the 1960s. Studies of norepinephrine, dopamine, and serotonin are reviewed in turn, and then evidence of interactions among these amines and other transmitters and neuromodulators—acetylcholine and γ-aminobutyric acid, for example—are considered. It is this most recent research into the relative balance of neurotransmitter function that shows the most promise of explicating the mechanisms of antidepressant and antimanic drug action. Enzymes involved in the degradation of neurotransmitters are then considered, followed by studies of the wide array of specific receptors with which the neurotransmitters interact.

Studies of neuroendocrine abnormalities are reviewed next. These abnormalities, inferred from the pathological mood states that can be associated with endocrine disorders, were originally expected to clarify the regulatory functions of neurotransmitters. Hormones released by the hypothalamus, such as cortisol, interact with central neurotransmitters. The hypercortisolemia consistently found among a significant proportion of patients with major depression is examined for its relevance to neurotransmitter functioning and for its own effect on the brain. Thyroid abnormalities, also common in depression, are explored as well.

Next we turn to the neuropeptides, substances involved in long-term regulation of behavior, cognition, and emotion. Although sketchy, the clinical evidence on peptides suggests that they may be involved in the pathophysiology of manic-depressive illness.

One of the oldest biochemical literatures on recurrent affective illnesses deals with electrolytes and changes in body water that accompany phase changes. Work on cations involved in nerve function—sodium, potassium, calcium, and magnesium—was given new emphasis when lithium, a similar cation, was found to be therapeutic and prophylactic in manic-depressive illness. This research is considered, with special emphasis on the role of calcium in bipolar illness.

The closely related studies on membranes are

reviewed next. We review studies demonstrating abnormalities in membrane transport systems that merit further exploration as potential genetic markers. Then miscellaneous biochemicals are studied for their relevance to manic-depressive illness.

Whereas the bulk of the chapter is devoted to a system-by-system review of our knowledge base, the final three sections reframe the data in terms of the enduring clinical realities of the illness. Thus, we review attempts to understand the recurrent nature of the illness, with a focus on studies of the switch process and of the kindling–sensitization hypothesis. That section is followed by a review of biological data from patients who have recovered, a strategy that might well uncover clues to trait markers of manic-depressive illness. Finally, in the last section, we consider from a cross-sectional perspective what we have learned about the clinical meaning of this enormous biochemical literature, that is, clinical correlates.

NEUROTRANSMITTER SYSTEMS

The Amine Hypotheses

The monoaminergic systems of the brain, briefly introduced in Chapter 16, were an early focus of biological hypotheses of manic-depressive ill-ness. The initial impetus for the amine hypothesis came from observations of the clinical effects of drugs subsequently shown to alter central amine function in animals. Reserpine, which depletes central amines, was found to be associated with the onset of depression in susceptible individuals, whereas monoamine oxidase inhibitors, which increase levels of amines in the brains of animals, were reported to have some antidepressant activity. Later, the tricyclic antidepressants were shown to block the presynaptic reuptake of amines, thereby increasing their availability at the postsynaptic receptor. These synaptic interactions and sites of drug action are illustrated schematically in Figure 17-1. Although the amine hypotheses of affective disorder were initially proposed as single-transmitter theories, subsequent developments in neuroscience highlighted the complex interrelationships among neurotransmitter systems. Here we present each amine transmitter system separately and discuss relationships between them throughout.

Catecholamine Hypothesis

The catecholamine hypothesis postulates that depression is associated with a functional deficit of one or more neurotransmitter catecholamines at critical synapses in the central nervous system (CNS) and that mania is associated with a functional excess of these amines. The early inves-

Figure 17-1. Presynaptic and postsynaptic mechanisms showing the known sites of action of mood-altering drugs (adapted from Potter, 1986).

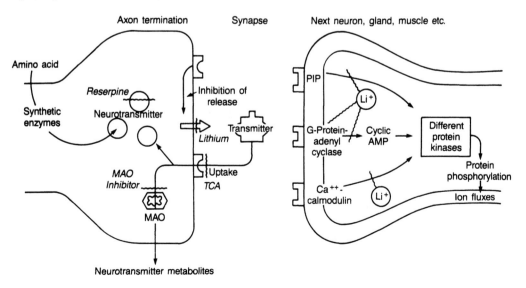

tigations of the biochemistry of manic-depressive illness focused on catecholamines (norepinephrine and dopamine) rather than indoleamines (serotonin). This was because reserpine sedation in animals is reversed by a catecholamine precursor (L-dopa), but not by an indoleamine precursor (5-hydroxytryptophan). The catecholamine hypothesis, a dominant force for nearly 15 years (especially among American investigators), was based on the assumption that mania and depression are biochemically opposite states. The early focus of this hypothesis was on norepinephrine rather than on dopamine, because dopamine's reuptake is not blocked by the tricyclic antidepressants.

Norepinephrine. Human neurons containing norepinephrine (NE) are organized into anatomically and functionally discrete nuclei in the upper brainstem. The most discussed of these in the neuropharmacological literature is the locus coeruleus (LC), the major source of noradrenergic innervation to higher cortisol structures. Several other brainstem NE nuclei appear to be more important than the LC for regulating the peripheral autonomic nervous system. In addition to projections, NE neurons are also organized into ganglia in the peripheral sympathetic nervous system (SNS). Stimulation of the LC in animals can cause peripheral NE release (Crawley et al., 1978), and alterations of SNS activity generally are accompanied by parallel changes in central noradrenergic activity (for review, see Leckman and Maas, 1984). Conversely, substances that inhibit the LC also reduce peripheral NE release (e.g., clonidine).

The overall function of NE systems in intact organisms is clearer when they are examined from another perspective. Many electrophysiologists view NE in the CNS as a modulator of other signals rather than as the primary signal transducer that it seems to be in the SNS. In the cerebellum, the release of NE following LC stimulation decreases the spontaneous firing of Purkinje cells, thereby increasing the relative signal from exogenous stimuli (Woodward et al., 1979). In other words, NE increases the signal/noise ratio in this area of the brain, thereby increasing the sensitivity to stimuli. Analogously, projections from the LC to other areas, such as the hypothalamus or cortex, may contrib-

ute to the overall functional role of NE by rendering these brain regions more responsive to any number of exogenous stimuli. This mechanism may be critical in the noradrenergic response to various stresses. Many antidepressants show marked effects on these NE systems and presumably also on their functions.

Both in vitro and in vivo experiments have demonstrated conclusively that tricyclic antidepressants (TCA) increase the amount of NE available at the synapse by inhibiting the reuptake of NE. Regardless of the TCA used, NE reuptake probably approaches its minimum after administration of therapeutic doses. This is true even for TCAs that appear to inhibit serotonin reuptake selectively (e.g., fluoxetine) and do not inhibit NE uptake in vitro. When administered in chronic doses in humans, these serotonergic TCAs produce equivalent effects on NE reuptake, either by achieving high enough concentrations or by being converted to active metabolites that do affect NE. Nonetheless, since the NE and serotonin systems are highly interdependent, the overall effect on NE may be different with TCAs that inhibit both serotonin and NE reuptake than with those that affect only NE (e.g., desipramine). Initially, after the administration of TCAs, intrasynaptic NE rises, and this primary effect is responsible for the compensatory down-regulation of β-receptors (seen in animal studies) and α_2-receptors (seen in both animal and clinical studies).

Monoamine oxidase inhibitors (MAOI), by blocking the principal route of amine degradation, probably also increase intrasynaptic NE (or the amount released per impulse), and they produce the same compensatory receptor changes as do the TCAs.[1] Studies of receptor regulation are consistent with numerous animal and clinical studies showing that chronic treatment with TCAs and MAOIs reduces the turnover of norepinephrine (Potter, 1984; Potter et al., 1985, 1987).

Many of the second-generation antidepressants with novel biochemical structures do not have a primary effect on the NE system. Nonetheless, in animals, chronic treatment with these agents usually reduces either β-receptor number or the β-receptor-mediated stimulation of 3',5'-cyclic adenosine monophosphate (cyclic AMP, cAMP), a postsynaptic second messenger, by isoproterenol. Moreover, primary serotonin uptake inhibitors, like their noradrenergic cousins, also reduce NE turnover in humans and may facilitate NE transmission.

Lithium's effects on norepinephrine are less clear. Early reports using high concentrations in vitro noted a stimulation of NE uptake, thereby decreasing functional norepinephrine. More recent studies done with therapeutic concentrations provide no evidence that lithium has a direct effect on intrasynaptic NE. On the other hand, both preclinical and clinical studies indicate that the ion does alter the regulation of the postsynaptic β-receptor complex by preventing the development of β-receptor supersensitivity following NE depletion by reserpine. Lithium also blocks the cAMP stimulation produced by adrenergic agonists, an effect that is beyond the receptor itself, interacting with the cell's second messenger machinery (Ebstein et al., 1987; Belmaker, 1981; Belmaker et al., 1982).[2] The ability of lithium to slow the formation of phosphatidylinositol-4,5-biphosphate (PIP_2, a second messenger for α_1-muscarinic and possibly serotonergic receptors analogous to cAMP for β-receptors) may ultimately prove to be a major mechanism by which lithium influences a range of neurotransmitter systems at postsynaptic sites. As Berridge and colleagues (1982) comment:

This implies that the action of Li^+ *in vivo* may be rather selective in that it will be maximally effective against those cells whose inositol phospholipid-linked receptors are being abnormally stimulated. Thus, Li^+ could preferentially affect those receptor pathways that are abnormally active, and this may account for its equal effectiveness in controlling both mania and depression. (p. 594)

The net functional consequences of these lithium-induced changes in receptor sensitivity are not yet well understood. Perhaps the receptor desensitization and stabilization associated with chronic lithium administration, coupled with its lack of an acute, direct stimulatory or inhibitory effect on NE, might explain the clinical observations that this drug precipitates neither mania nor depression, treats both phases slowly and often incompletely, and is most effective in preventing episodes. Considerable interest was generated by the report that the decrease in total NE turnover produced by chronic lithium administration occurred in bipolar patients but not in normal controls, a finding that suggests that decreasing

functional NE may be involved in the clinical stabilization produced by lithium. This finding has not yet been replicated, however.

The pharmacological bridge—the bridge between the pathophysiology of an illness and the mechanisms of action of drugs that treat it—is bolstered by other drugs that affect NE as well. Amphetamine and cocaine both have mixed acute effects. They inhibit NE uptake and promote its release, actions consistent with increased intrasynaptic NE. Acute L-dopa also can generate noradrenergic stimulation, presumably by transiently augmenting the synthesis of NE before compensatory mechanisms are activated.

Carbamazepine is structurally related to imipramine, and in clinical concentrations, it produces about 25 percent of the NE uptake inhibition seen with imipramine (Purdy et al., 1977) while stimulating firing of the locus coeruleus in the rat. In contrast, tricyclics, which are more potent NE uptake inhibitors, acutely inhibit firing of the LC, presumably as a result of increased availability of NE. The potentially more interesting effects of chronic carbamazepine administration on NE function have not been investigated extensively, and results so far are conflicting.

Dopamine. Central dopamine (DA) is most concentrated in the nigrostriatal region, and its involvement in movement disorders (e.g., parkinsonism) is closely related to alterations in these areas. There are also important mesolimbic and mesocortical DA systems, which play a major role in the facilitation of reward-motivated behaviors through the so-called behavioral facilitation system (Milner, 1977; Iversen, 1978). Finally, there is the dopaminergic tuberoinfundibular tract (regulated independently of the nigrostriatal system), which plays a central role in regulating prolactin and influences growth hormone release. A wide variety of studies have linked central dopamine to reinforcing, motivational, and psychomotor processes. In a recent theoretical article, Depue and Iacono (1989) review an impressive body of evidence linking central dopamine function, behavioral facilitation, and bipolar illness. Anatomical evidence supports a serotonin input onto DA-containing neurons, but not the reverse. This hypothesized relationship is consistent with the interpretation that dopamine is necessary but not sufficient for the behavioral states discussed by Depue and Iacono.

The multiple complex systems involving dopamine neurons may be independently regulated under certain circumstances. For example, in both naturally occurring and drug-induced parkinsonism, a selective loss of nigrostriatal and mesolimbic DA occurs that involves motor dysfunction but not the type of hormonal dysregulation expected if hypothalamic dopamine were also depleted. In the nigrostriatum, a reciprocal inhibitory relationship exists between dopaminergic and cholinergic neurons, a relationship that may explain why anticholinergic drugs are helpful in parkinsonism.

As noted, the catecholamine hypothesis focused on the noradrenergic system in part because the first tricyclic antidepressants did not appear to affect DA systems (i.e., did not affect DA uptake). The development of novel antidepressants that do have major effects on DA turnover has now sparked interest in the possible role of dopamine in affective illness. Pharmacological observations have led to several versions of a relatively simple DA hypothesis of bipolar illness:

• The DA precursor L-dopa almost uniformly produces hypomania in bipolar patients (Goodwin et al., 1970; Murphy et al., 1971a; Van Praag and Korf, 1975).
• Amphetamine, which promotes DA release and inhibits its uptake, can precipitate hypomania in bipolar patients, induce a hypomania-like state in normal people (Jacobs and Silverstone, 1986), but is not generally considered an antidepressant in unipolar patients (Goodwin and Sack, 1973).
• The direct DA agonists, bromocriptine and piribedil, seem to be effective antidepressants in some bipolar patients and able to precipitate mania (Silverstone, 1978, 1984; Gerner et al., 1976). Interestingly, antidepressant response to piribedil has been associated with low pretreatment levels of the dopamine metabolite homovanillic acid (HVA) in the cerebrospinal fluid (CSF) (Post et al., 1978a).
• Neuroleptics that selectively block DA receptors (such as pimozide) are effective against severe mania.
• Chronic administration of classic antidepres-

sants, such as imipramine and desipramine, decreases presynaptic DA autoreceptor sensitivity, and presumably reduces negative feedback on DA turnover (Chiodo and Antelman, 1980). Thus, activation of central dopaminergic neurotransmission is predicted during chronic, but not acute, administration of most antidepressants.

Moving toward a type of balance hypothesis, Goodwin and Sack (1974b) analyzed the effects of drugs selectively on the dopamine or on the norepinephrine systems in relation to the relative efficacy of the drugs against different symptoms of mania. Their analysis led them to suggest that DA abnormalities are primarily involved in the hyperactivity and psychosis associated with the more severe stages of mania, whereas norepinephrine might be implicated in the euphoria-grandiosity more characteristic of hypomania. They envisioned a cascade in which the initial noradrenergic dysregulation of hypomania gives way to the hyperdopaminergic state of mania. Antelman and Caggiula (1977) provided a more precise elaboration of the relative roles of DA and NE in the brain and the implications for each neurotransmitter in bipolar illness. They reasoned from behavioral and neuroanatomical studies that there is an inhibitory noradrenergic modulation of DA-mediated functions through serotonergic neurons in a midbrain region called the *raphe nucleus* or through direct projections from the locus coeruleus to the substantia nigra. If the inhibitory connection through the raphe were of major importance, reduced NE associated with bipolar depression could produce hyperactivity of the dopaminergic system, which would ultimately lead to a switch into mania. This would be consistent with the clinical observation that the switch is more likely to occur from a depressed state than from euthymia. The mania-precipitating action of a DA agonist provides the critical pharmacological bridge to this DA/NE balance hypothesis. Interestingly, destruction of the locus coeruleus may protect against DA-induced increases of locomotor activity seen after at least one antidepressant treatment: electroconvulsive therapy (ECT) (Green and Deakin, 1980).

As noted previously, a role of DA in the action of the major mood-altering drugs (TCAs, MAOIs, lithium, carbamazepine) is, in contrast, more difficult to establish. It can be argued that tricyclic antidepressants, as well as several new drugs that are potential antidepressants, do block dopamine uptake in concentrations that may be reached in the brains of patients receiving antidepressants (Willner, 1983). On the other hand, acute antidepressant treatment has highly variable effects on DA synthesis (Carlsson and Lindqvist, 1978) and does not affect selected DA-mediated behaviors (Schechter, 1980). Moreover, chronic antidepressant treatment does not produce consistent changes in DA turnover. Karoum and colleagues (1984a), however, showed decreased DA turnover in rat hypothalamus and caudate after both an NE uptake inhibitor and a serotonin uptake inhibitor, a finding consistent with the model suggested by Antelman and Caggiula described previously. The antidepressant MAOIs potentiate synaptic DA by inhibiting metabolism. The mood stabilizers lithium and carbamazepine, in therapeutic concentrations, have complex effects on DA (see reviews on lithium by Bunney and Garland-Bunney, 1987, and on carbamazepine by Post, 1987).

Studies of the effects of mood-altering drugs on more indirect measures of DA function, such as the behavioral effects of the direct DA agonist, apomorphine, have produced conflicting reports in the literature. More convincing evidence of altered dopaminergic function comes from behavioral responses in animals, showing increased sensitivity of the mesolimbic DA system after chronic antidepressants (Fibiger and Phillips, 1981).

In clinical studies, measures of prolactin (PRL) response to DA agonists provide a neuroendocrine window into central DA function. Response has been reported to be either unchanged or increased after antidepressants or electroconvulsant therapy. In one report (Coppen and Ghose, 1978), amitriptyline enhanced the bromocriptine-induced PRL decrease, suggesting that the TCA has augmented DA function. There are at least two reports that ECT treatment potentiates the PRL response to apomorphine or L-dopa in a way consistent with an effect on DA. Antidepressant effects on growth hormone response to DA agonists have not been investigated except after a monoamine oxidase inhibitor (Koulu and Lammintausta, 1981).

Biochemical studies of receptor density are not consistent with increased postsynaptic DA sensitivity after TCAs, MAOIs, or ECT. The reported stabilizing effect of lithium on postsynaptic DA receptor supersensitivity (induced by denervation or haloperidol) in rat striatum or mesolimbic regions (Pert et al., 1978) has not been consistently found in subsequent studies.[3] The case for lithium attenuation of haloperidol-induced presynaptic DA autoreceptor supersensitivity appears more straightforward (Pittman et al., 1984). Carbamazepine may decrease DA-stimulated production of cAMP (Post et al., 1984a), although it has not so far been found to affect DA receptor density. In high doses, it can decrease DA turnover. Thus, a primary role for DA in the action of antidepressants seems to be not as well supported as is a role for NE.[4] On the other hand, dopamine's involvement in the action of drugs that either induce or relieve mania is well supported by the data. As noted previously, there is no reason to assume that the mechanisms involved in turning mania on or off need to be the mirror image of what happens during depression. The reversal of bipolar depression might involve a more complex biochemical process than the induction of mania in a vulnerable individual at a vulnerable phase of a cycle.

Serotonin—The Permissive Hypothesis

The indoleamine serotonin (5-hydroxytryptamine or 5-HT) is classified as a neurotransmitter, although there is no well-defined link between neuronal firing, 5-HT release, and binding to specific receptors. In fact, even for NE, such relationships have only been demonstrated in the SNS. Overall, 5-HT appears to play a critical modulatory role in the CNS. Its depletion is associated with activation or disinhibition of a wide variety of behaviors. Major serotonin-containing cell bodies in the brain are located in the raphe nucleus, with widespread projections, including those to the cortex, septum, hippocampus, and various hypothalamic nuclei.[5] Animal studies have shown that moderate increases of 5-HT input will either cause or facilitate the release of certain pituitary hormones, especially prolactin, through unknown hypothalamic mechanisms. Moreover, an intact 5-HT system may be necessary to obtain chronic effects of antidepressant drugs on noradrenergic β-receptors and to achieve clinical antidepressant effects.

The permissive hypothesis of serotonin function anticipated later developments in neurobiology by focusing on the interaction of amine systems. According to this theory, both the manic and the depressive phases of bipolar illness are characterized by low central 5-HT function. Extensive data from a variety of animal species suggest that brain 5-HT systems dampen or inhibit a variety of functions subserved by other neurotransmitters. The permissive hypothesis postulates that defective serotonergic dampening of other neurotransmitter systems (perhaps especially the norepinephrine and dopamine systems) permits the wide excursions between depression and mania.

This hypothesis was based, in part, on earlier reports of low CSF levels of the serotonin metabolite 5-hydroxyindoleacetic acid (5-HIAA) in both mania and depression and their persistence after recovery.[6] Also consistent with the permissive hypothesis are findings suggesting that chronic lithium administration enhances or stabilizes central 5-HT systems (Mandell and Knapp, 1979), as well as clinical reports of successful prophylaxis with 5-HT precursors, either alone or in combination with lithium. The permissive hypothesis represented an advance over the earlier single-amine too much/too little hypotheses, because it could encompass the clinical reality that manic and depressive states are not in all respects opposite (see Chapter 2).

The ability of antidepressant treatments to influence the 5-HT system has been extensively evaluated. The most widely used TCAs inhibit 5-HT as well as NE uptake, as evidenced by both animal and clinical studies (e.g., platelet 5-HT uptake). Even drugs, such as desipramine, that are initially selective for NE uptake inhibition may affect 5-HT after chronic treatment by producing down-regulation, as reflected by reduced 5-HIAA in human CSF—a reduction that presumably reflects reduced turnover (Potter et al., 1985).[7] Despite common effects on 5-HT turnover, TCAs do not appear to down-regulate 5-HT receptors consistently in all species (Chuang et al., 1980),[8] and another antidepressant treatment, ECT, actually increases these receptors in certain brain regions. Like TCAs, MAOIs increase 5-HT concentration at the synapse but by a different mechanism—inhibiting the amine's breakdown. Thus, chronic treatment

with MAOIs does down-regulate 5-HT$_1$ (presynaptic) receptors. The effects of chronic *lithium* on 5-HT receptors are regionally specific: 5-HT receptor sites are reduced in the rat hippocampus but not in the cortex (Maggi and Enna, 1980; Treiser et al., 1981). Furthermore, at least in classic animal studies, chronic lithium administration decreases both whole brain 5-HT turnover and the activity of its rate-limiting synthetic enzyme, tryptophan hydroxylase, in the midbrain (Knapp and Mandell, 1973).[9]

As a group, antidepressant treatments either reduce or fail to change 5-HT receptors after chronic administration. On the other hand, behavioral and electrophysiological studies indicate an enhancement of 5-HT-mediated responses following the same antidepressant treatments (see review by Sugrue, 1983).[10] This discrepancy between measures of serotonergic receptor number and in vivo response measures reflecting activation suggests that the functional organization of 5-HT systems is different from that of the NE systems. A close link apparently exists between the presynaptic neuron, the transmitter itself, and postsynaptic receptor activity in the norepinephrine system, but not in the serotonin system.

Summary of Drug–Monoamine Interactions

Table 17-1 summarizes the antidepressant–monoamine receptor interactions (later we return to the issue of the interactions between amine systems). The chronic application of a wide variety of antidepressant treatments—classic tricyclics, atypical antidepressants, MAOIs, and ECT—demonstrates receptor effects that are, by and large, consistent across these treatments. They all down-regulate (that is, decrease the number of) postsynaptic β-adrenergic receptors while enhancing response to serotonergic and α-adrenergic stimulation. Chronic lithium also can decrease β-receptor function, down-regulate serotonin receptors in some regions, and perhaps enhance the stability of dopamine systems and of midbrain serotonin systems by improving synthetic capacity (through increased synthesis of tryptophan hydroxylase), while narrowing the range of fluctuation by decreasing tryptophan uptake into the nerve ending. Later we return to the subject of just how, or indeed whether, these pharmacological effects in animals relate to the

Table 17-1. Effects of TCAs, MAOIs, Lithium, and Carbamazepine
on Neurotransmitter Systems in Animals and Humans

	TCAs	MAOIs	Lithium	Carbamazepine
Chronic Biochemical Effects in Animals				
NE uptake	↓	=	= - ↑	↓
5-HT uptake	↓ - ↓	=	=	?
Monoamine oxidase	↓	↓	=	=
Chronic Effects on Receptor Density or Coupling to Cyclic AMP in Animals				
Beta-adrenergic	⇓	⇓	= - ↓	=
Alpha₁	= - ↑	=	=	?
Alpha₂	↓	⇓	= - ↓	?
5-HT₁	=	⇓	= - ?↓	?
5-HT₂	⇓	⇓	= - ↓	?
Dopamine-2	=	= - ?	= - ↓	?
GABA-B	⇑	= - ↑	?	?
Human Studies of Neurotransmitter Turnover				
MHPG in urine or CSF	⇓	⇓	= - ↓	=
"Sum" of metabolites in urine	⇓	↓	= - ↓	?
5-HT via 5-HIAA in CSF	⇓	↓	= - ?	=
Dopamine via HVA in CSF	=	↓ - ⇓	= - ?	= - ↓
Responses Related to Neurotransmitter Function in Humans				
Norepinephrine (NE)				
Plasma NE increase on standing	⇑	=	?	?
Heart rate	⇑	= - ↓	=	?
Blood pressure response to clonidine	⇓	= - ↓	?	?
Blood pressure response to phenylephrine	= - ↓	↑	?	?
Growth hormone response to NE agonists	↓	↓	?	?
Melatonin output	↑	↑	?	?
Serotonin (5-HT)				
Prolactin response to L-tryptophan	↑ᵃ	?	↑	↑
Cortisol response to 5-HTP	↓ᵃ	↑	↑	?

Entries indicating a range of effects reflect variability in the literature dependent on brain region studied, etc.

= = no effect
↓ = slight decrease, ⇓ = moderate decrease, ↓ = marked decrease
↑ = slight increase, ⇑ = moderate increase, ↑ = marked increase.
? = data unavailable or unclear

a Magnitude of response is indicated only as slight, since it is a normalization of response rather than enhancement or suppression

clinical actions of these drugs in manic-depressive patients.

Acetylcholine

Acetylcholine (ACh) is one of the most ubiquitously distributed neurotransmitters in the peripheral and central nervous systems. It acts on at least two types of presynaptic and postsynaptic receptors, the so-called muscarinic and nicotinic receptors, reflecting the action of the classic agonists. The net effect of cholinergic alterations can be either inhibitory or stimulatory, depending on the system with which it interacts. Unlike the case for norepinephrine, serotonin, and dopamine, there is no high-affinity (re)uptake system; deactivation of ACh depends primarily on hydrolysis by either neuronal acetylcholinesterase or non-neuronal (glial) pseudocholinesterase. This is the basis for using cholinesterase inhibitors as indirect cholinergic agonists. In the CNS, the major collection of ACh neurons is designated the magnocellular nuclei of the basal forebrain (MNBF).[11] Specific portions of the MNBF project to both cerebrocortical and limbic areas, which may be implicated in the affective and vegetative symptoms of depression. There is also a dopaminergic input to the tractus, the major cholinergic nucleus in the MNBF. Such connections suggest that models for central ACh function need to include variants of the well-known balance of peripheral autonomic control between the parasympathetic (acetylcholine) and sympathetic (norepinephrine) systems.

Some investigators have postulated a bridge from ACh to manic-depressive illness (increased ACh associated with depression, decreased with mania) because of the mood and behavioral effects of cholinergic agonists and antagonists. This association initially stemmed from observations that industrial poisoning with cholinesterase inhibitors (which enhance ACh function by inhibiting its degradation) produced a depression-like clinical picture (Rowntree et al., 1950). Janowsky and co-workers (1973c) noted that physostigmine, a central cholinesterase inhibitor, caused brief but dramatic decreases in manic symptoms, a finding replicated by Modestin and colleagues (1973 a,b) and Davis and associates (1978). Because physostigmine made the patients sick, questions were raised about the specificity of the finding. Proponents of the ACh hypothesis point out that generally the effect—inhibition of behavior and reduction of mania—precedes the nonspecific nausea and vomiting. Physostigmine administration can also precipitate depression in euthymic bipolar patients maintained on lithium (Oppenheim et al., 1979) and in normal volunteers (reviewed by Janowsky and Risch, 1984). The direct muscarinic agonist arecoline also produces depressive symptoms in euthymic bipolar patients off lithium and in normal volunteers (Nurnberger et al., 1983a, 1989).

The relationship between central ACh systems and the actions of standard antidepressant and antimanic drugs is less clear. Clinically, the anticholinergic effects of antidepressant drugs do not correlate with their potency. Central muscarinic

receptor densities are unaltered by chronic treatment with TCAs, MAOIs, or various second-generation antidepressants.

Studies of lithium's effects on muscarinic receptors have been interpreted as showing both that it stabilizes them by preventing up-regulation[12] and, conversely, that it additively increases the up-regulation that follows chronic treatment with a cholinergic antagonist (Lerer and Stanley, 1985). The more general notion that lithium may exert an effect only on selected components of variably disrupted or particularly active neurotransmitter systems remains attractive whatever the direction of change.

The initial theory formulating a role for ACh in mood regulation was cast in terms of the balance between noradrenergic and cholinergic systems (Gjessing, 1938; Janowsky et al., 1972). According to this hypothesis, mania involves a relative predominance of noradrenergic over cholinergic tone, and depression represents the reverse. An extension of the balance hypothesis involves dopamine. It has been suggested that the anticholinergic properties of some antidepressants may facilitate at least one apparent dopamine-mediated effect: locomotor stimulation by amphetamine (Martin-Iverson et al., 1983). Anticholinergic action could remove some degree of tonic inhibitory input to dopamine neurons and perhaps thereby contribute to the mania-inducing potential of antidepressants. Furthermore, the ability of lithium to prevent supersensitivity of peripheral and central ACh receptors (as induced by denervation or atropine) (Belmaker et al., 1982) may contribute to its mood-stabilizing properties. This stabilization apparently can be overcome by a physostigmine challenge, since, as noted, depression can be precipitated this way in euthymic patients on lithium.

γ-Aminobutyric Acid

γ-Aminobutyric acid (GABA), widespread in the CNS, is the major inhibitory neurotransmitter, diminishing the activity of its many target neurons. GABAergic neurons are much more diffusely located than catecholaminergic neurons, with similar GABA concentrations found in diverse brain regions. Functions of GABA include a general inhibitory role on brain excitability.[13] One version of a GABA hypothesis of affective illness is based on the fact that specific GABA neurons provide an inhibitory input to several dopamine systems and perhaps also to some norepinephrine systems.

Drugs that have been shown to reduce mania—lithium, carbamazepine, valproate, and propranolol—enhance GABAergic transmission (Bernasconi, 1982). This effect suggested the hypothesis that a GABA deficiency, perhaps in limbic structures, may be involved in the pathogenesis of manic syndromes (Bernasconi, 1982).

It has also been proposed that GABA is involved in the mechanism of action of antidepressant drugs and ECT (Lloyd et al., 1989). This group notes that in animal models of depression, GABA-mimetic drugs show antidepressant activity, and this activity is blocked by bicuculline, a selective GABA receptor blocker. Furthermore, Lloyd and colleagues report that chronic treatment with a wide variety of antidepressant drugs and ECT is similar to treatment with GABA-mimetic agents in their capacity to up-regulate GABA receptors[14] while down-regulating β-adrenergic receptors. Thus, the apparent pharmacological enhancement of GABA transmission has been associated with both antimanic and antidepressant effects; this would be consistent with some mood–behavior modulating role for GABA systems and may relate to the kindling–sensitization models described in Chapter 16.

Evidence in Manic-Depressive Illness

Postmortem Brain Studies of Monoamine Function

The most direct attempts to evaluate amine disturbances in depression have examined postmortem brain tissue from depressed patients (usually suicide victims). The initial studies were of brainstem or hindbrain; subsequently, more discrete areas were assayed. Table 17-2 perhaps suggests a pattern of decreased serotonin and its metabolite 5-HIAA in the depressed (suicide) group. However, the neurotransmitter specificity of this association is difficult to evaluate from these studies, since half of them dealt only with serotonin and its metabolites. Decreases in catecholamines (and metabolites) also have been noted in a few reports. Studies in which brains from suicides are examined for differences in imipramine-binding sites (which label serotonergic neurons) are reviewed later, in the section on receptor studies.

The use of brains from suicide victims was seen at first as an opportunistic approach to the biochemical study of depression. Evidence is

Table 17-2. Postmortem Brain Studies of Monoamine Function

Study	Subjects N Depressed	Control	5-HT	5-HIAA	NE	DA	MHPG
Shaw et al., 1967	11	17	↓				
Bourne et al., 1968	16	15	NC	↓	NC		
Pare et al., 1969	23	15	↓	NC	NC	NC	
Lloyd et al., 1974	5	5	NC[a]	NC			
Baskow et al., 1976	11	62	NC	NC[b]	NC[b]	NC	
Cochran et al., 1976	10	12	NC				
Crow et al., 1984	15	22		NC			NC

NC = no change

[a] 5-HT significantly reduced in 2 (dorsal raphe and central inferior nuclei) of 14 structures examined

[b] NE reduced in 2 of 3 structures examined and 5-HIAA reduced in 6 of 8 structures examined, but significance attributed to time lapse until autopsy

Adapted from Crow et al., 1984

now emerging, however, that these and related findings may be more specific to suicide (reflecting personality factors, such as impulsivity and aggression) than to depression per se. This important issue is discussed later in this chapter in the section on clinical–biological correlates.

Cerebrospinal Fluid Amines and Amine Metabolites

Methodological Issues. Cerebrospinal fluid provides a major route of access to the hypothesized amine systems dysfunction in manic-depressive illness. HVA, 5-HIAA, and 3-methoxy-4-hydroxyphenylglycol (MHPG) are the major CSF metabolites of brain dopamine, serotonin, and norepinephrine, respectively. Dihydroxyphenylacetic acid (DOPAC) and vanillylmandelic acid (VMA) are minor metabolites of dopamine and norepinephrine.

An important concern in research on CNS metabolites is the relative proportion removed from brain tissue by the CSF. Some metabolites are undoubtedly removed directly by the bloodstream, but because of the periventricular location of many important aminergic nuclei and terminals, a substantial proportion of transmitter metabolism in these systems is likely to be reflected in spinal fluid. For clinical studies, another major question is the extent to which amine metabolites are derived from amine turnover in the cord rather than in the brain, presumably the more critical information.

The origins of the three monoamine metabolites in lumbar CSF are reviewed elsewhere (Post and Goodwin, 1978). The findings, in summary, are: Lumbar HVA predominantly reflects brain dopamine turnover; for 5-HIAA, both spinal cord and brain sources contribute, whereas for MHPG, the major source is the spinal cord and the peripheral nervous system. However, even though MHPG and, to a lesser extent, 5-HIAA reflect substantial nonbrain contributions, alterations in CSF levels of these metabolites may still reflect brain functioning, since many of the serotonin and norepinephrine axons and nerve terminals in the cord originate in functionally important higher brainstem nuclei.[15]

Various methodological difficulties confound the interpretation of CSF metabolite data, such as length of time off medication, description of patient samples, nature of the control group, age and sex contributions, and the impact of diet, activity level, time of day, time of year, and body height (Table 17-3). One variable that is virtually never controlled for is the phase of illness. It is axiomatic in psychopharmacology that biochemical effects of a drug change as a function of time; that is, the effects of acute administration differ from the effects of chronic use. We suggest that parallel phenomena occur in the course of affective illness. Biochemical measurements early in an episode may be very different from those taken later in the episode, and changes seen after a first episode may not parallel those following later episodes, when the process being measured may have been substantially altered by repetitions. These issues are discussed extensively elsewhere (Cowdry et al., 1983a; Goodwin and Post, 1983; Jimerson and Berrettini, 1985).

Depression. Tables 17-4A, B, and C summarize controlled, baseline (i.e., nonprobenecid) studies

Table 17-3. Factors Contributing to Variability in CSF Metabolite Studies

- Age
- Sex
- Height
- Weight
- Drugs (specific and nonspecific effects)
- Withdrawal status
- Menstrual status and hormonal state
- Motor activity
- Acute stress/anxiety
- Personality variables
- Phase of illness
- Other physical illness
- Diurnal variation
- Seasonal variation
- Assay methodology
- Position of patient for lumbar puncture
- Site of lumbar puncture
- CSF aliquot
- CSF storage conditions
- Probenecid level
- Diet
- Nature of control group
- Diagnostic criteria

of CSF MHPG, HVA, and 5-HIAA, expressed as a percentage of control values. Primarily because they were published before the bipolar–unipolar distinction became accepted, most of these studies (similar to the postmortem studies) do not distinguish between the subgroups. Table 17-5 depicts those studies that investigated bipolar–unipolar differences.

CSF MHPG. Of the 16 studies reporting CSF MHPG findings in depressed patients and control subjects (Table 17-4A), two groups, using mass spectroscopy assays, reported significantly higher levels of MHPG in depression,[16] whereas two of the older studies found significantly lower levels. The majority of the studies found no significant differences or trends, however.[17] Considering only studies in which the patients were off drugs for 10 days or more does not alter the con-

Table 17-4A. Controlled Baseline Studies of CSF MHPG in Depression and Mania

	Patients N			Control Mean %		
Study	Control	Depressed	Manic	50	100	150
Med-free ≥ 10 days						
Post et al., 1973	10	25	9	◆a	◇ 16.3	
Shaw et al., 1973	13	22 UP			◆ 10.8	
Berger et al., 1980	23	13			◆ 9.2	
Koslow et al., 1983	61	99	14		◆b 8.0	◇b
Jimerson et al., 1984b	11	20			8.1	◆a
Widerlöv et al., 1988a	10	22			◆ 9.6	
Potter et al., unpublished data	48	101			◆ 7.6	
Med-free < 10 days						
Wilk et al., 1972	19	5	6		◆ 15.0	◇
Shopsin et al., 1974	18	8	13		◆ 15.9	◇a
Subrahmanyam, 1975	12	24		◆a	20.6	
Ashcroft et al., 1976	11	7	5		◆ 13.0	◇b (223%)
Vestergaard et al., 1978	21	27	4		◆ 10.4	◇
Oreland et al., 1981	42	18			◆ 9.1	
Träskman et al., 1981	45	7			◆ 9.7	
Gerner et al., 1984	33	34	14		◆◇a 7.7	
Åsberg et al., 1984	60	26 UP 2 BP I 6 BP II		◆	◆ 9.5	

The mean metabolite level (ng/ml) for the control group in each study appears in the 100% column. The shaded bar indicates standard error (expressed in percentage points) around the control mean expressed as 100%. (Data not available in Shopsin study.)

◆ = Mean for depressed group expressed as % of control mean
◇ = Mean for manic group expressed as % of control mean

a *p* < .05 vs. controls
b *p* < .01 vs. controls

Table17-4B. Controlled Baseline Studies of CSF HVA in Depression and Mania

| Study | Patients N | | | Control Mean % | | |
	Control	Depressed	Manic	50	100	150
Med-free ≥ 10 days						
Papeschi & McClure, 1971	18	17		◆[b]	50.0	
Brodie et al., 1973	6	7		◆[b]	51.0	
Goodwin et al., 1973	28	53	16		◆ 22.4 ◇	
Koslow et al., 1983	30 M	49 M	9 M		◆[b] 40.1 ◇	◇[a]
	32 F	43 F	5 F		◆ 43.7	
Roy et al., 1985b	41	27			◆ 28.2	
Widerlöv et al., 1988a	10	22			◆ 37.0	
Potter et al., unpublished	49	101			◆ 32.8	
Med-free < 10 days						
Van Praag & Korf, 1971	12	20			◆ 42.0	
Wilk et al.,1972	19	5	6	◆	◇ 18.0	
Van Praag et al., 1973	12	28			35.8 ◆	
Takahashi et al., 1974	30	30 UP			◆ 37.5	
Subrahmanyam, 1975	12	24			◆ 40.2	
Ashcroft et al., 1976	31	11 UP	11	◆[a]	◇	
		9 BP			◆ 41.0	
Banki, 1977	32 F	71 F	10 F		◆[b] 33.4	◇[b]
Vestergaard et al., 1978	23	29	4		◆ 45.0	◇[a] (256%)
Oreland et al.,1981	28 M	6 M			◆ 39.1	
	14 F	14 F			◆ 47.8	
Träskman et al., 1981	45	8			◆[b] 44.5	
Kasa et al., 1982	16	13		◆	41.8	
Gerner et al., 1984	37	38	13		◆ 28.6	◇
Åsberg et al., 1984	66	43 UP			◆[b]	
		4 BP I			◆	
		11 BP II			◆ 44.7	

The mean metabolite level (ng/ml) for the control group in each study appears in the 100% column. The shaded bar indicates standard error (expressed in percentage points) around the control mean expressed as 100%. (Data not available in Wilk study.)

◆ = Mean for depressed group expressed as % of control mean
◇ = Mean for manic group expressed as % of control mean

[a] $p < .05$ vs. controls   [b] $p < .01$ vs. controls

Table 17-4C. Controlled Baseline Studies of CSF 5-HIAA in Depression and Mania

Study	Patients N			Control Mean %		
	Control	Depressed	Manic	50	100	150
Med-free ≥ 10 days						
Ashcroft et al., 1966	21	24			19.1	
Papeschi & McClure, 1971	10	12			28.0	
Brodie et al., 1973	6	7			35.0	
Goodwin et al., 1973	29	58	16		27.3	
Berger et al., 1980	23 M	13 M			27.7	
Banki et al., 1981	32 F	33 F			27.0	
Koslow et al., 1983	29 M	49 M	9 M		20.1	
	29 F	43 F	5 F		21.0	
Roy et al., 1985b	41	27			13.0	
Widerlöv et al., 1988a	10	22			15.0	
Potter et al., unpublished data	49	100			15.6	
Med-free < 10 days						
Bowers et al., 1969	8	8	8		39.5 42.8	
Van Praag & Korf, 1971	11	14			40.0	
Coppen et al., 1972b	20	31	18		42.3	
Wilk et al.,1972	19	5	6		29.0	
Van Praag et al., 1973	12	28			29.0	
Takahashi et al., 1974	30	30			30.4	
Subrahmanyam, 1975	12	24			40.2	
Ashcroft et al., 1976	30	11 UP 9 BP	11		16.0	
Banki, 1977	32 F	71 F	10 F		27.5	
Vestergaard et al., 1978	22	28	4		28.0	
Curzon et al.,1980	5	20			16.4	
Oreland et al.,1981	28 M	6 M			16.8	
	14 F	14 F			22.8	
Gerner et al., 1984	37	38	13		22.2	

Continued

Table 17-4C Continued. Controlled Baseline Studies of CSF 5-HIAA in Depression and Mania

	Patients N			Control Mean %		
Study	Control	Depressed	Manic	50	100	150
Åsberg et al., 1984	66	60 UP			◆a ▩	
		8 BPI			◆ ▩	
		15 BPII			◆ 19.3	
Gjerris et al., 1987	10	21			20.4 ◆	

The mean metabolite level (ng/ml) for the control group in each study appears in the 100% column. Shaded bar indicates standard error (expressed in percentage points) around the control mean expressed as 100%. (Data not available in Wilk et al., 1972, and Gjerris et al., 1987.)

◆ = Mean for depressed group expressed as % of control mean
◇ = Mean for manic group expressed as % of control mean

[a]Depressed vs controls, $p < .05$
[b]Manics vs controls, $p < .01$

clusion. No bipolar–unipolar differences in MHPG were found in studies that examined the issue (Table 17-5).[18]

Methodological difficulties have so far limited the assessment of CSF levels of the amines themselves. There are no data on serotonin or dopamine, measured by validated assay, and only two studies of norepinephrine and two of epinephrine,[19] which together provide scant data on bipolar patients. Also, the likelihood that CSF norepinephrine could reflect plasma levels raises a question as to the importance of these studies.

CSF HVA. Of the 20 studies comparing depressed patients with controls (Table 17-4B), none reported significantly higher levels, whereas 7 reported significantly lower levels, and most of the others indicated a trend toward lower levels in depression. The majority of the probenecid studies also showed lower accumulations of HVA in depressed patients compared with controls. Of the 11 studies examining the bipolar and unipolar subgroups, only 1 found a significant difference (bipolar lower than unipolar). The probenecid studies also failed to uncover bipolar–unipolar differences (Table 17-5).

CSF 5-HIAA. Historically, 5-HIAA was the first CSF metabolite examined in depression (Ashcroft and Sharman, 1960). Is CSF 5-HIAA of depressed patients significantly different from that of controls? No simple answer can be given. Most of the 5-HIAA studies (Table 17-4C) involved the older fluorometric assay technique and were done under poorly described and variable

conditions. Seven of the 25 studies reported significantly lower levels, and only 1 showed a significantly higher level,[20] with the rest showing no consistent trends. Again separating out those involving longer off-drug periods did not clarify the data. The majority of probenecid studies reported lower accumulations in depressed patients than in controls.

Of the 10 baseline studies that specifically considered bipolar–unipolar differences (Table 17-5), 1 found higher levels in bipolar patients,[21] 4 noted a trend for lower levels in bipolar patients,[22] and the rest found no difference. However, one of the best controlled of these (Åsberg et al., 1984) showed no differences at all between bipolar-I, bipolar-II, and unipolar patients. Further, the cumulative intramural NIMH series involving only patients who had been off drugs at least 3 weeks found no difference in the CSF 5-HIAA of 54 unipolar patients compared with 47 bipolar patients (Potter et al., unpublished data).

CSF GABA. In four of six studies, significantly lower GABA levels were found in the CSF of patients with major depression (predominantly unipolar) compared with controls (Table 17-6). Three studies (Post et al., 1980b; Gerner and Hare, 1981; Joffe et al., 1986b) sampled a later aliquot higher up in the rostrocaudal gradient for GABA[23] and found no significant difference between depressed patients and controls. Berrettini and colleagues (1986) sampled euthymic bipolar depressed patients and found them not significantly different from controls.

Table 17-5. CSF Metabolites in Unipolar vs Bipolar Depressed Patients

Study	Patients N		UP Mean =		
	UP	BP	50%	100%	150%
MHPG					
Med-free ≥ 10 days					
Goodwin & Post, 1975	36	27 BP I			
		20 BP II		11.0	
Koslow et al., 1983	61	38		8.9	
Potter et al., unpublished data	54	47		7.6	
Med-free < 10 days					
Vestergaard et al., 1978	13	6		14.0	
Ågren, 1980	21	12		10.8	
Åsberg et al., 1984	26	2 BP I			
		6 BP II		9.4	
HVA					
Med-free ≥ 10 days					
Ashcroft & Glen, 1974	11	9		20.0	
Goodwin & Post, 1975	36	27 BP I			
		20 BP II		22.0	
Bowers & Heninger, 1977[c]	10	8		136.0	
Korf et al., 1983	17	17		100.7	
Koslow et al., 1983	26 M	23 M			
	32 F	11 F			
Potter et al., unpublished data	54	47		26.9	
Med-free < 10 days					
Banki, 1977	55 F	16 F	[b]	24.0	
Vestergaard et al., 1978	14	6		88.0	
Ågren, 1980	21	12		37.1	
Kasa et al., 1982	10	3		19.6	
Åsberg et al., 1984	43	4 BP I			
		11 BP II		36.7	
5-HIAA					
Med-free ≥ 10 days					
Ashcroft & Glen, 1974	11	9		10.0	[a]
Goodwin & Post, 1975	36	27 BP I			
		20 BP II		26.0	
Bowers & Heninger, 1977[c]	10	8		111.8	
Korf et al., 1983	17	17		65.2	
Koslow et al., 1983	26 M	23 M		19.1	
	31 F	12 F		24.7	
Potter et al., unpublished data	54	46		16.7	

Continued

Table 17-5 Continued. CSF Metabolites in Unipolar vs Bipolar Depressed Patients

Study	Patients N		UP Mean =		
	UP	BP	50%	100%	150%
Med-free < 10 days					
Banki, 1977	55 F	16 F		16.4	
Vestergaard et al., 1978	14	6		32.0	
Ågren, 1980	21	12		20.4	
Åsberg et al., 1984	60	8 BP I		17.1	
		15 BP II			

Mean metabolite level (ng/ml) for the unipolar group in each study appears in the 100% column. The shaded bar indicates standard error (expressed in percentage points) around the control mean expressed as 100%.

◆ = mean for bipolar depressed patients expressed as a percentage of the unipolar mean

[a] UP < BP, $p < .05$
[b] BP < UP, $p < .01$
[c] Study measured post-probenecid accumulations

Mania. Most data on amine-metabolite levels in mania are from the same studies just reviewed for depression. Here we note comparisons between manic patients and controls and between mania and depression. Studies comparing manic patients with controls are also summarized in Tables 17-4A, B, and C. Unfortunately, the mania-depression comparisons are difficult to interpret, since the depressed groups of earlier studies generally included both bipolar and unipolar patients.

CSF MHPG. As noted previously, advances

Table 17-6. Controlled Baseline Studies of CSF GABA in Depression and Mania

Study	Patients N			CV	C	D as % of C	S	M as % of C	S	Comments
	C	D	M							
Med-Free at least 1 week										
Gerner & Hare, 1981	29	24	6	34	183.2	73	$p < .01$	102	NS	D < M, $p < .01$ no BP-UP differences
Kasa et al., 1982	24	13		41	137.5	70	$p < .05$			UP > BP, NS
Gerner et al., 1984	36	37	12	14	190	74	$p < .05$	90	NS	D < M, $p < .01$
Med-Free at least 2 weeks										
Gold et al., 1980	20	15		53	218	56	$p < .01$			UP < BP, NS
Berrettini et al., 1986	34	15		35	127	102	NS			BPs only, some lithium treated
Joffe et al., 1986b[a]	41	42	8	17	233	88	NS	83	NS	

Control group mean metabolite levels in pmol/ml. Mean levels for depressed and manic patients expressed as a percentage of controls. Three separate assay techniques were used: Kasa et al., Gerner and Hare, and Joffe et al. used only fluorometric chromatography; Gold et al. and Berrettini et al. used only radioreceptor binding; and Gerner et al. used atomic absorption spectrophotometry. Gerner and Hare and Joffe et al. also took samples from the 15-28 ml and neither found D vs C differences.

C = controls, D = depressed, M = manic, CV = coefficient of variation = control group standard deviation divided by control mean, expressed as a percentage, S = significance of difference

[a]Reanalysis of Post et al., 1980b

in assay methodology for MHPG make cross-study comparisons difficult, but the literature is reasonably extensive, although less extensive than that concerning the acid metabolites. Four of seven studies found significantly higher levels of MHPG in manic patients than in controls. Control means vary by a factor of 2, with the later studies reporting lower means (perhaps reflecting more sensitive assay techniques). Three studies comparing manic patients with bipolar depressed patients reported CSF MHPG significantly higher in the manic than in depressed patients (O'Keeffe and Brooksbank, 1973; Vestergaard et al., 1978; Koslow et al., 1983), whereas one other (Gerner et al., 1984) gave insufficient data to make this comparison. Older studies with mixed depressed groups support this finding.

In studies of norepinephrine in the CSF of manic patients, Post and colleagues (1978b) found significantly increased levels compared with both depressed patients and controls.

CSF HVA. Compared with controls, the baseline levels of HVA in the CSF of manic patients have been reported as increased in four studies and not significantly different in three studies. When manic patients are compared with depressed patients, the results are more consistent: Five studies[24] separating bipolar depressed patients reported higher HVA in mania, and one other gave insufficient data to make this comparison (Gerner et al., 1984). These studies confirm the evidence from older studies with mixed depressed groups. Reports of significant differences in probenecid-induced accumulations of HVA are inconclusive. Sjöström (1973) was unable to replicate his own earlier finding of reduced HVA.

CSF 5-HIAA. Reports of baseline levels of 5-HIAA in the CSF of manic patients compared with controls do not reveal a consistent trend. Six studies showed no difference, two reported a significantly lower level in manic patients, and the NIMH collaborative study found CSF 5-HIAA to be significantly higher but only in women (Koslow et al., 1983).[25] Two of the six studies showing nonsignificant trends indicate lower 5-HIAA levels, however.

Reports comparing 5-HIAA in the CSF of manic patients with that of depressed patients have been remarkably consistent. All studies but one showed no significant difference between depression and mania. This is consistent with the proposition that 5-HIAA is independent of state but does not answer whether it is relevant to manic-depressive illness (see the discussion of well-state studies later in this chapter).

CSF GABA. The GABA level in the CSF during mania was examined by Post and colleagues (1980b), who found no difference between 8 manic patients and a mixed group of 16 depressed patients (Table 17-6). Joffe and co-workers' re-examination (1986b) of Post's original data likewise yielded no significant differences between manic and depressed or control patients. Two studies by the same group (Gerner and Hare, 1981; Gerner et al., 1984) indicate that a CSF gradient for GABA may affect the results. When the CSF was taken from a lower aliquot in the rostrocaudal gradient, a significant mania-depression difference was found, but not when taken from a higher aliquot, that is, in a way similar to Post's earlier study.

Mixed State, Well-State, and Longitudinal Studies. Mixed states (the simultaneous presence of manic and depressive symptoms) are now recognized as common (see Chapter 2), and it is likely that the biochemical studies already reviewed include such patients among subjects diagnosed as manic. To our knowledge, there is only one CSF study focusing on mixed states, that of Tandon and colleagues (1988), who compared mixed bipolar patients with pure manic and unipolar depressive patients. Whereas both HVA and 5-HIAA were higher in the patients with pure mania than in those with depression, the mixed group could be biochemically divided into two groups whose metabolite levels resembled the pure manic and pure depressive groups, respectively. In addition, these authors compared their metabolite data to published normal control values obtained by the same method and noted that all three groups had 5-HIAA levels that were significantly below normal, a finding they interpreted as consistent with the permissive hypothesis.

In a few of the CSF amine metabolite studies, the measurements were repeated after recovery in an attempt to assess the well state. As outlined in Chapter 15, abnormal findings in the well state (i.e., state-independent findings) may represent vulnerability markers, perhaps reflecting a genetic factor. In most studies of the well state, however, it is virtually impossible to tease drug effects apart from the recovered state itself. The study of spontaneous or ECT-induced recovery is one approach to this problem, but only preliminary data are available.

Coppen and colleagues (1972b), Ashcroft and co-workers (1973), and Van Praag and De Haan (1979) reported that their depressed patients with low levels of CSF 5-HIAA failed to normalize with recovery. Berrettini and colleagues (1985b), by contrast, found no difference in CSF 5-HIAA (and HVA) in recovered bipolar patients compared with healthy controls, although this study did not compare the well state to the illness phase in the same patients.[26] As in the case of the MHPG findings, the interpretation of these data depends on the nature of the control group. The persistence of low 5-HIAA levels reported by Coppen and by Van Praag is of interest in light of the suggestion that CSF 5-HIAA is similar in both the manic and depressive phases of the illness. Relevant to these questions are two small longitudinal studies of CSF 5-HIAA (Post et al., 1980a; Åsberg et al., 1973), which demonstrate reasonable stability of 5-HIAA levels over time. The issue of postrecovery metabolite data re-emerges when we review drug effects.

In a carefully designed study of CSF MHPG, Berrettini and colleagues (1985b) found no differences between normal controls and bipolar patients in the well state (2 weeks off lithium).

In a longitudinal study of one patient with rapid cycles, Joffe and co-workers (1986b) found CSF GABA significantly higher in the patient's five manic episodes than in the four depressed episodes. Two well-state studies of CSF GABA (Joffe et al. 1986b; Berrettini et al., 1986) produced conflicting results; the former noted lower levels compared with controls, and the latter did not.

To our knowledge, no group of bipolar patients has been studied with serial measurement of CSF metabolites through their depressive and manic phases. A few scattered cases of rapid-cycling patients have been presented, although it is not clear just how representative such patients are. Post and co-workers (1977) and Cutler and Post (1982b) followed CSF amine metabolites through seven depressive phases and eight manic phases in three patients. Baseline and probenecid-induced accumulation of 5-HIAA and HVA were not significantly different during mania and depression, but norepinephrine levels were significantly higher in mania. Additional longitudinal studies are discussed in the next two sections. The CSF amine and metabolite data are summarized at the end of this chapter when we evaluate biochemical correlates of clinical phenomena.

Plasma Amines, Amine Metabolites, and Amino Acids

Only a few studies of major depressive illness have examined amines and related compounds in plasma. These have focused on norepinephrine and its metabolite MHPG, and serotonin and its precursor, the amino acid tryptophan, along with two reports of the dopamine metabolite, HVA. Five of seven studies of supine plasma NE in unipolar patients reported increased levels compared with controls (Table 17-7). All four of the studies that made bipolar–unipolar comparisons found increased levels in unipolar patients. These same results generally can be found in the studies of upright plasma NE levels and NE response to a cold challenge (Roy et al., 1987b). Three of four studies found elevated levels in unipolar patients compared with bipolar patients and normal controls. It has been postulated that the increase in plasma NE may be specific to a subgroup of unipolar patients, namely, those with melancholia (Roy et al., 1985c).[27]

The few available studies of plasma MHPG in depression do not reveal an overall difference between primarily unipolar patients and controls, although three groups reported an increase in melancholic patients or those with a positive dexamethasone suppression test (DST) (Jimerson et al., 1983; Devanand et al., 1985; Roy et al., 1986). A greater variance in plasma MHPG has also been noted in patients with major depression (both bipolar and unipolar) than in controls (Siever et al., 1986). Wolkowitz and colleagues (1987) reported no significant differences between unipolar and bipolar patients. Plasma MHPG was followed longitudinally in two rapid-cycling bipolar patients (one with schizoaffective features) by Jimerson and colleagues (1981). All MHPG values during mania were higher than all values during depression, and the MHPG increase appeared to follow the switch from one state to another rather than precede it. Halaris

(1978) followed plasma MHPG longitudinally in a manic patient before and during treatment with lithium and noted a gradual decrease in MHPG, which only began after full clinical remission. However, other, more recent studies find no significant change in plasma MHPG after ECT (Linnoila et al., 1984; Devanand et al., 1989).

Plasma HVA was found to be increased above control values among female depressed patients with melancholic symptoms, especially among those with psychotic features (Devanand et al., 1985). Roy (1988) did not replicate this finding, however. As with their findings in MHPG, Linnoila and colleagues (1984) and Devanand and associates (1989) reported no difference in plasma HVA levels after ECT.

Data on blood levels of serotonin are difficult to interpret, since normally circulating serotonin

Table 17-7. Plasma NE (pg/ml)

Study	Control N	Control Mean ± SEM	UP N	UP Mean ± SEM	BP N	BP Mean ± SEM	Results
Supine							
Wyatt et al., 1971	22	200 ± 17.1	10	360 ± 25.3			C < UP (p <.01)
Esler et al., 1982[b]	17	225 ± 8.0	11	427 ± 49.4			C < UP (p <.05)
Lake et al., 1982[a,b]	22	270 ± 6.4	15	530 ± 33.6	30	420 ± 10.9	C < BP< UP (p <.05)[d] C < BP (p <.05)[d]
Veith et al., 1983[c]	8	390.8	14	304.5			UP < C (ns)
Roy et al., 1985c	41	147.2 ± 6.40	10	219.9 ± 40.7	7	121.8 ± 14.7	BP < C < UP (p <.05)
Rudorfer et al., 1985b	12	263.9 ± 33.8	12	233.5 ± 33.8	12	160.7 ± 25.4	BP < UP < C (p <.05)
Siever et al., 1986	21	232 ± 25.3	11	351 ± 81.1[e]	7	268 ± 29.9	BP < UP (p <.01)
Standing							
Lake et al., 1982	22	500 ± 8.5	8	780 ± 58.6	22	625 ± 13.9	C < BP (p <.05)[d]
Veith et al., 1983[c]	8	583.7	14	575.2			UP < C (ns)
Roy et al., 1985c	41	290.9 ± 17.4	10	444.9 ± 112.9	7	382.3 ± 69.7	C < BP < UP (p <.05)
Rudorfer et al., 1985b	12	463.6 ± 81.2	12	576.9 ± 69.4	12	438.2 ± 77.8	BP < C < UP (ns)

Summary:
   Supine NE levels of UP patients were significantly higher than controls in 4 of 7 studies; UP patients were significantly higher than BP patients in 3 of 4 studies

   Standing NE levels of depressed patients were generally elevated compared with controls; BP patients were consistently lower than UP patients

[a]NE levels (supine and standing) of BP patients tested during manic phase were higher than control levels (p <.05)
[b]Levels approximated from graphed data
[c]Adapted from Rudorfer et al., 1985b
[d]Combined supine and standing measures: C < D (p <.01)
[e]Depressed group variance significantly larger than control group variance (p <.005)

is stored in platelets. Two studies revealed no difference between depressed patients and controls (Gaylord et al., 1973; Kaneko et al., 1975), whereas one (Coppen et al., 1972b) showed lower levels in depressed patients. (Studies of platelet 5-HT are reviewed later in the chapter.)

Interest in the study of tryptophan levels in body fluids was stimulated by Tagliamonte and colleagues' observation (1971) that substantial changes in the levels of this serotonin precursor in plasma were followed by parallel changes in serotonin synthesis in the brain.[28] This finding is consistent with the observation that the rate-limiting enzyme in the synthesis of serotonin (tryptophan hydroxylase) normally is not saturated. In studies of depressed patients, Coppen's group (1967) reported reduced plasma tryptophan in a group of unipolar depressed females, similar to the more recent findings of Cowen and colleagues (1989). On the other hand, three groups (Moller et al., 1976; Wirz-Justice et al., 1975; Niskanen et al., 1976), using dietary controls, could detect no difference in a mixed group of depressed patients, including both bipolar and unipolar. Similarly, Garfinkel and colleagues (1976), studying a depressed group comprised primarily of bipolar patients (eight of ten), found that they did not differ from controls in total or free tryptophan. However, these investigators noted that, after administration of a peripheral decarboxylase inhibitor, the depressed patients, but not the controls, showed an increase in total tryptophan, an increase they interpret as a reduced flux of plasma tryptophan in (bipolar) depression.

The relationship between GABA in plasma and in CSF is not clear. In one small study, no correlation was found (Berrettini and Post, 1984). Petty and Sherman (1984) reported that GABA levels were significantly lower than normal in a group of 62 medicated depressed patients. Only 4 of these patients were bipolar, however, and their mean levels were very close to those of the controls. Combining data from their four previous studies, Coffman and Petty (1986) reported that manic and remitted bipolar patients had significantly higher levels of plasma GABA than those of control subjects, but when the patients were depressed, their plasma GABA levels did not differ from controls. Of the three studies of GABA in recovered bipolar patients, one, using lithium-treated patients, showed GABA levels significantly higher than normal levels (Petty and Sherman, 1984; Coffman and Petty, 1986), whereas the other two, using patients off all medication for 2 weeks, showed significantly lower than normal levels (Berrettini et al., 1983, 1985b). This apparent discrepancy might be explained by the longitudinal finding of the Berrettini group that plasma GABA levels fall significantly after lithium is discontinued. Interestingly, a small study of identical twins revealed that plasma GABA levels show a close intrapair correspondence (Berrettini and Post, 1984). However, it is too early to assess whether this measure will be useful as a trait marker for manic-depressive illness.[29]

Urinary Amines and Metabolites

Methodological Issues. Urinary 5-HIAA has not generally been studied in manic-depressive illness because a very large proportion of this serotonin metabolite appears to originate in the periphery. Urinary dopamine metabolites have not been systematically studied for the same reason. However, the evidence that a substantial portion of plasma HVA may reflect events in the brain (Bacopoulos et al., 1979; Swann et al., 1980) should increase interest in such studies.

The dominant focus of urinary metabolite studies has been on MHPG, the principal metabolite of norepinephrine in the brain. A central question is the extent of the brain's contribution to MHPG excreted in the urine. Initial estimates placed the brain's contribution as high as 60 percent (Maas et al., 1984), but studies using infusions of deuterium-labeled norepinephrine indicate that it is probably not more than 25 percent (Kopin et al., 1984; Márdh et al., 1983).

Despite important questions about the relative central or peripheral contribution to urinary amine metabolites, the study of such metabolites may still aid in understanding the pathophysiology of manic-depressive illness. The clinical symptoms suggest involvement of the peripheral autonomic nervous system, and there are important feedback regulatory interactions between the peripheral sympathetic system and the central aminergic systems.

Urinary metabolites other than MHPG initially were measured primarily as a way of controlling for what was thought to be peripherally contributed noise. One such attempt is Schildkraut and colleagues' (1978) development of the D score, derived from an equation that assigned empirically derived weightings to individual metabolites depending on their relative contributions to the overall difference between his depressed patients and controls.[30] Investigators now tend to study all of the major urinary metabolites of norepinephrine, so that total body norepinephrine turnover, as well as the rate of formation of individual metabolites, can be measured. The extent to which the individual metabolites correlate with each other (and with the amine itself) across patients is controversial.[31]

Interpretation of urinary amine metabolite data is colored by a wide variety of other methodological issues, such as sex and age differences and the effects of diet, activity, and stress. The contribution of these factors has been studied extensively by several groups (reviewed by Potter et al., 1983). Drug treatment is an especially important source of variance, and the standard 2-week washout period may not be long enough (Charney et al., 1981b; Ågren and Potter, 1986).

Urinary MHPG. Table 17-8 lists the studies of urinary MHPG in depression and mania. Although there is considerable variability from study to study, taken together, these studies indicate a lower level in depressed patients than in controls. Eight of nine studies that examined the bipolar and unipolar groups individually reported lower MHPG levels in bipolar patients, but in only four of these studies are the differences significant.

Longitudinal studies of bipolar patients have consistently shown higher levels of MHPG in the manic compared with the depressive phase.[32] Observations that increased urinary MHPG seemed to precede the switch into mania in one cycling patient (Jones et al., 1973) were not confirmed in two subsequent longitudinal studies of individual patients (Post et al., 1977; Muscettola et al., 1984).

Other Norepinephrine Metabolites. Applying their empirically derived formula, Schildkraut and colleagues (1978) found a widened difference (with no overlap) in D scores between their unipolar patients and the bipolar (and schizoaffective) depressed patients, who had significantly lower scores, and they suggested that these

other catecholamine metabolites are essentially noise, the measurement of which can enhance the signal. A later report by the same group (Schatzberg et al., 1989) again found D scores lower in bipolar-I patients than in any other depressive subtype, including bipolar-II patients. However, the D score findings of Schildkraut's group have not been replicated by an outside laboratory. Findings from the NIMH collaborative study (Koslow et al., 1983) suggest that the other metabolites might be more than just noise, since levels of urinary NE and essentially all of its major metabolites (with the important exception of MHPG) were increased over controls in both the bipolar depressed and the manic groups. However, the possibility that, as a group, the depressed patients were in a drug-withdrawal state makes this finding difficult to interpret. Commenting on these reports, Potter and Linnoila (1989) remarked that the D score formula used by Schildkraut, Schatzberg, and associates is unlikely to apply in other settings, mainly because of variation (and nonstandardization) in measurement. The urinary amine metabolite data are critically examined again at the end of this chapter when we evaluate clinical–biological correlates.

Trace Amines

More than 20 neuromodulatory trace amines have been identified in the brain. They are referred to as trace because they usually (but not always) exist in small quantities. Renewed interest in the neurobiology of these trace amines has been generated by new techniques for localizing them in the brain, as well as by the development of more sensitive and specific assays for clinical samples. Four trace amines have been studied clinically: phenylethylamine (PEA), tryptamine, tyramine, and octopamine. Data on the origins of these amines and their metabolites in body fluids are still fragmentary, as are the clinical data in most cases.[33]

Phenylethylamine. Among the trace amines, PEA has been the most extensively studied in biological psychiatry. It is of research interest because it is structurally similar to amphetamine and can produce behavioral stimulation. Like norepinephrine and serotonin, the level of turnover of PEA in the brain is decreased by reserpine and increased by TCAs and ECT, thus fitting into

Table 17-8. Urinary MHPG (mg / 24 hr)

Study	Controls		UP		BP		Manic		Results	Significance
	N	Mean ± SEM	N	Mean ± SEM	N	Mean ± SEM	N	Mean ± SEM		
Maas et al., 1968	11	1.52 ± .07	16	1.09 ± .13[a]					D < C	*p* <.05
Schildkraut et al., 1973			5	1.80 ± .09[b]	5	1.24 ± .16			BP < UP	*p* <.05
Deleon-Jones et al., 1975[c]	21	1.35 ± .06	16	1.07 ± .11[d]	5	.91 ± .15			*BP, UP < C*	*p* <.001
Garfinkel et al., 1977	10	1.60 ± .08			8	1.32 ± .19			BP < C	NS
Pickar et al., 1978	5	1.63 ± .10	10	1.18 ± .10[e]					D < C	*p* <.01
Taube et al., 1978	10	1.03 ± .09	14	.79 ± .05[f]					D < C	*p* <.05
Coppen et al., 1979	27	1.68 ± .12	23	1.58 ± .12[g]					D < C	NS
Beckmann & Goodwin, 1980	15	1.33 ± .12	21	1.82 ± .12	11 9	1.09 ± .12 BPI 1.44 ± .20 BPII			*BPI < C* *< BPII < UP*	*p* <.01
Edwards et al., 1980			32	2.07 ± .13[h]	3 2	1.31 ± .51 BPI 2.80 BPII			BPI < UP < BPII	NS
Ågren, 1982	16	3.00 ± .20	48	3.26 ± .16	19	3.02 ± .26			C < BP < UP	NS
Koslow et al., 1983	72	1.96 ± .09	74	2.11 ± .12	40	2.15 ± .18	17	2.45 ± .42	C < UP < BP < M	NS
Muscettola et al., 1984	27	1.85 ± .12	28	1.79 ± .11	19 19	1.44 ± .10 BPI 1.67 ± .13 BPII	13	2.11 ± .19	*BPI < BPII* *< UP < C, M*	*p* <.05
Siever et al., 1986	18	2.78 ± .19	10	2.53 ± .25	4	2.44 ± .36			BP < UP < C	NS
Zhou et al., 1987[i]	21	1.45 ± .10	25	1.35 ± .08	7	1.04 ± .19			*BP < UP, C*	*p* <.05

Summary: Levels of MHPG in manic patients were higher than in controls and depressed patients in all 3 studies reporting them. Eight of 11 studies found higher levels in controls than depressed patients and the other 3 found lower levels. In a comparison of UP - BP differences, 8 of 9 studies report higher levels in UPs, whereas the other found a nonsignificant increase in BP levels.

[a] Mixed depressed
[b] Chronic chronological depression
[c] Study included only females
[d] Includes 9 patients with recurrent depression and 7 with a history of 1 depressive episode

[e] Includes 8 UPs and 2 BPs for which separate scores were not given
[f] Patients with diagnosis of primary affective disorder
[g] Patients with primary depression
[h] Includes recurrent and nonrecurrent patients
[i] Urinary MHPG sulfate was tested

the amine hypothesis. Another reason for interest is that certain antidepressant MAOIs (of type B MAO or mixed A and B inhibitors) produce an increase in brain PEA that is nearly 100 times greater than the increase in the classic amines.

Although at least six studies have reported decreased excretion of PEA in patients with "endogenous" depression compared with controls (reviewed by Sabelli et al., 1978), many of them used assays of questionable specificity. Similarly, although both unipolar and bipolar patients were studied, data on bipolar illness are limited. The one study of mania (Fischer et al., 1972) cannot be interpreted because the specificity of the assay is problematic. Karoum and associates (1982) found increased urinary PEA excretion in five rapid-cycling atypical bipolar patients with episodic psychotic exacerbations; in two of these patients, the peaks in PEA levels corresponded to the psychotic episodes.

In a study of the PEA metabolite phenylacetic acid (PAA) in CSF, Karoum and associates (1984b) found PAA levels significantly higher than normal in eight depressed bipolar patients, and Sandler and colleagues (1979a) noted concentrations that were lower than normal in a mixed group of depressed patients (bipolarity not specified). Sabelli and co-workers (1986) reported no differences between unipolar and bipolar patients, but both groups had significantly lower PAA levels than normal controls. Significantly increased PAA levels in manic patients compared with controls also were reported by the Sabelli study. The authors note that this test is not specific and does not adequately differentiate types of affective illness. The confusion in this rather limited literature, therefore, may reflect assay variance.

Tryptamine. Like PEA, tryptamine has potent behavioral effects, and specific binding sites for this amine have been identified in brain. The principal metabolite of tryptamine is indoleacetic acid (IAA), formed primarily by the activity of MAO-B. Urinary IAA levels were reported to be low in depressed patients by McNamee and associates (1972) and by Rubin (1968), but the bipolar–unipolar distinction was not used. CSF IAA levels in depressed patients were found to have a unimodal distribution in another study, but a control group was not included (Åsberg et al., 1973).

A subsequent study showed significantly higher CSF IAA levels in a subgroup of retarded patients (Anderson et al., 1983), but the investigators did not differentiate bipolar from unipolar patients. At this point, it is difficult to know what to make of this sparse and apparently conflicting literature.

Tyramine. Tyramine first came to clinical attention when it was discovered to be responsible for the hypertensive reactions in some patients on MAOIs following the ingestion of tyramine-rich foods, especially aged cheeses. Levels of the major urinary metabolite of tyramine, parahydroxyphenylacetic acid, were found to be lower than normal in depressed patients, all of whom apparently were unipolar (Sandler et al., 1979b). Subsequent study of tyramine metabolism in patients led to the discovery that some individuals, including some depressed patients, were significantly impaired in their ability to conjugate tyramine, a normal route for its inactivation (Sandler et al., 1983; Harrison et al., 1984). The functional consequences of such a deficit are not yet clear.[34]

Octopamine. We are aware of only one relevant study of octopamine, that of Sandler and co-workers (1979b), who found a significant reduction in the urinary excretion of its major metabolite, hydroxymandelic acid, among a group of 23 unipolar depressed patients. Excretion levels were negatively correlated with severity as measured on the Newcastle scale.

In summary, it is unclear if any of these trace amines play a meaningful role in manic-depressive illness. Moreover, the interpretation of this literature is limited by the paucity of clinical data. Perhaps future clinical studies of trace amines in manic-depressive illness will benefit from a critical review of the classic amine literature and from studies of these systems in other illnesses where metabolic changes occur, such as hypothyroidism.

Neurotransmitter-Related Enzymes

Three major enzymes acting on amines have been under investigation: monoamine oxidase (MAO), catechol-*o*-methyltransferase (COMT), and dopamine-β-hydroxylase (DBH). MAO oxidatively deaminates norepinephrine, serotonin, dopamine, and other monoamines and is the principal degradational enzyme for these compounds. In neurons, MAO is located within the presynaptic terminal and is also found in glial mitochondria in the CNS. In this system, COMT is extraneuronal with respect to the presynaptic terminal—that is, it is located either on or in the postsynaptic membrane or associated gland elements. DBH is the final enzyme in the synthetic chain for norepinephrine, converting dopamine to norepinephrine. It is so highly localized in the storage vesicles of norepinephrine nerve terminals, both central and peripheral, that it has been used as a noradrenergic neuronal marker. When nerves in the peripheral SNS are stimulated, DBH is released along with norepinephrine (Smith and Winkler, 1972).

In clinical studies, MAO is obtained from blood platelets, which have a number of important similarities to nerve endings (Murphy et al., 1982b). The two species of MAO (A and B) have different substrate specificities. MAO-A, the principal species in neurons, metabolizes norepinephrine, serotonin, and dopamine, and MAO-B metabolizes phenylethylamine and dopamine. Since platelet MAO is of the B type, some questions arise about the interpretation of changes in the platelet enzymes in manic-depressive illness (Murphy et al., 1979). Peripheral COMT is found in association with red blood cell (RBC) membranes and is under genetic control. The relationship between RBC and neuronal COMT is not clear. DBH is a soluble enzyme in plasma, and its level is partly a reflection of peripheral sympathetic tone. MAO and DBH are by far the most extensively studied enzymes in manic-depressive illness. Both are relatively stable within a given individual but are widely variable across individuals (especially DBH). As noted in Chapter 15, family and twin studies indicate that the activity of both enzymes is highly heritable. The very large genetically determined variation among individuals (especially for DBH) has complicated attempts to examine relationships between enzyme levels and illness groups. So far, differences in these enzymes have not been found among first-degree relatives of manic-depressive patients.

Monoamine Oxidase. The numerous MAO studies in affective illness (reviewed by Murphy et al., 1982a) vary considerably, not only in the clinical groups studied but also in the assay methods employed. Most of the studies of bipolar depression, including those with the largest patient samples, demonstrated significantly lower enzyme activity compared with controls, a pattern not reflected in the studies of unipolar patients.[35] The lower activity seen in bipolar patients appears to be restricted to bipolar-I patients, since in the four studies that identified the bipolar-II patients, they were not different from controls.[36] Longitudinal studies of bipolar patients indicate that platelet MAO is state independent.

Catechol-o-Methyltransferase. RBC COMT was initially reported to be significantly lower in a group of women with primary affective disorder than in controls (Cohn et al., 1970). In a later study from the same laboratory, the enzyme was reported to differentiate bipolar and unipolar depressed patients (Dunner et al., 1977a). However, several subsequent attempts to replicate these findings have failed to produce a consensus (Fähndrich et al., 1980). Many factors might explain the discrepancies, including sex differences (Gershon and Jonas, 1975), assay differences, and genetic subgroups (Karege et al., 1987).

Dopamine-β-Hydroxylase. As noted above, it is difficult to evaluate diagnostic group differences in plasma DBH levels because of very large variation among individuals. DBH differs from MAO and COMT in that its level in plasma is partly determined by a dynamic process—the rate of transmitter release from sympathetic nerve endings. Most studies of plasma DBH in depressive illness (few of which have applied the bipolar–unipolar distinction) have been negative or inconclusive. Relatively lower levels of plasma DBH in bipolar depressed patients compared with unipolar patients or controls would be consistent with the previously reviewed data on norepinephrine and its metabolite, which suggests a lower noradrenergic tone in bipolar depressed patients. Thus, Strandman and colleagues (1978), studying 89 affectively ill patients, some in the depressed and others in the recovered phase, noted that in bipolar patients, DBH levels were somewhat lower than in unipolar patients, a difference that just achieved statistical significance.

Levitt and associates (1976), Rihmer and co-workers (1983), and Kjellman and colleagues (1986) also reported bipolar depressed patients as significantly lower than controls. In a group of 25 bipolar patients, Puzynski and colleagues (1983) noted that the mean DBH level was 25 percent lower than the unipolar patients or the controls, but the very large variance precluded statistical evaluations. Among these depressed patients, the lowest DBH level—nearly 50 percent lower than in the controls ($p < 0.05$)—was in the group with a family history of affective illness. Ikeda and co-workers (1982) reported on a longitudinal study of four cycling manic-depressive patients in which DBH was consistently higher in the manic phase than in the depressive phase. However, the extent to which DBH (released from sympathetic nerves and adrenal medulla into plasma) can reflect noradrenergic tone may be obscured by large, genetically determined variation from one individual to another.[37]

Other Enzymes. Several other enzymes of interest have been measured in manic-depressive patients. Studies of acetylcholinesterase (AChE) in erythrocytes of patients with affective disorders generally support the previously discussed cholinergic–adrenergic balance theory postulated by Janowsky and colleagues (1972). Four studies[38] found significantly reduced RBC AChE in both bipolar and unipolar patients compared with controls. These findings were reported independent of the patients' present state, and a low level of RBC AChE was, therefore, proposed by Mathew and associates (1982) as a possible trait marker for affective illness. A later study by Fritze and Beckmann (1987), however, did not replicate these findings.

GABA transaminase (GABA-T) was studied by Berrettini and co-workers (1982c) in euthymic bipolar patients in another effort to determine biological markers in the affective disorders. They reported lower GABA-T levels in patients compared with controls, a finding that has not yet been replicated. Although evidence supporting GABA-T and AChE as trait markers is inconclusive, both enzymes deserve attention. We return to a summary of the peripheral enzyme literature when we evaluate clinical biochemical correlates at the end of the chapter.

Receptor Studies

Receptor-mediated processes are central to the earlier discussion of drug studies, as well as to the neuroendocrine data that follow.[39] Here we focus on direct approaches to receptor function. Predictably, most of these direct studies in patients have used readily available peripheral tissues, such as blood elements (leukocytes and platelets) or skin fibroblasts. As in the many studies of neurotransmitter-related enzymes from peripheral tissues, the question of whether the physiological regulation of a given peripheral receptor resembles that of the corresponding brain receptor remains largely unanswered. Table 17-9 catalogs the major neurotransmitter–receptor subtypes.

Neurotransmitter–receptor sensitivity in manic-depressive illness can also be studied by administering selective receptor agonists and antagonists to patients and controls, followed by careful measurement of the physiological events (e.g., changes in hormone secretion, blood pressure, and pulse) known to occur after stimulation by such compounds. A critical issue in these studies concerns the exact location of the receptors (e.g., central or peripheral) mediating the various physiological responses. In some cases, such as the neuroendocrine challenges discussed later, such effects appear to be mediated by receptors within the CNS, but with other agents, such a distinction cannot be made unequivocally.[40] Direct approaches to receptors are not available to assess dopamine or serotonin function, except for some neuroendocrine strategies. Indeed, virtually all of these approaches focus on α-adrenergic and β-adrenergic receptor function, with the exception of a small literature beginning to examine acetylcholine receptors in patients. Despite this and other limitations, studies of receptors and response to receptor agonists are useful strategies in clinical research. They have uncovered several intriguing biological differences between manic-depressive patients and healthy controls.

Peripheral Tissue Receptors. The peripheral tissues most commonly used in clinical studies of receptor function have been the formed blood elements, including platelets and leukocytes. Platelets share several properties with neurons and

Table 17-9. Catalog of Amine Receptor Types and Drugs Used to Study
These Receptors in Laboratory Animals and Humans

	Agonist	Antagonist
Adrenergic		
α_1	Phenylephrine	Phenoxybenzamine
	Methoxamine	Thymoxamine
α_2	Clonidine	Yohimbine
		Idazoxan
β_2	Isoproterenol	Metoprolol
β_2	Salbutamol	Propranolol (nonspecific)
Dopaminergic	Apomorphine	
	Bromocriptine	
DA_1	Fenoldopam	SCH-23390
	SKF-38393	
DA_2	RU-24213	Pimozide
		Sulpiride
Serotonergic	m-CPP[a]	
5-HT_1	5MeODMT	Metergoline
	Buspirone	(no well-defined selective
		5-HT_1 antagonists)
5-HT_2	DOI[b]	Ketanserin
	DOB[b]	Ritanserin
5-HT_3	2Me5-HT	MDL-72222
Cholinergic		
Muscarinic	Betanechol	Atropine
	Oxotremorine	Scopolamine
	Arecoline	Quinuclidinyl benzilate (QNB)
Nicotinic	Nicotine	α-Bungarotoxin
Opiate[c]	Morphine	Naloxone
GABAergic		
$GABA_A$	Muscimol	Bicuculline
	THIP	Picrotoxin
	Benzodiazepines	
	(indirect)	
$GABA_B$	Baclofen	

[a] m-CPP = m-chlorophenylpiperazine

[b] Ring-substituted phenylisopropylamines. See Shulgin, 1981. For a general overview of serotonergic receptors, see Peroutka, 1988.

[c] Many subtypes with regional specificity. See review by Pert and Snyder, 1973

have even been proposed as a peripheral model of the serotonergic neuron (Stahl and Meltzer, 1978). For some biochemical events, such as serotonin uptake, platelets do behave like neurons, but for others, such as serotonin release, they are quite different. Human platelets also contain a well-characterized α_2-adrenergic receptor (i.e., a receptor related to catecholamines, such as norepinephrine) that inhibits the production of cyclic cAMP stimulated by prostaglandin E_1 (PGE_1) (U'Prichard et al., 1982).[41]

Early work by several groups failed to find differences between normal controls and bipolar depressed patients in the function of these receptors in platelets (Murphy et al., 1974c; Wang et al., 1974). Subsequent studies (Kafka et al., 1980; Siever et al., 1984a), in which unipolar patients predominated, revealed a significant blunting of both the PGE_1 stimulation of cAMP formation and its inhibition by norepinephrine in platelets from depressed patients. These observations are consistent with findings from several groups studying unipolar patients that show decreased physiological responsiveness to the α_2-adrenergic receptor agonist clonidine when compared with healthy controls or bipolar depressed patients. Therefore, alterations in platelet α_2-adrenergic receptors may be confined to unipolar patients.

Other studies of platelet adrenergic receptors used the binding of radioactive ligands to quantify directly the number (and affinity) of the receptors (Kafka et al., 1977; Daiguji et al., 1981a). Studies using receptor agonist ligands (i.e., clonidine, dihydroergocryptine, or paraminoclonidine) found more receptors in depressed patients,[42] whereas those employing antagonists (yohimbine and rauwolscine) did not (U'Prichard et al., 1982; Pimoule et al., 1983).[43] Thus, agonists and antagonists may label different populations of receptors. Along with the increased number of α_2-adrenergic receptors, U'Prichard and co-workers (1983) also found a decrease in the α_2-adrenoceptor-mediated inhibition of cAMP formation. Although these two findings (i.e., decreased inhibition of cAMP formation with an increase in density of receptors) seem paradoxical, previous studies showed that desensitization of α_2-adrenergic receptors results in decreased stimulation by agonists, along with an increase in the number of high-affinity receptors. Thus, there appears to be an emerging consensus that at least one type of platelet α_2-receptor may be desensitized in some depressed patients.

The most parsimonious explanation for such a finding would be the previously discussed increase in circulating catecholamines in depression. If this is the explanation for desensitized receptors, one would expect this receptor change to be found among unipolar rather than bipolar patients, since it is among the unipolar patients that the elevations in circulating catecholamines are found (see review by Kafka and Paul, 1986). Given that bipolar patients have not been separately identified in the receptor studies, this remains an assumption. To the extent that the receptor changes simply reflect increased sympathetic tone, they would not contribute to our understanding of pathophysiology. Nevertheless, the possibility cannot yet be ruled out that a defect is present in either the α_2-adrenergic receptor recognition site itself or in its coupling mechanism to adenylate cyclase. García-Sevilla and associates (1981) reported a decrease in platelet α_2-receptors following chronic antidepressant treatment but did not distinguish between bipolar and unipolar patients. Further work will be needed to clarify whether the changes seen in platelet α_2-receptors are state or trait markers and whether the decrease in these receptors following chronic treatment with antidepressants is a cause or effect of recovery.

β-Adrenergic receptors are present on human leukocytes (Parker and Smith, 1973). Several studies have measured β-receptor function in leukocytes from depressed patients and healthy controls.[44] In general, the depressed patients show a significantly decreased cAMP response to the β-receptor agonists norepinephrine and isoproterenol. Although the bipolar–unipolar question is not sharply defined in all of these studies, the decreased receptor response seems predominantly a characteristic of the unipolar patients. Compatible with this interpretation is the finding that a measure of coupling of the β-receptor to cAMP is lower in unipolar than in bipolar patients (Buckholtz et al., 1988).

Another possible peripheral source for a variety of neurotransmitter and hormone receptors is the skin fibroblast, which, unlike platelets and leukocytes, can be cultured almost indefinitely. An initial study by Nadi and co-workers (1984) suggested the presence of a relatively high-affinity muscarinic–cholinergic receptor on cultured human fibroblasts using [3H]-quinuclidinyl benzilate (QNB), a potent muscarinic–cholinergic antagonist. However, subsequent studies failed to replicate this finding.[45] Lymphoblasts (virally transformed lymphocytes) may also be cultured. Wright and colleagues (1984) noted decreased β-adrenergic receptors in lymphoblasts from bipolar patients and ill relatives, a provocative finding that was not replicated by Berrettini and colleagues (1987b). Methodological problems associated with the use of transformed cells for receptor studies are discussed elsewhere (Ebstein et al., 1986). The outlook on findings in peripheral tissue is understandably bleak, since no clear pattern has emerged, and such factors as morphology, age, and subtype of platelet or lymphocyte cell population have not been adequately controlled.

Drug Challenge Paradigms. Drug challenge paradigms have been increasingly used to assess neurotransmitter receptor function in depressed patients. In many cases, the drugs have been characterized on the basis of their interactions with specific receptor populations under controlled conditions in the test tube, conditions that are not generally feasible in humans (e.g., apomorphine and pituitary dopamine receptors, clonidine and vascular α_2-adrenergic receptors). In other cases, the actual receptor mechanism(s) mediating a given agent's physiological effects are not even clear in preclinical studies (e.g., amphetamine's action in increasing growth hormone). In this section, we review clinical studies that do not involve neuroendocrine measures, which are covered in the section that follows.

Peripheral adrenergic receptor activity in depressed patients was first studied by administering either sympathomimetic compounds that act indirectly, such as tyramine, or agonists that act directly, such as phenylephrine and norepinephrine (Ghose and Turner, 1975; Friedman, 1978). This literature is characterized by a lack of consensus,[46] which may be due, in part, to hidden bipolar–unipolar differences, since none of studies directly compared the two subgroups. Nevertheless, several different strategies suggest that the functional activity of peripheral α-adrenergic and β-adrenergic receptors is decreased among predominantly unipolar depressed patients and that such an effect might be due to receptor desensitization resulting from high circulating levels of catecholamines, as previously discussed (Kafka and Paul, 1986).

Consistent with this notion are the differing behavioral and biochemical responses of the two patient groups to amphetamine challenge. Amphetamine, an indirect-acting sympathomimetic, releases a predominantly extravesicular pool of catecholamines. Patients with low urinary MHPG, as seen in bipolar depression, respond to amphetamine with significant behavioral activation and, in many cases, even the induction of mania (Gerner et al., 1976). For example, when Nurnberger and Gershon (1981) administered

amphetamine to medication-free, well-state bipolar patients, those with low baseline plasma–urinary MHPG became significantly more activated than those who had high plasma MHPG. In the same study, healthy volunteers had virtually the opposite response (i.e., high plasma MHPG tended to be associated with enhanced activation in response to amphetamine). These results are supported by those of Silberman and co-workers (1981), who demonstrated a euphoric response to amphetamine in virtually all bipolar depressed patients but in only 40 percent of unipolar patients. Also, as discussed later in the section on clinical–biological correlates, the extent of the tricyclic-induced activation of bipolar patients (hypomania vs mania), and the latency of the response, were correlated with levels of pretreatment MHPG in bipolar patients. Lower levels predicted quicker and more serious reactions (Zis et al., 1979). Thus, compared with unipolar depressed patients, bipolar depressed patients, as a group, display a lower level of SNS activation and are more sensitive to adrenergic agonists.

Cholinergic receptor function has been rather extensively studied in predominantly bipolar groups of depressed patients by using the pharmacological challenge strategy. Centrally acting cholinergic agonists are administered to either ill or remitted patients and healthy controls, and dependent physiological variables, such as sleep or hormone secretion, are monitored. Specifically, Sitaram and colleagues (1980, 1982) showed that, in normals, the onset of rapid eye movement (REM) sleep was advanced in a dose-dependent fashion after infusion of either direct-acting cholinergic agonists, such as arecoline, or indirect-acting cholinesterase inhibitors, such as physostigmine, during non-REM sleep (see Chapter 19). Conversely, cholinergic receptor antagonists, such as scopolamine, delayed REM onset and also blocked the action of arecoline. Moreover, arecoline infusion causes depressed patients to enter REM sleep much faster than healthy controls do, suggesting a supersensitive response to cholinergic agonists in depression. This same phenomenon occurs during remission, indicating that muscarinic–cholinergic receptor supersensitivity may be a trait marker. This work has been confirmed in both unipolar and bipolar patients, albeit less robustly[47]; but definitive conclusions are still premature. Nevertheless, monozygotic twin concordance of arecoline REM induction response (Nurnberger et al., 1983c) and a report by Sitaram and colleagues (1987) of an association of supersensitive cholinergic REM induction and affective illness within pedigrees suggest, but do not prove, a possible role for ACh in genetic predisposition.[48]

Although most of the above data are from bipolar patients,[49] unipolar patients may show a similar phenomenon. The finding that scopolamine (which results in up-regulation of cholinergic receptors in brain), when given to normal volunteers, can produce depression-like sleep abnormalities (e.g., a shorter time to the first period of REM and reduced total sleep time) suggests that such changes are not specific to bipolar illness but rather are part of the pathophysiology of depressive symptoms. Consistent with this are related experiments by these same investigators, who found physiological evidence that enhanced cholinergic receptor sensitivity is related to the depressogenic effects of catecholamine depletion in a group of healthy volunteers (Sitaram et al., 1984). Furthermore, the same group (Dubé et al., 1987) found that patients with a primary panic disorder or generalized anxiety did not show a speedier REM induction after arecoline challenge, suggesting that cholinergic abnormality may be specific to depressive states, although not necessarily manic-depressive illness per se. A summary of the amine receptor studies is included as part of our discussion of clinical–biological correlates at the end of the chapter.

Construction of the Neurotransmitter Bridge
The evaluation of the pharmacological bridge analogy discussed in Chapter 16 may now be extended to embrace the possibility of several interacting building materials, including dopamine, serotonin, norepinephrine, acetylcholine, and GABA. Referring back to Figure 16-4 and the four types of drugs identified in Table 17-1, note the capacity of MAOIs to have both multiple effects on manic-depressive illness and substantial effects on NE, 5-HT, and DA turnover and function. TCAs are more clearly promoters of NE and 5-HT systems, with somewhat more indirect effects on DA systems. Lithium influences membrane regulation in some as yet poorly understood way, with modest, inconsistent, and diffuse

effects on either supersensitivity or cAMP stimulation at several types of receptors (those involving components of the NE system being the most studied). For all of the evidence supporting dopamine's role in mania, carbamazepine (an antimanic agent) has thus far been found to have more direct effects on NE and GABA than on DA, although indirect effects on DA are likely.

It now seems obvious that neurotransmitters interact and that the relative balance of these substances may be more important than their absolute amount. To quote Marie Åsberg (personal communication, 1985): "The central nervous system can be likened unto a net. If you pull any single mesh in the net, the shape of every other mesh will change." Unfortunately, we do not yet have sufficient data on the CNS relationship of so many neurotransmitter systems to define and predict the parameters of these interactions reliably. Nevertheless, we can apply what we know clinically about manic-depressive illness and its response to drugs as a means of conceptualizing functional consequences of shifts in the interactions between systems.

In attempting to select from among possible system balances that may be relevant to manic-depressive illness, we follow an implicitly hierarchical model that views some systems as more central than others. Neuroanatomical, functional –neurochemical, or electrophysiological studies all show that systems are not completely reciprocal. One example is the direct functional projections found from 5-HT to DA neuronal cell bodies, but not vice versa. Moreover, since the three monoamine systems (NE, 5-HT, and DA) are neuroanatomically and functionally better delineated than the cholinergic and GABAergic ones, they currently provide a richer and more solid basis for the construction of models.

Dopaminergic systems (as shown in Figure 17-2, opposite page 458) are relatively simple and discrete. Because of the involvement of the limbic system and prefrontal cortex in mood regulation, the DA system that projects to these areas (principally from the A10 nucleus of the central tegmental area) may have the most direct relevance to manic-depressive illness (see, e.g., Depue and Iacono, 1989). It is unclear to what extent TCAs and MAOIs directly alter dopamine function, but indirect effects may be just as important. For example, stimulation of the serotonergic system in the dorsal raphe area (see review by Soubrié et al., 1983) produces inhibition of dopamine neurons in the substantia nigra. Similarly, projections from the medial raphe to DA terminals in the median eminence may provide the basis for the decreased DA release following serotonergic agonists. Perhaps relevant to this functional interplay between 5-HT and DA (illustrated in Figure 17-3) is the observation that antidepressants with primary effects on the 5-HT system appear to be less likely to precipitate mania when compared with more noradrenergic tricyclics.

Figure 17-2 (opposite page 458) also adds NE to the schematic representation of 5-HT and DA pathways. As is readily apparent, NE projections from the locus coeruleus (NE$_6$) or other midbrain nuclei (NE$_1$-3) impinge on both the cell bodies and terminations of 5-HT and DA neurons. Acute increases of 5-HT may either facilitate or inhibit NE depending on the region studied. The pathways from NE to 5-HT neurons provide a neuroanatomical basis for the increasing evidence of norepinephrine–serotonin interactions involved in the effects of antidepressants, particularly chronic effects. These interactions between 5-HT and NE are outlined in Table 17-10.

With respect to the interaction between NE and DA, specific models are lacking because available evidence points to different functions: a timing cue for NE and a switching cue for DA (Oades, 1985) that may operate more in parallel than on each other. Nonetheless, since NE projections are more diffuse than those of DA, the interpretation of much pharmacological evidence that NE modulates DA in an inhibitory way (Antelman and Caggiula, 1977) has had considerable influence. However, subsequent evidence does not support this interpretation but suggests instead a facilitatory role of NE on DA-mediated functions (Archer et al., 1986). A recent interpretation of dopaminergic–noradrenergic interac-

Table 17-10. Antidepressant Effects: The Interaction Between Noradrenergic and Serotonergic Neurotransmitter Systems

- Down-regulation of β-adrenoceptors by antidepressants (TCAs) requires serotonergic input (Brunello et al., 1982; A. Janowsky et al., 1982)

- Electroconvulsive-shock potentiation of the serotonin-behavioral syndrome requires noradrenergic input (Green and Deakin, 1980)

- Serotonin-mediated behaviors are potentiated by β-adrenoceptor agonists (Cowen et al., 1982)

- β-adrenoceptor antagonists reduce brain serotonergic activity (Hallberg et al., 1982)

- "Serotonergic" antidepressants (zimelidine) down-regulate β-adrenoceptors (Sethy and Harris, 1982) or the β-adrenoceptor coupled adenylate cyclase system (Mishra et al., 1980)

- Serotonergic (zimelidine) and noradrenergic (desipramine) antidepressants decrease CSF 5-HIAA and MHPG (Potter et al., 1983)

tions is that NE's role is dependent on the type of DA-mediated process being studied. For instance, in an untreated animal involved in carrying out discrimination tasks, it is argued that NE maintains stimulus control of behavior, whereas DA increases both the rate and speed of responding (Cole and Robbins, 1987). Thus, we return to the notion that the systems act in concert. Interestingly, there is relatively little recent information on the consequences of DA-mediated events enhancing NE output. In this respect, the experience in humans with medications may provide some clues for future preclinical research.[50] Teleologically, since DA is a precursor of NE, it seems reasonable that the latter would have evolved as the more developed system modulating its antecedent, the more primitive one.

The interactions of most interest to manic-depressive illness are summarized in Figure 17-3, which illustrates three types of relationships: (1) pharmacological facilitation of the norepinephrine–serotonin axis is associated with antidepressant response; (2) facilitation of the norepinephrine–dopamine axis is associated with a tendency to precipitate mania or induce rapid cycles, and (3) facilitation of the serotonin–dopamine axis is associated with no obvious clinical effect.

Figure 17-3. Primary neurotransmitter vs clinical effects (adapted from Goodwin and Sack, 1973).

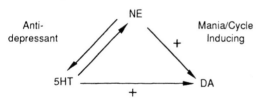

As should be obvious from the discussion thus far, models for explaining the clinical effects of drugs on manic-depressive illness are based on an understanding of the relationships between interacting biochemical systems (Potter et al., 1985). In addition to the animal literature, biochemical data from human studies also lend support to the concept of amine interactions. Thus, when CSF amine metabolite data from drug-free manic-depressive patients are subjected to a statistical technique based on relative probabilities and causal analysis, the results are consistent with 5-HT affecting DA (Ågren et al., 1986). The effect of pharmacological manipulations on CSF metabolites is also consistent with a 5-HT influence on NE, and vice versa (Potter et al., 1985; Stockmeier and Kellar, 1986). Under the influence of drug treatment, the dopamine system may initially shift modestly in either direction but generally compensates quickly, retaining its pretreatment relationship to 5-HT (i.e., correlations of HVA with 5-HIAA are sustained). With this model, certain clinical effects occur because the impact of the drug exceeds the compensatory capacity of the DA system. Thus, dopamine must be kept under control lest the bridge lead to manic psychosis. Acetylcholine and GABA can be invoked to provide needed weight, but too much could bring the whole structure down. Serotonin is perhaps the chemical surveyor, doing the fine tuning and measurements so that the bridge ends up where it is supposed to, leaving NE as the most versatile transmitter, which can be extruded or compressed into whatever shape and consistency is necessary.

As discussed extensively by Potter and colleagues (1988; Potter, 1986), norepinephrine remains the neurotransmitter most consistently implicated in the action of the most established agents with the widest range of effects in manic-depressive illness. Potter and colleagues (1988) make the additional interesting point that a major functional role of the NE system may be to increase the signal/noise ratio in a variety of brain areas that receive and modulate reactions to exogenous stimuli. The pharmacological probes used to study serotonin, dopamine, acetylcholine, or GABA systems generally can be shown to interact with the norepinephrine system on one level or another. However, a caveat is in order: the monoamines in general and nor-epinephrine in particular now have a long track record of extensive study, having been discovered decades ago. As new transmitters and modulators emerge, existing models will no doubt need to be revised, enlarged, or rejected outright.

NEUROENDOCRINE SYSTEMS

The contribution of altered endocrine function to pathological mood states was among the earliest themes in biological psychiatry. Clinically, it had been observed that hypothyroidism was often associated with depression. Less frequently, hyperthyroidism (or the administration of thyroid hormone) was associated with euphoric states, including full manic reactions. Depression and, rarely, mania were observed in patients with Cushing's disease, and exogenous steroids were noted to precipitate either mania or depression in some individuals.

In pioneering studies during the 1930s, Gjessing substantially ameliorated periodic catatonia in some patients with sustained use of hypermetabolic doses of thyroid hormone, one of the earliest prophylactic treatments in psychiatry. In his classic monograph, Gjessing speculated that reduced or poorly regulated thyroid function is important to the pathophysiology of various cyclic mental disturbances, including manic-depressive illness. Although his work did not have widespread influence at the time, recent developments have resurrected it.

The modern era of interest in the interactions between the nervous and endocrine systems began in the early 1960s, spurred by the development of simple, reliable assay methods for hormones in the blood and urine.[51] Neuroendocrine investigators began to focus their attention on depression as it became increasingly apparent that hypothalamic function was intimately involved in many of depression's core symptoms, such as poor regulation of appetite and sleep and decreased sex drive (Gold et al., 1988). Among patients with major depressive illness, especially those with endogenous features, elevated cortisol secretion was the first major neuroendocrine disturbance to become firmly established.

With the isolation of the specific peptide factors responsible for release of individual hormones from the pituitary, clinical endocrinology has developed increasingly sophisticated challenge tests for assessing the dynamics of hypothalamic–pituitary function. As a result, neuroendocrine research in depression has exploded. More recently, knowledge has developed rapidly on the hypothalamic neurotransmitter systems that regulate the release of trophic factors to the pituitary. This growing knowledge has increased the potential of neuroendocrine strategies as a window into midbrain neurotransmitter function, particularly of the biogenic amines. It is fair to say that the amine hypothesis is still the major conceptual prism through which neuroendocrine data in affective illness are viewed.

Most neuroendocrine researchers view the phenomena they study as secondary to disturbances in brain neurotransmitters—occurring downstream in a cascade of neuronal events. A major exception to this view is the relationship between decreased thyroid function and rapid cycling in bipolar patients. Here, the endocrine dysfunction itself may cause the increased cycling. This hypothesis led to evaluation of high-dose thyroid as a treatment for rapid cycling, and some amelioration has been reported (see Chapter 23).

The examination of neuroendocrine function is today one of the most prolific research arenas in biological psychiatry. Recent refinements of radioimmunoassays for most of the known pituitary, thyroid, and adrenal hormones have catalyzed literally thousands of studies of possible neuroendocrine abnormalities in the affective disorders. This section focuses on the peptide hormones of the hypothalamic–pituitary axis as they are measured in body fluids under both baseline and challenge conditions. The emerging animal data on the effects of neurohormones on brain function (i.e., the brain as a gland) provide added impetus to the trend toward evaluating neuroendocrine findings in their own right, not simply as reflections of amine neurotransmitter changes. The actions of a single neurohormone peptide on a wide range of brain receptors characteristically span a much longer time period than the action of monoamines. The influence of neurohormones on neurons may have been elaborated for teleological reasons. The possibility that one substance effectively commands and organizes multiple coordinated physiological and behavioral responses is consistent with the importance of

certain peptides in the long-term phasic changes typical of manic-depressive illness. One new and intriguing approach to interpreting neuroendocrine data in manic-depressive illness is to assess their variability, either within individual patients or across patient groups. The study of neuroendocrine variability may bring us closer to the pathophysiology of bipolar affective illness.

In summary, the neuroendocrine literature can be divided into two distinct but overlapping categories. The first includes studies that have used baseline neuroendocrine measures and provocative challenge tests to unravel subclinical endocrine abnormalities in depressed patients. The second encompasses studies in which neuroendocrine measures have been used as a window into central neurotransmitter function (e.g., as a measure of receptor activity or neurotransmitter turnover).

Hypothalamic–Pituitary–Adrenal Axis

Elevated cortisol secretion, hypercortisolemia, is a consistently replicated finding in studies of depressed patients. The anatomical sites and neurohumoral mediators involved, largely defined in the past decade (Figure 17-4) are among the best characterized of all neuroendocrine systems (for reviews see Martin and Reichlin, 1987, and Stokes and Sikes, 1988; Holsboer, 1988; and Charlton and Ferrier, 1989). Discovery of the physiological regulation of human cortisol secretion was soon challenged by further evidence

Figure 17-4. The HPA axis. Neurotransmitter control of corticotropin-releasing factor secretion.

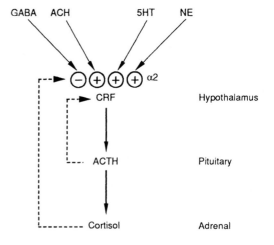

clarifying interactions between adrenal steroids, neuropeptides, and catecholamines. These interactions, which determine the absolute level and periodicity of cortisol secretion from both the hypothalamus and the pituitary, are considerably more complex than was previously suspected (Axelrod and Reisine, 1984). Such complexity must be kept in mind when relating clinically observed abnormalities in the function of the hypothalamic–pituitary–adrenal (HPA) axis to a specific neuroendocrine defect. Despite these complexities, the HPA abnormalities reviewed can probably be traced to central (i.e., hypothalamic) rather than peripheral dysregulation of cortisol secretion (Gold et al., 1984b).

In brief, the secretion of cortisol from the adrenal cortex is initiated in the CNS through a neurotransmitter-mediated release of hypothalamic corticotropin-releasing factor (CRF), which in turn stimulates pituitary corticotropin (ACTH) secretion. Various neurotransmitters and neuromodulators, including acetylcholine, norepinephrine, serotonin, and GABA, have been implicated in stimulating CRF release (Pepper and Krieger, 1984). Different ones predominate at different times, depending on environmental stress, circadian periodicity, and other physiological conditions. Human cortisol secretion can be inhibited by corticosteroids, such as dexamethasone, and this feedback inhibition can be readily demonstrated at both central and pituitary locations. Preliminary data indicate that the central components of the axis are ordinarily more sensitive to glucocorticoid negative feedback than are those in the pituitary (P. Gold, unpublished observations). Such distinctions become important in interpreting clinical data on cortisol secretion (with and without dexamethasone).

The earliest studies showed that depressed patients had elevated plasma cortisol levels, which decreased after recovery in most, but not all, patients (Board et al., 1957; Gibbons, 1964). By and large, these studies included a mixed population of depressive patients and used rather primitive techniques for assaying cortisol. More recent studies that have used highly specific radioimmunoassays, more frequent sampling of cortisol (to take into account the well-known diurnal rhythm in cortisol secretion), and more homogeneous groups of patients, including children (Weller and Weller, 1988), have consistently shown significant cortisol hypersecretion in many, but not all, depressed patients. Although cortisol hypersecretion has been reported in both bipolar and unipolar patients (Sachar et al., 1973b), whether it occurs with the same frequency in both groups is still open to question.

Several investigators examined bipolar patients longitudinally and observed significant hypercortisolemia (and/or elevations of urinary cortisol metabolites) during the depressed, but not manic, phase (Rizzo et al., 1954; Bunney et al., 1965; Kennedy et al., 1989). These results were confirmed and extended by Rubinow and colleagues (1984a), who found that both unipolar and bipolar depressed patients have higher urinary free cortisol levels than patients in the manic phase or healthy controls. The urinary free cortisol levels in Rubinow's manic patients were significantly lower than those of normal controls.

Investigators have found conflicting evidence of CSF cortisol levels in unipolar and bipolar depressed patients.[52] Gerner and Wilkins (1983) found that CSF cortisol values in manic patients were significantly lower than in any of the subgroups of depressed patients examined.

Indices of HPA axis activation correlate with levels of depression across several diagnostic groups, including major affective disorder (Reus et al., 1983), obsessive-compulsive disorder (Insel et al., 1983), and cyclothymia (Depue et al., 1985), and also in normal controls (Ballenger et al., 1980).

Dexamethasone Suppression Test

In addition to cortisol hypersecretion, other state-dependent abnormalities in HPA function have been reported in affective illness. The most common finding is an early escape, or rebound, of cortisol from the suppression induced by dexamethasone (Carroll et al., 1968; Stokes et al., 1975). This phenomenon, the basis of the DST, has been used extensively in psychiatric patients (for reviews, see Insel and Goodwin, 1983; Baldessarini and Arana, 1985; APA Task Force, 1987). The DST is an indicator of the sensitivity of the HPA axis to feedback suppression by exogenously administered steroid (dexamethasone). Approximately 40 to 50 percent of endogenously depressed patients respond abnormally to the DST (W. A. Brown et al., 1979; Carroll et al.,

1980). The specificity of the test in depression is questionable, however, since several confounding variables, such as weight loss and various medications, can produce false-positive (abnormal) results. Also arguing against specificity is evidence that other psychiatric disorders (particularly in their acute phases) may be associated with an abnormal DST. Nevertheless, even a conservative analysis of the many DST studies must conclude that positive tests occur far more frequently among severely depressed patients than among those with other major psychiatric diagnoses, even when the known confounding factors are taken into consideration. Among depressed patients, correlations have been found between the DST, levels of anxiety, somatization (Greden et al., 1984), guilt, anorexia, and weight loss (Feinberg and Carroll, 1984).

At first glance, an abnormal DST would seem consistent with the hypercortisolemia seen in depression, which might down-regulate functional receptors for glucocorticoids at either the hypothalamic or pituitary level.[53] However, hypercortisolemia and DST nonsuppression are apparently independent—one can be present without the other (Asnis et al., 1981). This finding suggests that the two phenomena may not be causally related or may be separate phenomena stemming from the same process but separated in time. For example, DST may persist for a short time after a brief episode of hypercortisolemia has passed.[54]

The DST has been relatively well studied in bipolar illness. During depression, between 25 and 60 percent of bipolar patients have abnormal DST results.[55] According to some (Carroll et al., 1976a; Greden et al., 1982) but not all (Godwin, 1984; Graham et al., 1982) investigators, these results revert to normal during the hypomanic or manic phases. The large variability in the rates of abnormal DST results among bipolar patients is also seen in unipolar patients (discussed in detail by Stokes et al., 1984). Most investigators have found no significant difference in the rates of abnormal DSTs among bipolar and unipolar depressed patients, but some do report that unipolar depressed patients have significantly higher postdexamethasone cortisol values than do bipolar patients (see, for example, Rothschild et al., 1982), primarily because of the very high values in psychotic unipolar patients.

In the initial DST findings in manic patients,

the rate of nonsuppression was not significantly greater than those reported in normal controls (Carroll et al., 1976a; Greden et al., 1982), but subsequent studies indicate that variable proportions of manic patients fail to suppress (Arana et al., 1983; Stokes et al., 1984; Woodside et al., 1989). In fact, in some studies, nonsuppression in mania is as frequent as it is in bipolar depression (Arana et al., 1983; Godwin et al., 1984; Graham et al., 1982).

How can we account for these discrepancies? Patients with dysphoric manias—that is, mixed manic-depressive states (see Chapter 2)—frequently have abnormal DST results (Evans and Nemeroff, 1983; Krishnan et al., 1983). If the proportion of such manias differed substantially from one study to another, variable nonsuppression in the manic groups might be expected. However, some of the reports of DST nonsuppression in mania specify that the patients were not simultaneously depressed (Arana et al., 1983; Graham et al., 1982). Of special interest is a small group of longitudinal studies in which the DST was used during both phases of the illness in the same patient. In one of these (Godwin et al., 1984), most of the bipolar patients showed a similar DST response (either abnormal or normal) in both the manic and depressive phases. This suggests that there may be a subgroup of bipolar patients in whom HPA axis dysregulation underlies both phases of illness.

When the entire literature on the DST in manic-depressive illness is examined critically, it becomes clear that nonsuppression occurs more frequently in the depressive and mixed phases of the illness, but it is also not at all uncommon in mania (Table 17-11). Clearly, if one considers all studies measuring some aspect of cortisol secretion in manic-depressive patients, the evidence indicates that hypercortisolemia occurs more frequently in the depressed phase than in the hypomanic, manic, or euthymic phases. But why, when cortisol hypersecretion clearly differentiates depression from mania, does the DST not do the same? Studies by Meltzer and colleagues (1982), H.E. Klein and associates (1984), and Atkinson and coworkers (1986) may shed some light on this question. These investigators showed that dexamethasone administration also decreases pituitary prolactin secretion and that, in a series of psychiatric patients with affective symptoms, there was a sig-

Table 17-11. Comparison of Neuroendocrine Findings in Bipolar Patients with Control Values

| | Response Compared with Controls | |
	Depressed	Manic
Plasma cortisol	↑	Normal
DST	Nonsuppression	Variable
CRF stimulation of ACTH	↓	Normal
5-HTP stimulation of cortisol	↑	↑
TRH stimulation of TSH	↓	↓
Melatonin	↓	↑
Prolactin	↓	?
GH	↓	↓

nificant association between nonsuppression of both cortisol and prolactin.[56] Thus, an abnormal DST could indicate a nonspecific abnormality in the feedback sensitivity of the pituitary gland rather than a specific limbic system disturbance, as was previously postulated. This interpretation is not, however, consistent with recent studies employing CRF infusions (Gold et al., 1984b, 1986a; Gold and Chrousos, 1985), which found normal feedback at the pituitary level.

Virtually all studies agree that both hypercortisolemia and the DST results become more normal after recovery from manic or depressive episodes (Carroll, 1982; Joyce and Paykel, 1989). Such evidence indicates that the abnormalities are state dependent and do not provide a marker for the underlying vulnerability to manic-depressive illness. Also, the fact that these HPA axis abnormalities are not specific to bipolar illness or even to major affective illness means that they probably reflect downstream physiological concomitants of depression and arousal. It is possible that manic-depressive illness involves some episodic vulnerability in these systems, perhaps initially requiring activation by stress.

Provocative Challenge Strategies

Endocrinologists use provocative challenge techniques widely to test the integrity of a given neuroendocrine system. Provocative neuroendocrine tests usually are reserved for the more subtle endocrine disorders or for determining the exact anatomical site(s) in a given axis responsible for the pathological changes in hormone production.

Since Vale and colleagues (1981) isolated and sequenced CRF, the hypothalamic peptide that regulates pituitary ACTH secretion, several laboratories have used a CRF-stimulation test to further examine the HPA axis in the affective disorders. Gold and colleagues (1984b) showed that both unipolar and bipolar depressed patients have a blunted ACTH response to intravenously infused CRF but that the cortisol response is not blunted. The blunted ACTH response to CRF is consistent with elevated plasma cortisol levels exerting normal negative feedback at the level of the pituitary. These investigators hypothesized that, since depressed patients have a "functionally and anatomically hypertrophied adrenal cortex," they probably undergo an exaggerated cortisol response to ACTH, which compensates for the blunted ACTH response to CRF. In fact, two groups of investigators (Amsterdam et al., 1983a, 1988a; Jaeckle et al., 1987) showed that depressed patients secrete significantly more cortisol in response to a given dose of ACTH than do healthy controls. These studies point to a central disturbance in CRF release as the cause of hypercortisolemia because the adrenal cortex, even though hypertrophied, would not secrete large amounts of cortisol autonomously and must be driven by ACTH and CRF.

In the study by Gold and colleagues (1984b), the CRF-induced release of ACTH was normal in a group of manic and euthymic bipolar patients, further supporting the previously mentioned findings of normal or low HPA axis function in manic patients as reflected by urinary free cortisol. Apparently, the central mechanisms responsible for the hypersecretion of CRF in depression revert to normal following the switch to mania or euthymia.

As mentioned previously, several major neurotransmitter systems (noradrenergic, adrenergic, serotonergic, cholinergic, GABAergic) have been implicated in the regulation of CRF release from the paraventricular nucleus of the hypothalamus. In studies of CRF release by hypothalamic organ culture, Gold's group showed that GABA is inhibitory, whereas norepinephrine, acetylcholine, and serotonin are excitatory (Calogero et al., 1988a,b,c, 1989).

Meltzer and colleagues (1984b) administered 5-HTP orally to depressed patients and controls and measured changes in serum cortisol. Previous studies in both laboratory animals and humans had implicated central serotonergic systems in the regulation of ACTH and cortisol secretion, presumably through regulation of hypothalamic CRF release (Fuller, 1981). The oral administration of 5-HTP induced a significantly greater increase in serum cortisol in depressed patients than in controls (Meltzer et al., 1984c). Of special interest, this supersensitive response, presumably reflecting decreased serotonergic activity, was more pronounced in the bipolar than in the unipolar depressed patients and also was observed in manic patients. In fact, there was no significant difference in the response during depression or mania. Thus, these data differ from baseline cortisol findings in the unchallenged state, in which elevated cortisol is seen only in the depressed phase.[57] In related studies (Meltzer et al., 1984c), the exaggerated cortisol response to 5-HTP was shown to be positively correlated with both depressive and manic symptoms, significantly greater in psychotic and in suicidal patients, and, interestingly, significantly more variable in bipolar than unipolar patients, suggesting perhaps greater instability of this system in bipolar illness. This group also found a negative correlation between CSF levels of 5-HIAA and the magnitude of the cortisol response to 5-HTP in depressed patients, a finding that offers further evidence that enhanced cortisol response to serotonergic agents reflects a decrease in central serotonergic activity in depression (Koyama et al., 1987). The results of these studies seem to indicate that bipolar (and some unipolar) patients

may have decreased central serotonergic activity, resulting in serotonin receptors that are more sensitive (and perhaps less stable). Further, this abnormality seems to occur during both depression and mania. Such data are compatible with the previously discussed hypothesis of Prange and co-workers (1974c) and of Kety (1971) that a decrease in serotonergic activity plays a permissive role in the pathogenesis of both depression and mania. It is notable that chronic lithium treatment was associated with a marked augmentation of the 5-HTP-induced secretion of cortisol (Meltzer et al., 1984a), a finding consistent with the previous reports that lithium facilitates serotonergic activity in animals.[58]

Several caveats should be considered, however, in assessing the findings of Meltzer and colleagues: First, the findings have not yet been replicated. Second, the exact anatomic site(s) at which 5-HTP stimulates cortisol secretion is unknown.[59] Further, the effects of other antidepressant drugs (TCAs and MAOIs) on the 5-HTP-induced release of cortisol in depressed patients are difficult to reconcile with a simple normalization of supersensitive serotonin receptors in both depression and mania. MAOIs enhance and TCAs inhibit the 5-HTP-induced increase in cortisol secretion (Meltzer et al., 1984a), yet both drugs can induce mania in bipolar patients. Perhaps this difference could relate to the suggestion made by some investigators (see Chapter 22 and the earlier discussion of the pharmacological bridge) that, in lithium-treated bipolar patients, MAOIs are superior to TCAs as antidepressants and that MAO-A inhibitors have anticycling effects in some lithium-resistant patients.

Drugs that mimic the actions of acetylcholine have been reported to increase ACTH/cortisol secretion in animals and humans, and there is evidence that cholinergic agonists work on the HPA axis through a receptor-mediated release of hypothalamic CRF. In animals, atropine (a muscarinic-cholinergic antagonist) has been shown to block both stress-induced elevations of ACTH and cortisol (Hedge and Smelik, 1968; Hedge and de Wied, 1971) and the normal circadian rhythm of cortisol secretion (Krieger et al., 1968; Ferrari et al., 1977). The previously discussed depressive-like behavioral effects of physostigmine (a reversible AChE inhibitor) are highly correlated with increased blood levels of

ACTH, β-endorphin, cortisol, and prolactin (Risch et al., 1980, 1981a). These same investigators also report that depressed bipolar and unipolar patients secrete significantly more ACTH/β-endorphin after physostigmine administration than do controls (Risch et al., 1983a). A rigorous comparison of physostigmine-induced changes in HPA axis function has yet to be carried out in bipolar and unipolar depressed patients. The use of centrally active cholinergic agents should help to determine whether increased cholinergic receptor sensitivity is, in fact, a genetic trait marker for depression and, if so, for what form of the disorder. These findings cannot yet be related to the data discussed previously demonstrating cholinergic receptor supersensitivity in depressed patients as measured by arecoline-induced REM.

Hypothalamic–Pituitary–Thyroid Axis

Of all the endocrine systems hypothesized to be linked to manic-depressive illness, the hypothalamic–pituitary–thyroid (HPT) axis is a prime candidate. In 1864, Graves noted that patients with endemic goiter often showed a markedly "morbid and melancholic turn of mind." Since that time, it has been repeatedly noted that disorders of thyroid function frequently are accompanied by changes in mood (Prange, 1974b), and bipolar patients (particularly those with rapid cycles) frequently have HPT axis abnormalities (reviewed by Wehr et al., 1988). Thyroid hormones reportedly alter the clinical course of some forms of cyclic depressive illness,[60] potentiate the actions of various antidepressants (Goodwin et al., 1982), and can precipitate mania in bipolar patients (Josephson and Mackenzie, 1979; Wehr and Goodwin, 1987a,b). The more recent and carefully controlled reports of HPT axis function in depressed patients have, in fact, revealed subtle but significant abnormalities in many manic-depressive patients. Finally, both lithium and carbamazepine have been shown to alter HPT axis function, and some investigators have suggested that the therapeutic effect of these drugs may correlate with their effects on this axis.

The regulation of thyroid hormone secretion—triiodothyronine (T_3) and thyroxine (T_4)—is initiated by the release of a hypothalamic tripeptide, thyrotropin-releasing hormone (TRH) (Figure 17-5). TRH is released into the portal circulation

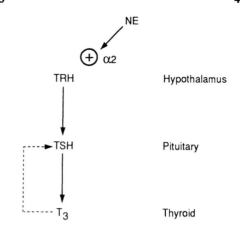

Figure 17-5. HPT axis. Neurotransmitter input.

from axons that originate in the median eminence of the hypothalamus. It is then transported to the pituitary, where it binds to specific thyrotropic cells, which release thyroid-stimulating hormone (TSH). This hormone, in turn, is released into the general circulation and stimulates the thyroid gland to synthesize and release T_3 and T_4. Thyroid hormones have widespread metabolic effects and can directly alter many aspects of peripheral nervous system as well as CNS function. (Several comprehensive texts review the physiology of the HPT axis, e.g., Demeester-Mirkine and Dumont, 1980; Ingbar and Braverman, 1986; Martin and Reichlin, 1987.)

Despite the existence of numerous studies, the status of peripheral thyroid indices in affective illness remains unclear. As reviewed by Bauer and Whybrow (1988a), among the 17 reports of T_3 and T_4 in major depression (predominantly unipolar), 8 noted no difference from normals, and only 2 found decreased T_4 (total and/or free). On the other hand, 7 studies reported that these indices were actually above normal, and, consistent with this, 9 of 10 longitudinal studies found a significant decrease with treatment. Bauer and Whybrow concluded that the most frequent thyroid abnormality associated with major depression (although not specific to this diagnosis)[61] is a relative increase in plasma T_4 without accompanying changes in its active (T_3) or inactive (rT_3) metabolites. In contrast, M. Gold and colleagues (1981) found mild hypothyroidism in 9 percent of their large unipolar sample (usually reflected by slight increases in TSH), and antithyroid antibodies have been reported in up to 20 percent of patients with depression (Nemeroff et al., 1985; M. Gold et al., 1982).

If T_4 actually is increased in depression, disagreement exists as to whether this is part of the pathophysiology of the depressive symptoms (Joffe et al., 1984) or is a compensatory peripheral increase[62] in order to "allow delivery of more thyroxine to a brain whose homeostatic mechanisms have gone awry—an effect achieved without subjecting the organism to increased metabolic demands due to increased circulating levels of T_3" (Bauer and Whybrow, 1988a, p. 82).

This latter interpretation may be most applicable to bipolar illness, where there is some evidence of a subtle decrease in thyroid function, especially among those with rapid cycles (Cho et al., 1979; Cowdry et al., 1983b),[63] although not all studies agree (Joffe et al., 1988a). Evidence of thyroid dysfunction in bipolar illness may have emerged because of the antithyroid effects of lithium, in effect unmasking subtle preexisting thyroid pathology. The association between lithium-induced hypothyroidism and rapid cycling is observed predominantly in women.[64] As noted in Chapter 22, women are also more sensitive to the cycle-inducing effects of TCAs.

If hypothyroidism (either in the presence or absence of lithium treatment) is related to the development of rapid-cycling bipolar depression, it is not yet clear how they are related. Several individual case reports have described cyclical mood disturbances developing in patients following subtotal thyroidectomy (Hertz, 1964). However, thyroidectomy per se is not sufficient for the development of rapid cycling; clearly, other predisposing factors must be present. In Chapter 19, we suggest that the effects of thyroid hormones on the periodicity of biological clocks in animals, coupled with altered circadian pacemaker function in bipolar patients, may explain the apparent inductive effect of hypothyroidism in rapid-cycling patients. Almost all rapid-cycling bipolar patients are female (Wehr et al., 1988a). Likewise, thyroid dysfunction, including the antithyroid effects of lithium, is much more common among women (Joffe et al., 1988). These observations link female sex, hyperthyroidism, and rapid cycling.[65] Hatterer and colleagues (1989) have proposed that relatively reduced thyroid function among bipolar patients on lithium may be associated with poor outcome. They report

that plasma T_3 levels were significantly lower among patients who relapse on lithium, although all values remained in the normal range (see Chapter 23).

Gjessing (1938) described a group of patients with periodic catatonia who, when given large doses of thyroid hormone, responded with rapid (less than 1 week) and long-lasting improvement. In a somewhat larger group of patients with periodic psychoses, Wakoh and Hatotani (1971) reported similar beneficial effects of treatment with large doses of thyroid hormone. As we note in Chapter 5, these patients share many clinical features with rapid-cycling bipolar patients and probably represent the same illness. In a later study, Stancer and Persad (1982) gave hypermetabolic doses of T_4 (300 to 500 μ/day) to ten rapid-cycling bipolar patients. Of the seven women, five responded dramatically, whereas two men and an adolescent did not. Consistent with this are reports that thyroid hormone in combination with standard mood-stabilizing drugs can attenuate cycles in bipolar patients (Goodwin, 1986; Bauer and Whybrow, 1988a).

Another approach to the HPT axis involves the study of circadian patterns of TSH release. Normally, TSH secretion peaks during the night (Weeke, 1973), but this peak is absent in some patients with affective disorder (Weeke and Weeke, 1978; Golstein et al., 1980; Kjellman et al., 1984), including those with rapid-cycling bipolar disorder (Sack et al., 1988b; Kasper et al., 1988). Sleep deprivation represents another challenge test, in that it is associated with an increase in nocturnal TSH. Both bipolar (Sack et al., 1988b) and unipolar depressed patients (Kasper et al., 1988) have been shown to have blunted TSH response to total sleep deprivation. Souêtre and colleagues' excellent review (1986) of this area is discussed further in Chapter 19.

Provocative Challenge Tests

The stimulation of TSH secretion by intravenously administered TRH (the so-called TRH test) is frequently used by endocrinologists to diagnose disorders of the HPT axis. The test has been applied more and more extensively to populations of depressed patients (studies of endogenous TRH are reviewed later in the section on neuropeptides). Prange and co-workers (1972) and Kastin and colleagues (1972) were the first to report a blunting of the TSH response to TRH in depressed patients. This finding has been replicated by many investigators, and, in most studies, approximately 30 percent of depressed patients show an abnormal TSH response. The TRH test, although relatively insensitive, may uncover a trait marker, since TSH blunting was seen more often in unaffected individuals with a family history of depression or alcoholism than in individuals with no such family history (Loosen et al., 1987; Loosen, 1988). Extein and colleagues (1981b) and Baumgartner and associates (1988), examining the relationship between the TRH test and the DST, found the abnormalities distributed in separate but overlapping subgroups of depressed patients. In the Extein study, the patients with abnormalities in both tests appeared to be sicker, at least as reflected in more frequent referral for ECT. Since sleep deprivation has been shown to augment the TSH response to TRH, depression-associated sleep changes may represent a source of variance in the TSH response. In addition, seasonal factors may contribute to variance in this measure. For the most part, too few depressed patients have a blunted TSH response to make the test of routine diagnostic or screening value.[66] Furthermore, its specificity for depression has been called into question (Baumgartner et al., 1988).

Several investigators have reported a different response to TRH in bipolar than in unipolar depressed patients, with the bipolar group showing an augmented response and the unipolar group a blunted response (Chazot et al., 1974; Sørensen et al., 1974). Not all investigators found this difference, however, and it has been suggested that the augmented response might reflect a carryover of mild hypothyroidism from the previous lithium treatment (P. Gold et al., 1977).[67]

The TRH test in mania has produced more consensus. At least five independent groups have reported a blunted TSH response in manic patients.[68] These results are especially noteworthy since many of the patients received neuroleptics, which have been shown to increase the TSH response to TRH (Kirkegaard et al., 1977). Two of these studies compared depression with mania in the same bipolar patients. They found that the TSH response was opposite in the two phases of illness—augmented during depression, blunted during mania. Extein and co-workers (1980b) emphasized the differential diagnostic value of an abnormal TRH test in mania (and schizoaffective mania), since they and others (Loosen et al., 1977; Kirkegaard et al., 1978; Kiriike et al., 1988) found a normal response in schizophrenic patients. Other studies (Extein et al., 1984b; Kirkegaard et al., 1977) suggest that continuation of a blunted TSH response to TRH after apparent clinical recovery from depression may signify a poor prognosis. Further, when both TSH response and the DST fail to return to normal, the patient is more likely to relapse than if either test alone remained abnormal.

Growth Hormone

Growth hormone (GH) is another anterior pituitary hormone that has been widely studied in psychiatric patients. Regulation of GH secretion is considerably more complex than that of most pituitary hormones because a variety of neurotransmitter systems are known to influence its secretion (Martin and Reichlin, 1987; Matussek, 1988) (Figure 17-6). Somatostatin, a hypothalamic peptide, inhibits the release of GH, whereas the catecholamines dopamine and norepinephrine, as well as the hypothalamic peptide growth hormone-releasing hormone (GRH), stimulate it. Growth hormone is sleep dependent in that the onset of sleep provides a major physiological stimulus to its secretion (see Chapter 19). Among patients with major depression, the sleep-dependent increase in GH is blunted, and this abnormality may persist after recovery (Steiger et al., 1989; Jarrett et al., 1989).

Clinical studies show that a variety of drugs and neurotransmitter receptor agonists alter GH secretion. Since the hormone can also be released

Figure 17-6. Neurotransmitter input to growth hormone-releasing factor (GRF) secretion.

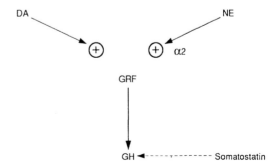

in response to environmental stress, some of the changes noted after drug administration may have been due to the stress of the injection itself (Martin and Reichlin, 1987). Despite this and other methodological problems of clinical studies, it is clear that human GH secretion is activated by α_2-adrenergic receptors in the hypothalamus and perhaps also in the pituitary. Agonists of these receptors, such as clonidine, are potent releasers of GH, whereas antagonists, such as yohimbine and piperoxane, block GH secretion induced either by drugs or by insulin-induced hypoglycemia (Lancranjan and Marbach, 1977). Clonidine-induced GH secretion has been studied extensively in depressed patients. The first studies (Matussek et al., 1980; Checkley et al., 1981) demonstrated a blunted GH response in depressed patients compared with controls, a finding now widely replicated and extended by others.[69] In general, the blunted GH response is seen most consistently in unipolar depressed patients,[70] whereas bipolar patients have normal (Siever and Uhde, 1984) or even exaggerated GH responses to clonidine (Siever and Uhde, 1984; Matussek et al., 1980).[71]

L-Dopa also increases GH secretion in humans, an effect apparently mediated by α_1-adrenoceptors.[72] Several investigators have demonstrated a blunted GH response to L-dopa in depressed patients, and some have suggested that this blunting may be confined to unipolar patients (Sachar et al., 1972).[73] Blunted GH response to amphetamine and methylamphetamine has generally been reported among depressed patients, although the findings may not be specific to depressive illness.[74] Gold and colleagues (1984b) found a GH response to CRF in bipolar depressed patients, which does not occur in healthy controls, and Lesch and colleagues (1988b) report the same thing among patients with major depression, suggesting some disintegration of hypothalamic–pituitary function in the patients.

Insulin-induced hypoglycemia reliably elevates plasma GH. This response also appears to be mediated via α-adrenergic receptors (Blackard and Heidingsfelder, 1968). There are many independent reports of an attenuated GH response to insulin-induced hypoglycemia among depressed patients (reviewed by Amsterdam et al., 1987). This attenuation has been reported for both premenopausal and postmenopausal patients and

does not seem related to the extent of hypoglycemia. On the other hand, the NIMH collaborative study failed to replicate the finding (Brunswick et al., 1988), and among bipolar patients, some investigators have observed normal (Amsterdam et al., 1983b) or a trend toward exaggerated (Sachar et al., 1973a; Koslow et al., 1982) GH responses to insulin-induced hypoglycemia, as in the studies with clonidine and L-dopa.[75] A study by Casper and colleagues (1977) reported that the response was blunted in manic patients.

The release of GH by the dopamine (DA) receptor agonist *apomorphine* is inhibited by selective DA receptor blockers (Rotrosen et al., 1976; Lal and Martin, 1980) and therefore represents a reasonable way to assess central DA receptor function, at least in the tibulo infundibular system, which releases DA from the hypothalamus into the hypothalamic-hypophyseal portal system down to the pituitary, where it participates in the release of GH. Given the fact that the dopamine hypothesis of depression has focused on bipolar disorder, it is somewhat surprising that there are no studies of GH release by apomorphine specifically in this population. Although the initial four studies[76] in major depression were negative, a recent study employing a lower dose of apomorphine (and, therefore, more likely to pick up relative hyposensitivity of receptors) did find a blunted response among unipolar depressed patients. This difference could reflect either a decreased sensitivity of hypothalamic DA receptors or perhaps a primary deficit in pituitary GH production or secretion.[77] However, a suprapituitary origin for the blunted GH findings seems more likely, given the fact that when depressed patients are infused with growth hormone releasing factor, there is apparently a normal pattern of GH release (Thomas et al., 1989). Lesch and colleagues (1988a) reached a similar conclusion from a more complex experimental design.

Prolactin

Prolactin is another pituitary hormone whose release is known to be influenced by several different neurotransmitter systems, prominent among them being a DA system exerting tonic inhibition. Studies of baseline PRL levels in major depression have not achieved a consensus, perhaps because a variety of factors influence it, especially the menstrual cycle. The three studies that have focused on bipolar depression all reported decreased resting levels (Garfinkel et al., 1979; Mendlewicz et al., 1980c; Joyce et al., 1988), which, considering only the DA input, would not be consistent with a functional DA deficit in bipolar depression. Such a conclusion is premature, however, given the variety of other neurotransmitters influencing PRL relapse. For example, PRL is increased in normal controls by the administration of the serotonin precursor L-tryptophan. This response was found to be blunted or attenuated in a mixed group of depressed patients, some of whom were bipolar (Heninger et al., 1984). In a more recent study of major depression (both bipolar and unipolar), Price and colleagues (1989) found that a tryptophan-induced increase in PRL was enhanced after 1 week of lithium, but under chronic lithium administration (3 weeks), the response returned to baseline. Since such an attenuation of response had not been seen in other studies of chronic lithium in normals, the authors concluded that "the homeostatic responses of the 5-HT system to long-term lithium treatment may differ in patients with affective disorders and healthy subjects." The serotonergic anorectic agent, fenfluramine, also increases serum PRL, and Siever and colleagues (1984b) reported that, compared with controls, this response was blunted among a group of predominantly bipolar depressed patients.[78] It is interesting that lithium has been reported to augment the fenfluramine-induced release of PRL (Slater et al., 1976), thus adding to the consensus that lithium potentiates functional serotonergic activity in a variety of systems.[79]

Depue and colleagues (1989b), studying PRL secretion in premenopausal women with seasonal affective disorder, found consistently lower basal PRL levels in depressed patients than in controls during summer and winter periods, although the patients' Hamilton depression scores were significantly higher in winter. They suggest that low PRL levels may be a trait characteristic of seasonal affective disorder, which overlaps considerably with bipolar-II disorder.

Pineal Melatonin Secretion in Manic-Depressive Illness

The pineal gland has been called a neuroendocrine transducer (Axelrod, 1974), since the output of its major hormone, melatonin, is regulated by neural (sympathetic) innervation. Moreover, the outflow of this sympathetic pathway is directly under the control of the endogenous circadian pacemaker located in the suprachiasmatic nucleus of the hypothalamus (Moore and Klein, 1974). Melatonin synthesis is stimulated through a β-adrenergic receptor located on the pinealocyte membrane. When norepinephrine is released from pineal sympathetic nerve endings, a β-receptor-mediated increase in cAMP results in an increase in the de novo synthesis of N-acetyltransferase, the rate-limiting enzyme in melatonin synthesis (Axelrod, 1974). In rodents and humans, melatonin synthesis increases at night, but light, which activates the retinohypothalamic tract, profoundly inhibits nighttime melatonin secretion.

A great deal is known about pineal melatonin secretion and its relationship to circadian rhythms from studies in laboratory animals (Moore and Klein, 1974; Lewy, 1984), but only recently has such work been extended to humans. These studies have been further stimulated by the development of reliable and sensitive methods for determining melatonin in plasma. Chapter 19 deals with melatonin as it relates to circadian or seasonal rhythms and their possible disturbance in manic-depressive illness. Here, we limit our consideration of melatonin to its possible use as an index of the activity of the β-adrenergic receptor in the pineal gland and, therefore, as an in vivo measure of receptor activity in an important norepinephrine-mediated system.

Lewy and co-workers (1980), using a sensitive gas chromatographic–mass spectrometric assay, systematically examined melatonin secretion around the clock in normal volunteers and in bipolar patients. Total 24-hour melatonin excretion was significantly higher in the manic than in the depressive phase, both within each individual and from one individual to another, whereas values for the normal controls were intermediate. A state-dependent increase during mania was also noted in a single-case longitudinal study by Kennedy and colleagues (1989), and Rosenthal and colleagues (1986b) reported a significant decrease among patients with winter depression (see Chapter 19). On the other hand, Thompson and associates (1988), in a carefully controlled study of depressed patients and age- and sex-

matched normal controls, could not confirm reduced melatonin secretion in a predominantly
unipolar group. Studies of the 24-hour urinary
excretion of 6-hydroxymelatonin, the major metabolite of melatonin, reported reduced excretion
in depressed patients compared with controls.[80]
These data are consistent with a relative increase
in pineal β-receptor activity in mania and, with
the exception of the Thompson study, a relative
decrease in bipolar depression.

The initial attempts in humans to suppress the
nighttime rise in melatonin secretion with light
were unsuccessful, even though light has a rapid,
strong effect on nighttime melatonin in a variety
of animals (Reiter et al., 1982). Later, as described in Chapter 19, Lewy and colleagues
found that very bright light ($\geq$ 2,500 lux) could
inhibit melatonin secretion in humans. They then
studied the effects of various intensities of light
on melatonin secretion in bipolar patients, who,
regardless of their clinical state (manic, depressed, or euthymic) or medication status, were
found to be more sensitive to light than normal
controls, experiencing nighttime melatonin suppression at light intensities (500 to 1,500 lux)
well below the normal threshold (Lewy et al.,
1981, 1985a).[81]

The supersensitivity to light might reflect a
trait or vulnerability marker in manic-depressive
patients. This possibility is intriguing, since it is
known that cholinergic stimulation of the suprachiasmatic nucleus of rats mimics the effects
of light on melatonin secretion (Zatz and Brownstein, 1981), and it has been suggested previously
that excessive cholinergic tone may be involved
in the pathophysiology of bipolar depression and
may perhaps also be an element in vulnerability to
this disorder. However, attempts to suppress
melatonin secretion with cholinergic agonists
have thus far been unsuccessful in humans.

Pituitary-Gonadal System

Several features of manic-depressive illness suggest possible abnormalities in the pituitary-
gonadal system: Changes in libido are prominent
symptoms, menstrually related exacerbations of
the illness have been noted in case reports, both
estrogens and androgens have been reported to
potentiate antidepressant drugs in some patients,
and certain conditions related to gonadal hormone output may be more frequent in bipolar

patients (see, e.g., the report by Lewis et al.,
1987, on endometriosis). Yet the literature on
gonadal hormones or their pituitary trophic factors, such as luteinizing hormone or follicle-
stimulating hormone, in manic-depressive illness
is very limited. Some, but not all, studies report
modest reductions in serum testosterone among
depressed patients, but the bipolar–unipolar distinction has not been made (reviewed by Rubin,
1981). Mason and colleagues (1988) found significantly higher serum testosterone levels among
paranoid schizophrenic patients than in manic patients hospitalized on the same ward. They suggested that this measure might prove useful in the
differential diagnosis of mania and schizophrenia. Given the very high incidence of mania
during the immediate postpartum period, when
high estrogen levels are falling dramatically,
Cookson (1985) suggested that increased estrogen during pregnancy leads to a phenothiazine
-like dopamine receptor inhibition, accompanied
by a compensatory increase in receptor number.
He hypothesizes that the sudden fall in estrogen
exposes a new supersensitive mesolimbic dopamine receptor system, which serves as a trigger to
a manic episode.

Conclusion

Neuroendocrine studies have provided a limited
window into the brain (see Table 17-11), but
they have not yet contributed fundamental new
insights into the pathophysiology of manic-
depressive illness, primarily because interactions between various neurotransmitters and
hypothalamic-releasing hormones are not fully
understood. For instance, the hypercortisolemia
that occurs in unipolar and bipolar depression appears to be centrally mediated via hypersecretion
of CRF, but exactly what is causing the CRF
hypersecretion remains a mystery. In patients
with major depression, challenge tests with
yohimbine produce an abnormally large increase
(L.H. Price et al., 1986) and clonidine an abnormally large decrease in cortisol secretion (Siever
et al., 1984c). These effects imply an alteration in
the sensitivity of α_2-adrenergic receptors in depression. Interpretation of these results is complicated by the fact that such adrenergic drugs have
sites of action in the brainstem, hypothalamus,
and the pituitary—all of which could influence
cortisol secretion. Furthermore, norepinephrine

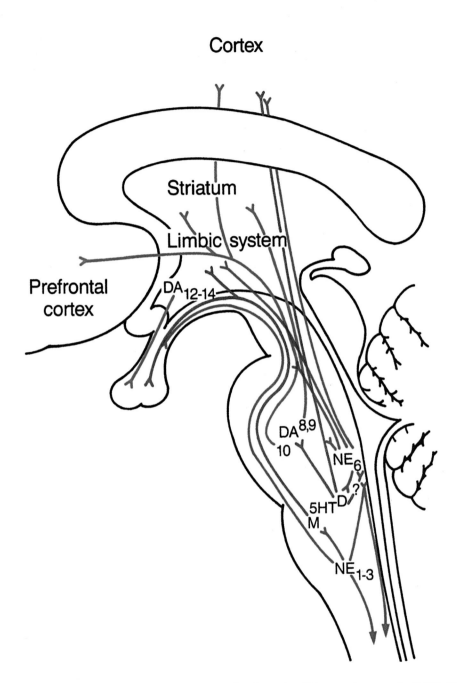

Figure 17-2. Limbic system: Schematic section illustrating dopamine (DA, green), serotonin (5-HT, blue), and norepinephrine (NE, red) systems in the brain. Numbers refer to groups of catecholamine neurons (NE and DA) according to the nomenclature of Dahlström and Fuxe (1964). The termination of a given axon projection is indicated by a >. D, dorsal raphe; M, medial raphe. The ? refers to evidence that the projection may be to the region most adjacent to the locus coeruleus (NE_6) and not directly on it. For text discussion, see pages 445 and 446; cf. page 409.

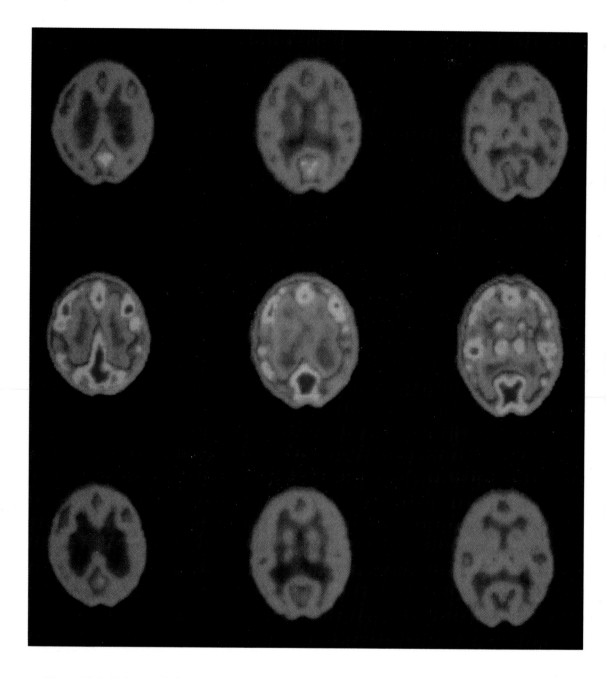

Figure 18-1. Positron emission tomographic scans of the brain of a drug-free rapid-cycling manic-depressive patient. The colors in the scans correspond to glucose metabolic rates, with the lowest rates associated with the coolest end of the color spectrum (blue) and the highest rates with the warmest (red). PET scans in the top row were made on May 17, when the patient was depressed. The second row shows the identical planes scanned the next day, when the patient had become hypomanic. The third row shows the scans on May 27, when the patient was again depressed (adapted from Baxter et al., 1985). For text discussion, see page 521.

was originally thought to inhibit hypothalamic CRF secretion, but recent animal studies (Guillaume et al., 1987) suggest a stimulatory effect. Therefore, until more is known about the site of action and the exact effect of these neurotransmitters on hypothalamic–pituitary function, the ability of the neuroendocrine approaches to illuminate the various amine hypotheses will be limited. Neuroendocrine data nevertheless suggest that norepinephrine and serotonin are dysregulated in affective disorder. For example, the blunted GH response to clonidine challenge and changes in melatonin secretion controlled by β-adrenergic receptors implicate norepinephrine and increased cortisol response to 5-HTP suggests serotonin involvement.

One explanation for discrepancies among studies of bipolar patients may be found in a study by Amsterdam and colleagues (1983b), who administered a battery of neuroendocrine tests to 22 bipolar patients (14 depressed and 8 hypomanic) and healthy controls.[82] Almost 80 percent of the patients had at least one abnormal hormonal response, compared with only 40 percent of controls. Further, over half of the patients, but none of the controls, had two or more abnormal hormonal responses. There were no differences in the number of abnormalities during depression or hypomania. The investigators concluded that the variability in hormonal responses in both bipolar and unipolar patient groups is greater than in healthy subjects and that abnormal test results in patients are more likely than in controls. They suggest that this increased hormonal variability may be responsible "for the conflicting results reported from a large number of previous studies that examined individual endocrine axes" (p. 521).

The variability in neuroendocrine function in bipolar patients is probably not surprising for several reasons. First, it is likely that whatever produces the mood swings in manic-depressive illness might also produce great variations in hormone secretion over the course of the illness. Second, a bipolar patient undoubtedly experiences great stress, especially when psychosis or a dysphoric mood is prominent. Individual variation in stress tolerance would be reflected in the magnitude of the endocrine responses. Stress causes the release of growth hormone, prolactin, and epinephrine, and cortisol inhibits somato-

statin and TSH secretion. Third, those patients who have a unique pattern, such as the same abnormalities in both the manic and depressed phases, may belong to a subgroup. It would be naive to assume that one pathophysiological chain underlies all bipolar illness. Clearly, there is a significant genetic heterogeneity in the familial transmission of the illness (see Chapter 15), and this could be reflected in specific neuroendocrine abnormalities.

Many have interpreted the neuroendocrine literature as a one-way view into the brain's neurotransmitter systems, neglecting the profound effects of hormones on the brain itself. Steroids and thyroid hormones are particularly relevant to affective illness because clinical syndromes involving altered function in these hormones are associated with both depression and mania. Thyroid abnormalities in rapid-cycling bipolar patients may be intrinsic to the pathophysiology of the illness. The identification of brain-specific thyroid receptors may have relevance to manic-depressive illness (Thompson et al., 1987). Thus, neuropeptides and peripheral hormones may be as important in the etiology of manic-depressive illness as the traditional neurotransmitters thought to control their production.

NEUROPEPTIDES

Neuropeptides comprise a large portion of the active substances in the CNS and have been found in brain regions regulating emotion. Neurons that secrete a particular peptide may also secrete classic neurotransmitters or other peptides. The synthesis, processing, release, and degradation of neuropeptides are controlled by enzymes, pathways, and processes different from those of the classic neurotransmitters.

As already alluded to in the discussion of neuroendocrine systems, peptides are of particular interest in behavioral disorders because they regulate behavior, physiology, and cognition that characteristically occur over relatively long periods of time. Their actions on different levels of functioning are often coordinated. Gonadotropin-releasing hormone, for example, enhances reproduction by increasing libido, stimulating reproductive hormone secretion, and enhancing sperm and ova production. It is even conceivable that a specific peptide abnormality could underlie the entire syndrome of manic-depressive illness.

Research on neuroactive peptides has exploded in the past decade. Dozens of endogenous peptides have been discovered, and more than 30 of them have been characterized as "neuromodulators" in brain.[83] New peptide neurotransmitter or neuromodulator candidates emerge with increasing frequency as methods for their isolation, characterization, and synthesis become more and more sophisticated and efficient. Their location within individual neurons has been elegantly and extensively mapped, and molecular genetic techniques will produce an even larger harvest of new peptides in the future (Bloom, 1987).

Not surprisingly, possible neuropeptide alterations in affective illness are now being actively explored. Questions about peptide system involvement in the pathophysiology of manic-depressive illness have followed logically on the heels of other discoveries, such as the existence of an endogenous opiate receptor and the apparent dual function of peptides in the neuroendocrine system—both as hormones acting on distant targets and as chemical messengers released close to their site of action (Matussek, 1988). To date, the clinical literature on peptides is relatively sparse. Nevertheless, we have chosen to develop this area in some detail in the expectation that it will assume increasing importance in the near future.

The Endogenous Opiate System

The discovery of the opiate receptor and its endogenous ligand provided the tools for characterizing endogenous opiate systems involving the endorphins and enkephalins. The fact that these systems modulate behavior related to mood, such as pleasure, pain, and self-stimulation, suggests that they are involved in affective illness. One straightforward formulation hypothesized decreased endogenous opiate function in depression and increased opiate function in mania. Such alterations might occur either in the endogenous opiate neuromodulator or in the density or sensitivity of opiate receptors. Evaluation of these hypotheses has been approached through several experimental paradigms, such as administrating opiate agonists or antagonists to patients, assessing endorphins and related opiate-binding activity in spinal fluid and plasma, conducting neu-

roendocrine tests following a challenge with exogenous opiates, and examining the effects of mood-altering drugs on opiate systems (see, e.g., Stengaard-Pedersen and Schou, 1982).

Trials of Opiate Antagonists in Mania

Endorphins have been studied more extensively than any other group of peptides, not only because they were among the first peptides localized in brain after the discovery of their receptors (Pert and Snyder, 1973) but also because the availability of the relatively pure opiate antagonist naloxone facilitated clinical dissection of the opiate system's function in manic-depressive illness. Despite this scientific activity, however, only tenuous links have so far been made between opiate systems and manic-depressive illness.

In light of morphine's obvious effects on mood and motor activity in animals and humans, the strategy of blocking endogenous opiate receptors with naloxone in manic patients was viewed with considerable anticipation. The initial study (Janowsky et al., 1978) showed small but significant decreases in manic symptoms following a daily 20-mg intravenous infusion of naloxone, but subsequent studies have not been as positive. In Janowsky and colleagues' 1979 report, only 2 of 7 manic patients were dramatically calmed, whereas Judd and his colleagues (1980) found observable decreases in manic symptoms in 4 of 12 manic patients with the same dose and route of administration. Davis and co-workers (1979) noted some apparent antimanic effects in 4 patients receiving up to 30 mg, but the changes were not sufficiently robust to reach statistical significance. Later, this same group (1980) gave 20 mg subcutaneously to 10 manic patients and reported no improvement in rated mania. These negative results were later replicated by the World Health Organization Collaborative Study (Pickar et al., 1982b), a well-controlled, double-blind, placebo-crossover study of 26 manic patients, although this group observed significant naloxone-associated reduction in psychotic symptoms in schizophrenic patients concurrently treated with neuroleptics. Emrich and co-workers (1979) actually reported exacerbation of manic symptoms in 1 of 2 bipolar patients.

Thus, the initial observations of antimanic effects with high-dose naloxone have not held up to more extensive efforts at replication. Naloxone-sensitive mania, if it exists, appears to be relatively rare and may require very large doses. It should be noted that several opiate-receptor subsystems in the brain are relatively resistant to blockade by naloxone, so that, even with high doses, the naloxone strategy does not provide an unequivocal test of the theory that mania is associated with excess function of some endogenous opiate system in a localized region of the brain.

Trials of Opiates and Opiate Analogs in Depression

The complementary strategy—administering opiates to depressed patients—has also been pursued. Synthetic opiates were among the earliest drugs used in the treatment of depression (see Chapter 22), and this area has been opened anew with trials of the endogenous opiate-like peptides, β-endorphin, and enkephalin analogs. The bipolar–unipolar distinction was, understandably, not used in the classic opiate literature. Surprisingly, some recent peptide studies also failed to distinguish these groups. In an open trial that included several depressed patients, Kline and Lehmann (1979) noted marked activation in one patient and some improvement in depression in two patients receiving intravenous β-endorphin. The effect occurred within minutes and lasted for several hours. Angst and colleagues (1979a) reported that when six depressed patients (four bipolar and two unipolar) received an intravenous infusion of β-endorphin, all improved in energy, mood, anxiety, and restlessness during the first 20 to 30 minutes, an effect that persisted for 2 hours. Four subsequently relapsed. Three patients switched into mania or hypomania during or soon after the trial, an outcome the authors suggested might have been caused by drug withdrawal, sleep deprivation, or stress. In a double-blind trial, Gerner and colleagues (1980) also observed significant improvement following intravenous β-endorphin in ten depressed patients, who then relapsed the day after the infusion; no hypomania was noted. Similar positive results were noted by Chazot and colleagues (1985) in a randomized placebo controlled double-blind trial involving 20 patients hospitalized for major depression (primarily unipolar). On the other hand, two other double-blind trials were negative, one involving des-tyrosine γ-endorphin (Fink et al., 1981), the other β-endorphin (Pickar et al.,

1981). Extein and colleagues (1979a,b) administered an analog of metenkephalin (FK 33824) to nine medication-free depressed patients (predominantly bipolar) and observed no clinical improvement. In sum, initial open studies (and one double-blind study) suggested that intravenous β-endorphin or related endogenous opiate substances may improve depression. More recent trials, including active placebo to mimic the flush, have shown less consistent evidence of improvement.

Several studies have investigated the effects of chronic opiate administration on mood and behavior in depressed patients. Krebs and Roubicek (1979) reported improvement in three of four depressed patients given repeated injections of FK 33824 (2 to 5 mg intramuscularly for 3 to 8 days), and Emrich and associates (1982b) noted antidepressant effects with the mixed opiate agonist–antagonist buprenorphine in 5 of 10 depressed patients. Earlier Fink and colleagues (1970) had reported moderate improvement in 8 of 10 "psychotically depressed" patients treated with the mixed opiate agonist–antagonist cyclazocine (1 to 3 mg/day).

A case report from a different patient population is of note here. Pickar and co-workers (1984b) observed the late onset of an activated, confusional, manic psychosis in a patient receiving intrathecal β-endorphin for intractable pain associated with cancer. Two other case reports also mention the induction of euphoric or confusional states (Foley et al., 1979; Oyama et al., 1982). The fact that large amounts of an endogenous opiate substance administered directly into the CNS can produce a manic-like state does not, however, really bear on the question of whether disturbances in the endogenous opiate systems are involved in the pathophysiology of manic-depressive illness.

Not surprisingly, acute or chronic naloxone has little positive effect in depressed patients (Janowsky et al., 1979; Davis et al., 1979; Terenius et al., 1977). Cohen and colleagues (1984) reported increased depression and anxiety in six patients (five unipolar, one bipolar) given intravenous naloxone (2 mg/kg).

Measurement of Opiates in Body Fluids

The role of opiate substances in manic-depressive illness has been assessed by measuring their concentrations in CSF. CSF may be a more appropriate substance for investigation than plasma, since evidence suggests that direct brain stimulation or acupuncture in animals or humans can produce differential and selective release of opiates into CSF. Terenius' group (1976) initially reported that CSF from manic and depressed patients showed alterations in binding to an opiate receptor preparation. Many of these patients were not studied under medication-free conditions, however, and it is also not clear how many of the depressed patients were bipolar.

Gerner and Sharp (1982) found no significant differences in CSF β-endorphin concentrations among medication-free unipolar or bipolar patients or normal subjects. Likewise, in a well-controlled study of bipolar illness, Pickar and associates (1982a) reported no overall relationship between manic or depressive mood state and total CSF opiate activity measured by binding in the radioreceptor assay, although all four patients studied in both phases had significantly higher opiate receptor activity during mania than during depression.

The opioid peptide precursor proopiomelanocortin (POMC) is cleaved to form various fragments, including β-endorphin, β-lipotropin, α-MSH, ACTH, and the N-terminal fragment of POMC (N-POMC). Berrettini and colleagues (1985a, 1987d) measured the five fragments in CSF and plasma in 30 normal volunteers and 40 euthymic bipolar patients (15 unmedicated, 25 lithium treated). None of the five peptides was different in either group of well-state patients compared with controls.

In summary, the trials of opiate agonists and antagonists in depression and mania have so far failed to produce any convincing evidence that these systems are significantly involved in the pathophysiology of affective illness. The same can be said about the study of these peptides in body fluids. Since opiates were virtually the only agents available for the treatment of serious depression for centuries, further exploration of these systems seems unlikely to produce new insights or new treatments.

Somatostatin

Somatostatin, a gut peptide now also identified as a neuromodulator in the brain, appears at first to be an unlikely candidate for a substance specifically involved in affective illness. Unlike the opiate systems, which can be analyzed with agonists and antagonists, the somatostatin system has not yet yielded to such pharmacological dissection. Several pieces of indirect data do, however, suggest its potential importance in affective illness. Somatostatin is widely distributed in the CNS, including cortical, limbic, and hypothalamic regions. It exerts inhibitory control over the HPA axis, which, as noted earlier, is often disinhibited in depression and perhaps in some manic states as well. Somatostatin is depleted in temporal cortex and CSF of patients with Alzheimer's disease. It is sometimes reduced in patients with other conditions often accompanied by cognitive impairment, including parkinsonism, multiple sclerosis, and anorexia nervosa. Somatostatin inhibits endocrine responses to a variety of hormones and alters appetite, pain, sleep, and motor activity (Rubinow et al., 1983), all of which are often abnormal in affective illness. Somatostatin affects a variety of the classic neurotransmitters (NE, 5-HT, DA, GABA, and ACh) and coexists in neurons containing norepinephrine, acetylcholine, or GABA, suggesting important regulatory functions in these systems.

Five of six studies of CSF somatostatin of depressed patients ($n = 167$), compared with normal controls or other patient populations, showed significantly lower levels among depressed patients (Table 17-12). In the study by Rubinow and co-workers (1983), lowered somatostatin levels were observed in both unipolar and bipolar depressed patients. Low somatostatin levels in depression appear to be state-dependent. Thus, Rubinow and associates (1983) observed that, with improvement to a euthymic state or a switch to mania, somatostatin increased to normal levels. These findings are consistent with those of Berrettini and colleagues (1987d), who reported that in 30 euthymic bipolar patients (10 free of medication and 20 receiving lithium), somatostatin levels in the CSF did not differ from those of 20 normal volunteers. Initial studies (Doran et al., 1986), confirmed by Rubinow (1986), suggest that somatostatin is lower in patients who have abnormal DST results regardless of diagnosis, a finding consistent with a role for this peptide in the regulation of ACTH secretion (Reisine, 1984). Also, somatostatin in CSF is

Table17-12. CSF Somatostatin in Depression and Mania

Study	Control	Depressed	Manic	50	100	150
Gerner & Yamada, 1982	29	28	10	♦a	15.0 ◊	
Rubinow et al., 1983	39	25 (18 BP, 7 UP)		♦a	62.8	
Berrettini et al., 1984	20	10 unmedicated BP / 20 Li-treated BP			♦ 33.1	♦
Bissette et al., 1986	10	17		♦b	116.1	
Black et al., 1986	46	18	a	♦	55.5	
Rubinow, 1986	47	49 (26 BP, 23 UP)	9	♦a	◊ 62.1	

Control group mean somatostatin level (pg/ml) appears in the 100% column. Shaded bar indicates standard error (expressed in percentage points) around the control mean expressed as 100%.

♦ = Mean for depressed group expressed as a % of control mean
◊ = Mean for manic group expressed as a % of control mean

a p <.05 vs. controls
b p <.01 vs. controls

lower in patients with Cushing's disease (Kling et al., 1986), suggesting that elevated cortisol levels may suppress somatostatin release.

The anticonvulsant carbamazepine, which has both acute and prophylactic effects in some manic-depressive patients (particularly those not responsive to lithium), is associated with significantly decreased levels of somatostatin in the CSF compared with medication-free values (Rubinow, 1986). Whether this lowered level of somatostatin is in any way related to the clinical effects of carbamazepine is not clear. Lithium and antidepressants do not appear to have this effect.

Vasopressin

Extensive animal data indicate that central vasopressin is involved in regulating memory, pain sensitivity, sleep, the synchronization of circadian rhythms, and fluid and electrolyte balance. Noting the parallel between these functional roles of vasopressin and the syndrome of affective illness, Gold and Goodwin (1978) hypothesized that a deficiency in central vasopressin function is involved in the pathophysiology of depression, especially alterations in cognitive functioning, circadian rhythms, and fluid and electrolyte balance. Clinical evaluations of this hypothesis have used the measurement of CSF vasopressin, plasma vasopressin response to saline infusion challenge, and the behavioral response of depressed patients to a vasopressin analog.

P. Gold and co-workers (1981), Gjerris and associates (1985), and Sørensen and colleagues (1985) observed that nonpsychotic bipolar depressed patients had significantly lower levels of vasopressin in CSF than had manic patients, with normals falling in the middle. Gold's group (1984a) also found that vasopressin levels in CSF were significantly correlated with plasma vasopressin responses to hypertonic saline. There appeared to be differences in vasopressin levels across manic and depressive states in the small number of patients receiving hypertonic saline infusion. These findings suggest that there may be subtle vasopressin changes across manic and depressive mood states that are relevant to alterations in cognitive functioning. However, two studies of euthymic bipolar patients (Berrettini et al., 1982b, 1984) found no abnormalities in platelet vasopressin uptake and arginine vasopressin levels in CSF.

As noted, animal research suggests that vasopressin is important in memory processes (De Weid, 1980), and several studies have reported that administration of vasopressin (or its analogs) to normal volunteers, depressed patients, or amnesic subjects improves some aspects of memory and cognition (Weingartner et al., 1981b). Gold and colleagues (1979) reported that mood improved in two of seven hospitalized, medication-free depressed patients given 1-desamino-8-D-arginine vasopressin (DDAVP), but even more significant was the uniformity of the memory improvement. However, Zohar and associates (1985) did not find a therapeutic effect of lysine vasopressin on mood in 12 severely depressed, treatment-resistant patients in a double-blind crossover study.

Two important drugs for manic-depressive illness, lithium and carbamazepine, affect vasopressin function in apparently opposite directions. Lithium is associated with the induction of diabetes insipidus, presumably by inhibiting renal vasopressin-induced adenylate cyclase activity, and carbamazepine has been used in treating hypothalamic diabetes insipidus (even though it will not reverse the condition when it is induced by lithium) (Post et al., 1984a).[84] These findings are of clinical interest because lithium and carbamazepine may have differential therapeutic effects. In addition, they differ in certain side effects; for example, lithium has been linked to certain subjective and objective measures of memory impairment (particularly recall mechanisms), an effect that could relate to inhibition of vasopressin function. To that extent, carbamazepine, which actually potentiates vasopressin function, would not be expected to produce the side effect (see Chapter 23). A study of the effects of ECT on vasopressin levels in depressed patients showed a sharp rise in plasma vasopressin levels after treatment, which continued in most patients 4 to 8 days thereafter (Devanand et al., 1987).

Oxytocin

Oxytocin is similar to vasopressin in its structure, anatomical distribution, and wide-ranging effects in the CNS. Secretion of these peptides into CSF has been demonstrated to be independent of their secretion into plasma (Kalin et al., 1985; Perlow et al., 1982). Thus, CSF measures may provide a window into the brain that cannot be obtained by peripheral sampling. Demitrack and Gold (1988) measured oxytocin in CSF of patients with affective illness and normal volunteers, with findings

roughly reciprocal to those of vasopressin: Manic patients had lower levels of oxytocin than depressed patients. If this interesting finding is replicated, it may be relevant to the opposite effects of oxytocin and vasopressin on learning and memory in animals; that is, oxytocin produces effects resembling amnesia (Bohus et al., 1978).

Other Peptides

MIF-1

Melanocyte-stimulating hormone release-inhibiting factor (MIF-1), a hypothalamic tripeptide with the structure of prolyl-leucyl-glycinamide, is identical to the C-terminal portion of oxytocin. MIF-1 increases the rate of synthesis of central dopamine, but not of norepinephrine or serotonin, and shows antidepressant activity in certain animal screening tests. In double-blind studies with depressed patients (bipolar–unipolar distribution not specified), MIF-1 had antidepressant effects greater than placebo; their magnitude and time course were similar to those of imipramine (Ehrensing and Kastin, 1974; Levy et al., 1982). Beyond 1 or 2 weeks, however, more than half the patients relapsed, so that the antidepressant effect of MIF-1 apparently is transient and of questionable clinical value. In contrast, Van der Velde (1983) reported a rapid and robust antidepressant effect of MIF-1 in 20 depressed patients randomly assigned in a double-blind study to either daily MIF-1 (60 mg orally) or imipramine (75 mg twice daily). After 2 weeks, the difference between MIF-1 and imipramine was not significant, suggesting that MIF-1 does have some value. However, about one third of the initial responses deteriorated during the first week, and the question of later relapse is not considered.

Calcitonin

Animal studies indicate that calcitonin is involved in regulating a variety of functions, including motor activity, appetite, and pain. It is for this reason and for its effects on calcium metabolism that calcitonin is an interesting candidate for study in affective disorders. Carman and coworkers (1984) observed significantly lower levels of immunoreactive calcitonin in the CSF of manic than in bipolar depressed or euthymic patients or normal controls. Carman's team followed its preliminary CSF investigations with a double-blind clinical trial of calcitonin in mania and observed a significant and substantial reduction in hyperactivity in 85 percent of the manic patients. To our knowledge, these interesting leads have not been pursued by others.

Substance P

Substance P, originally discovered in 1931 by Von Euler and Gaddum and later identified as a decapeptide, is found throughout the CNS, especially in the substantia nigra, caudate, amygdala, hypothalamus, and cortex. When applied to cells, it generally produces prolonged excitation. Rimón and colleagues (1984) reported significantly increased substance P in the CSF of depressed and schizophrenic patients over normal controls, with depressed patients showing significantly higher levels than schizophrenic patients. However, Berrettini and associates (1985c) failed to show any significant difference in CSF substance P between normal controls and a group of medication-free bipolar patients in depressed, euthymic, and manic phases. Further, the peptide was not affected by treatment with lithium. This negative finding is consistent with those of Kleinman and colleagues (1985), who found no significant alteration in substance P concentrations in the caudate nucleus of 19 suicide victims compared with 18 normal postmortem controls.

Cholecystokinin

The peptide cholecystokinin (CCK) is of interest in affective illness primarily as a potential mediator of appetite disturbance, since it can produce anorexia in various animals. Moreover, in light of the previously reviewed evidence that dopamine may be involved in manic-depressive illness, it is of interest that CCK has been found to coexist with dopamine in individual neurons. Some, but not all, clinical trials of CCK or its analogs in psychotic patients suggest that these peptides can alter psychotic symptomatology.

Gerner and Yamada (1982) and Gjerris and associates (1984) found no significant differences among normal volunteers and depressed or manic patients in CSF levels of CCK. In contrast, Verbanck and colleagues (1984) reported a significant decrease in CCK in the CSF of patients with bipolar depressive illness compared with controls. However, in examining the range of values

in their control group, it appears that the bipolar patients were well within the normal range, although they lacked the relatively greater high tail of values observed in the normal volunteers.

Thyrotropin-Releasing Hormone

TRH is a tripeptide, widely distributed in brain, suggesting a functional importance beyond its role as a trophic factor for the release of thyroid-stimulating hormone. In animals, TRH administration has been associated with various activating effects, including the reversal of barbiturate sedation (Prange et al., 1974a). Consideration of these findings led Prange and others to test TRH as an antidepressant. Although these initial clinical trials were promising, subsequent experience has not sustained the initial promise (see reviews by Extein et al., 1984a; Joffe et al., 1984). On the other hand, evidence exists showing that T_3 produces clinically important potentiation of antidepressant response in some patients and that T_4 treatment can enhance the prophylactic efficacy of lithium. The mechanism of these potentiations, as well as their relationship to observed abnormalities of TRH-stimulated TSH, were discussed previously. To our knowledge, there is only one direct study of TRH levels in the CSF of depressed patients, that of Banki and colleagues (1988), who reported higher levels than in controls. The bipolar–unipolar distinction was not made. Clearly, more studies of CSF TRH are needed, especially given the evidence that it probably reflects a different TRH pool from that which participates in the HPT axis.

Neurotensin

Neurotensin has complex interactions with mesolimbic dopaminergic systems and displays neuroleptic-like properties in some animals, making it an interesting peptide for study in affective illness. Unfortunately, to date, the clinical studies of neurotensin in CSF have not included meaningful numbers of manic-depressive patients. (For a detailed discussion of this important peptide, see the excellent review of Nemeroff et al., 1983.)

Vasoactive Intestinal Polypeptide

Vasoactive intestinal polypeptide (VIP), a peptide with very high concentrations in the cerebral cortex, is thought to have important interactions with muscarinic-cholinergic receptors (Hedlund et al., 1983). VIP is also of interest because it is an agonist in the release of ACTH cortisol secretion. Gjerris and colleagues, in two separate studies (1981a, 1984), found that VIP levels in the CSF of patients with endogenous depression or mania did not differ from those of controls. However, they found decreased levels in patients with nonendogenous atypical depression characterized by dysphoric hysterical features, reversed diurnal variation, and lack of clearly circumscribed past depressive episodes. Berrettini and colleagues (1984) reported no difference in VIP levels between euthymic bipolar patients and normals.

Corticotropin-Releasing Factor

CRF is a newly sequenced 41-amino acid peptide first isolated from the hypothalamus in sheep and thought to be a principal mediator for activation of the HPA axis. Earlier we reviewed studies of the CRF challenge test as a probe into the mechanisms of HPA activation in manic-depressive patients. CRF has also been studied directly in CSF. Although Nemeroff and collaborators (1984) reported significantly increased CRF in the CSF of depressed patients compared with normal controls, two other groups did not replicate these findings (Davis et al., 1984, Gold et al., 1984b). Given the probable transient nature of any increase, however, negative findings are not unexpected. Roy and colleagues (1987c) did find a positive correlation between CRF in the CSF and postdexamethasone plasma cortisol concentrations, suggesting that increased hypothalamic CRF secretion is the driving force for escape from dexamethasone. In a small study of manic patients, Banki and associates (1987) found CRF in the CSF to be in the same range as the normal controls.

Neuropeptide Y

Neuropeptide Y (NPY), a 36-amino acid peptide belonging to the pancreatic polypeptide family, is widely distributed in the CNS, in various regions coexisting in neurons containing norepinephrine, GABA, or somatostatin (reviewed by Widerlöv et al., 1988b). Its possible relevance to manic-depressive illness is suggested by the fact that, when injected into the hypothalamus, it can produce circadian phase shifts or hypercortisolemia

depending on the site. Although it can be measured reliably in human CSF, at this writing there is only one study in patients with major depression, who had significantly lower levels of NPY than schizophrenic patients or normal controls (Widerlöv et al., 1988b). Additional studies of this interesting peptide are awaited.

Conclusion

Although the data are still preliminary, they suggest that several peptides may be involved in the pathophysiology of some manic-depressive symptoms (Table 17-13). Decreased somatostatin and increased CRF are now established as state dependent. One reasonable hypothesis is that the CRF changes are more upstream and are responsible for the secondary changes in somatostatin and perhaps other neuroendocrine measures, such as vasopressin and the blunted TSH response to TRH. New classes of peptides are rapidly being discovered and confirmed as neuromodulators. These substances have a slower and more sustained action than that of the classic neurotransmitters, perhaps consistent with slow and sustained mood changes and the lag in onset of antidepressant response. Uncovering the regional neuroanatomy of putative discrete peptide dysfunction in affective illness and its potential pharmacological amelioration should

Table 17-13. CSF Peptide Levels in Depression and Mania Compared with Normal Controls

Peptide	Depression	Mania
ß-endorphin	=	=[a]
α-MSH	=	
Somatostatin	↓	=
Vasopressin	↓	= or ↑
Oxytocin	↑	= or ↓
Calcitonin	=	↓
Substance P	= or ↑	=
CCK	=	=
VIP	= or ↓	=
CRF	= or ↑	=
Y	↓	

[a] ß-endorphin levels were reported to be higher in mania than depression in cycling patients

provide an exciting and potentially rewarding challenge to neuroscientists and clinical investigators.

ELECTROLYTES

Some of the earliest physiological studies of manic-depressive illness revealed changes in body water related to the phase of the illness. Electrolytes, too, received research attention several decades ago, especially sodium and potassium in blood and urine (reviewed by Colt et al., 1982). In the 1960s, the study of total body water and electrolyte balance in manic-depressive patients was revitalized by growing appreciation for the importance of sodium, potassium, calcium, and magnesium in nerve cell excitation and synaptic transmission. Interest in electrolytes was further spurred by the discovery that lithium—a simple cation, closely related in physical and chemical properties to the cations involved in nerve function—is an effective pharmacological treatment for manic-depressive illness. The current focus on the possible role of neuropeptides in mood disorders adds a new reason to explore this subject, since some of these peptides, such as vasopressin, have a direct regulatory influence on fluid and electrolyte physiology.

Although the early studies suggested that intracellular sodium may be higher than normal in both depression and mania, the isotope-dilution methods employed were cumbersome, and artifacts were difficult to control. Perhaps because of these methodological problems, initial efforts at assessing total-body electrolyte status were never thoroughly followed up. But they did provide important background information for later work on membrane ion transfer mechanisms.

Independent of the work on the monovalent cations, interest in sodium and potassium stimulated the exploration of the possible pathophysiological significance of derangements of other divalent cations, magnesium and calcium. It was noted, for example, that altered plasma and CSF calcium were found in mania and depression. The now extensive body of calcium data in manic-depressive illness has been variously interpreted.

Given the established importance of lithium therapy, as well as the fundamental role of ions in neuronal function, it is curious that the study of electrolytes in manic-depressive illness has now all but disappeared from the research scene. There is no mention of electrolytes in most of today's major edited books on affective illness.[85] One contemporary monograph (Whybrow et al., 1984) devotes only two paragraphs to the topic but at least includes electrolyte disturbances in an integrated model of the psychobiology of affective disorder. The scant attention paid to this subject is even more curious when one notes that in an important edited book relevant to bipolar illness, *Basic Mechanisms of Lithium Action* (Emrich et al., 1982a), 8 of the 18 chapters focus primarily on electrolytes. It would seem that this particular pharmacological bridge lacks a clinical shore.

Specific Electrolytes

Studies on the four main cations—sodium, potassium, magnesium, and calcium—are described here. Research on the transport of these ions is reviewed later as part of the discussion of membranes.

Sodium

Moderate hyponatremia or hypernatremia is generally not associated with significant behavioral changes, perhaps reflecting the efficacy of homeostatic mechanisms in the CNS. When such changes do occur, they are not specific to affective symptoms. Several longitudinal studies of manic-depressive patients in the 1940s and 1950s, including the classic work of Gjessing on periodic catatonia (published posthumously, 1976), noted phase-related shifts in urinary sodium. In these studies, there was no control for the many factors that can affect urinary sodium, such as diet, activity, weight loss, sleep disturbance, and, especially, changes in excretion of adrenal catecholamines and steroids (particularly aldosterone, which directly affects sodium excretion in the kidney). The occasional reports of an abnormality in plasma sodium in manic-depressive illness have not been replicated, and CSF sodium levels in depressed and manic patients have not yielded consistent results (Bech et al., 1978; Jimerson et al., 1979; Tandon et al., 1988).

In studying the transport of radioactive sodium, Coppen (1960) reported that sodium transfer from plasma to CSF in depressed patients occurred at only half the rate seen in controls (the bipolar–unipolar distinction was not used). This interesting finding was replicated by Baker (1971), who showed the same deficit in a group of manic patients. Later, Carroll (1972), pooling his data with those of Coppen and Baker, concluded that, compared with controls, both depressed and manic patients had a significantly lower rate of sodium transfer into CSF. In a related study, Glen and associates (1968) noted a decrease in salivary sodium transport in manic-depressive patients. These interesting early observations, although never pursued directly, pointed to the subsequent transport studies reviewed in the next section.

Using an isotope-dilution technique with radioactive sodium infusions, Gibbons (1960) calculated that total exchangeable sodium decreased following recovery from depression, and Coppen and colleagues (Coppen and Shaw, 1963; Coppen et al., 1966) noted the same decrease following recovery from either depression or mania. The latter investigators estimated that residual sodium, assumed to be predominantly intracellular (calculated by subtracting the extracellular sodium from the total exchangeable sodium), was increased in both depression and mania and returned to normal with recovery. Subsequent small-scale attempts to replicate these findings were equivocal. Questions were raised both about the methods used to estimate the extracellular space (i.e., the bromine space) and about the possible effects of dehydration, hyperactivity, muscle/fat ratios, and drugs. Because residual sodium is derived by subtracting two large numbers, small variations, especially in the estimates of extracellular space, could lead to large errors in residual sodium. (These studies have been extensively and critically reviewed by Gibbons, 1963, and Murphy et al., 1971b.)

In 1982, Colt and colleagues, using a more reliable measure of extracellular space, reported significantly higher residual sodium values in bipolar depressed patients compared with controls. In addition, the ratio of intracellular/extracellular water was higher in these patients. The residual sodium story is still incomplete. Yet to be pursued are the interesting and careful balance studies of Hullin and co-workers (1976), in which sodium retention (positive sodium balance) was

noted in the depressed phase followed by normalization with recovery or a switch into mania.

Red blood cells (erythrocytes or RBCs) provide a direct measurement of intracellular sodium. Unlike the neuron, the RBC lacks a nucleus, and its energy production comes from glycolysis rather than respiration. Its active transport system for sodium is, however, quantitatively similar to that of nerve cells (Post et al., 1967). Initially, Frazer and Mendels (1977) reported a significantly higher level of erythrocyte sodium in bipolar patients (both manic and depressed) than in patients with either unipolar or secondary depression. More recently, Esche and colleagues (1988) found increased intracellular sodium in depressed and manic patients compared with those in the recovered phase, whose RBC sodium levels were significantly lower than those of normal controls. Taken together, these findings are consistent with the earlier reports of state-dependent increases in intracellular sodium (residual sodium) in both depression and mania. On the other hand, the NIMH collaborative study of plasma and erythrocyte electrolytes in affective disorder (Frazer et al., 1983) has failed to demonstrate any difference in erythrocyte sodium between normal controls and unipolar and bipolar depressed or manic patients. (Sodium transport in RBCs from manic-depressive patients is reviewed later in this section).

Given the negative studies and the obvious methodological limitations of the earlier positive studies, the suggestion that bipolar illness may be accompanied by intracellular sodium retention is still neither established nor adequately refuted. Further research progress will probably require the evolution of more reliable and less cumbersome methods.

Potassium

Specific mood alterations have not been associated with medically induced alterations in body potassium (Baer et al., 1973). As in studies of sodium, some of the earlier uncontrolled urinary studies had noted mood-related fluctuations in potassium secretion. But in subsequent well-controlled balance studies, Russell (1960) and Coppen and Shaw (1963) found no changes when patients shifted from depression to recovery. Later sophisticated measurement of total body potassium (Murphy and Bunney, 1971; Murphy et al., 1971b; Colt et al., 1982) also found no difference in potassium secretion between depressed or manic patients and controls. (Both of these research groups point out the importance of controlling for differences in body fat.) While potassium levels in the CSF of depressed and manic patients do not differ from those of controls (Bech et al., 1978; Jimerson et al., 1979), one study of erythrocyte potassium levels found significantly higher levels in depressed patients (both ill and recovered) than in controls (Joffe et al., 1986a). Later, the same investigators found the same abnormality associated with a variety of other psychiatric disorders (Esche et al., 1988).

Magnesium

The magnesium ion plays an important role in several processes involved in synaptic transmission, including the function of certain ionic membrane pumps (ATPases), as well as postsynaptic receptor and second messenger coupling mechanisms (e.g., the binding of guanosine triphosphate to G proteins). Although high doses of exogenous magnesium can depress CNS activity, specific mood alterations have not been noted in clinical states of hypermagnesemia or hypomagnesemia. There are several conflicting studies of urinary, plasma, RBC, or CSF magnesium in various groups of (mostly hospitalized) depressed patients; in these studies, unipolar and bipolar are not generally differentiated. The NIMH collaborative study[86] reported significantly higher plasma magnesium in both depressed (bipolar and unipolar) and manic patients compared with hospitalized controls (Frazer et al., 1983). However, levels of the ultrafiltrable (ionized) fraction, considered to be the physiologically active ion, did not differ among any of the groups. Studies of RBC magnesium generally have failed to reveal differences between depressed patients and hospitalized controls (Frazer et al., 1983). Likewise, studies of CSF magnesium have not found any differences among depressed patients, manic patients, and controls (Jimerson et al., 1979). The effects of lithium on magnesium levels and the possible relationship between CSF magnesium and suicide (Banki et al., 1985) are discussed later.

Calcium

In contrast to the findings for sodium, potassium, and magnesium, pathological changes in extracellular calcium (usually due to parathyroid abnormalities) have been shown to produce mood alterations. In general, moderate alterations in calcium cause mood disturbances, whereas more severe changes lead to organic brain syndromes. The most common association occurs between hypercalcemia and depressive symptoms. Hypocalcemia, on the other hand, is associated with mood instability, irritability, and hyperactivity (see Katzman and Pappius, 1973, for a comprehensive review).

A link between calcium and manic-depressive illness was first suggested by Weston and Howard (1922), who found CSF calcium increased in depression and decreased in mania. Subsequent attempts to evaluate the link usually measured calcium in the blood. This literature never achieved a consensus. Some studies found higher levels in depressed patients than in controls; others did not. It should be noted that the reported calcium changes in manic-depressive patients do not generally fall outside the broad normal range, so the link between these findings and mood changes secondary to pathological calcium levels is tenuous (see reviews by Jimerson et al., 1979; Mellerup and Rafaelsen, 1981; Bowden et al., 1988).[87] Since blood studies do not measure ionized or free calcium, they probably do not account for potential changes in calcium-binding proteins.

Studies using measures of CSF calcium, which are less confounded by protein binding, are somewhat more consistent with the original findings of Weston and Howard. Five of nine studies found a general increase in the CSF calcium levels of depressed patients compared with controls,[88] although only two of these studies noted a significant difference. Three studies comparing manic patients to depressed patients and controls found lower or normal levels in mania (Ueno et al., 1961; Bech et al., 1978; Jimerson et al., 1979). No bipolar–unipolar differences were observed in two studies (Bech et al., 1978; Jimerson et al., 1979). Five groups studied levels of CSF calcium before and after ECT treatment; three reported a decrease or trend toward normalization (Flach and Faragalla, 1970; Faragalla and Flach, 1970; Carman et al., 1977), and two found no difference (Björum et al., 1972; Mellerup et al., 1979). Jimerson and co-workers (1979) reported a significant decrease in CSF calcium following lithium treatment and found a striking correlation ($r = 0.92$) between improvement in depression at 3 weeks and decrease in CSF calcium. (The CSF calcium literature has been reviewed well by Jimerson et al., 1979.)

Calcium changes have also been reported during the switch into mania. Following up on four earlier reports in which transient increases in serum calcium and phosphorus were associated with the abrupt onset of mania or recurrent episodes of psychoses, Carman and Wyatt (1979a) conducted a longitudinal study of nine rapid-cycling medication-free patients who had repeated episodes of mania or psychotic agitation. Subjects included typical manic-depressive patients as well as schizoaffective patients with periodic episodes of catatonia. In each patient, most switches were associated with a transient increase in serum calcium levels. Overall, there was a highly significant association between the switch and increased calcium.[89] Paired analysis of CSF calcium obtained from six patients during depression (or stupor) and mania (or excitement) revealed a significantly higher CSF calcium level in depression than in mania. Thus, serum and CSF calcium levels changed in opposite directions in association with the switch. The investigators hypothesize that the transient calcium increase in serum triggers the decrease in CSF, which in turn activates the illness.[90]

Carman and Wyatt (1979b) extended these studies by direct pharmacological manipulation of calcium using both dihydrotachysterol (DHT), which increased serum calcium levels, and calcitonin, which decreased them. During DHT administration, the three patients who had experienced spontaneous exacerbations during the placebo period had shorter cycles accompanied by more severe manic or agitated episodes. Conversely, when the same three patients were given calcitonin, their cycles lengthened, and their agitated episodes became less severe. Among the other patients (in whom changes in cycle length could not be evaluated), DHT was also associated with increased agitation, and calcitonin had the opposite effect. Unfortunately, these interesting

observations have not been followed up by other investigators, although Mussini and associates (1984) did report antidepressant effects of calcitonin in a small group of unspecified treatment-resistant depressed patients.

The relationship between these serum and CSF findings to intracellular calcium has been the focus of some hypotheses. One version posits increased intracellular calcium in mania, with an even greater increase in some depressions (Dubovsky and Franks, 1983). Alternatively, Jimerson and colleagues (1979) interpreted the CSF calcium data to mean that intracellular calcium is decreased in depression and increased in mania. Two more recent studies measured intracellular calcium in platelets. Dubovsky and associates (1989) found a continuum, with the highest levels in mania, intermediate levels in bipolar depression, and the lowest levels in unipolar depression and the control condition. Following stimulation with a platelet activating factor, both bipolar groups (manic and depressed) had higher levels of intracellular calcium than controls, who, in turn, had higher levels than the unipolar patients. Bowden and colleagues (1988) also found significantly higher platelet calcium among bipolar depressed patients than in unipolar patients or controls. These changes are hypothesized to lead to presynaptic and postsynaptic membrane changes either facilitating or inhibiting aminergic transmission.

Calcium channel blockers inhibit the influx of calcium into the cell and dampen calcium-dependent neurosecretory processes. An increasing number of reports indicate that these drugs may have antimanic and perhaps antidepressant and anticycling properties.

In summary, the calcium story appears more interesting in bipolar than unipolar illness, especially the possible longitudinal changes associated with mood shifts. If more specific pharmacological probes become available, perhaps these scattered observations can coalesce into robust testable hypotheses.

Effect of Drug Treatments on Electrolytes

Lithium

No meaningful changes in serum sodium or potassium have been observed in association with the lithium treatment of healthy individuals.

However, metabolic balance studies indicate that sodium and potassium diuresis occurs during the first day or two on lithium, followed by 2 to 5 days of sodium and potassium retention (accompanied by a concomitant rise in aldosterone secretion), with a subsequent return to normal by the second or third week of drug treatment (Trautner et al., 1955; Baer et al., 1970; Fann et al., 1969). In depressed patients, total body potassium levels were decreased in the first 2 weeks of lithium administration but were slightly increased by lithium in manic patients (Murphy and Bunney, 1971). The different responses in depression and mania could not be explained by differences in weight or electrolyte intake or output, and the meaning of this finding is not clear.

Most, but not all, studies show an increase in serum magnesium levels during lithium administration. Apparently persisting over time, the increase may reflect displacement of intracellular magnesium and, as such, may be an index of the intracellular lithium influx. The level of increase reportedly predicts both acute antidepressant responses (Carman et al., 1974) and prophylactic responses to lithium (Smigan, 1985). In a similar vein, 10 of 12 studies found a slight increase in serum calcium levels during lithium treatment (reviewed in Baastrup et al., 1978), with the peak effect seen at 5 to 7 days (Davis et al., 1981). Smigan (1985) maintains that this increase significantly predicts prophylactic response. Consistent with the notion that a serum increase might reflect displaced intracellular calcium is the finding that bone mineral content, a correlate of total-body calcium, is significantly decreased in patients receiving long-term lithium. This effect is seen in bipolar but not unipolar patients (Baastrup et al., 1978).

Carbamazepine

Joffe and associates (1986c) found a significant decrease in serum sodium and calcium levels, but not in potassium or magnesium, in bipolar patients treated with carbamazepine for 4 weeks. The sodium effect may be related to the antidiuretic effects of this drug. In vitro carbamazepine can stabilize sodium channels under conditions of rapid neural firing (Post, 1988).

Conclusion

Disturbances in sodium and calcium are the most consistently reported electrolyte changes in manic-depressive illness. Intracellular sodium retention, although not firmly established, continues to be reported by some and could be consistent with the membrane transport changes reviewed in the next section. Most of the studies of CSF calcium (but not plasma calcium) find a state-dependent increase associated with depression. The bipolar–unipolar issue is not often considered in the electrolyte literature, although most of the interesting leads on the role of calcium have come from work with bipolar patients.

MEMBRANE STUDIES

Spurred by advances in molecular biology, the study of membrane function has today evolved into an active research area in manic-depressive illness and has become one focus of contemporary genetic investigation (Egeland et al., 1984).[91] Historically, membrane abnormalities in manic-depressive illness were formulated to explain abnormalities in electrolyte dysfunction. For example, a deficiency in the membrane-bound sodium pump was postulated to explain the finding of increased intracellular sodium, which had been derived indirectly as described previously (Naylor et al., 1971; see also reviews by Naylor and Smith, 1981, and El-Mallakh, 1983).

Later, studies of lithium transport across erythrocyte membranes from patients provided a strategic advance toward unraveling membrane dysfunction in manic-depressive illness at the molecular level. The lithium–sodium counterflow mechanism in the RBC has been characterized, and preliminary biophysical studies suggest protein structural differences between patients and controls (Mallinger and Hanin, 1982). As reviewed in Chapter 15, characterization of this system allowed population studies employing segregation analysis to evaluate the mode of genetic transmission for this trait and its possible linkage to manic-depressive illness, including the vulnerability to the illness in families of patients.

Membrane studies occupy a special place in research on manic-depressive illness, not only because they offer the opportunity for a possible biological handle for unraveling the genetic vulnerability but also because membrane transport mechanisms are vitally involved in transmitter function at the synaptic level. Indeed, it has been suggested that the pathophysiology of manic-depressive illness may ultimately be explained by some membrane abnormality, either localized or generalized. An implicit assumption of membrane studies is that a genetically transmitted abnormality found in peripheral tissue, such as the RBC or platelet, will also be expressed in other tissues, including the CNS. Although such generalizability for manic-depressive illness is by no means clear, for some CNS disorders involving membrane disturbances (e.g., Huntington's disease), it has been suggested that parallel changes occur in peripheral tissues and could reflect the underlying genetic abnormality (Butterfield and Markesbery, 1980).

We first discuss approaches to the study of ion transport across membranes and then review direct studies of the major enzymatic ion transport systems in the membrane—the ATPases. Finally, we explore some attempts to evaluate possible abnormalities in the biophysical properties of membranes from manic-depressive patients.

Ion Transport Studies

Red Blood Cell/Plasma Lithium Ratio

After 2 to 3 weeks of lithium treatment, the concentration of lithium in RBCs of manic-depressive patients stabilizes at about 50 to 60 percent of the plasma concentration. Substantial interindividual variation has been noted that apparently reflects a strong genetic contribution (Dorus et al., 1975, 1980; Mendlewicz et al., 1978). The initial study of lithium ratios in bipolar and unipolar patients showed no significant difference (Elizur et al., 1972). Another early study (Mendels and Frazer, 1973) reported that, among depressed patients treated with lithium, responders showed a significantly higher lithium ratio than did nonresponders. Subsequent studies comparing bipolar patients with controls were of two types: (1) in vivo studies comparing RBCs from patients on maintenance lithium with those from normal controls placed on lithium for 2 to 3 weeks, and (2) studies in which lithium was added in vitro to RBCs from drug-free controls and from bipolar patients off lithium for 2 weeks or less. Although most of the studies showed that bipolar patients had significantly higher lithium ratios than normals, not all agreed (reviewed in Mallinger and Hanin, 1982). Furthermore,

Nurnberger and co-workers (1983b) have suggested that high-ratio patients in the bipolar group could be a treatment artifact. They had found (albeit with relatively few subjects) that the ratio was higher than normal only among bipolar patients off lithium for less than 2 weeks. Among those off lithium for more than 3 weeks, the ratios did not differ from those of normal controls.[92] The pharmacokinetic study of Goodnick and associates (1979) is also consistent with this conclusion, and Richelson and colleagues (1986) found no differences in lithium ratio or sodium–lithium countertransport comparing randomly selected blood donors with manic-depressive patients.

Another approach that offers some control of treatment variance is to compare lithium ratios in lithium-treated bipolar and unipolar patients. Table 17-14 displays 12 studies in which this approach was used. Bipolar patients showed a higher ratio than unipolar patients in nearly every study; this difference is significant in 5 studies. However, this bipolar–unipolar difference might still be an artifact if there were systematic differences in the levels of lithium used in the two patient groups, since blood levels can affect the lithium ratio (Dunner et al., 1978; Mallinger et al., 1987). Bipolar–unipolar differences in sex ratios are unlikely to contribute to a bias in these results because in most studies women (who should be overrepresented in the unipolar sample) have higher ratios than men.

Another factor that may contribute to variable results is the stability of the lithium ratio over time. Most, but not all, workers have found this measure to be relatively stable and to persist through ill and well states. Certainly, among more rapidly cycling patients, lithium ratios can show substantial instability (Ostrow et al., 1982).[93] In an interesting but preliminary study of in vitro lithium incorporation into fibroblasts from cultured skin cells, the cells from manic-depressive patients accumulated 20 percent more lithium than did cells from controls, but the difference did not achieve statistical significance in this relatively small sample (Breslow et al., 1985).

Studies of Lithium Transport Across Membranes

The suggestion that bipolar illness may involve a state-independent alteration in lithium distribu-

Table 17-14. RBC/Plasma Lithium Ratio

Study	BP ± SEM (N)	UP ± SEM (N)	Control ± SEM (N)	Significance
Elizur et al., 1972	0.31 ± 0.02 (16)	0.28 ± 0.03 (9)		NS
Rybakowski et al., 1974	0.54 ± 0.02 (28)	0.55 ± 0.04 (11)		NS
Soucek et al., 1974	0.47 ± 0.02 (36)	0.45 ± 0.03 (12)		NS
Cazzullo et al., 1975	0.60 ± 0.04 (11)	0.44 ± 0.04 (12)		$p < .01$
Albrecht & Müller-Oerlinghausen, 1976	0.34 ± 0.02 (19)	0.33 ± 0.02 (9)		NS
Lyttkens et al., 1976	0.45 ± 0.03 (37)		0.37 ± 0.02 (16)	$p < .05$
Frazer et al., 1978	0.54 ± 0.04 (24)	0.41 ± 0.04 (12)		$p < .05$
Kim et al., 1978	0.51 ± 0.02 (64)	0.39 ± 0.05 (15)		$p < .02$
Mendlewicz et al., 1978	0.59 ± 0.07 (3)	0.62 ± 0.07 (3)		NS
Rybakowski et al., 1978	0.52 ± 0.02 (79)	0.47 ± 0.03 (34)	0.43 ± 0.01 (49)	NS
Ramsey et al., 1979	0.52 ± 0.02 (49)	0.41 ± 0.03 (23)		$p < .001$
Szentistvanyi & Janka, 1979	0.50 ± 0.02 (52)	0.38 ± 0.02 (32)		$p < .001$

tion across the cell membrane has stimulated interest in the possible biochemical mechanisms underlying this abnormality. Although most lithium enters the cell by passive diffusion, it leaves mainly by a sodium–lithium countertransport system that actively carries the ion against an electrochemical gradient in exchange for the sodium entering the cell (reviewed by Ehrlich and Diamond, 1980, and Mallinger and Hanin, 1982).

Some investigators have identified a lithium efflux, or lithium pump, system that is probably closely related, if not identical, to the lithium–sodium countertransport system, since both can be inhibited by the drug phloretin. Several studies in bipolar patients show a correlation between the countertransport system measured in vitro and the in vivo lithium ratio.[94] Thus, it is not surprising

that some studies report lower lithium–sodium countertransport in lithium-treated bipolar patients than in lithium-treated normals.[95] One longitudinal study of patients starting treatment with lithium reported a slowly developing inhibition of this system, a time frame corresponding to the clinical effects of the drug (Goodnick et al., 1979).[96] Like the lithium ratio, the lithium–sodium countertransport system appears to be state-independent and relatively stable, although among rapid-cycling bipolar patients, it shows significant variability, analogous to that reported for the lithium ratio by Ostrow and colleagues (1982) and for the sodium–potassium and calcium–ATPases by Linnoila and colleagues (1983a).

Dorus and co-workers (1983) initially presented family data (segregation analysis) suggesting that abnormal countertransport function in bipolar patients may be associated with a genetic polymorphism in an autosomal major gene locus. However, she and others have not been able to replicate this (Gibbons et al., 1984; Egeland et al., 1984, Waters et al., 1983).

If some bipolar patients do have an abnormality in the membrane processes responsible for the movement of sodium into the cell and lithium out of it, it is not necessarily intrinsic to the membrane. For example, RBCs of patients undergoing hemodialysis show an acute reduction in sodium–lithium countertransport. A similar reduction occurs when RBCs are preincubated with plasma that has been dialyzed. These findings could reflect a dialyzable factor in plasma necessary to maintain full activity of this transport system (Woods et al., 1983).

Anion Transport

Anion transport in manic-depressive illness has received very little attention. One study showed that the rate of phosphate transport into erythrocytes was significantly lower than normal in bipolar and recurrent unipolar depressed patients (Szentistvanyi et al., 1980).

Other Transport Systems[97]

Studies of choline, glycine, and histamine are discussed here because reported differences in manic-depressive illness involve their relative concentrations in RBCs or platelets and hence may involve transport mechanisms. Choline and glycine differences may result from lithium treatment. Choline, glycine, and histamine are also of interest in their own right, since they function as neuromodulators and because choline and glycine are important in 1-carbon metabolism (reviewed in Deutsch et al., 1983).

Choline

The putative role of cholinergic mechanisms in manic-depressive illness led to clinical studies of plasma and RBC choline, which is known to be transported actively across the RBC membrane (Martin, 1974; Mallinger et al., 1984). Initial reports of significantly increased RBC choline in manic patients never exposed to lithium (Jope et al., 1980; Hasin et al., 1980) were not confirmed (Shea et al., 1981; Domino et al., 1981; Hasin et al., 1982; Kuchel et al., 1984). More consistent

are the many reports of very large (10- to 40-fold) increases in RBC choline levels with lithium treatment. Although they develop very early in treatment, these increases may be greatest in patients on long-term lithium administration (Haag et al., 1984).[98] The lithium-induced choline increase appears to be unrelated to clinical state; whether it can predict lithium response is controversial.

Glycine

The initial report of elevated RBC glycine levels in bipolar patients (Rosenblatt et al., 1979) was subsequently shown to be a result of lithium treatment (Shea et al., 1981; Deutsch et al., 1981). Compared with choline, lithium's effect on RBC glycine is relatively modest and develops more gradually. Although the mechanisms of this effect are not well understood, attention has focused on the processes responsible for the diffusion of this amino acid out of the RBC. However, the finding that lithium can increase brain glycine in the rat suggests that other mechanisms may be important (see, e.g., Hunt et al., 1983, and review by Deutsch et al., 1983).

Histamine

Histamine, a monoamine in the CNS, is not yet well understood (Schwartz et al., 1980), but the fact that it interacts with mood-altering drugs has stimulated some interest in its possible role in manic-depressive illness. Wood and co-workers (1983) found that the accumulation of histamine into platelets from depressed women (both bipolar and unipolar) was significantly lower than in normal controls, with very little overlap between the two populations. This preliminary finding, although repeated by the same investigators (Wood et al., 1984), requires independent confirmation.[99]

Serotonin

The uptake of 5-HT into platelets is an active process, coupled to sodium,potassium-ATPase (Stahl, 1977). Various aspects of this uptake process—total uptake, rate of uptake, affinity (K_m), and maximal velocity (V_{max})—have been reported to be altered in depressed patients. Eighteen of 23 studies[100] reported less 5-HT uptake by platelets in depressed patients than in controls (Table 17-15). Most of these studies have also

Table 17-15. Summary of Platelet 5-HT Uptake Studies Findings of Depressed Patients vs Controls

	Decrease N	No Difference N	Increase N
Studies	18	3	2
Depressed	399	43	27
Controls	379	79	110

shown that bipolar depressed patients have significantly lower uptake than unipolar patients or show a trend in that direction. The issue of whether platelet 5-HT uptake depends on the state of illness is less clear. Modai and associates (1984) found no significant difference in uptake matching euthymic bipolar patients and healthy controls, whereas Coppen and colleagues (1980b) noted that bipolar patients still showed low uptake in the drug-free, recovered phase but did show increases in uptake in association with lithium treatment. Rausch and co-workers (1988) reported increased 5-HT uptake levels in depressed patients following ECT. Manic patients have been reported to have either normal or elevated uptake values.[101] A related parameter reflecting platelet membrane function is uncoupler-induced 5-HT efflux from platelets. Two studies both found 5-HT efflux to be greater in bipolar patients than in normal controls or unipolar patients (Wirz-Justice and Pühringer, 1978; Stahl et al., 1983).

The Serotonin Transporter as Reflected by [³H]-Imipramine Binding

Specific high-affinity binding (or recognition) sites for [³H]-imipramine have been demonstrated in brain tissue from a variety of species (Briley et al., 1979), including humans (Rehavi et al., 1980). These binding sites are also present on human platelets, and the characteristics of [³H]-imipramine binding are quite similar in both human brain cell and platelet membranes (Paul et al., 1980). Although its physiological significance is not yet fully known, there is good evidence that [³H]-imipramine binding is intimately associated (both structurally and functionally) with the 5-HT uptake site (Paul et al., 1980; Innis et al., 1987). Thus, changes in [³H]-imipramine binding may reflect changes in neuronal serotonin transport mechanism(s).

Table 17-16A outlines some potential sources of variance among clinical studies of platelet [³H]-imipramine binding. Despite some variability in these parameters, most studies (summarized in Table 17-16B) showed fewer binding sites in platelets from depressed patients than from age-matched and sex-matched controls, although substantial overlap exists. In the earlier studies, the decrease in binding appeared to persist even after recovery (Briley et al., 1980; Paul et al., 1981); later studies, however, demonstrated "normalization" of platelet [³H]-imipramine binding when the sampling time is extended to several weeks or months following recovery (Berrettini et al., 1982a; Suranyi-

Table 17-16A. Sources of Variance in [³H]-Imipramine Binding Studies

Diagnostic heterogeneity

Age: positive correlation with B_{max} (Schneider et al., 1985)
inverse correlation with B_{max} (Langer et al., 1980)

Prior use of psychotropic drugs: imipramine ↓ B_{max} (Briley et al., 1982)

Season: B_{max} highest in January, lowest in September (Whitaker et al., 1984; Kanof et al., 1987)

Time of day (Lemmer et al., 1977)

Method of platelet separation (discussed by Kanof et al., 1987)

Method of platelet membrane preparation (discussed by Mellerup et al., 1982)

Method of measuring [³H]-imipramine binding (Lemmer et al., 1977)

Protein concentration used in binding assay (Friedl et al., 1983)

Table 17-16B. Platelet [^{3}H]-Imipramine Binding in Depressed Patients
(Drug Free at Least 2 Weeks) vs Controls

Study	Patients N	Control N	Patients v. Controls		Comments
			K_d	B_{max}	
Asarch et al., 1980	23	16	=	↓	
Briley et al., 1980	16	21	=	↓	Female patients
Paul et al., 1981c	14	28	(trend ↓)	↓	
Suranyi-Cadotte et al., 1983	6	17	=	↓	
Langer & Raisman, 1983	48	70	=	↓	
Baron et al., 1983a	15	15	↓	trend ↓	Female patients
Whitaker et al., 1984	16	17	=	=	
Gentsch et al., 1985	8	11	=	=	
Schneider et al., 1985	16	10 EL	=	↓	Elderly depressed vs elderly
	16	12 YO	=	=	controls; no diffs. compared with younger controls
Lewis & McChesney, 1985a	45	20	=	↓	
Wägner et al., 1985	63	53	=	↓	
Nankai et al., 1986	13 UP	28	=	↓	UPs had signif. lower binding;
	4 BP	28	=	=	BPs not diff. from controls
Carstens et al., 1986	29	20	=	=	
Muscettola et al., 1986	9	31	=	=	
Baron et al., 1986	34	58	=	=	
Innis et al., 1987	9	22	↓	↓	
Kanof et al., 1987	38	30	=	=	Signif. seasonal effect for all subjects
Roy et al., 1987a	38	43	=	trend ↓	
Schneider et al., 1988	18	14	trend ↓	↓	Elderly depressed vs elderly controls

EL = elderly controls, YO = young controls

Two-thirds of the studies (13/19) found a significant decrease in or trend toward decreased binding-site density (B_{max}) in depressed patients compared with controls. Significant data showing a change in apparent dissociation constants (K_d) in depression derives from only 2/18 studies, both with UP patients.

Cadotte et al., 1982). This question has been further clarified by a study by Langer's group (1986b), who found that among depressed patients who recovered after ECT, the binding returned to normal within two half-lives of the platelets. Thus, the changes in this binding are probably related more to the depressive episode itself than to a genetic predisposition. Most studies have not, however, found a relationship between the magnitude of the changes in binding and the severity of depressive symptoms. In this regard, the observation of Roy and co-workers (1987a) of an association between reduced binding and hypercortisolemia is of interest.

Although most studies failed to reveal any significant differences in binding between unipolar and bipolar depressed patients (Table 17-16C), in five of seven studies mean binding sites were lower in bipolar patients.[102] Lewis and McChesney (1985a), using family history and illness course to identify well-specified subgroups of their unipolar patients, indicated that the de-

Table 17-16C. Bipolar-Unipolar Differences in Platelet [^{3}H]-Imipramine Binding

Study	N / DX	$K_d \pm$ SEM	$B_{max} \pm$ SEM	Comments
Briley et al., 1980	3 BP	2.03 ± 0.25	348 ± 54	NS
	5 UP	2.40 ± 0.51	237 ± 31	
Lewis & McChesney, 1985a	6 BP	0.68 ± 0.15	754 ± 61	B_{max} of BPs and FPDDs signif. lower than that of
	39 UP:			DSDs, SDDs (and 20
	15 DSD	1.05 ± 0.15	$1,236 \pm 62$	controls), $p < .05$
	13 SDD	0.82 ± 0.09	$1,188 \pm 90$	
	11 FPDD	0.60 ± 0.18	870 ± 73	
Gentsch et al., 1985	2 BP	not given	1,555	Range 1,230-1,880
	9 UP		1,628	Range 1,160-2,540 NS
Wägner et al., 1985	7 BP	not given	958 ± 52	NS
	48 UP		$1,020 \pm 47$	
Nankai et al., 1986	4 BP	1.41 ± 0.23	$1,143 \pm 317$	NS
	13 UP	1.74 ± 0.22	$1,051 \pm 61$	
Baron et al., 1986	33 BP	3.23 ± 0.33	755 ± 44	NS
	34 UP	3.25 ± 0.31	821 ± 54	
Roy et al., 1987a	5 BP	0.94 ± 0.21	528 ± 39	NS
	26 UP:			
	13 MC	0.94 ± 0.12	533 ± 30	
	13 NMC	1.29 ± 0.37	552 ± 30	

Differences in BP Depressed (D) Compared with Manic (M) Patients

Lewis & McChesney, 1985b	6 D	0.68 ± 0.37	754 ± 149	B_{max} of DBPs signif. lower
	15 M	0.54 ± 0.17	$1,112 \pm 248$	than that of MBP (& of
	25 controls	0.71 ± 0.37	$1,237 \pm 201$	controls), $p < .05$
Muscettola et al., 1986	9 D	0.90 ± 0.15	885 ± 155	NS
	10 M	0.76 ± 0.06	924 ± 138	

K_d values expressed in nM; B_{max} values expressed in fmole/mg protein.
FPDD = familial pure depressive disease, DSD = depression spectrum disease, SDD = sporadic depressive disease, MC = melancholic, NMC = nonmelancholic, DBP = depressed bipolar, MBP = manic bipolar

creased binding was confined to bipolar patients and those with familial pure depressive disease. The data tend in the same direction as the previously mentioned platelet serotonin uptake data, which in most studies showed that bipolar depressed patients had the greater reduction in uptake.[103] If these findings hold up, they may mean that the presynaptic transport of 5-HT is altered during bipolar depression. Recall that within the large and somewhat confused CSF amine metabolite literature, the principal indication of a trend was a tendency for lowered 5-HIAA (the principal 5-HT metabolite) levels among bipolar depressed patients.

In light of the permissive hypothesis, which posits decreased functional serotonin in both bipolar depression and mania, it is of interest that among the bipolar patients studied by both Lewis and McChesney (1985b) and Muscettola's group (1986), decreased imipramine binding was associated with the depressed but not the manic phase. Thus, the serotonin uptake findings do not support a unidirectional change in both depression and mania.

ATPases

The membrane ATPases (adenosine triphosphatases) have been the focus of considerable study because they play an important role in maintaining the ionic gradients across cell membranes. In nerve cells, critical transmitter functions, such as reuptake and release, depend on the maintenance of these gradients. The principal species of this enzyme in the membrane is sodium,potassium-ATPase (Na^+,K^+-ATPase), often referred to as the "sodium pump," since its principal function is to pump sodium out of the cell against an electrochemical gradient.

ATPase derives its energy from adenosine triphosphate, is stimulated by sodium and potassium, is dependent on magnesium, and is inhibited by cardiac glycosides, such as ouabain. Although the sodium and lithium transport functions previously reviewed reflect the function of Na^+,K^+-ATPase, here we review studies in which the enzyme has been measured directly by assaying release of phosphate from ATP.

Clinical investigators have again turned to the erythrocyte as a rich, easily available source of the enzyme. It is encouraging that studies comparing the characteristics of ouabain binding in human erythrocytes and brain cells (Hauger et al., 1985) suggest that the erythrocyte enzyme may be closely related, if not identical, to that in brain. Studies of this enzyme in erythrocytes from manic-depressive patients are summarized in Table 17-17. As can be seen, no consistent overall pattern emerges. Na^+,K^+-ATPase levels are generally lower than normal in depression and higher in the recovered and manic states, but few of the reported differences were significant. Comparisons across individual bipolar groups and controls likewise present a confused picture. A bare majority, five of eight studies that compared depressed bipolar patients and controls found lower levels in patients. Linnoila and co-workers (1983a), who failed to find any differences between bipolar depressed patients and controls, did note significantly more day to day variability in the bipolar group, as previously noted by Naylor and colleagues (1976a). No overall difference was evident between manic patients and controls, with three studies finding higher and two finding lower levels in manic patients. Only one of the two studies comparing bipolar depressed and manic patients found significant elevations in mania. Five of seven studies reported increases in the Na^+,K^+-ATPase of euthymic patients compared with controls, whereas four of five found higher levels compared with depressed patients, but rarely were these differences significant. The general state changes alluded to above apparently reflect changes in enzyme activity rather than in the number of

enzyme molecules, since ouabain binding does not change with mood (Naylor et al., 1980). In light of these discrepancies, Na^+,K^+-ATPase may not be particularly useful as a trait (genetic) marker for the illness. Indeed, despite the report by Nurnberger and colleagues (1982) of slight increases in Na^+,K^+-ATPase levels in euthymic bipolar patients, the failure to find significant differences supports this conclusion.

Treatment effects on Na^+,K^+-ATPase levels are also inconsistent. Five studies from two independent laboratories[104] showed that lithium treatment was associated with increased Na^+,K^+-ATPase levels in manic-depressive patients,[105] but two later studies failed to replicate this (Nurnberger et al., 1982; Linnoila et al., 1983a). Choi and colleagues (1977) reported that low Na^+,K^+-ATPase levels in depressed patients returned to normal after ECT, a finding Whalley and associates (1980) failed to replicate.

Since vanadium ions can inhibit ATPase activity in vitro (Cantley et al., 1977), the Naylor group examined the levels of this element in the plasma of a small group of manic and depressive patients and found them significantly higher than in controls (Dick et al., 1982). Later, this same group and others (Ali et al., 1985) were unable to replicate the original finding, but Naylor and associates (1984) did report significantly higher vanadium levels in hair samples from manic patients compared with controls. However, others have found no relationship between erythrocyte Na^+,K^+-ATPase activity and membrane vanadium concentrations in manic-depressive patients (MacDonald et al., 1982; Linnoila et al., 1983a). The Naylor group also evaluated the therapeutic potential of several compounds that can decrease vanadium content in the tissue: vitamin C, methylene blue, and the chelator, ethylenediaminetetraacetic acid (EDTA).[106] They reported that each treatment was associated with some improvement. Methylene blue improved both mania and depression in a group of treatment-resistant bipolar patients (Narsapur and Naylor, 1983), and EDTA and vitamin C improved depression but not mania (Kay et al., 1984). This latter observation seems problematic for the vanadium hypothesis, since increased tissue (hair) vanadium had been found in mania but not in depression. A more recent report that serum vanadium is significantly lower in patients

Table 17-17. Erythrocyte Na$^+$, K$^+$-ATPase Activity Summary Table

Study	BP Depressed	BP Euthymic	BP Manic	Control	Results	Significance
Naylor et al., 1973	283 ± 44[a] (8)	63 ± 27[a] (3)			EBP < DBP	*p* <.02
Hokin-Neaverson et al., 1974		197 ± 14[b,c] (6) 210 ± 15[b,d] (12)	179 ± 13[b] (5)	229 ± 10[b] (20)	*MBP < EBP* < *C*	*p* <.05
Hesketh et al., 1977	263 ± 42 (12)			342 ± 42 (10)	DBP < C	NS
Scott & Reading, 1978			263 ± 57 (8)	323 ± 96 (10)	MBP < C	NS
Akagawa et al., 1980		336 ± 25[e,f] (4)	504 ± 36[e,f] (11)	324 ± 26[e,f] (15)	*C* < EBP < *MBP*	*p* <.01
Sengupta et al., 1980	399 ± 20 (2)			305 ± 27 (43)	C < DBP	*p* <.005
Rybakowski et al., 1981	233 ± 15 (8)	318 ± 17 (8)		319 ± 13 (16)	*DBP* < EBP < *C*	*p* <.05
Numberger et al., 1982	120 ± 18[g] (20)	200 ± 26 (17)	240 ± 31 (7)	190 ± 60 (16)	*DBP* < C < EBP < *MBP*	*p* <.01
Thakar et al., 1985	210 ± 32 (27)	240 ± 27 (36)		210 ± 21 (28)	C < DBP < EBP	NS
Alexander et al., 1986		696 ± 65 (23)		633 ± 61 (24)	C < EBP	NS
Reddy et al., 1989	270 (4)	660 (19)	510 (21)	420 (22)	DBP < C < MBP < EBP	NS

Summary: Five of 8 studies (including Choi & Linnoila, see below) reported control values higher than those of depressed patients. Of those reporting euthymic-depressed differences, 4 of 5 studies found greater activity in euthymic patients, while 5 of 7 studies found this same result comparing euthymics with controls. Of the 5 studies of manic patients, 3 found higher activity levels compared with controls, 2 of 4 found higher levels compared with euthymics, and 1 of 2 studies comparing manic and depressed patients found significant increases in manics.

Unless otherwixe stated, values are in nM/mg/hr.

Two other studies (Choi et al., 1977; Linnoila et al., 1983) were not included in this table because the data needed to compile this table were not given in these papers. Choi and colleagues found DBP < C (*p* <.005). Linnoila's group found no significant difference between depressed patients and normal controls.

DBP = depressed BP, EBP = euthymic BP, MBP = manic BP, UBP = untreated BP, C = control

[a] All patients psychotic
[b] Activity pg/g protein/2 hours
[c] On phenothiazines but not on lithium
[d] On lithium but not on phenothiazines
[e] Activity pg/g protein/minute
[f] Med-free or medicated 1 month or less
[g] 2 UP, 10 BP II

on long-term lithium than in controls (Campbell et al., 1988) appears to be consistent with the vanadium hypothesis. All of this work has originated from a single group, and evaluation of its significance must await independent replication.

There are several other ATPases that are of interest: magnesium (Mg^{2+}) ATPase, calcium (Ca^{2+}) ATPase, and calcium,magnesium (Ca^{2+}, Mg^{2+}) ATPase. The literature on each of these is scanty and the results are mixed.

Mg^{2+}-ATPase has been the most investigated of the three but the results are not consistent. Glen (1978), Whalley and colleagues (1980), and Rybakowski and associates (1981) found lower levels in depressed patients compared with normal controls, the latter two finding significant differences. By contrast, a later study (Linnoila et al., 1983a) reported no difference between these groups. Similarly, Choi and co-workers (1981) found no difference in levels between depressed and manic patients. Finally, two studies of euthymic bipolar patients (Thakar et al., 1985; Alexander et al., 1986) found elevated levels compared with controls.

Data on Ca^{2+}-ATPase are likewise scanty, and the results are even more varied: One study reported increased levels in depressed patients (Linnoila et al., 1983a), another found decreased levels, which normalized after ECT treatment (Choi et al., 1977), and a third reported no difference (Whalley et al., 1980)—all compared with controls. These inconsistencies could reflect bipolar–unipolar differences, since Bowden and colleagues (1988) found that bipolar depressed patients had significantly higher levels than unipolar patients or controls. Both Linnoila's and Bowden's groups found elevated levels among manic patients as well. The status of the enzyme among euthymic bipolar patients is still unclear. Higher levels were found in patients than in controls in both studies (Linnoila et al., 1983; Bowden et al., 1988), but lower levels were found by Alexander and associates (1986). Ca^{2+}-ATPase, which is primarily responsible for calcium transport out of the cell, is regulated by calmodulin, a protein (Cheung, 1980). Meltzer and Kassir (1983), therefore, used calmodulin stimulation of Ca^{2+}-ATPase in a study of bipolar outpatients (the clinical state was not described). They observed greater activation in lithium-treated patients than in controls. In a subsequent study, Meltzer and colleagues (1988) found greater concentrations of Ca^{2+}-ATPase in membranes of bipolar-I and bipolar-II patients than in controls. MacDonald and co-workers (1984) could not find this difference between manic or depressed patients and normal controls but did note substantially greater variability in the bipolar patients, similar to that noted for Na^+,K^+-ATPase.

Three studies (Glen, 1978; Whalley et al., 1980; Rybakowski et al., 1981) of Ca^{2+},Mg^{2+}-ATPase all reported lower levels in depressed patients compared with controls. Only the findings of the last study were significant. As with the Ca^{2+}-ATPase data, bipolar–unipolar differences might explain this variance. Bowden and colleagues (1988) found higher levels in bipolar patients than in unipolar patients or controls. Although the hypotheses of deficient ion pumps are attractive and have been vigorously pursued by some investigators, the direct studies of the ATPase enzyme have certainly not yielded the consensus that appears to be developing in the ion transport or serotonin transport studies. This is a curious discrepancy, since the relevant transport systems intimately involve the ATPases.

Biophysical and Biochemical Studies of Membranes

Studies of biophysical and biochemical properties, although still preliminary, may turn out to be a promising approach to evaluating membrane abnormalities in manic-depressive illness. Pettegrew and colleagues (1982), using two fluorescent probes with known affinity for specific regions of cellular membranes,[107] studied erythrocytes and lymphocytes from bipolar patients[108]. Compared with age- and sex-matched controls, the patients' erythrocytes showed a significant restriction of the probes' rotational mobility in the hydrocarbon core but not at the cell surface. In the lymphocytes, the core was normal, but the cell surface demonstrated restricted rotational mobility. It was striking that there was almost no overlap between the patients and controls, so that the differences were highly significant ($p < 0.001$) even though the sample size was relatively small. Both findings were state independent and were not altered by the presence of drugs, including lithium. Subsequently, Pettegrew and colleagues (personal communication, 1985) extended this work to include 25 additional patients, with similar results. The abnormality in the hydrocarbon core (demonstrated in the erythrocyte) could significantly affect the function of membrane protein channels, such as ionophores. The investigators point out that the presence of altered membrane dynamics in two very different types of cells, if confirmed independently, would be consistent with a more generalized membrane deficit in manic-depressive illness, as has already been established for some neurological and neuromuscular disorders (Butterfield and Markesbery, 1980).

Another biophysical approach is to examine electron microscopic images of freeze-etched erythrocytes. When such cells are washed under acidic conditions (pH 5.6), elevations occur in the membrane surface. Although the mechanisms responsible for such elevations are not clear, they do not occur if the cells are washed at physiological pH (7.4). Patients with major depression (but not schizophrenia) showed a significant decrease in the number of elevations observed at pH 5.6, and two thirds of them (including all six of the bipolar patients) fell below the normal range (Butterfield and Markesbery, 1980). Since some agents that inhibit anion permeability through erythrocyte membranes decrease elevations in normals, these results may suggest a disturbance in anion exchange systems in major depression. Indeed, as noted previously, Szentistvanyi and colleagues (1980) reported reduced transport of an anion, phosphate, in erythrocytes from depressed patients.

Phosphatidylcholine (PC), a membrane phospholipid, has been studied by Hitzemann and co-workers (1984) using an erythrocyte membrane preparation (ghosts) obtained from a group of 48 patients with mixed psychotic diagnoses, including 15 with mania by DSM-III criteria. Mean PC levels in the manic patients were not different from those of controls, but they tended to cluster in the upper one fourth of the PC distribution, whereas those of a group of schizophreniform patients clustered in the lowest one fourth. The patients from the highest quarter of the PC distribution had lithium–sodium counterflow values that were significantly higher than the lowest-quarter PC patients. Increased PC levels in manic patients, again nonsignificant, were reported in a subsequent study (Hitzemann et al., 1986). Although of potential interest, this work is preliminary, and its relevance to affective disorder is still unclear.

Finally, the apparent antidepressant effects of the methyl donor S-adenosylmethionine (SAM) draws attention to the possibility that membrane phospholipid methylation, which has been implicated in the process of receptor activation by monoamine neurotransmitters (Hirata and Axelrod, 1978), may be involved in mood disorders.

Jesberger and Richardson (1985b) have suggested that antidepressants may work by altering membrane fluidity. They go on to suggest that the lipid alterations known to be involved in a wide range of disease states, including inborn errors of metabolism, may be central to the pathophysiology of affective disorders, perhaps reflected in pathologically altered membrane fluidity.

Conclusion

Membrane transport and biophysical studies continue to represent an important area of investigation, with increasing technical sophistication. Although no single finding is as yet firmly established, the results of different approaches have converged to suggest some abnormality in cellular ionic transport mechanisms. If such abnormalities do in fact exist, they might explain alterations in amine neurotransmitters or neuroendocrine function since the integrity of these systems depends on the integrity of a variety of membrane-dependent processes (e.g., ion transfer receptor function). The indication that some of these measures may be state independent has stimulated considerable interest in them as possible genetic markers.

MISCELLANEOUS BIOCHEMICAL STUDIES

Tetrahydrobiopterin

Tetrahydrobiopterin is the principal cofactor for the rate-limiting hydroxylation steps in the synthesis of norepinephrine, dopamine, and serotonin. Biopterin levels in urine (Duch et al., 1984)[109] and in plasma (Hashimoto et al., 1990) from patients with major unipolar depression show a state-dependent elevation over normal. In studies of bipolar-II patients, Hashimoto and colleagues (1988) found elevations of plasma biopterin in both the depressed and hypomanic phase with a return to normal following recovery. On the other hand, Blair and associates (1984), examining urinary biopterin, found that recovered bipolar (but not unipolar) patients had lower than normal levels. Coppen's group (1989) found a positive correlation between urinary biopterin and plasma folate, suggesting that a folate deficiency might explain lower biopterin through impaired synthesis. Although the origins of plasma biopterins are unclear, those in the urine probably derive from peripheral tissues rather than brain, since in Parkinson's disease, a condition in which CSF biopterins are known to be low, urinary levels are not (Nagatsu et al., 1981).

CSF biopterin levels in affectively disordered patients have been examined in two studies (Van Kammen et al., 1978; Kellner et al., 1983a). Both studies reported nonsignificant decreases in levels of depressed patients compared with controls. However, as Levine and Lovenberg (1984) point out, with the advent of high-pressure liquid chromatography (HPLC), which neither of these early studies used, a more accurate indication of total biopterin levels is now possible.[110] This interesting area merits further exploration, especially in light of reports that some depressed patients respond to the administration of biopterin-like cofactors (Curtius et al., 1982, 1983).

Folic Acid

Folic acid (folate), an important methyl donor in the CNS, is required for the synthesis of S-adenosylmethionine (S-AMe), the principal intermediary in a wide variety of methylation reactions in the brain, particularly those involving amine neurotransmitters and certain membrane proteins and phospholipids important in neuronal signal transmission (Reynolds and Stramentinoli, 1983). Folate-deficient states have been associated with depressive symptoms. In a group of 100 patients admitted for primary depressive diagnoses (no bipolar–unipolar distinction given), 24 percent had serum folate below the normal range (Reynolds et al., 1970). Among 107 bipolar and recurrent unipolar patients on long-term lithium, those with low plasma folate had significantly higher levels of psychiatric morbidity. This was independent of lithium level or other known treatment variables (Coppen and Abou-Saleh, 1982).[111]

S-AMe reportedly has antidepressant effects in some patients and can precipitate hypomania or mania in bipolar patients (Carney et al., 1989) (see Chapter 22).[112] However, it is not clear that the clinical effects of this methyl-donor compound are specific to manic-depressive illness. Folic acid is important because of its general role in a wide range of brain processes that sustain normal functions, including mood, cognition, and psychomotor state. Whether folic acid and related methylation reactions are involved in the

pathophysiology of manic-depressive illness is not as clear.

Carbohydrate Metabolism

Abnormalities in carbohydrate metabolism were among the earliest biological findings in psychiatry, with reports dating back to 1919. Although most of these early studies focused on depression and manic-depressive illness, a variety of other psychiatric diagnoses were found to be associated with abnormalities in glucose metabolism. Most older studies, which used either the oral or intravenous glucose tolerance test (GTT), showed reduced glucose use in depressed patients, suggesting decreased sensitivity to endogenously released insulin. Many of these studies, particularly those using the oral test, were confounded by many sources of variance, such as glucose uptake, other dietary factors, activity, and the usual problems of diagnostic imprecision. The development of the insulin tolerance test (ITT) in the 1960s gave clinical investigators a more precise tool for exploring one aspect of carbohydrate metabolism. Insulin resistance, defined by a less than normal reduction in blood glucose following intravenous insulin, has been found consistently among medication-free severely depressed patients.[113] Only the NIMH collaborative study has differentiated bipolar and unipolar patients (Koslow et al., 1982). It showed that, after correcting for age and sex, the extent of insulin resistance is greater among unipolar than bipolar patients.[114]

Carbohydrate metabolism in mania has not been studied as extensively. Employing both the glucose and insulin tolerance tests, Heninger and Mueller (1970) reported increased sensitivity to insulin in mania. These investigators attributed its reduction by lithium treatment to the clinical change. On the other hand, Shopsin and co-workers (1972), who also found decreased glucose tolerance (i.e., decreased insulin sensitivity) in various patient populations receiving lithium, concluded that it was a direct pharmacological effect. The effects of lithium on carbohydrate metabolism are undoubtedly complex, an issue discussed again in Chapter 23, since it bears on the important clinical problem of weight gain associated with lithium administration.

As reviewed in Chapters 19 and 20, the suprachiasmatic nucleus of the hypothalamus has been implicated in affective illness, primarily because of its involvement in circadian rhythms. Therefore, it is of interest that the suprachiasmatic nucleus has been proposed as the locus for the regulation of glucose homeostasis (Yamamoto et al., 1984).

In summary, changes in carbohydrate metabolism (insulin resistance in depression, and perhaps increased insulin sensitivity in mania) are clearly related to the state of illness. To what extent such changes might be specific to affective illness is not as clear, since other diagnoses have not been extensively studied with the newer techniques. In the last section of this chapter we review the extensive literature associating low levels of the serotonin metabolite 5-HIAA with impulsivity and violence and suicide. Linnoila and colleagues (in press) expanded this concept by suggesting that disturbed carbohydrate metabolism is linked to both low serotonin, which regulates appetite, and violence and impulsivity.

Other Biochemical Studies

Here we take note of various biochemical parameters that have been examined in manic-depressive illness but that have not yet developed into a systematic literature. Sixteen trace elements from several tissues (hair, whole blood, serum, urine) were assayed from depressed patients, manic patients, and recovered depressed patients by Naylor and associates (1985). The scattered differences noted are difficult to interpret because diet and drug intake were not controlled. The amino acid serine was examined in a mixed group of "psychotic" patients, including those with schizophrenia, mania, and major depression with and without psychosis (Waziri et al., 1984). Elevations were found with a very high frequency in the psychotic groups, including all of the manic and schizophrenic patients. Niklasson and Ågren (1984) suggested that creatine and creatinine levels in the CSF may reflect brain energy metabolism. Later, these authors (Ågren and Niklasson, 1988) reported that bipolar depressed patients had significantly lower levels of both compared with unipolar patients (no controls were included).

In addition to the amine-related enzymes previously discussed, several others have been examined in patients with affective disorders. The most extensive literature has developed around the study of serum levels of muscle kinase enzymes, especially creatine phosphokinase (CPK), originally reported to be elevated in acute psychosis (Meltzer, 1968). Over the years, Meltzer extended these original observations to a wide range of psychotic disturbance, including schizophrenia, major depression, and mania, and has consistently found that patients with psychotic symptoms, such as delusions, hallucinations, and bizarre behavior, have a very high incidence of abnormally elevated serum CPK (65 to 75 percent), with median increases of two to three times the upper limit of normal (Meltzer et al., 1970, 1971; Meltzer, 1974). Various nonspecific causes for these striking elevations have been examined and ruled out. Clinical features associated with the elevations are hyperactivity, psychosis, hallucinations, and excitement. In related studies, Meltzer's group has found abnormalities in muscle fibers and subterminal motor neurons from a high percentage of psychotic patients, including those with manic-depressive illness. Although the incidence of muscle abnormality is higher in the elevated CPK group (72 percent), it is still substantial in the normal CPK group (60 percent). Associated with these muscle findings was histological evidence of excessive branching of the motor axons innervating the muscle fibers. The CPK, muscle, and nerve abnormalities also were found among a proportion of the non-ill, first-degree relatives of these psychotic patients. Although these interesting findings are not specific to manic-depressive illness, it is possible that the changes reflect some common underlying pathophysiological processes related to psychotic symptoms in both schizophrenia and manic-depressive illness (for a comprehensive review, see Meltzer, 1975). Limbic lesions in rats have been shown to produce increases in serum CPK consistent with suggestions that the peripheral neuromuscular changes observed clinically may in some way be related to so-called central atrophy. Whether comparable abnormalities in neuronal branching might occur in the CNS of psychotic individuals is an interesting speculation.

Another enzyme, glucose-6-phosphate-dehydrogenase (G6PD), a rate-limiting step in the hexose monophosphate shunt, also has been studied in manic-depressive illness following case reports associating G6PD deficiency with transient psychosis. Although most studies have found no significant differences in the incidence of G6PD deficiency among various psychiatric populations and normal controls, there is one study reporting a trend for an increased incidence of this deficiency in bipolar patients (Nasr et al., 1982).

The distribution of different ABO blood groups has been examined in manic-depressive patients, with some studies reporting a positive association between the illness and blood type O, although others did not find this association.[115] Later, Shapiro and colleagues (1977) reported a significantly higher frequency of type O in bipolar than in recurrent unipolar patients, but again subsequent reports yielded no consistent conclusion. Studies of the frequency of type A blood have also led to inconsistent results.[116] When considered together, bipolar and unipolar depressed patients have been reported to have type B blood more frequently than controls, but when the subgroups are considered separately, the difference disappears (Tanna and Winokur, 1968; Takazawa et al., 1988). Findings in unipolar patients have been similarly mixed.[117] Rihmer and Arató (1981), the only group to examine differences in bipolar-I and bipolar-II patients, noted a higher frequency of type O blood and a lower frequency of type A blood in bipolar-I patients. A careful review and reanalysis of the literature (Lavori et al., 1984) concluded that a differential distribution of ABO blood groups in manic-depressive patients has not yet been demonstrated.

Finally, in a preliminary study, high levels of negative air ions were reported to produce sedative and antimanic effects in eight of eight manic patients. In a subsequent double-blind phase of the study, four of the patients evidenced similar changes (Misiaszek et al., 1987). The authors speculate about the relationship between their findings and the reported effect of negative air ions on serotonin metabolism.

STUDIES OF PHASIC CHANGES

Most of the studies we reviewed have used biochemical measures associated with the state of depression (and less frequently of mania), reflecting the fact that biological data are usually collected from patients when they are ill and compared with a similar cross-sectional snapshot of

data from a comparison group, usually normal controls. Interpretation of state-dependent snapshots is difficult. Does a particular difference point upstream to pathophysiological mechanisms of symptom formation, or does it simply represent a biochemical symptom? In the alternative longitudinal strategy, a small number of patients is followed to reveal biological changes associated with shifts in clinical state between mania and depression—shifts that sometimes occur rapidly without obvious precipitants. By examining the switch process over time, investigators attempt to tease apart biological and clinical changes. If one can be shown to precede the other, a causal inference may be appropriate. As a corollary, by examining the subset of patients with frequent clinical state changes (rapid-cycling patients), investigators may learn more about the long-range cyclic process of which the switch is an integral part.

The Switch Process

Two prominent theories that deal with aspects of the switch process and the recurrent nature of manic-depressive illness—one involving electrical kindling or behavioral sensitization and the other circadian rhythms—are reviewed in Chapters 16 and 19 respectively. Since studies of the biology of the switch process are almost always confined to bipolar patients, the bipolar–unipolar distinction is not an issue.

Careful longitudinal studies of the switch process really began with the classic work of R.R. Gjessing (reviewed in Gjessing, 1976). His work focused on metabolic studies of nitrogen balance, and he was the first to experimentally alter the switch process by manipulating metabolism with hypermetabolic doses of thyroxine.

As noted previously, a variety of noradrenergic indices are higher in mania than in depression. In theory, longitudinal studies across the switch from depression into mania might shed light on whether this increased noradrenergic function precedes or follows the switch. Because this switch occurs abruptly, only a few studies have obtained a sufficient number of data points to assess temporal relationships meaningfully. Many of these longitudinal studies have been done in the intramural research program at NIMH. Bunney and colleagues (1972b) found an increase in urinary norepinephrine preceding the behavioral switch into mania, but Post and colleagues' finding (1977) of an increase in activity preceding the switch suggests that the increase in norepinephrine may merely be an epiphenomenon. Although Jones and colleagues (1973) suggested that an increase in the urinary norepinephrine metabolite MHPG, occurred before the switch, implying that some change in central noradrenergic activity was responsible for the behavioral change, Post and colleagues (1977) did not replicate this result. Further, Wehr and coworkers (1980) reported that the earliest changes preceding the switch were those of activity, time of awakening, and temperature, with changes in MHPG and REM sleep (increased REM latency) occurring somewhat later and appearing to be secondary. Although studies of naturalistic switches have not yet been able to pinpoint a biological trigger, evidence that norepinephrine-enhancing drugs can produce a switch into mania (see Chapter 22) continues to support some role for central catecholamines in the switch process. However, the neurotransmitter specificity cannot really be inferred for the phenomenon of antidepressant-induced switching, since a wide variety of antidepressant treatments (including sleep deprivation) have been implicated.

The role of dopamine in the switch, originally suggested by the ability of such dopamine agonists as L-dopa to induce a switch, has been approached in other ways. One patient longitudinally studied by Wehr and Goodwin (1981) showed an increase in CSF HVA levels just before the switch, but another pair of case studies showed that state-dependent dyskinesias occurred only in the depressed and not the manic state (Cutler and Post, 1982b). The latter finding seems to be inconsistent with a straightforward increase in dopaminergic tone preceding the switch to mania.

The longitudinal NIMH intramural studies suggest that ongoing changes within the depressed and manic phases may be important to an understanding of the switch. Several parameters, such as activity, temperature, and REM sleep, seem to differentiate the earlier phase of the depressed or manic state from the later phases. These relationships suggest that some biological variables involved in the behavioral states may rise and fall gradually (sine wave), whereas the behavioral states often appear to change abruptly (square wave) when a certain threshold is reached. To establish these relationships convincingly will require far more longitudinal biological data in association with careful behavioral observations.

Bunney and colleagues (1977) suggested that underlying biological oscillations occur in certain neurotransmitter receptors, which, in turn, mediate the switch in behavioral states. They hypothesized that during the depressed state, supersensitivity gradually develops in noradrenergic or dopaminergic receptors in response to deficient neurotransmitter function. When the supersensitivity reaches a critical threshold, small increases in noradrenergic or dopaminergic turnover can then trigger a dramatic behavioral change: the switch into mania. The model implies an exaggerated or sluggish receptor adaptation process in manic-depressive illness, resulting in an amplification of presynaptic changes. Although some evidence supporting this hypothesis has come from studies of sleep during the sequential administration of amine synthesis inhibitors and direct receptor agonists, clinical receptor data bearing directly on this interesting theory are not available.

Evidence for the role of other biological variables in the switch process is even more slender. Patients treated with cyproheptadine, a serotonin antagonist, sometimes switch from depression to mania after treatment. During the switch, excretion of urinary free cortisol decreases, a finding consistent with observations that the hypercortisolism of depression is generally reversed in the manic state. However, not all investigators agree that abnormal HPA axis regulation is confined to the depressed state. Further, this question is somewhat confounded by the presence of mixed states. Findings from one study suggested that an increase in cyclic-AMP levels in RBCs occurs in the manic state, and decrease occurs in the depressed state. These observations are consistent with a report by Bunney's group (1972b) of an early increase in urinary cyclic-AMP just before the manic switch. A study of mentally retarded manic-depressive patients showed cyclic alterations in erythrocyte sodium,potassium-ATPase and in the concentrations of sodium-ATP, but these changes were out of phase with the changes in clinical state (Naylor et al., 1976b). One of the earliest longitudinal studies of a cycling patient

(Jenner et al., 1967) showed, in association with mania, increased weight and extracellular fluid volume and decreased aldosterone and urine volume but no changes in biogenic amines in urine or plasma (perhaps because of limitations in assay sensitivity). This study is more noteworthy, however, for having introduced the notion of circadian rhythms and the environmental synchronization of rhythms. It is also remembered for its warning that a biological change could represent an effect, as well as a cause, of mood changes.

Rapid Cycling

The concept of rapid-cycling manic-depressive illness (defined as four or more episodes per year) is itself complex, as noted in Chapter 6. Issues include the distinction between drug-induced and spontaneous cycling and between continuous cycling (true cycling from depression to mania with no appreciable intervening normal phase) and frequent episodes of mania or depression but with normal periods in between. Also unanswered is whether the cycle length differences between individuals are evenly distributed across a spectrum or separated into discrete clusters.

Rapid cycling is, to date, still an enigma. Wehr and colleagues (1988) suggested that it is very closely analogous to typical bipolar illness both phenotypically and genetically, representing a dramatic form of the illness. If so, the intensive study of such patients should yield important insights about bipolar illness in general. Consistent with the notion that it is not a separate illness is the clinical observation that individual patients can shift from rapid to nonrapid cycling during the course of illness. In Chapter 18, we review the evidence that this phenomenon might be associated with seizure activity in the limbic system and the pathophysiology of these cycles may overlap with complex partial epilepsy. In Chapter 22, we discuss drug-induced cycling. Here, we summarize the neurotransmitter and neuroendocrine associations with such cycling. As described in the neuroendocrine section, some data suggest that thyroid abnormalities may be involved, consistent with animal studies in which thyroidectomized rats displayed rapid-cycling alterations in their pattern of rest and activity. Although some of the clinical data support an association with low thyroid function, rapid cycling may also involve destabilization of the HPT axis.[118]

Perhaps not coincidentally, most rapid-cycling bipolar patients with thyroid abnormalities are women, as are most rapid-cycling patients. Thus, female reproductive hormones may play a role in rapid-cycling manic-depressive illness, a suggestion consistent with evidence that estrogens can induce rapid cycling.

Finally, there is some preliminary evidence that elevations in phenylethylamine excretion occur in a subgroup of bipolar patients with rapid mood fluctuations within a single day (Semba et al., 1988). This finding is interesting in light of evidence that phenylethylamine seems to increase norepinephrine and dopamine release, as well as postsynaptic dopaminergic receptor sensitivity. These findings may be related in some way to the previously noted increases in noradrenergic activity associated with the switch from depression into mania.

Conclusion

The fact that manic-depressive illness tends to cycle from one phase to another and frequently displays a dramatic switch between opposite behavioral states offers investigators a rich natural laboratory for exploring the relationships between clinical and biological variables. Longitudinal studies of the switch process, although time-consuming and limited in numbers of subjects, are needed to answer questions that cross-sectional approaches simply cannot answer, no matter how large the number of patients. Observations of pharmacologically induced cycling have been important both practically and theoretically.

SUMMARY OF WELL-STATE STUDIES[119]

The study of biological abnormalities that persist once the patient has recovered from a depressed or manic episode—the euthymic or well state—can provide important clues about the nature of manic-depressive illness. Such abnormalities are presumably more central to the process underlying the illness than are those seen in the ill state. As discussed in Chapter 15, a well-state abnormality that is demonstrably heritable and appears only in family members who have the clinical illness may constitute a genetic marker for the illness. Well-state findings can also represent effects carried over from the ill state. An important source of variance not always specified in studies of euthymic patients is the time since recovery. Recently recovered patients may not, in fact, be well, and even biological abnormalities that persist long after recovery are not necessarily vulnerability markers. The term *vulnerability* should be reserved for biological abnormalities found in never ill subjects that can be used to predict the subsequent occurrence of the illness. Theoretically, any abnormality found after patients have been ill, no matter how long they have been in remission, may be a manifestation of latent illness. In this section, we summarize biological findings that constitute potential well-state markers for manic-depressive illness. They are reviewed more thoroughly in Chapter 15, along with potential linkage markers that are not related to hypothesized etiological factors.

Although findings are still too scant to support definitive statements, two lines of evidence have been advanced to support the hypotheses that supersensitivity of the cholinergic system exists during the well state. REM sleep induction by cholinergic agonists has been shown to be faster than normal,[120] and euthymic patients with manic-depressive illness appear to be supersensitive to the effects of light on nocturnal melatonin secretion.[121] Sitaram and colleagues (1987) showed a similar association between cholinergic supersensitivity and affective illness within pedigrees that had a member with affective illness and the cholinergic trait. However, these same findings might be explained by other factors, such as changes in noradrenergic or serotonergic tone, or they could be secondary to having had a prior episode of affective illness.

Evidence reviewed earlier suggested that abnormalities in HPA axis regulation, such as cortisol escape from dexamethasone-induced suppression, were state specific. As noted, such studies always examined patients at a single point in time (i.e., on a given day). Kathol (1985) departed from this by looking at 24-hour mean urinary free cortisol secretion intermittently over a period of a year in seven euthymic patients (two bipolar and five unipolar). He found an overall annual increase in mean urinary free cortisol secretion, particularly in the summer and fall months, with a loss of the normal circannual rhythm. If this interesting study is replicated, it would indicate that manic-depressive patients can manifest persistent signs of abnormal HPA axis regulation, even in the well state.

Evidence reviewed in the previous sections indicates that an important relationship exists between HPA axis regulation and central serotonin systems. Some, but not all, studies of CSF 5-HIAA suggest that abnormalities in serotonin systems may exist in bipolar illness and that they may persist in the well state. We have used the term *abnormality* to include the possibility of a persistent instability of the system, rather than a fixed deficit.

Although a presumed marker of the serotonin transporter (imipramine binding) was initially reported to remain decreased in manic-depressive patients after recovery, subsequent studies have shown normal binding in patients who have been well for a few months (Berrettini et al., 1982a). These studies underline the importance of timing, since, as noted earlier, patients studied soon after remission may continue to show abnormalities (which originated in the depressed state) for some time after recovery.

A similar question can be raised about studies of CSF GABA, which has been reported by some to be low during depression and immediately after recovery, but no longer low in patients who have been euthymic for at least 6 months.

The relatively small body of data on other substances from the CSF of bipolar patients in the well state has not yet revealed any significant differences between patients and controls, although the possibility of false negatives should be considered. These other substances include norepinephrine, MHPG, HVA, DOPAC, ACTH, β-endorphin, β-lipotropin, α-melanocyte stimulating hormone, neurotensin, adrenocorticotropin, corticotropin-releasing factor, substance P, arginine vasopressin, vasoactive intestinal peptide, somatostatin, calcitonin, neuropeptide Y, and calmodulin.

Evidence suggesting that blunted TSH responses to TRH may persist in the euthymic state in some individuals is inconsistent. Although 8 of 13 studies reported some persistent blunting, most presented group means, making it difficult to determine the proportion of patients who actually show persistence. Also disappointing is the fact that data are seldom reported separately for unipolar and bipolar patients, and in many studies the repeat testing was done soon after recovery.

As noted in Chapter 15, the most genetically relevant well-state biological abnormalities would be those involving or implicating the protein products of genes. Falling into this category are abnormalities of enzyme activity or of certain membrane transport functions in which enzymes interact with protein portions of membranes. Numerous studies over the years have suggested that platelet MAO activity is reduced in patients with bipolar manic-depressive illness, whether in the ill or well state. These same studies, which also suggested that MAO activity is heritable and that decreased MAO activity in patients is associated with an increased familial incidence of affective illness, prompted investigators to continue to pursue MAO activity as a genetic marker. However, MAO activity did not coaggregate with illness in families, and its activity has been found to be low in some schizophrenic patients, suggesting that decreased MAO activity is not specific to manic-depressive illness (see review by Gershon et al., 1977). In addition, studies of lithium ratio in RBC/plasma have shown a high ratio in patients with bipolar illness; some, but not all, studies find this to be state independent. Dorus and colleagues (1979a), attempting to combine both these factors, reported that all the relatives of patients with bipolar illness, who themselves had both low MAO activity and an increased lithium ratio, had a high vulnerability to affective illness. Combining two putative well-state markers together in an attempt to enhance their predictive power is a strategy that should be pursued further.

Studies of the enzymes DBH and COMT have failed to yield consistent differences in the well state. In the area of membrane function, one study (so far unreplicated) showed that euthymic manic-depressive patients cannot increase sodium-ATPase pump sites in response to a greater concentration of sodium and that euthymic patients may share some biophysical membrane abnormalities with patients in the depressed state.[122]

Conclusion

The results of many well-state studies have been confounded by medication effects, testing of patients too early after recovery from an episode, lack of good evidence that euthymic patients are not still significantly more depressed than controls, and failure to clarify the bipolar–unipolar

distinction. Another important gap is the paucity of longitudinal studies in which the same patients are studied during consecutive affective episodes and periods of remission. Cholinergic supersensitivity, melatonin supersensitivity to light, serotonin deficiency, low MAO activity, and a high lithium ratio have all been suggested as well-state markers. Whereas all remain to be established, the first two, which may be interrelated, are the most robust. As discussed in Chapter 15, the question of the diagnostic specificity of these findings is as important as whether they are state independent. Thus, low serotonin levels may be more closely associated with behavioral and personality traits than with manic-depressive illness per se. As emphasized in Chapter 16, future well-state studies should be combined with strategies testing the putative marker in first-degree relatives of well patients to delineate more clearly the heritable aspects of manic-depressive illness.

CRITICAL EVALUATION OF CLINICAL–BIOLOGICAL CORRELATES

Sources of Variance

In this section, we offer a critical summary of the clinical–biological correlates previously discussed. The clinical meaning of biological findings depends first on their diagnostic specificity. Although our focus is on bipolar and recurrent unipolar illness, we must range beyond the evidence pertaining to these forms of affective illness to analyze diagnostic specificity. Otherwise, we would forgo using biological variance to explore the relationship of recurrent to nonrecurrent depression. In addition, of course, biological variance is a useful approach to exploring the meaning of various clinically or genetically derived subgroups within either the unipolar or bipolar category.

In addition to diagnostic imprecision, other sources of variance can confound efforts to interpret biological findings. The factors identified in our earlier review of CSF studies (see Table 17-3) are for the most part applicable generally. They include possible nonspecific effects of changes in activity, appetite, or sleep, the influence of diurnal and seasonal rhythms (see Chapter 19), environmental temperature, variable levels of stress, and the phase of the illness (Wehr and Goodwin, 1977).[123]

Determining whether deviations from the norm are intrinsic to the illness or merely incidental may be difficult. For example, weight loss—an apparent side effect of the illness—could be centrally related to some biological process responsible for it. Even if certain phenomena separable from the illness have biological correlates, the nature of these relationships may differ in patients and normal subjects. This, in turn, might reflect some important biological differences between the two groups (Cowdry and Goodwin, 1978). It is possible that a particular biological variable may modulate traits or behaviors rather than the illness per se. Or the variable may be more strongly associated with response to treatment than with diagnosis. We will consider these questions by separately exploring how biological findings relate to the general diagnosis of manic-depressive illness, to the bipolar–unipolar distinction, to certain symptom clusters or personality traits, to the phenomena of suicide, impulsivity, and aggression, and to treatment response.

Diagnostic Specificity

Most biological research on manic-depressive patients compares them with psychiatrically well control subjects. There is a major flaw in this strategy. Demonstrating that manic-depressive patients differ significantly from normal subjects on some biological measure tells us more about the biology of psychiatric illness in general than about the specific biological correlates of manic-depressive illness. To achieve the needed specificity, one needs to determine whether, for each variable, manic-depressive patients differ from, for example, patients with schizophrenia. In this section, we limit our use of the term *specificity* to psychiatric illness. Although some biological changes found in manic-depressive illness may also occur in neurological or other medical illnesses, there is virtually no comparative literature on this question.

Although studies of CSF amine metabolites comprise a substantial literature, only reductions in CSF dopaminergic indices (i.e., HVA) appear to consistently characterize an otherwise indistinguishable subgroup of depressed patients, whether bipolar or unipolar. However, it is unlikely that low HVA is specific to affective illness, since similar findings have been reported for subgroups of schizophrenic patients (Bowers et al., 1969; Post et al., 1980a). Combining baseline and probenecid data, a majority of studies of CSF 5-HIAA have found decreases among some subgroups of depressed patients, but where the low 5-HIAA patients fit into the bipolar–unipolar spectrum is not clear. Indeed, the well-replicated association between low 5-HIAA and suicide and/or impulsivity seems to obtain for every diagnostic group examined except bipolar illness. A much smaller number of studies has looked at CSF GABA,[124] an indicator that is not specific for depression, since low levels of CSF GABA have also been found in some subgroups of schizophrenic patients. Findings on urinary metabolites, enzyme studies, or receptor studies are all insufficient to assess their diagnostic specificity. For example, low platelet MAO distinguishes bipolar from unipolar groups, but it can also be found among subgroups of schizophrenic patients.

The question of diagnostic specificity has been most extensively considered through neuroendocrine strategies, particularly the DST and TRH test. Although the DST was originally proposed as a specific test for the diagnosis of depression, its widespread use revealed that cortisol escape from dexamethasone-induced suppression also occurred in patients with certain forms of schizophrenia, dementia, primary anorexia nervosa, bulimia, obsessive-compulsive disorder, and borderline personality disorder. To suggest, on the basis of the DST results, that all of these patients have a forme fruste of major depressive illness is circular. More likely, the abnormal cortisol response to dexamethasone reflects some more generalized state—possibly limbic activation—that may occur across diagnostic lines, although most frequently associated with major depression. Within the depressed group, the relationship between a positive DST and melancholia may in part reflect the contribution of overall severity. The DST abnormality is generally state dependent, reverting to normal following recovery.

Other measures of HPA axis activity, such as the corticotropin-releasing hormone (CRH)-stimulation test, also seem to be relatively nonspecific, since blunted ACTH responses to CRH have been found not only in depressed patients but also in any psychiatric patients whose illness is characterized by hypercortisolism, including patients with primary anorexia nervosa and panic disorder (Roy-Byrne et al., 1985b; Gold et al., 1986b). The TSH response to TRH has proven to be relatively nonspecific for the diagnosis of manic-depressive illness, occurring as well in some patients with remitted alcoholism, bulimia, primary anorexia nervosa, borderline personality disorder, and panic disorder, and even in some cases of schizophrenia. In addition, it appears to be less state dependent than the DST. Blunted growth hormone response to several stimuli, a well replicated finding in depression, has not been extensively evaluated in other diagnostic groups.

Other biological variables, such as changes in electrolytes, membranes, neuropeptides, urinary melatonin metabolites, and light sensitivity, have not been examined enough to permit conclusions about diagnostic specificity.[125]

Bipolar–Unipolar Differences

Although many biological studies of affective illness do not report bipolar and unipolar data separately, some replicated biological differences between the two forms of manic-depressive illness have emerged. Table 17-18 summarizes the biological variables for which replicated differences between the two subgroups have been found and those for which no differences are evident. It should be remembered that a particular finding might simply be due to greater clinical heterogeneity among the unipolar group, especially differences between more and less recurrent forms. This heterogeneity was undoubtedly a factor in the earlier studies and may still be one. As previewed earlier, most differences seem to cluster into two groups: one involving enzyme activity and membrane function and one involving the noradrenergic system.

Numerous studies have shown reduced MAO activity in the platelets of bipolar patients, whereas MAO activity in unipolar patients is similar to or occasionally higher than that of controls, perhaps as a function of anxiety. Although these findings apparently are independent of the state of illness, the usefulness of MAO as a genetic marker is questionable (see Chapter 15). Of relevance to catecholamine theories, some studies found

lower plasma DBH activity in bipolar patients than in unipolar or control groups. The hypothesis that bipolar illness involves reduced serotonergic function (the permissive hypothesis) received support in a majority of the studies of platelet 5-HT uptake, which found lower levels in bipolar than in unipolar patients. On the other hand, the evidence is still weak that low [³H]-imipramine binding, which reflects fewer serotonin transporter sites than is normal, differentiates bipolar from unipolar patients. Two studies reported that the efflux of 5-HT from platelets was greater in bipolar patients, but further replication is needed to confirm this. Finally, the RBC/plasma lithium ratio generally has been found to be higher in bipolar than in unipolar patients. These enzyme and membrane findings all show state-independent differences involving proteins. As such they offer opportunities for the application of molecular probes, that is, restriction fragment length polymorphisms, to explore for genetic differences.

Most studies have demonstrated that bipolar-I patients have lower levels of urinary MHPG than do unipolar patients. In plasma, where norepinephrine has been the focus, differences between the two subgroups are not as consistent as the urinary findings. Nevertheless, bipolar patients do have lower levels if compared only with melancholic unipolar patients. This subtle difference again highlights how both diagnostic and phenomenological heterogeneity of the unipolar (and bipolar) groups can obscure the clinical meaning of biological findings. Previous failures to find lower MHPG in the CSF of bipolar than in unipolar patients may be due to the confounding effects of variability in blood–brain barrier permeability, since a study controlling for this found lower CSF MHPG in bipolar patients. The possibility that bipolar patients have lower noradrenergic activity is consistent with the finding that they have lower DBH activity (DBH converts DA to NE and is released into plasma from sympathetic nerve endings).

Findings that bipolar patients have increased or normal growth hormone response to several stimuli that exert their effects through the noradrenergic system (L-dopa, insulin, clonidine), whereas unipolar patients have reduced responses, also may be consistent with reported differences in noradrenergic function, whatever

Table 17-18. Summary of Biological Differences

Biological Correlate	Depressed vs Normal	Bipolar vs Unipolar
Neurotransmitters, Metabolites, and Related Enzymes		
CSF HVA	↓	=
CSF MHPG	=	↓
Plasma NE	↑	↓
Urinary MHPG	↓	↓
Platelet MAO	↓	↓
Neurotransmitter Receptors		
Platelet α_2 receptors	↑	?
Platelet α_2 sensitivity	↓	?
Lymphocyte β-receptor sensitivity	↓	↑
Neuroendocrine Output and Response		
Cortisol (plasma, urine, and CSF)	↑	=
Cortisol postdexamethasone (DST)	↑	=
Growth hormone responses	↓	↑
TSH to TRH	↓	= or ↑
Peptides		
Somatostatin (CSF)	↓	=
Electrolytes		
Calcium in CSF	↑	?
Membrane Transport		
RBC/Plasma lithium ratio	↑	↑
5-HT uptake by platelets	↓	↓
[^{3}H]-Imipramine binding in platelets	↓	↓

↑ = increased, ↓ = decreased, = no differences, ? = data unavailable or unclear,
↑ or ↓ = trend toward increase or decrease, but data preliminary or questionable

Adapted from Potter et al., 1987

the source. Reduced responses in unipolar patients may indicate that receptors are in a state of desensitization due to increased noradrenergic activity (as might occur if the patients were chronically anxious). Also consistent with these noradrenergic findings is evidence that virtually all bipolar patients become more active following a single intravenous dose of D-amphetamine, whereas only about 40 percent of unipolar patients show this type of response. This finding suggests that bipolar patients have relatively increased receptor sensitivity secondary to their lower levels of presynaptic norepinephrine, and unipolar patients have relatively decreased sensitivity secondary to higher levels. In euthymic bipolar patients, the extent of activation following D-amphetamine seems to be inversely proportional to plasma MHPG level. Thus, patients with lower levels of noradrenergic activity seem to become more activated following this infusion.

Among studies in which bipolar–unipolar comparisons are made or can be derived, most involve the two widely used neuroendocrine challenge tests, the dexamethasone suppression test and the TRH-stimulation test. Although initial studies suggested that the rate of dexamethasone nonsuppression was similar in unipolar and bipolar patients, some subsequent studies indicated a higher postdexamethasone levels of cortisol in unipolar patients. These findings, along with evidence of a positive correlation between levels of postdexamethasone cortisol and plasma catecholamines, support previous suggestions that unipolar patients have higher noradrenergic activity than bipolar patients. In addition, evidence that patients with higher platelet MAO activity had higher rates of nonsuppression may also suggest that bipolar–unipolar differences in both these variables are related. At any rate, the interpretation of bipolar–unipolar differences in the HPA axis will depend on studies that adequately control for the major factors known to contribute to activation of this axis, including age, weight loss, intense anxiety, and differential metabolism of dexamethasone. The initial reports of differential bipolar–unipolar TSH responses to TRH have not been well replicated.[126]

Most other biological variables have not consistently differentiated bipolar and unipolar groups. These include CSF amine metabolites, other amine-related enzymes, plasma amino acids and metabolites, CSF neuropeptides, and intracellular and extracellular electrolytes. Unfortunately, there are not yet enough well-designed studies of most of these variables to permit a clear conclusion.

Diagnosis vs Symptoms

In the foregoing sections, we raised the question of specificity, noting some abnormalities that appear to cross diagnostic lines and occur in several psychiatric conditions. We know too that several symptoms or clusters of symptoms, such as anxiety, psychomotor retardation, and psychosis, occur in a variety of psychiatric conditions. These facts raise the possibility that some apparently nonspecific biological abnormalities may indeed be related to limited aspects of manic-depressive illness rather than to its core pathophysiology. Further, it is likely that some biological variables modulate certain behaviors or traits in both the ill and well states. More careful study of the relationships between biological variables and symptoms, traits, and behaviors within and across homogeneous diagnostic groups is needed to resolve these questions.

Several lines of evidence suggest that the three principal monoamine metabolites found in CSF may be related to certain aspects of manic-depressive illness. For example, several studies have shown that central dopamine activity, as measured by CSF HVA, is related to the psychomotor state of the depressed patient, with motorically retarded patients having lower levels of HVA. In addition, there is evidence that central noradrenergic activity may be positively correlated with anxiety level, since the level of CSF norepinephrine is correlated with anxiety in both depressed and manic patients, and CSF MHPG is correlated with state anxiety in normal volunteers. Peripheral measures of noradrenergic function, such as levels of plasma norepinephrine and MHPG, also are correlated with anxiety in depressed patients. Evidence that serotonin and its CSF metabolite 5-HIAA are linked to suicide, aggression, and impulsivity is robust and extensive and is described later.

Despite the lack of diagnostic specificity of the DST, several studies support some relationship between HPA axis hyperactivity and symptom (or syndrome) severity, using a variety of cortisol measures (DST and urine and CSF cortisol) in a wide spectrum of subjects, both patients and normal controls.[127] Another important correlate of dexamethasone nonsuppression is psychosis, with psychotic unipolar depressed patients having the highest rate of nonsuppression in numerous studies of clinical psychiatric samples. The presence of psychosis may explain why a small subgroup of schizophrenic patients also shows nonsuppression (i.e., despite phenotypic differences, there may be underlying biological similarities). However, this association with psychoses does not seem to hold true for bipolar patients. Because few studies used DST results as the independent variable to explore clinical correlates, the data are limited. Nonetheless, the relationship between psychosis and DST responses is provocative and requires further inquiry.

Some emerging evidence suggests that certain state-related biological variables may be strongly correlated to aspects of the prior course of manic-depressive illness. Some studies have shown that both CSF norepinephrine and GABA are correlated with the number of previous depressive episodes and that cortisol nonsuppression following dexamethasone is more frequent in those patients with a relatively long history of illness but a short index episode. Could this reflect the fact that the patient experiences each successive episode as yet more stressful? Such a cumulative impact would be consistent with the kindling–sensitization notions discussed elsewhere or, more simply, could reflect the cumulative psychological scarring with each successive episode. This laudable research strategy has been too seldom used. The extent to which findings from other studies result from variation in the prior course of illness is impossible to determine. Perhaps some bipolar–unipolar differences are related to the fact that bipolar patients generally have had more episodes of illness.

Suicide, Impulsivity, and Aggression

One of the most replicated findings in biological psychiatry today is the association between suicide and low CSF 5-HIAA, the serotonin metabolite (reviewed by Brown and Goodwin, 1986, and Van Praag, 1984).[128] The suicide-serotonin metabolite relationship has been observed in a variety of diagnostic groups other than depressed patients, including those with schizophrenia, adjustment disorders, various personality disorders, and neurotic depression, but its relevance to bipolar patients is unclear. The few negative studies in this area seem to be unique in having included a large proportion of bipolar patients (Vestergaard et al., 1978; Berrettini et al., 1985b), and two studies (Ågren, 1983; Roy-Byrne et al., 1983), which analyzed bipolar and unipolar patients separately, found that 5-HIAA was related to suicide only in unipolar patients.[129]

The association between serotonin and suicide has been further supported by postmortem studies of 5-HT receptors in the brains of patients who had killed themselves (reviewed by Arora and Meltzer, 1989). Consistent with the notion of lowered serotonin neurotransmission in suicides, these studies showed increased postsynaptic serotonin receptors (presumably supersensitive from decreased exposure to serotonin neurotransmitter) and decreased presynaptic autoreceptors (presumably decreased to attenuate negative feedback, which normally constrains neuronal firing).

Some of these and other studies further suggest that low 5-HIAA levels are associated with particular kinds of suicide—those in which the attempt is violent and impulsive. This hypothesis is reinforced by the findings that 5-HIAA levels are inversely correlated with psychometric and behaviorally derived measures of aggression and impulsivity[130] and that low 5-HIAA levels have

been found in murderers without a suicidal history. Studies suggesting that homicidal urges are more common in depressed patients than previously appreciated provide an additional clue to the meaning of these findings. It is possible that a low 5-HIAA level is correlated with a tendency to act impulsively and violently while in acute emotional or psychiatric turmoil. However, an important source of variance must be considered. Low 5-HIAA levels have also been found in alcoholics well after they cease drinking (Ballenger et al., 1979) and in subgroups of depressed patients with a family history of alcoholism (Rosenthal et al., 1980a). Since suicide, homicide, aggression, and impulsivity are all frequently associated with both alcoholism and alcohol intoxication, which in turn are associated with manic-depressive illness, all of these variables need to be explored more systematically in future studies.

Other studies have found suicide strongly associated with states of hypercortisolism as measured in urine, plasma, and blood or after dexamethasone challenge. Because these studies have usually been confined to depressed patients, it is not yet established that the hypercortisolism is specific to the suicidal behavior per se rather than reflecting the greater vulnerability to suicide among severely depressed patients. There is now evidence that patients with mixed affective states, characterized by rapid dysphoric fluctuations in mood, have high rates of both dexamethasone nonsuppression and suicide. This finding may help to explain the lack of a relationship between suicide and 5-HIAA in bipolar patients because their rapid mood alterations and the associated hypercortisolism might override the contributions of the serotonin system. Also to be considered in interpreting the apparent lack of an association of 5-HIAA and suicide in bipolar patients is the possibility that the illness itself may involve serotonergic dysfunction perhaps overriding the contribution of personality variance.

Preliminary neuroendocrine evidence, currently less well replicated than the findings cited, supports an association between suicide—particularly violent suicide—and blunted TSH response to TRH. This finding is interesting in light of earlier studies suggesting that patients with blunted TSH responses to TRH may have lower CSF levels of 5-HIAA. There is preliminary evidence that, across diagnostic boundaries, patients who kill themselves may have low CSF magnesium levels in association with their low 5-HIAA levels (Banki et al., 1985). Two studies by Ostroff and associates (1982, 1985) found a significantly lower ratio of urinary norepinephrine to epinephrine in suicidal subjects compared with patients having no history of suicide attempts. These results cannot be readily generalized to patients with manic-depressive illness because mixed diagnostic groups were incorporated in these studies.

Predictors of Treatment Response

Initial enthusiasm for using biological markers to predict response to antidepressant drugs has been tempered by greater appreciation of the sources of variance in such studies (Goodwin et al., 1978a). Again, a major problem in most studies is their failure to distinguish between bipolar and unipolar illness. Several earlier studies suggested that low urinary MHPG levels were selectively associated with antidepressant response to noradrenergic antidepressants such as imipramine and nortriptyline, and decreased 5-HIAA levels were selectively associated with antidepressant response to predominantly serotonergic antidepressant drugs. Related to these findings is one study showing that the lower the urinary MHPG value in bipolar patients, the shorter the latency of an antidepressant-induced hypomanic switch— that is, the more rapidly the switch occurred after exposure to the drug. In addition, several studies showed that the antidepressant response to psychostimulants, such as D-amphetamine or methylphenidate, is related to the antidepressant response to imipramine.

The NIMH multicenter collaborative study presented evidence that low urinary MHPG levels may be selectively associated with response to antidepressants only in bipolar patients (Koslow et al., 1983; Bowden et al., 1987), whereas low CSF 5-HIAA levels are selectively but not significantly associated with response to antidepressants only in unipolar patients (Maas et al., 1984). This is consistent with the notion that a noradrenergic deficit may differentiate bipolar and unipolar patients. Furthermore, an increase in urinary metanephrine, a measure of adrenal medullary activity, was also found to be associated selectively with antidepressant response only in unipolar patients. This is interesting in light of data suggesting greater HPA axis activation and higher peripheral measures of catecholamines in unipolar than in bipolar patients. While these bipolar–unipolar subgroup differences are intriguing, the overall evidence does not provide consistent support for the ability of amine metabolites to predict antidepressant response among patients with major depression in general. This is not surprising, since most antidepressant drugs, even those whose initial actions are serotonergic or noradrenergic, lose that specificity after a week or two of administration. The subgroup findings must be viewed with great caution, however, since more potentially confounding variables are common in multicenter studies and since this study in particular failed to replicate certain rather well-established findings, such as low noradrenergic function in bipolar patients.[131]

Several authors have suggested that a higher RBC/plasma lithium ratio is associated with short-term acute or prophylactic response to lithium. (Recall that a higher lithium ratio and a positive response to lithium are both found more frequently in bipolar than in unipolar patients.) More recent evidence suggests that extremely high or low lithium ratios may be associated with responses to lithium in psychotic patients who do not have manic-depressive illness. Other investigators have measured sodium,potassium-ATPase activity in the RBCs of manic-depressive patients and have noted that this activity may also be related to lithium response. These various findings, however, do not produce a clear message concerning prediction of lithium response.

Several neuroendocrine tests have been used to predict antidepressant response. Numerous studies have looked at the DST, but on the whole no association between treatment response and the DST was found. However, since no separate data analysis was performed for subgroups of unipolar and bipolar patients or subgroups of patients with potential differences in treatment-response rate (such as delusional and nondelusional depressed patients), the question remains open. In this arena, the best substantiated finding is that patients with persistent cortisol nonsuppression following successful treatment are more likely to relapse with drug discontinuation than are patients whose DST results become normal. A parallel finding has emerged for the TSH response to

TRH. Following successful treatment and repeated TRH testing, those patients who failed to increase their TSH response by 2 μIV/ml were particularly likely to relapse. These two neuroendocrine predictors of relapse may offer some promise for enhancing treatment.

Conclusion

There is a relative paucity of data on the contributions of personality traits, individual symptoms, and certain behaviors to biological findings in the bipolar population. Drawing analogies from data obtained in unipolar patients is problematic, since the two groups have been shown to differ on such markers as that tying suicide to the serotonin metabolite. The bipolar group is more homogeneous than the various unipolar groups studied, and essentially no separate data are available for the recurrent unipolar group. Thus, studying the issues we have just reviewed in large cohorts of bipolar and recurrent unipolar patients is likely to help resolve the inconsistencies seen in previous studies of clinical–biological correlates.

NOTES

1. Reviewed by Siever et al., 1982b; Charney et al., 1981b; Sugrue, 1983; Stone, 1983a.
2. Ebstein et al. (1987) point out that individual differences in adenylate cyclase sensitivity to lithium may account for the occasional polyuria and hypothyroidism that some patients experience during lithium prophylaxis.
3. Staunton et al., 1982; Reches et al., 1982; Pittman et al., 1984; Banay-Schwartz et al., 1982.
4. Several studies with ECT provide evidence for alteration of DA function in animals and humans, but since ECT also shares with antidepressant drugs the reduction of β-receptors, it is not clear that the DA action is related to the antidepressant effect.
5. The septohippocampal serotonergic neurons appear to be critical to the function of a CNS behavioral inhibition system, which interacts with and, in a sense, balances the behavioral facilitation system. This area has been elegantly reviewed by Depue and Spoont (1986).
6. More recent CSF literature has not consistently replicated earlier findings in bipolar patients. The database for the conclusion that low 5-HIAA levels persist after recovery is especially scanty. On the other hand, recent studies are problematic because many of the patients were referred to research centers after resisting conventional treatments and may, therefore, reflect an increasingly atypical group. Also, the relatively short off-drug periods complicate the interpretation of some contemporary CSF studies.
7. Concentrations of 5-HIAA in human CSF provide our only current measure of 5-HT turnover in living humans. A validated assay for 5-HT in human CSF has yet to be developed. More direct turnover measures in animals do show reductions after chronic tricyclic administration.
8. 5-HT$_2$ (postsynaptic) receptors are reduced in animal brain after chronic TCA administration (Chuang et al., 1980), but this does not appear to be the case for 5-HT$_1$ (presynaptic) receptors.
9. Knapp and Mandell (1973) found that chronic lithium had two seemingly opposite effects: A decrease in 5-HT synthetic capacity and an increase in 5-HT uptake into the neuron. Together, these changes could provide more stability by ensuring that the rate-limiting enzyme remains saturated, i.e., that its level actually controls how much 5-HT is synthesized, thereby making the system resistant to fluctuations in intraneuronal 5-HT content, and thus more stable.
10. Antidepressant treatments appear to activate the serotonergic system, whatever effect the variable down-regulation of 5-HT$_2$ and 5-HT$_1$ receptors (as measured by number of antagonist binding sites) might be presumed to have on function. It is interesting that certain endocrine responses used as possible probes of serotonergic function are differentially altered by treatments. Thus, according to Meltzer (1986), the cortisol response to 5-hydroxytryptophan (5-HTP, a precursor that increases CNS 5-HT) is decreased after TCAs but increased after lithium and an MAOI. In contrast, PRL response to tryptophan (the amino acid precursor of 5-HT) may be augmented by TCAs, and the PRL response to 5-HTP may be augmented by lithium (see Meltzer et al., 1984a).
11. The magnocellular nuclei are so diffusely located that inclusive lesions to study all projections are not feasible.
12. Pestronk and Drachman (1987) report that their findings (that lithium reduces the number of ACh receptors in skeletal muscle) suggest that lithium selectively reduces ACh receptor synthesis and insertion into the surface membrane.
13. Many anticonvulsant drugs appear to act by enhancing GABAergic transmission.
14. Antidepressant drugs affect the type B GABA receptors but not type A.
15. Brain amine metabolism has also been studied by measuring CSF metabolites after the administration of probenecid, which inhibits active transport of acidic metabolites (5-HIAA and HVA) out of the CSF but does not affect the passive diffusion of the neutral metabolite MHPG. Animal studies indicate that the rate of acid metabolite accumulation is proportional to the turnover rate of the parent amine, as measured directly. The probenecid technique measures a dynamic

event (metabolite accumulation) rather than a static baseline level alone. In addition, by attenuating the steep, downhill ventriculolumbar gradient normally maintained by the acid transport system, probenecid reduces the relative proportion of the spinal cord contribution to lumbar CSF. Evidence for the validity of this technique in estimating CNS amine turnover was obtained by studying alterations in the probenecid-induced accumulation of 5-HIAA and HVA produced by amine precursors and synthesis inhibitors. Thus, L-tryptophan and L-dopa (precursors of 5-HT and DA, respectively) increase the corresponding amine metabolite accumulation on probenecid, whereas the synthesis inhibitors parachlorophenylalanine and α-methylparatyrosine virtually eliminate the respective amine metabolite accumulation in the CSF (Goodwin et al., 1973). Metabolite accumulation depends on probenecid levels, however, and this level might be affected by illness-related factors, such as transport system changes. The utility of the technique is thus limited, and it is generally no longer employed. Probenecid studies are impossible to interpret without determining probenecid levels because both probenecid and the acid metabolites are transported by an energy- and ion concentration-dependent mechanism. Both ATPases and ion concentrations may be affected by mania or depression. Thus probenecid levels may be affected as well (state dependently).

16. In the NIMH collaborative study (Koslow et al., 1983), the elevated MHPG among the depressed patients could be accounted for by very high levels in the subgroup of postmenopausal females.

17. Since plasma MHPG can diffuse into CSF (Kopin et al., 1983), it is important to evaluate whether reported differences in CSF MHPG reflect altered plasma MHPG, since the parent amine, NE, has been found to be elevated in the plasma of some depressed patients. In a study by Jimerson and associates (1984b), however, simultaneous measurement of MHPG in both fluids indicated that diffusion from plasma did not account for the increase in CSF MHPG.

18. VMA is a minor metabolite of NE in the CNS. We are aware of only one relevant study of CSF VMA, that of Jimerson and associates (1975), who found it significantly lower among depressed patients than in other psychiatric or neurological controls.

19. Post et al., 1978b, 1984c; Christensen et al., 1980; Gjerris et al., 1981b.

20. These higher levels were unique to women (Koslow et al., 1983).

21. This study (Ashcroft and Glen, 1974) involved patients who were in drug withdrawal, that is, 5 days after discontinuation of neuroleptics, and the proportion of patients on drug was different in the bipolar and unipolar groups (the latter being treated primarily with ECT).

22. Banki, 1977; Vestergaard et al., 1978; Ågren, 1980; Korf et al., 1983.

23. Wood et al. (1980) found significantly different GABA levels between higher and lower aliquot samples in the rostrocaudal gradient.

24. Goodwin et al., 1973; Bowers and Heninger, 1977; Banki, 1977; Vestergaard et al., 1978; Koslow et al., 1983.

25. Roos and Sjöström (1969) found significantly higher 5-HIAA levels in their manic patients, but these were compared with a mixed control group that included neurotic depressed and schizophrenic patients, and medication status was not controlled.

26. Data from Rudorfer and colleagues (personal communication) indicate that both 5-HIAA and HVA are elevated within 3 to 4 weeks after ECT as compared with the depressed state, although it is not clear how these recovery levels compare with those of normal controls.

27. Higher NE in unipolar than in bipolar depressed patients would be consistent with some (but not all) studies of the HPA axis, suggesting that elevations are more likely among unipolar patients. This fits with the known association between elevated noradrenergic measures and hypercortisolemia.

28. The relationship between rates of 5-HT synthesis in the CNS and serotonergically mediated functions is, however, not clear.

29. The preliminary findings that CSF GABA levels are associated with measures of chronicity, whereas plasma GABA levels are associated with well-state differences, require replication in a larger number of bipolar patients, with careful attention to minimizing such sources of variance as differences in assays, age and sex distribution, and the CSF aliquots used.

30. The equation essentially subtracts the peripheral metabolite VMA and the ratio of normetanephrine plus metanephrine over VMA from MHPG.

31. Linnoila and colleagues (1982) reported positive correlations of 0.83 or better for NE and any of its three major metabolites (MHPG, VMA, and normetanephrine) among 12 depressed patients. Based on these findings, they suggested that any one of the individual metabolites could be used to estimate total NE metabolism. However, the correlation between metabolites among the large sample in the NIMH collaborative study (Koslow et al., 1983) is not nearly as robust, leading these investigators to suggest that the whole family of metabolites be measured in clinical studies. Koslow et al.'s patients were in various states of withdrawal and thus not under steady state.

32. Greenspan et al., 1970; Jones et al., 1973; Bond et al., 1974; Post et al., 1977; Koslow et al., 1983; Muscettola et al., 1984. In the cross-sectional NIMH collaborative study (Koslow et al., 1983), MHPG in male manic patients was 23

percent higher than in male bipolar depressed patients, but among the small group of six female manic patients, mean levels of MHPG were no higher than in bipolar depressed females.

33. For a comprehensive review of this subject, see *Neurobiology of the Trace Amines* (Boulton et al., 1984).

34. In one report (to our knowledge not yet replicated), Bonham-Carter and colleagues (1978) note that the tyramine conjugation deficit persists after recovery from depression.

35. The elevated MAO reported in some unipolar patients seems to reflect atypical or secondary depressions with high levels of anxiety.

36. In a group of bipolar and unipolar depressed patients, Murphy and colleagues (1979) noted differences between low-MAO and high-MAO subjects. The low-MAO patients had more manic (but not depressive) episodes, earlier age of onset (in men), more thought disorder when ill, and more suicide attempts (in men). The first three of these associations would be expected on the basis of a greater frequency of bipolar patients in the low-MAO group. The increase in suicide attempts is interesting, since it is similar to the findings of Buchsbaum and colleagues (1977) in a large sample of college students.

37. To our knowledge, there is only one study of DBH levels in the CSF (Lerner et al., 1978). The lowest levels were observed in 13 manic patients. DBH levels in bipolar depressed patients were significantly higher than in controls or unipolar patients.

38. Milstoc et al., 1975; Mathew et al., 1982; R.H. Perry et al., 1982; Deutsch and Campbell, 1984.

39. The use of neuroendocrine measures as a window into CNS receptor function is discussed in the subsequent section in neuroendocrine systems.

40. Mendelson and co-workers (1983), for example, showed the total abolition of sleep-related growth hormone surge by a peripheral anticholinergic (methscopolamine).

41. The inhibition of PGE_1-stimulated cAMP accumulation by α_2-adrenoceptor agonists, such as NE, is reversed by α_2-adrenoceptor antagonists, such as phentolamine, but not by α_1- or β-adrenoceptor antagonists. These findings support the specificity of this response to the α_2-adrenoceptor subtype.

42. García-Sevilla et al., 1981; Kafka et al., 1980; U'Prichard et al., 1983; Siever et al., 1982d. Although most of the studies include some bipolar patients, the samples are predominantly unipolar.

43. Heninger and colleagues (1988) employed in vivo indices of α-adrenergic receptor function—pulse, blood pressure, and the plasma NE metabolite MHPG—as well as behavioral measures; response of the depressed patients (unipolar) to the α_2-antagonist yohimbine was similar to that of the controls.

44. See, for example, Pandey et al., 1979c; Extein et al., 1979c; Mann, 1985; Halper et al., 1988.

45. The subsequent replication attempts failed on a number of levels. Van Riper and associates (1984), for example, failed to detect the presence of muscarinic receptors on human skin fibroblasts. There is also a rather large discrepancy (almost a 20-fold difference) between B_{max} values obtained by Nadi and colleagues (1984) and those of Lin and Richelson (1985) and Lenox and co-workers (1985). If the muscarinic receptors are indeed present, there remains a probable lack of their functional significance, since classic second-messenger responses, such as increases in $[^3H]$-GMP or inhibition of cAMP, were notably absent with carbachol addition (Lin and Richelson, 1986). Given all of the above, the failure to note patient-control differences by Lin and Richelson (1986) and indeed by the original group headed by E.S. Gershon (Lenox et al., 1985) compels an unequivocal refutation of any abnormality of skin fibroblast muscarinic receptors in affective illness.

46. Early tyramine studies, using predominantly unipolar patients, suggested that depressed patients are more sensitive to tyramine's pressor actions than are healthy controls (Ghose et al., 1975; Friedman, 1978), but the later, better controlled studies had opposite results. Pickar and co-workers (1979), for example, found that a greater dose of tyramine was needed to raise blood pressure by 30 mm Hg in a group of predominantly unipolar depressed patients than in healthy controls. However, tyramine induced a greater release of NE in the patient group, perhaps related to their larger preinfusion plasma catecholamine levels, consistent with previous literature. Several studies, using direct-acting sympathomimetic amines showed an increased pressor response to both phenylephrine and NE in depressed patients, whereas others showed a decreased response. Whether these discrepancies can be traced to hidden bipolar–unipolar differences in the populations studied is not clear. In a study by Prange's group, the pressor responses of predominantly unipolar patients to NE were compared during both depression and remission and found to be significantly decreased during depression (Prange et al., 1967).

47. Jones et al., 1985; Nurnberger et al., 1983c; Gillin et al., 1987; Dubé et al., 1985.

48. Nurnberger et al. (1989) recommend that cholinergic REM induction not be considered as a clinical test because of difficulties with test-retest reliability and overlap between groups. For the same reasons they do not recommend its use in high-risk studies. They still believe that increased responsiveness of muscarinic-cholinergic receptors is related to genetic vulnerability to affective illness, however.

49. Many of the bipolar patients included in well-

state studies are taken off lithium for only 2 weeks. This raises the question of whether a medication withdrawal state could contribute to some of the reported receptor findings.

50. With regard to biochemical measures in animals that parallel those in humans, drug-induced enhancement of NE neuronal activity in the rat leads to increased production of the DA metabolite HVA in CSF (Scheinin, 1986).

51. For a nice review of this subject see Rubin and Mandell (1966) and Selye (1973).

52. They were found to be elevated by Carroll et al., 1976b; Träskman et al., 1980; Gerner and Wilkins, 1983, but not by Coppen et al., 1971a; Jimerson et al., 1980b; López-Ibor et al., 1985.

53. Corticosterone down-regulates steroid receptors in the hippocampus but not in the pituitary or hypothalamus in rat (Sapolsky et al., 1984).

54. Rubin and colleagues (1987) examined cortisol secretion before and after dexamethasone administration in unipolar depressed patients and normal controls. They found a positive correlation between the average 24-hour serum cortisol concentration before dexamethasone and the serum cortisol concentrations after dexamethasone in both controls and patients. This would suggest that the two phenomena are related in unipolar depression. DST nonsuppression also correlates with rapid metabolism of dexamethasone (see, e.g., Holsboer, 1983, and Stokes, 1975). Meltzer and colleagues (1984) found that desensitization or down-regulation of lymphocyte corticosteroid receptors occurs in many depressed patients, although, again, the relationship of this phenomenon to DST nonsuppression is unclear.

55. A study of patients with anergic bipolar depression (characterized by motor retardation, hypersomnia, weight gain, etc.), in which only 13 percent exhibited nonsuppression (Thase et al., 1989), suggests that clinical indicators of arousal are associated with nonsuppression.

56. The relevance of cortisol/prolactin data to bipolar depression is unclear, since Joyce et al. (1988) found that the correlation between baseline and afternoon cortisol and prolactin levels does not hold for bipolar patients.

57. Incidentally, Meltzer's group found no apparent relationship between the magnitude of a patient's cortisol response to 5-HTP and that patient's ability to suppress cortisol following dexamethasone administration. This is curious, since the DST findings, like those with 5-HTP and cortisol secretion, have tended to cut across both depression and mania.

58. However, Goodnick (1986) reported decreased 5-HTP cortisol response following chronic lithium administration.

59. 5-HTP can be decarboxylated to form 5-HT by the nonspecific aromatic L-amino acid decarbox-

ylase that is present in many monoamine systems and other cells. There are some reports that serotonin may act directly on the pituitary rather than the hypothalamus (Spinedi and Negro-Vilar, 1983). In fact, Westenberg and colleagues (1982), who failed to find an effect of 5-HTP on cortisol secretion in depressed patients, used a peripheral decarboxylase inhibitor, which may have prevented the formation of 5-HT at the level of the pituitary.

60. Gjessing, 1938; Wakoh and Hatotani, 1973; Stancer and Persad, 1982; Bauer and Whybrow, 1988a.

61. Stress-induced increases in thyroid indices have been reported, as well as correlations with anxiety and with stress-related hormones (i.e., cortisol). Elevations have also been reported in other major diagnostic groups, such as acute schizophrenia.

62. Through autoregulatory mechanisms, the brain is able to maintain remarkably stable thyroid hormone levels despite large peripheral changes (Dratman et al., 1983). However, these mechanisms may be disturbed in depressed patients (Loosen et al., 1980), which could explain why subtle peripheral changes may produce CNS-mediated mood and behavioral alterations.

63. In their retrospective study of bipolar patients, Wehr and co-workers (1988) found similarly high rates of "thyroid disease" (25 percent) in both the rapid-cycling and the nonrapid-cycling groups. Thyroid dysfunction among bipolar patients may be unmasked by the antithyroid effects of lithium.

64. O'Shanick and Ellinwood (1982) found elevated TSH levels in a group of affectively ill women with rapid cycles but normal thyroid function.

65. For an excellent review of thyroid abnormalities in women, with emphasis on depression, see Reus (1989).

66. Weller and Weller (1988) reviewed the use of the TRH test in children with affective disorder and concluded that the data are too sparse to evaluate its diagnostic utility.

67. Even though the patients in these studies had been off lithium for more than 2 weeks, this explanation may still be tenable, since the antithyroid effects of lithium are known to persist for some time.

68. Gold et al., 1977; Loosen et al., 1977; Kirkegaard et al., 1978; Extein et al., 1980b; Kiriike et al., 1988.

69. For example, Siever et al., 1982a,c,d; Mitchell et al., 1988; Ansseau et al., 1988.

70. However, Gelernter and colleagues (1987) reported a blunted GH response to clonidine among euthymic bipolar patients.

71. Krishnan and associates (1988b) reported that GH response to GRH was significantly higher in depressed patients than in controls and suggested

that the blunted GH response to clonidine reported in unipolar depressed patients is not due to a pituitary deficit in GH secretion.

72. Mediation by α_1-adrenoceptors is inferred from the fact that it is blocked by phentolamine, an α_1-receptor blocker (Kansal et al., 1974) and not pimozide, a DA-receptor blocker (Masala et al., 1977).

73. In fact, two independent studies (P. Gold et al., 1976; Sachar et al., 1973a) reported an enhanced GH response to L-dopa in bipolar compared with unipolar depressed patients, with intermediate responses in the healthy controls. A subsequent study failed to replicate this bipolar–unipolar difference (Maany et al., 1979).

74. Amphetamine blunting of the GH response has been reported by Langer, 1976, and Arató et al., 1983, but found to be nonspecific by Feinberg et al., 1981b, and Checkley, 1979. Checkley and Crammer (1977) observed no difference in the GH response to methylamphetamine in depressed patients in either ill or remitted state. Later, this group found no difference in the GH response to methylamphetamine between depressives and other groups of psychiatric patients (Checkley, 1979). Mendlewicz and co-workers (1986) presented data that GH is hypersecreted in depression, particularly in late evening before sleep. This group speculates that the blunted GH responses to a variety of stimuli in depression could reflect the restraining influence of this GH hypersecretion on the somatotroph's response to subsequent pharmacological or physiological challenge. Compatible with this hypothesis is the observation by Khan and associates (1987) of blunted GH responses to the recently sequenced GRH in depression. They reported that such blunted responses occurred in the presence of increased plasma somatomedin C levels; it is known that somatomedin C production is dependent on GH stimulation and that somatomedin C exerts potent negative feedback effects on GH release from the pituitary. Although there are no definitive data on the mechanism of the putative GH hypersecretion in depression, this defect could reflect a deficiency of somatostatin, which restrains the somatotroph, or hypersecretion of GRH, which stimulates it. Recent data suggest that the somatostatin deficiency in depression is a consequence of hypercortisolism (Kling et al., 1986), whereas hypersecretion of GRH could reflect the chronically unrestrained activation of the stress response in depression, as postulated by Gold and associates (1988).

75. Results of GH studies with depressed children are mixed. Some studies report significant GH hypersecretion, whereas others report significant hyposecretion (reviewed by Weller and Weller, 1988).

76. Casper and Davis, 1977; Maany et al., 1979;

Jimerson et al., 1984a; Meltzer et al., 1984d.

77. GH-releasing factor (GRF) was found to be normal in the CSF of bipolar patients (Berrettini et al., 1987c).

78. These results seem at variance with those of Meltzer's group (1984c) on 5-HTP-induced cortisol secretion. However, the lack of information concerning the exact site(s) of action of these various serotonergic probes (CNS or periphery) or their precise mechanisms(s) in altering hormone release makes direct comparisons futile.

79. Linnoila and colleagues (1984) found significant increases in plasma prolactin after ECT, but Devanand and associates (1989) failed to replicate the finding.

80. Beck-Friis, 1984; Brown et al., 1985; Claustrat et al., 1984; Lewy et al., 1979; Mendlewicz et al., 1979a; Sack and Lewy, 1986.

81. These studies did not include patients with seasonal affective disorder (see Chapter 19), who might be expected to show a different light-sensitivity profile.

82. The neuroendocrine battery administered by Amsterdam et al. (1983b) included the TRH test, gonadotropin-releasing-hormone test, insulin-tolerance test, and the DST.

83. How many of these peptides will fulfill the strict criteria for a neurotransmitter in the CNS remains to be seen.

84. Compared with medication-free conditions, the vasopressin response to hypertonic saline infusion is increased by lithium treatment and by carbamazepine (Gold et al., 1984a).

85. Paykel, 1982a; Angst, 1983; Usdin et al., 1984; Davis and Maas, 1983.

86. This study included 57 well-characterized, medication-free unipolar depressed patients, 41 bipolar depressive patients, and 18 manic patients, along with 32 hospitalized controls and 47 nonhospitalized controls.

87. Bowden and colleagues (1988), reporting on the NIMH collaborative study, found that both unipolar depressed and manic patients had significantly lower levels than controls, whereas bipolar depressed patients were not different from controls.

88. Scholberg and Goodall, 1926; Harris and Beauchemin, 1956; Ueno et al., 1961; Hakim et al., 1975; Bech et al., 1978, found higher levels in depressed patients, and Katzenelbogen et al., 1939; Breyer and Quadbeck, 1965; Björum et al., 1972; Jimerson et al., 1979, did not.

89. In a separate group of 26 bipolar-I depressed patients, transient hypomania developed during the first 10 days of lithium treatment in the 12 patients who had the largest increase in serum calcium (Carman et al., 1979).

90. The observed calcium-level changes could not be related to activity levels, nonspecific stress, or

dietary changes. The possible role of sleep loss or circadian phase shifts is not clear.

91. Although many studies of amine function, for example, uptake, release, receptor binding, involve the study of membrane-mediated processes, that literature is included in the sections dealing with amine findings.

92. Also in the in vivo studies, the normal controls were on lithium for only 2 to 3 weeks, which may not have been sufficient time to test for a chronic drug effect.

93. The report by McCoy and co-workers (1982) of a correlation between a low lithium ratio and hypertension in bipolar patients could not be confirmed by Ghadirian and colleagues (1989).

94. Pandey, 1979a; Ostrow, 1978; Dorus, 1979b; Ehrlich and Diamond, 1979.

95. Ostrow, 1978; Pandey, 1979a; Szentistvanyi and Janka, 1979; Zaremba and Rybakowski, 1986.

96. One mechanism that might explain the effect of lithium treatment on its countertransport system is the observation of Amsterdam and co-workers (1988b) of a decrease in the lithium affinity of the transport carrier during chronic lithium administration.

97. One indirect indication of altered membrane function in manic-depressive illness comes from CSF studies using probenecid to inhibit transport of the acid metabolite from CSF into blood (Goodwin et al., 1973). Cowdry and colleagues (1983) noted that the correlation between metabolite accumulation and CSF probenecid levels was significantly different across diagnostic groups, being highest in the bipolar group and lowest among schizophrenic patients. These investigators suggested that differences might reflect a membrane transport abnormality, especially in bipolar patients.

98. In one study of patients receiving lithium, higher RBC/plasma choline ratios were associated with poorer prophylactic response to lithium (Haag et al., 1984), but others have not found this (see, e.g., Kuchel et al., 1984).

99. In the second study by Wood and colleagues, patients on long-term lithium showed histamine accumulation rates that were intermediate between normals and untreated depressed patients. Of interest in this study is an inverse relationship between histamine accumulation (expressed per platelet) and platelet count. In the presence of fewer platelets, there is greater histamine uptake per platelet. These interesting preliminary findings require replication as well as further studies to evaluate questions of specificity.

100. Hallstrom et al., 1976; Mulginigama, 1976; Tuomisto et al., 1976; Coppen et al., 1978; Scott et al., 1979; Tuomisto et al., 1979; Born et al., 1980; Coppen et al., 1980b; Ehsanullah et al., 1980; Mirkin and Coppen, 1980; Malmgren et al., 1981; Meltzer et al., 1981; Kaplan and Mann, 1982; Raisman et al., 1982; Rausch et al.,

1982; Healy et al., 1983; Modai et al., 1984; and Rausch et al., 1986, found decreased platelet 5-HT uptake in depressed vs controls, whereas Shaw et al., 1971; Wirz-Justice and Pühringer, 1978; and Stahl et al., 1983, found no difference, and Oxenkrug et al., 1979; and Zemishlany et al., 1982, found an increase.

101. Scott et al., 1979; Meltzer et al., 1981; Zemishlany et al., 1982; Modai et al., 1984; Rausch et al., 1986.

102. Patients with seasonal affective disorder (winter depression often followed by summer hypomania) appear to be part of the bipolar spectrum (see Chapter 19). Thus, it is of interest that [^{3}H]-imipramine binding has been reported to be low among patients with winter depression, a deficiency that is normalized after successful treatment with high-intensity light (Szódóczky et al., 1989).

103. It is worth noting that in the only two studies reporting significantly reduced dissociation constants (K_d) the depressed patients were all unipolar.

104. Naylor et al., 1974; Dick et al., 1978, Hesketh, 1977; Glen, 1978; Johnston et al., 1980.

105. The Naylor group, the major source of positive findings in this area, reported that lymphocytes from euthymic bipolar patients showed a significantly reduced ability to produce new sodium pump sites in response to experimentally induced increases in sodium concentration or to decreases in extracellular potassium.

106. In addition, Whyte (1981) has suggested that a glutathione-rich diet, which should reduce intracellular vanadium, might be useful in treating manic-depressive illness.

107. One of the probes, fluorescamine, covalently binds to primary amines on the cell surface, and the other, anthroyl stearate, inserts the anthroyl portion into the deep hydrocarbon core of membranes.

108. The 14 bipolar patients (depressed, hypomanic, or euthymic) were studied on at least four occasions. Five of the patients were studied off all medication and, in fact, had never received lithium or antipsychotic medication.

109. Data from nine bipolar patients also studied by these investigators cannot be interpreted, since the authors lumped together those in the depressed, manic, and euthymic phases.

110. In the plasma biopterin study by Hashimoto and colleagues (1988), the HPLC was used.

111. A later report from this same group of patients (Abou-Saleh and Coppen, 1989) indicated that the lower than normal folate levels occurred principally among the unipolar patients.

112. Cantoni and co-workers (1989) postulate that methylbarinine (formed from the S-AMe-dependent methylation of barinine) may be responsible for the mood-elevating effects of S-AMe. They go on to speculate that a deficit of

endogenous methylbarinine may underlie depressive states, and excesses could be involved in the pathophysiology of mania.

113. Mueller et al., 1969; Carroll, 1969; Nathan et al., 1981; Koslow et al., 1982; Menna-Perper et al., 1984.

114. The unipolar–control comparison for insulin resistance was significant at the 0.001 level, and the bipolar–normal comparison just missed significance at the 0.05 level. Some relationship to severity was suggested by the fact that the unipolar patients who were excluded because of inadequate glucose response had significantly higher Hamilton depression ratings than those included in the study.

115. Parker et al., 1961; Irvine and Miyashita, 1965; Masters, 1967; Mendlewicz et al., 1974.

116. Four studies reported that bipolar manic-depressive patients had type A blood significantly less frequently than normal populations (Masters, 1967; Mendlewicz et al., 1974; Shapiro et al., 1977; Rinieris et al., 1979). Two others reported a trend in that direction (Parker et al., 1961; Takazawa et al., 1988). Two other studies, however, reported significantly increased frequencies of type A blood (Flemenbaum and Larson, 1976; Rihmer and Arató, 1981).

117. Shapiro et al., 1977; Rinieris et al., 1979; Lavori et al., 1984; Takagawa et al., 1988.

118. A circadian study of TSH (Sack et al., 1988b) showed that in rapid-cycling patients in the depressed phase, the nocturnal rise of TSH was attenuated, possibly resulting from insufficient hypothalamic TRH secretion. This finding is consistent with the high TSH values seen in lithium-treated rapid-cycling patients, since the lithium-induced lowering of T_4 would feedback more strongly at the pituitary in the absence of TRH and cause greater increases in TSH. Thus, in rapid-cycling patients, the HPT axis might be somewhat more easily perturbed than in patients with slower cycles.

119. The bulk of the data reviewed in this summary section is covered earlier, along with the appropriate references.

120. Euthymic patients do not have the shortened REM latency characteristic of depressed patients. Sitaram and colleagues (1980) were able to unmask this hidden tendency, however, by administering intravenous arecoline during sleep. This cholinergic challenge caused REM sleep to occur far more quickly in patients who had been euthymic for at least 3 months than it did in normal control subjects.

121. In one study that awaits replication, euthymic manic-depressive patients (predominantly bipolar) were found, like their depressed counterparts, to be supersensitive to bright light, as manifested by a greater suppression of nocturnal plasma melatonin levels than in normal controls (Lewy et al., 1985a). These patients had been euthymic from 1 month to 7 years, but the degree of suppression was unrelated to duration of euthymia. Since there is a cholinergic receptor in the suprachiasmatic nucleus that may mediate the effects of light on melatonin levels, this abnormality may also represent a kind of cholinergic supersensitivity. Another study including both bipolar and unipolar patients in the euthymic phase (Beck-Friis et al., 1984) found lower than normal nocturnal plasma melatonin levels (without artificial light exposure), suggesting a tonic increase in cholinergic tone, resulting in greater suppression of basal levels of melatonin. These decreases were of the same magnitude in unipolar and bipolar patients.

122. Nurnberger (personal communication) was unable to find increases in Na^+-ATPase pump sites in four of four normals.

123. Clinical evidence suggests that some biological abnormalities that are present early in an episode may either attenuate or reverse (in a compensatory fashion) later in the episode.

124. Preliminary evidence suggests that low GABA levels may be related to the depressed state within given individuals (i.e., they increase with recovery or the switch into mania).

125. One interesting finding that has raised the specificity issue involves patients' responses to tyramine, an amino acid that may be involved in the neuromodulation of noradrenergic synapses. In this research area, the conflicting results of early studies measuring responses to tyramine challenge have been supplanted by a newer one demonstrating that only depressed patients with melancholia, whether unipolar or bipolar, manifest characteristic deficits in tyramine metabolite excretion following a tyramine challenge. The specificity question here relates to medical states: Would hypothyroid patients also show this metabolic change?

126. The augmenting effect of lithium on the TSH response to TRH might persist beyond the traditional 2-week drug washout period used in most studies. Assuming that lithium is used more frequently in bipolar patients, this could explain the association between bipolarity and augmented TSH responses previously reported.

127. With any of these behavioral correlates of HPA activation, it is important to consider the possibility that caffeine intake may constitute the critical intervening variable, since Uhde et al. (1985) demonstrated a relationship between high caffeine intake and escape for dexamethasone. Thus, the possibility that certain clinical states (psychomotor retardation, fatigue, anxiety, psychoses) resulting in increased caffeine intake could produce an abnormal DST.

128. In retrospect, early European suggestions that low 5-HIAA is diagnostically specific for depression may have resulted from very restrictive hos-

pital admission policies that virtually required depressed inpatients (i.e., the participants in CSF studies) to be suicidal.

129. Low 5-HIAA is not totally independent of low HVA, since (as shown in the analysis by Gibbons and Davis, 1986), individuals belonging to a low 5-HIAA subgroup also tend to belong to a low HVA subgroup.

130. Depue and Spoont (1986) review that evidence supporting a role for serotonin in what they term a "generalized behavioral constraint system," the function of which depends substantially on the context.

131. Like other recent studies, the NIMH multicenter collaborative study depends on referrals to university-based research centers. Given the success of contemporary treatments for manic-depressive illness, it is likely that the patient pool available for study has become more atypical, at least with respect to a higher rate of treatment resistance.

18

Anatomical, Physiological, and Medical Studies

This chapter combines three different areas of inquiry—neuroanatomical localization, electrophysiologically measured functions, and immunological and viral factors implicated in manic-depressive illness. Clearly, the first two bodies of data are interrelated. Laterality of hemispheric functioning is assessed by both anatomical and electrophysiological approaches, for example, and the anatomical locus of disturbances is inferred from the electroencephalogram and other central electrophysiological measures. Neuroanatomical and electrophysiological studies of manic-depressive illness are similar in another important respect: In neither field have investigations been as systematic and sustained as in the search for biochemical correlates of manic-depressive illness, reviewed in the preceding chapter.

Interest in the neuropathology and anatomy of manic-depressive illness grew out of the observation that lesions of the central nervous system (CNS) are often accompanied by signs of abnormal cognitive, behavioral, or motor functioning. Such observations may not seem relevant to manic-depressive illness, since most patients experience discrete episodes followed by recovery. A substantial minority do not recover, however, and others improve only partially between episodes. At the very least, then, a neuropathological approach may prove fruitful in the study of chronic cases, and we believe it may have a wider relevance as well—for several reasons.

First, in some disorders, demonstrable organic lesions are associated with the signs and symptoms of manic-depressive illness, including mood, cognitive, psychomotor, behavioral, and physiological manifestations. In other disorders, periods of asymptomatic remission can occur despite the presence of fixed neuropathological lesions. These episodic disorders resulting from fixed structural lesions are especially relevant (Jeste et al., 1988).[1] A prime example is multiple sclerosis, which, at least early in its course, has clear episodes. (The association of multiple sclerosis with manic-depressive illness in the same families has been of some interest.) As discussed in Chapter 20, one could hypothesize that manic-depressive cycles result from a lesion or defect in an area (or system) of the brain responsible for modulating or dampening oscillations.

A second reason to investigate neuropathology is that pharmacological agents can resolve manic-depressive symptoms without apparently altering an underlying neuropathological deficit. Indeed, manic or depressive symptoms that result from—that is, are secondary to—known brain lesions often will respond to pharmacological intervention. This response challenges common beliefs about the mechanism of drug effects. It is generally assumed that when an episode of manic-depressive illness remits (spontaneously or in response to treatment), the clinical changes reflect a resolving or normalizing biochemical diathesis. Less conventional explanations are possible, however. Perhaps damaged cells are regenerated, or collateral circuits are mobilized, or a toxin disappears. Thus, the reasoning that correction by a drug indicates a purely biochemical problem is not airtight. Parkinson's disease, for example, responds to pharmacological treatment despite a clearly demonstrable lesion in the substantia nigra.

Third, clues to the pathophysiology of primary manic-depressive illness may emerge from understanding the neuropathology of depressions and manias secondary to CNS lesions caused by cerebrovascular accident, tumors, head injuries, Alzheimer's disease, Huntington's chorea, acquired immunodeficiency syndrome (AIDS) dementia (Buhrich et al., 1988; Schmidt and Miller, 1988), or other conditions. Secondary affective syndromes may arise from specific neurochemical changes set in motion by the primary damage, and tracing the chain of effects may help to locate the CNS regions involved in the expression of these syndromes or their various individual symptoms. Secondary depressions were shown to be phenomenologically "highly similar" to primary cases in a study by Lipsey and associates (1986), who conducted structured clinical interviews of 43 patients with poststroke depression and 43 with primary major depression.[2] Another strategy is to examine those cases in which severe depressive or manic symptoms have been alleviated by neurosurgical intervention (e.g., cingulotomy).

It is this third reason that may be the most useful in understanding possible neuropathological correlates of manic-depressive illness. Clues from the study of secondary states will become important in directing and applying the new technologies for regional imaging of the brain in primary manic-depressive illness and for orienting postmortem studies of the illness. (For a full discussion of the concept of secondary affective states, see Chapter 5.)

A caveat is in order here. As noted by Wexler (1986):

After prolonged study of brain-injured patients, A.R. Luria decided that the neural substrate of a particular behaviour or function is to be found in a series of brain regions, in the relationships among these regions, and in the processes that link them, rather than in a specific anatomical location. The brain processes and regions that together are associated with a particular cognitive process or behaviour constitute a cerebral functional system. . . . The same function may be subserved by different combinations of neural components at different times. (p. 358)

Here we focus on the neuroanatomical studies themselves. In Chapter 20 we return to Wexler's caution, as we consider the neuroanatomical data from the perspective of broader models of brain function.

APPROACHES TO LOCALIZATION

Neuropathological Studies

Primary Depression and Mania

Little research attention has been given to the neuropathology of primary affective disorder. In a careful literature review, Jeste and colleagues (1988) were able to identify only six such studies in the world literature, all focused on schizophrenia. Manic and depressed patients were included only as controls. As a result, important variables (e.g., prior treatment) were not reported. Because of methodological problems in these studies and the small total number of patients (61 unipolar, 51 bipolar), Jeste and co-workers refrained from drawing conclusions about specific cerebral lesions in unipolar and bipolar illness.

Secondary Depression and Mania

I have seen a case of melancholia in which the patient had been accidentally wounded with a sword, fracturing his skull. Now, just so long as the wound was open, he remained quite well, but if the wound were allowed to close, then mania appeared, and I think that if the wound were kept open for a sufficient time, and during that period the proper remedies were employed, a cure would be effected.   — Gordonius (ca. 1300)[3]

Most of the relevant neuropathological literature concerns patients whose depressive or manic symptoms appear to be secondary to lesions of the brain. Our update of the review by Jeste and colleagues (1988) examines 29 large-scale prevalence studies of secondary affective disorders involving 3,087 patients (Table 18-1). In the 20 studies that gave quantitative information, 39 percent, or 540 of 1,395 patients, had affective symptoms.

Using criteria developed by Krauthammer and

Klerman (1978) for secondary mania and the DSM-III criteria for major depressive disorder, Jeste and associates (unpublished data) reviewed individual case reports of depression and of ma-

Table 18-1. Large-Scale Prevalence Studies of Secondary Affective Disorders

Study	Patients N	Lesion Type/Location	Affective Disorder
Feuchtwanger, 1923	400	Gunshot wounds, frontal lobes in 200 patients	Euphoria common with frontal lobe injuries, depression less common
Kolodny, 1928	38	Tumor, temporal lobes	8 patients with affective symptoms (depression euphoria)
Kleist, 1931 Tow, 1955	300	Trauma, frontal lobes in 105 patients	Euphoria more common with orbito-frontal damage. Depression less common
Minski, 1933	58	Tumor, frontal and temporal lobes	14 patients were depressed, 7 "excited." Of depressed patients, 9 had frontal tumors (8 left, 1 right). Of "excited" patients, 5 had frontal (3 left, 2 right) and 2 had temporal (both left) tumors
Strauss & Keschner, 1935	85	Tumor, frontal lobes	13 patients depressed, 5 manic or hypomanic
Keschner et al., 1936	110	Tumor, temporal lobes	21 with depression, 6 hypomanic. Depression more common with left-sided tumors
Keschner et al., 1938	530	Tumor, different regions	46 percent with affective disturbances. No localizing value
Assal et al., 1957	35	Tumor, posterior fossa	3 patients depressed
Pool & Correll, 1958	25	Tumor, mainly supratentorial	14 depressed; 7 with right-sided tumors, 4 left-sided, 3 bilateral or diffuse
Lishman, 1966, 1968, 1978	670	Penetrating head injuries, different regions	Affective disorders (mainly depression) more localized to right frontal lobe
Flor-Henry, 1969	100	Psychomotor epilepsy, temporal lobes	Association of bipolar symptoms with right hemisphere lesion
Direkze et al., 1971	25	Tumor, frontal lobes	5 patients with depression
Folstein et al., 1971	20	Stroke, left hemisphere in 10; right hemisphere in 10	5 right-sided and 4 left-sided stroke patients belonged to "depression category"
Gainotti, 1972	160	Different types lesions, left hemisphere in 80; right hemisphere in 80	Depressive-catastrophic reactions more frequent with left-sided lesions. Indifference-euphoria more frequent with right-sided lesions
Kanakaratnam & Direkze, 1976	56	Tumors, frontal lobes	12 with initial diagnosis of depression

Continued

Table 18-1 Continued. Large-Scale Prevalence Studies of Secondary Affective Disorders

Bear & Fedio, 1977	27	Psychomotor epilepsy, temporal lobe (12 left, 15 right)	Right foci associated with depression and mood lability
Gasparrini et al., 1978	24	Different types, mainly temporal lobe (16 left, 8 right)	43.8% of left-hemisphere group had depression-scale score on MMPI $\geq$ 70, all of right-hemisphere group had scores < 70
Heath et al., 1979	31	Pathology on CT scan, cerebellar vermis	3 patients were depressed
Robinson & Szetela, 1981	29	Stroke (18), trauma (11), left hemisphere	61% of stroke & 18% of trauma patients were at least moderately depressed. Positive correlation between degree of depression & proximity to left frontal lobe
Sackeim et al., 1982	19	Hemispherectomy, right hemispherectomy in 14; left in 5.	12 of 14 with right hemispherectomy showed euphoria. 3 of 5 with left hemispherectomy had normal mood with 1 depressed and 1 euphoric
Lipsey et al., 1983	15	Stroke or trauma, different regions	Patients with left anterior lesions were significantly more depressed
Robinson et al., 1984	103	Stroke, different regions	30 with depression, 7 of 18 depressed patients with left-hemisphere stroke had major depressions. Only 1 of 4 with right hemisphere stroke had major depression
Shukla et al., 1987	20	Trauma, different regions	Manic episodes were irritable, not euphoric. Psychosis occurred in 15%; 70% had no depressive episodes; most had negative family histories. Most BPI
Starkstein et al., 1988a	12	Different types, right hemisphere in 7; with bilateral in 4; left in 1	All developed mania. Apparent association damage to structures functionally connected to obitofrontal cortex
Starkstein et al., 1988b	26	Stroke, different regions	13 developed major depression. Depressed group also had higher VBRs and greater cognitive impairment, 11 had lesions in the left hemisphere
Robinson et al., 1988a	59	Stroke, different regions	31 experienced depression associated with left hemisphere, particularly anterior cortical and subcortical regions
Robinson et al., 1988b	17	Tumor or trauma, different regions	All developed mania associated with areas in right hemisphere connected to limbic system. They had significantly greater frequency of positive family history of affective disorder compared with post stroke depression (above)
Starkstein et al., 1989	93	Stroke, right hemisphere	19 developed "undue cheerfulness;" 17 developed major depression. Among those who developed depression there was significantly more family history of major psychiatric illness and more parietal lesions.

Update of Jeste et al., 1988

nia following injury to the CNS. Their review and two reports published since (Nizamie et al., 1988; Yatham et al., 1988) have identified 24 cases of secondary depression and 15 cases of secondary mania. Jeste and colleagues warn, however, that limitations in the data[4] make it impossible to de-determine if the cases represent de novo emergence of affective syndromes or the precipitation of an affective syndrome in vulnerable individuals,[5] a point made also by Stasiek and Zetin (1985) and by Cummings (1986). In their review of poststroke affective syndromes, Starkstein and Robinson (1989) conclude that, although depression is much more common than mania, it is the manic reactions that are more frequently associated with a preexisting personal or family history of affective disorder.[6] Taken together, these observations suggest that poststroke depression is a somewhat heterogeneous and unspecific syndrome and perhaps, therefore, of limited usefulness for general modeling of the depressive phase of manic-depressive illness (Goodwin, 1983).

Despite these limitations, it is useful to note some tentative anatomical patterns. Most frequently associated with depression or mania were lesions located in the frontal or temporal lobes. Left-sided lesions tended to be associated with depressions and right-sided lesions with symptoms suggestive of mania (Cummings, 1986; Starkstein and Robinson, 1989). The left–right differences may be reversed in regions closer to the posterior. Thus, depression tends to be associated with left frontotemporal or right parietooccipital lesions, and manic-like symptoms are more likely to follow right frontotemporal or left parietooccipital lesions.[7] Robinson and Szetela (1981), in studying stroke patients, noted a positive correlation between the degree of depression and the proximity of lesions to the left frontal pole.[8] Earlier, Gainotti (1972) compared an equal number of left-sided and right-sided lesions and found a higher frequency of depressive reactions associated with the left-sided lesions and "indifference euphoria" more frequently associated with right-sided lesions. It is clear, however, that not all of the neuropathological data are consistent with such lateral or anterior–posterior specialization. (Neurophysiological tests of lateralized dysfunction in manic-depressive patients are discussed later in this chapter.)

Most of the secondary cases refer to single epi-sodes of depression or mania. A few reports of true (i.e., cycling) bipolar disorders secondary to brain lesions have appeared.[9] These case reports involve diverse areas of the brain, confounding any simple neuroanatomical explanation of their bipolar disorders. Cook and co-workers (1987) compared 39 patients whose bipolar illness was preceded by some organic factors with age- and sex-matched bipolar controls. The patients with preexisting organicity were older and had relatively more manic episodes and less family history of bipolar disorder. When manic, the organic patients were more assaultive and irritable. It is of interest that Jeste and colleagues (1988) were unable to find reports of recurrent unipolar depression secondary to structural brain lesions.

Indirect Studies of Localization

Neurological Correlates

Huntington's disease, which is characterized by atrophy of the striatum and cerebral cortex, occurs together with affective disorder too often for the association to be explained by chance. Of 80 Huntington's patients studied by Heathfield (1967), 10 had endogenous depression (recurrent in 4), and 4 had hypomania with delusions of grandeur. The affective symptoms usually appeared early in the course of the illness and responded to "appropriate" treatment, including antidepressant drugs. Folstein and colleagues (1983) studied 88 patients with Huntington's disease and found 36 (41 percent) with a history of major affective disorder (28 unipolar and 8 bipolar). In almost all of the cases, the affective syndrome was present early in the course of the disease and responded well to standard treatments. Another disease involving the basal ganglia, Parkinson's disease, is also frequently associated with depression, although apparently not with mania. As discussed later in the section on immune factors, the incidence of manic-depressive illness among patients with multiple sclerosis (MS) is significantly higher than would be expected by chance. The fact that the families of MS patients apparently do not have an excess of affective disorder (Joffe et al., 1987a) suggests that the manic and depressive symptoms are secondary to the MS.

Several investigators have commented on the association of depression with neurological abnormalities that disappear when moods become normal. For example, Staton and co-workers (1981) and Freeman and associates (1985) identified depressed patients in whom focal left-sided neurological signs resolved with improvement in depression. Keshavan and Goswamy (1983), by contrast, reported the case of a rapid-cycling bipolar patient in whom dyskinesia was less severe during depression than during euthymic states. Yet another pattern was reported by Cutler and Post (1982b): two bipolar patients had dyskinesia during their depressions but not during their manias.

Cox and Ludwig (1979) compared patients with bipolar and unipolar major affective disorders (by Feighner criteria), schizophrenia, alcoholism, and character disorders for specific neurological soft signs[10] thought to reflect diffuse cortical dysfunction. There were substantially more temporal lobe and total cortical signs in patients with bipolar and unipolar disorders than in normal controls, although the number of subjects with affective disorders was not large enough to evaluate statistical significance or bipolar–unipolar differences. Nasrallah and colleagues (1983) assessed DSM-III-diagnosed manic, schizophrenic, and control men for 30 neurological soft signs. They noted that patient groups had significantly more soft signs than did controls, but the manic and schizophrenic patients showed no overall differences. A treatment artifact could not be ruled out, however, since both patient groups were on antipsychotic drugs at the time of the study.

Walker and Green (1982) compared the neuromotor performance of 20 patients with affective disorder (11 manic and 9 major depressive, type not stated) with that of 20 schizophrenic patients. They measured stereognosis, successive finger-thumb opposition, hand pronation–supination, and grip strength. For every motor test, the patients with affective disorders performed at a level between that of schizophrenic patients and normals. Their performance was significantly worse than that of the normal subjects only in the case of finger–thumb opposition. Mukherjee and colleagues (1984) administered graphaesthesia[11] and face–hand tests to 75 DSM-III-diagnosed bipolar patients. The investigators noted a tendency toward left hand errors, but only in patients who had been treated with neuroleptic medications for long periods. Unfortunately, information was not provided separately for depressed and manic states, nor were any control groups studied. Merrin (1984) noted greater superiority in right hand than in left hand grip strength in 21 bipolar and 12 unipolar patients diagnosed by research diagnostic criteria (RDC) than in normal controls and nonpsychotic schizophrenic patients. The findings, thought to be consistent with frontotemporal impairment (particularly in the nondominant hemisphere), were primarily associated with the presence of psychotic symptoms. These findings were not specific to affective disorder—that is, psychotic schizophrenic patients were not significantly different from bipolar patients.

In summary, although there is some evidence that neurological symptoms may be associated with affective disorders, they do not appear to be specific. It is unclear whether such symptoms are useful for locating specific brain sites associated with affective disorders. Further, since most of the affective patients were studied as controls for schizophrenic patients, some important information was omitted, for example, medication effects, differences between mania and depression, and differences between bipolar and unipolar depression.

Laterality

Thanks to the pioneering work of Sperry on split-brain preparations (1968), it is now established that the left and right cerebral hemispheres subserve different (albeit overlapping) aspects of information processing and cognitive function. The left hemisphere is more specialized for language and logical, linear thinking—the right for imagery and visuospatial, musical, and holistic, gestalt processing. Some studies in normal volunteers indicate that the right hemisphere plays a major role in processing and responding to emotional stimuli,[12] a dominance that is, however, not as absolute as that of the left hemisphere for language (reviewed in Tucker, 1981; Tucker et al., 1981; Coffey, 1987). The whole concept of dominance has been qualified considerably with growing knowledge about the complexity of the interactions between right and left hemispheres, including the capacity for lateralization patterns to shift under certain circumstances (Tucker, 1981; Tucker et al., 1981).

Laterality of function in manic-depressive illness has been studied by several approaches. In addition to the analysis of lateralized lesions already discussed, these include dichotic listening and handedness among mood-disordered patients, electrophysiological and brain-imaging studies of hemispheric function (literature reviewed in the second part of this chapter), comparison of the effects of unilateral electroconvulsive therapy (ECT) administered on the dominant or nondominant side, and exploration of neuropsychological differences. These latter studies have been central to the laterality literature and are detailed in Chapter 11.

In general, the laterality research field is still clouded by controversies over basic interpretations. The same experimental observation, for example, can be understood as right-sided overactivation or left-sided underactivation, and a given outcome may be seen as release of ipsilateral or contralateral cortical control of subcortical processes.

Dichotic Listening. In dichotic listening tests, different information is presented simultaneously to each ear through headphones. In normal subjects, verbal sounds are better perceived by the dominant hemisphere, nonverbal by the nondominant hemisphere. The dominant hemisphere's advantage with verbal tasks was reported to be below normal in untreated depressed (predominantly unipolar) patients (Johnson and Crockett, 1982) but exaggerated in manic and depressed patients undergoing treatment (Lishman et al., 1978; Yozawitz et al., 1979). In dichotic listening tasks involving nonverbal material, bipolar patients (both manic and depressed) showed a reversal of normal processing, in effect demonstrating a nondominant hemisphere disadvantage (Yozawitz et al., 1979; Bruder et al., 1981, 1989). Patients with unipolar depression, on the same tasks, lost lateralized functioning; neither hemisphere was dominant (Johnson and Crockett, 1982; Bruder et al., 1981). Although it is difficult to interpret these findings definitively, the abnormalities noted on dichotic listening tasks in bipolar disorder suggest impaired functioning of the nondominant (i.e., generally right) temporal lobes.[13]

Studying both affective disorder and schizophrenia, Wexler and Heninger (1979) noted in both diagnostic groups an inverse relationship be-

tween the extent of laterality on verbal dichotic listening and the overall degree of psychopathology. This finding would suggest that, at least as measured in this study, the loss of normal lateralization of function is nonspecific, perhaps reflecting a breakdown of interhemispheric inhibition that is associated with major psychopathology.

Handedness Studies. The literature on handedness in affective illness, which usually focuses on unipolar illness, suggests a relatively normal distribution of left and right handers, controlled for gender.[14] However, one study of "manic-depressives and schizoaffective" patients indicates that they are more likely to be left handed than are normal controls (Lishman and McMeekan, 1976). There are two case reports of bipolar patients who changed handedness from left to right when switching from depression to mania (Bruce, 1895; Flor-Henry, 1979).

Other Studies of Laterality. Some investigators have observed that when intracarotid sodium amytal is injected in brain-damaged subjects, left-side injections seem to produce depressive symptoms, and right-side injections produce euphoria, giddiness, or a manic state (Terzian, 1964; Rossi and Rosadini, 1967; Gainotti, 1972). Others have not replicated these results, although Milner (1967) and Hommes and Panhuysen (1971) noted an elevation of mood following injection of sodium amytal into either hemisphere of depressed patients (type not stated).

Clinical observations on differences in the effectiveness of ECT administered to either the left or right hemisphere also have contributed to our understanding of laterality. Deglin and Nikolaenko (1975) administered unilateral ECT to opposite hemispheres on alternate days in a group of patients with various types of depression. Compared with baseline levels, more initial depression was associated with left-sided (dominant) application, and more euphoric responses followed right-sided (nondominant) application. In treating depression, unilateral nondominant ECT is generally as effective as bilateral ECT but unilateral dominant ECT is not (Janicak et al., 1985; Weiner, 1984). Consistent with this is the finding of Kronfol and co-workers (1978) that the treatment of depression[15] with either right-sided or left-sided ECT is associated with normalization of the pretreatment right hemisphere neuro-psychological dysfunction. In treating mania, however, unilateral nondominant ECT seems to be less effective than bilateral treatment. Of possible relevance to these ECT data are studies of unilateral temporal lobe epilepsy (Bear and Fedio, 1977) in which left-sided seizures were characteristically associated with negative or depressive affect, whereas right-sided seizures were associated with more positive affect or indifference.

Summary. In general, the studies reviewed, along with the neuropsychological studies reviewed in Chapter 11, suggest that relative functional deficits in the nondominant (generally right) hemisphere can be found in both phases of manic-depressive illness. Later, we attempt to integrate these indirect measures of laterality with the neuropathological and imaging data. Such integration is limited not only by the methodological problems noted earlier but also (and perhaps especially) by the lack of fundamental consensus concerning the proper interpretation of the various tests or conditions used to infer laterality. Some conclusions about laterality depend on the assumption that normal depressed mood and the mood of depressive illness are strictly parallel. In fact, it is likely that each hemisphere contributes differentially to various aspects of mood and cognition. In the syndrome of depression, dysfunction or activation of each hemisphere may contribute to specific symptoms (Tucker, 1981).

Additional clarification of these important questions will no doubt be provided by direct assessment of brain function in manic-depressive patients using brain-imaging strategies under various behavioral conditions. Such studies should enlarge our understanding of overall patterns of dysfunction as well as help to specify particular areas (e.g., temporal vs frontal lobe) and the predominant side. Clarification of the laterality question is important for a number of reasons, not the least of which is the emerging evidence of hemispheric differences in the distribution of important neurotransmitter substances (Oke et al., 1978; Mandell and Knapp, 1979; Robinson, 1983).

Brain Stimulation and Psychosurgery

Animal studies have shown that stimulating or lesioning the brain, especially the amygdala, can result in a variety of mood changes, including withdrawal, anger, rage, apparent depression, and excitement. These findings are difficult to extrapolate to humans, however, since quite different effects result from stimulating or lesioning the same brain area in humans and in animals (Brazier, 1972). Stevens and colleagues (1969) reported lesioning experiments on patients with seizure foci located in the temporal lobe. In one patient, a lesion in the right amygdala was followed by a severe depression lasting a week, and a lesion in the left amygdala was followed by a longer depression eventually requiring pharmacological treatment. Of related interest are reports of four patients with right-sided and one with left-sided temporal lobe epilepsy who became hypomanic following an increase in complex partial seizures (Barczak et al., 1988; Humpheries and Dickinson, 1988; Morphew, 1988). We return to these laterality issues when we review the EEG literature.

Lesions in the anterior cingulate gyri can sometimes relieve depression and perhaps mania as well. Two studies reported that 65 to 75 percent of 188 depressed patients who underwent bilateral cingulotomy subsequently improved (Ballantine et al., 1977; Corkin et al., 1979). In contrast, very few patients with schizophrenia benefited from this operation (Ballantine and Giriunas, 1979). It is not clear how many of the subjects in these studies, depressed patients who were presumably resistant to other treatments, met standardized diagnostic criteria for bipolar or unipolar depression.

Ballantine and colleagues (1977) have suggested that cingulotomy may exert its effects through secondary neurochemical alterations, since postoperative improvement is delayed. Corkin and co-workers (1979), however, interpret the effects as being directly related to an interruption of fibers traveling through the cingulate gyrus. In other words, they view serotonergic and dopaminergic fiber disruption as the principal mechanism. Interestingly, neuropathological studies of postcingulotomy patients indicate that lesions must extend into the most superficial part of the corpus callosum for psychiatric improvement to occur (Bernad et al., 1979), implying that interruption of interhemispheric transmission may play a role in producing therapeutic results. Another procedure reported to be effective with bipolar patients is stereotactic subcaudate tracto-tomy. The relatively recent articles on this pro-cedure report mixed results among bipolar pa-tients, with about half the patients experiencing clinically significant benefit. Two of the groups believed that manic episodes responded better than depressive episodes (Lovett and Shaw, 1987; Poynton et al., 1988), but the other did not (Sachdev et al., 1988). These investigators sug-gested that the procedure be considered only for severely ill patients who do not respond to other treatments.

Regional Neurochemistry

The large body of literature on neurochemical abnormalities in bipolar disorders is reviewed in Chapter 17. Here we focus only on the question of localization. The literature is scant. We could find only one investigative group doing regional neurochemistry; they studied the brains of four "endogenous" depressed patients and compared them to age-matched controls (Birkmayer and Riederer, 1975). Their main findings[16] can be summarized thus: In "endogenous depression" the loss of drive may be related to dopamine defi-ciency, sleeplessness to serotonin deficits, and other signs and symptoms to norepinephrine deficiency.

Neuroendocrine Studies

As reviewed in Chapter 17, a variety of neuroen-docrine abnormalities have been described in the major affective disorders. They involve primarily the hypothalamic–pituitary, adrenal, and thyroid axes but also include possible abnormalities in vasopressin, enkephalin, somatostatin, and oth-ers. In general, the neuroendocrine abnormalities tend to implicate dysfunction of the hypothala-mus and its connections.

Other studies have examined melatonin secre-tion as a marker of pineal adrenergic activity and, more generally, of circadian rhythms and their possible pathophysiological role in the cyclical characteristics of affective disorders (see Chapter 19). This work also indirectly implicates regions in the anterior hypothalamus, principally the su-prachiasmatic nucleus. Of course, one can only speculate whether these hypothalamic changes are involved in the primary pathology of the ill-ness or themselves are downstream.

Structural Brain-Mapping Studies

The past two decades have witnessed the devel-opment and refinement of computer-assisted techniques for visualizing the structure and func-tion of the living brain. The structural imaging techniques include computed tomography (CT) scans and magnetic resonance imaging (MRI), and the functional techniques include positron emission tomography (PET) scans, regional cere-bral blood flow (rCBF), and single photon emis-sion computed tomography (SPECT). The avail-ability of these approaches has spurred interest in neuropathological studies of many mental dis-orders, including manic-depressive illness.

In this section, we discuss studies of structural abnormalities in manic-depressive illness using CT scans and MRI. In a later section of this chap-ter, we examine functional abnormalities as re-vealed by PET scans and rCBF and SPECT.

Computed Tomography

In contrast to the limited data available from classic postmortem studies of the brains of manic-depressive patients, CT scanning offers the op-portunity to study neuroanatomical structure at different stages of the illness and also in the well state. The most frequently reported CT scan mea-sure is the cerebral ventricle/brain ratio (VBR). When measured in patients with such diagnoses as schizophrenia and Alzheimer's disease, an in-crease in the VBR (reflecting enlargement of the lateral cerebral ventricles) is presumed to reflect cell loss, that is, degeneration.

Studies of VBR measures in patients with af-fective disorders have relied on single measures rather than on repeated tests, perhaps reflecting assumptions about fixed, stable lesions. Such re-liance on one test is unfortunate, since, given the interindividual variability of this measure, mean-ingful comparisons of symptomatic–asymptoma-tic states across patients will require longitudinal studies. As reviewed by Jeste and colleagues (1988), a bare majority of studies reported that VBR measures were somewhat larger in patients with affective illness than in controls (matched for age and alcohol use) (Table 18-2). Some of the studies failed to find a significant differ-ence between patients with affective illness and those with schizophrenia, an illness with a well-established association with enlarged ventricles

Table 18-2. CT-Scan Abnormalities: Ventricular Enlargement

Study	Affective Disorders			Schizophrenia			Other Controls			Comments
	N	VBR	% Abnl	N	VBR	%Abnl	N	VBR	%Abnl	
Von Gall & Becker, 1978	37 UP	?	13.5	45	?	2.2	20[a]	?	0	Affectives different from schizophrenics, other controls
Jacoby & Levy, 1980; and Jacoby et al., 1980, 1981, 1983	2 BP[b] 39 UP[b]	?	22				50[c]	14.2 ± 3.9	16	Affectives different from no group. Large VBR associated with delusions and hallucinations
Pearlson & Veroff, 1981	16 BP + UP	6.5 ± 3.3	12.5	22	7.5 ± 2.9	23	35[a]	3.6 ± 2.6	?	Affectives different from other controls
Nasrallah et al., 1982b	24 BP	7.5 ± 3.2	29.2	55	8.7 ± 4.0	34.5	27[c]	4.5 ± 2.6	7.4	Affectives different from normals. Large VBR associated with decreased hospitalizations
Weinberger et al., 1982	23	3.8 ± 2.9	0	17	6.0 ± 4.2	23.5	35 SF 27[a] 26[d]	5.3 ± 3.6 3.2 ± 2.9 2.9 ± 2.9	20 0 0	Affectives different from schizophrenic and schizophreniform
Rieder et al., 1983	19 BP	5.3 ± 3.7	10.5	28	3.7 ± 3.4	7.1	15 SA	3.9 ± 3.8	6.7	
Scott et al., 1983	10 UP	9.5 ± 3.4					10[c]	4.2 ± 2.9		Affectives different from normals.
Targum et al., 1983	9 BP 29 UP: 20 D 18 ND	5.1 ± 3.3 3.6 ± 2.0	25 0				26[c]	2.9 ± 2.9	0	Delusionals different from nondelusionals and normals. Large VBR associated with delusional depression & lower IQ scores
Shima et al., 1984	2 BP 44 UP	11.2 ± 3.5					46[c,e]	9.1 ± 2.4		Affectives different from normals. Large VBR associated with late onset, 1 episode, no melancholia, and poor outcome
Pearlson et al., 1984	27 BP	6.6 ± 3.4	31	19	6.2 ± 2.6	?	46[d]	4.7 ± 2.0	?	Affectives different from normals. Large VBR associated with negative symptoms, increased hospitalizations, persistent unemployment

Reference	Patients (n)	VBR	(n)[a]	VBR	%	Normals (n)	VBR	Def.	Comments
Luchins et al., 1984; Meltzer et al., 1984e	22 BP+ UP	4.5 ± 2.7	18	45 4.1 ± 2.7	10.9	62[e]	3.0 ± 3.2	?	Affectives different from other controls. Large VBR associated with psychotic features, low CSF-DBH
Nasrallah et al., 1984	19[f]	7.5 ± 3.2	42			27	4.5 ± 2.6		Affectives different from normals. Large VBR associated with decreased hospitalizations
Dolan et al., 1985	74 BP[g] 27 UP	7.3 ± 4.6				52	5.6 ± 3.3		Affectives different from normals. Large VBR associated with aging in both groups
Sacchetti et al., 1987	108 MAD	6.1 ± 3.7	20			66	4.7 ± 2.5	?	Affectives different from normals. Large VBR associated with age, age of onset, delusions, anxiety, no family history, and poor response to lithium
Schlegel & Kretzschmar, 1987a	21 BP 27 UP 5 SA	7.4 ± 2.4				60	6.9 ± 2.6		No affective/normal difference and no BP/UP difference
Iacono et al., 1988	18 BP 16 UP	6.2 ± 1.9 6.4 ± 3.0	31	6.7 ± 2.6		44	6.4 ± 2.8		No significant BP/UP differences or differences between any groups of patients
Dewan et al., 1988a,b	26 BP	6.9 ± 2.9				22 SA	6.3 ± 1.9		No significant differences between BP patients and SA control
Roy-Byrne et al., 1988b	47 BP 12 UP	4.9 ± 1.8 5.9 ± 3.0							No significant BP/UP differences. VBR not positively associated with course. When analyzed by sex, VBR was inversely related to chronicity

Definition of abnormal VBR varies from a decision by a neuroradiologist to a standard deviation of two.
SA = Schizoaffective, SF = Schizophreniform, VBR = Ventricle brain ratio, D = Delusional patients, ND = Not delusional patients, MAD = Major affective disorder

[a] Other psychiatric patients
[b] All were 60 or older
[c] Normals
[d] Neurologic patients
[e] Headache patients
[f] Manic patients
[g] Depressed patients

Update of Jeste et al., 1988

(Weinberger and Kleinman, 1986). Of the 18 VBR studies of major depression, only 3 (Schlegel and Kretzchmar, 1987a; Iacono et al., 1988; Roy-Byrne et al., 1988a) reported data separately for the bipolar and unipolar subgroups. No bipolar–unipolar differences were observed.

Is it now established that, compared with appropriately matched controls, manic-depressive patients have, on average, significantly larger ventricles? A recent analysis by Depue and Iacono (1989) suggests that such a conclusion may be premature. They found that those studies reporting ventricular enlargement in major affective disorder used control groups whose average ventricular size was significantly smaller than that among the control groups in the studies reporting no difference between patients with affective disorders and controls. They conclude that "control group selection may have an important influence on the outcome of CT investigations of lateral ventricle size" (p. 482).

The search for clinical correlates of ventricular size is still inconclusive. Of the various features examined, including medication history, family history, and cognitive deficit, only psychotic symptoms and poor outcome have been associated with VBR by more than one investigator, and in both these instances the association is far from well established (see, e.g., Dolan et al., 1985, Roy-Byrne et al., 1988a, and the review by Depue and Iacono, 1989). Biochemical or endocrine correlates of larger VBRs include increased urinary free cortisol (Kellner et al., 1983b), hypothyroidism (Johnstone et al., 1986), increased levels of CSF 5-HIAA (the principal serotonin metabolite) (Standish-Barry et al., 1986), and decreased plasma dopamine beta-hydroxylase (DBH)[17] activity (Meltzer et al., 1984e). The association between a relatively larger VBR and hypercortisolemia may reflect acute changes in ventricle size associated with the hemodynamic effects of increased cortisol secretion (i.e., diuretic central effects leading to reduction in brain mass and secondary enlargement of the ventricles). Although the association with hypothyroidism requires replication, it is nevertheless intriguing, given the association between thyroid function and affective illness, as reviewed in Chapter 17.

Sulcal widening, also revealed by CT scan, is an important measure that reflects some loss of cortical mass and possible atrophy. Table 18-3 summarizes nine studies totaling 321 patients with affective disorder (132 bipolar), comparing them with schizophrenic patients or various control groups (six studies). Of these six studies, half found widening, half did not. On average, widening was identified in 17 percent of the patients with affective disorder compared with about 4 percent of the controls. Studies of bipolar patients tended to show more frequent sulcal widening than did studies of unipolar patients, but Dolan and associates (1986) and Iacono and colleagues (1988) both compared the bipolar and unipolar groups directly and found no difference.

Another measure derived from CT scanning is cerebellar vermian atrophy. A summary of eight studies (Table 18-4), totaling 244 affective patients (100 bipolar), indicates such atrophy in about 26 percent of affective patients, 19 percent of schizophrenic patients, and less than 4 percent of normal controls. Only one direct bipolar-unipolar comparison is available. Yates and colleagues (1987) found atrophy in 8 percent of their bipolar patients but in none of their unipolar patients; this difference was not statistically significant, perhaps because of the relatively small numbers. Comparing the two groups across the remaining studies, the percentages with cerebellar vermian atrophy are roughly the same.

Table 18-5 includes seven studies of other CT parameters. Schlegel and Kretzschmar (1987b) found normal VBRs among a group of 53 patients with major affective disorder, but they noted increases in the distance between the tips of the frontal horns, the bicaudate distance, and the size of the third ventricle. Discriminate function analysis indicated that these abnormalities could be attributed to the older, unipolar, psychotic male patients. Schlegel and Kretzschmar (1987a) also found higher brain density values in two regions among the bipolar patients compared with unipolar patients and with age- and sex-matched controls. The higher values could not be attributed to differences in ventricular size. Also notable is the Dewan and associates study of 26 bipolar patients (1988a), which found normal VBR but an increase in third ventricle size and increased density in a variety of brain areas, especially on the right (nondominant) side (temporal lobe and diencephalic nuclei, in particular). These authors suggested that the enlargement of the third ventricle

Table 18-3. CT-Scan Abnormalities: Sulcal Widening (Cortical Atrophy)

Study	Affective Disorders N	% Abnormal	Schizophrenia N	% Abnormal	Other N	% Abnormal	Comments
Von Gall & Becker, 1978	37 UP	10.8	45	6.6	21 OP	5.0	Moderate-to-severe cortical atrophy
Jacoby & Levy, 1980	39 UP 2 BP	?			50 NC 40 D	?	Elderly patient and control groups. No significant differences between affectives and controls
Pearlson & Veroff, 1981	16 BP	12.5	22	18.0	35 OP	?	
Weinberger et al., 1982	23	13.0	17	0.0	35 SP 53 OPN	14.0 0.0	
Nasrallah et al., 1982b	24 BP	25.0	55	40.0	27 NC	3.7	No significant differences between schizophrenic and manic patients
Rieder et al., 1983	19 BP	21.0	28	17.9	15 SA	33.0	No significant differences between schizophrenics, schizoaffectives, and BPs
Dolan et al., 1986	74 UP[a] 27 BP[a]	?			52 NC	?	Patients had significantly greater sulcal widening, especially frontotemporal correlation with VBR
Dewan et al., 1988a	26 BP				22 HP		No significant differences between bipolars and controls
Iacono et al., 1988	18 BP 16 UP		31		44 NC 30 MC		No significant differences between groups; no BP/UP differences

OP = Other psychiatric, NC = Normal controls, D = Dementia, SP = Schizophreniform, OPN = Other psychiatric & neurologic, SA = Schizoaffective, HP = Headache patients, MC = Medical controls

[a]Depressed patients

Update of Jeste et al., 1988

Table 18-4. CT-Scan Abnormalities: Cerebellar Vermis Atrophy

Study	Affective Disorders		Schizophrenia		Other		Comments
	N	% Abnormal	N	% Abnormal	N	% Abnormal	
Heath et al., 1979	31 FP	29.0	85	40.0			No significant difference between the two groups
Nasrallah et al., 1981	15 BP	27.0	43	12.0	36 NC	3.0	Cerebellar atrophy significantly greater in manics (but not schizophrenics) than controls
Heath et al., 1982	64 FP	53.1	50	50.0	1,541 NP	3.7	Affectives and schizophrenics different from controls.
Weinberger et al., 1982	23	9.0	17	12.0	88 SP	0.0	Affectives and schizophrenics similar; both significantly different from other groups
Lippmann et al., 1982	18 BP	28.0	54	17.0	79 NC	4.0	Both patient groups significantly different from controls
Nasrallah et al., 1982b	24 BP	20.8	55	9.1	27 NC	3.7	
Rieder et al., 1983	19 BP	10.5	28	7.1	15 SA	6.7	No significant difference among schizophrenics, schizoaffectives, and BPs
Yates et al., 1987	24 BP 26 UP	8.3 BP 0.0 UP	108	3.7	74 NCA	2.7	No significant difference among groups, although BP-UP trend is of interest

FP = "Functional psychosis other than schizophrenia", NP = Nonpsychotic, nonepileptic, NC = Normal controls, NCA = Normal controls — age & sex matched, SP = Schizophreniform, other psychiatric & neurologic, SA = Schizoaffective

Update of Jeste et al., 1988

Table 18-5. CT-Scan Abnormalities: Other Findings

Study	Affective Disorders N	Other N	Comments
Tanaka et al., 1982	9 BP 31 UP	40 HP	Below age 50, left septum-caudate distance was lower in affectives Over age 50, there was a significant enlargement of the width of the interhemispheric fissure and between the sylvian fissure and inner skull in the affective group
Jacoby et al., 1983	37 UP	36 NC 23 D	Lower CT density in affective and demented patients
Schlegel & Kretzschmar, 1987a	22 BP 33 UP 5 SA	60 NC	Affectives had significant ↑ 3rd ventricle width than controls; no significant differences when BPs compared to NCs alone
Schlegel & Kretzschmar, 1987b	21 BP 27 UP 5 SA	60 NC	Frontal horn distance and bicaudate distance abnormally large among affective patients, especially older and psychotic
Dewan et al., 1988a	26 BP	22 SA	BPs had ↑ 3rd ventricle width
Dewan et al., 1988b	26 BP	22 HP	↑ density in several areas including right temporal lobe. No correlates with neuropsychological tests, family history, psychotic symptoms, or response to lithium
Iacono et al., 1988	18 BP 16 UP	44 NC 30 MC	No significant BP-UP differences, UPs had ↑ 3rd ventricle width than MCs. No significant BP or UP differences from NCs

SA = Schizoaffective, NC = Normal controls, D = Dementia, HP = Headache patients, MC = medical controls

is probably not specific to bipolar illness but that the increased right temporal lobe density is. One other CT parameter, cerebral asymmetry in brain width,[18] was reported to be not significantly greater in bipolar patients than in controls.[19]

In interpreting the CT scan literature, it is important to note that these are all relatively recent studies with variable methodology and as yet no agreed upon standard for assessing and dealing with methodological artifact. The most important limitation, noted earlier, is the variability among the control groups. In addition, the patients are hospitalized. Given the considerable success of contemporary treatments for bipolar illness, inpatient samples now available to investigators are likely to be skewed toward sicker, more

treatment-resistant patients. With the exception of one study that found a strong relationship between a high VBR and poor response to maintenance lithium (Sacchetti et al., 1987) and one that found no relationship to other CT measures (Dewan et al., 1988b), treatment response has not generally been examined in these studies (unlike the schizophrenia literature), perhaps because it was not particularly variable in these populations. Possibly some of the apparent CT scan similarities between these affective patients and schizophrenic patients are consistent with more schizophrenic or organic features among contemporary (largely treatment-resistant) hospitalized patients with affective illness.[20] Obviously, before the specificity question can be evaluated, we will need carefully standardized CT scan data from a broad spectrum of outpatients undergoing successful treatment for recurrent affective illness.

Magnetic Resonance Imaging

MRI is the new terminology for nuclear magnetic resonance (NMR) imaging, a change instituted to enhance patient compliance by shedding any connotation of radioactivity that might be conveyed by the word *nuclear*. MRI depends on the behavior of nuclei with an odd number of protons or neutrons (i.e., they are electrically charged), which, because of their inherent properties of spinning, generate tiny magnetic fields. When an external magnetic field is applied, the individual endogenous magnetic fields line up parallel to the external field, and they emit a characteristic signal, depending on such factors as the extent of molecular motion resulting from solid or liquid states. MRI gives a neuroanatomical definition at least as good as CT scans while allowing cross-sectional images along multiple axes. It is thus more flexible than the CT scan for visualizing brain structure in three dimensions. MRI does not involve ionizing radiation, an important feature for clinical studies.

As a relatively new technology, MRI has been used in only a few studies of manic-depressive patients. Rangel-Guerra and colleagues (1983) studied the effect of lithium on T_1 relaxation time of the water proton, a measure thought to reflect the ratio of free to bound water. In 17 of 20 drug-free bipolar patients, T_1 in the frontal and temporal lobes was greater than in normals. Following 10 days of lithium treatment, the T_1 relaxation in the bipolar patients was reduced to the normal range. Lithium treatment had no effect on this measure in the normal controls. These data suggest that the higher T_1 in these bipolar patients before treatment reflected a relative edematous state in the frontal and temporal lobes that was corrected by lithium. In an MRI study of erythrocytes of bipolar patients before and during lithium treatment (J. Rosenthal et al., 1986), a similar pretreatment increase in T_1 time was noted among the patients compared with controls, and this increase normalized after 1 week of lithium treatment. Thus, at least in this study, a peripheral change associated with lithium reflected one seen centrally.

MRI signal hyperintensities involving subcortical white matter have been reported among elderly depressed patients (Coffey et al., 1988; Krishnan et al., 1988a); since such abnormalities can be nonspecifically associated with advanced age and particularly with ischemic brain disease, the lack of age-matched control groups makes these findings difficult to interpret. Of more interest are the results of Dupont and colleagues (1989), who found state-independent subcortical white matter abnormalities in 8 of 14 young bipolar patients. No abnormalities were found among age-matched normal controls. A similar trend was seen by Andreasen (1989) in her study of 50 bipolar patients. In a follow-up study involving six additional patients, Dupont and colleagues (1990) reported that bipolar patients with MRI abnormalities had significantly more previous hospitalizations and were more impaired on certain cognitive tests than bipolar patients without such abnormalities.

We are aware of two studies employing MRI tomography to explore the temporal lobes. Hauser and colleagues (1988) determined that the ratio of temporal lobe to hemisphere area was significantly smaller in affectively disordered patients compared with controls. On the other hand, examining a group of bipolar patients, Johnstone and colleagues (1989) found no temporal lobe differences compared with controls, although there were differences between schizophrenic patients and controls.

Functional Brain-Imaging Studies

Perhaps no other area of technological development has so captured the imagination of psychiatric researchers as the family of techniques referred to as functional brain imaging, which includes rCBF, PET, and SPECT. Deriving from fundamental scientific advances ranging from tracer methodology to computer technology, these techniques promise, at last, to give us access to the functional anatomy of the living brain.

Regional Cerebral Blood Flow

In the 19th century, some believed that mental diseases might be caused by disturbances in brain nutrition, and Meynert (1885) suggested that melancholia might result from decreased blood flow to the brain, with mania resulting from increased flow. The direct study of cerebral blood flow (CBF), pioneered by Kety and Schmidt with the development of the nitrous oxide technique in 1945, was a monumental advance, since this measure is linked to metabolic activity in the brain. Later, Marcus Raichle made many important contributions that have enhanced the application of CBF techniques (see, e.g., Raichle et al., 1976).

The ability to measure blood flow over specific regions of the cerebral cortex was first demonstrated by Ingvar and Lassen in 1961, using a radioactive tracer. (Recall that a tracer is a physiological substance altered so as to emit a detectable signal, usually radioactivity, without compromising normal physiological processing and function.) As developed by Obrist and colleagues (1967), the tracer used in regional CBF studies today is a radioactive isotope of xenon, a biologically inert gas. Xenon-133 emits low-energy gamma-rays, which are measured by multiple scintillation detectors positioned around the head. The brain is first saturated with radioactivity through inhalation of the freely diffusible xenon-133 gas. The calculated rate of disappearance of radioactivity (washout) is a measure of blood flow to that region.

Compared with the PET technique, rCBF measures are only two-dimensional and primarily reflect the surface of the brain. Also, rCBF measures lack the spatial resolution of PET. However, the xenon-inhalation method has certain advantages for measuring cerebral blood flow: (1) it is noninvasive and is nonthreatening to the patient, minimizing cerebral activity produced by the procedure itself, (2) because the isotope has a long half-life and its production does not require a cyclotron, it is easier to work with, and (3) it is cleared rapidly, assuring minimal radiation exposure and allowing repeated studies and the capacity to follow rapidly changing events. Under normal conditions, glucose metabolism and blood flow are correlated, so that one might expect a rough correspondence between PET and rCBF data from the same area.

Reviewing the rCBF studies of affectively ill patients, Mathew and associates (1985) and Silfverskiöld and Risberg (1989) noted considerable variability in results, perhaps related to methodological problems, such as relatively small sample sizes, lack of standardized diagnostic criteria in some instances, differences in age and/or sex distribution between the patients and the controls, uncontrolled medication effects, and lack of a control for the effects of anxiety[21] on regional blood flow. Of the seven studies comparing patients with major depression in the resting state with a control group, three found reduced CBF in the patients (Mathew et al., 1980; Warren et al., 1984; Sackeim et al., 1987), and four found no difference (Gur et al., 1984; Goldstein et al., 1985; Silfverskiöld and Risberg, 1989; Berman, 1989). There is considerable variation in absolute blood flow values, particularly from the various control groups, making an overall conclusion difficult. In one of the positive studies (Mathew et al., 1980), there was a not unexpected negative correlation between depression ratings and CBF. In their negative study, Silfverskiöld and Risberg (1989) found a positive correlation between depression ratings and CBF. Both of the studies that distinguished bipolar and unipolar patients[22] (Sackeim et al., 1987; Silfverskiöld and Risberg, 1989) reported higher flow among the bipolar patients, a small difference that may not be subgroup specific because it was also noted among the psychotically depressed unipolar patients in the Silfverskiöld and Risberg study. Regional differences were suggested by Mathew and colleagues (1980), who reported that reduced CBF was limited to the left hemisphere, but there were no regional trends among the four negative reports. The activation of CBF by a cognitive task was found to be greater than normal in the left anterior and right posterior regions among depressed patients by Gur and colleagues (1984). On the other hand, Guenther and co-workers (1986) reported that severely depressed patients failed to show the normal increase in blood flow in the contralateral motor area in response to right handed motor tasks, but this occurred among some schizophrenic patients as well, and medication effects could not be excluded. Comparing depressed and schizophrenic patients with normal controls on the Wisconsin card sort task (WCS), Berman (1989) found no difference between the depressed patients and the controls and replicated the WCS-specific hypofrontality among the schizophrenic patients.

In a single-case study of a rapid-cycling patient, Mukherjee and colleagues (1984) noted that the manic state was accompanied by a global increase in blood flow compared with the euthymic or depressed state, with most of the increase in the frontal lobes. However, two cross-sectional studies of mania have not found any differences from controls (Sackeim et al., 1987; Silfverskiöld and Risberg, 1989).

Single Photon, Emission-Computed Tomography

SPECT is another technique that is being applied to the study of regional cerebral blood flow. It measures photons emitted by relatively long half-life isotopes of heavy elements, such as xenon-127, thallium-201, and iodine-123. Using SPECT in a comparison of a mixed group of affectively disordered patients with controls, Rush and co-workers (1982) reported that cortical blood flow was decreased during depression but was higher than normal in mania or mixed states. Unfortunately, statistical comparisons were not given. In the newest version of SPECT, an array of detectors continuously rotate in multiple planes, a technique that produces three-dimensional pictures of blood flow that include deep structures. Using thallium-201 diethyldithiocarbamate as tracer, Van Royen and co-workers (1987) found a higher ratio of nondominant/dominant frontal cortex activity in three patients with major depression than in three with hypomania and in controls. As this technology becomes more widely applied, new insights regarding rCBF in manic-depressive illness should emerge, but at this writing, no definitive conclusions are possible, either for SPECT studies or for the CBF studies using xenon-133.

Positron Emission Tomography

PET is essentially a three-dimensional quantitative tracer technique, unique in its capacity to visualize tracers because of the extreme sensitivity, high spatial resolution, and uniform quantification that can be obtained with the use of positron-emitting radionuclides as tags. Such radionuclides decay by emitting a positron as a proton is converted to a neutron. The emitted positron travels only a few millimeters before it meets its antiparticle, the electron. This collision results in the annihilation of both particles and the production of two 511-kiloelectron-volt photons emitted at a 180-degree angle from one another. A scanner makes use of the simultaneous detection of photons in opposite direction to achieve a quantitative imaging power possible only with PET. The PET image represents the spatial location of the isotope as reconstructed by computer from measurements by a ring (or several rings) of photon detectors positioned around the head in a way analogous to the generation of a CT scan. Positron-emitting isotopes, in general, have short half-lives and high specific activities. This allows for maximum resolution and specificity for the tracers with a minimum of ionizing radiation exposure for the subject.

The application of PET to the study of brain metabolism in three dimensions was made possible by Louis Sokoloff of NIMH, who pioneered the development of the 2-deoxyglucose (2-DG) method. Since glucose is the primary (and usually the only) energy source for cerebral metabolism, its use is indeed crucial to cerebral activity and function. Sokoloff took advantage of the fact that the glucose analog, 2-DG, is transported into the brain and its cells and is metabolized through the first intracellular step in a fashion identical to that for glucose itself, but then is metabolized no further. Thus, 2-DG serves as a marker for both glucose uptake and metabolism. Sokoloff has shown, on both theoretical and experimental grounds, that normally the uptake and metabolism of glucose by brain cells provide the best reflection of brain activity under the widest range of conditions. The 2-DG technique is adapted for use in PET procedures by using ^{18}F-labeled 2-DG. Clinical applications have been advanced by the contributions of many others, especially David Kuhl, Michael Phelps, Michel Ter-Pogossian, and Martin Reivich.

Cortical Metabolism. The application of PET to the study of psychiatric disorders is in its infancy, and important methodological problems remain (Cohen and Nordahl, 1988). Until very recently, PET studies employed scanners with limited resolution, that is, above 1 cm. As has been the case with CT, most of the early PET studies in psychiatry focused on schizophrenia. Some found a relative hypofrontality but others have not. As defined initially by Ingvar and Franzén (1974) in their studies of cerebral blood flow under resting conditions, normally the frontal cortex (i.e., the association areas) shows greater functional activity than the more posterior areas involved in the initial input and processing of sensory stimuli. Thus, relative hypofrontality reflects an attenuation of the normal frontal dominance.

Three groups have published PET studies of glucose metabolism in major affective illness—one initially at NIMH and later at the University of California at Irvine (Buchsbaum et al., 1984, 1986), another at the University of California at Los Angeles (Phelps et al., 1983, 1984; Baxter et al., 1985, 1989; Schwartz et al., 1987), and a third at NIMH (Cohen et al., 1989). Each group studied patients when they were moderately depressed (or manic) and were off medications for at least 1 week (average of 8 weeks for UCLA patients and 5 weeks for Buchsbaum's patients). In the initial UCLA studies (Baxter et al., 1985, 1987), the glucose metabolic rate for the whole cortex was significantly lower in bipolar depressed patients than in unipolar depressed patients, manic patients, or normal controls. Even though the number of subjects in the various groups was relatively small, there was almost no overlap in the data. Thus, each of the subgroup differences was highly significant. The global hypometabolism associated with bipolar depression was state dependent, since in each of the six bipolar depressed patients studied longitudinally, normalization (i.e., an increase) of the metabolic rate occurred during mania or euthymia. For example, in the two rapid-cycling patients studied longitudinally, global metabolic rates for the "hypomanic day" were 38 and 34 percent higher than for the "depressed day." Regional analysis indicated that metabolism in the frontal lobe of the bipolar depressed patients was 40 percent below normal, and occipital lobe metabolism was 29 percent below normal. These differences, although not statistically significant, suggest that a modest degree of relative hypofrontality may be associated with bipolar (but not unipolar) depression.

Bipolar patients also showed more differences in laterality. Although all groups showed a greater reduction of metabolic activity in the left frontal lobe than in the right, this difference was largest among the bipolar depressed patients. Moreover, for the entire hemisphere, the bipolar depressed patients showed a slightly (but significantly) larger reduction on the left. In an extension of this study, Baxter's group (1987, 1989)

identified an area on the left dorsal anterolateral prefrontal cortex in which reduced metabolism[23] was common to both depressive subgroups and positively correlated with global depression ratings. This finding was state dependent, since metabolism was higher in mania than in bipolar depression (Figure 18-1, opposite page 459). It would appear for the UCLA data that the most anatomically localizable abnormality (left dorsal anterolateral prefrontal cortex) is similar in all of the depressive subgroups, whereas the more global abnormalities in metabolism (whole cortex, frontal lobes, left frontal lobe) are more specific to the bipolar subgroup. If this is so, it raises interesting questions.

In the NIMH/UC-Irvine studies (Buchsbaum et al., 1984, 1986), patients (predominantly bipolar) received mildly painful somatosensory stimulation to the right forearm, a procedure chosen because it increases blood flow to the frontal cortex (Ingvar, 1975). However, such somatosensory stimulation confounds a straightforward interpretation of the PET results or meaningful comparisons with studies using resting conditions, since manic-depressive patients have been shown to have less pain sensitivity than normal controls. Three slices were chosen for analysis of anterior–posterior gradients and cortical lateralization (Buchsbaum et al., 1984). Overall glucose metabolic rate in the slices was 28 percent higher in the bipolar depressed patients than in the controls, and the overall rate in the depressed patients showed a significant positive correlation with severity of depression and psychosis ratings. In agreement with the initial UCLA data, the frontal/occipital ratio was significantly lower for the bipolar depressed patients. This difference reflects frontal decreases more than it does occipital increases. By comparison, the small sample of four unipolar depressed patients showed relative hyperfrontality. This bipolar–unipolar difference was highly significant. With regard to laterality, the bipolar depressed patients showed a loss of the normal left predominance in the most frontal section and a "somewhat greater than normal" asymmetry (right greater than left) in the posterior section.

In a recent report from NIMH (Cohen et al., 1989), bipolar and schizophrenic patients were studied while performing an auditory discrimination task. Both groups showed reduced metabolic rates in the middle prefrontal cortex. The normal controls had prefrontal metabolic rates that were positively correlated with performance on the discrimination task. Neither patient group showed such correlations. Cohen and colleagues suggest that both disorders may share a common pathophysiology of impaired sustained attention.

Subcortical Metabolism. Although overall glucose metabolism rates for the UCLA unipolar depressed patients were not different from those of normal controls, they did show markedly lower metabolism in the head of the caudate relative to the hemisphere on the same side, a ratio that normalized with recovery. The authors speculate that this might reflect a relative hypodopaminergic state in unipolar depression. The bipolar depressed patients had a normal caudate/hemisphere ratio (albeit with high variance), whereas the manic and mixed-state patients actually tended toward a lower ratio, one closer to that of the unipolar group (Baxter et al., 1985). These data are interesting in light of inferences from the pharmacological data reviewed in Chapter 17, specifically that decreased dopamine function may be more characteristic of bipolar than of unipolar depression. As interpreted by Baxter and colleagues (1985), these preliminary caudate metabolic data would not support that differential. Schwartz and co-workers (1987) have speculated that the metabolic differences between bipolar and unipolar patients may be related to differences in depressive symptoms, such as agitation and retardation. Whatever their ultimate meaning for pathophysiology, the bipolar–unipolar differences reported by the UCLA group are of interest and require replication and extension.

In line with the work of Baxter and colleagues at UCLA (Baxter et al., 1985; Schwartz et al., 1987), Buchsbaum and co-workers (1986) used the ratio of metabolic activity in the basal ganglia to that in the whole slice as a measure of subcortical metabolic activity. In Buchsbaum's study, both bipolar and unipolar depressed patients had significantly decreased caudate metabolism as measured by this ratio, and the relative reduction was more pronounced on the right side, especially in the bipolar patients. (Recall that the UCLA

investigators had found reduced caudate metabolism only in the unipolar patients.)

Overall, the differences among these studies point to the need for standardization of the PET procedures, especially with regard to the presence or absence of sensory stimulation. It would appear that differential patterns (i.e., ratios) of metabolic activity may be more informative than absolute values from individual regions.

Another PET study from the NIMH group (Post et al., 1987a) focused on glucose metabolism in the temporal lobes to evaluate the hypothesis that temporal subictal events may be involved in the pathophysiology of manic-depressive illness. Thirteen patients with DSM-III major affective illness, medication-free for at least 2 weeks, were studied with a somatosensory stimulation procedure during clinical states ranging from "moderately severe depression" to "mild hypomania." Relative metabolic rates in the temporal lobes of the affectively ill patients were not significantly different from those of controls. In fact, temporal lobe metabolic activity in the depressed group was actually lower than in controls, especially on the right side. However, these results are inconclusive, since PET studies of epileptic patients with complex partial seizures show the expected increase in temporal lobe metabolism during the seizures but a decrease in metabolism in postictal or interictal periods. This reduced interictal metabolism is of interest, since in patients with complex partial seizures, the interictal period is associated with a moderately high incidence of depression (Robertson and Trimble, 1983; R.M. Post et al., 1986b).

A new and exciting application of PET is the in vivo quantification of neuroreceptors using isotope-labeled ligands (Wagner et al., 1983; Wong et al., 1987; Cohen and Nordahl, 1988). In a preliminary study, Wong and colleagues (1987) found that some bipolar patients show large increases in the apparent density of dopamine receptors in the caudate, as reflected in the caudate/cerebellum ratio. Although the meaning of such studies is still unclear (since schizophrenic patients show similar increases), the approach is promising.

[11]C-glucose, which labels the amino acid pools, was used in a small PET study, and the results indicated globally increased labeling in

manic patients and decreased labeling in unipolar depressed patients, both compared with normal controls (Kishimoto et al., 1987). The pattern of changes was different from that of schizophrenic patients.

Critical Evaluation

The literature bearing directly and indirectly on the neuroanatomy of manic-depressive illness is more extensive than we had initially expected, but it is still relatively unsystematic. All too often, the affective patients are of secondary interest (as controls for a schizophrenia study), and there is sometimes disturbing variability from one control group to another. Another limitation is that methods are generally still evolving and, therefore, not standardized. Finally, few investigators have attended to the bipolar–unipolar distinction. Trends can nevertheless be discerned that could help guide future imaging research.

No clear findings emerge from the few postmortem studies of primary manic-depressive illness. A slight majority of the neuropathological studies of secondary affective syndromes suggests an association between depression and left frontotemporal or right parietooccipital lesions, and secondary manic-like symptoms are more frequently seen following right frontotemporal or left parietooccipital lesions. For understanding primary manic-depressive illness, the more uncommon secondary manic syndromes may be more useful than the secondary depressions, since the former are generally associated with a prior history of affective illness, whereas the latter are not (Starkstein and Robinson, 1989).

In imaging studies of manic-depressive illness, a focus on specific regions and the ratios between them would be worthwhile. One approach is to focus on quadrants. Consistent with such an approach are the findings of Robinson and colleagues (1985, 1986) on poststroke mania/hypomania, in which patients with nondominant-sided anterior strokes were especially vulnerable to these reactions, whereas those with dominant anterior or nondominant posterior strokes were prone to secondary depressions.

Consideration of brain quadrants also could clarify some discrepancies in the laterality literature. For example, findings implicating left hemispheric dysfunction in depression and right

hemispheric dysfunction in mania may have predominantly reflected characteristics of the frontotemporal regions. Thus, when depression follows amytal injection in the left carotid artery and mania follows right-sided injections, it is worth noting that the more anterior areas of the brain are being affected, since they are the areas supplied by the carotid arteries. If differential quadrant patterns for mania and bipolar depression do indeed emerge, they could provide a useful basis for enlarging our understanding of pathophysiology. Sackeim and co-workers (1982) have proposed that quadrant differences reflect inhibitory effects of one brain region on another. Of interest here are the reports of gradients and asymmetries in the distribution of neurotransmitters in the brain. Thus, in rhesus monkey brains, dopamine concentrations in the neocortex diminish from front to rear (R.M. Brown et al., 1979), left–right asymmetries have been noted for serotonin in rat brains (Mandell and Knapp, 1979), and in humans, norepinephrine shows opposite bilateral asymmetries in different regions of the thalamus (Oke et al., 1978). Dysfunction in one major area might result in a loss of the normal relationships between neurotransmitter concentrations reflected in anterior–posterior or left–right gradients. Such instances could be expressed in depression or mania.

What might be inferred about lateralization of mood function from the study of patients with unilateral lesions? The traditional view is that a cortical lesion would diminish normal cortical inhibition of lower centers in the same hemisphere, increasing the relevant behavior or state mediated by that same hemisphere. This concept provides one way to reconcile the lesion data (pointing to left-frontal dysfunction in depression) with the various lateralized physiological and performance measures (pointing to right-sided dysfunction in depression and mania), although just how this reconciliation is formulated can depend on whether one subscribes to an ipsilateral or contralateral release hypothesis. Indeed, virtually the same evidence has been marshaled to argue that depressive symptoms are associated with a right (Coffey, 1987) or a left hemisphere defect (Robinson, 1983).

Baxter and associates (1987), integrating PET and rCBF studies of primary manic-depressive illness with others' observations of secondary depression,[24] argue that the left (i.e., dominant) prefrontal cortex is a key locus for cerebral activity mediating the expression of depression. The prefrontal cortex is complex, interconnecting extensively within the ipsilateral cortex. Baxter's PET data suggest that in bipolar and unipolar depression, there is both prefrontal involvement (perhaps nonspecifically associated with depressive symptoms) and a more global left-sided dysfunction, which, ironically, may be more specific to bipolar depression. We concur with Baxter in cautioning the reader not to infer causal relationships from any of these findings. Thus, although these early PET data and some of the blood flow data point to left-sided dysfunction in bipolar illness, neuropsychological tests, by and large, implicate the right. Whether these can be reconciled by positing contralateral release remains to be seen.

There is another factor to consider in attempting to reconcile the lesion and imaging data with the physiological and performance measures (the former pointing to left and the latter to right anterior dysfunction). The lesion and imaging approaches study the brain in its resting state, whereas the physiological and neuropsychological approaches measure the active functioning of the brain in response to a task demand. What is needed are imaging studies that integrate a variety of performance measures.

Since dysfunction in the left prefrontal area in schizophrenia also has been the focus of considerable interest, the question of specificity remains open. We find it difficult to conceptualize a core of clinical manifestations common to major depression and to schizophrenia that could correspond to a common CNS localization of dysfunction. However, the concept of biological changes common to psychotic illness has been proposed.

Here we should return to Wexler's caution (1986) regarding the importance of focusing on integrative systems that are defined both functionally and anatomically. Although particular cells, cell clusters, or brain regions do have specialized characteristics, behavior is not subserved by any one site. Instead, specific behaviors, according to Wexler,

. . . are represented by an integrated ensemble of such regions, as words are represented by composites of letters. Such a system is much more powerful and versatile than one in which specific behaviours are located in specific specialised regions, just as a phonetic alphabet in which a relatively small number of letters can be arranged in a large number of different words is more powerful and versatile than a pictographic language with the same number of characters, each representing a specific word. (p. 359)

One such integrative system is the isodendritic core of the brainstem (IDCB), a network of neurons containing dopamine, serotonin, norepinephrine, and acetylcholine. Jeste and associates (1988) proposed that the IDCB could link diverse areas of the brain, including the cortex, in the pathophysiology of manic-depressive illness.[25]

The literature reviewed here deals with relatively large regions of the brain, but it is possible (although unlikely) that manic-depressive illness involves neuropathology in a discrete area, even a small group of specific cells. Future postmortem studies will require both quantitative neuropathological and histochemical techniques, including computed neuronal imaging. The specific neurochemical information obtained from such studies can be used in conjunction with findings from in vivo brain-imaging techniques, such as PET, to map specific neurotransmitters and receptors. Such an integration will be necessary if we are to make meaningful progress in defining and understanding the neuropathology of manic-depressive illness.

We close this section by returning to the question of specificity. Some of the studies that included both manic-depressive and schizophrenic patients found no significant differences between the two groups. In part, this may be explained by type II errors (false negatives with small sample sizes) or by biased patient selection (e.g., over-inclusion of manic-depressive patients with a chronic course). Although nonspecific findings usually are dismissed, we should remain open to the possibility that, at some level, important and relevant pathophysiological mechanisms may be common to more than one major disorder. Freedman (1975) proposed that there may be "a general biology of psychosis that would cut across traditional diagnostic lines," (p. vii) a concept echoed by Meltzer (1982) and by Liberman (1982). However, this very broad concept has not yet been formulated into specific testable hypotheses. We return to this issue in Chapter 20.

ELECTROPHYSIOLOGY

Among the oldest approaches used in psychobiological research are clinical electrophysiological techniques. Changes in electrical activity in the nervous system have been measured both in the brain, through various forms of the electroencephalogram (EEG), and in the periphery (somatic and autonomic), through a variety of techniques, including measures of skin conductance, cardiovascular function, and salivary flow. This technology has been used to study basic sensory, cognitive, and affective functions and to provide both diagnostic and etiological clues to neuropathy and psychopathology. In theory, evaluating the functional state of the autonomic nervous system (such as the relative activity in sympathetic and parasympathetic subsystems) may provide electrophysiological markers for neurochemical process in the CNS. However, that promise remains unfulfilled. For a comprehensive review of this very large literature, see Zahn (1986).

Electrophysiological evidence about manic-depressive illness is fraught with problems. Usually, the illness has not been the focus of study, serving instead as a comparison for schizophrenia. Data that do exist are difficult to interpret, since they were usually not collected to test a specific hypothesis. The lack of a coherent theory about electrophysiological activity in manic-depressive illness further clouds the meaning of these data. As with other traditional approaches, most electrophysiological research predates the practice of distinguishing between bipolar and unipolar disorders. This literature suffers from other limitations as well. Techniques, terminology, and interpretations vary widely from laboratory to laboratory, possible medication effects often are not controlled, longitudinal data are rare, and trait characteristics are often confused with measurements that may merely reflect clinical state, which frequently is not noted. In addition, studies that do collect separate data from depressed and manic patients often do not indicate whether the depressed group consists purely of bipolar patients or a mix of bipolar and unipolar patients. By thus confounding polarity and state, these investigations have produced data that could reflect either differences between bipolar and unipolar disorder or between depression and mania. This literature is of interest, then, primarily for whetting rather than satisfying the appetite for electrophysiological information.

Somatic and Autonomic Measures

Electrodermal Activity

Among the oldest physiological studies in psychopathology are those that have attempted to measure overall emotional arousal by recording changes in the skin's resistance to an electrical current passing through it. Despite its longevity, however, the presumed relationship between electrodermal activity and emotional response (an assumption that provides the rationale for using the polygraph as a lie-detector test) remains controversial. Originally called the galvanic skin response (GSR), the measurement of electrodermal activity is now referred to by more precise terms. Skin conductance, the reciprocal of the skin's resistance to conducting electrical current, is given as the skin conductance response (SCR), which can be either spontaneous (SSCR) or elicited in response to a specific experimental stimulus. Animal studies indicate that SCR is decreased following lesions of the frontal lobes (Pribaum, 1969) or following specific lesions of the limbic system, such as amygdalectomy (Bagshaw et al., 1965). Studies of skin conductance were reviewed by Christie and associates (1980), who found that reductions in electrodermal activity were reported often in depressed patients (bipolar–unipolar differences not specified).

In a series of studies conducted after publication of that review, Iacono and collaborators (1983, 1984) were the first to separate bipolar and unipolar patients and, at the same time, consider whether measured changes reflected an underlying trait or the patients' clinical states. Baseline measures of skin conductance (skin conductance level or SCL) and response to tones were measured in three groups: 26 recurrent unipolar patients, 24 bipolar patients who were well at the time of the study but had a history of at least three prior episodes of depression, and 46 controls. On average, the patients with unipolar disorder showed the least skin conductance, the normal controls showed the most, and the bipolar patients were intermediate in response and varied among themselves more than did the unipolar patients.[26] However, there was no significant bipolar–unipolar difference, and nearly identical proportions of bipolar and unipolar patients showed no electrodermal response to a variety of stimuli.

In a subsequent study of 27 unipolar and 9 bipolar patients while they were depressed, this same group (Williams et al., 1985) noted no bipolar–unipolar differences in SCL or SCR, although the patients with psychomotor retardation had significantly lower SCLs than those with a normal psychomotor state. The association between retardation and lower SCL might explain why depressed bipolar patients, who show more psychomotor retardation than do unipolar patients (see Chapter 2), also have SCLs that are 15 percent lower in this study.[27] Of possible relevance to these bipolar findings is the study of unipolar patients by Ward and associates (1983), who found the lowest SCL levels among a subgroup with recurrent depression (which is perhaps genetically closer to bipolar depression)— levels that were significantly lower than those of patients with nonrecurrent unipolar depressions. Unfortunately, no control group was included in this study. (Electrodermal studies of laterality are discussed at the end of this section.)

SCR also has been used to study the habituation of the autonomic nervous system (ANS). Habituation refers to the decrease in ANS responsiveness to a particular stimulus that is presented constantly or repeatedly. In most studies of depressed patients, habituation of the SCR decreased as anxiety and agitation increased. In other words, as anxiety and agitation increased, responses to a repeated stimulus were less likely to decrease. Not surprisingly, reduced habituation was most pronounced in patients with high cortisol levels (Deakin, 1979) that were not suppressed by dexamethasone (Reus et al., 1985), findings that are associated with anxiety/agitation and may in addition reflect the negative effects of cortisol on selective attention processes (Kopell et al., 1970). The apparent link to hypothalamic–pituitary axis dysregulation (suggested by the relationship to cortisol levels and to dexamethasone responses) is consistent with the possibility that nonspecific factors, such as arousal, contribute to disturbed ANS habituation in manic-depressive illness.

To our knowledge, habituation has not been compared in bipolar vs unipolar patients or in depressed vs manic patients. But in an interesting study of a diagnostically mixed group of suicide attempters (the majority of whom had major depression), Edman and colleagues (1986) found a bimodal distribution in the habituation rate. Further, all of the violent attempters, as well as four who later completed suicide, were in the group that habituated quickly. Fast habituation probably reflects low anticipatory state anxiety (perhaps contributing to suicide risk in the presence of other factors) and also stable individual characteristics such as impulsivity (Schalling et al., 1983). If the SCR reflects the initiation of central processing of a stimulus (Ohman, 1979), then rapid habituation might reflect a more cursory processing of new information, that is, less anticipation, more impulsivity (Edman et al., 1986).

Cardiovascular Measures

Cardiovascular measures assessed in the affective disorders include heart rate, systolic and diastolic blood pressure, and forearm blood flow. In none of the fairly sparse studies examining such measures in manic-depressive illness have bipolar or unipolar patients been reported separately. Even in the studies of major depression, the results are difficult to interpret because of the known effects of tricyclic antidepressants on measures of cardiovascular function. As with some of the skin conductance studies, the abnormalities that have been detected are difficult to interpret because the contribution of the depressive state per se cannot be teased apart from the effects of anxiety, agitation, retardation, and other symptoms. In general, anxiety and agitation have been associated with increased heart rate, blood pressure, and forearm blood flow, but the value of this knowledge for understanding bipolar illness is debatable (Zahn, 1986).

Other Measures

Salivary flow, taken as a reflection of activity of the parasympathetic nervous system, is generally lower in depressed patients than in controls, especially among retarded depressed patients (Noble and Lader, 1971). To our knowledge, no systematic bipolar–unipolar comparisons have been reported, although in 1939, Strongin and Hinsie used salivary flow to discriminate "manic-depressive patients" in the depressed phase, who salivated less than "other depressed patients." Among bipolar patients, salivary flow has been found to be higher in the manic than in the depressive phase (Strongin and Hinsie, 1938).

Electromyography (EMG) also has been used as a measure in depressed patients.[28] Most studies have reported specific patterns of facial musculature activity as well as an overall increase in resting activity compared with controls. The degree of activity is positively correlated with severity of the depression (Greden et al., 1986) and may predict treatment outcome (Carney et al., 1981). No bipolar–unipolar comparisons have been made, however.

Very early in this century (see, e.g., Diefendorf and Dodge, 1908), extensive and sophisticated quantitative studies of eye movements were conducted in hospitalized psychiatric patients, and some differences were noted between mania and depression, on the one hand, and schizophrenia on the other. The study of smooth pursuit eye movements (SPEM), which has become considerably more technologically sophisticated since then, has focused primarily on schizophrenic patients, who show poor tracking both when ill and when in remission. Similar deficits have been found in first-degree relatives of schizophrenic patients, an observation that has led some investigators to suggest that SPEM may be a genetic marker for schizophrenia (Holzman et al., 1977). The neurobiological processes involved in SPEM have not yet been elucidated.

Some earlier studies of depressed patients reported no SPEM abnormalities (Couch and Fox, 1934), although more recent studies found abnormalities in depression and mania that were similar to those in schizophrenia (Shagass et al., 1974; Lipton et al., 1980; Levin et al., 1981). None of these studies separated bipolar and unipolar patients or distinguished trait from state. In a SPEM study of 25 bipolar and 24 unipolar patients in the well state, Iacono and colleagues (1982) found no overall significant difference from controls, although error rates in the bipolar group were closer to those of the schizophrenic group than to the control group. Among the bipolar patients, the tracking errors were greater for patients receiving lithium and for those with a higher frequency of prior episodes. As far as we know, pupillography (the recording of pupillary actions) and eye blink rates, although relatively well studied in schizo-

phrenia, have not been pursued in the study of affective disorders.

Endicott (1989) has noted some interesting psychophysiological correlates of bipolarity. He studied 400 outpatients with major affective disorders, grouping them according to their lifetime intensity, frequency and duration of high energy–positive mood states. Approximately half the sample met RDC criteria for bipolar-II disorder (n = 138) or bipolar-I disorder (n = 49). Ratings of bipolarity showed a significant positive correlation with a cluster of disturbances, including classic migraine headache,[29] the peripheral vascular disturbance of Raynaud's disease, enuresis, vague episodic phenomena similar to migraine prodromata, fingernail biting, and learning disorders. Interestingly, most of the psychophysiological conditions showed their highest incidence in the bipolar-II groups, a finding that is not consistent with a straightforward continuum for unipolar disorder through bipolar-II disorder to bipolar-I disorder. Aside from the bipolar-I patients, a continuum model appears to fit the data. Of relevance to our discussion of the fundamental stability dimension in Chapter 20, Endicott interprets his data as reflecting the relative balance of regulation and dysregulation. These interesting concepts should be further operationalized. Comprehensive reviews of somatic and autonomic measures in manic-depressive illness can be found in Lader (1975) and in Zahn (1986).

Central Measures

In recent years, psychophysiological study of mental disorders has shifted from measuring peripheral autonomic activity to measuring brain activity (L.C. Johnson, 1974).

Resting EEG

As Perris and co-workers observed (1978), the clinical electroencephalograph has contributed disappointingly little to the understanding of nonorganic mental disorders despite its origins in a psychiatric institute. The literature on EEG studies of affective illness is quite variable and difficult to synthesize because of the variety of diagnostic terms and EEG techniques[30] used and the frequent failure to account for age differences, medication artifacts, or potential contributions of associated neurological conditions. Much of the EEG literature concerning depression suggests that changes correlate with the relative weighting of individual symptom clusters, such as anxiety, depression, agitation, or retardation, rather than with the diagnosis or diagnostic subgroups per se. Well-replicated findings are, unfortunately, not the rule.

Some studies have reported that manic-depressive patients differ from controls in the overall frequency of EEG abnormalities. Abrams and Taylor (1979) reported that, among a large number of patients with schizophrenia and manic-depressive illness (including bipolar and unipolar), the rate of abnormalities was lowest in depression (6.5 percent), intermediate in mania (16.8 percent), and highest in schizophrenia (25.9 percent). The differing EEG abnormality rates in mania and depression are difficult to interpret, since the bipolar and unipolar data are not reported separately. Perris (1966d) examined the EEGs of 109 patients with recurrent affective illness (39 bipolar and 70 unipolar) and noted "slight nonspecific abnormalities" in 43 percent but found no clear bipolar–unipolar differences.[31] Others have noted that the alpha frequency is higher in mania than in depression (Davis, 1941; Hurst et al., 1954). Manic patients also have been reported to have a higher incidence of paroxysmal activity (Chabanier et al., 1964) and of the mitten pattern, a slow-wave-and-spike pattern that occurs only in sleep. These findings may reflect disturbed vigilance in mania and may underlie the delirious features of severe mania (Van Sweden, 1986).

In his original 1966 study, Perris reported a bipolar–unipolar difference in the EEG response to activation by photic stimulation. The bipolar response suggested a slower neuronal recovery time. This increased activation by repetitive photic stimuli may be analogous to kindling. In light of the importance of the kindling hypothesis of manic-depressive illness (see Chapter 15), this approach should be pursued further, especially in studies of rapid-cycling patients.

The relationship between temporal lobe epilepsy (psychomotor seizures, complex partial seizures) and manic-depressive illness is discussed in Chapters 5, 16, and 20. Given the symptom overlap among some forms of bipolar illness (perhaps especially rapid cycling) and these temporal lobe disorders, some of the discrepancies in the EEG literature may result from the inclusion of some patients with temporal lobe disorders in bipolar samples. Alternatively, findings of temporal lobe EEG abnormalities could reflect the actual pathophysiology of at least some forms of manic-depressive illness. For example, Levy and colleagues (1988) and Drake (1988) report temporal lobe paroxysms among rapid-cycling bipolar patients.

Abnormal EEGs in bipolar patients are significantly related to a negative family history of manic-depressive illness (Dalén, 1965; Kadrmas and Winokur, 1979; Cook et al., 1986). This association suggests that at least some of the abnormalities may occur in patients who have organic conditions with secondary mood disturbances. Small and colleagues (1975), however, in reporting that 43 percent of their sample of bipolar patients had "transient small sharp spikes," noted that among the women, these EEG features were significantly associated with a history of mental illness on the maternal side. Unfortunately, most of the remaining EEG literature does not provide data on family history. Knott and co-workers (1985) examined a group of identical twins, one of whom had been diagnosed with bipolar illness. Individuals with bipolar illness (who were well and for the most part off medication at the time of the study) had significantly more alpha-frequencies than their well co-twins. This finding suggested to the authors that "CNS overarousal" may be a trait characteristic of bipolar illness.

Only a few scattered studies have attempted to correlate EEG changes with biological measures. For example, Miller and Nelson (1987) found that among inpatients with major depression, those with EEG abnormalities had a significantly higher incidence of nonsuppression on the dexamethasone suppression test (DST) compared with those without EEG abnormalities (61 percent vs 19 percent). The authors speculate that both the EEG changes and the DST abnormality could reflect cortical dysfunction (resulting in a disinhibited hypothalamic–pituitary–adrenal axis).

Event-Related Potentials

Event-related potentials, or evoked responses, are changes in the electrical activity of the CNS that occur in response to sensory stimulation, in association with psychological processes, or in preparation for motor activity. Since these individual events are usually lost in the background variation of the EEG, their study depends on computer-assisted, signal-averaging techniques. Early evoked-potential events (less than 100 msec) probably reflect transmission of information, and later events reflect information processing and level of attention.

Unlike the neurophysiological study of the periphery, in which the principal theoretical focus has been on schizophrenia, evoked potentials in the affective disorders have received considerable attention. Because these studies are relatively recent, they are more likely to employ modern diagnostic criteria and to distinguish between bipolar and unipolar patients. Nevertheless, like the studies using peripheral electrophysiology and EEG measures, attention to age and sex differences and to clinical state and treatment effects is all too often lacking. Some studies, while attending to differences in diagnostic subgroups, have failed to consider the contribution of individual symptoms to the variance in evoked-response measures. Interpretation of this rather large literature is also hampered by important differences in experimental approach, such as the sensory modality being examined (i.e., visual, auditory, or somatosensory evoked responses), the particular component of the evoked response being studied, and the location of the recording leads. Evoked responses show considerable interindividual variability, principally of genetic origin. This variability, combined with the contributions of nonspecific noise, leaves relatively little potential for detecting differences specific to a particular diagnostic group.

One kind of evoked response, the EEG alpha-blocking response to visual stimuli, generally has been reported as prolonged in depression, perhaps suggesting increased activity in the reticular systems. The degree of alpha-blocking correlates positively with the degree of psychomotor retardation.

Studies of affective illness have variously examined the amplitude of the various components of the evoked response, the latency between stimulation and response, the relationship between stimulus intensity and response amplitude (in augmenters the amplitude of the response increases with increasing stimulus intensity, whereas in reducers, the response amplitude increases less or decreases), the topographical or

regional distribution of the evoked responses, the evoked-response variability from one averaging sequence to another, and the recovery functions using paired stimuli.[32]

The extensive literature on evoked responses in affective disorders has been reviewed by Shagass (1975), Perris (1980, 1988b), and Zahn (1986). Most studies focus on the amplitudes or the latencies of evoked-response components but fail to replicate the same conditions with respect to sensory modality, component examined, topographical location, or the nature of the requirements of attention and the task. Indeed, using multiple modalities in the same subjects, Shagass and colleagues (1980) showed that the degree of similarity between the evoked-response amplitude in psychotically depressed patients and in controls depended on the choice of sensory modality and electrode location. In general, among the more severely depressed patients (often referred to as "psychotically depressed"), the earlier peaks (both auditory and somatosensory) tend to be larger than in controls, and the later peaks are smaller (Shagass et al., 1980; Lader 1975). In the study (referred to earlier) of identical twins discordant for bipolar illness, Knott and colleagues (1985) found that, compared with the normal twin, the co-twin with the illness (albeit in the well state) showed a significantly larger peak in the auditory evoked response, a finding interpreted as consistent with CNS overarousal as a trait marker, although presumably not a genetic marker.

Evoked-response recovery is a measure of the effect of an initial stimulus on the response to a second, slightly delayed, identical stimulus. In some parts of the CNS, the operation of inhibitory feedback systems set in motion by the first stimulus is normally reflected in a slightly reduced response to the second stimulus. Acutely manic patients show decreased inhibition similar to that seen in schizophrenia (a deficit in sensory gating), but in manic patients (unlike schizophrenics), this function apparently returns to normal during euthymic periods (Franks et al., 1983).

Like most of the clinical neurophysiology of affective illness, the classic evoked-response literature is largely atheoretical. Thus in the early 1970s, the introduction of the concept of evoked-response augmenters and reducers was a breath of fresh air in that it suggested a way to distinguish bipolar and unipolar patients in a theoretically interesting way. In the initial series of studies by Buchsbaum and colleagues at NIMH (Borge et al., 1971; Buchsbaum et al., 1971, 1973), bipolar patients showed increased response amplitude to increasing intensities of auditory stimulation (i.e., they were augmenters), whereas unipolar patients had a more modest response increase or a decreased response (i.e., they were reducers). Of special interest was the finding among the bipolar patients that these response patterns appeared to be relatively independent of illness state. Thus, the investigators initially thought that evoked-response augmentation might reflect part of a trait marker for bipolar illness. The fact that administering lithium to bipolar patients appeared to decrease the tendency toward augmentation (Borge et al., 1971) reinforced the belief that this measure might convey something specific about the illness. Further, Buchsbaum hypothesized that evoked-response reduction reflected an adaptive protective mechanism for dealing with sensory overload. Although some replicated the work of Buchsbaum's group (Baron et al., 1975), others did not (Von Knorring et al., 1974; Von Knorring, 1978).[33]

Of possible relevance to the interpretation of the somatosensory evoked response literature are findings of altered subjective pain sensitivity. In general, hospitalized depressed patients have been found to be *less* sensitive to experimentally induced pain (see, e.g., Von Knorring and Johansson, 1979) in spite of their tendency to report a higher than normal level of somatic discomfort. Davis and Buchsbaum (1981) found some bipolar–unipolar differences among the depressed patients, depending on the pain measure used. The lowest pain sensitivity was found in the manic patients. In general, the somatosensory evoked responses are consistent with the subjective responses: lower than normal amplitude/intensity slopes in the depressed patients (reducers) and lower still in the manic patients.[34]

Following these initial studies in affective disorders, extensive methodological research (reviewed by Prescott et al., 1984) raised questions about the technique. The issue focuses on the infrequent control for eye movement artifacts in studies of visual evoked responses and on the low correlation between different methods of assess-ing augmentation and reduction (e.g., when different components of the evoked response are measured, even using the same sensory modality, or when different regions are used for recording the response). This lack of generalizability not only complicates the theoretical meaning of particular results but also renders replication difficult.

Another event-related potential of sorts is contingent negative variation (CNV), defined as slow negative potentials (expectancy waves) that develop mainly over the frontal regions in anticipation of either motor or mental performance during the time between a preparatory stimulus and the signal to respond (Black and Walter, 1965; Perris, 1980). CNV, although reflecting genuine cerebral phenomena, is quite vulnerable to artifacts. Small and colleagues (1971b), reporting that CNV amplitude was lower in patients with affective disorder than in controls, noted that this amplitude was further reduced by lithium treatment. The difference between depressed patients and controls was later replicated by Timsit-Berthier and associates (1984). In one longitudinal study of five bipolar patients during both manic and depressive phases, Rizzo and colleagues (1979) noted a modest voltage decrease in the depressive phase and a more conspicuous decrease in the manic phase. They interpreted this finding as reflecting a decrease in attention. Ansseau and colleagues (1985b) showed that among endogenously depressed patients there is a significant inverse correlation between CNV and rapid eye movement (REM) latency (the time between sleep onset and the first REM episode). They suggested that both phenomena may depend on cholinergic mechanisms. (For a discussion of REM latency, see Chapter 19.)

Evoked potentials have been examined during task performance in studies of such mental processes as attention. For example, Kaskey and co-workers (1980) found that in manic-depressive patients, lithium treatment increased the late positive component evoked by a continuous performance task and improved task performance. The authors concluded that the attention-enhancing effects of lithium made patients less likely to respond to random stimuli, and thus their performance was enhanced. (Other performance studies are reviewed in Chapter 11.)

Electrooculography and Electroretinography

Electrooculography (EOG) is, in a sense, a variation of the electrodermal studies reviewed earlier. Eye potentials (measured from the eyeball during a shift from darkness to bright light) are thought to reflect alterations in the functional state of pigment epithelium in the retina. Dopamine, which is abundant in the retina, is thought to be involved in the process of light and dark adaptation (Makman et al., 1975; Bitensky et al., 1975), and, as discussed in Chapters 16 and 17, this catecholamine transmitter may be involved in the pathophysiology of manic-depressive illness. Economou and Stefanis (1979) reported that EOG ratios (light/dark) were lower than normal in retarded bipolar depressed patients and higher than normal in manic patients. The EOG changes were observed only when patients were ill; they became normal after recovery. These investigators had previously reported low EOG ratios in patients with parkinsonism (associated with a dopamine deficiency), which became normal after treatment with the dopamine precursor, L-dopa (Economou and Stefanis, 1978). Hanna and colleagues (1986) showed electrooculographic changes in association with the switch process in a patient with 48-hour cycles of mania and depression. These changes may reflect alterations in dopaminergic tone.

Electroretinography (ERG), which assesses function of the neural retina, has not generally been applied to the study of manic-depressive illness. Steiner and colleagues (1988) found no ERG differences between controls and depressed patients hospitalized for ECT. However, following ECT-induced remission, the ERG response to light showed a significant decrease in amplitude and an increase in latency. As discussed in Chapters 19 and 20, the possibility that a treatment for depression might reduce light sensitivity is of interest, given that increased sensitivity to light has been reported in manic-depressive patients.

Electrophysiological Approaches to Laterality

The issue of laterality, introduced in the preceding section on anatomical studies, has been studied also electrophysiologically. Only a few studies of electrodermal activity have considered the question of lateralized dysfunction, and they are generally consistent with the neuropsychological studies in finding right-sided dysfunction. Thus, Gruzelier and Venables (1974) found skin conductance orienting response lower on the right than on the left among depressed patients, as did Myslobodsky and Horesh (1978) and Toone and associates (1981). These authors did not separate bipolar and unipolar illness. To our knowledge, there are no electrodermal laterality data available specifically for depressed bipolar patients, although among a group of college students with cyclothymia (or "subsyndromal bipolar disorder"), Lenhart and Katkin (1986) did find lower electrodermal activity in the right than in the left hand. Studying skin conductance response in *recovered* patients, Iacono and Tuason (1983) found no consistent bilateral asymmetries in a group of 50 depressed patients (24 bipolar and 26 unipolar) compared with controls.[35] More recently, Zahn and colleagues (1989) studied electrodermal activity in a group of 22 young adults at high risk for bipolar illness (each had a bipolar parent). They found that electrodermal activity elicited by mild stress (a reaction-time task and mental arithmetic) was significantly more lateralized to the left hand in the high-risk group than in a low-risk control group, a finding consistent with the laterality evidence in bipolar patients themselves.

The literature on EEG laterality, which is considerably more extensive and complex than that on the electrodermal response has been reviewed by Zahn (1986). Flor-Henry and colleagues (in Flor-Henry, 1983) examined a large number of EEG parameters, with subjects both at rest and under various forms of activation. One interesting finding from these complex studies was an abnormality in the EEG activity over the temporal lobe, as measured by power spectral analysis (Flor-Henry and Koles, 1984). This activity was greater in the nondominant (right) hemisphere in bipolar patients and in the dominant hemisphere in schizophrenic patients. It was symmetrical in normal subjects. According to the authors, bipolar depression involves a nondominant temporal lobe abnormality, whereas mania appears to affect both hemispheres.

D'Elia and Perris (1973) examined EEGs in 18 patients with psychotic depression (mainly recurrent unipolar) before and after treatment with medications. They noted that, following treatment, the variance of the EEG signal on the dominant side significantly decreased, whereas the nondominant hemisphere remained unchanged. Abrams and Taylor (1979) compared EEG abnormalities in the parietooccipital region on the nondominant side in a group of patients with affective disorders (101 manic, 31 depressed, type not stated) with those of schizophrenic patients. They found a higher frequency of such abnormalities in the affective groups than in the schizophrenic patients. The number of EEG abnormalities did not differ between the depressive and manic groups. Abrams and Taylor did not consider the issue of possible differences in specific types of abnormalities. As noted previously, in most of the cases of secondary mania and depression reviewed by Jeste and colleagues (1988), depressive symptoms were associated with left (i.e., dominant) frontotemporal and right parietooccipital lesions, and manic-like syndromes were associated with right frontotemporal lesions and left parietooccipital lesions. This observation, as well as others noted earlier in this chapter, suggests that the concept of laterality may need to be expanded to include the concept of anterior and posterior quadrants.

An extension of computer-assisted quantitative EEG strategies (neurometrics) involves the analysis of individual profiles of deviation from normal values measured over different brain regions (John et al., 1977, 1983). Using this technique, Prichep and colleagues (1986) compared 20 bipolar and 31 unipolar medication-free patients hospitalized for major depressive illness (diagnosed by RDC) with normal controls. A discriminate function classification was derived that correctly separated 83 percent of the depressed patients and 89 percent of the normal controls. In a replication using a separate sample, 85 percent of the unipolar and 87 percent of the bipolar patients were classified correctly (John et al., 1988).[36] The discriminating pattern reflected disturbed interhemispheric relationships as noted previously by Perris' group and others. Because the bipolar–unipolar differential was dependent on the multivariate combination of diffuse weak trends rather than on any individual measures, further independent replication of this study is especially important. Topographical approaches to brain electrical mapping may provide important new knowledge

if they can be integrated with the new generation of brain-imaging studies reviewed earlier in this chapter. In considering the many benefits of these techniques, however, it is important to emphasize, as Kahn and colleagues have (1988), that great care must be given to methodology.

Event-related potentials (evoked responses) also have been employed in laterality studies of affective illness. For bipolar manic-depressive illness, no clear right or left predominance can yet be stated (reviewed by Zahn, 1986). Evoked-response topography of depressed patients may also deviate in other respects, particularly in the greater amplitudes in the posterior regions, primarily among the somatosensory modalities (Shagass et al., 1980).

Critical Evaluation

Major methodological difficulties mar the literature on electrophysiology, both peripheral and central. Techniques vary considerably and modalities measured range widely, limiting attempts to integrate the findings. The frequent failure to account for sex and age effects, the inconsistency of diagnostic terms and criteria, and especially the lack of clarity about drug status and clinical state all reflect a literature dominated by older studies or studies in which manic-depressive patients were not the main focus. To these difficulties we could add the intrinsic problems associated with obtaining electrophysiological measurements in disturbed patients, particularly in the manic phase. Virtually all of the studies of peripheral measures fail to take the bipolar–unipolar distinction into account. In the more recent evoked-response literature, this distinction has been given considerable attention, in some cases at the expense of examining the contribution of symptoms or symptom clusters that cut across the bipolar–unipolar subgroups.

There are too few longitudinal studies or data on patients in the well state, particularly when they are not taking medications. Since state variables, such as anxiety and level of depressive symptoms, affect many of these measures, the fundamental question of specificity will remain unanswered until a sufficient number of well-state studies are performed. Given the scattered evidence of considerable genetically determined interindividual variability in some of these measures, large numbers of patients will need to be studied to avoid type II errors (false negatives) in studies of characteristics that are highly variable in the population. Any contributions of electrophysiology to the laterality literature depend primarily on the central measures, principally the EEG. Among bipolar patients, abnormalities on the right side are the ones most often cited.

IMMUNOLOGICAL AND VIRAL FACTORS

As is evident from the mortality data reviewed in Chapter 6, affective illness has long been associated with certain medical disorders, notably cardiovascular disease, some allergic disorders and cancers, and perhaps some infectious diseases. In the years before mania and depression could be treated effectively, the ravages of repeated episodes and the conditions of chronic hospitalization must have contributed to many of these associated illnesses. But even now, the links between manic-depressive illness and medical illness persist, although they are attenuated.

The relationship between endocrine abnormalities and affective states is covered in Chapter 17. This section pulls together a scattered, somewhat unsystematic, and often preliminary literature, very little of which focuses specifically on bipolar disorder. Our review highlights immune function and viral illnesses, two areas in which hypotheses have been developed.

Immune Function

In recent years, it has become increasingly clear that the CNS plays a subtle but important role in the regulation of immune function (Fauman, 1982; Besedovsky et al., 1983a; Stein et al., 1987). Pioneering work by Ader and Cohen (1975) demonstrated that immune responses could be behaviorally conditioned, and both afferent and efferent links between the CNS and the immune system have been demonstrated. We now know that lymphocytes and neurons share many of the same surface antigens (Pert et al., 1985; Ruff et al., 1989). Specific CNS lesions, particularly of the hypothalamus, can interfere with immune responses (Keller et al., 1980; Cross et al., 1980), and, conversely, activation of an immune response can be associated with brain neurotransmitter changes (Besedovsky et al., 1983b; Hall et al., 1985). The immunosuppressive effects of

stress are largely mediated through CNS mechanisms (S.E. Keller et al., 1981).

Immune responses involve the close linkage of cellular and humoral mechanisms, each mediated by its own type of lymphocyte. Cellular immunity is provided by T lymphocytes, whereas humoral immunity is provided by circulating antibodies formed from B lymphocytes.[37] For a brief review of immune mechanisms see Stein and colleagues (1987).

A literature is emerging on disturbances in immune function in patients with major depression, and most studies have found decrements using one or another standard measure. For example, the lymphocyte response to various mitogens is commonly used as a measure of general immune responsiveness. Kronfol and associates (1983) reported a substantial reduction of this in hospitalized depressed patients compared with other psychiatric patients and controls—a finding replicated by three groups of investigators (Schleifer et al., 1984, 1985; Linn et al., 1984; Van Dyke et al., 1984) but not by a fourth (Albrecht et al., 1985). The question of specificity is complex. Schleifer and associates (1985) found that the differences in mitogen response among depressed patients were not related to sex or to hospitalization but were related to severity of depression and to age. On the other hand, Senger and associates (1982) found no differences in similar measures between recovered depressed patients and normal subjects. Kronfol and House (1988) reported impairments of cellular immunity in a small group of manic patients.[38]

Levels of circulating immunoglobulins have been reported to be lower in patients with major depressive illness than in controls (DeLisi et al., 1984; Wood et al., 1986), but this decrease may be confined to the unipolar group (Wood et al., 1986). These authors also noted lower than normal immunoglobulins in a group of recovered patients maintained on lithium (predominantly recurrent unipolar illness).

Some depressed patients are reported to have decreased numbers of circulating lymphocytes (see, e.g., Kronfol et al., 1984) and the extent of decrease correlates with depression ratings (Darko et al., 1989). This decrease, too, may be greater in unipolar than in bipolar depressed patients (Murphy et al., 1987)—a finding consistent with decreased immune response, but not invariably linked to it. Elevated neutrophil counts have also been noted in patients with major depression (Kronfol et al., 1984; Darko et al., 1989) and with mania (Kronfol et al., 1986), but at this writing, these observations have not yet been replicated independently.

Prostaglandin E_2 (PGE_2), which is known to be involved in immune regulation (Goodwin and Webb, 1980), has been found to be elevated among patients with major depression,[39] a finding which could be linked to deficient immune function.

Another aspect of immune regulation involves the hypothalamic–pituitary–adrenal axis. Indeed, the known tendency for some forms of depressive illness to be associated with hypercortisolemia has been offered as an explanation for the observed alterations in immune response. Although the relationship between adrenal cortical function and immune state has not been studied extensively in depressed patients, there is reason to believe that immune changes cannot be explained entirely on this basis (Zacharski et al., 1967).

The possibility that certain affective disorders might be associated with an abnormally increased immune response also has been raised, that is, manic-depressive illness might involve autoimmune phenomena. Increased antinuclear antibodies (which may reflect an autoimmune phenomenon) have been found in depressed patients by some but not all investigators (reviewed by Legros et al., 1985), and the possible contribution of medications has not been determined. Multiple sclerosis is a remitting CNS disorder that is probably autoimmune in nature (Antel et al., 1978; Dick and Gay, 1988). There is now good reason to conclude that the coexistence of MS and bipolar illness frequently noted in case reports cannot be explained by chance alone. Joffe and colleagues (1987b) found that 13 percent of their MS patients met strict RDC criteria for bipolar disorder, more than 10 times the chance expectation. Whether the affective disorder is simply secondary to the neurological disease or the two illnesses share some common pathophysiological mechanism(s) (perhaps involving autoimmune phenomena) is not yet known. It seems unlikely, however, that the bipolar illness reported by Joffe's group was merely secondary since there was no association between the degree of MS-induced functional impairment and the presence of bipolar disorder. Using an epidemiological approach, Schiffer and colleagues (1986) found the MS–bipolar association to be nonrandom and possibly linked genetically (Schiffer et al., 1988). However, in a formal family history study of the first-degree relatives of a large number of patients with MS, Joffe and colleagues (1987a) did not find an increased incidence of affective disorder.

Two studies have reported an increased association between major affective disorders and allergic phenomena such as asthma and hay fever (Baldwin, 1979; Nasr et al., 1981), and there are scattered case reports suggesting that lithium treatment improves these conditions. Indeed, at clinically meaningful levels, lithium has been noted to have a variety of effects on the immune system in both directions (perhaps more stimulatory than inhibitory), and there are anecdotal reports that patients on maintenance lithium often note reduced vulnerability to colds and flu-like symptoms (see Chapter 23). Horrobin and Lieb (1981) have hypothesized that lithium's biphasic effects on the immune system are analogous to its effects in manic-depressive illness (i.e., beneficial in both manic and depressive phases). They hypothesize that lithium modulates the formation of PGE_1 by limiting the mobilization of its precursor, dihomogamma-linolenic acid (DGLA), and prevents subsequent excess PGE formation and DGLA depletion. In their view, since PGE may be an important determinant in both mood regulation and immune regulation, lithium should be evaluated as a treatment for recurrent or relapsing disorders that involve immune dysfunction, such as MS.

Viral Factors

Linked closely to the question of dysfunction in the body's immune defenses in manic-depressive illness is the possibility of viral involvement. As reviewed by Crow (1984, 1987), the possibility that viruses may be involved in the pathophysiology of some major mental disorders was first noted over 60 years ago by Menninger (1926), who described the very close similarities between postinfluenza psychosis and typical schizophrenia. Several years later, Goodall (1932) formally outlined a viral hypothesis of schizophrenia.

The recent resurgence of interest in viral etiologies of mental disorders is probably related to three developments: (1) the discovery by Gajdusek (1977) and others of very slow-growing neurotropic viruses associated with degenerative diseases of the CNS, such as kuru, (2) the discovery of retroviruses that transcribe viral RNA into DNA, which can then become integrated into the genetic material of the host, substantially enlarging the possibilities of viral–gene interactions in illnesses with known genetic components, and (3) of special relevance to manic-depressive illness, the increasing recognition that many viruses with a predilection for the CNS are associated with relapsing illnesses with long latency periods and well intervals.

The finding that more schizophrenics are born during the winter and early spring than during other seasons (reviewed by Boyd et al., 1986) has been cited as being consistent with a viral etiology (Hare, 1983; Crow, 1984). Among manic patients, an equally pronounced predominance of winter births has been shown (Hare, 1983). However, the smaller number of studies renders the conclusion somewhat less firm for mania than it is for schizophrenia (Boyd et al., 1986). Hare (1983) argues that the clinical distinction between schizophrenia and mania did not emerge until the end of the last century and that the distinction only became possible because the affective disorders gradually evolved toward forms with less serious clinical manifestations.

Although most of the work on viral factors in mental disorders remains focused on schizophrenia, several reports dealing with affective illness have examined evidence relating to cytomegalovirus, herpes, Epstein-Barr, and Borna disease virus. It is important to note that the presence of antibodies constitutes the evidence of a specific viral involvement, past or present. Thus, abnormal antibody levels could be a reflection of differences in the immune response (e.g., an exaggerated immune response to a normal virus in the host) rather than simply constituting evidence for a specific viral infection.

As part of a large study of 178 schizophrenic patients, Torrey and colleagues (1982) examined the cerebrospinal fluid (CSF) of 17 bipolar patients (diagnosed by RDC) for immunoglobulin M (IgM) antibody to cytomegalovirus, a neurotropic virus with an affinity for the limbic system. Eighteen percent of the bipolar patients were antibody positive, compared with 11 percent of the schizophrenics, 3 percent of the neurological controls, and none of the normal controls. The CSF-positive patients did not have antibody in their serum.

Herpes is another class of neurotropic virus known to be associated not only with acute CNS infections but also with lifelong latent infections characterized by periodic exacerbations, such as those experienced with herpes zoster. Experimental CNS herpes simplex infections in animals are associated with alterations in catecholamine function, an observation that provides additional impetus for examining the possible role of the virus in manic-depressive illness. Three studies report a significantly higher prevalence of herpes simplex antibodies among patients with major depressive disorders (Rimon and Halonen, 1969; Rimon, 1971; Cappel and Sprecher, 1983), and one does not (Pokorny et al., 1973). In two of the positive studies and the one negative study, the antibody prevalence was very high (greater than 70 percent) in both the patient and control groups. The Cappel and Sprecher study is of note because the control antibody prevalence was relatively low (45 percent) and because both the incidence of antibody and mean antibody titers were significantly higher among the depressed patients than among the controls. It is also of interest that none of their patients reported herpes simplex infection in the 6 months before hospitalization, increasing the likelihood that the antibody finding may relate to manic-depressive illness per se.[40]

Epstein-Barr virus (EBV), the active pathogen in infectious mononucleosis, has been shown to be associated with a chronic relapsing illness characterized by lymphadenopathy, fluctuating symptoms of severe fatigue, malaise, fever, and often depression. Allen and Tilkian (1986) reported a preliminary uncontrolled study of 12 depressed patients, all of whom had "serological evidence of a chronic or recrudescent viremia caused by the Epstein-Barr virus" (p. 133). Allen and colleagues (1987) claimed that among their bipolar patients, EBV antibodies were reduced (or even disappeared) during hypomania, only to increase again during the depressive phase. They explain this as the interaction of the prior viral infection with state-dependent fluctuations in immune function. This group subsequently reported similar findings based on what was apparently a new sample of patients: bipolar patients who became manic during the study changed from having typically abnormal EBV antibody panel to no detectable EBV antibodies (Pitts et al., in press). DeLisi and co-workers (1986b) studied 40 outpatients with affective disorders (predominantly bipolar) and found that, compared with controls, a significantly higher proportion of them had antibodies to the viral capsule, although, unlike the patients of Allen and co-workers, there was no correlation with severity of depression. However, other groups (King et al., 1985; A.H. Miller et al., 1986; Amsterdam et al., 1986) were unable to find any differences in EBV antibodies between depressed patients and controls. In each of these studies and in others, the incidence of EBV antibodies is quite high across all groups, especially among older individuals (Cooke et al., 1988). The negative study of Amsterdam was especially convincing because of its relatively large sample size and its careful design.

Finally, the Borna disease virus, a highly neurotropic agent with an affinity for the limbic system, has been of interest because, when injected into animals, it can produce a syndrome of hyperactivity–aggression alternating with passive apathy, a pattern somewhat suggestive of manic-depressive illness. In a large study, Amsterdam and co-workers (1985) found 12 depressed patients who were antibody-positive (4.5 percent of their sample) compared with none of the 105 healthy controls. Interestingly, virtually all of the antibody-positive patients had the recurrent or cyclic forms of affective illness, either unipolar or bipolar.

Given the increasing recognition of the neurotropic viruses and their ability to produce chronic and recurrent symptoms, this preliminary area clearly warrants further development.

Critical Evaluation

The role of immunological and viral factors in manic-depressive illness is an emerging area, dominated by preliminary reports and characterized by considerable knowledge gaps. Central to the interpretation of the data on immune dysfunction is whether the changes are merely secondary to altered CNS neurotransmitter/endocrine function (e.g., hypercortisolemia producing immune changes) or might reflect a primary cellular dysfunction involving elements common to both the nervous and immune systems. One fruitful approach to unraveling this puzzle may lie in epidemiological studies designed to examine the association between manic-depressive illness, on the one hand, and immune and viral disorders, on the other. At another level, answers to these compelling questions may only come with further advances in our understanding of the intimate and intriguing interactions between the nervous system and the immune system. If the receptor-like interactions that subserve both systems do indeed involve the same fundamental molecular processes, this similarity opens new approaches to exploring the functional specificity of these two systems and perhaps their respective roles in the pathophysiology of disease.

SUMMARY

Before the development and application of brain-imaging techniques, the search for neuroanatomical correlates of manic-depressive illness relied primarily on studies of affective syndromes secondary to CNS lesions. Initially, the two sides of the brain were the focus of attention, but interest gradually shifted to quadrants. Depressions tend to be associated with lesions in the left frontotemporal or right parietooccipital quadrants. The most common affective sequelae of brain lesions involve poststroke depressions, the severity of which increases the closer the damage is to the left frontal pole. Consistent with the trend in these findings is the brain laterality literature, which implicates left hemispheric dysfunction in depression, perhaps reflecting frontotemporal characteristics. On the other hand, secondary manic-like symptoms appear to be associated with right frontotemporal or left parietooccipital lesions, evidence that is consistent with laterality findings indicating right-sided dysfunction in mania. In contrast to the secondary depressions, the less common manic reactions probably are more relevant to primary manic-depressive illness, since they are much more frequently associated with a history of primary affective illness.

Differential quadrant patterns may reflect inhibitory effects of one brain region on another, and this possibility makes it difficult to know whether clinical symptoms associated with a localized lesion are the result of direct or indirect effects. Also, dysfunction in one major area might result in a loss of the normal anterior–posterior or left–right relationships between neurotransmitters, which also appear to vary by quadrant. What is increasingly apparent from this work is that it is unlikely that one manic-depressive site will be found in the brain. As we observed some years ago:

Topographic specificity of mood disorders results not so much from control of emotion in the lesioned area (centers of emotion), but rather that, within the area of lesion, certain neurotransmitter systems may be passing that may be important for drive and affect. (Goodwin, 1983, p. 42)

Integrating some preliminary PET and rCBF evidence with the data on secondary depressions has led one group to suggest that a disturbance in the left prefrontal cortex, accompanied by more general left-sided dysfunction, may mediate the expression of depression. However, there is as yet no satisfactory way to reconcile this with the evidence from physiological and neuropsychological performance studies, which points to right-sided dysfunction in both the depressive and manic phases of the illness. On the other hand, the data on secondary mania are consistent with the neuropsychological evidence. Both point to a right frontal disturbance, which is of interest given the observation that secondary manias appear to reflect the primary disorder more closely than do secondary depressions. Evidence of left prefrontal dysfunction in schizophrenia also affects data interpretation, since it reminds us that pathophysiological mechanisms may be common to more than one major psychotic disorder.

The question of specificity arises again in the CT scan studies, some of which show an incidence of abnormalities among manic-depressive patients similar to that reported for schizophrenic patients. We should recall both the control group problems and the fact that manic-depressive patients who currently participate in hospital-based studies are more likely to be treatment-resistant and have more organic features than the average patient. Thus, some caution should apply to the emerging data for cerebral blood flow and PET studies.

The literature on peripheral electrophysiology is so methodologically flawed that little can be concluded. Especially troublesome in this relatively old literature is the failure to account for clinical state and drug status. Central electrophysiological measures are a more promising area. Of particular interest are studies of evoked responses and computer-assisted quantitative EEG mapping, which suggests bipolar–unipolar differences. Right-sided abnormalities appear to predominate among bipolar patients.

Immunological and viral factors in manic-depressive illness have only recently been subjected to systematic study, but we anticipate that this work will evolve into a very fruitful area of inquiry. The central question is whether observed immune changes result from altered functioning in CNS neurotransmitter and endocrine systems or instead reflect primary dysfunction in elements common to both the nervous and immune systems.

NOTES

1. Even Alzheimer's disease, with its characteristic cell death, does not invariably show linear deterioration of CNS function. Much to the puzzlement of clinicians treating patients with this disorder, "good days" (sometimes even weeks) punctuate periods of deteriorating CNS function.
2. For comprehensive reviews of poststroke mood disorders, see Dupont and colleagues (1988) and Messner and Messner (1988).
3. Quoted by Whitwell, 1936, p. 198, from Gordonius Bernardus: *Opus, lilium medicinae inscriptum.* (Lugd.), 1559.
4. Jeste and colleagues noted six major limitations: (1) bias in reporting (i.e., lesions associated with affective symptoms are more likely to be reported than are uncomplicated cases), (2) lack of diagnostic precision, (3) lack of periodicity or cyclicity in clinical manifestation, with only five cases documented to have recurrent bipolar disorder and only two to have recurrent unipolar depression, suggesting that they may not have pathophysiology comparable to recurrent affective illness, (4) differences between the site of the gross lesion and the area associated with the secondary affective symptoms, (5) confusion between association and causality (given the relatively high prevalence of the affective disorders and neurological problems, chance associations are possible), and (6) lack of an adequate history of affective illness.
5. Two recent systematic studies consider this issue. Starkstein and colleagues (1987) compared 11 manic patients whose mania developed after brain injury with 25 manic patients without brain injury. Their type and frequency of symptoms were not significantly different. In the patients with secondary mania, the lesions usually involved limbic structures and were in the right hemisphere. Many

in this group had prior depressive episodes, and almost half had a family history of affective disorders. On the other hand, Hoff and colleagues (1988) found that manic patients with an antecedent history of presumptive neurological dysfunction (such as birth trauma, head trauma, encephalitis or convulsive disorder) evidenced more cognitive dysfunction on neuropsychological tests than did manic patients without such histories.

6. In their study of mood reactions following right sided stroke, Starkstein et al. (1989) note that the minority who experienced major depression tended to have a family history of psychotic illness.

7. Cummings (1986) has concluded that the lesions associated with secondary mania tend to be localized close to the ascending monoaminergic pathways.

8. The literature on poststroke depression has been reviewed by Dupont and associates (1988) and by Starkstein and Robinson (1989).

9. Cohen and Niska (1980) described a 59-year-old man with no prior personal or family history of affective disorder who had a right temporal lobe hematoma and three subsequent documented episodes of mania, each of which responded well to lithium. Oyewumi and Lapierre (1981) reported the case of a 21-year-old man with no prior personal or family history of affective disorder, who, following emergence of a tumor in the fourth ventricle, exhibited numerous episodes of alternating hyperactivity and depression that responded well to lithium. Trimble and Cummings (1981) described alternating periods of hyperactivity and hypoactivity in a 21-year-old woman following an intraventricular bleed with upper brainstem involvement. She was diagnosed as manic-depressive. Cummings and Mendez (1984) reported a case of a 61-year-old man who, 12 months after an apparent secondary mania, suffered a major depressive episode followed by a brief period of mania. Jampala and Abrams (1983) described two patients with long-standing histories of DSM-III bipolar affective disorder apparently secondary to vascular lesions of the left and right cerebral hemispheres, respectively; one responded to lithium, the other to carbamazepine. Forrest (1982) presented a case of a 45-year-old man with cerebral palsy whose unipolar depressions evolved into rapid-cycling bipolar illness. Twenty-seven years earlier, his right cerebral cortex was removed for epilepsy. His cycling responded poorly to lithium alone but responded well when carbamazepine was added. Pope and associates (1988) reported two cases of bipolar disorder following closed head injury. A chart review of 56 bipolar patients yielded eight more whose bipolar illness apparently was preceded by head injury. All 10 cases were poor responders to conventional treatment but responded when the anticonvulsant valproate was added.

10. According to Mukherjee and colleagues (1984),

soft signs imply a lack of specificity for neuroanatomical localization and pathological significance.

11. *Graphaesthesia* is the ability to recognize figures written on the skin.

12. Otto and colleagues (1987) reviewed the evidence suggesting that the right hemisphere preferentially processes negative affective experiences. They propose a feedforward cycle, in which negative stimuli activate the right hemisphere, which in turn leads to the perception of subsequent stimuli as negative. Such a process could enlarge cognitive theories of the onset of depression or, of more relevance to recurrent affective illness, could be integrated with the kindling–sensitization theories of Post.

13. Since most studies of depression involve unipolar patients, however, reported differences in laterality between mania and depression could reflect either clinical state or polarity.

14. Metzig et al., 1976; Fleminger et al., 1977; Chaugule and Master, 1981, Moscovitch et al., 1981; Nasrallah and McCalley-Whitters, 1982, Shan-Ming et al., 1985. However, these studies either do not include bipolar patients or do not indicate if they do.

15. The depressed patients in the study by Kronfol and colleagues (1978) were not specified as either bipolar or unipolar.

16. The major histochemical findings of Birkmayer and Riederer (1975) were as follows: (a) serotonin concentration was decreased in most brain areas studied, but especially in raphe, striatum, substantia nigra, amygdala, and hypothalamus; (b) Norepinephrine concentration was reduced in the red nucleus but not in basal ganglia, raphe, and limbic structures, although it was found to be reduced in the basal ganglia (striatum, globus pallidus, and substantia nigra) and hypothalamus of older patients; (c) Dopamine concentration was low in the striatum and red nucleus but not in the globus pallidus, substantia nigra, amygdala, or cingulate gyrus; (d) The concentration of 3-methoxy-4-hydroxyphenylglycol (MHPG, the major norepinephrine metabolite in brain) was reduced in the hypothalamus, substantia nigra, and raphe and to a lesser extent in the globus pallidus, mammillary bodies, and nucleus accumbens.

17. Changes in DBH activity in association with enlargement of the ventricles are difficult to explain, since in plasma, this enzyme comes from multiple sources, including peripheral adrenergic neurons and the adrenal medulla. In the CNS, DBH is localized in norepinephrine-containing neurons and serves as a marker for them. However, the contribution of CNS DBH to plasma levels of the enzyme is not clear.

18. Normally, the right frontal and left occipital widths are larger than their contralateral structures.

19. Dewan and colleagues (1987), Tanaka and co-

workers (1982), and Weinberger and associates (1982) reported nonsignificant differences between bipolar patients and controls, and Tsai and colleagues (1983) reported an increase in reversed brain asymmetry (occipital) in schizophrenic patients compared with bipolar subjects.

20. However, Dewan and colleagues (1988b) found no relationship between CT abnormalities (primarily third ventricle enlargement in this study; VBR was normal) and the presence of psychotic symptoms within a group of DSM-III bipolar patients.

21. For example, as noted by Silfverskiöld and Risberg (1989), habituation to the procedure (and, therefore, decreased anxiety) could contribute to the small decrease in rCBF that they observed following recovery from either depression or mania.

22. In a CBF study by Uytdenhoef et al. (1983), depressed unipolar patients were compared with bipolar patients in the well state. The latter group had rCBF values that were not different from those of normal controls, whereas the unipolar patients revealed increased blood flow in the left-frontal and right-posterior quadrants.

23. Baxter's results were expressed as the ratio of activity in the left anterolateral prefrontal cortex to that in the entire left hemisphere. The evaluation of this important study is difficult, since certain details concerning how the data were collected and analyzed are not provided.

24. Recall that the observations of secondary depressions are probably less specific than those of secondary manias, the latter being generally associated with a preexisting vulnerability, the former not.

25. The concept of the isodendritic core, although controversial, incorporates brain regions of interest to neuropsychiatry: the substantia nigra, substantia innominata, and lower layers of the superior colliculus, hypothalamus, raphe nuclei, and locus coeruleus (see Chapter 17). According to the IDCB hypothesis, the dendritic patterns in the isodendritic core, unlike those observed in most neurons, show a nonspecialized configuration. Parkinson's disease has been hypothesized to involve depletion in this region, and cholinergic deficits in the same region have been found in Alzheimer's disease. Similarly, serotonergic or noradrenergic dysfunction in the isodendritic core could be related to manic-depressive illness. The common involvement of the IDCB is consistent with the frequent coexistence of Parkinson's disease with depression and dementia and with the hypokinesia and pseudodementia that often accompany bipolar depression. Since this brainstem region sends extensive projections to the rest of the brain, especially the amygdala, cingulate gyrus, and frontal lobe, secondary involvement of these areas might be expected, or conversely, a primary lesion in one of these other areas could produce secondary changes in the IDCB (Pycock et al., 1980).

26. A median of 8 months had passed since the last episode, and 90 percent of the patients had been essentially asymptomatic for at least 2 months. For the unipolar group, the mean values for each individual response parameter were all significantly different from the control group. Although the majority of the patients were taking imipramine, lithium, or both, the authors concluded from their own data and those of others that these treatments did not contribute to any of the differences between patients and controls.

27. Although there are no significant bipolar–unipolar differences in the studies for the Iacono group, among the remitted patients the unipolars tended to be lower, whereas among the depressed patients the average for the bipolars was slightly lower.

28. Schwartz et al., 1976; Teasdale and Bancroft, 1977; Greden et al., 1986; Knott and Lapierre, 1987.

29. Another study using a different design did not find a significant association between bipolar depression and migraine headache (Marchesi et al., 1989).

30. For clinical descriptive purposes, EEG frequencies are divided into four wavebands: delta, less than 4 hertz (Hz); theta, 4 to 8 Hz; alpha, 8 to 13 Hz; beta, faster than 13 Hz.

31. In contrast to most U.S. studies, Perris' unipolar patients are clearly recurrent, with a minimum of three episodes required for the diagnosis. Thus, they are more likely to be closer to the bipolar group than would be the case with a more heterogeneous unipolar sample.

32. Recovery is measured by assessing the effects of an initial stimulus response to a second stimulus that immediately follows.

33. Von Knorring could not replicate either the bipolar–unipolar differences or the independence from clinical state noted by Buchsbaum and colleagues. In the original study (Buchsbaum et al., 1971), patients with simultaneous symptoms of depression and mania (mixed states) showed more augmentation than those with pure depressive states, and auditory evoked responses changed when the patient switched from depression to mania. These findings were consistent with the later work of Von Knorring (1978), who found that evoked-response reducing was correlated with severity of depression, whereas augmenting tended to occur in mania.

34. Von Knorring et al., 1974; Von Knorring, 1978; Buchsbaum, 1975; Buchsbaum et al., 1981.

35. Test–retest data indicated poor temporal stability for indices of lateral differences, although the baseline levels themselves were relatively stable over time. This indicates that bilateral asymmetry is not a trait characteristic of individuals prone to affective disorders.

36. In the Prichep study, the variables that contributed most to the bipolar–unipolar discrimination were beta-activity (especially in the left posterior re-

gion), left hemisphere alpha, and some measures of asymmetry in the distribution of the different wave forms. In general, bipolar patients had increased beta activity and decreased alpha-activity (indicating more power on the left), whereas unipolar patients had decreased beta-activity (indicating more power on the right). In both groups beta-distribution was asymmetrical.

37. T is for the thymus gland, a way station in the formation of T lymphocytes. B lymphocytes were first discovered in birds, and the B is for bursa of Fabricius, the structure in birds in which their pre-processing occurs.

38. Although 8 of 11 manic patients were on psychotropic medications, Kronfol and House present evidence suggesting that the immune changes are not likely to be due to a drug effect.

39. Calabrese et al., 1986; Abdulla and Hamadah, 1975; Lieb et al., 1983; Linnoila et al., 1983b.

40. It is still possible that the elevated titers could have reflected the patients' exposure to herpes simplex in the hospital.

19

Sleep and Biological Rhythms

Our body is like a clock; if one wheel be amiss, all the rest are disordered . . . with
such admirable art and harmony is a man composed.   —Robert Burton, 1628

I become possessed by an intense, overpowering sense of sadness, that in my then
sickly, nervous state produced a mental condition adequately to describe which
would take a great physiologist. I could not sleep, I lost my spirits, my favourite
studies became distasteful to me, I could not work, and I spent my time wandering
aimlessly about Paris and its environs. During that long period of suffering I can
only recall four occasions on which I slept, and then it was the heavy, death-like
sleep produced by complete physical exhaustion.   —Hector Berlioz, 1870

As surely as the sun rises in the morning and bears
hibernate in the winter, human functioning heeds
its own innate rhythms. Body temperature rises
and falls in oscillations, as do hormone secretion,
cell division, heart rate, urine flow, allergic reactions, mathematical finesse, activity, and—most
obvious of all rhythms—the need for sleep.
Mood also fluctuates, waxing and waning regularly even among the imperturbable but cycling
in months-long paroxysms of euphoria, irritability, or despair in manic-depressive patients.
The insistent reappearance of such disquieting
moods, the leitmotif of the illness, is accompanied by disruptions in the temporal distribution
of many bodily functions, especially in the ca-
dences of sleep.

Investigations into the biological rhythms of
manic-depressive illness grew from clinical recognition of these striking rhythmic irregularities.
Unlike cross-sectional studies of biological variables that correlate with the illness, research on
biological rhythms represents one important approach to understanding changes that occur over
time.

CLINICAL CLUES TO RHYTHMIC DISTURBANCES

The very earliest recorded observations of rhythmic disturbances are descriptions of seasonal patterns in the episodes of manic-depressive illness:

In the spring, mania, melancholia and epilepsy are apt
to occur. . . . Many diseases regarded as summer affections may also occur in the autumn, such as epilepsy, mania and melancholia. (Hippocrates, c. 400 BC)[1]

By the 16th century, specific patterns were more
discernible:

A certain woman of Buderic was every year disturbed by such a kind of melancholia, or rather mania. . . . the attack most frequently occurred about
Easter Day—that is, in the spring of the year. (Johann
Weyer, 1515–1588)[2]

And three centuries later:

There are individuals who pass the summer in a state of
prostration or agitation; whilst in the winter they are in
an opposite condition. (Esquirol, 1845, p. 32)[3]

In recent years, clinical investigators have established the existence of syndromes of depression
or mania that occur regularly at a certain season,
year after year.

Sleep disturbances also have been considered
as cardinal symptoms of both depression and mania for as long as these disorders have been recognized.[4] So profound is the insomnia of major depression that many patients experience the illness
primarily as a sleep disorder. Those in the depressed phase of bipolar illness are more likely to
sleep excessively, but even they are not rested.
Patients in the throes of mania sleep little or not at
all and, since they do not seem fatigued, apparently require less than usual. The pervasiveness

of sleep disturbances in affective illness suggests that they are not merely symptomatic but may be instrumental in the pathophysiology of the disorder.

Daily oscillations in mood, another common feature of affective illness, also have been noted clinically for centuries. In their classic textbook, for example, Mayer-Gross, Slater, and Roth (1955) discussed the diurnal pattern commonly observed in depressed patients:[5]

An important and significant symptom of the endogenous depression—but also of mania—is the *daily fluctuation* of mood and of the total state. Improvement of all symptoms usually occurs towards evening, the retardation and depressive mood particularly showing a change for the better. In the morning, however, the patient wakes direct from sleep into his characteristic sombre mood or is normal for a few minutes, before, as he says, the depression comes down "like a cloud". (p. 211)

The very cyclicity of recurrent bipolar and unipolar affective illness constitutes a type of rhythm. The episodic nature of the illness, together with its circadian disturbances, could indicate malfunctions in a master biological clock. Experimental treatments point in the same direction. Wehr and Goodwin summarized these inferences:

Because of its inherent cyclicity, the illness itself is a kind of abnormal biological rhythm spanning weeks, months, or years. Circadian rhythms are implicated in some of the symptoms of depression, such as early awakening and diurnal variation in mood. The possible importance of the circadian system in its pathogenesis is suggested by the capacity of experimental alterations in the timing of sleep and wakefulness to alter clinical state. (1983b, p. 5)

Biological rhythms range in frequency from milliseconds to months or years. Most rhythmic disturbances identified in the symptoms of affective illness occur over the course of a day—that is, they are *circadian* rhythms—and are most apparent in the daily rest-activity cycle. The episodic recurrences of the illness, on the other hand, are usually *infradian,* oscillating over periods of months or years.[6] (See the Appendix to this chapter for definitions of terms used in the study of biological rhythms.) To date, we lack a satisfactory comprehensive model for understanding the relationship between circadian abnormalities in the illness and the episodic recurrences:

The periodicity of affective disturbances suggests some relationship of biological rhythms to depressive and manic illnesses. . . . It is not immediately apparent how yearly, monthly, or even 48-hour rhythms in the occurrence of depressive and manic symptoms may be related to daily rhythms, but 24-hour rhythms are certainly disturbed in depressed patients. (Kripke, 1983, p. 42)

Episodic mania and depression may also reflect disturbances in *ultradian* rhythms, those that oscillate more than once a day, which are common at the cellular level and in hormone secretion, as well as in such autonomic functions as circulation, blood pressure, respiration, and heart rate and in the cycles of sleep. As Edmunds (1988) has pointed out:

It is important not to overlook the great number of biological and biochemical oscillations with ultradian periods. . . . [There is a] possibility that high-frequency ticks might generate lower-frequency, circadian tocks by the use of some sort of counter, by coupling among oscillators, or by other mechanisms. . . . circadian oscillations, in turn, might contribute to the generation of even longer periodicities, such as infradian estrous cycles and circannual rhythms. (p. 5)

THE EVOLVING INTEREST IN RHYTHMS

The rhythmic manifestations of manic-depressive illness have sometimes been dismissed as so much irritating noise requiring experimental control. Increasingly, this variability—from one part of the day to another, one season to another—is recognized as either part of the pathogenesis of the illness or, at least, as involved in the pathophysiology of important symptoms. In the study of affective illnesses, research on sleep per se preceded interest in basic biological rhythms, and traditionally the two have been largely independent fields of inquiry. Gradually, sleep researchers have extended their reach, recognizing that the sleep-wakefulness cycle is an integral part of an overall circadian system and that other biological rhythms are involved in both the mechanisms and the effects of sleep. We believe this broader approach is salutary, and consequently we combine our discussions of sleep and rhythms.

Disturbances in biological rhythms may have to be explained before the etiology of manic-depressive illness can be understood. Among the questions that need answering: Do the rhythmic features of the illness reflect the action of an endogenous mood-regulating oscillator or the coupling of such a system with other biological or environmental rhythms? Do disturbances in the timing and structure of circadian processes (such as the sleep-wakefulness cycle) trigger episodes of affective illness, or are the disturbed rhythms themselves simply a symptom of some primary CNS dysregulation accompanying the illness? Could desynchronization of one rhythm (e.g., cortisol secretion) from another (e.g., the sleep-wake cycle) actually cause recurrent episodes of illness? What is the source of the apparent instability of rhythmic processes in manic-depressive patients? What is the relationship of the very short (ultradian) rhythms to once-a-day rhythms and, in turn, the relationship of these circadian rhythms to recurrent episodes of illness? How are endogenous rhythms influenced by the environment—by the number of daylight hours, for example, or the time demands of advanced societies?[7] How do the very different behaviors associated with depression and with mania (e.g., level of activity) affect bodily rhythms?

Research reviewed in this chapter has so far focused more on describing the phenomena than on explaining mechanisms. Investigations directed at characterizing chronobiological disturbances in manic-depressive illness, understanding their significance, and explaining their mechanisms have demonstrated only that the reality of rhythmic processes involves a far more complex series of events than had originally been envisioned.

Studies of the mechanisms that control sleep and the physiological and biochemical changes that accompany it have spawned several testable hypotheses, some related to sleep itself, some to circadian rhythms in general. These, in turn, have suggested new types of treatment. Hypotheses about rhythm disturbances also have led to new treatment techniques. Before examining these developments, we briefly digress to review sleep and circadian rhythms in normal functioning. The methodological challenges of research into biological rhythms in clinical populations are discussed next. Then we review the bulk of the evidence—that describing the nature of sleep and other rhythm disturbances in affective illness. Next we examine the hypotheses that have been postulated to account for the mechanisms of cir-

cadian disturbances. Finally, turning to seasonal rhythms in affective disorders, we report what is known of the epidemiology of these disorders and explore their neurobiology, with a focus on the mechanisms that might explain the antidepressant effects of very bright artificial light in winter depression.

BIOLOGICAL RHYTHMS IN NORMAL POPULATIONS

Life is partitioned by time—years, months, days, minutes—into events that tend to recur at regular intervals, a periodicity as evident in the behavior of protozoa as it is in the sleeping habits and other schedules of human beings. Surely among the most abstract of concepts, the rhythmic organization of time is grounded in material reality. Biological functioning is itself organized into periods linked to the rotations of the earth around the sun and the moon around the earth (Figure 19-1). Although biological rhythms cycle in synchrony with these "celestial mechanics,"[8] they are clearly regulated by endogenous processes. These innate rhythms may have evolved as adaptations to rhythmic fluctuations in environmental light, heat, humidity—perhaps even the earth's electromagnetic fields. Such evolutionary explanations for the origins of biological rhythms are controversial, but there is little disagreement that oscillatory processes serve homeostatic regulation at the cellular, biochemical, physiological, and probably psychological levels.[9]

Sleep

The discrete stages of sleep are marked by variations in electroencephalogram (EEG) patterns, eye movements, and muscle tone. By convention, human sleep is divided into two major phases that alternate throughout the night; the phases are identified by the presence or absence of rapid eye movement (REM). Normal adults, on falling asleep, go into non-REM sleep, the period of rest and energy conservation, when the brain literally cools while respiration, blood pressure, heart rate, and other physiological processes slow down, eyes are still or move only slowly, and muscles are relaxed but not flaccid. This first phase is made up of four stages of progressively deeper sleep. On EEG recordings, the

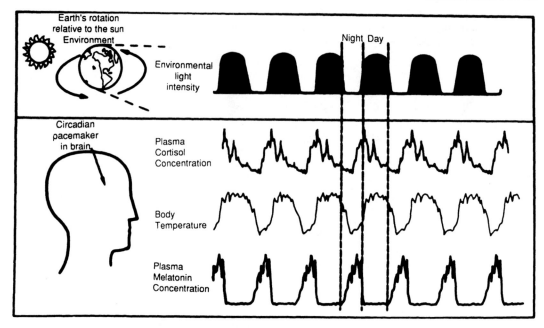

Figure 19-1. Circadian rhythms. Adaptation to the environment by internalization of the day/night cycle.

frequency of electrical waves decreases steadily from stage 1 to stage 4 while the amplitude—the energy discharged at each impulse—increases (Figure 19-2).

Following a complete cycle of these four stages of sleep comes the second major phase, REM sleep, a period marked by intense mental activity, when dreaming occurs, and cerebral metabolism is rapid and diffuse. Blood flow, most neuronal firing rates, and probably brain temperature are higher during REM sleep than during either non-REM or awake states, but the large muscles are virtually paralyzed. Bursts of rapid eye movements occur, pulse and blood pressure rise and fall, respiration becomes irregular. EEG activity shows a sawtooth pattern, low in amplitude (voltage) and variable in frequency, similar to stage 1 non-REM sleep, the brief transition period between wakefulness and sleep. Wehr has hypothesized (Wehr, submitted) that a function of REM sleep is to generate heat in the brain in order to maintain CNS temperature as the remainder of the body is cooling during sleep. REM sleep propensity is greatest when body temperature reaches its minimum near the end of the sleep period.[10]

In 1957, Dement and Kleitman observed that in normal individuals, the distribution of REM sleep during a night's sleep was skewed, with more REM occurring toward the end of the night than at the beginning. In a study of naps, Maron and associates (1964) found large amounts of REM sleep during afternoon naps but little during evening ones. Linking their own findings with those of Dement and Kleitman, Maron and colleagues proposed that the propensity for REM sleep is governed by a process that exhibits a circadian rhythm independent of sleep.

In the normal sleep of a young adult, the first period of non-REM sleep (through all four stages) is followed, after a period that averages about 90 minutes, by a 15 to 20 minute period of REM sleep. Slow-wave sleep (stages 3 and 4) predominates during the first part of the night, whereas REM sleep periods get progressively longer and are most concentrated in the hours before waking. An internal self-sustaining circadian pacemaker appears to govern the propensity for REM sleep. Homeostatic processes determine such other sleep patterns as the amount of slow-wave sleep, which is directly related to the length of time the person has been awake before sleep.

The duration and structure of sleep are, in addition, influenced by other endogenous rhythms, such as those governing certain neurotransmitters. In 1975, McCarley and Hobson elaborated

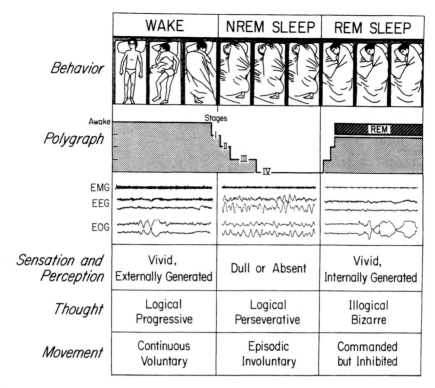

	WAKE	NREM SLEEP	REM SLEEP
Behavior			
Polygraph			
	EMG		
	EEG		
	EOG		
Sensation and Perception	Vivid, Externally Generated	Dull or Absent	Vivid, Internally Generated
Thought	Logical Progressive	Logical Perseverative	Illogical Bizarre
Movement	Continuous Voluntary	Episodic Involuntary	Commanded but Inhibited

Figure 19-2. Normal sleep. EEG patterns, distribution of non-REM and REM periods (from Hobson and Steriade, 1986).

and provided evidence for a sleep model based on the interaction of separate REM-enhancing and REM-inhibiting neuronal populations. This model postulates a balance between cholinergic and aminergic systems regulating REM sleep. Evidence strongly suggests that cholinergic mechanisms are involved in generating REM sleep. The direct application of cholinergic agonists to certain areas of the midbrain can produce a REM episode. In humans, REM latency can be shortened by the intravenous administration of an agent that enhances cholinergic mechanisms (i.e., a cholinergic agonist, such as arecoline) or a cholinesterase inhibitor (physostigmine), whereas a cholinergic antagonist (scopolamine) prolongs REM latency (reviewed by Gillin and Sitaram, 1984). There is also some evidence from animal studies that aminergic neurotransmission is inhibitory to REM sleep (see, e.g., Karczmar et al., 1970), although the data are not as extensive as those pertaining to cholinergic transmission.

As people age, sleep patterns change. Sleep disruptions increase, and the time spent in slow-wave sleep progressively decreases. These and other changes resemble, but are not as severe as, the sleep abnormalities that typically accompany depressions with endogenous or melancholic features. The effects of age can confound research on the sleep of depression, a possibility not always considered in study design (Thase et al., 1986).

Other Circadian Rhythms

Evidence that circadian rhythms are endogenous came from experiments in which people lived for weeks or months in caves, underground bunkers, or windowless, sound-proof apartments, isolated from external time cues (Chouvet et al., 1974; Siffre, 1975; Wever, 1979). In these conditions, the circadian rhythms ran according to their own intrinsic period, which in humans is usually slower (i.e., longer) than one cycle each 24 hours. Thus, by clock time, the experimental subjects gradually extended each day, falling asleep later each night and waking later the next morning. Their intrinsic human circadian period averaged about 25 hours, which in normal everyday life adjusts to 24 hours, synchronized with the environment by periodic factors that serve as 24-hour time cues, or *zeitgebers*. Light is probably the principal zeitgeber, entraining circadian oscillators, which in turn regulate some annual and seasonal biological rhythms.

Experimental results indicate that external time cues synchronize circadian rhythms not only with the day/night cycle but also with one another. When entrained by zeitgebers, homeostatic mechanisms ensure that the various circadian rhythms keep distinct phase relationships to the environment and to one another. In humans, for instance, the temperature minimum nearly always occurs during the last third of the night, just before dawn. Internally, circadian rhythms that are normally synchronized with each other can dissociate when one becomes disentrained from the zeitgeber. The temperature rhythm of a night-shift worker, for example, might continue to be entrained to the day/night cycle but dissociated from the sleep-wake cycle when the worker slept during the day. Or consider what would happen under free-running conditions (i.e., in the absence of zeitgebers). The two cycles, each following its own intrinsic pattern, would go in and out of phase with the other (Figure 19-3). This internal desynchronization can create what has been called a beat phenomenon, analogous to the audible beat produced by two tuning forks of slightly different frequencies (Halberg, 1968; Kripke et al., 1978). Such desynchronization,

observed in the early isolation experiments, suggested that the human circadian system is controlled by more than one oscillator.[11] In some experimental subjects, this desynchronization increased or impaired activity and performance, cycling every several days (Wever, 1977).

Although the nature and number of biological oscillators are subjects of controversy, prevailing opinion is that human circadian rhythms are regulated by multiple self-sustained, coupled oscillators, which probably are organized hierarchically. The overt rhythms themselves are believed to be controlled simultaneously by multiple oscillators, although one oscillator usually exerts the most influence on any one rhythm. The primary oscillators driving overt rhythms vary in strength, so much so that many investigators believe that only one truly endogenous circadian oscillator exists (for discussion, see Czeisler et al., 1987).

Weitzman and colleagues (1974) showed that the REM sleep rhythm is inversely related to the rhythm of body temperature, which, as mentioned, normally reaches its nadir in the latter half of the sleep period, when REM sleep is at its peak (Figure 19-4). The close association of REM sleep, body temperature, and cortisol secretion suggested that their respective circadian rhythms are controlled by the same oscillator. It is now generally believed that core body temperature, REM sleep propensity, alertness, cortisol secretion, urinary potassium excretion (and, no doubt, other biochemical rhythms), and cognitive and psychomotor performance are regulated by the strong oscillator—"strong" because it is almost impervious to environmental influence.[12] A much weaker circadian process, which under normal conditions appears to be linked to and driven by the strong oscillator and which readily responds to environmental influences, regulates the rest-activity, sleep-wake cycle, and sleep-dependent neuroendocrine activity.

The anatomy and physiology of the circadian pacemaker regulating the weak oscillator are fairly well understood, and the existence of a human pacemaker(s) regulating the strong oscillator is inferred from the dissociation or uncoupling of temperature, REM, and cortisol rhythms from the sleep-wake cycle under free-running conditions. Experiments in nonhuman animals, and recently in humans, have demonstrated that the su-

Figure 19-3. The beat phenomenon. This hypothetical model shows two circadian rhythms. Oscillator *A* is synchronized to the day/night cycle and always peaks during the day. Oscillator *B* free-runs slightly faster than one cycle per 24 hours and, therefore, goes out of phase with *A*. When *A* and *B* are in phase, their ratio is stable, but when out of phase, the ratio of *B/A* may become very high. This ratio indicates the cyclic beat phenomenon that occurs every few days (adapted from Halberg, 1968, and Kripke, 1978).

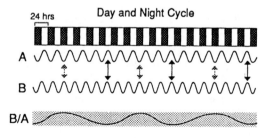

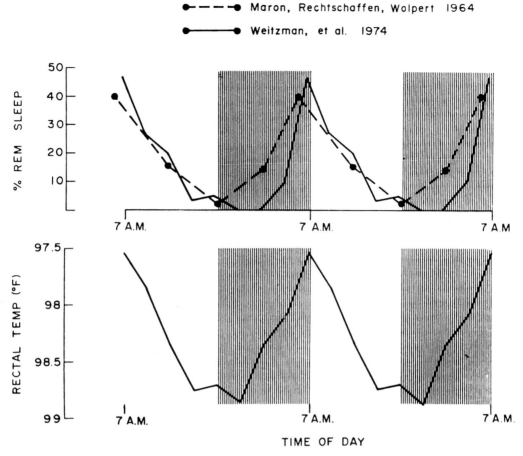

Figure 19-4. Circadian rhythms of REM sleep and (inverse) body temperature. Note that REM sleep is greatest when body temperature reaches its minimum at the end of the sleep period. There is preliminary evidence that the rapid eye movements themselves generate increased temperatures in a venous plexus that bathes parts of the brain, thereby providing one mechanism by which temperature and REM might interact (from Wehr and Goodwin, 1981).

prachiasmatic nucleus (SCN) of the anterior hypothalamus is the location of an autonomous circadian pacemaker that appears to drive the weak oscillator.[13] It, in turn, is influenced by the light/dark cycle. Light activates the retina, which sends signals through the retinohypothalamic–retinogeniculohypothalamic tract into the SCN.[14] Because light must be considerably brighter to elicit a response in the oscillator in humans than in other animals, humans are able to discriminate between the brightness of ordinary artificial light and natural light. This ability may have evolved after human beings discovered fire hundreds of thousands of years ago so that random artificial light would not interfere with natural entrainment of the circadian system.

Proper functioning of the human circadian system depends on continuous sensory input from the environment. This feature may be particularly relevant to understanding circadian disturbances in manic-depressive illness. Equally important, behavior regulates biological rhythms by subjecting a person to the entraining zeitgebers or shielding him from them—it serves a gating function. The depressive patient who hides under the covers is certainly less likely to be exposed to light and other zeitgebers than is the manic patient who races through the day and sleeps little at night.

The normal phase relationships between circadian oscillators and their overt rhythms can be temporarily disturbed during rapid transmeridian travel, as well as experimentally. As demonstrated in the isolation experiments, the oscillators may spontaneously dissociate and oscillate with unequal periods when humans are experimentally deprived of external time cues. The timing of circadian rhythms relative to the day/night cycle and to one another is homeostatically controlled and partly reflects the period of the intrinsic rhythm of their driving oscillators. Such a system may be altered by disease and treatment interventions. Alterations can occur in the intrinsic periods of the oscillators, in the coupling between oscillators, or between the oscillators and the external day/night cycle. Such changes might affect the phase position of circadian rhythms entrained to the day/night cycle and even their capacity to be entrained at all (Aschoff, 1981b,c).

METHODOLOGICAL CONSIDERATIONS IN CLINICAL STUDIES

Clinical studies of circadian rhythms are difficult because they require long-term, around-the-clock monitoring of multiple variables. Their results are confounded by the masking of overt rhythms, particularly the tendency for experimental procedures themselves (such as blood drawing or even behavioral assessment) to serve as unexpected zeitgebers distorting the rhythm. Differences in the statistics used and the method applied to plot the data into phases can also mask rhythms.[15] Unlike the familiar sleep-wake cycle, other circadian rhythms can be detected only with special measurement techniques. Among the most striking patterns are those that occur in the various secretions of the endocrine system, but they can be observed only when plasma is sampled several times an hour for 24 hours and then analyzed with sensitive radioimmunoassay procedures.

One problem that can compromise findings is the masking of oscillator-driven rhythms by external or internal influences that can change the apparent phase or amplitude of, for example, hormone or temperature levels. Such factors include sleep schedules, environmental temperature, physical activity, dietary habits, and lighting conditions.[16] Masking is a particular problem in research with manic-depressive patients because apparent differences in rhythms could actually reflect the distorting effects of such characteristic symptoms as weight loss, disturbed sleep, and hypoactivity or hyperactivity. To control for masking in circadian rhythm studies, Minors and Waterhouse (1984a,b) advocated using constant routines, keeping subjects at bedrest, giving them equal hourly feedings, and keeping them awake throughout the study.[17] These conditions have made it possible to describe what is believed to be normal intrinsic circadian rhythms in cortisol, urinary electrolytes, and mental performance, but comparable work that could clarify differences found in manic-depressive patients[18] is in its early stages (Sack et al., 1987). Masking can also influence the results of sleep studies. Most sleep laboratories impose schedules on patients, waking them at certain times in the morning and thus interfering with the hypersomnia that characterizes many patients with bipolar illness. Or the procedure might call for interrupting sleep to sample blood or perform other tests, thus introducing time cues that confound experimental results.

Two other sources of variance that often go unrecognized in circadian studies are differences that occur as a function of the stage of the episode and the time of the year. As reviewed subsequently, the available longitudinal studies indicate that the phase position of some circadian rhythms is significantly different in the early stages of a depressive or manic episode than in later stages. Considerable unrecognized variance in the literature may be due to this factor, since the stage of illness is rarely reported in cross-sectional studies. Season of the year is another factor that should be controlled in circadian rhythm studies, since the length of the photoperiod (which varies dramatically throughout the year in temperate latitudes) is an important determinant of circadian phase position and amplitude.

Even more formidable than research on circadian rhythms are studies of longer periodicities, such as monthly or yearly cycles of mood. Assessment, itself troublesome because of problems associated with self-monitoring instruments, must usually rely on the compliance of subjects performing burdensome tasks over periods of a year or more. Further, advanced mathematical methods are required to analyze the data, and the results are difficult to interpret (Eastwood et al., 1985). Not surprisingly, studies of infradian rhythms are rare.

An alternative strategy that eliminates some of the compliance and accuracy problems associated with self-monitoring are hospital ward studies with rapid-cycling bipolar patients. Patients with rapid cycles offer the opportunity to trace the sequence of events preceding switches from depression to mania and back again. Some studies that have followed such patients over prolonged periods provide rich descriptions of the illness and clues to its pathophysiology. These studies are, however, expensive and time-consuming and consequently involve few patients. The results, although perhaps more reliable than self-monitoring studies, may be less generalizable, since rapid-cycling patients may not be, in all respects, representative of bipolar patients in general. (This question is discussed in Chapter 6.) Studies of rapid-cycling patients must be seen against the backdrop of short-term, cross-sectional studies of larger numbers of patients.

CIRCADIAN RHYTHM DISTURBANCES IN AFFECTIVE ILLNESS: DESCRIPTIVE EVIDENCE

After a quarter of a century of laboratory research, the pattern of sleep in major depression has now been reasonably well characterized. It is less clear for the bipolar subgroup because investigators generally have not distinguished depressed bipolar patients from those with unipolar disorders, and they find manic patients difficult to study. Despite this deficiency, other evidence has provided tantalizing leads to understanding the connection between sleep and the bipolar form of manic-depressive illness. Switches from depression to mania frequently occur after patients miss a night of sleep, for example. Those who resume sleep too soon after being therapeutically deprived of it may relapse into depression.

Sleep in Major (Predominantly Unipolar) Depression

Nearly all patients with major depressive illness experience disturbances in their sleep. These abnormalities, certain forms of which tend to become more pronounced with age, have been established over the past few decades by polygraphic EEG recordings (Reynolds and Kupfer, 1987; Reynolds et al., 1987; Gillin et al.,

1984). The sleep problems usually reported by unipolar patients with endogenous or melancholic depression include interruptions throughout the night, early morning awakening, and, for some, difficulty falling asleep; together these changes result in a reduction of total sleep. EEG recordings also demonstrate a shorter than normal interval between the onset of sleep and the first REM period, the so-called *REM latency*. This reduction in the initial period of non-REM sleep, which becomes much more common in elderly depressed patients (Kupfer et al., 1986), may be associated with the genetic form of unipolar disorder (Giles et al., 1989b).[19] Slow-wave sleep (stages 3 and 4) that normally occurs during this first non-REM period shifts into the second non-REM period, and total slow-wave sleep for the night is typically reduced. REM sleep is also distributed differently throughout the night, with more occurring in the first few hours of sleep than is normal. In addition, the frequency of eye movements during REM sleep is greater, a characteristic referred to as *increased REM density*.

Although some of the EEG abnormalities have been proposed as diagnostic markers of depression, most can also be found in other illnesses, psychiatric and nonpsychiatric, and, as noted, some of these changes also accompany normal aging. Gillin (1983) and Wehr and Sack (1988) conclude that sleep EEG findings in depression, like those related to the dexamethasone suppression test, appear to reflect abnormal functioning in sleep-related processes but lack diagnostic specificity. In their 1987 review, however, Reynolds and colleagues cite evidence that a certain cluster of abnormalities are more specific to endogenous depression than to Alzheimer's dementia, schizophrenia, and generalized anxiety disorder. These anomalies include the abbreviated first non-REM period, the redistribution of EEG delta activity (the deepest sleep) from the first to the second non-REM period, and the increased REM density in the first period. There are not yet enough replications of these findings, however, to convince us that these changes are indeed specific to major depressive disorder.

Another issue that awaits resolution is whether the sleep disturbances are traits of major unipolar depressive illness or merely concomitants of it. Rush and colleagues (1986a) found no significant changes in sleep variables 6 months after depressed patients became free of symptoms (2 to 5 weeks after they were no longer taking antidepressants), a finding that essentially replicates an earlier study by Avery and colleagues (1982) on a smaller number of patients. On the other hand, Reynolds and colleagues (1987) reported that a shortened REM latency persisted after remission from an acute episode.[20]

Sleep in the Bipolar Subgroup

The sleep of bipolar patients varies with clinical state and severity, and it probably changes as an episode progresses. During manic episodes, patients report that they sleep very little. During episodes of depression, they often report sleeping too much, but this hypersomnia appears predominantly in bipolar depression of mild to moderate severity. Sleep disturbances may be more pronounced when the bipolar depression is more severe, with endogenous or melancholic features. Complicating the picture are possible differences in the pattern of sleep in bipolar-I and bipolar-II patients. Unfortunately, most of the reports of sleep changes among bipolar patients do not distinguish bipolar I from II, possibly obscuring differences in bipolar and unipolar illness.

Much of the sleep research on bipolar patients, particularly that related to sleep duration, is confounded by artifact. Patients may be awakened, for example, to conform to hospital schedules. In the EEG literature, sleep duration in hypersomnic patients is almost certainly underestimated, since most sleep laboratories impose external constraints on patients' sleep schedules (e.g., patients are awakened at 7 AM). In a depressed bipolar patient who was permitted to sleep freely, daily sleep periods reached 12 hours and encompassed as many as nine cycles of REM and non-REM sleep (Wehr et al., 1985b). In settings where sleep was not disrupted by hospital routine, hypersomnia has been confirmed by EEG studies (Duncan et al., 1979).[21]

Although some studies have found that EEG sleep patterns in bipolar depressed patients are similar to those in unipolar depression (and different from normals), there are other reports of no differences between the bipolar patients and normal subjects. These included reports on normal REM sleep latencies,[22] the distribution of REM sleep throughout the night (Duncan et al., 1979; Thase et al., 1989). In some (Duncan et al., 1979;

Mendelson et al., 1987), but not all studies (Thase et al., 1989), the REM sleep of depressed bipolar patients is found to be significantly less efficient (more fragmented REM periods) than that of unipolar patients or normal individuals.[23]

The discrepancies in the sleep EEG literature on depressed bipolar patients may be due to different levels of clinical severity, variable proportions of bipolar-I and bipolar-II patients, and age differences (bipolar patients tend to be younger, and sleep abnormalities are most pronounced in older depressed patients). Thus, Giles and colleagues (1986) found no differences between bipolar-I and unipolar depressed patients (matched for age, sex, and severity), but they did find differences between the unipolar patients and the bipolar-II patients, who had longer REM latencies, more non-REM time, and hypersomnia.[24] Ansseau and colleagues (1984, 1985a) noted that depressed bipolar-II patients had more variability in REM latency ($p < 0.05$), as well as a trend toward more sleep-onset REM periods ($p < 0.07$), than did those with bipolar-I illness. Their findings are merely suggestive, however, since they were based on only a few patients.

As reviewed in Chapter 16, a critical question is whether the sleep differences reported among bipolar patients are state dependent or are trait (perhaps vulnerability) markers. At this writing, there is only preliminary information available. Knowles and colleagues (1986) studied ten remitted bipolar depressed patients for five nights. Although the patients showed slightly more sleep disturbance, there were no significant differences from age-matched controls. On the other hand, Sitaram and colleagues (1982) found increased density and percentage of REM among bipolar patients in the well state compared with normal controls. More striking, however, was their finding that when infused with arecoline (an acetylcholine agonist that can produce a shortened REM latency), the recovered bipolar patients in the well state were more sensitive to its effects on REM architecture than were the normal controls.

Sleep in mania is difficult to monitor polygraphically because patients may be uncooperative or sleep so little that monitoring is difficult. Until 1986, nearly all reports on unmedicated manic patients were single-case studies.[25] In general, they showed disturbances in sleep continuity, decreased time asleep, and reduced time spent in each stage of sleep. The percentage of time spent in stages 1, 2, and REM appear to be normal, but some studies showed less time spent in stages 3 and 4. Findings on REM latency and REM density are conflicting in these case reports.

Van Sweden (1986) studied two unmedicated severely manic patients who had been hospitalized after 2 and 3 weeks of mania. He found that, contrary to the common assumption and other reports that manic patients are unable to sleep, the EEGs of both patients showed stage 2 sleep within seconds of closing their eyes. In a more extensive study of six unmedicated manic men, Linkowski and colleagues (1986) found that REM latency, as well as the percentage of time spent in any stage of sleep, was no different than it was in age-matched normal men, although the patients took longer to fall asleep and spent less time asleep. In a slightly larger study, however, Hudson and colleagues (1988) found shorter REM latencies and higher REM densities in nine unmedicated manic patients than in normal controls. The patients showed hyposomnia and sleep continuity disturbances very similar to those shown in major depression. Unlike patients with major depression, however, the manic patients in the Hudson study did not have disturbances in delta sleep (stages 3 and 4).[26]

Experimental Alterations of Sleep in Affective Illness

After observing the effects of sleep on severely depressed patients, clinicians have from time to time concluded independently that sleep itself exacerbates depression. Ostenfeld (1986) reports that this clinical observation was one of several[27] that led him to try iatrogenic asomnia as a method for treating a bipolar manic-depressive patient in 1954, a time when the only available treatment known to be effective was electroconvulsive therapy. Since then, investigators using sleep deprivation and many other experimental manipulations of sleep have produced a body of evidence that suggests that the dramatic changes in the timing and duration of sleep during manic and depressive episodes are not mere epiphenomena.

It is now well established that total sleep deprivation (Pflug and Tölle, 1971) and partial sleep deprivation in the second half of the night (Schilgen and Tölle, 1980) can induce temporary remissions in depressed unipolar and bipolar patients (for reviews, see Gillin, 1983; Joffe and Brown, 1984; Wehr, in press). Of the nearly 1,500 depressed patients who have participated in sleep deprivation trials, the overall improvement rate is approximately 60 percent (see Chapter 22). Although patients usually relapse after sleeping again, even briefly, some observer ratings have shown that the depression may not be as deep as it was before the sleep deprivation. Wehr and Sack (1988) emphasize the importance of the sleep deprivation studies:

The single most important argument that sleep is an important factor in mental illness is the observation that sleep deprivation rapidly induces remissions in the majority of depressed patients, and induces mania in bipolar patients, and that recovery sleep after sleep deprivation rapidly induces depression in the majority of patients who have responded to sleep deprivation. (p. 208)

The therapeutic effect of sleep deprivation does not depend on the loss of sleep per se but is associated with not being asleep in the second half of the night. Thus, Sack and colleagues (1988a) compared an equivalent amount of sleep loss (4 hours) distributed either in the first or second half of the night. Improvement was associated only with being awake in the second half. In addition, advancing the entire sleep period by 6 hours has been shown to produce antidepressant effects (Wehr et al., 1979; Sack et al., 1985), further indicating that the clinical effect depends not on the amount of sleep, but rather on its timing. These relationships are illustrated in Figure 19-5. Unlike sleep deprivation, the improvement seen with ongoing phase advance treatment generally persists for about 2 weeks, presumably reflecting the time it takes for the circadian clock to fully reset itself. The link between the clinical effects of sleep deprivation and the phase advance hypothesis of depression is discussed subsequently.

Other Circadian Rhythm Disturbances

Early clinical studies of circadian rhythms in depression carried out in England in the 1950s and 1960s were inspired by Lewis and Lobban's discovery (1957) that placing a subject on unusual schedules during the Arctic summer alters the relative timing of his various circadian rhythms. The English clinical studies (see, e.g., Lobban et al., 1963; Palmai and Blackwell, 1965) were de-

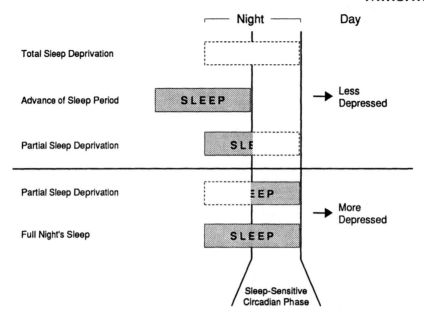

Figure 19-5. Relationship between the timing of sleep and the antidepressant effect of sleep deprivation (from Wehr and Goodwin, 1981a).

signed to explore whether early morning awakening in depressed individuals is related to an analogous but pathological internal phase disturbance. Early studies of circadian rhythms sometimes showed dramatic phase disturbances in depressive patients, but no consensus emerged about the significance and pattern of these changes. That situation appears to be changing. Until the 1970s, normal circadian physiology remained largely unexplored, so that no context was available in which to place findings on depression. Investigative groups studying circadian rhythms were distant from one another, their studies widely separated in time. Now an immense amount of work is being done on basic mechanisms of biological rhythms, and investigators at several centers have simultaneously constructed hypotheses using rhythmic processes to link biological findings in depression to behavioral, social, and environmental phenomena.[28] Specific studies dealing with circadian rhythms in manic-depressive illness—their phase position, stability, and amplitude—are integrated into the discussion of mechanisms that follows.

HYPOTHESIZED MECHANISMS OF CIRCADIAN DISTURBANCES

Early efforts to relate the sleep abnormalities of depression and mania to the pathophysiology of

the illness have evolved rapidly. Models that attempted to account for sleep anomalies were, shortly after their formulation, supplemented by circadian hypotheses that borrowed from concepts being developed in the broader field of chronobiology. An appreciation for the influence of longer, sometimes seasonal, cycles soon led investigators to examine yet another set of variables. What seems to be emerging from all of these conceptual endeavors is a dawning appreciation for the central, possibly integrative and regulatory, role played by rhythmic processes and the interconnection of mood, sleep, and energy. Given that the concept of cyclicity is inherent in these formulations, it is no wonder that rhythm models are attracting increasing attention among those interested in understanding the pathophysiology of this fundamental characteristic of manic-depressive illness.

Before discussing specific models of alterations in the timing of daily circadian rhythms and then possible homeostatic mechanisms, it is important to place the mechanism of circadian rhythm disturbances in a broader context. Figure 19-6 illustrates schematically a hypothesized relationship among genetic vulnerability, stress, circadian rhythm disturbances, neurotransmitter-neuroendocrine dysregulation, and the symptoms of manic-depressive illness. As discussed in Chapter 15, of the known vulnerability factors for

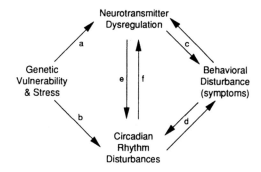

Figure 19-6. Hypothesized relationship among genetic vulnerability, stress, circadian rhythm disturbances, neurotransmitter–neuroendocrine dysregulation, and the symptoms of manic-depressive illness.

manic-depressive illness, the genetic ones are dominant. Thus, the recent identification of a specific mutation of the circadian system in golden hamsters is of considerable interest (Ralph and Menaker, 1988). The mutation, involving a single autosomal locus, is associated with a shortening of the intrinsic period of the circadian locomotor rhythm (i.e., a faster than normal clock) and an inability to entrain. There is preliminary evidence suggesting a similar speeding up of the circadian clock in rapid-cycling bipolar patients under free-running conditions. Further, a decreased capacity for entrainment in manic-depressive patients has been hypothesized to explain some of the clinical findings.

Implicit in the preceding discussion is the hypothesis that the genetic defect in some forms of manic-depressive illness involves the circadian clock. Stress is capable of producing both neurotransmitter-neuroendocrine dysregulation and circadian rhythm disturbances (Stroebel, 1969). Siever and colleagues (1987) have suggested that the circadian rhythm disturbances are secondary to neurotransmitter dysregulation. It is equally important to consider this alternative: that the circadian clock, by providing for the temporal ordering of CNS function, represents a principal organizing and regulating force, so that a primary circadian disturbance would produce widespread secondary neurotransmitter dysregulation (Wehr and Goodwin, 1983c; Healy, 1987).

The link between circadian rhythm disturbances and clinical symptoms (perhaps through neurotransmitter-neuroendocrine intermediaries) is, in our opinion, likely to be a closed loop, with rhythmic disturbances producing symptoms, which reinforce or exacerbate abnormal rhythmic processes—or vice versa, the arrows of causation going in both directions.

The Free-Running Hypothesis of Cyclic Mood Disorders

Among the first hypotheses of abnormalities in the biological rhythms of depressed individuals was Georgi's suggestion (1947) that the rhythms are out of synchrony. He proposed that the patient's own circadian rhythms are desynchronized either with one another (internal phase disorder) or with the entraining day/night cycle (external phase disorder).

Later, Halberg (1968) formulated a more specific version of a desynchronization hypothesis. He suggested that some circadian rhythms in affectively ill patients (perhaps particularly those with rapid cycles) may not be entrained to the 24-hour day cycle but free run, gradually going in and out of phase with other circadian rhythms that remain synchronized with the day/night cycle. According to Halberg, such phase disturbances leading to affective episodes would occur periodically every few days or weeks.

In support of Halberg's hypothesis, Kripke and associates (1978; Kripke, 1983) found that five of seven rapid-cycling manic-depressive patients had some circadian rhythms that appeared to free run with periods shorter than the 24-hour day/night cycle. Wehr's group (1985b) studied four patients under free-running (isolation) conditions (three bipolar and one unipolar).[29] One bipolar patient experienced an abnormally short intrinsic period, as predicted by the hypothesis of a fast circadian pacemaker. Unlike Kripke's group, Pflug and colleagues (1983) failed to detect free-running circadian rhythms in patients living on normal schedules, that is, entrained to the environment.[30]

The behavioral consequences of living under conditions without zeitgebers are not well understood. Although major mood disorders have not been reported among the normal subjects in these experiments, they have not often been looked for, and anecdotal accounts suggest that mood disturbances may occur (reviewed by Kripke, 1983). In contrast, the few manic-depressive patients studied in isolation, if anything, have shown improvement. Thus, one of the three bipolar patients studied by Wehr and colleagues (1985b) switched into mania and the one unipolar patient improved.

As observed by Wehr and Goodwin (1983c) and Kripke (1983), stable depression might occur in patients in whom an overly fast, intrinsic pacemaker rhythm causes circadian rhythms to become abnormally but stably advanced relative to the day/night cycle. Cyclic depression, on the other hand, may result from an overly fast rhythm that escapes from entrainment and free runs, advancing repeatedly through 360 degrees relative to the day/night cycle.

In a study by Wehr and colleagues (1982), most of the patients who had rapid (1 to 6 week) manic-depressive cycles experienced one or more double-length (48-hour) sleep-wake cycles at the onset of each manic phase of their mood cycle. Before switching from the depressed to the manic phase, they often have alternate nights of total insomnia. It is conceivable that these recurring escapes of the sleep-wake cycle from its primary (1:1) mode to its secondary (1:2) mode of coupling to the day/night cycle result from its driving oscillator having an overly long intrinsic period. Because the sleep-wake oscillator is weak, its oscillations remain relatively well coordinated with the day/night cycle and other circadian rhythms. Thus, the dissociation of its oscillations is expressed only in the periodic 24-hour phase jumps associated with the double-length sleep-wake cycles. Normal individuals in free-running circadian rhythm experiments sometimes experience similar 48-hour, sleep-wake cycles in conditions where all external time cues have been eliminated (Wever, 1979, 1983; Wehr et al., 1982; Weitzman et al., 1982). Thus, 48-hour sleep-wake cycles in manic patients may reflect normal sleep-regulating mechanisms under free-running conditions, perhaps associated with uncoupling of oscillators that are normally linked.

The possibility of free-running circadian rhythms has far-reaching implications for research on manic-depressive illness. Not only could such a mechanism drive the dramatic cyclicity observed in some bipolar patients, but it could also result in epiphenomena that are misinterpreted as biological correlates of changes in the mood cycle. If, for example, a biological variable is sampled at a fixed time of day, its level appears to change cyclically as the rhythm goes in and out of phase with the sampling time, even if its mean 24-hour level never changes.

Longitudinal studies with hamsters indicate that antidepressant drugs can slow the intrinsic rhythm of circadian oscillators and lead to the sleep-wake cycle lengthening and temporarily escaping from the primary mode of entrainment (Wehr and Wirz-Justice, 1982). Clinically, this drug effect might lead to the frequently recurring escapes and double-length (48-hour) sleep-wake cycles found naturalistically to be associated with switches into mania (Wehr et al., 1982). This mechanism might help to explain the observation of Wehr and Goodwin (1979, 1987a) (reviewed in Chapter 22) that maintenance tricyclics can induce rapid cycling in bipolar patients. Most of these patients experienced 48-hour sleep-wake cycles at the beginning of each manic phase. Based on carefully timed sleep deprivation experiments in patients with rapid cycles, Wehr and colleagues concluded that the insomnia associated with these 48-hour cycles probably helps to trigger switches into mania or exacerbates switches that have just begun. Thus, a drug-induced slowing of the intrinsic rhythm of circadian oscillators, leading to more frequent escapes from the primary mode of entrainment, may be a mechanism underlying the drug-induced rapid manic-depressive cycles.

Abnormalities of Phase Position

The Phase Advance Hypothesis

In his original formulation of the desynchronization hypothesis, Georgi linked depression to a phase disturbance:

In the true endogenous depressive we see a shift in the 24-hour rhythm, a phase shift, that can express itself from a slight phase shift to a complete reversal—the night becomes day. Anyone knowing the material would look for the CNS origin in the midbrain, where the entire vegetative nervous system is controlled by a central clock whose rhythmicity . . . regulates and balances the biological system. (1947, p. 1267)[31]

As noted earlier, the link between the patterns of REM sleep and nonsleep circadian processes was made in 1964 by Maron and colleagues. The following year, in one of the first EEG studies of sleep in depressed patients, Gresham and colleagues (1965) found that the normal pattern of REM sleep was altered. Depressive patients had more REM sleep than controls in the first third of the night and less REM sleep in the last third of the night. Most subsequent EEG sleep studies of depression are variations on this theme. All the changes in the temporal distribution of REM sleep in depressed patients may result from a phase advance of the circadian rhythm governing the propensity for REM sleep. If the rhythm were advanced, its maximum, instead of occurring near dawn, would occur nearer to the beginning of sleep (Papousek, 1975; Wehr and Goodwin, 1981).

In addition to REM propensity, the most extensively studied circadian rhythms among depressed patients are those of temperature and plasma cortisol. In 1981, Wehr and Goodwin reviewed all of the studies in which the circadian pattern of a biological or physiological variable in depressed patients was considered. They concluded that in the majority of studies, compared with control subjects, the phase position among the depressed patients (as reflected in the peak, nadir, or both) was variably advanced, generally occurring 1 to 4 hours earlier. Later, Aschoff observed (1983) that "phase advances of autonomic functions relative to the sleep-wake cycle seem to be among the best documented abnormalities in psychiatric research" (p. 37).

Souêtre and colleagues (in press), in a review of the literature on circadian rhythms in depression, found 80 studies involving a total of 1,061 patients. The reviewed studies showed considerable variability in their findings on cortisol, temperature, thyroid-stimulating hormone (TSH), melatonin, various neurotransmitter markers, heart rate, and motor activity. In 7 of 14 studies on temperature (185 patients) and 14 of 24 on plasma cortisol (350 patients), a phase advance was found, but statistically significant differences were infrequent (with 2 of the 13 cortisol studies and none of the 11 comparable temperature studies reporting statistics). However, reports of a phase delay were strikingly less frequent than would be expected by chance: only 1 of 10 studies, with none reporting a significant difference. We might conclude from this that if the phase position of one or more circadian rhythms is abnormal in a depressed patient, it is more likely to be advanced than delayed; that is, in general, circadian rhythms in depression appear to be unstable and variable, but with a tendency toward assuming a phase advanced position some of the time. This tendency is most clear in the case of the cortisol rhythm.

Distorting or masking factors may compromise the validity of description of circadian rhythms measured in the usual clinical setting. Whether the variable in question is the acrophase (peak) of a rhythm or its nadir (trough) may also be critical. Studies in normal subjects (e.g., Czeisler et al., 1980) have suggested that the acrophase of the cortisol circadian rhythm may be controlled by different physiological processes than its nadir and that the latter may be a better marker of circadian phase. Age is another factor that must be controlled in circadian studies, since studies of normals have shown that the phase of some rhythms advances with increasing age (e.g., Linkowski et al., 1985b,c for cortisol).[32] Other important variables are diagnostic: whether the patients are unipolar or bipolar, cyclic or relatively noncyclic. Thus, Linkowski and associates (1985b,c) found a significant phase advance in the cortisol nadir among unipolar patients but only a trend among the bipolar patients. However, of the four cortisol studies involving predominantly bipolar patients reviewed by Souêtre and associates (in press), three reported a nonsignificant phase advance, and none reported a delay. Of the six studies of temperature among predominantly bipolar patients, four noted a nonsignificant advance, and none reported a delay.

The phase advance hypothesis may be compatible with some evidence that tricyclic and monoamine oxidase inhibitor (MAOI) antidepressants, as well as lithium, delay the phase position of circadian rhythms in experimental animals (reviewed by Wehr and Wirz-Justice, 1982; Tamarkin et al., 1983; Duncan and Wehr, 1988). Although not all the animal findings are consistent, when an effect of these mood-altering drugs is seen, it is in the direction of phase delay. Thus, it is conceivable that a common mechanism of action might involve correction of the putative abnormal phase advance of depressed patients' circadian rhythms. Comparable studies in humans (i.e., under free-running conditions) are quite rare. The few that exist have failed to show "a uniform effect of psychoactive compounds on formal properties of the human circadian system" (Duncan and Wehr, 1988, p. 141).

One clinical antidepressant treatment that does appear to support the phase advance hypothesis is the sleep schedule shift described earlier (Wehr et al., 1979; Sack et al., 1985; Souêtre et al., 1985), although additional studies with more controls are needed. Figure 19-7 illustrates how depriving patients of sleep in the second half of the night or advancing their sleep may help to synchronize the abnormally advanced strong oscillator controlling REM sleep, temperature, and cortisol with the oscillator controlling sleep and wakefulness. By advancing sleep (or eliminating its second half), the abnormal phase relationship in the second half of the night would be corrected.

However, there are as yet no studies directly examining the relationship between circadian phase position and response to phase advance treatment, and other mechanisms may account for the effects of these sleep manipulations. For example, since REM sleep usually is more concentrated in the second half of the night, sleep deprivation during this phase would preferentially reduce REM sleep. Indeed, Vogel and colleagues (1980) have shown that selective REM deprivation has antidepressant effects. The suggestion that a selective reduction of REM might be important to the antidepressant effect of sleep deprivation also comes from a study of naps. Patients whose depressions lifted after losing a total night's sleep and who were allowed to nap the following day relapsed only if those naps contained REM sleep (Wiegand et al., 1986). These issues are discussed later under "Sleep Deprivation Hypotheses."

Figure 19-7. Hypothesized correction of abnormally advanced oscillator by partial sleep deprivation or phase advance treatment (from Wehr and Wirz-Justice, 1981a).

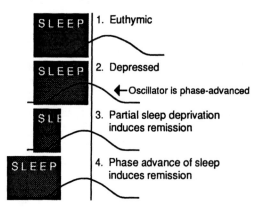

1. Euthymic

2. Depressed

←Oscillator is phase-advanced

3. Partial sleep deprivation induces remission

4. Phase advance of sleep induces remission

Phase Instability: Evidence From Longitudinal Studies of Temperature and REM Propensity

Longitudinal studies are used to investigate questions about phase stability as well as phase position. This literature, involving only a few patients, is dominated by studies of temperature[33] and REM.

Wehr and Goodwin (1983c) investigated sleep EEG and temperature for 240 days and nights in a 48-year-old manic-depressive woman, whose total mood cycle lasted about 6 weeks (Figure 19-8).[34] Transitions from mania to depression, or vice versa, usually occurred within the course of a single day or night; that is, they fit a square wave pattern. On the other hand, the temporal distribution of REM sleep and temperature shifted gradually; that is, their circadian phases advanced and delayed progressively over many days, following a sine wave pattern. Thus, REM latency became progressively shorter until the switch into depression and then became progressively longer until the switch from depression into mania, while, as expected, the length of the first REM period followed the inverse pattern. The peak of the temperature rhythm progressively advanced during the course of the 24-hour day until the time of the switch into depression, then progressively delayed until the time of the switch out of depression into mania.[35]

Pflug and associates (1976, 1981) measured oral temperature every 3 hours from 7 AM to 10 PM during depressive episodes in three manic-depressive patients. In two of them, the time of the daily temperature maximum advanced during each depressive episode, shifting back during nondepressed periods. Kripke and colleagues (1978) found in three of seven rapid-cycling manic-depressive patients that peaks in temperature rhythms progressively advanced 24 hours as the patients passed through their mood cycle. In other words, the temperature rhythm was no longer strictly entrained to the 24-hour day/night cycle but continually ran faster and went in and out of phase with it. These findings are similar to those of Wehr (1977): The temperature cycle is relatively advanced at one phase of the manic-depressive cycle and relatively delayed at another.

In general, changes in REM sleep variables

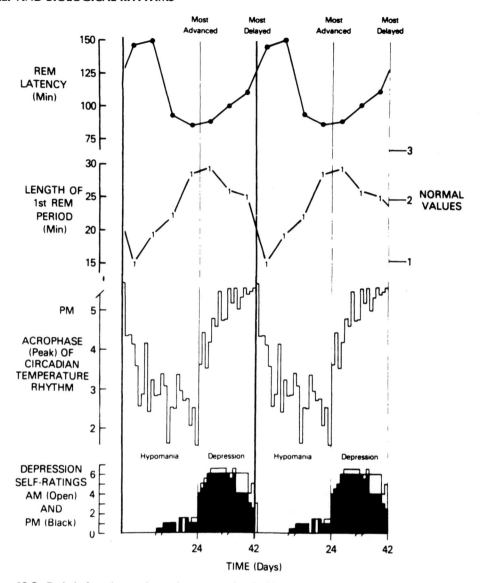

Figure 19-8. Period of maximum phase advance associated with switch into depression. Period of maximum phase delay produced switch out of depression (from Wehr and Goodwin, 1981).

and slow-wave sleep reportedly characteristic of depression are more accentuated during the depressive than the manic phases in rapid-cycling patients. In some cases, sleep EEG changes appear to anticipate the switch into depression (Post et al., 1976; Wehr, 1977; Cairns et al., 1980).

In summary, a few longitudinal case studies suggest a dramatic correspondence between changes in the circadian temperature rhythm and manic-depressive cycling. In two cases (Pflug et al., 1976, 1981; Wehr and Wirz-Justice, 1982), the temperature rhythm advanced several hours

during the switch into depression. In two other cases (Pflug et al., 1981), temperature rhythms advanced, then later delayed during the course of depressive episodes. In three cases (Kripke et al., 1978), the temperature rhythm advanced continually through all phases of the manic-depressive cycle. Only one study monitored both sleep EEG and temperature in the same patient (Wehr and Wirz-Justice, 1982). In that study, before the patient switched into depression, advances occurred in the phase position of the temperature rhythm that were accompanied by advances in the temporal distribution of REM sleep within the sleep period. Although not inconsistent with a circadian rhythm, phase advance model of depression, these data suggest that in cycling patients the circadian phase position may be more related to the stage of the episode than simply to the state of depression or mania per se.

Apparent instability of phase position may also characterize depression in noncycling patients. In their study of a mixed group of unipolar and bipolar depressed patients, Wehr and Goodwin (1983c) found a bimodal distribution in the time of the temperature minimum with many of the patients falling in both modes (early and late) when sampled on different days. Thus, there may be, on the one hand, a certain phase instability inherent to depression, perhaps reflecting poor entrainment by environmental zeitgebers, and, on the other hand, a phase instability linked to shifting phases of bipolar illness.

Amplitude of Circadian Rhythms

Schulz and Lund (1985) hypothesized that alterations in the timing of REM sleep could be explained by a "flattening of the arousal cycle . . . indicators of this hypothetical arousal cycle are measures of subjective sleepiness and body core temperature" (pp. 70–71). They based this hypothesis on their finding (Schulz and Lund, 1983) that subjects with sleep onset REM periods (perhaps reflecting phase advanced REM) had significantly reduced amplitude of the circadian temperature curve (peak to trough difference) compared with those without sleep onset REM periods. In their extensive review of the circadian literature in major depression, Soûétre and colleagues (in press) note that the majority of studies report some reduction in amplitude (blunting) of various measures. Overall, 75 percent of the studies (60 of 80) found reduced amplitude, reflecting considerably more consistency than the literature on phase position. Of the studies reporting statistical analyses, the reduction in amplitude was significant in 63 percent (36 of 57) and was most consistent for motor activity (4 of 4 studies), TSH (8 of 9 studies), and melatonin (9 of 12 studies), and less so for cortisol (3 of 12 studies). None of the 80 studies reported any increase in amplitude, even a nonsignificant one.

Like measures of phase position, amplitude estimates are not always straightforward. Although the peak to trough difference is a direct reflection of amplitude for smooth rhythms, such as temperature, it cannot be used for cortisol, with its many secretory pulses superimposed on the underlying circadian rhythm. Meaningful analysis of the cortisol rhythm requires some kind of curve fitting, which probably contributes to the greater variability in this literature.

A variety of antidepressant treatments have been reported to increase circadian amplitudes of temperature, cortisol, or TSH in patients, including tricyclic antidepressants, ECT, bright light, sleep deprivation, and phase advance treatment.[36] In addition, increased amplitudes of neurotransmitter-receptor rhythms have been observed in animals after chronic administration of tricyclic antidepressants but not after an MAO inhibitor (Wirz-Justice, 1983).

Critical Summary and Integration

The circadian literature is subject to all the methodological problems inherent in clinical studies (e.g., diagnostic heterogeneity, variable medication status, age and sex differences) and has special problems of its own. In addition to masking (particularly the impact of sleep and activity levels on the underlying circadian rhythms), the principal problem is the overreliance on cross-sectional snapshot studies, which, with the exception of a handful of case studies of temperature and REM, rarely involve more than a single 24-hour period of observation. Indeed, the available longitudinal data indicate considerable within-patient variability in phase position of the temperature and REM rhythms—a variability that reflects, at least in part, circadian shifts in association with the evolving stages of depressive and manic episodes.

Although the methodological problems described suggest caution in drawing sweeping conclusions, some integrative suggestions might be helpful in the design of future studies. The challenge is to link (1) decreased amplitude, (2) phase instability with a tendency toward phase advance over delay, and (3) a faster than normal clock in some of the few rapid-cycling manic-depressive patients who have been studied. Let us consider each of these individually.

If relatively low amplitude rhythms were somehow intrinsic to depression or manic-depressive illness, we would expect such rhythms to be more vulnerable to perturbation by internal or external influences, since the stability of a circadian system is positively correlated with amplitude (Wever, 1980; Aschoff, 1980). Not only do the frequency and timing of environmental zeitgebers vary considerably under normal conditions, but also the dramatic behavioral shifts associated with manic-depressive illness multiply this variability. Thus, blunted amplitudes associated with affective disorder would be expected to produce phase instability.

One explanation for a decreased circadian amplitude is poor entrainment by external zeitgebers (Aschoff and Wever, 1981), as observed in normal individuals isolated from time cues under free-running conditions. Such reduced or irregular entrainment—initially the consequence of depression (due, e.g., to loss of social zeitgebers during withdrawal)—could then feed the depression through the resulting disturbance in rhythms (Ehlers et al., 1988). In this context, it is necessary to consider a paradox. Lewy and colleagues (1981; 1985a) found that, compared with normal controls, manic-depressive patients are supersensitive to light, as reflected by a lower threshold required to reduce nighttime plasma melatonin levels, and this supersensitivity appears to be state independent. If increased sensitivity to light is a trait marker of manic-depressive illness, how can one posit decreased entrainment of zeitgebers? First, although light is indeed important to entrainment, it is hardly the only influence, since activity and temperature are each important. Second, one could view the increased sensitivity to light as compensatory, that is, an attempt to offset the reduced entrainment due to either the compromising of other zeitgebers (e.g., activity) by the illness or to an intrinsic defect in the clock mechanism. The latter possibility is particularly interesting in light of evidence that monkeys with lesions in the SCN can compensate by becoming more sensitive to certain zeitgebers (Van Cauter and Turek, 1986).

It is also possible to consider the inverse relationship—that the phase instability is primary, producing the *appearance* of a low amplitude when individual data are averaged for a group. We might refer to this as a smearing effect. In the extreme, if individuals' phase positions were randomly distributed along the time axis, the group mean would exhibit no circadian rhythm. If the pattern were simply smeared by interindividual variability, the average amplitude for the group would appear decreased (Wehr and Goodwin, 1983c).

The preceding discussion is relevant only to phase instability. What about the apparent tendency for this instability in phase position to express itself as a phase advance? One situation that might produce both instability and a bias toward advance would be a clock with an intrinsic period length of about 24 hours. That is faster than the normal period of the rest-activity cycle in humans when measured under free-running conditions, which is about 25 hours. Basic research on the factors that determine circadian phase position under conditions of entrainment (Pittendrigh and Daan, 1976; Wever, 1979) indicates that the faster the intrinsic period of the pacemaker or clock, the earlier is its phase position relative to the entraining schedule—that is, it is relatively phase advanced. Furthermore, if the intrinsic period of the clock is just fast enough so that it happens to coincide with the external day/night cycle (i.e., 24 hours), it might be expected to wobble, that is, to be unstable. This is so because, under normal conditions, the intrinsic period is slower than 24 hours, a discrepancy that produces constant tension in the system—the 24-hour environmental light/dark cycle continuously pulls forward the intrinsic 25-hour clock. This constant tug of the environment on the internal circadian mechanisms would be expected to provide stability. Under conditions where the intrinsic period of the clock is very close to the external day/night cycle, little or no tug or tension exists, and the clock is free to wobble. This mechanism would tie together the evidence of a faster than normal clock in some patients with the findings of phase instability and the tendency toward advance.

Another possible explanation for phase advance is an increased sensitivity to zeitgebers. Given that in humans the intrinsic period of the circadian pacemaker is slower than that of the environment, environmental zeitgebers tend to pull it closer to 24 hours, and a pacemaker that is more sensitive to zeitgebers might be expected to assume a relatively more advanced phase position (Wever, 1979). Relevant to this observation is the finding that manic-depressive patients show an increased sensitivity to light, which appears to be independent of the state of illness (see Chapter 20).

Obviously, the many gaps and even some apparent contradictions in the circadian literature prevent a complete synthesis. Clinical heterogeneity is a major confounding variable and may well explain seeming contradictions. Thus, much of the cross-sectional data on phase amplitude and position are from unipolar patients, whereas the data on a faster than normal clock are from rapid-cycling patients and the increased light sensitivity has been found in bipolar patients. The suggestion that unipolar patients are more phase disturbed than are bipolar patients[37] simply may reflect more consistency in the unipolar literature; that is, there may be greater variance among bipolar patients, because of the impact of variable stages of illness on circadian phase, particularly among those with rapid cycles.

Throughout this discussion, we have referred, explicitly or implicitly, to the concept of a closed loop involving the circadian system and the phenomenology (and biochemistry) of depressive and manic episodes. We return to this subject here because it remains the most significant conceptual challenge in interpreting the circadian literature. Until we have more data from manic-depressive patients studied under free-running conditions, we will not be able to answer the question of whether a disturbance in the function of the circadian clock is primary and, therefore, driving the symptoms or is itself simply a physiological symptom secondary to the large shifts in mood, sleep, and behavior that characterize the illness. This possibility deserves further consideration in light of recent evidence showing that behavioral arousal may feed back directly on the circadian pacemaker's behavior (Mrosovsky, 1988).

OTHER RELATED MECHANISMS OF SLEEP DISTURBANCES

Other mechanisms have been proposed to account for the disturbed sleep of affective disorders and the clinical effects of sleep deprivation. Although not, strictly speaking, circadian, they are closely related to and overlap with the observations of circadian physiology just reviewed.

As previously discussed, the McCarley-Hobson model of separate REM-enhancing and REM-inhibiting neuronal populations is consistent with the concept that REM sleep might be controlled by the balance of cholinergic (agonistic) and noradrenergic (antagonistic) neurotransmission. The relevance of this observation to the pathophysiology of sleep disturbances in manic-depressive illness is suggested by its fit to the cholinergic-noradrenergic balance hypothesis of Janowsky and colleagues (1972), which is reviewed in Chapters 15 and 17. If depression is associated with a relative increase in cholinergic tone (or decrease in noradrenergic tone), this might be associated with an increase in REM propensity and shortened REM latency. However, since the clinical data focus on changes in REM latency, which could reflect either an overall change in REM propensity or a phase shift, it is difficult to use these data to compare circadian and noncircadian models.

Homeostatic Models

Homeostatic models posit that the onset and maintenance of sleep are regulated by the interaction of two processes, a circadian process, C, and a sleep-dependent process, S (Borbély, 1982). This model envisions that a sleep-inducing process or substance (process S) gradually accumulates during wakefulness and eventually results in sleep. The amount of slow-wave sleep, which depends largely on the duration of prior wakefulness, has been considered the primary reflection of this homeostatic process. In one explanation of depressive sleep, Borbély and Wirz-Justice (1982) attribute decreases in sleep duration and in the amount of slow-wave sleep to a deficiency in the sleep-inducing, homeostatic process during wakefulness. Process S represents a need for non-REM sleep, while process C reflects the circadian variation in the threshold for the onset of sleep (Van den Hoofdakker and Beersma, 1985).

The hypothesis consists essentially of the proposition that the build-up of Process S during waking is deficient in depressives and therefore does not rise to its usual level. As a consequence, its level in depressive patients is below that of normal controls throughout the major part of the sleep period. It was further proposed that the pathologically low level of S can be normalized by the prolongation of waking time, an effect that is considered to underlie the antidepressant action of sleep deprivation therapy. (Borbély et al., 1984, p. 28)

In quantitative analyses of sleep EEG data, the level of process S is presumed to be reflected by a certain portion of the EEG spectrum. Kupfer and colleagues (1986) found the predicted low levels of delta sleep measured with an automated analyzer, and Borbély and associates (1984) found correspondingly low levels of power density of the EEG in patients. However, two studies in which EEG spectral analysis was performed (Van den Hoofdakker et al., 1986; Mendelson et al., 1987) yielded the somewhat surprising finding of no difference in EEG power density between depressed and normal subjects, even when conventional manual scoring of EEG records showed reduced slow-wave sleep in the depressed patients. These findings imply that although the amount of slow-wave activity in sleep EEG recordings during depression may be normal, slow waves are dispersed or attenuated and thus escape detection by manual scoring criteria.

The process S deficiency hypothesis is consistent with the antidepressant effects of sleep deprivation. Since S rises during wakefulness and falls during sleep, sleep deprivation extends the wakeful period during which S can accumulate. With added time to build up S levels, depressive patients can compensate for their low S accumulation rate. The process S model is intended to explain the loss of sleep in depression. Given that many bipolar patients exhibit hypersomnia (albeit perhaps of lower quality), the application of this hypothesis to bipolar illness may be different. Presumably the shorter duration of wakefulness that accompanies hypersomnia would lead to a reduced buildup of S, which in turn would produce less slow-wave sleep. Thus, although bipolar depressed patients may sleep long hours, the sleep may still be deficient in its deeper stages.

Sleep Deprivation Hypotheses

The mechanisms of the clinical effect of sleep deprivation implied in the phase advance or process S deficiency hypotheses are not the only ones to have been proposed. Early sleep investigators observed that changes in REM sleep are a late complication of depression. Snyder (1972) noted that most patients are studied during a late phase of illness, and he suggested that at this time the initial severe insomnia is improving and sleep is rebounding. In normal subjects, REM sleep rebound after REM sleep deprivation is associated with short REM latency and increased REM density. Normal subjects, unlike depressed patients,

have increased total REM sleep, which shows the normal temporal distribution. Some prospective longitudinal studies of sleep during the switch into depression fail to show a period of decreased REM sleep during the initial phase of the episode (Post et al., 1974a; Cairns et al., 1980).

As noted earlier, the observed benefits of sleep deprivation in depressed patients and the mania associated with loss of sleep in some manic-depressive patients (Wehr, et al., 1986, 1987a,c) not only has suggested new treatments but also has pointed to new approaches to understanding etiology. Reducing REM may be one mechanism by which sleep deprivation has its effect. Vogel and associates (1980) noted a similarity between the sleep of depressed patients at the beginning of the night and that of normal people who slept later than usual in the morning. In both situations, successive REM sleep periods tend to grow shorter, and REM density is increased. Thus, depressed patients appear to begin sleep with a pattern normally typical of its end. Vogel suggests that in normal individuals some factor inhibits or postpones REM sleep at the beginning of the night but is exhausted during the course of the night's sleep, and, further, that this factor is deficient in depression.

Nocturnal Temperature and Endocrine Changes

In depression, nighttime temperatures are higher than normal,[38] the principal factor producing the reduced amplitude of the circadian temperature rhythm in depression. As noted previously, although non-REM sleep is associated with heat loss, one function of REM may be thermogenesis, that is, to maintain brain heat while the sleeping body cools. In depression, the increased REM in the second half of the night could overheat the brain, and this excess brain heat, occurring at a critical circadian period, may be associated with depressive symptoms (Wehr, in press,a). Consistent with this formulation is the recent preliminary observation by Wehr (in press,b) that the antidepressant effects of sleep deprivation depend on environmental temperature. Clinical improvement was seen at a cool room temperature (21°C) but not at a warmer temperature (32°C).[39]

TSH is released from the pituitary in response to its trophic hormone, TRH, from the hypothalamus and other areas of the brain. As reviewed in Chapter 17, TSH has been of interest in affective illness because its release of TRH has been reported to be blunted in depression. Following its normal circadian rhythm, plasma levels of TSH are highest at night (Weeke, 1973), although this nocturnal increase is partially masked by sleep (Parker et al., 1976). Among patients with major depression, the circadian rhythm is blunted; that is, there is a loss of the normal nocturnal increase (reviewed in Sack et al., 1987), a finding that may be secondary to the elevated nocturnal temperatures in depression. In depressed patients, sleep deprivation produces an increase in nocturnal TSH, an effect that may reflect both release of the sleep inhibition and an interruption of REM, with the attendant decrease in brain warming. Consistent with this formulation is the observation that the sleep deprivation-induced rise in nocturnal TSH, like the antidepressant effect, is blunted in the presence of high environmental temperature (Wehr, personal communication). Thus, sleep deprivation may produce its clinical effect by activating TSH changes. This possibility and others can be investigated with pharmacological probes, such as TRH, that might mimic or block the effects of sleep deprivation.

In addition to its powerful effects on TSH, sleep deprivation also inhibits prolactin (Parker et al., 1974) and growth hormone[40] (Takahashi et al., 1968), and it increases cortisol (Weitzman et al., 1982).

SEASONAL PATTERNS

Melancholy occurs in autumn whereas mania in summer.
—Posidonius, 4th Century AD[41]

Repeatedly I saw in these cases moodiness set in in autumn and pass over in spring, "when the sap shoots in the trees," to excitement, corresponding in a certain sense to the emotional changes which come over even healthy individuals at the changes of the seasons. (p. 139)   —Emil Kraepelin, 1921

. . . the gloom of the Arctic night sets in, and although the Eskimos spent their time telling stories and legends and tried hard to amuse us, I could notice a depression among ourselves, as well as among the people . . . that reached its climax at Christmas. . . . we were all very blue.   —Frederick A. Cook, M.D., 1894, Surgeon to the Peary Arctic Expedition[42]

As noted at the beginning of the chapter, the clinical lore surrounding affective disorders has alluded to their seasonal nature since ancient times. Seasonal trends emerge in the epidemiology of populations of patients, and seasonal patterns become evident in the course of manic-depressive illness in individual patients. Onsets of episodes tend to cluster in the spring and fall, especially among those who tend to have annual recurrences. As Wehr and Rosenthal (1989) point out, these patterns imply that environmental changes can both cause and ameliorate episodes of affective illness.

In the 19th century, unlike today, psychiatrists had the opportunity to observe the course of untreated manic- depressive illness for long periods. Several leading psychiatrists of the era, including Esquirol (Baillarger, 1854b), Griesinger (1867), Falret (1890), and Kraepelin (1921), recorded many cases in which the pattern of recurrences was seasonal. In one pattern, depressions began in spring and summer. In another, the onset of depression occurred in fall or winter, then mania or hypomania appeared in the summer. These patterns also show up in longitudinal data published by Baastrup and Schou in their now classic lithium studies (1967) and, more recently, by Kukopulos and Reginaldi (1973). Analysis of the frequency distribution of the cycle lengths of episodes drawn from a longitudinal study of 105 bipolar patients (Zis et al., unpublished data) shows a very large peak at 12 months, with smaller peaks at subsequent multiples of 12 (Figure 19-9A). Although reporting bias may account for some of this, it is probably not sufficient to explain the size of this effect.

Slater (1938a) was the first to apply systematic statistical analysis to the study of seasonal patterns among manic-depressive patients. He noted that for each patient, recurrences were significantly more likely to occur at the same time of the year than at random; that is, variability in the month of onset for any one patient was less than half the variability between patients. The study of seasonality did not resurface in the literature for nearly half a century. In the early 1980s, a specific syndrome, winter depression, one form of seasonal affective disorder, was identified and since has been extensively investigated in the United States, Europe, Great Britain, Australia, and South America.

Wehr and Rosenthal (1989) attribute the long hiatus in psychiatric interest in seasonality to changing fashions in theory—from the ancient humoral theories that emphasize seasonal influences to contemporary theories that emphasize

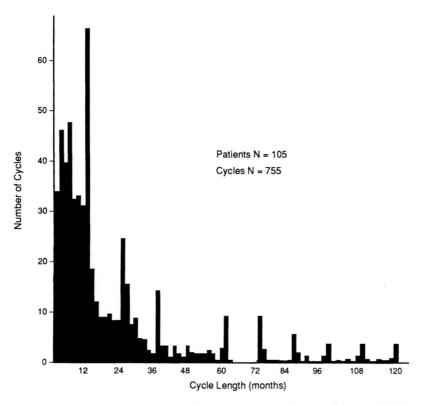

Figure 19-9A. Seasonal variation in the length of the photoperiod and in its rate of change: Relationship to seasonal peaks in depression, mania, and suicide.

internal psychological and biological processes. Another possible reason for this recent neglect, according to Wehr and Rosenthal, may be that modern life has so shielded psychiatric observers from environmental influences that they no longer consider seasonal patterns, which in addition have become obscured by modern treatments. They also note that both psychiatrists and patients may now tend to see episodes of affective illness as linear rather than cyclical, a shift in thinking about time that may be general in the culture.

Epidemiology of Seasonality

It is striking how few of the modern studies of major affective illness have examined seasonality, despite its clinical and theoretical importance and the fact that seasonal components in depression and mania have been observed for centuries. Many sources of variance bedevil the collection of seasonality data. For example, hospital admission dates, although likely to be meaningful markers for the onset of manic episodes, are unlikely to reflect the true onset of depressive

episodes. In fact, hospitalizations for depressions are more likely to reflect severity or lethality of illness than onset. Voluntary admissions and hospital schedules (rotation of physician staff or holidays) may affect seasonal patterns, and diagnostic criteria vary from hospital to hospital. Despite these methodological problems, the consistency of findings in the seasonality studies of both affective episodes and suicide is noteworthy (Eastwood and Peter, 1988). The evidence gains further weight from the fact that virtually all the studies were carried out after the widespread use of lithium had begun, which may have dampened the natural pattern of seasonal variability. A familiar problem in studies of the seasonal incidence of depression is that results for bipolar patients usually are not reported separately from those for unipolar patients.

Certain patterns emerge from an examination of the studies of seasonality. Two broad peaks are evident in seasonal incidence of major depressive episodes: spring and autumn. This pattern tends to parallel the seasonal pattern for suicide—a

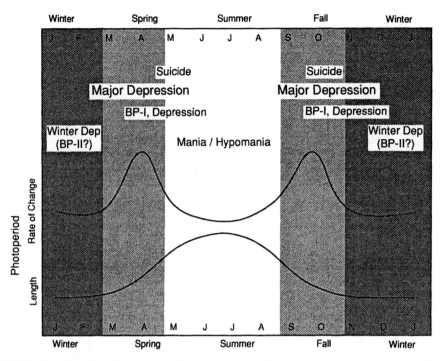

Figure 19-9B. Frequency distribution of cycle lengths among bipolar patients, showing 12-month peaks (data from Zis et al., unpublished observations).

large peak in the spring, a smaller one in October (see Chapter 10).

The data on mania are somewhat more scarce and, therefore, a bit less compelling, but the peak incidences occur in the summer months. Myers and Davies (1978) and Carney and colleagues tients show an increased sensitivity to light, (1988) showed significant correlations of admissions for mania with monthly total hours of sunshine and average monthly day length, but their results differ with respect to environmental temperature.[43]

Figure 19-9B displays these spring and fall peaks in major depression and suicides and also includes the more recently reported seasonal affective disorder (SAD) predominantly characterized by regularly recurring atypical depressions in the winter, often with hypomania in the summer. The light/dark cycle shown in Figure 19-9B is the principal seasonal variable of interest. Note that the overall length of the photoperiod has two extremes, longest in summer and shortest in winter, whereas the rate of change in the ratio of light to dark has two peaks, one in late winter/early spring, the other in late summer/early fall.[44]

Thus if manic-depressive patients were abnormally sensitive to seasonal light changes, this could be reflected either by opposite behavioral patterns at the two extremes (winter and summer) or behavioral disturbances in early spring or early fall reflecting the period of rapidly increasing light and rapidly decreasing light, respectively.

Another factor to be considered in interpreting the more recent studies is seasonal variation in the effects of drugs, particularly lithium (Garver and Hutchinson, 1988). The seasonality literature has been extensively reviewed by Wehr and Rosenthal (1989) and by Eastwood and Peter (1988).

Seasonal variations in mood and behavior appear to be common in the general population as well as in individuals with affective disorders. Eastwood and colleagues (1985) compared the infradian rhythms of mood, sleep, anxiety, and energy over a period of 14 months in 30 patients with affective illness (25 of whom were bipolar) and 34 healthy control subjects matched for age and sex. They found that the majority of patients and many of the healthy subjects had infradian rhythms in mood, energy, and sleep,[45] and about half of these were seasonal.

The principal difference between patients and control subjects is the amplitude of cycles, and hence, affective symptoms may be considered a variant of normal hedonic states. . . . Affective symptoms seem to be universal, with a periodic component that differs in degree rather than kind; the pattern of cycles for ill persons is defined by amplitude. This makes affective disorder akin to hypertension and diabetes, wherein a physiological variable shades into a pathological variant. (Eastwood et al., 1985, p. 298)

Eastwood's group hypothesizes that, because half of the rhythms are seasonal, "some infradian mood cycles may be driven or timed by meteorologic factors" (p. 298). They further suggest that a "familial tendency toward depression may be the factor that determines the amplitude of the cycle."

In a recent survey based on a random sample of one Maryland county, Kasper and colleagues (1989b) noted that seasonal changes were reported as problematic by more than a quarter of the sample, and for 4.3 percent, the seasonal depression was severe enough to meet criteria for major affective disorder. In general, depressed mood is not prominent in the subsyndromal forms that are dominated by lethargy, increased need for sleep, increased appetite, and functional impairment.

Patterns of Seasonal Affective Disorder

In the contemporary literature, recognition of a syndrome characterized by the regular reappearance of affective episodes at certain seasons of the year came as recently as 1984, when Rosenthal and colleagues, studying recurrent winter depressions, often with summer hypomania, published the original criteria for seasonal affective disorder. By 1987, criteria for a seasonal pattern of mood disorders had been incorporated into DSM-III-R. Table 19-1 compares the original criteria of Rosenthal and colleagues with the broader criteria of DSM-III-R, which encompass other seasonal patterns. This rapid acceptance of SAD may be due to the accompanying discovery that very bright light is an effective treatment for the condition in many patients with winter SAD (see Chapter 22).

Recurrent Winter Depression

Winter depression, the best studied of the recently identified seasonal affective disorders, has been observed primarily in women, although the

Table 19-1. Criteria for Seasonal Affective Disorder and Seasonal Pattern

Seasonal Affective Disorder Rosenthal et al., 1984	Seasonal Pattern DSM-III-R, 1987
1. Recurrent fall-winter depressions	1. Regular temporal relationship between onset of episode of affective disorder and a particular 60-day period of the year
2. No seasonally varying psychosocial variables that might account for the recurrent depressions	2. Do not include cases in which there is an obvious effect of seasonally related psychosocial stressors, e.g., regularly being unemployed every winter
3. Regularly occurring nondepressed periods in the spring and summer	3. Full remissions (or a change from depression to hypomania or mania) within a 60-day period of the year
4. At least two of the depressions occurred during consecutive years	4. At least three episodes of mood disturbance in three separate years that demonstrated the temporal relationship defined in 1 and 3; at least two of the years were consecutive
5. At least one of the depressions has met Research Diagnostic Criteria (Spitzer et al., 1978a) for major depression	5. The corresponding criterion is implicit here as "seasonal pattern" is provided as a modifier of other DSM-III-R diagnoses, bipolar disorder or recurrent major depression
6. No other Axis I psychopathology	6. Seasonal episodes of mood disturbance outnumbered nonseasonal episodes by more than 3 to 1

From Rosenthal et al., in press

percentage of identified male patients is increasing. Onset most often occurs in the second and third decades of life, but several cases in children also have been reported. The presence of winter depression increases as the latitude gets closer to the pole (Potkin et al., 1986; Lingjaerde et al., 1986; Rosenthal et al., 1988b). Around Washington, DC, the area where the first studies were done, depressions usually begin in October or November (Figure 19-10A, B); in the southern hemisphere, winter depressions generally begin in April or May (Boyce and Parker, 1988). They are characterized by hypersomnia, hyperphagia, anergia, carbohydrate craving, and weight gain, symptoms considered atypical in unipolar depression but common in bipolar patients. Other symptoms include the usual features of depression, especially decreased libido, and hopelessness, suicidal thoughts, and social withdrawal. Depressions usually end by March and may be followed by hypomania, mania, or normal mood in the spring and summer. True winter depression can be associated with considerable functional impairment,[46] apparently representing one end of a spectrum of seasonal variation.

Because 50 to 60 percent of patients with winter depression have first-degree relatives with major affective illness, this form of SAD is probably part of the general spectrum of major affective disorders that includes manic-depressive illness. Rosenthal and colleagues (in press) note that most patients with winter depression are sensitive to decreased ambient light even when it occurs during other seasons:

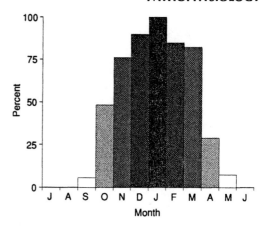

Figure 19-10B. Percent of subjects experiencing depression each month (from Rosenthal et al., 1984).

Thus patients may become depressed during a spell of cloudy weather at any time of the year and at any latitude. Similarly, patients may be symptomatic even in sunny weather if they are confined indoors in dark environments for much of the day. This situation can produce a type of perennial SAD, which may be light responsive. A clue to diagnosing such cases is a report of chronic depressions with winter exacerbations. In some cases symptoms can be improved by light throughout the year, whereas in others only the winter component of the problem may be light responsive.

Reports in the literature vary considerably in the proportion of patients with recurrent winter depressions who also meet criteria for hypomania or mania in the summer (Table 19-2). Differences in the threshold for the diagnosis of hypomania no doubt account for some of these differences. For example, Rosenthal and colleagues (1987) originally reported that 89 percent of their patients with winter depression were bipolar (predominantly bipolar II). When the same group was subsequently rediagnosed according to the very stringent DSM-III-R criteria using the SCID[47] instrument, the bipolar portion had dropped to 57 percent (Rosenthal et al., in press). However, diagnostic criteria are probably only part of the reason for this inconsistency. Climate and latitude also may affect the expression of polarity. Those areas with more extreme swings in ambient light may be associated with more bipolar cases.[48] Another possible influence is the phototherapy that patients are receiving in some of the prospective studies of winter depression. If light treatment successfully flattens out one phase of the cycle by eliminating the winter trough, the

Figure 19-10A. Average daily photoperiod for Rockville, MD (from Rosenthal et al., 1984).

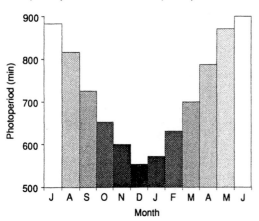

Table 19-2. Relationship Between Seasonality and Polarity

Study	Patients with SAD N	Bipolar %
Rosenthal et al., 1985b	125	90 (82 BPII, 8 BPI)
Wirz-Justice et al., 1986	22	77 (BPII)
Yerevanian et al., 1986	9	11
Rosenthal & Wehr, 1987	220	89 (83 BPII, 6 BPI)
Garvey et al., 1988	18	56
Depue, 1989[a]	50	100
Lewy et al., 1989[a]	40	8 (5 BPII, 3 BPI)
Terman et al., 1989[a]	112	28 (26 BPII, 2 BPI)
Thase et al., 1989[a]	18	17
Hellekson, unpublished data	17	82 (BPII)
Rosenthal et al., unpublished data	23	57

[a] Cited as personal communication by Hellekson (1989)

subsequent phase (summer hypomania) might be flattened out as well. From a theoretical point of view, what is probably most important is that the syndrome is essentially bipolar in that the mood and behavior are opposite in the two seasons even though they may not pass a certain threshold in the summer.[49]

Recurrent Summer Depression

Wehr and colleagues (1987b, 1989) identified a reverse pattern of SAD with regular summer depression (usually beginning in May and ending in September), often accompanied by hypomania in the winter (half of the patients in the Wehr et al. study). A similar pattern was identified in the southern hemisphere (Australia) by Boyce and Parker (1988). This pattern, which in the Washington, DC, area is only 20 to 25 percent as prevalent as winter SAD, is characterized by depressions that differ substantially from winter depression. Typical endogenous symptoms predominate: insomnia, decreased appetite, weight loss, and agitation or anxiety.[50] Such patients often have histories of summer trips to the north, where they find relief from their depression in cold climates. Generally, normal air conditioning is not sufficient. One patient, for example, only found relief by regularly swimming in a cold New Hampshire lake.

Spring and Fall Peaks

The substantial spring peak and a smaller fall peak for the onset of major depression (and suicide) are evident in epidemiological surveys that vary considerably in their diagnostic methodology and criteria for determining onset. How to relate these phenomena to descriptions of regularly recurring winter and summer SAD is not yet clear. Wehr has hypothesized that this specific form of summer depression may be similar to the much larger universe of typical endogenous (predominantly unipolar) depressions with a late spring peak of onset. Likewise, he views the fall peak as corresponding to the onset of winter SAD.

The Neurobiology of Winter and Summer SAD

Mechanisms of Artificial Light in Winter Depression

As noted earlier, seasonal variation in the timing and duration of daylight triggers changes in animal behavior and physiology. Food producers have exploited this well-established phenomenon by using artificial light to coax animals to breed and plants to bloom out of season. Seasonal patterns in affective illness led clinical investigators to question whether changes in natural light might be involved and subsequently to explore the use of artificial light to treat winter depression (Lewy et al., 1980, 1982; Rosenthal et al., 1984) (see Chapter 22). Treatment with very bright artificial light has so far been significantly beneficial in approximately 80 percent of patients with winter depression (see Chapter 22).

An important question relates to the specificity of the therapeutic effect: Is bright artificial light beneficial to depressed patients who do not fit the criteria for winter SAD? Yerevanian and colleagues (1986) found that bright light was not effective in patients with nonseasonal depression, although Kripke and colleagues (1986) reported modest activation in such patients. In normal subjects with little or no seasonal variation, bright light did not show beneficial effects (Kasper et al., 1989a) but did produce improvement in individuals with mild SAD-like symptoms.

Three principal hypotheses have been advanced to explain the mechanism of phototherapy (Wehr and Rosenthal, 1989). From studies in animal models, N.E. Rosenthal and associates (1986b) hypothesized that phototherapy ameliorates SAD by suppressing nocturnal pineal melatonin secretion.

. . . changes in the length of the day (photoperiod) trigger winter depression by modifying the pattern of nocturnal melatonin secretion, which acts as a chemical signal of darkness. According to this model, phototherapy should be effective only when it is administered before dawn or after dusk, thus interrupting the long winter night and abbreviating the phase of active melatonin secretion. Phototherapy should be ineffective when it is administered after dawn and before dusk, leaving the photoperiod and the pattern of melatonin secretion unchanged. (Wehr and Rosenthal, 1989, p. 834)

Three observations mitigate against this hypothesis: (1) Although administration of melatonin to remitted patients during light treatments reproduces some of the atypical symptoms of depression, such as fatigue, hypersomnia, and hyperphagia, it fails to induce relapses with typical symptoms as reflected in the Hamilton Rating Scale for Depression (N.E. Rosenthal et al., 1986b). (2) Administration of atenolol, a beta-adrenergic antagonist that suppresses melatonin secretion, is relatively ineffective in the treatment of winter SAD (Rosenthal et al., 1988b). (3) Light administered in the middle of the day, which has little effect on the already low daytime levels of melatonin, is an effective treatment for winter SAD (Wehr et al., 1986; Jacobsen et al., 1987b).[51]

The second hypothesized mechanism of phototherapy, proposed by Lewy and colleagues (1985b, 1987a,b), is based on experimental evidence that phototherapy administered in the morning appears to advance the phase of circadian rhythms. According to the hypothesis, this shift corrects the timing of circadian rhythms, which are abnormally delayed in winter depression. Evidence conducted by other groups has

been inconsistent, with some finding superior effectiveness of morning light, others failing to show such a superiority, and still others finding positive effects of light in the middle of the day or evening.[52] It is possible, as suggested by Terman (1988), that some patients respond selectively to morning light, which may represent the beneficial effect of a circadian phase correction or may reflect a circadian rhythm in responsivity to light.

A third hypothesis postulates that winter depression is associated with a reduced amplitude in circadian rhythms, a reduction that is predicted to be corrected by phototherapy (Czeisler et al., 1987; Skwerer et al., 1988). Since light administered in the middle of the day increases the amplitude of the temperature rhythm (Czeisler et al., 1987) and light in the night decreases it, light in the day should improve winter depression. Although no specific test of this hypothesis has been done so far, the evidence of reduced amplitude of circadian rhythms in depression is not specific to winter depression (Souêtre et al., 1989) whereas the therapeutic effect of light generally is.

Evidence reviewed earlier suggests that supersensitivity to light may be a trait marker for bipolar disorder. Further supporting this hypothesis are findings by Nurnberger and colleagues (1988) that young adults (ages 15 to 25) with affectively ill parents also show more suppression of melatonin when exposed to light at night (Table 19-3). This supersensitivity may be corrected by lithium and by antidepressant treatments, including ECT.[53]

We might hypothesize that the increased sensitivity to light in bipolar patients would amplify the normal behavioral response to the greater intensity and duration of light during the summer and that this amplification could be expressed in mania or hypomania. As illustrated in Figure 19-11, the subsequent depression in the fall or winter would follow as a compensatory response in order to conserve the total seasonal energy output. This model implies a continuum between normal seasonal variation in mood, subsyndromal seasonal affective disorder, full seasonal affective disorder, and at least some forms of bipolar illness.

Biological Correlates of Winter Depression

Several biological correlates of winter SAD have been observed that could lead to better under-

Table 19-3. Relationship Between Morbid Risk of Affective Disorder and Light Sensitivity as Reflected by Melatonin Suppression

Group	Estimated Morbid Risk %	High Melatonin Suppression (0.84 SD above control mean) %
Screened controls	5-9	15
Unscreened controls (Lewy et al., 1985a)	10-15	21
One parent ill	18-25	33
Two parents ill	35-55	57
Patients (Lewy et al., 1985a)	100	91

Adapted From Nurnberger et al., 1988a

standing of the pathophysiology of the syndrome. Sleep EEG recordings confirmed patients' reports that they slept more in winter than in summer (Rosenthal et al., 1984). Compared with normal persons, patients with winter SAD showed reductions in slow-wave sleep in winter, but none of the other features usually associated with endogenous depression, such as reduced REM sleep latency or increased REM density. The atypical nature of the EEG sleep changes in winter depression is not surprising given the predominance of atypical features and the tendency to be bipolar.

Results of the dexamethasone-suppression test (DST) and TRH test are both normal in patients with winter SAD (Rosenthal et al., 1984; James et al., 1986), whereas prolactin levels have been reported as both higher (Jacobsen et al., 1987a) and lower than those of a control group (Depue et al., 1989b).[54] Skwerer and associates (1988) speculate that the hypothalamic–pituitary–adrenal axis, which is overactive in typical depressions, might be underactive in winter SAD, with its atypical vegetative symptoms. A possible mechanism is suggested by the fact that seasonal variation normally occurs in some biological variables, among them, cortisol, which is generally lower in winter. Because of this biological difference, winter depressions might be expected to be atypical symptomatically as well.

Dysregulation in neurotransmitter systems may be present in winter SAD. Skwerer and colleagues (1988), who reviewed the literature on this question, noted that the seasonal variation in serotonin metabolism observed in normal sub-

jects may be exaggerated in patients with SAD. This possibility is inferred from their craving and overeating of carbohydrates, which may represent attempts to regulate concentrations of brain serotonin.[55] Although there is some evidence consistent with a dysregulation of serotonin in winter SAD, it is still far from conclusive. On the other hand, a strong case for the involvement of a central dopamine deficiency has been made by Depue and colleagues (1989b). These issues are reviewed in the report of the NIMH workshop on SAD (Blehar and Rosenthal, 1989). Our understanding of the neurobiology of winter SAD should be enhanced by additional basic research on the biological effects of light.[56] We return to these issues in the Chapter 20.

Mechanisms of Summer Depression and Its Treatment

As we discussed earlier, scattered indirect evidence is beginning to suggest an association between elevated brain temperatures and depression. To date, there is very little systematic study of patients with summer SAD. The principal support for an association between elevated temperature and the depressive syndrome comes from clinical studies comparing the therapeutic effect of artificial cooling (40°C) with that of light deprivation using dark goggles (Wehr et al., 1989). Although significant improvement was observed under both experimental conditions, several factors point to cooling as the more important variable. Principal among these is the fact that when these patients were reexposed to summer

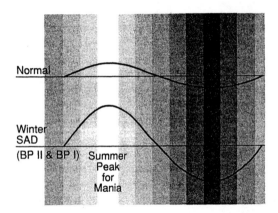

Figure 19-11. Seasonal energy conservation model.

conditions—either high temperature or bright light—during the late winter, they relapsed in response to the high temperature but not the bright light ($p < 0.02$). So far these preliminary results are relevant only to patients with clearly defined summer SAD. Further work will be needed to determine if artificial cooling might have broader applicability to the much larger number of typical endogenous depressed patients who are more likely to experience episodes in the hot months of late spring or summer.

In Chapter 20, we suggest that a comprehensive understanding of seasonal influences will have to consider not only the extremes of temperature and light in the winter and summer, but also the extremes in the daily rate of change in these environmental conditions (Figure 19-9B), which have very sharp peaks at the two equinoxes that mark the beginning of fall and the beginning of spring.

SUMMARY

Rhythmic disturbances in manic-depressive illness are clinically obvious: diurnal variations in mood, distressful and pervasive disruptions in sleep, and seasonal recurrences of episodes. The illness is itself a kind of rhythm. Increasingly, the research has evolved from disruptive studies to explorations of the pathophysiology of these disruptions.

Chronobiological studies in clinical populations are beset by methodological problems that can limit the interpretation of findings. Among the most serious are the overreliance on cross-

sectional studies and the problem of masking of oscillator-driven rhythms by external or internal influences (e.g., diet, sleep schedules) that can change the phase or amplitude of the rhythm. Masking is a particular problem in research on manic-depressive illness because apparent differences in rhythms could actually reflect the distorting effects of such characteristic symptoms as weight loss, disturbed sleep, and hypoactivity or hyperactivity.

Sleep disturbances in unipolar depression are more extensively described than they are in bipolar depression and mania. The sleep of bipolar patients varies with clinical state and severity, and, perhaps, the stage of the episode. When depressed, bipolar patients may sleep too much. When manic, they sleep little or not at all. Bipolar-I and bipolar-II patients may show different patterns.

Among the very few relatively consistent findings in bipolar patients is the tendency for sleep loss to precede, and perhaps trigger, manic episodes. Experimental evidence on the processes responsible for switches into mania or depression suggests that in some cases mania can be prevented and depression treated by appropriate manipulations of the sleep-wake cycle. Related to this is the antidepressant effect of sleep deprivation, which has been shown to be associated with being awake in the second half of the night. Circadian research on affective illness has so far shown the presence of decreased rhythm amplitudes, phase instability with a tendency toward phase advance over delay, and a faster than normal clock in some of the few rapid-cycling manic-depressive patients who have been studied.

The phenomenon of seasonal variation in the occurrence and expression of affective disorder recently has been rediscovered. It appears that the patterns of seasonality reflect both the extremes of light and temperature (winter and summer) and the extremes in the rate of change of these parameters, perhaps especially the ratio of light to dark (spring and autumn). The onset of major depression and suicide has its principal peak in the late spring and a smaller peak in the autumn, whereas mania peaks in the summer. A specific syndrome of regularly recurring winter depressions often associated with hypomania in the summer has been identified and linked to changes in the photoperiod. These winter depressions are characterized by atypical symptoms, and the larger group of spring onset depressions are characterized by typical endogenous symptoms. In addition, a specific pattern of recurrent summer depressions often with winter hypomanias has been identified.

Application of basic research in seasonal biological rhythms to clinical investigations of seasonality in manic-depressive illness is leading to the manipulation of light and temperature as experimental treatments for these two seasonal patterns. Better understanding of the psychophysiology of both bipolar and unipolar disorders is likely to come from studies of the mechanisms of treatments and the neurobiology of winter and summer depressions.

APPENDIX: BIOLOGICAL RHYTHMS GLOSSARY

Acrophase The peak of a sine function fitted to the raw data of a rhythm.

Advance To move earlier. When a rhythm advances, its peak and trough occur earlier.

Amplitude The range of the oscillation; the difference between its maximum or minimum value and the mean.

Beat phenomenon The alternating coordination and interference between two uncoupled oscillators.

Circadian rhythms Rhythms with a period of about a day. The intrinsic period of a circadian rhythm (approximately 25 hours in humans) is expressed and can be measured only when it free runs in constant conditions.

Delta sleep Slow-wave sleep, which occurs during stages 3 and 4.

Desynchronization The uncoupling of a biological rhythm from a zeitgeber or from another endogenous rhythm

Entrainment The synchronization of endogenous biological rhythms to an environmental cycle.

Free run The activity of a nonentrained circadian rhythm.

Infradian rhythms Rhythms with a period of more than a day.

Masking External or internal influences that can change the phase or amplitude of rhythms that distort true, oscillator-driven rhythms.

Period The duration of one complete cycle; under conditions of entrainment to the day/night cycle, the period of a circadian rhythm is ordinarily 24 hours.

Phase The timing of the rhythm (e.g., the timing of its peak) relative to phases of other circadian rhythms or time of day.

Power density The brain's electrical potential per cycle per second ($\mu V^2/Hz$), an expression of electrical energy.

REM latency Time slept before the onset of the first REM period.

Sleep architecture The percentage of time spent in each of four sleep stages.

Sleep efficiency The ratio of time spent asleep to total recording period.

Sleep latency The time from lights out until the appearance of stage 2 sleep.

Ultradian rhythms Rhythms with a period of less than a day.

Zeitgebers From the German: *Zeit* (time) *geber* (giver). Periodic signals in the environment that serve as time cues that entrain biological rhythms (e.g., dawn light, social cues).

Sources: Aschoff, 1981d; Kripke, et al., 1978; Kripke, 1985; Wever, 1979; Kupfer et al., 1988c.

NOTES

1. Quoted by Whitwell, 1936, p. 157.
2. Quoted by Whitwell, 1936, pp. 222–223. Weyer, greatly admired by Zilboorg, was a Dutch physician, who was pious and conventional, yet courageously fought against witchcraft. He had "great intellectual penetration and daring," was a serious practitioner, an empiricist, whose major interest was mental illness.
3. Wehr and Rosenthal (1989) say that Esquirol, the "father of modern research on seasonality of affective illness," may have been the first to delineate the two opposite patterns of recurrence, as reflected by this quote, from Esquirol, 1845, pp. 31–33, 226, 227.
4. For reviews of the subject, see Detre et al., 1972; Kupfer et al., 1972; Rosenthal et al., 1984; Taub et al., 1978; Garvey et al., 1984; Gillin and Borbély, 1985; Reynolds et al., 1987; Reynolds and Kupfer, 1987; Wehr et al., 1987a.
5. These classic descriptions do not differentiate the bipolar and unipolar subtypes.
6. Assessment of whether a recurrent pattern reflects a true infradian rhythm goes beyond whether it is regular in any obvious way. Oscillations can be expressed as regular irregularity, in which the pattern can be quantified and predicted only by harmonic analysis. For example, if a patient has had successive cycle lengths of 3, 2, 1, 2, and 3 years, the regularity would only become apparent after harmonic analysis.
7. As methods develop, new environmental factors (other than light and temperature) will no doubt be evaluated (Wilson, 1988). For example, it has been suggested that exposure to extremely low frequency electromagnetic fields can alter circadian rhythms (Wever, 1970) and that such alterations may contribute to depression (Anderson and Phillips, 1985).
8. The felicitous terminology is borrowed from Pittendrigh (1981).
9. For further discussion of the fundamental charac-

teristics of biological rhythms and their relationship to behavior, see Aschoff, 1981a; Wever, 1979, 1983; Mendlewicz and Van Praag, 1983; Wehr and Goodwin, 1983b; Van Cauter and Turek, 1986.

10. Wehr and colleagues have obtained preliminary clinical data consistent with this hypothesis. Core body temperature (as reflected by rectal temperature) continues to decline throughout sleep, but temperatures on the forehead, eyelids, and tympanic membranes increase during REM. Also, volunteers who simulate the rapid eye movements of REM sleep can increase periorbital temperatures in the venous plexus that bathes the hypothalamus and surrounding brain structures. This mechanism could explain how REM activity could increase brain temperature.

11. The data supporting the existence of two separate oscillators have recently been challenged. This issue is well reviewed by Van Cauter and Turek (1986) and reported by Mrosovsky (1986).

12. Some animal studies have been interpreted as challenging the conclusion that temperature and REM density are controlled by the same oscillator (Czeisler et al., 1980).

13. A study by Reppert and colleagues (1988) suggests that the human strong oscillator is also located in the SCN. Reppert's group identified melatonin binding sites in the SCN but not elsewhere in the hypothalamus. Melatonin has been shown to modulate the entraining of rhythms in rats (among other species). The existence of SCN melatonin binding sites in humans, like the similar ones in rats, suggests that melatonin's effects on human circadian rhythms are, like the rat's, mediated by direct action on a hypothalamic biological clock.

    For state-of-the-art reviews of evidence pertaining to the anatomy and physiology of circadian rhythms, see Wever, 1979, 1983; Moore-Ede et al., 1982; Wehr and Goodwin, 1983a; Turek, 1985; Rosenwasser and Adler, 1986; Minors and Waterhouse, 1986; Czeisler et al., 1987.

    According to Kripke (1985), evidence disputing the theory that the human strong oscillator is anatomically located in the SCN is as strong as evidence supporting the theory. "It appears there could be other oscillatory areas in the hypothalamus. In addition, mammalian adrenal glands display circadian rhythms of cortisol secretion *in vitro*. Thus, the adrenal might be an important independent oscillator" (p. 9).

14. The pathways by which light affects the mammalian circadian clock have been well described by Kripke (1985):

    In rodents and probably also in primates, light is sensed by retinal cells. Responses to illumination are conveyed to the brain through the retinohypothalamic tract, which leaves the optic chiasm to enter the hypothalamus, terminating in the suprachiasmatic nucleus and adjacent structures. Light stimulation to the retina produces an increase in the firing of suprachiasmatic nucleus cells and an increase in their uptake of glucose. Through a multisynaptic pathway passing through the spinal cord, the suprachiasmatic nuclei inhibit sympathetic neurons in the superior cervical ganglia, the peripheral sympathetic ganglia located in the neck. Noradrenergic ganglion cells send their fibers up along the cerebral arterial tree, where they synapse on cells of the pineal gland. The effect of norepinephrine upon the pinealocyte is to activate metabolic enzymes that convert serotonin to the hormone melatonin. The melatonin is promptly released into the blood. Thus, melatonin secretion is facilitated in the dark and inhibited by light. (p. 9)

    As noted by Jacklet (1984), the cell bodies of ocular neurons are necessary for the activity of the pacemaker, but only a few of these neurons are necessary. Edmunds (1988) has observed that the circadian pacemakers in the brain constitute the driving oscillators in a hierarchically ordered system providing temporal coordination of physiological function, either by direct neural connections or by hormonal secretion.

15. For a more detailed discussion of these methodological issues, see Wehr and Goodwin (1981, 1983b).

16. For further discussion of these factors, see Minors and Waterhouse, 1984a,b, Wever, 1979.

17. However, efforts to control all variables may themselves be problematic. For example, keeping patients awake throughout a circadian study is a form of sleep deprivation, which can be associated with physiological change.

18. This work involves efforts to evaluate whether the rest-activity cycle or the temperature cycle runs inherently faster or slower than normal in manic-depressive patients under nonentrained, free-running conditions.

19. Giles et al. (1989b), examining secular trends in unipolar depression, found that reduced REM latency was associated with a similar (high) rate of depression in two successive generations (siblings and parents of the probands), whereas the depressed subjects with normal REM latency had higher rates of depression than their siblings but not their parents, suggesting the predominance of nongenetic factors in this group.

20. The many issues involved in the interpretation of so-called well-state studies are discussed extensively in Chapter 17.

21. Another confounding variable for sleep studies is the tendency for some depressed patients to take brief naps during the day, which generally go undetected by staff.

22. Linkowski et al., 1985b,c; Jernajczyk, 1986; and Mendelson et al., 1987; Thase et al., 1989. Jernajczyk attributes the findings in his study to the mildness of symptoms in the patients.

23. The study by Thase and colleagues (1989) in Pittsburgh differed from two others (Duncan et al., 1979; Mendelson et al., 1987) in that the Pittsburgh patients were predominantly bipolar II.

24. Bipolar-II outpatients are often less depressed than

bipolar-I patients or the hospitalized bipolar-II patients originally described by Dunner and colleagues (1970, 1976d). In the study by Giles and associates, which did control for severity, sleep differences between the bipolar-II and bipolar-I patients did not achieve statistical significance, although uncontrolled factors may have accounted for this failure (bipolar-I patients were somewhat younger, more depressed, and more likely to be female than the bipolar-II patients).

25. Hartmann, 1968; Mendels and Hawkins, 1971; Post et al., 1976; Gillin et al., 1977.

26. The interpretation of sleep changes in mania is complicated by the observation that in normal subjects increased activity throughout the day is associated with increased delta sleep (Horne and Moore, 1985).

27. Many patients, Ostenfeld observes, experience their depressive low point early in the day and their high point close to bedtime, when they consciously and perhaps biologically rebel at the prospect of sleep. Second, many with mild conditions learn that they are night people, working and socializing at night and sleeping in the day, which is the most unpleasant for them. Third, depressive dreams, reinforced by pessimism, make sleep even more disagreeable. Fourth, winter depressions seem to demonstrate the same ill effects as dark periods. Finally, Ostenfeld contends that people with a predisposition to manic-depressive illness are susceptible to weather changes even between episodes and often feel restless and ill at ease and experience outbreaks of rheumatism in joints and muscles before such changes occur: ". . . weather conditions, in particular extreme cases of barometric pressure, have an influence on the sleep rhythm and . . . this is especially evident in cyclically disposed persons" (p. 45).

28. See, for example, Wehr and Goodwin, 1981; Kripke, 1984; Healy, 1987; Wehr and Rosenthal, in press; Ehlers et al., 1988.

29. Of the bipolar patients, one was depressed, one manic, and one rapidly cycling between the two states. The unipolar patient was depressed.

30. Of Pflug's four patients (Pflug et al., 1981), one had rapid cycles, one clearly did not, and two were intermediate—that is, they had two to three episodes during an investigative period of approximately 1 year. The patients of Lund and colleagues (1983) did not have rapid cycles.

31. From Wirz-Justice (1983b, p. 235), who quotes Georgi, 1947.

32. However, in their review of circadian cortisol studies, Sack and colleagues (1987) found that the results remained inconsistent after controlling for age.

33. Since the long-term studies have usually relied on oral temperature measures, no measurements were made during sleep, and consequently no data were gathered on the minimum temperature, which usually occurs between 3 and 6 AM.

34. The patient was on a constant dose of lithium and amitriptyline throughout the study. Her manic phase never became more severe than a hypomania, in which she was energetic, outgoing, euphoric, and excessively talkative. In her depressed phase, she was quiet and withdrawn; her physical activity, thought processes, and speech were slowed down, and she felt pessimistic and sometimes suicidal. Welsh and colleagues (1986) conducted a similar but shorter term study on a 35-year-old woman who showed a persistent 48-hour pattern of hypomania and mild depression. For 2 months before and 2 months after the study, she adhered to her normal routine and kept a sleep diary and recorded her mood twice a day. The study itself lasted for 16 days, during which her body temperature, activity, and heart rate were recorded by a small portable monitor. Sleep EEG, electrooculogram (EOG), and electromyogram (EMG) were recorded the last 11 days, the final 9 of which she was observed while isolated from time and social cues. Following lithium administration, which began on the 7th day of isolation and continued throughout follow-up, the period of the circadian rest/activity rhythm shortened—a result that is inconsistent with lithium's effect in animal and some human studies. The drug attenuated the mood cycles, which may have resulted from its effect on the circadian period, although other interpretations cannot be ruled out. Data from the study confirmed the regular alternating long and short sleep episodes the patient had reported. This pattern coincided with unusual phase jumps in the circadian rhythm of body temperature. On nights of short sleep, the temperature minima occurred closer to bedtime than on nights of long sleep.

35. Recall that the circadian rhythm of REM is roughly reciprocal to that of temperature, and both have been thought to be controlled by the same oscillator, at least until recently.

36. The studies on tricyclic antidepressants were by Linkowski et al., 1987, Souêtre et al., 1986, and Kjellman et al., 1984, on ECT was by Avery and Casey, 1987, on bright light by Dietzel et al., 1986, Rosenthal et al., 1987, and Lewy et al., 1987b, on sleep deprivation by Yamagushi et al., 1978, Gerner et al., 1979, and Sack et al., 1988b, and on phase advance treatment by Wehr et al., 1979, and Souêtre et al., 1985.

37. See, for example, Linkowski et al., 1985b,c; also, Kupfer et al., 1986, did not find abnormalities in the timing of REM sleep among patients with recurrent depressions.

38. Wehr et al., 1980; Pflug et al., 1981; Avery et al., 1986; Smallwood et al., 1983; Souêtre et al., 1988.

39. In a study of 33 endogenously depressed unipolar patients who were on clomipramine, Elsenga and Van den Hoofdakker (1988) found that antidepressant response to sleep deprivation was associated

with a higher minimum in nocturnal rectal temperature during the procedure. Although this study seems at variance with the observation of Wehr and colleagues, it is difficult to interpret because of the presence of a tricyclic antidepressant with thermoregulatory effects of its own. Perhaps it is not simply the cooling of the brain that is involved, but the overall difference between the brain temperature and the environmental temperature (i.e., lower environmental or higher brain temperature).

40. Growth hormone is a sleep dependent hormone. The onset of sleep is a powerful stimulus to its secretion.

41. Quoted by Roccatagliata, 1986, p. 143.

42. From Cook, 1894. Our thanks to D. Oren and N. Rosenthal for calling our attention to this quotation.

43. Myers and Davies (1978) suggest that the amount of environmental light acts as a coarse adjustment determining which months the vulnerability to mania is greatest, whereas temperature changes (which are more variable) provide fine-tuning, determining when a manic episode (admission) actually occurs.

44. These peaks occur because of the elliptical orbit of the earth around the sun.

45. In the Eastwood et al. study, 60 percent of patients and 41 percent of controls had "significant and sustained" mood cycles. Comparable figures for sleep cycles were 50 percent and 44 percent, for energy cycles 63 percent and 44 percent, and for anxiety cycles 57 percent and 59 percent. The patients' cycles were apparently attenuated but not eliminated by the lithium, tricyclic antidepressants, or neuroleptics they were taking.

46. In evaluating published studies of the syndrome, it is important to keep in mind that the Hamilton Rating Scale for Depression underestimates the severity of this type of depression, since increased sleep and weight and improvement in these symptoms after treatment are scored negatively.

47. SCID is the acronym for Structured Clinical Interview for DSM-III-R.

48. They note that the highest proportions of unipolar disorder have been reported in Oregon and Rochester, two areas with considerable year-round cloud cover.

49. Of course, from the point of view of pathophysiology, it would be of interest if some cases of SAD showed swings of equal magnitude in each direction while others showed a predominance of depression or of mania. This variability is, of course, characteristic of nonseasonal manic-depressive illness.

50. The pattern of seasonal disorders can take several other forms. Ironically, the first patient identified with SAD (Rosenthal et al., 1983) showed an atypical pattern, with depressive and hypomanic episodes occurring 3 to 4 months earlier than in most patients with winter SAD. In this patient, decreasing or increasing light seemed to serve as a switch that touched off mood changes lasting for months. For further discussion of this interesting case, see Rosenthal et al., in press.

51. It is possible that melatonin plays an important role in a subgroup of SAD patients, since three patients responded very well to atenolol for three consecutive winters (Rosenthal et al., 1988b).

52. Hellekson et al., 1986; Terman et al., 1987; Wehr et al., 1986; Jacobsen et al., 1987b; Yerevanian, 1987; Isaacs et al., 1988; Terman, 1988; Avery et al., 1988; Wirz-Justice et al., 1987. In the studies that found morning light superior, evening light still showed some beneficial effect.

53. Seggie and colleagues (1989b) found that the Dark Adaptation Threshold was significantly greater in a group of manic-depressive patients stabilized on lithium than it was in normal controls, a finding that the authors interpret as lithium-induced subsensitivity to light. In a companion paper (Seggie et al., 1989a), they reported that among patients with major depressive disorder, antidepressant treatment (with doxepin) reversed the patients' increased sensitivity to light. Also, a preliminary study (Steiner et al., 1988), employing electroretinograms to assess function of the neural retina in response to light, reports decreased light sensitivity following a successful course of ECT in depressed patients. However, before treatment, the depressed patients did not differ from normals on this measure.

54. Depue and colleagues (1989b) cite several differences between their study and that of Jacobsen and associates (1987a), including the lack of menstrual cycle control in the latter study and sex differences.

55. This unproven hypothesis was questioned by Fernstrom (1987). Also, Depue and colleagues (1989b) note that a serotonin deficiency should produce hyposomnia rather than the hypersomnia more typically seen in winter SAD.

56. For example, Dilsaver and Flemmer (1988) report that bright light blocks the capacity of experimental stress to supersensitize a central cholinergic/muscarinic mechanism in the rat. This may be of interest given the acetylcholine hypothesis of mood disorders.

20

Pathophysiology: Critical Evaluation, Integration, and Future Directions

Stability, the most important predictive aspect of the dynamics of complex systems [i.e., the brain], has never been a significant descriptive parameter in any formal psychopharmacologic program of basic or clinical research. (p. 3)

—Mandell, 1985

This chapter, a coda to the pathophysiology section, is divided into two parts. The first is a selective summation and general critique of the evidence reviewed in the section; the second highlights several areas of developing theory and data that to us seem best to reflect and respect the clinical realities of the illness. Taking off from these areas of study, we direct our attention to the future, identifying emerging directions for research.

Eric Kandel (1979) reminds us that "psychology and psychiatry can illuminate and define for biology the mental functions that need to be studied if we are to have a meaningful and sophisticated understanding of the biology of the human mind" (p. 1029). Recent interest in the history of descriptive psychiatry (Jackson 1986; Wehr et al., 1989) encourages us that scholarly attention to phenomenology, together with careful clinical observation, is increasingly influencing investigators in this field.

Manic-depressive illness is not only a subject of interest in its own right but also one that lends itself to research into biological processes. It is, first, the most homogeneous of the major mental disorders. It does take different forms, and it varies along several dimensions—polarity, severity, cyclicity—yet the forms and dimensions of the illness are better characterized than, for example, the schizophrenias.

Manic-depressive illness could become a model for the long-elusive goal of reconciling disagreements about the roles of nature and nurture in the etiology of mental illness. It is intriguing to consider the impact of environmental stress on an illness in which the case for a biological substrate is so compelling. The course of illness may provide the key. Evidence gathered in the era before prophylactic treatment was available shows a striking pattern in the way the illness unfolds. Averages calculated from hundreds of individual patients indicate a decreasing cycle length with each successive episode for the first several episodes, after which the illness ceases to accelerate further. It seems to settle in to an average cycle length of approximately 1 year, a pattern that is consistent with a seasonal influence on the illness.[1] In some patients, the pattern of recurrence evolves into one of clocklike regularity, precluding the operation of random psychological or social precipitants. Nevertheless, a precipitating event can often be identified for the first two or three episodes; then with each succeeding episode, environmental stress becomes less and less necessary as the pattern of recurrence takes on a life of its own.

575

Although this tendency to recur is among the most distinguishing features of manic-depressive illness, in both its bipolar and its unipolar forms, it is poorly described and not well understood. As a subject of scientific investigation, recurrence has been largely ignored. One aspect of the pattern of recurrence, seasonality, was often discussed in the classic literature on manic-depressive illness but, until recently, had virtually disappeared in modern formulations. Are such patterns found in other illness? To explore the pathophysiology of recurrence, bipolar disorder offers the advantage of symptoms that appear, to some extent, predictably and episodes that recur more frequently than in unipolar illness. Within the bipolar spectrum itself, recurrence is even more predictable in rapid-cycling patients. For that reason rapid cycling is and will continue to be the subject of pathophysiological investigations and hypotheses out of proportion to its incidence.

CRITICAL EVALUATION

In each of the preceding chapters in this section, critical evaluation was by and large limited to first-order or immediate interpretations of the data being reviewed. Here we consider more general issues. Some were alluded to earlier, but they bear repetition.

Biogenic Amine Hypotheses: Old and New

Is the brain more properly regarded as a precisely wired, chemically transmitted switchboard, or as a collection of loosely bounded chemical ponds acting on shifting cellular shores? (p. 1687)—Bloom, 1987

Since the biogenic amine neurotransmitter systems have been central to contemporary theories of the biology of affective disorders, we begin with an evaluation of the data generated in support of the amine hypotheses. We consider whether they can be used to frame questions that pertain to the underlying pathophysiology of manic-depressive illness, or if their relevance is limited to the state of depression (or mania) or particular symptoms associated with these states. We also ask whether this area of research can identify what is distinctive about the biology of manic-depressive illness when compared with the broader spectrum of the affective disorders. Can the amine data, for example, help to understand cyclicity and the relationships between bipolar

and recurrent unipolar illness and between more and less recurrent forms of affective illness?

A relatively impressive body of animal data and some clinical data link the effects of mood-altering drugs to the effects on brain aminergic systems or the balance between them. For clarifying the etiology of the affective disorders, however, the amine hypotheses seem to be at a juncture analogous to a paradigmatic crisis as outlined by Kuhn (1970), albeit on a smaller scale. These hypotheses originally energized and organized clinical data collection, but in recent years observations relevant to amine function seem to be spawning more and more subgroups that do not readily correspond to clinically derived distinctions. Notable for its absence in these analyses is the more salient clinical reality of forms of illness that are more or less recurrent. The practice of creating these new amine subgroups, furthermore, does a disservice to the original hypotheses, generating doubt that an amine system could be central to the core pathophysiology of the illness. At times, it seems that those who create new subgroups to account for biological heterogeneity (the splitters) take the amine hypotheses as a given—an edifice against which new data are to be measured and into which it must be made to fit. On the other hand, the lumpers, who would be true to Kraepelin's notion that the enormous clinical variability of manic-depressive illness[2] reflects but "a single morbid process," have yet to offer alternative hypotheses that can match the scope and heuristic power of the amine formulations.

Too many interpretations of the animal pharmacology data bridging drug effects to neurotransmitters still treat the central nervous system (CNS) as a homogenized soup. In formulating animal models and in other attempts to understand the mechanism of action of mood-altering drugs, many investigators continue to ignore the abundant new knowledge about the functional neuroanatomy of the brain and the relationship among behavior and specific neuronal pathways, neurotransmitter networks, and receptor fields. Paul Willner registers a similar complaint:

Beginning with the catecholamine hypothesis, a number of empirical generalizations have been proposed, but . . . there has been almost no attempt to discuss changes in neurotransmitter or neuroendocrine status in relation to the functioning of the brain. As a result, instead of moving forward into a period of theory testing, research has reverted to what in many cases amounts to little more than a random trawling through the body or brain in the hope of netting anything that will be statistically significant at a level sufficient to satisfy a journal referee. (1985, p. 420)

A related issue concerns the relatively unsophisticated way that the concept of causality has been applied. All too often, pathophysiology is taken as etiology, at least implicitly. Other reductionistic fallacies are not uncommon. Familiar examples include reasoning backward from the effects of drugs to pathophysiology and the (usually implicit) assumption that understanding the components is tantamount to understanding the whole. Any attempt to understand the biological basis for disorders with behavioral and psychological components must go beyond an understanding of the biological machinery. For example, it must include models that clarify the specific way in which environmental factors can alter the system in a manner that produces particular symptoms. It must develop models that can account for enormous variability in symptom expression over time.

Mandell (1985) argues that the reductionistic linear constructs that dominate contemporary neuroscience will not prove adequate for an understanding of brain function. To him, a neuroscience that is dominated by molecular biology "suffers from an unawareness of the beauty, generativity, and clinical relevance of the great premolecular biology [that is] the more molar brain theories . . . modern molecular biological dogma has eclipsed this rich history of integrative ideas" (pp. 4-5). Chaos theory, developed recently in the physical sciences, provides one glimpse into what may be the future of clinical neuroscience (Skarda and Freeman, 1987; Gleick, 1987; Pool, 1989). Gray (1982) emphasizes the need to define psychological processes precisely before attempting to evaluate the usefulness of a given neurobiological construct: " . . . if the psychological component [is] wrong, there can be no success in finding neuronal processes to match its supposed functions" (p. 4).

Before the formulation of the amine hypothesis, Schou (1963) had already raised an issue that would later become a criticism of the hypothesis. He suggested that attempts to understand

manic-depressive illness should build on the observation that some drugs (he cited lithium and imipramine) can have similar therapeutic effects in both mania and depression. Also at that time, Klein (1965) suggested that a cybernetic model might best describe the interactions between mood-altering drugs and the central nervous system. Later, Court (1968, 1972), Whybrow and Mendels (1969), and Goodwin and Sack (1973), implicitly building on Schou's and Klein's earlier formulations, offered alternatives to the "too much/too little" bipolar catecholamine hypothesis. These formulations focused on processes that might underlie both manic and depressive episodes. Whybrow and Mendels (1969) emphasized CNS arousal mechanisms, whereas Goodwin and Sack (1973) focused on regulatory mechanisms, particularly those that respond to stress. These early revisionist ideas did not challenge the notion that biogenic amines were involved in the pathophysiology of the depressed and manic states. Rather, they tried to redirect the etiological focus to underlying disturbance. Ten years later, Carroll (1983) was more sweeping in his criticisms:

The biogenic amine theory now more closely resembles a venerable flag that the field salutes than a tool we can work with effectively. The theory has been modified, qualified, inverted and decorated with such baroque reverses that it is exhausted as a source of new insights. (p. 164)

Carroll, in turn, proposed a three-dimensional (albeit still bidirectional) model that builds on the earlier work of Klein (1974) and that attempts to relate signs and symptoms of depression and mania to known behaviorally defined brain systems.[3] The model posits that almost all of the classic features of mania and depression can be understood as opposite disturbances of three systems: (1) central pleasure or reward, (2) central pain disturbance, and (3) psychomotor regulation disturbance.[4] One interesting aspect of this model is that it provides an explanation for lithium-modified breakthrough depressive episodes (see Chapter 23); that is, that lithium acts primarily by dampening the disinhibited central pain mechanism. Although this model lacks neuroanatomical specificity, it is a useful step in the direction of supplying it. As its author acknowledges, however, the model fails to account for either the biology of recurrence or preexisting vulnerability. Another problem with this and similar formulations, as pointed out by Healy (1987), is that they are implicitly derived from models of depression based on behavioral psychology (depression comes from a deficiency of reward or reinforcement mechanisms or from an excess of punishment mechanisms) and, therefore, carry the limitations of these models.

Traditional Approaches to Clinical Biology

Viewed in its entirety, the pathophysiology literature is clearly wanting in longitudinal studies. This deficiency is especially unfortunate, since two fundamental realities of manic-depressive illness, genetic vulnerability and inherent cyclicity, can best be studied longitudinally:

"Cyclicity" denotes a tendency for a sequence of symptoms to recur regularly, implying an underlying process that is continuous over time. The term is usually used in connection with illnesses with frequent episodes, but in theory it is applicable to periods spanning years. *To view an illness as cyclic rather than episodic requires a fundamental reorientation in thinking. Cyclicity implies that the illness is continually evolving and remissions no less than relapses are expressions of the disease process.* An apparent discontinuity in cyclic mood disorders, the behavioral switch process, can be regarded as a threshold phenomenon that occurs when an underlying continuous process exceeds or falls below certain limits or "set points." (Wehr and Goodwin, 1977, p. 292) [Emphasis added]

Table 20-1 outlines the major conceptual approaches that have guided clinical biological research in the affective disorders. The approaches are listed roughly in the order of prominence in the existing literature. The first five are essentially cross-sectional; the last four are longitudinal.

The biological effects of antidepressant and antimanic drugs—the so-called pharmacological bridge—are listed first for two reasons: (1) Historically, this area has been the incubator for the major attempt to define the pathophysiology of manic-depressive illness—the amine hypotheses. (2) The proposed role of amines in the action of mood-altering drugs is the most straightforward aspect of these hypotheses. In most work in this field, depressed or manic states have been considered separately.[5] Another problem with the traditional pharmacological bridge is the implication that depression and mania are in all respects opposite states, with antidepressant and

Table 20-1. Conceptual Approaches to the Biology of Affective Illness

Cross-Sectional Approaches
- Biological effects of antidepressant or antimanic drugs (e.g., the amine hypotheses)
- State-dependent changes (e.g., amine metabolites)
- Contributions to clinical topology (e.g., DST)
- Predictors of treatment response (e.g., MHPG)
- Intersection of normal variance with illness (e.g., CSF 5-HIAA)

Longitudinal Approaches
- State-independent abnormalities (the biology of vulnerability)
- Biological correlates of natural course variables (e.g., age of onset, number of episodes, cycle length)
- Focus on within-patient variance
- Mechanisms of cyclicity (the biology of recurrence)
  Effects of drugs on cycle length
  Kindling and sensitization
  Biological rhythms, circadian and seasonal

antimanic drugs presumed to have opposite mechanisms of action. For an elaboration of this critique, see Goodwin and Sack (1973) and Himmelhoch and associates (1976a). Finally, the fact that antidepressant and antimanic treatments can also be effective in depressed or manic states that are secondary to nonspecific organic factors (see Chapter 18) suggests that they might be working downstream from the core pathology in primary manic-depressive illness.

Chapters 16 and 17 discuss drug–neurotransmitter interactions in terms of hierarchical models, with a focus on the monoamine systems, which are relatively well characterized functionally and neuroanatomically compared to other transmitters, such as acetylcholine, γ-aminobutyric acid (GABA), and glycine. Multiple bidirectional interactions occur between norepinephrine and serotonin, each of which has opposite effects on dopamine systems, that is, facilitation by norepinephrine and inhibition by serotonin. Pharmacological facilitation of the norepinephrine–serotonin axis may be associated with antidepressant response, facilitation of the serotonin–dopamine axis is not associated with any clear clinical effect, and facilitation of the norepinephrine–dopamine axis can precipitate mania or accelerate cycles of the illness. Norepinephrine serves an important function as a modulator of incoming signals, a process that increases the signal/noise ratio by suppressing random, spontaneous lower level firing. The result is that the norepinephrine-modulated neuron is better able to recognize relevant input, and its firing is more linked to its functional output (Potter, 1986). In this way, drug-induced enhancement of noradrenergic function (increasing efficiency) could be critical to the clinical efficacy of mood-altering drugs (Stone, 1983b; Potter, 1986), even though the noradrenergic systems were not themselves the locus of the pathological disturbance.

In direct biological studies of patients, the great majority have focused on state-dependent changes. Although this literature covers a wide range of subjects, from neuroendocrine measures to electrolytes to neuropeptides, the bulk of it represents efforts to clinically evaluate the amine hypotheses derived from animal pharmacology. This essentially cross-sectional work has generated several derivative areas, among them biological correlates of clinical topology (e.g., the DST), treatment response (e.g., MHPG), and personality variables in manic-depressive patients (e.g., 5-hydroxyindoleacetic acid, 5-HIAA, correlation with impulsivity and aggression).

State-independent biological abnormalities, the focus of clinical genetic studies, are often identified as predisposing but in fact are derived from studies of recovered patients. For example, there is evidence that the low CSF levels of the serotonin metabolite (5-HIAA) found in some depressed patients persist after recovery. However, this finding in no way establishes that low 5-HIAA is a vulnerability marker in these patients. The confirmation of a vulnerability marker would depend on its identification in subjects who have not yet been ill but who later become depressed. To do this requires a longitudinal evaluation of populations at risk, that is, first-degree relatives of depressed patients. The putative markers derived from studies of pathophysiology include the enzymes involved in the function of amines (monoamine oxidase, catechol-o-methyltransferase, dopamine-β-hydroxylase, the imipramine-binding site) and electrolytes (ATPases, lithium transport), various amine metabolites (e.g., 5-HIAA), and responses to pharmacological challenge (decreased REM latency with arecoline, growth hormone responses to amphetamine). None of these has as yet fulfilled

the requirement of an illness marker: that it covary with the illness in pedigrees. The concept of a vulnerability marker suggests that exploration of challenge paradigms might be more revealing than resting measures, although ethical limits are an issue here. An example of one of those challenges is stress activation, such as the learned helplessness paradigm of Breier and colleagues (1987). Later, we discuss the promising area of genetic linkage studies in manic-depressive illness.

Clues to the biology of recurrence are more likely to be found when biological measures are systematically examined for their relationship to natural course variables. Similarly, the study of within-patient variance could provide clues to factors involved in the underlying instability that characterizes the illness. Although the literature on biological correlates of natural course variables (such as cycle length, age of onset, and number of episodes) is sparse, there are some fascinating leads. For example, Post and colleagues (1984c) have reported that CSF norepinephrine levels are positively correlated with the number of prior episodes, a finding that might be interpreted as reflecting the accumulated stress of multiple relapses.

Approaches that focus on mechanisms of cyclicity are listed last because, indeed, they are relatively new on the scene and are only beginning to work their way into the mainstream of thinking about the pathophysiology of affective disorders. Two independent, but perhaps interrelated, hypotheses attempt to clarify mechanisms of cyclicity. The first posits that manic-depressive cycles reflect a disturbance in the regulation of biological rhythms, especially circadian rhythms (see Chapter 19), and the second posits that the inherent cyclicity may involve a process analogous to electrical kindling or sensitization (see Chapter 16). Because we believe that both these areas have considerable promise for providing new and perhaps unifying insights into the pathophysiology of manic-depressive illness, they are discussed further below.

Cautions in Interpreting Clinical Data

Sources of Variance

The complex issues of sources of variance have been discussed in detail in Chapter 17. When patient groups cannot be matched for comparison on a particular variable, the appropriate statistic may be an analysis of covariance. The parameter must be shown to be independent of the illness. Even age matching can introduce distortions. For example, in age-matched unipolar and bipolar depressed patients, the bipolar group's earlier age of onset means their average duration of illness would have been longer, and this parameter should be evaluated independently, despite the general homogeneity of the population (Goodwin et al., 1978b).

Of special interest to the pathophysiology of manic-depressive disorder is the variance contributed by diurnal and seasonal rhythms. Not only are data collected at different times of the day (or seasons) not comparable, but a free-running rhythm could produce epiphenomena that may be misinterpreted as correlates of the mood cycle. These problems are of more than passing interest, since rhythm disturbances have been hypothesized to be central to the pathophysiology of the illness. The 1982 Dahlem conference on depression (Angst, 1983) produced an important group of consensus recommendations for a standardized approach to biological studies of depression (Kupfer and Rush, 1983). These are outlined in Table 20-2.

Importance of Normative Data

Unfortunately, studies of patients often outpace or attempt to reach beyond the available base of normative data. Clinical data on sleep neuroendocrine measures, or PET imaging, are difficult to interpret when these parameters and the relationships between them have not been carefully characterized in normal people. As we develop new hypotheses of affective disorders, such as those based on the interactions of mood with temperature regulation, energy metabolism, and light, we would do well to make our principal initial investment in a very careful study of these mechanisms in normal subjects.

The availability of data for normal controls may be especially fruitful for understanding the meaning of particular drug effects. For example, Wehr and Goodwin (1977) noted differential norepinephrine metabolite responses to induced activity in depressed patients (predominantly bipolar) compared with controls, and Rudorfer and colleagues (1985a) found that certain effects of

lithium on peripheral cardiovascular function occur only in manic-depressive patients but not in normal controls. Such differential effects may represent important clues to the differences that characterize the vulnerability of certain systems in manic-depressive patients.

The Question of Biological Specificity and Subgroups

Biological specificity refers to the degree to which the evidence in affective illness favors a single discrete neurobiological system or a pattern of alterations in more than one system, with emphasis on the largest body of data, that involving the biogenic amines.[6] These systems may be involved in etiology of illness or symptoms. Even if amine disturbances are far down the pathophysiological chain (to the point of being considered simply biochemical symptoms), it is still important to ask whether the evidence favors the involvement (at whatever level) of one amine over the others. Although what we know about the complex functional interrelationships between multiple amine neurotransmitter systems should give us pause in asking this question, one approach is to ask whether there might be a more specific relationship between a given amine change and a particular symptom or group of symptoms.[7]

Another issue in interpreting clinical biological data, noted earlier, is the often casual way in which biological subgroups are created. Frequently, this seems like no more than a device for assigning biological meaning in the face of heterogeneity. For any such subgroup to be meaningful, it would have to be validated against independent clinical and pharmacological response parameters (Cowdry and Goodwin, 1978). These relationships are illustrated in Figure 20-1. Most convincing would be an association in which the biological variable shows a statistically significant bimodal (or not normal) distribution, and there is a clinically (or pharmacologically) defined subgroup corresponding closely to each cluster of biological data on the distribution. A further refinement involves the validation of a biological or pharmacological response measure against genetically meaningful subgroups. For example, Smeraldi and colleagues (1984) could not find a correlation between lithium response and a particular genotype. This might be obtained

Table 20-2. Methodological Recommendations from the Dahlem Conference

Methodological Issues:
- If the sample or part of the sample was *previously reported* in another study, this fact should be noted
- The degree to which the clinical and laboratory findings were made *independently and blindly* to each other should be stated
- The process of patient *recruitment* or referral should be specified
- How many patients were *excluded*, and why, should be noted
- *Exclusion* and *inclusion criteria* for subgrouping patients should be clearly stated
- *How is the diagnosis made?*

Patient Variables:
- The *age and gender descriptions* of the full sample and the gender distributions within each decade of life should be noted
- The *severity* of illness should be reported using at least one clinician-rated method with proven reliability and validity
- The *diagnostic composition* of the group should be noted and the criteria used for diagnosis stated
- The number of *psychotic* (hallucinating and/or delusional) depressions should be reported
- The *length* of the current clinical (syndromatic) episode should be reported
- Some description of degree of *chronicity* should be given, in the form of total length of illness, number of episodes, or amount of time in the previous 5 or 10 years that the patient was not symptomatic
- The *medication status* both during the study and within 30 days prior to the study should be reported
- The patients' immediately *previous treatment* and response to it should be stated to inform others of the extent of "treatment-resistant" patients in the sample
- If female, the patients' *ovarian status* should be noted by reporting either time from last menstrual period, or where necessary by measuring gonadotropins and steroids
- The *inpatient or outpatient status* at the time of the study should be reported

On behalf of the Dahlem workgroup, these recommendations were published by Kupfer and Rush (1983).

Additionally we would recommend that investigators note the time of day and the month of the year for their clinical and biological data points so that circadian and circannual rhythms can be analyzed.

if lithium were acting downstream from the genetic defect(s), alleviating both genetically and nongenetically related affective syndromes.

One reason subgroup findings are often not replicated is that clinical variability over time may reflect variations within the same episode or between different episodes. For example, some patients can shift from rapid cycles to regular cycles during the course of illness. If such clinical variability is also reflected in biological variability, it is not surprising that subgroups generated from cross-sectional snapshots of a particular biological system may be difficult to reproduce.

A related issue is how differences (or nondifferences) between group means are to be interpreted in the face of differences in variance. For example, not infrequently, all of the individual values in the ill group fall within the control range, but the mean for the ill group is lower because there is an insufficient number of patient values corresponding with the upper range for the control group—as if the illness were exerting a ceiling on the system. Or, conversely, the patients might not be significantly different from controls with respect to group means but will show significantly more (or less) variance. Rarely are differences in variance considered when pathophysiological inferences are drawn from group comparisons.

In studies of recurrent affective disorder, the burden of proof ought to be on those who propose that biological subgroup findings support the existence of various and different pathophysi-

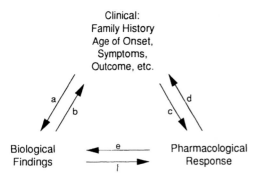

Figure 20-1. Approaches to the validation of subgroups. The model draws attention to several issues. First, although it may appear that moving in opposite directions between two spheres (e.g., arrows a and b) is really asking the same question, in fact the answer to one does not always predict the other. This is so because we are dealing with a series of partial correlations in which considerable portions of the variance are not accounted for. Second, it is clear that difficulties can arise when the relationship between any two of the spheres is examined independently of the third. For example, unipolar and bipolar depressed patients (a clinical parameter) may be found to have significant differences in both a biological parameter, x, and a pharmacological response parameter, y. If one examines the relationship between x and y in the entire depressed population and does not consider the unipolar–bipolar difference in x and y, misleading conclusions are likely to be drawn (from Cowdry and Goodwin, 1978).

ologies, each leading to a different clinical variant of illness. On the face of it, this inference is not in keeping with the principal of parsimony and is contrary to Kraepelin's notion that the wide variety of different clinical forms of manic-depressive illness represent but "a single morbid process." As noted previously, the subgrouping that may ultimately convey the most meaning will be that between cross-sectional and longitudinal data, the latter being more likely to shed light on the morbid process.

Shifts in the Precision of Diagnostic Boundaries

The evolution of diagnoses based on cross-sectional criteria (RDC and DSM-III-R) carries with it the risk of losing some of the original meaning of a diagnosis informed by the pattern recognition of experienced clinicians.[8] As Carroll (1983) has noted,

A conceptual drift of alarming proportions has occurred in the name of diagnostic reliability. This drift threatens to retard the field by increasing the variance present in clinical populations and by obscuring historical insights that helped us construct the amine paradigm 20 years ago. As a result, new problems of epistemology and methodology have been created. How is a theory of depression to be developed, how is it to be tested, and how is an antidepressant drug effect to be recognized if the clinical entity (or independent variable) no longer corresponds to the original?

. . . the legitimate pressure for diagnostic reliability, coupled with the new criteria, has changed the training and behavior of a new generation of clinicians. In the United States we are no longer transmitting psychiatry's historical tradition of phenomenology, clinical skill, discriminative judgement, and diagnostic pattern recognition based on interview, observation, family history, and natural history. The diagnostic criteria are being used *in practice* as sufficient rather than merely necessary for the diagnosis of depression. In practice, the criteria have proved to be so elastic that, when used in stand-alone fashion without a prior clinical diagnosis, they can accommodate an extremely heterogeneous group of patients under the rubric [of major depressive disorder]. (p.165)

Fortunately, this problem is less serious in work on bipolar-I illness, since the presence of mania renders it less vulnerable to boundary diffusion. Nevertheless, the boundary, or heterogeneity, problem afflicting the major depressive disorder category has an important impact, especially when one attempts to interpret bipolar–unipolar differences, or, as we have done in the preceding chapters, to glean from the biological literature on major depression some insights relevant to bipolar illness. A particularly glaring deficiency of the DSM-III-R criteria for major affective disorder is the omission of any reference to natural course.

A more fundamental conceptual problem for biological theory is the way that DSM-III-R is organized. By separating bipolar disorder and major depressive disorder at the outset, the system arbitrarily reinforces the bipolar–unipolar dichotomy and complicates the development of biological theories that posit underlying commonalities. A neutral system would start with major depressive disorder and then subdivide into bipolar and unipolar forms. This would be far better for the development of unbiased biological theory. At least with the issue of polarity, DSM-III-R sides with the splitters over the lumpers. It need not be so.

Another problem in the clinical biological literature represents a paradox: at a time when our techniques are becoming increasingly sophisticated (e.g., brain imaging), there is a distinct possibility that the clinical characteristics of the patients available for study are becoming more atypical. This may be especially likely in the case of manic-depressive illness because the large majority of such patients can be successfully treated in the community, leaving a population available to research centers that is likely to be overrepresented by treatment-resistant patients. This inherent limitation of contemporary studies must be kept in mind when a new set of data is at odds with a previously established conclusion derived from earlier studies. Thus, although the biological methodology has improved, the representativeness of the clinical population may be going in the opposite direction. What can be done about this problem? Unfortunately, the straightforward application of diagnostic criteria is not enough, given the broad range of clinical phenomena encompassed by a single category. Other possibilities include investigators reporting separately the (pretreatment) biological data for those patients who went on to show a clear-cut response to standard drug treatment, and greater use of large private practice clinic samples, such as those reported by Kukopulos in Rome.

Scientific Fads

Another impression that one gets from the literature is a certain unfortunate tendency toward scientific fads. It is unfathomable why certain areas of literature simply drop out as others capture our attention and take over. For example, the relatively robust literature on electrolyte disturbances died out rather abruptly in the late 1960s for no apparent reason. Certainly, there was not a rash of nonreplications to explain the curious disappearance of this trail. As we have noted earlier:

Legitimate concerns are now being expressed that too many of us who work in the field of clinical-biological studies have tended to jump immediately from the classical transmitter studies to every new peptide modulator or transmitter that comes along, that we are likely to repeat the mistakes made in the early studies of classical transmitters, and that consequently the field isn't going to progress very quickly. Needless to say, there is no shortage of examples of these new studies, which attract considerable attention even though they lack the most rudimentary attention to sources of vari-

ances and issues of specificity. On the other hand, we can ill afford to ignore the potential clinical significance of a newly discovered substance or system because it might be the very discovery that could unlock existing mysteries and clarify our confusion. Clearly we need both: to continue our pursuit of the classical neurotransmitters and to be ready to exploit the new neurobiology. But we must insist that the latter be done with the same rigor that we require from the former. (Goodwin, 1984, p. 11)

Illness Specificity

We have in front of us a fruit called psychosis, and we don't know whether it's a citrus that will divide itself into separate sections or an apple that we must divide along arbitrary lines.   —Belmaker and Van Praag, 1980b, p. 4

Chapters 5, 15, and 16 deal with the disease models that underlie diagnostic concepts, focusing especially on the clinical and genetic findings related to the question of whether the two major psychoses (major affective illness and schizophrenia) are discrete illnesses or variations of some unitary generic psychotic illness on different parts of a continuum. Specifically, we note that the genetic data relating to affective illness in general do not support the unambiguous separation of the two and, therefore, could be consistent with the continuum model of Crow (1986). However, the data do support the independence of bipolar disorder from schizophrenia, with unipolar being nonspecifically expressed in association with either.[9] Crow cites earlier observations of "one-way movement between generations from affective disorder to schizophrenia" (p. 423) in building his interesting hypothesis that "quantum changes in a variable gene" (p. 425) produce transgenerational movement from a less to a more severe position along the spectrum (unipolar—bipolar—schizoaffective—schizophrenia). He further speculates that the link between creativity and productivity, on the one hand, and manic-depressive illness, on the other (see Chapter 14), provides the genetic advantage needed to offset the survival disadvantages associated with the illness.[10] Although Crow prefers a genetic hypothesis to account for an etiologic core common to both groups of the major psychoses, it is also conceivable that nongenetic etiologic factors could be common to psychotic illness (e.g., a slow virus). Under these circumstances, the illness specificity would come from this common environmental factor interacting with two different sorts of genetic vulnerabilities to produce either schizophrenia or manic-depressive illness.

The fundamental clinical phenomenology by which Kraepelin originally separated manic-depressive illness from schizophrenia still seems valid. That is, the characteristic clinical presentation of manic-depressive illness—specific episodes, periods of remission, opposite states of activation and inhibition, and seasonal patterning of episodes—distinguishes it from schizophrenia.

The efficacy of pharmacological treatments of the psychoses is characterized by both specificity and nonspecificity. Lithium is effective in the acute and prophylactic treatment of both mania and depression, whereas neuroleptics, the treatment of choice for schizophrenia, are also useful in mania and some cases of agitated depression. In addition, it has been emphasized that some drugs, for example, stimulants, are capable of producing both affective and schizophreniform alterations and thus may be useful in imagining a continuum along which the same drugs or the same transmitter systems may mediate both euphoric and dysphoric as well as schizophrenic-like processes.

Unfortunately, the individual biochemical, physiological, and anatomical studies reviewed in the preceding chapters were rarely designed as well-matched direct comparisons between schizophrenia and carefully defined subgroups of affective illness. Thus, it is not yet possible to assert beyond a doubt that a given finding in manic-depressive illness is clearly specific to that diagnosis. Nevertheless, a tentative case for specificity has been made for hypothalamic–pituitary–adrenal (HPA) axis activation (hypercortisolemia, decreased CSF somatostatin), altered serotonin transport (decreased platelet uptake, decreased imipramine binding), and some sleep abnormalities and circadian rhythm disturbances. One problem in assessing the diagnostic specificity of these findings is that a given measure may differ among subgroups of patients with affective illness, or the finding may vary across different phases of the illness.

There is some suggestion of a rough similarity in some anatomical measures between manic-depressive illness and schizophrenia. In both diagnostic groups, for example, enlarged ventricular/brain ratios (VBR), sulcal widening, and metabolic hypofrontality are present. However, since these anatomical studies are of relatively recent vintage, we must recall our earlier caution concerning the possibility that the more recent research populations are more biased toward treatment-resistant patients. Moreover, since the resolving power of these techniques is still relatively crude, one cannot make too much of this nonspecificity. The currently evolving techniques for in vivo imaging of receptor fields and neurotransmitter pathways should allow clarification of these specificity questions in the near future.

Summary

In this section, we offered broad philosophical critiques of existing biological hypotheses and reviewed more specific limitations of the clinical biological data. We noted that the amine hypotheses have not yet taken us beyond models for the clinical effects of mood-altering drugs. In other words, we still cannot say whether the amine changes associated with these drugs are specific to or necessary for the clinical effects. We do not know if the observed amine effects reflect a correction of an abnormality or whether they are incidental, that is, biochemical side effects. Likewise, the literature on state-dependent and state-independent biochemical, physiological, and anatomical findings has not yet yielded an abnormality that has been conclusively established as specific to manic-depressive illness. We have taken note of a variety of problems in the design and conceptualization of clinical research that may account for the failure to answer the specificity question. Although further testing of existing hypotheses is no doubt called for (especially if the lessons already learned are applied), it is obvious that fresh thinking is needed. As Willner has pointed out in his comprehensive review of the neurobiology of depression (1985), what is needed are paradigms that allow us to integrate huge amounts of data. This challenge is all the more daunting because the different fields (e.g., pharmacology, neuroanatomy, physiology) approach the illness with vastly different assumptions and conceptual frames of reference, and each has made little effort to reach out to the others. In the section that follows, we review some areas of evolving theory and data that in our view hold promise for furthering an understanding of the pathophysiology of manic-depressive illness, some of which offer new approaches to integration.

FUTURE DIRECTIONS

To serve as an outline for this section we review once again what an adequate hypothesis of the illness should embrace:

- Genetic vulnerability
- Spontaneous remissions and exacerbations (inherent cyclicity)
- Environmental stressors; these may be more important in the precipitation of early episodes or less important in later ones
- Seasonal patterns in the timing of episodes
- The similarities between depression and mania as well as their differences
- The observation that some treatments (e.g., lithium, ECT, and perhaps also carbamazepine) can benefit both manic and depressive phases of the illness.

Genetic Vulnerability

In addition to the extensive use of genetic studies to elucidate questions of illness specificity,[11] genetic epidemiology, particularly pedigree studies, should be expanded to clarify whether genetic factors determine variability in the fundamentally recurrent nature of the illness—that is, is cyclicity genetically determined? A few data suggest that rapid-cycling bipolar disorder shares the same genetic substrate with nonrapid-cycling disorder. Winokur and Kadrmas (1989), on the other hand, found a strong relationship between many episodes in bipolar patients (three or more) and a history of bipolar illness and remitting affective disorder in first-degree relatives. They suggest that what is inherited may be an episodic course, not bipolar illness per se (see Chapter 6). Thus, whether individual differences in cyclicity are genetically influenced is not yet settled. Since pharmacological treatment can affect cycle length, prior treatment represents a contaminant in any study aimed at characterizing covariates of this parameter. Information on the genetics of recurrence independent of polarity could help clarify the genetic relationship between the bipolar and unipolar subgroups.

Another important question related to recurrence in manic-depressive illness is the genetics of circadian and seasonal rhythms. Animal data indicate that the frequency of circadian oscillators and seasonal photoperiodic mechanisms are under genetic control. It would be of interest to know whether genetic factors contribute to variability in the phase position of circadian rhythms among manic-depressive patients. With regard to seasonality, retrospective data indicate that individuals with seasonal and nonseasonal mood disorders appear to have roughly similar numbers of first-degree relatives with major affective disorders, and there are anecdotal data suggesting that seasonality per se may be inherited. However, systematic interview-based family history studies have not been reported. Some of the hypotheses concerning the impact of seasonal influences on manic-depressive illness will benefit from a more quantitative estimation of the genetics of seasonality and of light sensitivity and whether any genetic variability in these features exists independent of affective illness.

Future genetic epidemiology might also consider the capacity for kindling and sensitization. The genetically epilepsy-prone rats (Riegel et al., 1986) may provide a useful model, since the development of kindled seizures is accelerated in these animals (Savage et al., 1986). Other animal data indicate that certain rodent strains can be bred for sensitivity to cocaine-induced seizures (Post et al., 1988b) or audiogenic seizures (Vergnes et al., 1987). Clinically, there is increasing recognition that the genetic contributions to epilepsy are substantial (Newmark and Penry, 1980) and may be as important as they are for manic-depressive illness. As the clinical delineation of the various epilepsies has evolved, it is becoming possible to examine the question of genetic overlap between various forms of epilepsy and recurrent affective disorder. In addition, the relative importance of precipitating events in the onset of initial manic or depressive episodes could be examined within families, an approach that could shed light on the genetics of kindling and sensitization.

Finally, other physiological parameters possibly involved in recurrence in manic-depressive illness might be explored in a family history context using both formal interview-based family history methodology and pedigree analysis. An important example is thyroid function.

The potential offered by recent advances in molecular genetics is discussed in Chapter 15. At this juncture, it is not possible to predict reliably whether new advances will come first from the exploration of candidate genes or from applying linkage strategies in informative pedigrees, without starting from a hypothesis. The chromosome 11 linkage initially reported in the Amish (Egeland et al., 1987b) has not been replicated in the recent reanalysis of the same pedigree (Kelsoe et al., 1989). Thus, the interest in the genetic loci for tyrosine hydroxylase and tryptophan hydroxylase, the rate-limiting enzymes in the synthesis of the major amines hypothesized to be involved in manic-depressive illness (located on the same short arm of chromosome 11), is somewhat deflected. In preliminary studies, Ginns and associates (unpublished data) have been unable to find any abnormalities in the nucleotide sequence in the coding regions of the tyrosine hydroxylase gene from affected vs unaffected members of the Amish pedigree.

In medicine in general, a success story has yet to come from a host of efforts to identify a specific genetic locus by starting with a candidate gene suggested by pathophysiological studies. For example, the early excitement generated by the apparent identification of a linkage between the amyloid gene and the hereditary form of Alzheimer's disease was dimmed when it was found subsequently that the linkage could not be established. On the other hand, the alternate molecular genetic model is represented by a success story—that involving muscular dystrophy, which resulted in identification of a new protein inferred from the nucleic acid sequence of the identified genetic locus. This offers the hope that molecular genetic approaches may lead to identification of new proteins specific to psychiatric disorders (Bloom, 1987). Also, as more and more of the human genome is mapped, it will be possible to employ molecular genetic strategies in the evaluation of previously proposed linkage markers, such as those associated with the X chromosome.

The discovery of entirely new proteins based on the analysis of gene sequences shown to be linked is not incompatible with efforts to build on existing pathophysiological clues. For example, if studies of pathophysiology point to an abnormality in the regulation of a particular neurotransmitter system (e.g., serotonin), it is quite possible that the genetic defect could reside in a protein modulating this system.

In considering the potential contribution of molecular genetic strategies, it is important to keep in mind that there can be considerable genetic heterogeneity in the face of relative phenotypic homogeneity, or vice versa. For example, multiple separate genetic defects can produce mental retardation syndromes that are clinically indistinguishable, whereas Huntington's disease, caused by a single dominant gene defect, can occur with a confusing array of different clinical pictures.

Spontaneous Remissions and Exacerbations

The Effects of Drugs on Stability

As noted earlier, the amine hypotheses were formulated by linking the effects of drugs on brain amine systems in animals to their clinical effects on the depressed or manic state, that is, the pharmacological bridge. In Chapter 17, we proposed a new bridge, the clinical shores of which would be the effects of drugs, not on episodes, but on cycle length, an emphasis that incorporates the inherent cyclicity of the illness. Figure 20-2 schematically illustrates the ways in which antidepressant treatments might interact with the natural course of the illness. The natural tendency of both depressive and manic episodes is to evolve toward remission either into a euthymic phase or into an episode of opposite polarity. An antidepressant that reverses a depressive episode has in effect accelerated the natural tendency of the episode toward remission. By the same token, it may accelerate the next sequence in the natural

Figure 20-2. Postulated interactions of antidepressant treatments with the natural course of illness.

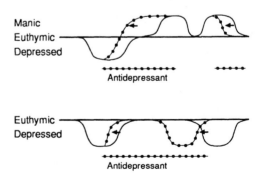

course, that is, the onset of a manic episode. The drug-induced acceleration of a manic episode may result in the mania coinciding with the natural course of a depressive episode, resulting in a mixed state, a not infrequent outcome of tricyclics in bipolar patients. The top line of Figure 20-2 illustrates how the ability of antidepressants to accelerate bipolar disorder can also translate into a paradoxical (albeit controversial[12]) observation—the antimanic effect of imipramine, as reported many years ago by Akimoto and colleagues (1962, 1963).

We have suggested that this same process should be considered when evaluating the impact of antidepressant treatments on recurrent unipolar illness, as illustrated in the bottom half of Figure 20-2. If the natural sequence of recurrent unipolar illness goes from depression to recovery and then eventually to the next episode, treatments that accelerate recovery of the index depression could also accelerate the onset of the next episode. As noted in Chapter 22, there is less evidence for this possibility than there is for the impact of antidepressants on the course of bipolar illness. Nevertheless, we should recall that, in his review of the controlled prophylactic studies, Schou (1979b) noted that the relapse rate among the recurrent unipolar patients treated with tricyclics was 50 percent higher than among those treated with lithium (35 percent vs 22 percent).[13]

At this point, we might speculate more generally about the effect of drugs on the behavior of the highly regulated neurotransmitter systems that characterize the CNS. Under normal conditions, the operation of compensatory responses generates oscillations as the system maintains its capacity to respond flexibly to random perturbations—that is, the normal compensatory oscillations provide a kind of fluidity that can absorb transient perturbations in the milieu. Under conditions in which the oscillatory range becomes narrowed, the system loses its give—the set point triggering the compensatory response is too close to midline conditions. When the system becomes more brittle in this way, a strong perturbation can trigger a response that breaks out of the oscillatory range and becomes an uncompensated and, therefore, disruptive perturbation in the system. It is roughly analogous to a suspension bridge. A certain amount of flexibility is built in so that in a strong wind it will sway rather than break.[14]

The capacity of antidepressant drugs to down-regulate neurotransmitter receptors and to increase the signal/noise ratio in some systems (i.e., increase efficiency) could result in more tightly regulated systems with narrowed compensatory response capacity. It is thus conceivable that the association between antidepressant treatment and an increased rate of switches into mania (and perhaps into depression as well) might be explained in this way—that is, the more tightly regulated system being more likely to break out when perturbed, perhaps by environmental stress. Indeed, the increased efficiency produced by antidepressants means that the normal random background noise is reduced. Perhaps it is this noise that conveys the system's fluidity and flexibility, enabling it to more easily absorb environmental stresses. Thus the same mechanisms that might explain the ability of antidepressants to alter the steady state from a stable depression to a stable recovery may also explain their propensity for inducing increased cycling in certain vulnerable individuals. We should consider also the possibility that antidepressant-enhanced signal/noise ratio could render the system more sensitive to environmental inputs (signals), including light serving as a perturbation. On the other hand, the ability of lithium to function as a normalizer may relate to the fact that its effect on an important and ubiquitous postsynaptic second messenger system is proportional to the level of activation of the system above its normal baseline.

The new pharmacological bridge must also incorporate the kindling–sensitization models to be discussed. Applying these models, Post has suggested that lithium should be more effective in preventing earlier episodes, while the anticonvulsants become more important in later phases of the illness. Although we lack studies of differential pharmacology based on direct comparisons of lithium and anticonvulsants at different stages of illness, the fact that rapid cycling (lithium resistant, anticonvulsant responsive) usually develops later is consistent with Post's prediction. Post and colleagues (1988c) have also hypothesized that "conditioned tolerance" may account for the recent observation that the prophylactic efficacy of carbamazepine is attenuated over time in some patients with rapid-cycling illness (see Chapter 23). According to Post's model, this phenomenon may require the occurrence of an episode off medication in order to regain prophylactic responsiveness.

Another aspect of the new pharmacological bridge, discussed in Chapter 19, is the effect of antidepressant, antimanic, and mood-stabilizing drugs on biological rhythms. Tricyclic and monamine oxidase inhibitor antidepressants can slow the underlying circadian oscillator, producing a phase delay in its position relative to the activity–rest cycle. This fact has been hypothesized as important to the mechanism of antidepressant activity. Furthermore, this clock slowing, phase-delaying effect of antidepressants has been linked to the capacity of these drugs to produce an acceleration of manic-depressive cycles, perhaps operating through an uncoupling of internal oscillators. The effects of mood-altering drugs on seasonal rhythms[15] are an important consideration, as is the possibility of seasonal variability in pharmacological action and clinical efficacy. Finally, hypotheses regarding the role of energy metabolism, temperature, and thyroid function in manic-depressive illness point to the need for more study of the effects of mood-altering drugs on these important fundamental physiological parameters.

Kindling and Sensitization

That manic-depressive illness in general and rapid-cycling illness in particular may represent the clinical outcome of a process analogous to electrical kindling or sensitization to pharmacological stimuli is discussed in Chapter 16. Although how precisely one can translate the specific experimental paradigms of kindling and sensitization to the variable clinical phenomena of manic-depressive illness is problematic, these models highlight two important general principles: (1) environmental causality and biological vulnerability need not be viewed as opposing hypotheses, and (2) the temporal dimension can be critical both in determining the degree to which environmental influences can activate genetic vulnerabilities and in explaining the way in which prior episodes may themselves constitute a form of stress that increases the likelihood of subsequent episodes. The kindling–sensitization hypotheses provide one important way to link environmental influences with the natural course of

the illness, including its tendency to accelerate and then level off.

These models thus provide a way to understand Kraepelin's classic observation that the illness often seems to require stress activation in its early phases. This should have profound implications for clinical management, giving special emphasis to the earliest possible detection and treatment intervention. Indeed, the importance of early treatment was emphasized by the American psychiatrist Benjamin Rush nearly a century before Kraepelin's observations:

> In all forms and combinations of madness that have been described, the duration of the disease, after it is completely formed, seems to be as much fixed by nature as the duration of any autumnal fever. It may be weakened, and life may be preserved during its continuance, but, *unless it be overcome in its first stage*, it generally runs its course, in spite of all the power of medicine. (1812) [Emphasis added]

It is likely that stress activation of bipolar illness involves a pathological reaction to the normal stresses associated with adolescence. As discussed in Chapter 16, if early pharmacological treatment, combined with psychological support, could protect the vulnerable CNS from the impact of environmental stressors, the kindling hypotheses would predict that very early treatment (even before the first episode) should diminish the likelihood of subsequent episodes or at least reduce the chances of developing the more disabling rapid-cycling form of the illness (see Figure 16-1). This prevention strategy depends on the ability to identify vulnerability before the illness has expressed itself, a possibility that awaits the discovery of biological or genetic markers applicable to the general population of manic-depressive patients. A further interesting challenge is to link kindling–sensitization models with recently reaffirmed seasonal influences on the illness.

The relevance of kindling models raises important questions about the neurochemical substrates of this phenomenon. General amine depletion by reserpine augments kindled seizures in the amygdala, and this effect is reversed by monoamine oxidase inhibitors (Wilkinson and Halpern, 1979). Specifying the role of a particular amine in kindling may be more complex and may involve regional specificity. Generally, chemical or physical lesioning of serotonin neurons in the midbrain raphe area increases kindled seizures in the amygdala (Racine and Coscina, 1979), and chemical or electrical stimulation of these serotonin neurons decreases cortical kindled seizures (Kovacs and Zoll, 1974; Siegel and Murphy, 1979). Similarly, there is some evidence associating decreased norepinephrine function in some regions with an increased susceptibility to kindled seizures. With respect to the neurotransmitter effects of anticonvulsants that are clinically effective in manic-depressive illness, the role of the GABA system appears to be most prominent in the two drugs with established clinical efficacy, carbamazepine and valproic acid. For the monoamines as well as for GABA, the fundamental relationship to kindled seizures appears to be inhibitory, so that a functional decrease in one or more of these transmitter systems might be expected to increase the likelihood of kindling. The relationship between kindling phenomena and the stress-sensitive neuroendocrine changes that have been associated with affective illness is very well reviewed by Kling and associates (1987).

Biological Rhythms: Circadian and Seasonal

We can introduce our discussion of circadian rhythms and manic-depressive illness by proposing a hypothesis: **The genetic defect in manic-depressive illness involves the circadian pacemaker or systems that modulate it.**

The clinical evidence consistent with this hypothesis is discussed in Chapter 19, and major highlights are outlined in Table 20-3. Here we focus on (1) the link between a primary circadian defect and CNS dysregulation, (2) the ways in which seasonal patterns might derive from circadian disturbances, (3) a possible link between seasonality and an increased sensitivity to light, a biological finding that is apparently independent of the state of illness, and (4) a brief review of what is known about the neurochemistry of the circadian systems, an area that may be fruitful for studies of manic-depressive illness.

As noted earlier, the various neurotransmitter and neuroendocrine abnormalities in manic-depressive illness might better be described as reflecting dysregulation rather than a straightforward deficiency or excess. Also, one interpreta-

Table 20-3. Clinical Evidence Consistent with the Hypothesis that the Genetic Defect in Manic-Depressive Illness Involves the Circadian Pacemaker, and/or Systems That Modulate It

- Many symptoms show disturbed diurnal variation
- Circadian abnormalities can produce long-term rhythmic or periodic disturbances, perhaps including mood cycles
- Circadian systems serve a major regulatory role in the CNS, and the reported biological changes in the affective illness appear to reflect dysregulation
- Most, if not all, state-dependent biological changes could reflect disturbed circadian rhythms
- Seasonal rhythms in the illness might be expected if the circadian pacemaker is disturbed
- The major state-independent finding involves the circadian system (i.e., increased sensitivity to light)

tion of the laterality findings reviewed in Chapter 18 is that they reflect an overall breakdown in integration of the CNS, particularly of the two hemispheres. Understanding the underlying pathophysiology of deterioration of regulation or integration in the CNS requires knowledge about systems that potentially organize or coordinate disparate aspects of brain function. A primary candidate for such an overriding organizing function is, of course, the temporal organizers, the biological clocks. Sir Francis Crick (1979) anticipated this function when he made the following observation:

. . . if a breakthrough in the study of the brain does come, it is perhaps likely to be at the level of the overall control of the system. If the system were as chaotic as it sometimes appears to be, it would not enable us to perform even the simplest tasks satisfactorily. To invent a possible, although unlikely, example, the discovery that brain processing was run phasically, by some kind of periodic clock, as a computer is, would probably constitute a major breakthrough. (p. 232)

Now let us consider the connection between disturbed circadian rhythms and seasonality of the illness. Among seasonal animals there are certain phases of the circadian period that are more sensitive to light (photosensitive interval). These phases are windows through which the animal reads the length of the photoperiod and thus senses the season of the year. Disturbances in circadian rhythms could disrupt this light-sampling mechanism. For example, if a phase advance resulted in a longer sampling period for dawn light, it might make certain patients more sensitive to seasonal shifts in the light/dark ratio. Of course, the extent of seasonal variation can also affect circadian rhythms (Wehr and Goodwin, 1983c; Wirz-Justice and Richter, 1979; Arató et al., 1986). As reviewed in Chapter 19, seasonal patterning in the occurrences of manic and depressive episodes and related phenomena, such as suicide, was recognized extensively in the classic literature on manic-depressive illness. However, in the modern era, seasonality has received very little attention until recently.

In Chapter 6, we discuss the relationship between cycle length and episode number drawn from three large longitudinal studies of manic-depressive illness conducted in the era before prophylactic treatment. We note the strong tendency for cycle length to shorten with each successive episode until a limit point is reached after the fourth or fifth episode. What is apparent from these data is that, on average, this limit point approximates 12 months. That is, the illness starts out slowly, gradually accelerates with each episode, and finally settles into a recurrence pattern that appears to be, on average, annual. Does this mean that the imposition of a seasonal rhythm after several episodes is a characteristic of manic-depressive illness or that a seasonal subgroup pulls the average into 12 months? Findings reviewed in Chapter 19 suggest a seasonal subgroup. It is also of interest that the cycle lengths for earlier episodes may tend to cluster around multiples of 1 year. This pattern would be consistent with seasonal influences operating from the beginning, with the initial one to three episodes involving the input of random environmental stresses, perhaps amplified by a seasonal signal in such a way that the coincidence of a random stress with a seasonal signal results in an episode every second, third, or fourth year. As the episodes recur, perhaps a kindling-like process is underway (seasonal influences may themselves represent stressors that can kindle) such that the recurrences become progressively more endogenous. One important endogenous factor would be the disturbed circadian clock, which renders the patient increasingly more vulnerable to seasonal variations.[16]

This defective buffering from normal environmental (seasonal) perturbations could result in exaggerated reactions to seasonal changes. The photoperiod has four times of interest: the beginning of summer and winter are the longest and shortest days, respectively, and the beginning of spring and fall are the two periods of maximum rate of change in the ratio of light to dark.[17] Abnormal sensitivity to light could express itself clinically either by opposite states during the two extremes of light (e.g., winter depression, summer mania) or similar disturbances in association with maximum change in light, that is, early spring or early fall, the peaks for major depression and suicide.

Relevant to these issues is the finding reviewed in Chapter 19 that manic-depressive patients show increased sensitivity to light, as measured by suppression of plasma melatonin. Not only was this increased sensitivity found in both the ill and well states, but it was also found in children who were at higher risk for manic-depressive illness by virtue of having either one or two parents with the illness. This is an important study, since it suggests that increased sensitivity to light may be part of the genetic vulnerability to manic-depressive illness and that abnormal light sensitivity in manic-depressive patients is probably not simply a result of the illness but may be a predisposing causal factor. Whether this finding can be related to the somewhat controversial reports of augmentation in the visual evoked response of manic-depressive patients (see Chapter 18) remains to be seen.

How might this increased sensitivity to light be related to the rhythm disturbances reviewed in Chapter 19? It could affect the circadian disturbances by compensating as the system attempts to overcome oscillators that, because they are poorly regulated internally, need stronger zeitgebers in order to perform their time setting, gating, regulatory role. Or, as a primary abnormality, increased light sensitivity could explain the phase advance of the strong oscillator observed in many depressed patients (and apparently also in some manic patients) (Wehr et al., 1980). Can we reconcile the state-independent increase in light sensitivity among bipolar patients with the fact that phase advances, when found, are state dependent? This might be understood in the following way. A state-independent increase in light sensitivity could produce a tendency toward phase advance that would be manifest only when the system was otherwise destabilized; that is, the phase advance would only be apparent during some periods of the depressed or manic state and would normalize with recovery. In the discussion of phase shifts occurring among rapid-cycling patients (see Chapter 19), we note progressive advances through hypomania up to the switch into depression and then progressive delays through the depression until the switch back into hypomania. Thus, maximum phase advance occurred at the end of hypomania and the beginning of depression, whereas the maximum delay occurred at the end of depression and the beginning of hypomania. (However, in trying to reconcile this with the phase advance in both depression and mania, it is important to remember that the data from rapid-cycling patients involve only hypomanic episodes.) Recall also our conclusion that phase instability may be more characteristic of manic-depressive illness than is phase advance per se.

Concerning seasonal rhythms in some forms of manic-depressive illness, we hypothesize in Chapter 19 that a vulnerability trait of increased sensitivity to light in bipolar patients could amplify the normal behavioral response to the greater intensity and duration of light during the summer, producing mania or hypomania,[18] followed by increased vulnerability to a subsequent depression in the fall or winter, reflecting a compensatory response to conserve the total seasonal energy output. Critical to the further evaluation of the light sensitivity–seasonality hypothesis would be the exploration of any similarities and differences between seasonal affective disorder patients and regular manic-depressive patients with regard to light sensitivity. Here we have only preliminary data. Lewy (personal communication) found normal light sensitivity among a group of six patients with winter SAD.

It is obvious that this model is limited, given the fact that the seasonal peaks for the onset of major depressive episodes and for suicide appear to coincide with the peaks in the rate of change in light, that is, the beginning of spring and fall. Unfortunately, the data on seasonality generally have not separated unipolar and bipolar depression, and it is difficult to avoid treatment artifacts, particularly in the data from the last 40

years. Also, some reports are based on the month of initial onset of symptoms, whereas others record hospitalizations, presumably reflecting the end stage of an episode that probably began some weeks or months earlier.

Wehr and colleagues (1989) have hypothesized that there are fundamentally two types of recurrent seasonal affective disorder, one involving winter depressions, the other summer (or late spring) depressions. Their studies indicate that the summer depression pattern displays more typical vegetative symptoms, is more severe, and is more frequently associated with suicide and with a family history of suicide. On the other hand, winter depressions are characterized by reverse neurovegetative symptoms (atypical) and may be less severe. How these distinctions generalize to a large unselected population of depressed patients is unknown. Furthermore, it is not entirely clear where bipolar patients fit in this scheme. For many, perhaps particularly those with bipolar-II disorder, atypical symptoms are generally the rule rather than the exception. On the other hand, for bipolar-I patients, it appears that typical and atypical neurovegetative symptoms may occur in the same person at different times and may vary across individuals, perhaps as a function of severity (greater severity being associated with more typical symptoms). Another interesting aspect of the seasonal specificity of symptoms is the parallel between typical melancholic depression and mania, as illustrated in Table 20-4. Thus we might visualize spring/summer activation expressing itself as mania/hypomania or as an agitated depression depending on the vulnerability of the individual.

Table 20-4. Parallels Between Typical Melancholic Depression and Mania

	Typical Depression (Melancholia)	Mania/ Hypomania	Bipolar Depression (Atypical)
Sleep	↓	↓	↑
Activity	↑	↑	↓
Mood	↓	↑	↓
Seasonal Peak	Late spring, Late summer/fall	Summer	Fall/winter

One interesting question about the seasonality of affective disorders is whether it has any bearing on the increased incidence of affective illness in the cohort born since the mid-1940s (see Chapter 7). In addition to a variety of other environmental changes that may have occurred in these last 40 years, it is worth considering that the advent of central air conditioning has altered seasonal temperature variation and has perhaps resulted in decreased exposure to natural light and greater demands for sudden adaptation to profound temperature gradients. The impact of seasonality on the epidemiology of manic-depressive illness has not been fully clarified. Seasonal influences could contribute to broad geographic differences or to variation in rural and urban locales. Unfortunately, the cross-national epidemiology data are not sufficiently precise to answer such relevant questions as whether the incidence of manic-depressive illness is lower at the equator or whether the light pattern there would simply eliminate the seasonal subgroup, leaving the overall incidence the same.

Although possible neurotransmitter or neuroendocrine contributions to seasonal rhythms in manic-depressive illness are not well established, there are some intriguing leads. As reviewed in Chapter 19, human studies of seasonal variations in neurobiological parameters are scattered and far from conclusive, with a dearth of data for normal controls. So far, the most convincing case can be made for the serotonin metabolite, which apparently is normally at its lowest point in late winter-early spring, corresponding to the principal seasonal peak in suicide, major unipolar depression, and perhaps mixed states among bipolar patients. If certain patients are already vulnerable to the destabilizing effects of the rapid change in the light/dark ratio at this time of year, having one of the buffering systems of the CNS (i.e., serotonin) at its natural seasonal low could enhance their vulnerability. Whether seasonal patterns in neurotransmitter and neuroendocrine functions in manic-depressive patients are different from normal is not known.

Patients with winter SAD, which may be analogous to bipolar-II disorder, are different from typical endogenously depressed patients because they generally do not show abnormalities in the dexamethasone suppression test, thyroid-stimulating hormone response to thyroid-releasing hor-

mone, or shortened REM latency. In reviewing the still very incomplete biological data in winter SAD, O'Rourke and co-workers (1987) and Skwerer and colleagues (1988) point to a possible dysregulation of serotonin systems. It is not clear whether or how this might be related to the apparent normal seasonal variation in central serotonin noted previously. A case can also be made, however, for the dysregulation of catecholaminergic systems in winter SAD, given its similarity to bipolar-II disorder, in which decreased dopaminergic or noradrenergic tone during the depressive phase has been suggested. Depue and colleagues (1988, 1989b) hypothesize a state-independent reduction in central dopamine activity in winter SAD. They base their hypothesis on their careful studies of abnormalities in prolactin secretion, spontaneous eyeblink rates, and thermal regulation, each of which is partly regulated by dopamine systems.

Extensive animal studies continue to define the various neurotransmitter pathways involved in the function of the circadian clock.[19] Dopamine is the principal neurotransmitter in the retina (Hadjiconstantinou and Neff, 1984), its production therein being stimulated by bright light but not by dim light (Brainard and Morgan, 1987). The suprachiasmatic nucleus (SCN) is made up of different populations of neurons containing acetylcholine, vasopressin, GABA, somatostatin, and vasoactive intestinal polypeptide. Projections to the SCN include a monosynaptic pathway from the retina (the retinohypothalamic tract), an important serotonergic pathway from the midbrain raphe region, and a visual projection from the lateral geniculate nucleus of the thalamus (an important waystation in the processing of light from the retina), which contains two closely related neuropeptides, avian pancreatic polypeptide and neuropeptide Y (NPY). Microinjections of NPY into the region of the SCN produce phase shifts in circadian rhythms in hamsters (Albers and Ferris, 1984). In light of this, it is especially interesting that NPY recently has been reported to be significantly lower in the CSF of patients with major depression than in controls or schizophrenic patients (Widerlöv et al., 1988b).

As the resolving power of the brain-imaging strategies improves, it should become possible to study the SCN region clinically using both metabolic tracers and specific neurotransmitter receptor ligands. At this point, we simply note with interest the coincidence that the neurotransmitter-neuromodulatory substances apparently involved in the modulation of the clock (especially serotonin, acetylcholine, somatostatin, vasopressin, and perhaps NPY) have each been independently suggested as being involved in the pathophysiology of manic-depressive illness, with serotonin having perhaps the longest standing indications of some role.

A Generic Hypothesis

A broad and generic hypothesis would ideally link much of the literature reviewed in the pathophysiology section and also be congruent with the clinical realities of the illness. Our hypothesis might start with a genetic vulnerability expressed as altered membrane proteins (or lipids) localized in a widely distributed system that subserves the selective integration of cognitive, emotional, and motoric functions, particularly in response to stress. The defect might be in the system(s) responsible for gating stimuli and dampening unwarranted oscillations, thus providing a kind of regulatory stability while maintaining necessary flexibility. From the point of view of known neurotransmitter systems, there are several appealing candidates, including serotonin, norepinephrine, and GABA. Primarily for purposes of discussion, we prefer to focus on central serotonin and on the systems that modulate serotonergic function (some perhaps yet undiscovered) because, at this writing, several findings in manic-depressive illness seem to converge here.[20] Some of the neuroendocrine parameters point in the direction of serotonin. For example, serotonin systems exert a phasic modulatory influence on the HPA axis, and serotonin inhibits kindled seizures. In addition, perhaps the most cohesive explanations for the mechanism of action of lithium focus on the drug's ability to enhance and stabilize central serotonin function. The fact that there may be a similar convergence around the serotonin systems in seasonal affective disorders adds impetus to further explorations of this general area. At this juncture, the preliminary neuroanatomical evidence reviewed in Chapter 18 can provide scant leads as to which system or systems might be involved. This is primarily because the neuroanatomical data have been analyzed almost exclusively from the perspective of a search for

some discrete localized lesion to explain a symptom or syndrome, rather than as an approach to evaluating potential dysfunctions in the integration of diverse regions. As noted previously, the laterality findings have been interpreted as reflecting some loss of the normal integration of the hemispheres.

Specifying the nature of the dysfunction related to this neurotransmitter system might require a focus on membrane uptake mechanisms, since this process involves proteins (the likely expression of a genetic defect), and at least some of the platelet uptake and binding data suggest reduced serotonin transport in bipolar patients. A generalized disorder of membrane transport function might produce a particular clinical syndrome through its effect on discrete systems especially vulnerable to the generalized defect. Even a small defect in a system that regulates other systems could become amplified into a cascade of events, resulting in a perturbation leading to a switch into an episode. One candidate for such a vulnerable system is that comprising the serotonergic input to the regulation of circadian function.

Another membrane hypothesis is more generic in that it focuses on second-messenger systems that function postsynaptically beyond the neurotransmitter-specific receptors on the neuronal surface. Two of these second-messenger systems (cyclic AMP and polyphosphoinositide, PI) have been the focus of speculation concerning the mechanism of action of lithium. Depending on their presynaptic linkage, these systems serve to amplify either inhibitory or stimulatory signals. Down-regulation of these second-messenger systems by lithium could, therefore, correct an imbalance—dampening an overly excited system, stimulating an inhibited one, and having no effect on a system in normal balance. This is especially relevant to the PI system, since the effect of lithium is proportional to the level of activation of the system. Because this is consistent with the clinical profile of lithium, the second-messenger hypothesis is appealing, at least as an explanation for the mechanism of action of the key drug used in treating manic-depressive illness.

In a more general vein, we should reiterate what we said earlier concerning the need for greater focus on nonlinear stochastic processes, since they might ultimately yield a greater under-

Table 20-5. Clinical Implications of Instability Models

- Aggressive treatment early

- Bias toward prophylaxis

- Enhancement of circadian integrity
  - regular schedule of sleep, meals, exercise, etc.
  - intervene under special circumstances
    (jet lag, stress or event-related insomnia, etc.)
  - avoid substances which disrupt rhythms
    (alcohol, cocaine, etc.)

- Avoid intermittent stressors (including substances)
  with kindling potential, including episodic alcohol
  and drug abuse

standing of brain function. In a regulated system, such as the brain, normal compensatory processes lead to oscillations. If the system is too inflexible—that is, if it is overregulated—a strong stimulus might trigger oscillations that break out of the normal range, resulting in perturbations that can no longer be compensated. These sudden phasic shifts can then produce a disruption in the system that renders it more vulnerable to subsequent perturbations through a process analogous to kindling.

In general, we are referring here to models that postulate that instability is the fundamental dysfunction in manic-depressive illness.[21] The clinical implications of these instability models are outlined in Table 20-5 and have been developed more thoroughly in Chapter 23. Incorporation of these principles into clinical practice gives emphasis to a renewed focus on environmental psychiatry[22] (Wehr et al., 1988).

NOTES

1. As noted in Chapter 19, reporting bias may account for some of the clustering of cycle length around yearly peaks, although the magnitude of the effect seems too large to be fully accounted for in this way. The appreciation of seasonality characteristic of the classical literature on manic-depressive illness virtually disappeared in modern formulations.
2. Kraepelin's definition of manic-depressive illness includes bipolar and recurrent unipolar major affective disorder.
3. He did not consider what is known about the neurotransmitters subserving these systems.
4. These three dimensions are analogous to those originally formulated by Donald Klein and also

contain elements of the work of Stein (1962) and of Crow and Deakin (1981) regarding the neuroanatomy and neurochemistry of reward systems. Thus, according to this model, depression involves an inhibition of central pleasure mechanisms, generally but not always accompanied by disinhibition of central pain regulation and an "inhibited psychomotor facilitatory mechanism," as originally defined by Klein (1974). Mania, on the other hand, involves disinhibitions of central pain and disinhibited psychomotor facilitatory mechanism. Carroll accounts for mixed manic-depressive states as reflecting disinhibited pain regulation, disinhibited reinforcement reward function, and disinhibited psychomotor facilitatory mechanism. It should be noted, of course, that there is an extensive literature describing the prominence of the monoamine transmitters in these functionally defined systems.

5. In Chapter 17, we attempt to draw attention to the effects of drugs on cyclicity per se.
6. The subject of illness specificity, that is, how reliably biological abnormalities differentiate manic-depressive illness from other psychiatric illnesses such as schizophrenia, is discussed subsequently.
7. For example, when large doses of the catecholamine precursor L-dopa were administered to depressed patients, there was some activation of the psychomotor retardation but no improvement in mood, cognition, or the overall depressive syndrome (Goodwin et al., 1970). Similarly, L-tryptophan, the amino acid precursor of serotonin, has been shown to potentiate the effects of a tricyclic antidepressant on depressed mood and on anxiety but not on the level of psychomotor activity or arousal (Walinder et al., 1976). The model of amine abnormalities in other (nonpsychiatric) illnesses involving the CNS is noteworthy in this respect. For example, in parkinsonism, although degeneration of dopamine neurons is undoubtedly close to the basic pathology, optimal treatment might involve both dopamine replacement (with L-dopa) and anticholinergic agents. Here one aspect of the syndrome (akinesia) might reflect the primary pathology, and other aspects (perhaps tremor or rigidity) might reflect secondary neurochemical concomitants, such as disinhibition of acetylcholine neurons or compensatory overactivity of remaining dopamine neurons (Goodwin et al., 1977).
8. These issues were extensively discussed in Chapters 3, 4, and 5.
9. The fact that unipolar is broadly defined (i.e., as nonbipolar) may account for its relative nonspecificity in family history studies.
10. Crow has also speculated that laterality shifts (see Chapter 18) might be the pathophysiological expression of the "variable underlying psychoses" with left temporal dominance associated with schizophrenia and right dominance associated

with affective illness. He suggests "the possibility that the determinants of brain lateralisation and psychosis are related" (p. 425)

11. The complexity of the relationship between genotypic and phenotypic variance can be illustrated by the example of Huntington's disease. Although it is now established that it results from a defect in a single gene locus, the disease can occur with enormous phenotypic variation in age of onset, nature of symptoms, and course of illness. This variation presumably comes from the interaction of the specific genetic defect with other genetic or environmental sources of variance. With regard to the influence of environmental factors on the clinical expression of a genetic defect, the classic example is the autosomal dominant condition of phenylketonuria, the symptoms of which require the presence of certain substances in the diet.

12. In 1967, Klein conducted a random, double-blind comparison of imipramine and placebo in 13 manic patients and found no significant difference.

13. This tricyclic–lithium difference (which did not quite achieve statistical significance) could of course reflect simply that the tricyclics were less effective in preventing the natural occurrence of relapses or that their prophylactic efficacy among some of the patients was offset by the acceleration of the illness among others.

14. The role of variability (chaos) in maintaining the healthy function of complex, regulated, physiological systems is becoming an important new force in biology (see, e.g., Pool, 1984; Mandell, 1985; Glass and Mackey, 1988).

15. Drugs could exert their effects on seasonal rhythms directly by acting on oscillators or indirectly by affecting sensitivity to light (see, e.g., Seggie et al., 1989a,b) or to changing temperature.

16. Depue and colleagues (1987) have suggested that bipolar patients have an inherently greater variability in their level of "behavioral engagement" (BE). Among bipolar patients with a seasonal pattern, this excess variability is expressed as amplification of normal seasonal changes in BE.

17. These peaks occur because of the elliptical orbit of the earth around the sun.

18. It is interesting that one study of phase advance comparing depression and mania within the same bipolar patients (Wehr et al., 1980) indicated somewhat greater advance during mania, although the mania-depression difference does not reach statistical significance. A phase advance during mania could increase the duration of exposure to morning light in the summer, which, given increased sensitivity to light, could contribute further to the mania.

19. Rusak and Zucker, 1979; Moore, 1983; Albers et al., 1984; Johnson et al., 1988.

20. Of course, given the pervasive and functionally important linkages between the serotonergic, noradrenergic, and other neurotransmitter systems, one could just as well build a case around dysfunction of a central norepinephrine system or other systems.

21. Both Mandell and colleagues (1984) and Depue and associates (1987), each group approaching the issue from its own unique perspective, have suggested that variability per se may be a basic feature of bipolar illness.

22. In addition to light, temperature, and specific stressors, there are other environmental factors that may constitute the legitimate focus of study in the future as adequate methods are developed. For example, exposure to extremely low frequency (ELF) electromagnetic fields has been suggested as a factor to explain certain phenomena in the epidemiology of depression and suicide (Anderson and Phillips, 1985). Wilson has suggested (1988) that this association may be mediated through the disruptive effects of ELF fields on circadian rhythms. For example, Wever (1973) found that under free-running conditions, normal human subjects experienced a shortening of the normal circadian period (i.e., a faster clock) when exposed to ELF electrical fields. If manic-depressive patients were poorly entrained to zeitgebers (as some data suggest)—that is, if they had a tendency to free run—they could be vulnerable to having their clock accelerated by ELF fields in the environment.

PART FIVE

TREATMENT

Of all our conversations, I remember most vividly [Robert Lowell's] words about the new drug, lithium carbonate, which had such good results and gave him reason to believe he was cured: "It's terrible, Bob, to think that all I've suffered, and all the suffering I've caused, might have arisen from the lack of a little salt in my brain."
—Robert Giroux[1]

Until the middle of this century, manic-depressive illness had remained intractable, frustrating the best efforts of clinical practitioners and their forebears. This long history ended abruptly with the discovery of lithium's therapeutic benefits. In an ironic turn of events, the pharmacological revolution then mobilized a renaissance in the psychotherapy of manic-depressive patients. Substantially freed of the severe disruptions of mania and the profound withdrawal of depression, patients and therapists could sustain their focus on the many psychological issues related to the illness and also confront basic developmental tasks. To be sure, even the combination of drugs and psychotherapy cannot yield a completely satisfactory outcome for every patient. But the treatment approaches now available do allow most manic-depressive patients to lead relatively normal lives—lives that are less painfully interrupted by illness and less often prematurely ended by suicide.

This portion of the book departs from earlier sections in its emphasis on the application of accumulated knowledge to the pragmatic business of treating individual patients. This shift—from the concerns of clinical science to the concerns of clinical practice—calls for a different approach. As one medical sociologist and historian has observed:

While the aim of all sciences is the maximum of generality, that of medicine ought always to be *action* aimed at the maximum welfare of the *individual*. (Wightman, 1971, p. 14)

It is that principle that has guided the writing of these chapters.

The section discusses practical therapeutic choices faced by the clinician and summarizes the clinical research on the effectiveness of available treatments. With some exceptions, applying the treatment strategies outlined here does not require a highly specialized background in manic-depressive illness. However, consultation may be necessary in some situations: When the diagnosis is uncertain, when the decision to hospitalize is difficult, when the response to initial treatment is poor, when the patient fails to comply with a prescribed regimen, or, especially, when there is danger of suicide. Although bipolar illness remains the primary point of focus in this section, recurrent unipolar illness and its management are considered, especially in our discussions of prophylactic treatment.

STRUCTURE AND RATIONALE OF THE TREATMENT CHAPTERS

We chose a somewhat unconventional organization for these chapters, with clinical recommendations preceding the evidence that supports them. There were two reasons for this choice. First, our treatment recommendations are more than just a distillation of research findings. They are drawn from our reading of the literature and, we believe, represent the essential core of the evidence. Where we find the literature incomplete or equivocal, we supplement it with the seasoned judgments of our colleagues and opinions based on our own clinical experience. The second reason we organized these chapters as we did is our belief that the formal literature has more meaning when framed by clinical treatment issues. Although future research certainly will alter and add to our recommendations, we hope the fundamental principles will have lasting value for the clinical care of patients with manic-depressive illness.

The first three chapters are devoted to medical techniques—medication, electroconvulsive therapy, and manipulation of sleep and light. The use of these techniques for treating manic episodes is covered in Chapter 21, and their use in depressive episodes in Chapter 22. In both chapters, it is assumed that the patient is not already on a prophylactic regimen. Long-term maintenance treatment is discussed in Chapter 23; also covered in this chapter are the acute and long-term side effects of lithium and other medications and the management of breakthrough episodes during prophylactic treatment.

Chapters 24 and 25 deal with psychotherapy and related issues, major components of the clinical management of manic-depressive illness. Chapter 24 discusses the nature of psychotherapeutic work in treating manic-depressive illness, and Chapter 25 focuses on the special issue of compliance with medical treatments, especially lithium.

The coexistence of substance abuse is increasingly recognized as a complicating and limiting factor in the treatment of manic-depressive illness. Thus, successful management of the illness depends on the clinician's ability to recognize and treat alcohol and drug abuse, as reviewed in Chapter 26.

Far too many manic-depressive patients kill themselves, and clinicians must be astute in assessing suicide potential and sensitive to the special management issues raised by that potential. We consider these questions in Chapter 27.

STAGES OF TREATMENT

In reading this section, it is well to keep in mind the natural course of manic-depressive illness described in Chapter 6. Although many treatments can alter acute symptoms dramatically, the nature and logic of planning treatment should be shaped by respect for the course of the illness: its inherently, insidiously, recurrent nature. The tendency of the illness to worsen over time is another crucial point to remember.

Throughout these chapters, we use several terms to describe stages of medical and psychotherapeutic treatments that are linked conceptually to aspects of the natural course. We define them as follows:

- *Acute treatment* refers to treatment given during the period from the beginning of a manic or depressive episode to remission. For example, in the case of successful antidepressant drug treatment, acute treatment usually lasts from 6 to 12 weeks, far less time than the 9 to 12 month duration of an untreated episode of bipolar depression.
- *Continuation treatment* is the ongoing treatment of a depressive or manic episode from the point of clinical remission to the point at which spontaneous remission would be expected to occur in untreated patients. Although overt clinical symptoms of illness may remit rapidly, an underlying tail of vulnerability can remain for some time. The duration of continuation treatment is determined by the natural course of illness. In unipolar patients, antidepressants are usually recommended for a period of 6 to 12 months after remission,[2] but in bipolar patients, the continuation phase after a depressive episode should be kept much shorter because of the risk of antidepressant drugs pre-

cipitating mania or inducing rapid cycling (as reviewed in Chapter 22). The continuation phase of treatment after a manic episode can involve the management of a postmania depression or a sometimes protracted period of mood instability dominated by dysphoria (see, e.g., Fox, 1988) as the patient attempts to repair the external and internal damage wrought by the manic episode.

- *Long-term maintenance (prophylactic) treatment*[3] is intended to prevent or attenuate future episodes of manic-depressive illness, and it is used somewhat more selectively than are acute and continuation treatments. The treatment of breakthrough episodes, discussed in Chapter 23, requires an understanding of the principles of both acute and maintenance treatment.

GENERAL CLINICAL CONSIDERATIONS

Psychiatric Evaluation and Diagnosis

Evaluating the patient before treatment is the most important stage in managing the illness. As extensively as the patient's clinical condition permits, the evaluation should cover the pattern and duration of symptoms, the patient's exposure to possibly stressful life events, and the patient's suicidal potential, substance use, and personal and family history. If at all possible, the patient's spouse or a close family member should participate. Family members are almost always helpful in evaluating the patient, and their presence serves as an opportunity for the clinician to assess their attitudes about such issues as hospitalization. The situation also provides an occasion for evaluating the family's ability and willingness to participate further in treatment and follow-up.

Differential diagnosis, discussed fully in Chapter 5, most often involves:

- Patients who are in a hyperactive psychotic state and whose personal or family history is not available. In these cases, acute schizophrenia and organic and drug-induced psychoses must be ruled out.
- Patients with mild manic-like symptoms. Normal elevated mood must be differentiated from clinical hypomania.
- Patients with severe depressive symptoms whose history is unknown. The most important alternative diagnosis to consider is unipolar depression. Schizophrenia and schizoaffective illness, drug-induced states, and dementia also must be ruled out.
- Patients with moderate depressive symptoms. Major depressive illness, either unipolar or bipolar, must be distinguished from milder forms. Manic-depressive illness should be considered whenever recurrent, discrete episodes are present.

Medical Evaluation

The medical evaluation preceding treatment, like the psychiatric evaluation, should be shaped by the clinical situation. When lithium treatment is being considered, more emphasis must be given to thyroid and renal function, whereas when tricyclics or monoamine oxidase inhibitors are to be used, the cardiovascular history should receive more attention. Since pretreatment medical evaluation is most critical for long-term treatment, specific recommendations for laboratory tests are listed in Table 23-1.

A form on which patients can report necessary psychiatric and medical pretreatment data is useful when the patient's clinical condition permits. It can help the clinician structure questions during the actual evaluation session. Family members can provide supplemental information or may even fill out the form completely. Some clinicians may prefer to use full-scale diagnostic instruments, such as the Schedule of Affective Disorders and Schizophrenia or Structured Clinical Interview for Diagnosis, or rating scales such as the Hamilton.

Clinicians often discover previously undiagnosed medical problems in the course of their routine pretreatment evaluations. This potential dividend provides a further reason to exercise care in the initial phase of treatment.

The Therapeutic Alliance in Drug Treatment

Chapter 24 deals extensively with the relationship between psychotherapy and drugs (especially lithium) in treating bipolar patients. Here we pause briefly to underscore a fundamental truth in psychopharmacology: To achieve its full potential, any drug should be given in the context of a solid and positive clinician–patient relationship. Unfortunately, a working therapeutic alliance is not always achieved in the context of a busy practice.

The healing role of the clinician and the potentially life-saving influence of competent and compassionate psychotherapy are too often overlooked in an era of increasingly sophisticated psychopharmacology. The extraordinarily important role of this relationship in treatment and recovery was described by Morag Coate in *Beyond All Reason* (1964)[4]:

> A psychotic illness is the loneliest experience in the world, and a patient who writes bizarre, joking, enthusiastic, or possibly unintelligible letters may well not convey this simple fact. An occasional letter from the outside doctor, even if it is no more than two typed lines above a signature, will do more to help than a quart of tranquilisers. Even a message given through one of the other doctors can be of great value. The knowledge that he still cares to keep in touch may be the one thing that will make the prison-like impact of hospital endurable. But the recovered patient is not likely to say this; it is not easy to admit to having been so vulnerable. . . .
>
> Living as a patient in a mental hospital is an illuminating way of discovering what doctors are like and what their work can mean. The psychiatrists who are most concerned about their patients must suffer much stress and many disappointments, but they might well be warmed to know the tributes paid to them in those night-time discussions that they never hear. . . .
>
> Because the doctors cared, and because one of them still believed in me when I believed in nothing, I have survived to tell the tale. It is not only the doctors who perform hazardous operations or give life-saving drugs in obvious emergencies who hold the scales at times between life and death. To sit quietly in a consulting room and talk to someone would not appear to the general public as a heroic or dramatic thing to do. In medicine there are many different ways of saving lives. This is one of them. (pp. 209–214)

Nothing substitutes for clinical experience in applying the general principles and research knowledge to the drug treatment of manic-depressive illness. In most instances, we cannot predict with complete certainty that a given patient will tolerate and benefit from a particular drug. Nor can we predict the safest and most effective dose. Experimentation and adjustment are required when treatment begins, and the patient should be warned accordingly.

The patient is most likely to cooperate if the clinician approaches drug treatment as an investigative undertaking—one depending on active collaboration. Controlled double-blind studies of antidepressant drugs consistently show success rates substantially below those reported in open trials. Some of this difference certainly can be attributed to the positive expectations of the clinical investigator in the open trial, but much of it is probably due to better compliance and the positive and reinforcing effects of the therapeutic alliance.

Clinicians are in the best position to help a depressed or manic patient when they convey an attitude of serious concern for the individual's suffering and, at the same time, communicate confidence in their own ability and measured optimism about the ultimate outcome of treatment. It is important not to oversell a treatment. If the first approach fails without the patient's having been advised about the possibility of failure, not only is the patient's trust eroded, but the clinician feels defeated and discredited—feelings which, in turn, may be subtly conveyed back to the patient. When both clinician and patient view a treatment as an experiment, even a poor response can be seen as an important piece of new information that can contribute substantially to the rational choice of subsequent treatments. Patients who are prescribed drugs should be told that if they fail to respond to one class of drugs, they may, by that fact, be more likely to respond to an alternate class.

In summary, competent and compassionate treatment assumes a thorough knowledge of the diagnosis, clinical description, and natural course of manic-depressive illness, an understanding of the pharmacological and psychotherapeutic options available, and the ability to establish a good therapeutic relationship, as well as the ability and willingness to communicate clearly with patients and their families. With these general points in mind, we turn to the specifics of medical and psychological treatments of manic-depressive illness.

NOTES

1. In introduction to *Robert Lowell: Collected Prose,* 1987.
2. For the more recurrent forms of unipolar illness, it may be advisable to keep the continuation phase of antidepressant treatment shorter, as one would do for a bipolar patient.
3. We use the term *prophylaxis* to describe the effects of treatment on the long-term course of manic-depressive illness. These effects can range from complete prevention of future episodes to attenuation of their frequency, duration, and/or severity. For us, *complete prophylaxis* reflects the prevention of future episodes, and *partial prophylaxis* reflects attenuation but not full prevention.
4. Other patients' views of the importance of the clinician in their treatment are presented in Chapters 10, 24, and 25.

21

Medical Treatment
of Manic Episodes

No one predicts how long it will be before the drugs take hold & [Robert Lowell]
begins to be himself again. Meanwhile he writes and revises translations furiously
and with a kind [of] crooked brilliance, and talks about himself in connection with
Achilles, Alexander, Hart Crane, Hitler and Christ, and breaks your heart.
—William Meredith[1]

A patient in the throes of a manic episode can be intensely agitated, uncooperative, psychotic, aggressive, or dangerous. By the time the clinician is brought in, both patient and family are understandably confused and distraught. The bizarre, frightening behavior obviously must be controlled humanely, but the clinician has little time to ponder available choices. Which drugs are best for this patient in this situation? Should the patient be hospitalized? Should electroconvulsive therapy be used? Each decision calls for balancing the ravages of the illness against the consequences of intervention—a medication's potency against its side effects, for example, or the patient's safety against the stigma of hospitalization.

This chapter focuses on such issues in the medical management of acute manic episodes. Like others in this section, the chapter begins with a discussion of practical issues of clinical management, an approach to treatment drawn from the research evidence and our own clinical experience. The research literature is reviewed in the second part of the chapter, which some readers may choose to read first.

We are convinced that medical management is necessary for all patients who are truly manic or are hypomanic and likely to become manic. Based on that assumption, we devote the follow-

ing discussion largely to criteria for appropriate pharmacological treatment for acute mania. One important caveat is in order, however. Not all activated patients are necessarily manic, or even hypomanic, and not all mildly hypomanic patients inevitably progress to mania. The line between normal exuberance and clinical hypomania is sometimes difficult to discern, and clinicians must approach the task of differential diagnosis with care (see Chapters 4 and 5). Once the diagnosis has been made, skillful psychological management must accompany the drug treatment of emerging or acute mania, especially if the patient or family resists the idea of medications (see Chapter 25).

Lithium, the first of the modern antimanic agents, remains the most important. Its therapeutic value was discovered by the Australian physician John Cade (1949), whose post-World War II experiments with guinea pigs signaled a revolution in the treatment of manic-depressive illness. Several years were to pass before the importance of Cade's pioneering work was recognized. European psychiatrists began to take notice in 1954, when his observations were confirmed and extended by Mogens Schou in Denmark. Although a handful of American psychiatrists were among the pioneers, lithium was not widely used in the United States until the late 1960s. This slow acceptance was partly traceable to earlier adverse experiences with lithium as a salt substitute.

Chlorpromazine, the prototypical antipsychotic medication for controlling the symptoms of schizophrenia, was first used clinically for a psychiatric disorder in a manic patient (Schneider, 1951, cited in Swazey, 1974). More extensive clinical observations in acutely manic patients followed (Lehmann and Hanrahan, 1954). Since lithium was still essentially unknown at that time, particularly to American psychiatrists, chlorpromazine quickly became the treatment of choice for acute mania. Haloperidol, a butyrophenone that also controls psychotic symptoms, was introduced in the late 1960s and was found to control psychotic behavior as effectively as chlorpromazine while producing less sedation and hypotension. As a result, many clinicians now prefer haloperidol and other high-potency neuroleptics, such as thiothixene.

The use of anticonvulsant drugs to treat manic episodes dates back to the 1970s (Okuma et al., 1973). Some anticonvulsant drugs that have shown considerable therapeutic promise, particularly carbamazepine, clonazepam, and valproate, are already widely used with manic patients. Although not yet approved by the U.S. Food and Drug Administration for marketing as antimanic agents, they can, of course, be used by physicians at their own discretion.[2]

CLINICAL MANAGEMENT

Clinical Factors Influencing Drug Choices

Clinical decisions in managing mania are influenced by the treatment setting, the nature and overall severity of the symptoms, and the presence of medical complications. The following recommendations are based on findings of the studies reviewed later in this chapter, modified and amplified by our own clinical experience and that of colleagues we surveyed.

Symptoms

The most important consideration in choosing a treatment for manic symptoms is their nature and severity. Mild manic symptoms (hypomania or stage-I mania) usually respond well to lithium alone. Restoring a normal sleep pattern (Hudson

et al., 1989) can often avert escalation to more severe stages of mania. This might be accomplished by using an adjunctive sedative hypnotic, such as the benzodiazepines clonazepam or lorazepam, during the evening.

A neuroleptic may be needed to control severe symptoms, particularly gross hyperactivity and psychotic features. Whether to chose a neuroleptic of high potency (e.g., haloperidol, thiothixene) or low potency (e.g., chlorpromazine, thioridazine) is still an unsettled issue. High-potency drugs have a relatively low level of hypotensive and sedative side effects, a feature that allows more rapid initial dose escalation and, therefore, presumably more rapid control of the psychosis. Low-potency neuroleptics, on the other hand, are more sedating—actually an advantage in achieving early control of the acute mania. In addition, low-potency drugs carry less of a risk of extrapyramidal effects,[3] including tardive dyskinesia, and neurotoxic reactions, and also the rare neuroleptic malignant syndrome[4] (Casey, 1984; Pope et al., 1986).

Both the research literature and our own clinical experience suggest that the anticonvulsants and neuroleptics are superior to lithium in the early phase of treating severe mania, that is, during the first week or two. After the first 2 weeks, lithium and, perhaps, carbamazepine are more effective than neuroleptics. Because of their greater specificity, lithium and carbamazepine calm the patient with a minimum of sedation and nonspecific tranquilization. These drugs are also superior because they are less likely to be associated with postmania depressions and, even more important, carry no appreciable risk of tardive dyskinesia.

The proper role of the anticonvulsants in treating acute mania has not yet been fully established. As reviewed later, carbamazepine is clearly effective, even when used alone (although in most trials it was given in combination with lithium or neuroleptics). Existing data suggest that carbamazepine may be as effective in acute mania as lithium or neuroleptics, but its overall efficacy requires more study. Compared with lithium, carbamazepine is similar in its relative specificity against the affective core of mania and often faster in achieving its antimanic effects. Less clear is whether it can match the effectiveness of neuroleptics in the short-term control of the extreme hyperactivity seen in psychotic mania, although some evidence is encouraging.

As a treatment for manic-depressive illness, carbamazepine is best established as an alternative for patients who do not respond to lithium or cannot tolerate it.[5] Thus, carbamazepine is the treatment of choice for managing acute mania in patients with a history of lithium-resistant rapid cycles, lithium failure or intolerance, or kidney dysfunction. Because of its antidepressant properties, carbamazepine, alone or combined with lithium, may be particularly useful in the acute treatment of mixed states, which may not respond well to lithium alone (Secunda et al., 1985). Because it lessens aggression, carbamazepine may also be a good choice for suicidal patients. Until further information is available, the other anticonvulsants should generally be reserved for patients who do not respond satisfactorily to carbamazepine. A possible exception to this rule may be clonazepam, which, because of its sedative profile and safety, can be an important adjunct in the initial treatment of mania.[6]

Setting

The treatment setting also influences the choice of drugs or electroconvulsive therapy (ECT). Mania subsides more gradually with lithium than with neuroleptics, the anticonvulsants, or ECT. This lithium lag, 7 to 12 days when the mania is moderate to severe, might be tolerable in a well-staffed inpatient research unit, but very rapid control of symptoms has priority in most settings and is clearly a necessity in some, such as an emergency room without a closed psychiatric unit for backup.[7] In these settings, neuroleptics and/or anticonvulsants (or, selectively, ECT) are preferable for highly agitated patients. A decision tree outlining the choice of treatments for mania is illustrated in Figure 21-1.

Contraindications

Medical conditions or medication needs sometimes limit the choice of drugs.[8] Although we are concerned here with the short-term use of drugs in treating acute mania, the medical factors discussed subsequently are also relevant to discussions of long-term prophylactic treatment (see Chapter 23). Medical contraindications for antimanic drugs, although rare, must always be bal-

anced against the risks of untreated mania. Table 21-1 lists, in approximate rank order, contraindications to antimanic drugs. (The subjective and behavioral side effects of lithium and its effect on organ systems are fully reviewed in Chapter 23.)

Impaired kidney function is a relative contraindication for lithium treatment because lithium is eliminated principally through the kidney and can influence renal tubular activity. Lithium can be used for patients with moderate or stable impairment, but the blood level should be carefully monitored, since a therapeutic level usually can be reached with lower doses than those needed for patients with normally functioning kidneys. Carbamazepine can be substituted for lithium when severe renal impairment precludes its use.

Cardiac disease is another important consideration in treating mania. By virtue of its ionic properties and especially its ability to substitute for potassium, lithium produces changes in the electrocardiogram (particularly T-wave flattening) that are generally benign and reversible. There are, however, rare and scattered case reports of patients with certain kinds of cardiac pathology who experience lithium-induced complications (Jefferson et al., 1987).

Myocardial infarction requires a balancing of risks. Lithium can conceivably produce complications in an already compromised myocardium (primarily because it can increase irritability). This risk must be weighed against possibly even greater risks, such as the effect of the untreated manic patient's uncontrolled activity, psychophysiological stress, and uncertain compliance with cardiac medication, as well as the hypotension that may result from taking neuroleptics. Lithium should, therefore, be considered for managing a manic or hypomanic episode, even during or shortly after myocardial infarction. Carbamazepine or perhaps clonazepam may provide useful alternatives to lithium or neuroleptics in this situation. (For comprehensive reviews of the cardiac effects of lithium, see Albrecht and Müller-Oerlinghausen, 1980; Jefferson et al., 1987.)

Neurological conditions that influence treatment decisions in mania include epilepsy, parkinsonism, dementia, cerebellar disease, and myasthenia gravis. The risk of neuroleptic-induced tardive dyskinesia increases with age, particularly in women. In addition, the risk appears to be

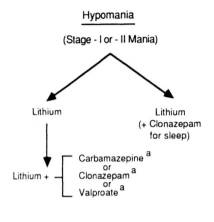

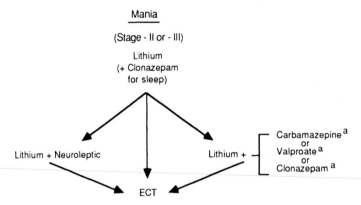

Figure 21-1. A treatment decision tree for mania. [a]The anticonvulsants are more likely to be indicated when there is a history of rapid cycles, lithium resistance, or temporal lobe–like symptoms.

substantially greater for patients with affective illness than for those with schizophrenia (Casey, 1984). Intermittent use of a neuroleptic, more typical in manic-depressive illness than in schizophrenia, may also be associated with a greater risk of tardive dyskinesia, but this association is controversial.

Neither lithium nor the neuroleptics are contraindicated for acute mania in patients with classic epilepsy, although both drugs can produce activation of the electroencephalogram (EEG). The obvious choice for treating manic-depressive illness in patients with seizure disorders is carbamazepine, which has anticonvulsant activity.

Lithium can aggravate preexisting Parkinson's disease, an effect that is not surprising, since lithium decreases dopamine synthesis in the brain (see Chapter 17) (Makeeva et al., 1974).[9] Carbamazepine, which does not markedly affect the

dopamine system, is preferable to neuroleptics in managing the mania that can emerge when parkinsonian patients are treated with L-dopa. It is also best for manic patients with preexisting tardive dyskinesia.

Neuroleptics or anticonvulsants may be better than lithium for manic patients with dementia, cerebellar disease, or other pathology of the CNS because lithium is more likely to intensify the underlying dysfunctions. However, some patients with dementia are particularly sensitive to the organic confusional effects of neuroleptics or anticonvulsants. In the neuroleptics, this effect is probably due to their potent hypotensive action.

The tendency of lithium to produce muscle weakness makes it unsuitable for treating manic patients with myasthenia gravis. It has been used successfully to treat the pathological mood lability associated with multiple sclerosis without

Table 21-1. Relative Contraindications
for Antimanic Drugs

Lithium

Usually contraindicated:
Renal function impairment
Acute myocardial infarction
Myasthenia gravis
Pregnancy - 1st trimester
Breast feeding
Compromised fluid or salt balance

Use with close medical supervision, including limited
dosage:
Other cardiac pathology
Parkinson's disease
Pregnancy - 2nd or 3rd trimester
Delivery
Epilepsy
Thyroid disorders

Use with caution, including limited dosage:
Cerebellar disorders
Dementia
Other CNS disorders
Diabetes mellitus
Ulcerative colitis
Psoriasis
Senile cataracts
Osteoporosis
Certain drugs (see text)

Neuroleptics

Myocardial infarction
Parkinson's disease
Compromised liver function
Porphyria
Hypotension
Tardive dyskinesia

Carbamazepine

Compromised liver function
Porphyria
Hematopoietic system abnormality
A-V block

Clonazepam

Neurological disorders affecting balance
CNS depression

A previous history of allergic reaction to any antimanic drug
would be a contraindication for that particular drug.

aggravating the neurological disorder (see, e.g., Kemp et al., 1977), although such patients may have a lower threshold for some of lithium's side effects in the CNS.

Other medical conditions also may be affected by drug treatments for mania. Neuroleptics and perhaps carbamazepine should be ruled out for patients with compromised liver function and porphyria, for example. Carbamazepine and the new atypical neuroleptic, clozapine, both have been associated with bone marrow suppression and should be avoided in patients with disturbed hematopoietic function. Although lithium is not contraindicated for patients with diabetes, the disease process should be monitored closely once the drug is started since it has been reported to exacerbate diabetes, especially in patients taking it for several years (see, e.g., Mellerup et al., 1983).

Thyroid disease can be aggravated by the chronic use of lithium, but in the relatively brief acute treatment phase, the administration of thyroid hormone can offset any effects of lithium. Hypothyroidism may also contribute to inadequate lithium response. One severely manic patient, for example, was unresponsive to a lithium–neuroleptic combination until after her hypothyroidism was corrected (Balldin et al., 1987). Similarly, postpartum mania may be associated with poor lithium response (Targum et al., 1979), which may be caused by a correctable low estrogen state (Wehr and Goodwin, 1981). Conditions in which electrolyte imbalance exists, such as severe diarrhea, complicate the use of lithium and perhaps also of carbamazepine, and neuroleptics might be favored. Any abnormality in the hematopoietic system may complicate the use of carbamazepine. To our knowledge, there are no medical contraindications to the use of clonazepam or other benzodiazepines.

Pregnancy

Birth defects, principally involving the cardiac system, occur at rates that are significantly higher than normal rates in babies whose mothers received lithium in the first 3 months of pregnancy. Thus, lithium should be avoided during the first trimester whenever possible. Mild manic episodes during pregnancy should probably be managed without drugs, but it is prudent to treat more severe episodes, since the possible consequences of an untreated episode (such as injury, psychophysiological stress, dehydration and malnutrition, profound sleep deprivation, and suicide) could pose a greater risk to the fetus than the side effects of lithium. The risk–benefit considerations for the use of lithium during pregnancy are thoroughly reviewed in Chapter 23. Clonazepam is not known to be associated with fetal abnormalities and, therefore, might be used in these circumstances. Another option is ECT, which can be used without special risk to the fetus. The clinical management of mania during pregnancy has been reviewed by Nurnberg (1980) and by Sitland-Marken and colleagues (1989).

Concurrent Medications

Although several drugs interact with lithium, neuroleptics, and the anticonvulsants, only a few combinations are contraindicated (see Table 23-5 and discussion in this chapter). Knowledge of these interactions will influence the choice of one drug over another, but potential drug interactions generally should not take precedence over the clinical indications outlined previously.

The concurrent use of lithium and diuretics deserves special attention. Loop diuretics, such as furosemide, do not substantially alter lithium excretion and can be administered together safely (Saffer and Coppen, 1983; Jefferson et al., 1987). The thiazide drugs are more problematic, since they decrease tubular reabsorption of sodium and indirectly increase lithium reabsorption and decrease its excretion. When these drugs are used, lithium should be started at a low dose and increased very gradually, with frequent monitoring of the blood level.

Other medical drugs with potential lithium interactions include anti-inflammatory agents, such as indomethacin and phenylbutazone, which increase lithium levels (Reimann et al., 1983); cardiovascular medications, especially the antihypertensive methyldopa, which decreases renal clearance; and digoxin, which has been shown to reduce the acute manic efficacy of lithium (Chambers et al., 1982). Finally, some antibiotics prescribed for lithium-associated acne have nephrotoxic potential.

Because they compete for hepatic metabolism, certain drugs may significantly increase carbamazepine blood levels and produce toxicity. Consequently, the combination of valproic acid and carbamazepine is contraindicated (Meyer et al., 1984; Lambert and Venaud, 1987; Meijer et al., 1984). Among the other drugs that should be used cautiously with carbamazepine for this same reason are verapamil, isoniazid, diltiazem, and erythromycin and related antibiotics (Berrettini, 1986; Sovner, 1988). By contrast, other drugs—phenobarbital, primidone, and phenytoin—can decrease carbamazepine blood levels, presumably by inducing hepatic metabolism (Post et al., 1985).

Concurrent administration of carbamazepine and neuroleptics has been reported in more than 100 patients. The two drugs produce some additive effects in the CNS, and there is some evidence that they enhance each other's effects. Carbamazepine does not appear to alter lithium levels. Additive CNS effects, especially sedation and cognitive and memory functions, should be kept in mind when deciding how fast to increase dosages and the ultimate dose level. Patients with preexisting CNS disease may be especially vulnerable to neurotoxicity with this combination (Shukla et al., 1984).

Determining Medication Dosage

Neuroleptics

Clinicians traditionally have used larger doses of neuroleptics for acute mania than for schizophrenia, but recent experience suggests that more modest doses can be effective. The lower dose is feasible if the patient is carefully monitored for early signs of improvement and takes lithium along with the neuroleptic. Chlorpromazine doses averaged more than 1 g per day in controlled studies, and comparably high doses have been reported for the high-potency neuroleptics, such as haloperidol and thiothixene. Blood level determinations for neuroleptics are not yet routinely available as they are for lithium. Clinical state, age, sex, and weight must be considered in setting dose levels; higher doses are required for more disturbed and highly active patients and for patients who are male, young, or heavy. Haloperidol is usually started at 5 to 15 mg intramuscularly (or 10 to 25 mg orally) every 4 to 6 hours. For chlorpromazine, the preferred dosage is 50 to 100 mg, which can be administered intramuscularly every 6 hours and then gradually replaced by oral doses.[10] The need for such high doses of neuroleptics should be reevaluated continually throughout treatment of the acute manic episode. To minimize the possibility of neurotoxicity, extrapyramidal side effects, or postmania depression, dosage should be reduced as soon as manic symptoms begin to subside.

Lithium

The gap between therapeutic and toxic levels of lithium is the narrowest of any drug routinely used in psychiatry. Fortunately, the level of lithium in plasma is readily determined, and dosage requirements have been studied extensively. In managing acute mania with lithium alone, it is best to use a dosage schedule that produces the highest plasma level consistent with acceptable side effects. These blood levels usually are higher than those considered necessary or safe for maintenance therapy. The dose/blood level relationship is influenced by the individual's sex, age, weight (especially muscle mass), salt intake, amount of sweat, intrinsic renal clearance capacity for lithium, and, as noted, other medications. A relatively higher dose/blood level ratio is associated with being younger, male, and heavier and having a higher salt intake.

In the lithium treatment of acute mania, the patient's clinical state is one of the most important factors affecting the dose/blood level relationship. Some patients, when manic, retain lithium in body pools outside the plasma, probably largely in bone (Greenspan et al., 1968; Almy and Taylor, 1973). In practice, more lithium is needed to achieve a given blood level during mania than during euthymia or depression (Goodwin et al., 1969; Serry, 1969; Kukopulos et al., 1985). When mania begins to subside, a dosage reduction usually is necessary to avoid lithium toxicity. Obviously, blood levels should be monitored more frequently when the clinical state is changing, especially from mania to euthymia or depression.

To predict dosage requirements, some investigators recommend a test dose of lithium followed 24 hours later by a plasma level determination (Cooper and Simpson, 1976; Perry et al., 1984). Fava and colleagues (1984) showed that, by using this technique, therapeutic levels were obtained faster, and fewer blood level determinations were required. Although this technique probably can be applied reliably when the mood state is stable, its practical value in treating acute mania is limited by the state-dependent kinetics of lithium. Errors in the predicted dose may, for example, be due to changes in patients' sleep and activity, which presumably cause changes in renal clearance (Perry et al., 1984). In addition, use of this method necessitates a 24-hour delay in treatment. Norman and colleagues (1982) proposed a faster technique that can also account for changes in renal clearance. This technique may be impractical, however, since it requires a 4-hour urine collection along with a blood sample.

The plasma level of lithium needed to produce a clinical response differs substantially from one manic patient to another. The same is true of toxicity. These differences are partly caused by variability in tissue sensitivity, a variability encountered with any drug. More important, however, are individual differences in the ratio of plasma lithium to intracellular lithium, as reflected in red blood cell (RBC) determinations. Toxic reactions reflect intracellular lithium, whereas serum levels reflect only the extracellular compartment.

These issues are important to treatment because increasing plasma levels of lithium (up to 1.4 mEq/liter) are associated with proportionately higher rates of therapeutic response (Stokes et al., 1976). Although there is reason to push the dose in patients who fail to respond, blood levels above 1.5 mEq/liter are not generally recommended, and even levels between 1.2 and 1.5 mEq/liter require considerable care to avoid toxicity. Indeed, an increase in the RBC/plasma lithium ratio often precedes the development of neurotoxicity (see, e.g., Dunner et al., 1978; Carroll and Feinberg, 1977). In most cases, blood levels in the therapeutic range can be achieved at doses between 900 and 1,800 mg daily of lithium carbonate.

In deciding the maximum lithium level to use with a manic patient, the clinician should keep in mind that the most important potential toxic effects are those involving the CNS. This task is made more difficult by the fact that the delirium-like symptoms that can occur in severe mania may be nearly indistinguishable from neurotoxic effects. (Specific neurotoxic effects of lithium are discussed in Chapter 23.)

Some authors have suggested using a loading dose strategy for treating mania with lithium,[11] both to achieve the maximum blood level quickly and to speed therapeutic onset. The value of this strategy is questionable, however, especially in light of animal and human data indicating that lithium is slow to enter the brain from the blood, even when plasma levels are high. In one study, CSF lithium levels increased 50 percent, on average, from the first to the third week on a constant lithium dose (Rey et al., 1979).

Lithium Plus Neuroleptics

The additive and possibly synergistic effects of lithium and neuroleptics must be considered when combining the two drugs. A severe encephalopathy syndrome was first reported in four manic patients treated with high doses of both lithium and haloperidol by Cohen and Cohen in 1974. Since then, some 50 additional cases of neurotoxic syndromes resulting from the combination of lithium and a neuroleptic have been reported. Most of these conditions are reversible. On the other hand, eight prospective and retrospective studies with a total of more than 600 patients have generally failed to find any special neurotoxicity with this combination.[12] This literature suggests that the risk of neurotoxicity is associated with pre-existing encephalopathy and high dose levels, especially of the neuroleptics.[13] Thus neuroleptics should be used in substantially lower dosages when combined with lithium than when used alone. We also recommend that the lithium level be kept below 1.0 mEq/liter, in part because neuroleptics increase the RBC/plasma lithium ratio (Von Knorring et al., 1982). Although lithium and neuroleptics generally can be combined safely and effectively when done in this way, it is important to monitor CNS function and, in hospital settings, to alert the staff to watch for symptoms of neurotoxicity. Patients in seclusion rooms, who can rapidly become dehydrated, require special caution, including temperature monitoring (see later discussion of seclusion and restraints). One report of a high frequency of neurotoxicity with lithium–neuroleptic combinations in people over 65 suggests caution in this age group as well (Miller et al., 1986).

Carbamazepine and Valproate

When carbamazepine is used alone, the starting dose is usually 200 to 400 mg, which is increased to the 800 to 1,000 mg range during the first week. Further increases (up to about 1,600 mg) are appropriate if no response is evident after the first 2 weeks and if not limited by unacceptable side effects. The blood level generally should be between 6 and 12 ng/ml. When carbamazepine is combined with lithium or neuroleptics, the dose and target blood level are typically somewhat lower. Over time, carbamazepine can induce its own hepatic metabolism, and blood levels can fall. This problem is more troublesome in prophylactic treatment (see Chapter 23).

Side effects are more likely to occur when dosages are increased rapidly in treating acute mania than when the dosage is built up slowly in the first phase of prophylactic treatment. These early side effects—drowsiness, dizziness, ataxia, confusion, double vision, and nausea—usually do not persist beyond the first week or two and often respond to temporary dosage reduction.

Carbamazepine produces side effects about as frequently as lithium and less often than neuroleptics. Skin rashes of varying degrees of severity are a frequent problem (10 to 15 percent of patients). Those that are unaccompanied by evidence of a systemic allergic response can be treated with 20 to 30 mg of prednisone administered daily for a few weeks, then gradually discontinued. Liver enzyme levels, complete blood count, and platelet count should be obtained before treatment and weekly for the first 3 to 4 weeks of treatment and then every 4 to 8 weeks.

Although transient suppression of white blood cells and platelets is common, it does not require discontinuation of the carbamazepine. Serious hematopoietic complications (agranulocytosis and aplastic anemia) are rare, occurring once in about 15,000 to 20,000 patients. Nevertheless, the drug should be discontinued if the white count drops below 3,000 or if the patient shows clinical signs of these complications, such as sores, infections, fever, easy bruising, or petechiae. In one report, the benign suppression of white blood count by carbamazepine was offset by the addition of lithium (Brewerton, 1986). Comprehensive reviews of the clinical pharmacology of carbamazepine (dosage, blood levels, and side effects) are now available.[14] Differences in the side effect profile of carbamazepine and lithium influence treatment choices for long-term maintenance; these profiles are compared in Chapter 23.

In treating acute mania with sodium valproate or valproic acid (generally used in combination with lithium), it is usual to start at 500 to 1,500 mg/day in divided doses, with peak doses ranging from 750 to 3,000 mg/day, corresponding to blood levels between 50 and 100 μg/ml (with a median of about 75 μg/ml). No serious adverse effects have been found in the 268 psychiatric patients reported in the literature, and side effects are minimal or absent. However, hepatic function should be monitored in light of rare reports of potentially fatal hepatitis in epileptic patients. Also, when valproate is combined with carbamazepine, blood levels should be monitored closely and dosages may need to be adjusted, since there are complex metabolic interactions between the two drugs.

Clonazepam

Clonazepam has become popular among some clinicians for the rapidly, albeit perhaps nonspecific, control of manic symptoms because it is relatively safe and easy to use (e.g., it requires no blood monitoring) (Santos and Morton, 1987). In high doses (10 to 15 mg), it may be well suited to emergency room or inpatient settings where the profound sedation presents a more manageable risk. For outpatient use, the dose-dependent sedative and related dissociative reactions may present problems, such as in driving a car or operating machinery. In these situations, it is wise to use the smallest possible dose needed to restore sleep and, it is hoped, abort an emerging manic episode (the 2 to 5 mg range). Experience to date indicates that clonazepam can be administered safely in combination with any of the other drugs discussed previously, and its effects are additive. Other sedative benzodiazepines, such as lorazepam, are also used for mania.

Strategies for Drug Treatment of Severe Mania

In the first few days of treating moderately severe to severe mania (stages II or III), the three choices are neuroleptics, carbamazepine, or clonazepam. Of the neuroleptics, haloperidol is generally preferred. After 3 to 4 days, or as soon as the acute hyperactive and psychotic symptoms begin to subside, the dose of neuroleptic can be reduced and lithium added—cautiously, since side effects are additive. By not giving the drugs concurrently, the clinician can assign the side effects to the appropriate drug. Careful monitoring of both clinical effects and side effects permits gradual decrease of the dose of neuroleptic and increase of the lithium dose. By the third week, most patients can be maintained on lithium alone, al-

though some will require modest doses of neuroleptics for a longer period. For patients with substantial schizoaffective features, adjunctive neuroleptics may have to be maintained indefinitely.

Carbamazepine, initially reserved for lithium nonresponders, is now being seriously considered as a first-choice alternative to neuroleptics as an adjunct to lithium. If additional studies continue to show that carbamazepine is at least as effective as neuroleptics without the same potential for tardive dyskinesia, postmania depression, or cycle induction, carbamazepine may be preferable.

Finally, for the reasons noted above, clonazepam and related benzodiazepines are being used increasingly for acute mania.

Electroconvulsive Therapy

ECT is a valuable alternative to medications in treating acute mania, a point that was underlined by two favorable comparisons with lithium, a randomized controlled trial (Small et al., 1988) and a large retrospective study (Black et al., 1987, 1989). ECT may be especially useful for severely manic patients, for those who have proven unresponsive to drugs, and for those in mixed states with a high risk of suicide. If ECT is to be used, lithium should not be administered simultaneously (even in reduced doses) because neurotoxic complications have been reported to occur with this combination (see, e.g., Small, 1980; Rudorfer and Linnoila, 1986). Some clinical investigators believe that bilateral electrode placement may be necessary to obtain the full antimanic effect of ECT (Small et al., 1985), whereas others find no difference between unilateral and bilateral placement (Black et al., 1987).

Hospitalization

Patients exhibiting fully developed psychotic (stage-III) mania almost always need to be hospitalized, often involuntarily. When their manic symptoms are still in the mild to moderate range, judging the need for and timing of hospitalization can be more difficult. The family's support and collaboration are essential when hospitalizing a patient. They are also needed to help control a patient who can stay out of the hospital by, for example, assuring compliance with medication.

In deciding whether to hospitalize a patient, the clinician must keep in mind that mild mania can progress to severe mania rapidly and unexpectedly. The possible social, occupational, or legal consequences of such extreme behavior must be weighed against the professional and personal consequences of hospitalization.

Since manic patients rarely recognize their need to be hospitalized, informed consent presents a dilemma, and involuntary commitment is often necessary. In some states, such legal procedures can be difficult and cumbersome, and commitment can result in stigmatization and loss of some legal rights for the patient. On the other hand, to acquiesce to the patient's refusal is to court disaster. A possible humane alternative to this no-win dilemma may be to obtain consent in advance, an application of the so-called Odysseus principle discussed in Chapter 24.

The hospital treatment of mania often requires decisions concerning the use of seclusion rooms and physical restraints. Seclusion substantially reduces the level of stimulation to a severely manic patient, thus ameliorating a factor that often seems to drive and perpetuate the episode. The potential for self-injury, including physical exhaustion, and the need for medical monitoring often necessitate the use of physical restraints. Indeed, failure to use restraints has been the basis for successful malpractice litigation.

Treatment of Mania in Children and Adolescents

Issues related to the treatment of mania in children and adolescents have become increasingly important with the growing recognition that mania and manic-like states occur frequently in adolescents and even in prepubertal children (see Chapter 8). Resolving these issues is more urgent if the early episodes alter the brain in such a way as to facilitate subsequent episodes—a prediction based on biological models of kindling and sensitization (see Chapters 16 and 20). Added to the already well-recognized psychological and social scarring that results from manic episodes, this possibility of an ever-worsening, accelerated course implies that the earlier the illness is treated the better the long-term outcome.

In general, the treatment of mania in children and adolescents follows the same principles that apply to adults.[15] Compared with manic episodes in adults, those in the young are more likely to involve delusions and psychotic disorganization, perhaps reflecting the impact of the manic process on a still developing nervous system (Ryan et al., 1987). Despite the severity of their symptoms, manic children and adolescents generally respond to lithium as well as do adults (see, e.g., DeLong and Nieman, 1983). Indeed, some evidence suggests that the young may actually respond better to lithium than adults with similar mood and psychotic symptoms (Van der Velde, 1970; Varanka et al., 1988), and supplemental neuroleptics may be less necessary. Within the adolescent group, however, those with a very early onset of disturbance may not respond as well to lithium as do those with symptom onset in adolescence (see, e.g., Strober et al., 1988, reviewed later in this chapter). It has also been suggested that very early onset bipolar disorder is more likely to involve mixed states and rapid cycling (Ryan and Puig-Antich, 1987), conditions that may require supplemental anticonvulsants.

Although controlled studies are lacking, open trials suggest that therapeutic blood levels for children and adults are about the same. When adjusted for differences in body weight, the lithium dosage required to reach these blood levels is somewhat higher in children than in adults, presumably due to the greater capacity of the young kidney to clear lithium (Weller et al., 1986). For the acute treatment of mania in children, side effect considerations appear similar to those in adults, although some investigators have noted fewer side effects in children. In dealing with medication compliance among the young, it is well to be aware of the special concerns experienced by this age group (body image, peer pressure, motor coordination, acne, to name a few). These issues are discussed in Chapter 25.

Treatment of Mania in the Elderly

As detailed in Chapter 5, mania in the elderly may be obscured by concurrent signs of organic brain syndrome or by prominent schizophrenia-like symptoms. Thus, before diagnosing mania in an elderly patient who has no history of manic episodes, the clinician should consider the possibility that the manic symptoms are caused by another medical condition or by medications (see Chapters 5 and 18 for a full discussion of secondary mania). If the identified primary factor cannot be corrected, pharmacological treatment of the manic symptoms is appropriate.

When using antimanic agents in an elderly patient, other medical problems and possible interactions with other drugs must be considered (Sargenti et al., 1988). Although systematic reviews generally do not support a direct correlation between age and overall side effects, there is an age-associated increase in moderate to severe side effects (Smith and Helms, 1982), perhaps related to important pharmacodynamic differences, such as reduced renal lithium clearance. Moreover, some case reports suggest an age-related increase in sensitivity to the neurotoxic effects of antimanic drugs (see, e.g., Strayhorn and Nash, 1977). This possibility must be kept in mind to avoid mistaking neurotoxic symptoms for the normal deficits of aging. Of special concern is the increased vulnerability among the elderly to tardive dyskinesia secondary to neuroleptics.

REVIEW OF THE LITERATURE

Lithium

Uncontrolled and Single-Blind Studies

In the earliest clinical trials of lithium, researchers did not define their diagnostic criteria for mania, notably failing to differentiate manic and schizoaffective states. Nor did they use a double-blind design or rating scales to evaluate clinical response. Despite these shortcomings, the early studies provide many rich clinical descriptions and give a good sense of patients' responses to the drug. In many reports from this period, for example, clinicians observed that typical manic patients were most likely to respond to lithium and that the patients with schizoaffective states did not appear to respond as well. Although conducted by many groups over several years, the uncontrolled studies consistently demonstrated a high rate of response, which usually began within about a week of starting lithium. When the results of these 10 early studies are combined, 334 of 413 patients (81 percent) showed lessened mania during acute lithium treatment (Goodwin and Ebert, 1973). This improvement did not necessarily mean complete remission, nor is it clear how much time it took for a full response to occur.[16]

More recent open studies of lithium appear to demonstrate its efficacy for mania in children. For example, Varanka and colleagues (1988), in a careful open study of 10 manic prepubertal children between the ages of 6 and 12, found that all patients responded well to lithium alone, with most of the improvement occurring in an average of 11 days. All of the patients exhibited mood-congruent psychotic symptoms that responded to lithium in about the same amount of time as did the mood symptoms.

Controlled Studies

The first controlled trial of lithium in mania (Table 21-2) was done in Denmark by Mogens Schou and colleagues in 1954. Almost a decade later, in 1963, Maggs, working in England, did a double-blind evaluation of lithium's effects on acute mania, the first such study to use formal rating instruments of manic behavior and to analyze the data statistically. The earliest American controlled study of lithium, done in 1968 by Bunney and co-workers at the National Institute of Mental Health (NIMH), offered longitudinal double-blind data on two patients, demonstrating the sensitivity of manic symptoms to temporary withdrawal of lithium medication. The NIMH group extended its study to 30 manic-depressive patients, of whom 12 were manic (Goodwin et al., 1969). A fourth study, by Stokes and his associates at the New York University and Cornell University Medical Colleges (1971), used a double-blind design with alternating 7 to 10 day periods on lithium or placebo in 38 manic-depressive inpatients.

Despite methodological differences, results of the four controlled studies are remarkably consistent. The overall response rate in the 116 patients is 78 percent, a figure very close to that derived from the open studies. Clearly, these four studies demonstrated that lithium is superior to placebo in the acute treatment of mania. They also revealed some characteristics of lithium discussed in the first part of this chapter. First, despite its demonstrated effectiveness, lithium is relatively slow to produce clinical changes, usually requiring a 2 week trial to reach maximum therapeutic effect. Second, although the diagnostic criteria used in these studies are not necessarily comparable to DSM-III, the lithium responders tended to be classic bipolar patients (manic phase), often in

Table 21-2. Lithium in Mania: Placebo-Controlled Studies

Study	Method	N	Response Rate %	Comments	Assessment
Schou et al., 1954	Random crossover[a]	30 typical	90	40% definite 50% probable	Global impression
		8 atypical	62	25% definite 37% probable	
Maggs, 1963	Random crossover	28		Lithium superior to placebo	Wittenborn scale
Goodwin et al., 1969	Nonrandom crossover	12	75	67% complete 8% partial	Modified Bunney-Hamburg scale
Stokes et al., 1971	Nonrandom crossover	38	75[b]	40% improved on placebo	Quantification of nurses' observations
Overall Response			78%		

[a] Not all cases included
[b] Refers to numbers of episodes

This table was originally produced by Goodwin & Zis, 1979, and reproduced by Tyrer, 1985.

stage I or II of mania, and nonresponders tended to be schizoaffective or in stage-III mania.

Once it had been unequivocally demonstrated that lithium did have antimanic activity, other questions could be asked: How does lithium alone compare with neuroleptics (major tranquilizers, antipsychotics)? Do the relative merits of these drugs differ with various manic symptom patterns? What sort of manic patients would benefit from lithium alone? When and how should lithium be used in combination with other drugs? The studies described subsequently partially answer these questions.

Case reports and controlled studies suggest that a relatively broad spectrum of clinical states in adolescents and children appears to respond to lithium. This diversity probably reflects, first, some lack of specificity in the action of lithium and, second, the variety of clinical presentations of mania in these age groups, as noted in Chapter 8. The reports of patients whose symptoms fit or approximate DSM-III criteria for mania[17] suggest that the efficacy of lithium is comparable to that reported for the treatment of mania in adults,[18] with the possible exception of children with very early onset of disturbance. Results are confounded, however, because in many of these reports, unlike the adult literature, lithium was given in combination with other drugs.

In one of the largest and most rigorous studies done on the subject to date, Strober and colleagues (1988) found that, when symptoms began after puberty, the rate of response to lithium was twice as great as when they began before puberty. Only 40 percent of bipolar adolescents with very early onset of symptoms responded to lithium, whereas 80 percent of those whose symptoms began in adolescence responded ($p < 0.02$).[19] Strober's group studied 50 adolescents with bipolar-I disorder who were treated with lithium and, as needed, neuroleptics and carbamazepine.[20]

. . . the poor lithium response in these probands is in accordance with data relating lithium failure to longer histories of illness preceding treatment . . . and greater overall personality disturbance. . . . Increased refractoriness to treatment in this group is also in line with theoretical speculation . . . that responsiveness to lithium carbonate may decrease over time in patients who experience a chronic, uninterrupted progression of their illness. (Strober et al., 1988, p. 265)

High-Potency vs Low-Potency Neuroleptics

In one of the few studies that directly compared the butyrophenone haloperidol with chlorpromazine under controlled conditions, Entwistle and colleagues (1962) noted that tranquilization was achieved more rapidly with haloperidol, requiring an average of 4 days for full effect, and that hyperactivity could be controlled even more rapidly, within 2 or 3 days. The more recent literature is reflected by the study of Janicak and colleagues (1988a), who found that chlorpromazine and thiothixene were similarly effective in manic patients who were also receiving lithium. As expected, the profile of side effects was different for the two drugs (extrapyramidal symptoms were significantly greater in the thiothixene group). Clozapine, a high-potency neuroleptic with a low incidence of extrapyramidal side effects, has not yet been fully evaluated in manic patients, but shows promise, perhaps especially for schizomanic patients.[21]

Lithium vs Neuroleptics

In most studies comparing lithium with neuroleptics, both manic and schizoaffective patients were treated (Table 21-3). With the exception of a Japanese study in which relatively low doses of lithium were used (Takahashi et al., 1975), lithium treatment was associated with marked improvement or remission in about two thirds of the patients in these comparison trials. These findings are in good agreement with the results of controlled studies of lithium alone and of open or single-blind studies. Furthermore, with the exception of the study conducted by the Veterans' Administration (VA) and NIMH (discussed later), lithium, over time, proved superior to chlorpromazine in treating acute mania, as judged by the proportion of patients showing marked improvement or remission. The evidence also strongly suggests that lithium ameliorates the very affective and ideational symptoms most specific to the manic syndrome. Chlorpromazine can match or exceed lithium in the initial control of psychomotor hyperactivity, but this effect may be due to nonspecific sedation. Comparisons of lithium and neuroleptics have been limited largely to chlorpromazine. The one study that did compare lithium with both chlorpromazine and haloperidol found that the latter neuroleptic has the most rapid action (Shopsin et al., 1975a).

The VA-NIMH study (Prien et al., 1972) warrants more extensive discussion because of its size—255 newly admitted manic and schizoaffective patients in 18 VA hospitals—and its unusual findings. Patients were differentiated not only by diagnosis but by activity level: "highly active" or "mildly active." Among the highly active patients who completed the 3-week treatment trials, both the lithium-treated and the chlorpromazine-treated groups improved significantly on a wide range of symptoms. However, 38 percent of the lithium-treated patients dropped out, compared with only 8 percent of those treated with chlorpromazine, in part reflecting more side effects attributable to lithium in this group, since the dose was pushed in an effort to control the hyperactivity. Both drugs produced significant improvement in the mildly active patients who completed the study, but in this group severe side effects were more frequent among the chlorpromazine-treated patients.

The investigators concluded that chlorpromazine was superior to lithium in the initial treatment of the highly active patients. The neuroleptic not only reduced motor activity, excitement, grandiosity, hostility, and psychotic disorganization, but it also sharply decreased the patients' need for ward supervision in the first week. By the end of 3 weeks, however, the two drugs were equivalent. Among the mildly active patients, there were fewer dropouts related to lithium than to chlorpromazine, primarily because lithium did not make them feel as "sluggish and fatigued."

Neither discharge rates nor overall improvement rates were reported in this study. In other studies, however, discharge rates and clinical impressions favor lithium over neuroleptics, thus underscoring the ultimate advantage of lithium. The dropout rate in the VA-NIMH study may reflect limitations in clinical management more than inherent limitations of the drugs in question.

Diagnosis is also a critical issue. Prien and associates did not specify how the differential diagnosis was made between the manic phase of manic-depressive illness and that of schizoaffective psychosis. Other investigators might have diagnosed their highly active patients as schizoaffective or "atypical." Although some studies have suggested that such patients do not respond as well to lithium as the more typical manic-depressive patients do (reviewed by Goodwin and Ebert, 1973), other investigators failed to find any difference in lithium response between the groups (reviewed by Goodnick and Meltzer, 1984). This discrepancy is probably more apparent than real. Goodnick and Meltzer (1984) have shown that compared with manic patients, schizoaffective manic patients require more than

Table 21-3. Lithium vs Neuroleptics in Mania

Study	Drug	N	Marked Improvement or Remission %	Qualitative Differences		Comments
				Hyperactivity	Normalization of Mood and Ideation	
Johnson et al., 1968	LI CZ	18 11	78 36	CZ > LI	LI > CZ	
Johnson et al., 1971	LI CZ	13 8	Not reported		LI > CZ	BPRS, CGI, NOSIE, TRAM, SCI
Spring et al., 1970	LI CZ	9 6	88 50	LI > CZ	LI > CZ	Target symptom assessment; N includes the crossover trials
Platman, 1970	LI CZ	13 10	Most None	?	LI > CZ	Quantified behavioral ratings
Prien et al., 1972	LI CZ LI CZ	59[a] 66[a] 69[b] 61[b]	Not reported	CZ > LI CZ > LI	CZ > LI LI > CZ	Multihospital study; BPRS, IMPS, PIP
Takahashi et al., 1975	LI CZ	37 34	32 12	CZ > LI	LI > CZ	Multihospital study; special rating scale; 5 weeks; low doses; higher incidence of depression with CZ
Shopsin et al., 1975a	LI CZ HAL	10 10 10	70 10 20	HAL > LI > CZ	LI > HAL > CZ	BPRS, CGI, SCI, NOSIE

Except as indicated, all studies were double-blind, random assignment, 3-week duration

CZ = chlorpromazine, LI = lithium, HAL = haloperidol
BPRS = Brief Psychiatric Rating Scale, CGI = Clinical Global Impression, NOSIE = Nurse's Observation Scale for Inpatient Evaluation
TRAM = Treatment Response Assesment Method, SCI = Structured Clinical Interview, IMPS = Inpatient Multidimensional Psychiatric Scale
PIP = Psychotic Inpatient Profile

[a]Highly active group; higher dropout rate with LI
[b]Mildly active group; higher frequency of severe side effects with CZ
This table was originally produced by Goodwin and Zis, 1979, and reproduced by Tyrer, 1985.

twice as long to achieve a full antimanic response to lithium alone (9 weeks against the 4 weeks for manic patients). Many of the reports of relatively poor lithium response rates among schizoaffective manic patients involve trials of 4 weeks or less. Again, from a practical point of view, this means that schizoaffective manic patients are likely to require other medications in addition to lithium for the acute treatment of mania.

Before lithium became available in the United States, the neuroleptics were the drugs of choice for treating mania. The willingness of many physicians to try lithium, a new and potentially toxic drug requiring careful monitoring, suggests that they found neuroleptics inadequate for many, if not most, patients. The fact that today virtually all clinicians include lithium in their treatment approach to mania is consistent with findings that this drug has an overall advantage over the major tranquilizers.

Neuroleptics still have a place in the treatment of acute mania, however. As we have seen, chlorpromazine is probably superior to lithium in the initial control of increased motor activity, and, as noted earlier, there are indications that haloperidol may act even more rapidly than chlorpromazine. Along with clozapine, another neuroleptic deserving further study as a rapid-onset treatment for acute mania is pimozide, a more or less specific dopamine blocker. In a 1980 study, Post and colleagues noted rapid control of manic symptomatology and behavior with this drug. Therapeutic effect with pimozide began within 24 hours, compared with a 5-day lag with lithium. Comparing pimozide and chlorpromazine in acute mania, Cookson and associates (1980) found that both were equally effective in controlling the syndrome but that pimozide produced less sedation.

Lithium–Neuroleptic Combinations

Surprisingly, no major systematic studies have been done comparing the combination of neuroleptics and lithium with either drug alone in treating acute mania, although such a comparison has been done for schizoaffective mania (as defined by the RDC). Biederman and associates (1979) found that both predominantly affective and predominantly schizophrenic schizoaffective patients did better on a combination of haloperidol and lithium than on haloperidol alone, but

the addition of lithium was more beneficial for the affective schizoaffective patients. In addition to producing a more satisfactory remission, lithium more often prevented the postmania depressions frequently experienced by patients whose mania is treated with neuroleptics alone.

Neuroleptics have been associated with the phenomenon of postmania depression (Kukopulos et al., 1980; Morgan, 1972), although at least one study did not observe this link (Lucas et al., 1989). In their longitudinal study of 434 bipolar patients over periods averaging 17 years, Kukopulos and colleagues (1980) also observed that treatment of manic episodes with neuroleptics contributed to a shortening of the intervals between episodes, thus worsening the long-term course of the illness. This finding, if validated in controlled studies, would underline the importance of limiting the use of neuroleptics in mania. Such a limitation contrasts with data showing improved long-term course in schizophrenic patients treated early and consistently with neuroleptics (Wyatt et al., 1988).

Anticonvulsant Drugs

The relationship between seizure disorders and manic-depressive illness is discussed in Chapter 5, and in Chapter 16, we suggest that kindling, a neural mechanism involved in seizures, provides a promising model for cyclic mood disorders.

Carbamazepine

Carbamazepine, which can prevent or reverse kindling, is an established treatment for temporal lobe epilepsy (Penry and Daly, 1975), a condition that not only is phasic but also is frequently associated with affective and other psychological changes. Reviewing 40 studies of the drug's effects in epileptic patients, Dalby (1975) estimated that carbamazepine showed a significant psychotropic effect in half of the patients, who reported feeling more alert and sociable and less anxious, irritable, and depressed than they had been before taking carbamazepine.

The first trial of carbamazepine in mania (Okuma et al., 1973) was a nonblind study of 64 acutely manic patients, half of whom were "markedly" or "somewhat" improved when the drug was added to the existing treatment regimen, which often included lithium or neuroleptics.

Later, Okuma and colleagues (1979) conducted a double-blind comparison of carbamazepine and chlorpromazine in 63 patients with acute mania. Marked to moderate improvement was seen in 70 percent of the carbamazepine group and 60 percent of the chlorpromazine group. In both groups most patients improved within the first week. Both drugs produced considerable sedation, although carbamazepine had fewer overall side effects.

At about the same time, Ballenger and Post (1978, 1980) reported positive antimanic results using a longitudinal double-blind crossover design with alternating periods of carbamazepine alone and placebo. The sample size was increased in succeeding years. To date, 12 of 19 acutely manic patients have responded to carbamazepine (Post et al., 1987). The time from administration of the drug to antimanic response was similar to that seen with neuroleptics and slightly shorter than with lithium. It is of interest that most of the patients who responded well to carbamazepine in this trial had previously not responded to lithium, although these authors did not conduct a direct comparison with random assignment. Strömgren and Boller (1985), in their review of 15 reports of carbamazepine treatment of 176 manic patients, note that a "marked or moderate" antimanic effect was reported in 55 percent (69 percent among the four double-blind studies). Among the 12 studies involving carbamazepine alone, 85 patients (61 percent) were reported to have "marked or moderate" improvement.

Only two studies have directly compared the efficacy of carbamazepine and lithium in mania. Placidi and co-workers (1986) found that both drugs were of equivalent efficacy in a mixed group of 83 manic and schizomanic patients, with about two thirds of the patients in each drug group showing a marked or moderate response. Among the schizoaffective patients with mood-incongruent psychotic features, those on lithium had a significantly higher dropout rate than those on carbamazepine, suggesting that the anticonvulsant might be superior to lithium for this group of patients. The authors also indicated that lithium may have been somewhat superior to carbamazepine among the "classical, pure" manic patients. Lerer and colleagues (1987) studied 28 manic patients, employing a randomized double-blind design, and noted a trend for lithium to be superior. The lithium effects were more uniform: 11 of the 14 lithium-treated patients showed a global improvement of two or more points on the Clinical Global Impressions scale, whereas only 4 of 14 carbamazepine patients showed that level of response ($p < 0.05$). Two of the three best responders to carbamazepine had rapid cycles, and all three had a prior history of lithium failure.

In the studies by Okuma's group and Post's group, as well as in several case reports, some of the patients received carbamazepine in addition to either lithium or chlorpromazine, and the anticonvulsant appeared to potentiate the antimanic effects of the other drugs without increasing toxicity. Likewise, many patients who fail to improve when taking carbamazepine alone do respond when lithium is added to the treatment regimen (Kramlinger and Post, 1989). Three direct studies of carbamazepine–neuroleptic combinations (Klein et al., 1984; Muller and Stoll, 1984; Möller et al., 1989) showed such potentiation, which was reflected in a reduced need for the neuroleptic after carbamazepine was added. The studies of carbamazepine in the treatment of mania are outlined in Table 21-4. Clinical predictors of the relative antimanic response to carbamazepine and lithium are discussed later.

Valproate

Another anticonvulsant drug, valproate, has attracted attention as a potential antimanic agent because, like carbamazepine, it reduces kindling and enhances the activity of γ-aminobutyric acid (GABA), a major CNS transmitter especially important in inhibiting central dopamine systems (see Chapters 16 and 17). Following the initial reports of antimanic effects by French investigators (Lambert et al., 1966, 1971), several studies have appeared, predominantly from Europe (reviewed by McElroy et al., 1987, 1989; Fawcett, 1989). More than half of the 181 manic or schizomanic patients in these studies had a therapeutic response to valproate, usually within 2 weeks, a response rate that was also noted in a large community based open trial (Brown, 1989). Most patients had previously failed to respond satisfactorily to lithium or lithium combined with neuroleptics, and in most cases the valproate was added to existing treatments. In the only two double-blind studies performed to date, however, 10 of 13 manic patients had a marked response to valproate alone after withdrawal of previous medications (Emrich et al., 1980; Brennan et al., 1984). The specificity of valproate for manic-depressive illness is suggested by the relatively poor results among 63 schizophrenic patients. In a study from the McLean Hospital group in Boston (McElroy et al., 1987), marked or moderate responses among the manic patients (11 of 17, or 64 percent) were initially associated with the presence of nonparoxysmal EEG abnormalities, but this relationship lost statistical significance as the sample size was increased. Among the four patients with rapid cycles, three showed a marked response to valproate.

The therapeutic profile of valproate appears similar to that of carbamazepine. Whether valproate will be useful in carbamazepine nonresponders or vice versa remains to be seen. So far, Post and colleagues have reported one patient with an antimanic response to carbamazepine but not to valproate (1984) and one with the opposite profile (1987). The prophylactic effects of valproate are discussed in Chapter 23. The widely used anticonvulsant, diphenylhydantoin, which has been tried as a treatment for mania with only very scattered responses (Himmelhoch, personal communication), has not been studied systematically.

Clonazepam

The benzodiazepine anticonvulsant clonazepam shows promise as an effective antimanic agent, at least for the initial phase of treatment. Chouinard and co-workers (1983; Chouinard, 1987) conducted double-blind crossover trials, one with lithium. Clonazepam, in daily doses ranging from 4 to 16 mg, was significantly more effective, with patients on clonazepam requiring less haloperidol to control agitation.[22] The specificity of the antimanic response to clonazepam remains unresolved, although the drug's sedative effects undoubtedly contribute to its efficacy.

Lorazepam

In a related finding, Modell and colleagues (1985; Modell, 1986) found that parenteral lorazepam 2 to 4 mg intramuscularly every 2 hours could be substituted for neuroleptics as an adjunct to lithium in the early phase of treating acute mania. In four cases, doses of 10 to 30

mg/day were used over the first 3 to 5 days to control manic agitation while lithium was being given. The response occurred after 1 week, a period similar to that of lithium–neuroleptic combinations, but side effects (e.g., extrapyramidal effects, delirium, akathisia) were fewer. This preliminary observation, coupled with the clonazepam and carbamazepine data, suggests that even patients in severe stage-III mania might be managed effectively without neuroleptic drugs.

Experimental Treatments

As noted in Chapters 15 and 17, pathophysiological theories of mania have focused primarily on disturbances in neurotransmitter function, especially the monoamines dopamine, norepinephrine, and serotonin. More recently, other transmitters have been considered, including those of the cholinergic, GABAergic, and endorphin systems. In this section, we briefly review experimental treatments developed to test various pathophysiological hypotheses.[23]

Serotonin-Related Drugs

Methysergide and *cinanserin,* drugs that block postsynaptic serotonin receptors, were tried therapeutically to test the old hypothesis that mania represented serotonin overactivity (Lapin and Oxenkrug, 1969). Two trials of methysergide (Dewhurst, 1968; Háskovec and Soucek, 1968) produced clear antimanic effects, particularly when given intramuscularly. These results could not be replicated in three controlled clinical trials using an oral preparation (Coppen et al., 1969; McCabe et al., 1970; Fieve et al., 1969), and no further trials have been conducted. Like methysergide, cinanserin was also noted to have antimanic properties (Itil et al., 1971; Kane, 1970), but these preliminary observations did not stimulate further clinical trials.

Para-chlorophenylalanine (PCPA), a potent inhibitor of central and peripheral serotonin synthesis both in animals (Koe and Weissman, 1966) and in humans (Goodwin and Post, 1972), was also used to test the hyperserotonin hypothesis of mania. In the human study, PCPA evidenced no specific antimanic effects at doses up to 4 g daily. No further trials of this drug have been conducted with manic patients, in part because of concern over such side effects as retroperitoneal fibrosis.

Table 21-4. Studies of Carbamazepine in Acute Mania

Study	N	Diagnosis	Design	Dose of CBZ (mg / day) (blood level)	Other Drugs	Duration	Results
Controlled Studies							
Okuma et al., 1979	30 CBZ 25 CZ	MD psychosis	Double blind	300-900 (2.7-11.7 μg/ml)	Bedtime hypnotics	3-5 wk	21/30 improved on CBZ 15/25 improved on CZ
Grossi et al., 1984	11 CBZ 15 CZ	MD	Double blind with CZ (150-800 mg/day)	300-1,600	Bedtime hypnotics	21 day	10/15 improved on CBZ; 13/15 improved on CZ
E. Klein et al., 1984	23	Excited psychoses[a]	Blind with PBO	600-1,600 (6-18 μg/ml)	HAL	5 wk	18/23 improved on CBZ + HAL
Müller & Stoll, 1984	6	MD	Blind with PBO	600-1,200	HAL+ hypnotics	3 wk	CBZ better than PBO (p <.01)
	10	MD	Blind with PBO (15-50 mg/day)	600-1,200 OXCBZ	HAL+ hypnotics	2 wk	OXCBZ = HAL
Emrich et al., 1985	7	Manic psychosis	Double blind with PBO	1,800-2,100 OXCBZ		variable	6/7 (>25% improvement on IMPS)
Brown et al., 1986	8	Manic	Double blind with HAL (20-80 mg/day)	400-1,600	CZ to 3 pts (only 1 after 2nd day)	42 day	5/8 marked improvement
Lenzi et al., 1986	11 CBZ 11 LI	MD or other	Blind with LI (900 mg/day) double PBO with CZ	1,200 (7-12 μg/ml)	CZ	3 wk	Equal efficacy in CBZ and LI groups; less CZ required in CBZ group
Desai et al., 1987	5	Manic	Blind with PBO in addition to LI	400 fixed dose		4 wk	CBZ + LI p <.05 better on BRMS than LI alone by 2nd week

				Dose Range	Duration	
Lerer et al., 1987	14 CBZ 14 LI	MD	Blind with LI (900 mg/day)	600 (8-12 µg/ml)	4 wk	11/14 improved on LI; 4/14 improved on CBZ
Post et al., 1987b	19	MD psychosis	Double blind	600-2,000 (7-15.5 µg/ml)	11-56 day	12/19 improved - time course similar to neuroleptics; frequent relapses on PBO substitution
Möller et al., 1989	10 CBZ + HAL 10 HAL	Manic or schizomanic	Double blind	600 levome-promazine	35 day	Compared to HAL alone, CBZ + HAL required significantly less supplemental neuroleptic
Summary	176[c]					71% improved[c]

Summary of open studies

	Dose Range	Duration	
N = 331	200-1600[b] CBZ was coadministered with LI or neuroleptics in most studies (one study compared CBZ and CZ and reported that CZ was better)	1-26 mos	53% improved

Overall rate of moderate to marked improvement among 507 patients (controlled and open): 60%[c]

CBZ = carbamazepine, CZ = chlorpromazine, LI = lithium, PBO = placebo, HAL = haloperidol, OXCBZ = oxcarbazepine, IMPS = Inpatient Multidimensional Ratings Scale, BRMS = Bech - Rafaelsen Mania Scale, MD = manic-depressive

[a]11 excited manics, 7 excited schizoaffectives, 5 excited schizophrenics
[b]One study administered 2.1-3.06 mg of OXCBZ / day
[c]Does not include studies which did not give number of improved (Müller & Stoll, Lenzi, and Desai)

Adapted from Post & Uhde, 1988; Post et al., 1987b; and Strömgren & Boller, 1985

In contrast to the excess serotonin hypothesis, the idea that mania (and perhaps bipolar illness itself) may involve diminished functional activity of brain serotonin systems (Coppen et al., 1972; Prange et al., 1974; Kety, 1971) has had more staying power. Pharmacological evaluations of this deficiency hypothesis have involved a serotonin-receptor agonist, fenfluramine, and the amino-acid precursor of serotonin, L-tryptophan. The limited evidence on fenfluramine is equivocal, but the L-tryptophan results are encouraging. When oral doses of 1 to 4 g are accompanied by pyridoxine and niacin, L-tryptophan produces an increase in serotonin synthesis in the CNS (Dunner and Goodwin, 1972). However, further use of L-tryptophan will have to await resolution of a major problem that surfaced in 1989: More than 1,000 cases of eosinophilia myalgia syndrome (EMS) were linked to the ingestion of gram quantitites of L-tryptophan, and, as of this writing, it has been withdrawn from the market. This syndrome may depend on concomitant suppression of the HPA axis, as occurs, for example, with certain benzodiazepines (E. Sternberg, personal communication).

L-Tryptophan in the treatment of mania has been studied in four double-blind clinical trials: Three have had positive results (Prange et al., 1974; Murphy et al., 1974; Chouinard et al., 1985), and one had negative results (Chambers and Naylor, 1978). Prange and colleagues compared the amino acid to chlorpromazine and found it "slightly superior to CPZ in all regards," whereas the other studies compared L-tryptophan to placebo. Murphy and colleagues found that L-tryptophan was more effective against moderate than against severe manic symptoms.

One double-blind study assessed L-tryptophan as an adjunct to lithium in the treatment of mania (Brewerton and Reus, 1983). The amino acid was added to lithium or placebo in 16 bipolar or schizoaffective patients, who received concomitant neuroleptics as needed. Although the L-tryptophan and lithium combination produced significantly greater improvement, the results were confounded by the greater, although nonsignificant, doses of neuroleptics in the L-tryptophan group.

Taken together, the studies of L-tryptophan in mania are encouraging, especially those in which the drug was combined with another antimanic agent. Further studies are warranted if the EMS puzzle can be solved and as long as caution is paid to the finding that large doses can produce ultrastructural changes in the liver of rats (Trulson and Sampson, 1986). Also, in 1989, several hundred cases of eosinophilia were associated with L-tryptophan.

Catecholamine-Related Drugs

Pharmacological and biochemical data have suggested that the manic syndrome reflects increased function of catecholamines, such as norepinephrine and dopamine. α-*Methylparatyrosine* (AMPT) is a potent and specific inhibitor of dopamine and norepinephrine synthesis, centrally as well as peripherally. When Brodie and colleagues (1971) gave AMPT to seven patients hospitalized for mania, five showed a significant drop in mania ratings. Two of the five responders relapsed after the drug was discontinued; they subsequently improved when AMPT was started again. AMPT responders showed changes in manic thinking and behavior that seemed more specific than the sedative effects observed with large doses of barbiturates or phenothiazines. Nevertheless, sedative effects were more pronounced with AMPT than with lithium, and overall, its antimanic effects appeared to be somewhat less specific than with lithium.

AMPT does not differentiate between norepinephrine and dopamine, since the synthesis of both depends on tyrosine hydroxylase, the enzyme inhibited by AMPT. The enzyme that converts dopamine to norepinephrine and exists only in norepinephrine neurons is dopamine β-hydroxylase (DBH). Goodwin and Sack (1974), in a trial of a DBH inhibitor, fusaric acid, evaluated how manic patients are affected clinically when norepinephrine but not dopamine is decreased. They found that although these amine changes were in fact produced, as validated by the changes observed in CSF amine metabolites, fusaric acid had only a slight antimanic effect in hypomanic patients. In those with more severe mania, including psychotic features, DBH inhibition worsened their condition, shifting manic symptoms from more purely affective to schizoaffective.

Reserpine, a drug that depletes neuronal stores of amines (see Chapter 17), was used as an antipsychotic before the development of chlorpromazine. Bacher and Lewis (1979) and Telner and colleagues (1986) reported their clinical observations of manic or schizoaffective-manic patients who did not respond to lithium combined with unspecified neuroleptics. Most patients responded quite favorably to a combination of lithium and reserpine (average dose of 5 mg/day intramuscularly). This combination, rarely tried for lithium-resistant mania, merits further consideration.

Another way to test the hypothesis that elevated noradrenergic activity produces mania is to administer *propranolol* or related drugs that block the postsynaptic β-receptor for norepinephrine. Several studies in manic patients (Von Zerssen, 1976; Volk et al., 1972; Möller et al., 1979) demonstrated some improvement. Since one form of the drug, the D-isomer, which does not block the β-receptor, still had some clinical effect (Möller et al., 1979), it is possible that it acts partly by other mechanisms. From a clinical perspective, although the effects of propranolol seem to go beyond sedation or tranquilization, they require very high doses (in the range of 800 to 2,000 mg a day), which produce substantial side effects, such as hypotension and bradycardia; therefore this approach remains primarily of theoretical interest.

Clonidine is a drug that reduces the presynaptic release of norepinephrine by a direct agonist action on the inhibitory presynaptic α_2-adrenergic receptor. It has been found to have antimanic effects in several open trials and case reports in doses ranging from 0.2 to 1.2 mg/day.[24] Three double-blind studies (Giannini et al., 1983, 1986; Janicak et al., 1988b) have not been as encouraging, however, and even suggested that the drug might increase depression. Nonetheless, clonidine deserves further exploration, since its clinical effects occur at doses that do not produce debilitating hypotensive or sedative effects.

Catecholamine Agonists. Drugs that are presumably stimulatory (agonistic) to norepinephrine or dopamine systems have been reported to have paradoxical antimanic effects. Beckmann and Heinemann (1976) observed substantial suppression of the euphoric symptoms of mania (but not the aggressive symptoms) following intravenous *amphetamine*, whereas Brown and Mueller (1979) and Garvey and colleagues (1987) reported similar beneficial effects of oral amphetamine (45 to 60 mg/day). Decreased man-

ic symptoms were also reported after *methylphenidate*, administered both intravenously (Janowsky et al., 1973a) and orally (Brown and Mueller, 1979). These investigators also noted antimanic effects of oral L-dopa, a catecholamine precursor, and of *apomorphine*, a dopamine-receptor stimulant.

In a controlled study, Post and co-workers (1978) noted antimanic effects of low doses of another dopamine-receptor stimulant, *piribedil*. In a preliminary double-blind controlled study, however, Smith and colleagues (1980) found no antimanic effects with *bromocriptine*, a dopamine agonist with pharmacological effects similar to those of piribedil.

In 1962, Akimoto, a Japanese investigator, and his colleagues, reported the antimanic effects of large doses of the tricyclic antidepressants *imipramine* and *amitriptyline*. This finding, potentially the most interesting from a clinical viewpoint since it involves widely available drugs, was not verified by Klein (1967), however. The notion that drugs of the same class can both precipitate and alleviate mania seems counterintuitive. The nature of the effect, however, may depend on when in the natural cycle of the illness the drug is administered. A drug that accelerates or drives the underlying cycle might be expected to hasten the arrival of the next phase so that, when given during mania, it might bring on depression. These issues are discussed more thoroughly in Chapters 19 and 20.

Cholinergic Drugs

Neurobiological theories of affective disorder have evolved in recent years from models focusing on single transmitters to ones that consider how two or more transmitter systems are interrelated. Trials of the serotonin precursor L-tryptophan in both mania and depression, for example, were based on the permissive hypothesis that a serotonin deficiency underlies the vulnerability to both conditions. Studies of the therapeutic potential of cholinergic agents in mania evolved from the theory that mood regulation involves, in part, a balance between the adrenergic and cholinergic systems, the former subserving excitation and arousal, the latter, inhibition. According to this hypothesis, depression involves relative cholinergic predominance, whereas mania involves adrenergic predominance.

Physostigmine, a reversible, centrally active acetylcholinesterase inhibitor, enhances cholinergic function by interfering with its degradation. The first controlled study of physostigmine in mania was conducted by Janowsky and colleagues (1973b) in eight manic patients, two of whom also had schizophrenic symptoms. Pretreatment with methscopolamine, a peripherally active anticholinergic agent, partially blocked physostigmine's peripheral cholinergic effects. Physostigmine was administered intravenously (in doses up to 3 mg). Neostigmine, a potent cholinesterase inhibitor that essentially does not penetrate the brain, was used as an active placebo in six patients. Both drugs were administered through a continuous intravenous tube, and both were alternated with placebo.

In all eight patients, manic symptoms, assessed by the NIMH Beigel-Murphy mania scale (1971), diminished after physostigmine but not after the active or inactive placebos. A parallel increase in depression was seen in some patients. The antimanic effect began to appear within 15 minutes and, with repeated infusions, was substantial within an hour. Scaled reduction in individual manic symptoms ranged from 48 to 78 percent. The drug also produced a generally retarded, inhibited, and somewhat organic state in the patients, an observation that has led to questions about the specificity of its antimanic action. Two subsequent studies (Shopsin et al., 1975b; Davis et al., 1978) confirmed the original observations. Although a research tool of some interest, physostigmine is not likely to become a clinically useful alternative in the management of acute mania.

Cohen and co-workers (1980, 1982) also attempted to enhance cholinergic function in mania in a double-blind study. They gave six manic patients, who were already being treated with either lithium or neuroleptic, large amounts of *lecithin,* the dietary precursor of choline, which is in turn the precursor of acetylcholine. Five of the six improved rapidly, and three of them relapsed when the preparation was withdrawn. This observation could be of some clinical relevance, since no toxic effects were observed, but it still awaits confirmation.

Other Experimental Drugs

The following agents also have been employed in the evaluation of various hypotheses of mania.

Findings of alterations in serum and CSF calcium in mania (see Chapter 17) led Carman and Wyatt (1979) to administer synthetic *calcitonin,* a peptide hormone that lowers serum calcium, to 12 hospitalized patients with "psychotic agitation or mania." They reported an overall depressant or tranquilizing effect, which did not, however, appear to be a specific antimanic response.

Several studies using a theoretically related treatment strategy have suggested that the calcium-channel blockers, such as *verapamil* (160 to 240 mg/day), have antimanic effects (Dubovsky et al., 1982, 1985; Dubovsky and Franks, 1983). In a controlled study of manic inpatients, Höschl and Kozeny (1989) showed that verapamil was as effective as neuroleptics alone or a neuroleptic–lithium combination, without producing the sedative, hypnotic, or cataleptic effects associated with neuroleptics. Although an open study of verapamil was negative (Barton and Gitlin, 1987) and a controlled trial in 10 acutely manic patients (Emrich et al., 1983) yielded only modest results, other calcium-channel blockers deserve additional study as adjunctive agents in the treatment of mania. The need for additional data is highlighted by the fact that these clinically available drugs are now being rather widely used for mania by clinicians in practice.

In an open preliminary trial, Caillard (1985) administered the calcium antagonist *diltiazem* to five manic patients with bipolar illness and two patients with organic manic syndrome (some had additional neuroleptics). The five bipolar patients showed significant clinical improvement within 14 days (although three briefly required additional neuroleptics for extreme agitation), although the two patients with organic manic syndrome did not. Side effects were minimal. Calcium-channel blockers highly selective for the CNS are being developed. These drugs (e.g., nimodipine) will be of great interest as potential antimanic agents.

The opiate antagonist *naloxone* has been evaluated for antimanic effects. Reasoning from a very rough analogy between the euphoria seen in some stages of mania and the euphoriant effect of opiates, Janowsky and colleagues (1978) tested a daily dose of 20 mg of intravenous naloxone and found that it had an antimanic action, with the most dramatic effect seen in the most manic patients. However, Emrich and his colleagues (1979) saw no antimanic effect in two patients, one of whom had an exacerbation. Similarly, Davis and colleagues (1980) were unable to observe any antimanic effects following 20 mg of naloxone administered subcutaneously (Davis et al., 1980). These negative results were later replicated in a well-controlled double-blind, placebo crossover study of 25 manic patients (Pickar et al., 1982). Unlike Janowsky's patients, those in the two NIMH studies (Davis; Pickar) were able to remain in the normal ward environment during the trials, since the drug was given subcutaneously rather than intravenously.

The ability of the tetracycline-like antibiotic *demeclocycline* to inhibit adenylcyclase has led to the proposal that such drugs, by inhibiting this postsynaptic second messenger involved in a variety of neurotransmitter-mediated functions, might have antimanic properties. However, the one trial so far with this antibiotic has been negative.

Because of indirect indications that abnormalities in the Na^+-ATPase may underlie mania, Naylor and colleagues (1975) administered *digoxin,* an inhibitor of this enzyme, to mania patients but without effect. Conversely, treatments designed to correct a hypothesized deficiency of ATPase activity by reducing levels of an endogenous ATPase inhibitor, *vanadium,* have been reported as successful in mania. Since all of these reports (involving ascorbic acid, methylene blue, and low vanadium diets) originate from a single group (Naylor, 1983; Naylor et al., 1988), independent replication will be important.

Electroconvulsive Therapy

After ECT was introduced as a therapeutic modality in the early 1940s, there were several clinical reports of its efficacy in treating acute mania. As reviewed by Fink (1979, 1987), these early uncontrolled studies generally cited response rates of 65 to 75 percent but provided little or no systematic data on the characteristics of the patients or their responses to ECT. Later, as the efficacy of drugs became established, the use of ECT in mania virtually ceased. It remains today a treatment alternative that is, perhaps unfortunately, used only occasionally. In his 1979 and 1987 reviews, Fink pointed to the virtual ab-

sence of valid information on the efficacy of ECT in mania compared with drugs. In their 1987 naturalistic study of 438 manic patients, however, Black and colleagues attempted to answer this question directly. They found that a significantly greater proportion of the patients showed a "marked" response to ECT than to adequate lithium treatment—78 percent compared with 62 percent ($p < 0.05$).[25] This finding recently has been supported by a randomized double-blind trial in which ECT was found to be superior to lithium during the first 8 weeks, especially for severely manic patients and those with mixed states (Small et al., 1988). McCabe and Norris (1977) directly compared ECT, chlorpromazine, and no treatment in hospitalized manic patients and found that both active treatments were superior to no treatment. The advantage of ECT when mania is complicated by pregnancy has already been noted.

Clinical Predictors of Antimanic Response

We now turn to the clinical prediction of response to various antimanic agents, a problem implicit in the foregoing review of the literature on treatment efficacy but here brought into focus. Many of these issues were introduced in Chapter 17 in the discussion of biological and pharmacological correlates of treatment response.

One problem confounding attempts to evaluate predictors of antimanic response is the variability of treatment response in the same patient from one episode to the next (Stokes et al., 1971). This tendency may reflect the influence of state variables, such as the severity of the episode or the point in the natural course of the episode when treatment is initiated. A second problem, noted in our earlier discussion of the response to lithium among patients with pure mania as opposed to those with schizoaffective mania, is that an apparent differential response may actually reflect a difference in the time needed to achieve it (see Goodnick and Meltzer, 1984). A third problem concerns research design. For example, schizoaffective manic patients undergoing a controlled trial of lithium who happen to require a brief period of neuroleptics to control hyperactivity or psychoses are sometimes dropped from the study (see, e.g., Prien et al., 1972), making the response rate for lithium appear worse than it might otherwise be (Carroll, 1979).

Despite these difficulties, it is possible to delineate clinical features that correlate with response. In some cases, they simply reflect the features of the most responsive diagnostic group, bipolar illness. In others, they describe the characteristics of a subgroup within the bipolar diagnostic category that might be preferentially responsive (or unresponsive) to a particular treatment—for example, patients with rapid cycles responding to anticonvulsants. A third possibility is that they reflect personality or other variables that are independent of bipolar illness but that nevertheless bear on treatment response—for example, personality attributes that contribute to poor compliance or the presence of drug abuse or alcoholism. The relationship between personality variables and lithium response is discussed in Chapter 12 (see especially Table 12-9).

Factors that stand out as predictors of a poor acute antimanic response to lithium are the presence of a mixed state, substance abuse, and a history of rapid cycles (see Table 21-5 for a summary of the literature).[26] As we have seen, mixed states are quite common, characterizing approximately 40 percent of manic episodes. As discussed in Chapter 9, the alcohol and drug abuse frequently associated with mixed states may represent the patient's attempt to achieve symptomatic relief from the intensely dysphoric wired feeling state.

Clinical variables associated with the acute antimanic response to carbamazepine are summarized in Table 21-6 (Post et al., 1986). Many of the features that predict poor response to lithium appear to predict good response to the anticonvulsant. Although preliminary, these data are consistent with suggestions that carbama-

Table 21-5. Clinical Predictors of Antimanic Response to Lithium

Patient Characteristics	Prediction
Demographic	
Age	None
Sex	None, but lower compliance rates in males (Chapter 25)
Marital status	Not known
Clinical	
Diagnosis	Some note poorer response for schizomania, others do not (Goodnick & Meltzer, 1984); slower response in this group accounts for the difference
Family history	Not reported for antimanic response
Age of onset	None
Duration of illness	None
Severity of mania	More severe symptoms predict poorer response (Prien et al., 1972; Swann et al., 1986) but time to response may be important variable
"Reactive" mania	Less likely to respond (Aronoff & Epstein, 1970; Jones & Wilson, 1972)
Mixed manic and depressive symptoms	Poorer response (Swann et al., 1986; Himmelhoch et al., 1976a)
Predominance of paranoid over elated / grandiose symptoms	Poorer response in one study (Murphy & Biegel, 1974) but not another (Swann et al., 1986)
Rapid cycles	Poor response (Dunner & Fieve, 1974; Post et al., 1986d)
Initial response	Poor response in the first week predicts poor outcome at 3-1/2 weeks (Swann et al., 1986); early dropouts (due to personality factors?) may or may not have been responsive (Taylor & Abrams, 1981b)
Drug abuse	Poor response (Himmelhoch et al., 1976a)

Table 21-6. Clinical Predictors of Antimanic Response to Carbamazepine

Patient Characteristics	Prediction
Severity of mania	Responders significantly more ill
Mixed manic or depressive symptoms	Responders tended to be more dysphoric
Rapid cycles	Responders had significantly more episodes in year prior to trial
Family history of bipolar illness	Responders had significantly less family history

From Post et al., 1986d

zepine, and perhaps also valproate, may be especially useful in patients who have responded poorly to lithium.

SUMMARY

The choice of medical treatment for acute manic episodes should be based primarily on the nature and severity of the symptoms. Lithium, the most specific antimanic drug, remains the treatment of choice. Because sleep deprivation can contribute to the progression of the manic syndrome, it may be wise to use clonazepam, which has sedative properties, in addition to lithium early in treatment. When symptoms are more severe, the urgency of achieving behavioral control often requires that lithium be supplemented with neuroleptics (briefly) or with the anticonvulsants carbamazepine, valproate, or clonazepam. The anticonvulsants may be the treatment of choice for patients with rapid cycles or a prior history of lithium failure or intolerance to it. Whether the anticonvulsants are preferable for patients with mixed states remains to be seen.

Fully developed psychotic mania usually requires hospitalization. The possible stigma that may result should be weighed against the sometimes rapid progression of mania into a condition that is even more dangerous for the patient.

Children and adolescents also suffer from mania, and their treatment is similar to that for adults. Early recognition and treatment are imperative to minimize lifelong psychological, social, and possibly biological consequences.

NOTES

1. Cited in Hamilton, 1982, p. 285.
2. The appropriateness or the legality of prescribing

drugs for uses other than those listed in their official labeling is sometimes a cause of concern and confusion. The Federal Food, Drug, and Cosmetic Act does not, however, limit a physician's use of an approved drug. The *FDA Drug Bulletin* clarifies the issue as follows:

Once a product has been approved for marketing, a physician may prescribe it for uses or in treatment regimens or patient populations that are not included in approved labeling. Such "unapproved" or, more precisely, "unlabeled" uses may be appropriate and rational in certain circumstances, and may, in fact, reflect approaches to drug therapy that have been extensively reported in medical literature. . . . accepted medical practice often includes drug use that is not reflected in approved drug labeling. (*FDA Drug Bulletin*, 12(1):4–5, 1982).

3. One high-potency neuroleptic, clozapine, has a low incidence of extrapyramidal effects and may be effective among neuroleptic-resistant patients. It is discussed later in the literature review section.
4. The concurrent use of neuroleptics and lithium has been reported to result in lethargy, tremulousness, severe neuromuscular symptoms, hyperthermia, impaired consciousness, and even irreversible brain damage (Cohen and Cohen, 1974; Goldney and Spence, 1986).

Neuroleptic malignant syndrome is an uncommon reaction to neuroleptic medications, especially those with high potency (e.g., haloperidol). First identified in 1960 by French psychiatrists (Delay and Deniker, 1968), it is characterized by muscular rigidity, extremely high fever, autonomic dysfunction, and altered consciousness (Levenson, 1985). Although its pathogenesis is not understood, disturbances in the hypothalamic–adrenal axis have been hypothesized (Horn et al., 1988).

5. These issues are discussed further in relation to prophylactic treatment, in Chapter 23.
6. A potential complication of using clonazepam for mania is the emergence of depression early in treatment. The effect may depend on dose (Cohen and Rosenbaum, 1987).
7. In addition to the needs of the clinical setting, ethical considerations argue for early vigorous treatment of mania.
8. Psychiatrists treating manic-depressive patients

should be sufficiently knowledgeable about relevant medical issues to work closely with internists and other specialists. Patients are not well served when they are simply turned over to the nonpsychiatric specialist. For many issues—the subtle CNS effects of mild hypothyroidism, for example—the psychiatrist should provide the expertise for the collaborative management of the patient.

9. The interaction of lithium with dopamine systems has also been put to therapeutic use in managing the on–off phenomenon that complicates the use of L-dopa in Parkinson's disease.

10. In treating schizophrenia, a 20:1 chlorpromazine /haloperidol dose ratio has generally been used. However, recent data suggest that in mania a ratio of approximately 13:1 is more appropriate (Janicak et al., 1988a). A similar ratio applies when comparing other neuroleptics with low potency to those with high potencies.

11. Administering a loading dose means to start with a super maximal dose rather than building up to the usual therapeutic dose.

12. Baastrup et al., 1976; Juhl et al., 1977; Krishna et al., 1978; Garfinkel et al., 1980; Carman et al., 1981; Perényi et al., 1983; Goldney and Spence, 1986; Miller and Menninger, 1987.

13. For example, Miller and Menninger (1987) found neurotoxicity in 6 of 22 manic patients (27 percent) on a lithium–neuroleptic combination. The average neuroleptic dose was 563 mg (chlorpromazine equivalents) in the nontoxic group vs 1,780 mg in the toxic group, whereas lithium doses were not different.

14. See, for example, Trimble, 1981; Pisciotta, 1982; Hart and Easton, 1982; Tompson, 1984; Post et al., 1987.

15. Even ECT has been used successfully in the treatment of mania in children (see, e.g., Carr et al., 1983).

16. In psychopharmacology, nonblind studies such as these are often dismissed as essentially meaningless. In the case of mania, however, they can be informative, since clinical experience suggests that patients with this major psychotic illness are not responsive to the subtle environmental and interpersonal factors that contribute to high placebo response rates.

A greater difficulty in interpreting these open trials derives from the fact that mania is cyclic and, even without treatment, will generally remit spontaneously. It is unusual, however, for spontaneous remission to occur during any given period of 2 weeks. Thus, the disappearance of manic symptoms observed during lithium therapy in most patients was probably a real effect of treatment, not the result of spontaneous remission or a placebo effect.

17. In a double-blind study, for example, DeLong and Nieman (1983) studied 11 children who met DSM-III criteria for manic episodes. Given lithium alone and placebo alternately for 3 weeks each, they improved when on the lithium, as rated from parental reports.

18. Reviewed in Youngerman and Canino, 1978; Jefferson, 1982; Campbell et al., 1984.

19. The adolescents with prepubertal onset of behavioral pathology (before age 12) had significantly more first-degree relatives with bipolar-I illness. Strober and colleagues speculate that, despite reservations about the validity of some parental recollections of their children's early behavior, it is possible to hypothesize that the early-onset pathology represents very early, subacute expressions of a bipolar genotype, which may be more severe than adolescent-onset disorder. The investigators note, however, that lithium maintenance treatment is usually found to be more effective in patients with positive family history of bipolar illness. Their findings suggest, by contrast, that lithium response in the acute treatment of manic episodes in adolescents may be negatively correlated with family history of bipolar illness.

20. The children were diagnosed by RDC using the Schedule for Affective Disorders and Schizophrenia at admission and discharge, as well as ongoing review of the course of symptoms during hospitalization and previous medical records. Semistructured interviews were also done with parents to obtain qualitative information on the adolescents' childhood—the Schedule for Affective Disorders and Schizophrenia for School-Age Children and the Psychosocial Schedule for School-Age Children.

The children were first administered lithium carbonate (titrated to achieve plasma levels of 0.9 to 1.5 mEq/liter), as well as neuroleptic drugs as needed to control agitation and psychotic symptoms. Those who failed to respond satisfactorily in the first 4 to 6 weeks were also administered carbamazepine.

21. The demonstrated effectiveness of clozapine in schizophrenic patients who have responded poorly to neuroleptic drugs (Kane et al., 1988) is one of the most significant recent developments in the pharmacotherapy of serious mental illness. The drug is a prototype of antipsychotic neuroleptics called *atypical* because they produce little or no extrapyramidal side effects, selectively block some dopamine receptors (e.g., mesolimbic > nigrostriatal), or broadly affect other CNS neurotransmitter systems (e.g., antiserotonergic, antiadrenergic properties) (see Meltzer, in press). Although the use of clozapine in patients with bipolar illness has yet to be systematically examined, pilot data from intramural NIMH researchers suggest that it may be superior to typical neuroleptics in reducing persistent psychotic symptomatology in schizoaffective patients (D. Pickar, personal communication). Further, it is emerging as the neuroleptic of choice for patients who have tardive dyskinesia. The significant risk of agranulocytosis

(approximately 1 percent), however, limits its use to treatment-resistant psychotic patients, those who poorly tolerate extrapyramidal side effects of conventional neuroleptics, or those with tardive dyskinesia.

22. Subsequent case reports (Victor et al., 1984; Freinhar and Alvarez, 1985) documented clonazepam's antimanic efficacy when given alone in both bipolar and schizoaffective patients. Others showed an accompanying disinhibition of behavior (Binder, 1987).

23. In this context *experimental* simply means that the treatment is not currently considered to be part of the ordinary clinical armamentarium. The anticonvulsants are considered along with the standard drugs because they are widely used in practice.

24. Jouvent et al., 1980; Jimerson et al., 1980; Zubenko et al., 1984; Hardy et al., 1986; Maguire, 1987; Kontaxakis et al., 1989.

25. Whether the ECT treatment of mania requires bilateral electrode placement is controversial. In the study of Black and colleagues (1987), unilateral ECT was found to be as effective as bilateral. This is an important issue, since unilateral treatment is associated with a lower residue of memory impairment.

26. The study of Taylor and Abrams (1981) is cited frequently, albeit incorrectly, as having failed to find a variety of clinical variables associated with lithium response. Actually, this was a retrospective study of outcome in manic inpatients treated by physicians' choice. Of the 111 patients, only 14 received lithium alone. The others were treated either with lithium plus neuroleptics, neuroleptics alone, or ECT. Obviously, no conclusions should be drawn concerning treatment response prediction, since the individual clinicians may already have given different treatments to patients with different clinical profiles.

22

Medical Treatment of
Acute Bipolar Depression

As early as 1833 a certain melancholy made itself felt. . . . In the night between
the 17th and 18th of October I was seized with the worst fear a man can have, the
worst punishment Heaven can inflict—the fear of losing one's reason. It took so
strong a hold of me that consolation and prayer, defiance and derision, were equally powerless to subdue it. Terror drove me from place to place. My breath failed me
as I pictured my brain paralyzed. Ah, Clara! no one knows the suffering, the sickness, the despair, except those so crushed. In my terrible agitation I went to a doctor and told him everything—how my senses often failed me so that I did not know
which way to turn in my fright, how I could not be certain of not taking my own life
when in this helpless condition.   —Robert Schumann, 1838[1]

The progress that has been made in treating severe depression in the last few decades represents
one of the most important medical advances in
recent history. Effective medications have been
found, electroconvulsive therapy has been refined, and other somatic techniques have been
developed. Suffering and hopelessness—the paralyzing core of depression—can now be relieved
more quickly and completely than at any time in
the history of man's long struggle with mental
illness. Despite this progress, all too little effort
has gone into developing new medications for
bipolar depression. The pharmaceutical industry's energies continue to be dedicated to producing medications for nonbipolar depression.

In this chapter, we review the medical treatment of depression, with an emphasis on the bipolar patient.[2] We open with guidelines drawn
from the research literature and clinical experience. These relatively brief suggestions for practice are then fleshed out by an examination of the
studies of established and experimental treatments. Much of that literature, particularly older
material, does not distinguish bipolar from unipolar illness. Nevertheless, we attempt to extract
information specific to the bipolar patient whenever possible.

Despite its often dramatic response to treatment, depression in bipolar patients continues to
challenge both clinicians and investigators. Most
problematic is the tendency of antidepressant
treatments to induce mania or rapid cycling in
some bipolar patients. The magnitude of this risk
may be underestimated by some clinicians, but it
is probably the reason bipolar patients are excluded from most trials of new antidepressant
agents.

The tricyclic antidepressants, along with related and newer heterocyclic compounds, such as
fluoxetine and bupropion, are the most widely
prescribed drugs used to treat major depression.
The basic chemical structure of the tricyclics is
similar to that of the phenothiazine nucleus. Since
the initial discovery of their antidepressant properties (Kuhn, 1957), the tricyclic drugs have been
subjected to hundreds of controlled trials, and
their efficacy in treating major depression is now
firmly established. In almost all of the controlled
studies, a majority of depressed patients showed
improvement in affective, behavioral, and cognitive symptoms of depression. Such impressive
rates of improvement do not necessarily hold true
for bipolar depressed patients, however. Definitive studies examining this issue have yet to be
done.

Observations about another class of drugs,
monoamine oxidase inhibitors (MAOIs), actually
inaugurated the antidepressant era. Clinicians no-

ticed that iproniazid, at the time a treatment for tuberculosis, was associated with the onset of hypomanic-like states (Crane, 1956) and activation (Loomer et al., 1957). These observations led to clinical trials of iproniazid as an antidepressant. The enthusiasm for the MAOIs as antidepressants that followed gave way to skepticism as reports of unexpected hypertensive reactions began to occur. Even after the dietary factor causing these reactions was identified (foods rich in the amine tyramine, especially aged cheeses), MAOIs continued to be underused, particularly in the United States. As the limitations of tricyclic and related heterocyclic drugs have become more apparent, however, this interesting class of drugs has been undergoing a revival, with bipolar illness a major focus of renewed interest in the MAOIs.

John Cade's original report of the antimanic effects of lithium (1949) did not argue well for the drug's antidepressant effects. Three patients with chronic depression not only failed to respond after a brief trial, but Cade reported that he thought the lithium had actually worsened their depression.[3] A later study also found no improvement in a few depressed patients treated with lithium (Noack and Trautner, 1951). At the time, mania and depression were viewed as opposite states, both phenomenologically and biologically, so that investigators did not expect the same drug to improve both conditions.

For two decades after Cade's initial report, Mogens Schou, Poul Baastrup, and other European pioneers continued to explore primarily the antimanic and prophylactic potential of this new treatment. Several uncontrolled reports[4] on the ion's antidepressant effects led to the controlled studies in the late 1960s and early 1970s by Goodwin and colleagues at the National Institute of Mental Health (NIMH). This group found that depressed patients often did not begin to improve until 3 or 4 weeks after they began taking the drug, a characteristic that may account for the failure to find antidepressant effects in the earlier, shorter trials. Subsequent studies showed that about three of five bipolar depressed patients have a clinically significant (albeit not necessarily complete) response to lithium, approximately twice the rate for unipolar depressed patients.

Historically, the convulsive therapies were the first genuinely effective treatments for serious depressive illness, and today, despite controversy and misunderstanding among some segments of the public, electroconvulsive therapy (ECT) remains an important therapeutic option. Used judiciously, it may, in fact, pose less of a risk of altering the course of manic-depressive illness than some medications. The more recently developed techniques involving sleep manipulation and exposure to high-intensity light offer additional options for the treatment of bipolar depression.

CLINICAL MANAGEMENT

This section briefly outlines the practical management of depression, with a focus on bipolar patients not already on maintenance medication.[5]

Pretreatment Evaluation

In dealing with the acutely depressed (perhaps suicidal) patient, the clinician faces an urgent— at times, an emergency—situation. There often is great pressure to begin treatment immediately, perhaps before adequate information has been obtained. Adding to this difficulty is the fact that depressed patients may be too preoccupied by their symptoms or too confused or retarded to give a comprehensive history in the all too short time that many busy practitioners give them.[6]

Despite those pressures, a careful pretreatment evaluation, as outlined in Chapter 5 and in the introduction to this section, must be done if treatment is to be successful. The patient's functional and symptomatic state and key aspects of his or her history, particularly past episodes of mania or hypomania, should be determined in as much detail and with as much reliability as possible. Often this information must come from a spouse or other close family member or friend because a depressed patient frequently underestimates prior hypomanic or manic symptoms, assuming that the symptoms simply represent the patient's normal "best." Interviewing the spouse also provides a quick overview of the patient's marital and family relationships, factors that may be important in understanding a depressive episode and planning its treatment. In addition, the active collaboration of relatives and friends may help to keep a patient out of the hospital.

Among the important facts to watch for in the patient's history are the following:

- The age at which the first definable affective episode began (depression, mania, or hypomania)
- The general characteristics of each episode, such as severity, duration, nature of symptoms, and patterns of recurrence, including seasonal patterns
- Information bearing on the nature of past responses to mood-altering drugs, since sometimes the only evidence for what might be latent bipolarity is a brief hypomanic period following exposure to antidepressant drugs
- Data on the family history of response to drug treatment, since family members may respond similarly to lithium, tricyclic antidepressants, and MAOIs.

General Indications for Medication

Acute drug treatment for depression is probably necessary when the patient is functionally impaired, has symptoms that do not respond to external events, and has significant disturbances of sleep, appetite, or diurnal pattern. A history of mania or hypomania, by itself, suggests the existence of a biological dysfunction potentially responsive to drugs. By contrast, the presence or absence of convincing psychosocial precipitants is generally irrelevant to the question of whether pharmacotherapy is indicated. A corollary is that the indications for psychotherapy and drug therapy should be evaluated independently.

A Drug Decision Tree Approach

The sequence of drug trials we suggest for depressed patients who have bipolar-I illness (major depression with a history of mania) is illustrated in Figure 22-1 (ECT is discussed later). Before moving on to an alternative medication, the clinician must evaluate a host of factors that can contribute to a poor antidepressant response. These include poor compliance, coexisting alcohol or drug abuse, inappropriate blood level, and intercurrent psychological or social stress. Thyroid supplementation should be considered, especially in females, before going on to an alternative medication (see later discussion).

Most of the research literature, as well as clinical experience, suggests that antidepressant treatments can precipitate mania in bipolar-I patients. The literature is less clear concerning the susceptibility of bipolar-II patients to manic episodes when taking antidepressants. A higher frequency of hypomanic episodes has been reported. It is our clinical impression that the activation of bipolar-II patients by antidepressants is generally confined to hypomania; that is, such treatments do not appear to convert bipolar-II illness to bipolar-I. Since some bipolar patients with moderate depression respond to lithium alone, some clinical investigators consider it prudent to initiate treatment with lithium, although this is not standard practice. In our experience, some patients show a rapid response to lithium alone, improving within 7 to 10 days, but for many the benefits of lithium do not become apparent until the fourth or fifth week. Since most patients will subsequently take lithium for prophylaxis, a trial of this drug spares them the necessity of having to take another drug along with it.

With more severe bipolar depressions, an antidepressant (tricyclic, heterocyclic, or MAOI) will be needed at the outset, and generally treatment should begin with lithium and the antidepressant together. With bipolar-II patients, in whom the risk of full-blown mania is less, some clinicians prefer to start treatment with the antidepressant first, saving lithium for subsequent potentiation. Among the tricyclic antidepressants (TCAs), one of the drugs with effects that are initially more activating and less sedating (e.g., desmethylimipramine, imipramine, or nortriptyline) may be preferable, since psychomotor retardation often is prominent in the depressive phase of bipolar illness.[7] This practice also avoids the excessive sedation that can occur when an anxiolytic tricyclic (such as amitriptyline) and lithium are combined. Also available are the second-generation heterocyclic antidepressants (particularly fluoxetine and bupropion), which may be more suitable than standard tricyclics because of their favorable profile of side effects. Whether any of these drugs will, in the long run, match or outperform the tricyclics as antidepressants remains to be seen. Clinical experience suggests that fluoxetine may have some MAOI-like characteristics.

In the treatment of unipolar depression, MAOIs are often reserved for patients who do not respond to tricyclics. For bipolar patients, how-

Moderate Bipolar Depression

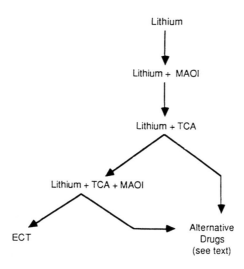

Severe Bipolar Depression

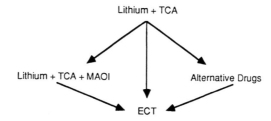

Figure 22-1. A treatment decision tree for bipolar depression (I or II). Adjunctive strategies may be employed at the various steps, for example, hormonal potentiation or sleep deprivation.

ever, many experienced clinicians prefer to use an MAOI before a tricyclic or heterocyclic, especially when the depression is characterized by less energy, hypersomnia, and excessive appetite. The differential efficacy of tricyclics and MAOIs in bipolar illness remains an unanswered question in psychopharmacology, and controlled studies are urgently needed. In our clinical experience (shared by many of the experts we surveyed), many bipolar depressed patients who do not respond to lithium alone do respond to the addition of an MAOI.

Some clinicians recommend the combination of a tricyclic and an MAOI when neither alone has produced a response.[8] Although we deal with this topic here because it logically follows the

discussion of tricyclics and MAOIs, in practice the use of such combinations would generally be reserved for patients who do not respond to the adjunctive or alternative strategies described later. It is still not clear whether TCA–MAOI combinations are associated with additional efficacy, but their safety is reasonably well established.[9] The safety of adding lithium to TCA–MAOI combinations has not been studied systematically, but clinical experience suggests that all three can be administered together, as long as dosages of each drug are kept to the minimum that is effective.

In using TCA–MAOI combinations, the sequence of administration is important. A tricyclic should not be given to a patient already established on an MAOI because of the risk of a hypertensive crisis. Either the two drugs should be started simultaneously (each at lower than usual doses), or the MAOI should be added when the patient is already taking tricyclics. In addition to the greater efficacy that may be possible with TCA–MAOI combinations, small doses of those tricyclics with more sedative effectiveness (25 to 50 mg at bedtime) fortuitously diminish the sleep disruptions associated with the MAOIs.[10]

The use of neuroleptics in the treatment of depression has been the subject of some confusion. Certainly, these drugs can ameliorate the agitation, anxiety, and sleeplessness experienced by some depressed patients, and they may also have antipsychotic effects in delusional depression. They are not, however, antidepressants. Among bipolar patients, they may be helpful in states characterized by a mixture of manic and depressive symptoms (see Chapter 21), but the possibility that manic-depressive patients may be at greater risk of neuroleptic-induced tardive dyskinesia than schizophrenic patients (Casey, 1984) argues for caution in the use of these drugs.

Dosage, Blood Levels, Length of Treatment

For the first administration of tricyclics (or MAOIs) with lithium, dosages should be lower than if each were used alone, since some side effects, such as sedation, may be additive. Once a patient has accommodated to the drug, the dose should be increased until the patient responds or experiences unacceptable side effects. Many treatment failures with tricyclics, MAOIs, or lithium result from inadequate dosage or duration of administration (Dunner et al., 1977; Klein et al., 1981; Quitkin, 1985).

Monitoring tricyclic blood levels may be helpful, especially with vulnerable individuals, such as elderly patients with cardiac pathology, or when no response is observed. The relationship to clinical response appears to be linear for imipramine and desmethylimipramine, whereas nortriptyline has a therapeutic window, that is, an optimal blood level range below or above which efficacy is reduced. Present knowledge about TCA blood levels, which comes primarily from studies of unipolar patients, has been the subject of several excellent reviews.[11]

The time patients need to take antidepressant medications before a response occurs may be longer than the 3 or 4 weeks recommended by many textbooks and review articles. Evidence suggests that some patients do not respond fully for 5 or 6 weeks (Quitkin et al., 1984), the same waiting period that can be encountered when lithium is used alone as an antidepressant.

Duration of Drug Treatment

If the patient responds to pharmacological intervention, how long should the drug or drugs be continued? Here we do not mean prophylactic treatment, aimed at preventing new episodes in the future, but continuation treatment. For unipolar depression, it is often recommended that antidepressants be continued for 6 to 12 months after remission of overt symptoms, a recommendation consistent with data showing an increased relapse rate when treatment is stopped within the first few months.

What is an adequate length of treatment for a depressive episode in a bipolar patient? If the patient has responded to lithium alone and is tolerating it well, it should be continued for 6 to 12 months after remission (as one would do with a unipolar patient who has responded to a tricyclic or MAOI), at which point the question of maintenance treatment can be considered, using the criteria outlined in Chapter 23. If a combination of lithium and another antidepressant has been effective, it is probably advisable to withdraw the tricyclic or MAOI gradually after the patient has reached a stable remission because of the risk of an antidepressant shortening the cycle. If treatment was started with a tricyclic or MAOI alone, lithium could be added or substituted as soon as the patient is in remission. As stated before, we do not recommend starting with an antidepressant alone (especially for the bipolar-I patient) because of the risk of drug-induced mania.

Adjunctive Use of Thyroid Hormone

In some patients, small doses of triiodothyronine (T_3) (25 to 50 μg) may accelerate or potentiate the antidepressant response to tricyclics, especially in women. As reviewed later, bipolar patients may be more responsive than unipolar patients. In light of this effect and the fact that subclinical hypothyroidism may first occur with depressive symptoms, thyroid potentiation should be considered when a depression is not responding to drugs. Hypothyroidism, as indicated by definite clinical or laboratory evidence, requires correction, regardless of the stage of decision making in treating the depression. When, as frequently happens, laboratory evidence indicates the thyroid is functioning in the low normal range but does not support a diagnosis of clinical hypothyroidism, the very persistence of the depression raises a question about thyroid function. If the lithium–antidepressant combination has failed, supplemental thyroid should be tried before going on to an alternate drug. T_3 potentiation is usually evident within 3 to 5 days; if it has not helped by 2 weeks it should be withdrawn. Although T_4 preparations are easier to use than T_3 because they do not interfere with the ongoing laboratory assessment of thyroid function, they may not potentiate antidepressants as effectively as T_3 (Joffe and Singer, 1988).[12]

Alternative Treatments

Today, the clinician can consider alternatives to the more or less standard approaches to acute treatment of bipolar depression outlined previously. This section highlights the major alternative or adjunctive approaches. Additional options are discussed later in the review of the literature.

Carbamazepine

In addition to its antimanic and prophylactic properties, carbamazepine has at least modest antidepressant effects, both when used alone and when used in combination with lithium. These effects may not begin until the second or third week and often do not reach their maximum until the fifth or sixth week. Studies have shown that the side effects of carbamazepine on the central nervous system are proportional to the rate of increase in the dose. When dose increments are kept small, such effects generally are mild and transient (see Chapter 23). For the acute treatment of depression, it is best to start with 100 to 200 mg at bedtime, increasing by 100 mg every 2 to 4 days until clinical response occurs (usually achieved at or below 1,200 mg) or until side effects become intolerable. At the higher dose levels, it is advisable to employ a twice daily dosage schedule. Another anticonvulsant, valproic acid, may also act as an antidepressant, but this effect is not as clear-cut as it is in carbamazepine.

Bupropion and Fluoxetine

Bupropion is a monocyclic antidepressant with virtually no anticholinergic effects. Some investigators suggest that it may be useful in treating bipolar depression because of three characteristics noted in the early trials: First, compared with classic tricyclics, bupropion may be associated with a somewhat lower incidence of mania. Second, it appears to be effective in some seriously depressed patients, especially against symptoms of psychomotor retardation. Third, bupropion (along with fluoxetine) is unusual among antidepressants in that it is not associated with increased weight (Feighner et al., 1984). The therapeutic range of bupropion is as high as 450 mg a day in divided doses (half-life is about 12 hours), starting at 75 to 150 mg a day and increasing by 75 mg every 3 to 5 days. The principal problem associated with this drug is the risk of seizures at doses moderately higher than the recommended range.[13]

Fluoxetine, another antidepressant reported to have few anticholinergic side effects, also has the considerable advantage of not being associated with weight gain, at least when administered alone. Because of its serotonergic effects, it has been thought that fluoxetine is less likely to precipitate mania than standard TCAs. Nevertheless, case reports of manic reactions have appeared, although the relative frequency of this phenomenon has not yet been evaluated. Most experience to date is with outpatients whose depressions are in the moderately severe range. Its use among severely depressed inpatients is not yet as well established. Treatment is started at 20 mg per day in a single dose, the timing of which is governed by the side effects, which are usually mild (nausea, nervousness, headache, daytime sedation, and, less commonly, insomnia). Although the standard dose is 20 mg/day, many patients require more; doses above 80 mg/day are not recommended.[14]

Partial Sleep Deprivation or Phase Advance Therapy

As reviewed in Chapters 19 and 22, adjusting the patient's normal sleeping patterns not only is interesting theoretically but also may offer a practical alternative to medications. A night of partial sleep deprivation—that is, wakefulness during the second half of the night (generally after 2 or 3 am)—can produce appreciable but transient anti-depressant effects in about 60 percent of patients with major depression. Unlike total sleep deprivation, it can be repeated on consecutive nights, a regimen that results in a more sustained clinical response. Related to partial sleep deprivation is the technique of phase advance, in which the patient is also awake during the second half of the night but can experience a normal amount of sleep by going to bed 4 hours earlier, that is, sleeping between 8 or 9 PM and 2 or 3 AM.

The repeated use of these techniques can produce a more sustained response than the day or two of improvement seen after a single night of sleep deprivation. Nevertheless, relapses are likely to occur after 10 to 14 days. This time frame suggests that sleep deprivation might be combined usefully with the initiation of pharmacological treatment, with the latter taking over after 1 or 2 weeks. At the very least, enlisting the patient in purposeful manipulation of what may be an already troubled sleep pattern (i.e., intentionally creating early-morning awakening) can decrease the anxiety and distress associated with disordered sleep.

High-Intensity Light

The syndrome of winter seasonal affective disorder (SAD) often has a bipolar-II pattern, with the onset of depressions in the late fall or winter followed regularly by remission in the spring or early summer, frequently progressing to hypomania in the summer (see Chapter 19). Controlled studies indicate that the majority of patients with this syndrome show rapid, substantial, and lasting improvement after exposure to several hours of bright artificial light during the short days of fall and winter—approximately 2500 lux or 225 foot-candles at 4 feet away, an amount sufficient to suppress plasma melatonin. (Further details of this approach are described later in the review of the literature section of this chapter.) Bright light also may be useful as an adjunct to medications when breakthrough depressions occur during the fall or winter in bipolar-I patients or recurrent unipolar patients without the pure SAD syndrome.[15]

Psychostimulants

Some clinicians experienced in the treatment of depression use modest doses of methylphenidate or dextroamphetamine in conjunction with tricyclics early in treatment. Although systematic data on this use are not available, experience indicates that these agents, used judiciously, can be helpful to some patients, primarily when the sedative effects of the tricyclic–lithium combination may interfere with antidepressant effects or discourage compliance. These drugs are not generally used in conjunction with MAOIs, although clinical experience and one report in the literature (Feighner et al., 1985) suggest that this combination may be safer than previously thought and may be particularly effective in cases of treatment-resistant depression. Satel and Nelson (1989), in their comprehensive review of the literature, make a compelling case for more controlled studies.

A cautionary note: To the extent that any of the alternate or adjunctive approaches is capable of producing an antidepressant response, some risk of mania generally will be present.[16] With the psychostimulants, the risk of tolerance or dependence must also be considered.

Electroconvulsive Therapy

ECT continues to have an important place in the treatment of some cases of bipolar depression and should be given consideration as the initial treatment if the patient is severely ill, especially delusional, at high risk for suicide, or has a history of good response to ECT. Reserving ECT only for drug failures ignores data showing that patients with delusional depression respond poorly to tricyclics but are remarkably responsive to ECT. Unfortunately, ECT is sometimes discounted because of misconceptions on the part of many clinicians and patients and, in some areas, because of legal barriers to its use. In the United States, many psychiatrists who treat depression have not learned how to use ECT, further limiting the likelihood of its being given balanced consideration as a treatment option. If ECT is to be used, it is probably best to discontinue lithium temporarily, since some investigators have noted an apparent increase in neurotoxicity with this combination (Small et al., 1980; Weiner et al., 1980; Mandel et al., 1980).[17] Unilateral ECT is generally preferred over bilateral because the latter is associated with more memory disturbance while not showing a clear advantage in efficacy.

Hospitalization

Most bipolar depressions can be managed on an outpatient basis, but hospitalization is sometimes advisable. Although there are no universal guidelines, the following evaluation of each patient's individual situation is useful:

- Is the patient likely to be suicidal? A personal or family history of serious suicidal behavior could provide a strong argument for hospitalization, although the absence of such a history does not imply a lack of risk. Often the beginning of a drug response is the most dangerous period; the patient experiences some return of energy and motivation but is still feeling hopeless and depressed. (The clinical assessment and management of suicide are discussed at greater length in Chapter 27.)
- Is the clinician readily available? The initial administration of any new drug requires frequent contact with the patient, often twice a week or more.
- Does the patient have reliable, willing, and available relatives or friends who can temporarily take on some of the responsibility of the hospital staff? Of course, the family's well-being and its future relationships with the patient also need to be considered.
- What are the social, economic, and occupational costs to the patient of hospitalization? What effect would hospitalization have on the patient's self-esteem? Conversely, what would it cost to be kept out of the hospital? For example, if an individual might lose his job by being hospitalized, more effort should be made to treat him on an outpatient basis. Conversely, in some cases, working while depressed might be more damaging to the patient's professional well-being. Depression per se tends to color patients' assessments of their ability to continue functioning at work. A clinician's hasty decision to hospitalize should not reinforce a patient's self-defeating attitude.
- How is hospitalization likely to affect a patient's response to drugs? Inpatients may respond to drugs they had not responded to as outpatients (Kotin et al., 1973a), perhaps because of enhanced compliance.

REVIEW OF THE LITERATURE

Tricyclic Antidepressants

An increasing variety of tricyclic (and related monocyclic, bicyclic, and tetracyclic) drugs is available to treat major depression. Although more than 25 such drugs are marketed worldwide, imipramine and amitriptyline have been used in most controlled studies. The efficacy of this class of drugs in treating major depression is clear. More than two thirds of the controlled studies (done largely with inpatients) demonstrate their superiority over placebo (reviewed in Morris and Beck, 1974). Improvement rates across different studies range from 50 to 85 percent, averaging 65 to 70 percent.[18] Still to be answered is the question of relative efficacy: Are tricyclic antidepressants as effective for bipolar depressed patients as they are for unipolar patients?

Throughout the history of the tricyclics, attempts to identify groups of patients most likely to respond have focused on the now-outdated endogenous-reactive dichotomy. Relatively high response rates generally have been found in patient groups predominantly characterized by so-called endogenous symptoms, particularly anorexia and weight loss, middle and late insomnia, psychomotor change, and lack of reactivity to the environment. Conversely, relatively low response rates have been noted among patients whose depressions are accompanied by overt delusions or are characterized in the old terminology as neurotic or reactive.

Despite its large size, the clinical literature dealing with tricyclics provides almost no information about the relative efficacy of this group of drugs in bipolar depression compared with unipolar depression. We carefully analyzed 77 studies (involving 3,226 patients), covered in an excellent review by Morris and Beck (1974) on the efficacy of tricyclics and by Bielski and Friedel (1976) on predictors of tricyclic response. Very few studies provide sufficient information to determine how many bipolar patients are included in the sample. Since the great majority of these investigations were performed before the bipolar–unipolar distinction became established, this oversight is at least partly understandable, but the extreme scarcity of even simple data on past manic or hypomanic episodes is less comprehensible.[19]

A small study of hospitalized bipolar and unipolar depressed patients showed that imipramine and amitriptyline are significantly less effective in bipolar than in unipolar depressed patients (Bunney et al., 1970). On the other hand, Goodwin and colleagues, in a larger sample, found only a slight and nonsignificant trend for bipolar depressed patients to respond less well to tri-cyclics (unpublished data, 1981), and results from the NIMH collaborative study indicate similar rates of response to imipramine among hospitalized unipolar and bipolar depressive patients (Katz et al., 1987). Avery and Winokur (1977), as part of a comparison of the efficacy of tricyclics and ECT in depression, presented data that also suggest similar rates of tricyclic response in both groups of depressed patients. Since the bipolar group comprised only 8 percent of the sample, however, no conclusion can be drawn.

In 1964, De Carolis described imipramine responses in 264 depressed patients, reporting an improvement rate of 47 percent in those with "manic-depressive psychosis" (bipolar) compared with 61 percent for those with "endogenous monopolar depression" (unipolar). The statistical significance of this difference could not be evaluated because only 15 patients were in the manic-depressive group.

Upon reanalysis, two of the studies reviewed by Bielski and Friedel shed light on this problem. Deykin and DiMascio (1972), studying the relationship between pretreatment background characteristics and response to amitriptyline in 163 depressed women, noted that "the absence of manic behavior was related to good drug response" (p. 214). No statistical comparisons were given, however. In a related study, Wittenborn and colleagues (1973) investigated the relationship between pretreatment symptoms and personality variables in response to amitriptyline or imipramine in 157 women hospitalized for depression. They reported that "six of the 10 criteria indicate that patients who have had a history of schizophrenia, or manic episodes . . . tend to be among those whose response is relatively poor" (p. 105). Unfortunately, no diagnostic criteria or statistical analyses were given. In the Deykin and DiMascio study (1972), a significant relationship ($p < 0.02$) was noted between a past history of multiple episodes and a poor response to tricyclic antidepressants. Wittenborn and colleagues (1973) reported a similar finding but did not evaluate their findings statistically. In their analysis of 76 inpatients with major depressive illness who were refractory to amitriptyline, Kupfer and Spiker (1981) identified bipolarity as a significant predictor of poor tricyclic response.

In summary, the controlled studies suggest that bipolar depressed patients (and perhaps also the more cyclic unipolar patients) may be less likely to show an acute response to tricyclics than patients with unipolar major depression, although this difference may not be true for patients with more severe depressions. Systematic studies of both polarity and cyclicity as predictors of tricyclic response are needed, but they would be difficult because of the widespread use of lithium prophylaxis. The very important related question of the effects of long-term tricyclic administration on the course of bipolar affective illness is discussed later in this chapter.

Monoamine Oxidase Inhibitors

Very few formal clinical investigations have been done of the efficacy of MAOIs for bipolar depression. Major reviews of the antidepressant efficacy of MAOIs (Quitkin et al., 1979; Pare, 1985; White and Simpson, 1985) do not contain sufficient information to estimate response rates among bipolar patients with depression. Quitkin's review of the placebo-controlled trials of phenelzine in endogenous depression is of interest in that two of the three studies reporting significant antidepressant effects of the MAOI specifically focused on "recurrent depression," whereas four negative studies and one positive study did not. Himmelhoch and co-workers (1972) reported an open study of 21 patients with "bipolar characteristics" who were on lithium and had not responded to tricyclics, either at that time or during previous trials. (Their reanalysis revealed that 13 were actually bipolar and 8 had recurrent depressions characterized by low energy and hypersomnia.) Sixteen of these 21 patients had an "excellent" response to the addition of the MAOI tranylcypromine. Quitkin and colleagues (1981a) reported an open trial of phenelzine in five bipolar patients who failed to respond to a tricyclic. Four of the five showed a "clear antidepressant response." These investigators also reported anecdotally that of the 40 bipolar depressed patients they treated in a 2-year period, approximately 75 percent appeared to respond adequately to tricyclic antidepressants (often given in addition to lithium). Like Himmelhoch and colleagues, they found that most bipolar patients who did not respond to a tricyclic did respond to an MAOI.

Himmelhoch and colleagues (1982) randomly assigned 59 anergic depressed outpatients (29 bipolar, 11 "pseudounipolar") to either tranylcypromine or placebo. They found "marked and rapid" improvement in the MAOI group, which was significantly better than in the placebo group—71 percent vs. 13 percent ($p < 0.001$). Following further tranylcypromine trials (Mallinger et al., 1986), this same group (Thase et al., 1988) compared tranylcypromine and imipramine in a randomized, double-blind trial (without lithium) in 49 anergic depressed bipolar patients (21 bipolar I, 28 bipolar II) who did not have rapid cycles. Of the 25 patients in the MAOI group, 84 percent were significantly improved after 6 weeks compared with only 46 percent of the 24 imipramine-treated patients ($p < 0.007$). Although both drugs were associated with similar rates of hypomania, seven of the imipramine-treated patients experienced a psychotic dysphoric mania necessitating discontinuation of the drug, and only one of the MAOI-treated patients failed to complete the trial.[20]

Unfortunately, the recent controlled studies of MAOIs in the acute treatment of depression, usually atypical depression, either have excluded bipolar patients or have not described the polarity of their sample.[21] Atypical depression, a subtype of unipolar depression, shares many clinical features with bipolar depression, such as hypersomnia, hyperphagia, profound psychomotor retardation, and a greater tendency to recur, but the relationship has not been formally explored.

Lithium

As noted earlier, Cade and the other pioneers in the use of lithium failed to demonstrate antidepressant effects. Three open trials during this period noted acute antidepressant properties, however. In 1969, Goodwin and colleagues reported the first placebo-controlled study that clearly demonstrated unequivocal antidepressant effects of lithium in bipolar compared with unipolar patients. The antidepressant response often did not become evident until the third or fourth week on the drug. Thus, the negative results from the earlier studies may have been due to their shorter periods of observation. By the time these studies were done, the conceptual models of affective illness had begun to evolve beyond the original too little/too much formulations. The in-

tellectual climate had slowly evolved to the point where investigators could entertain the possibility that a single drug could have both antidepressant and antimanic effects.

Later, this group replicated its earlier finding in a larger study involving 52 hospitalized depressed patients (Goodwin et al., 1972). Of the 40 bipolar patients, 32 showed complete or partial antidepressant responses (and more than one third relapsed when a placebo was substituted for lithium). Among the 12 unipolar patients, only 4 responded. The bipolar–unipolar difference was significant ($p < 0.02$). Similar bipolar–unipolar differences were later reported by other groups (Noyes et al., 1974; Mendels, 1975; Baron et al., 1975).

Table 22-1 outlines the placebo-controlled studies of lithium as an antidepressant; six confirm significant antidepressant effects. The one that does not (Stokes et al., 1971) is difficult to interpret because lithium was administered for only 10 days. Virtually all of the positive studies involved evaluation periods that lasted into the fourth and fifth week, beyond the period when antidepressants generally are evaluated. From these studies, one can calculate an overall response rate (complete and partial) of 79 percent for the bipolar patients, compared with 36 percent for the unipolar patients.[22]

Lithium vs Tricyclics

Five controlled studies have directly compared lithium and tricyclics as antidepressants. Most involved both bipolar and unipolar patients (Table 22-2). In the initial report by Fieve and coworkers (1968), imipramine was superior to lithium, whereas all of the subsequent studies either found lithium equivalent to tricyclics (Mendels et al., 1972; Watanabe et al., 1975; Khan, 1981) or superior to them (Worrall et al., 1979). Unfortunately, these studies did not consider the possibility of differential response in bipolar or unipolar patients.

Lithium Potentiation of Tricyclics or MAOIs

The literature on the interaction of lithium with tricyclics or MAOIs does not focus on bipolar depressed patients, but it may nonetheless be relevant to bipolar illness. We reviewed 12 studies of treatment combining lithium and antidepres-

Table 22-1. Lithium Treatment in Patients Hospitalized for Depression:
Placebo-Controlled Studies

Study	N	Patient Characteristics	Results
Goodwin et al., 1969	18	13 BP depression 5 "non-cyclic depression"	10 of 13 BPs showed some response; only 2 of 5 "non-cyclic" depressives did
Stokes et al., 1971	18	Manic-depressive	Lithium trial lasted only 10 days, showing a nonsignificant trend toward response
Goodwin et al., 1972	52	Primary affective disorder 40 BP (I or II), 12 UP	32 of 40 BPs responded vs 4 of 12 UPs ($p < 0.05$)
Noyes et al., 1974	22	Manic-depressive, depressed with "endogenous features"	6 of 6 BPs responded vs 7 of 16 UPs ($p < 0.05$)
G. Johnson, 1974	10	Endogenous depression with recurrent histories	5 showed "marked improvement"
Baron et al., 1975	23	Primary affective disorder (Feighner criteria) 9 BP (I & II), 14 UP	7 of 9 BPs responded vs 3 of 14 UPs ($p < 0.05$)
Mendels, 1975	21	Primary affective disorder 13 BP, 8 UP	9 of 13 responded vs 4 of 8 UP (6 of 7 unequivocal responses in BP group)
Totals	164	Response Rate (Complete & Partial)	BP 64/81 = 79% UP 20/55 = 36%

Table 22-2. Lithium Treatment of Patients Hospitalized for Depression:
Double-Blind Comparisons with Tricyclics

Study	Patients N	Design	Results
Fieve et al., 1968	21 BP	Imipramine comparison	Significantly more improvement on imipramine; lithium had "mild" antidepressant effects
Mendels et al., 1972a	12 BP & UP	Desipramine comparison	Lithium as effective as desipramine
Watanabe et al., 1975	45 Mixed	Imipramine comparison	Lithium as effective as imipramine
Worrall et al., 1979	29 BP & UP	Imipramine comparison with elimination of initial placebo responders	All 14 patients on lithium improved but not until 2nd week; patients on imipramine who improved did so during 1st week; response was significantly more uniform on lithium
Khan, 1981	30 Recurrent UP	Amitriptyline comparison	Lithium as effective as amitriptyline
Total N	137	Conclusion: 4 of 5 studies find lithium at least equivalent to the tricyclic	

sant therapy (tricyclics or MAOIs) that employed open as well as double-blind designs (Table 22-3).[23] All but 3 added lithium to an antidepressant regimen that had failed to produce a response in patients after at least 3 weeks. Taken together, these studies support the notion that lithium acts synergistically with tricyclics or MAOIs. The synergism is most clear when lithium is given to patients who are already established on a regimen of tricyclics or MAOIs. Of those who had not responded to the antidepressants, half responded when lithium was added. Response latency varied considerably, averaging about 10 days. L. Cohen and colleagues (1988) note that half of

Table 22-3. Effects of Lithium Combined With Antidepressant Drugs in Treatment-Resistant Depression

Study	Patients N	Design	Results
Antidepressant added to or coadministered with lithium			
Himmelhoch et al., 1972	13 BP 8 UP	Open trial of tranylcypromine added to LI	11 of 21 remitted and 5 others improved substantially
Lingjaerde et al., 1974	45[a]	Double-blind, multihospital study of TCA treatment augmented by LI or placebo. HDR and global improvement assessment	At 4 wk, HDR scores of LI + TCA group significantly improved vs TCA group. Marked global improvement in 82% of LI group, in 57% of TCA group ($p = .04$)
L.H.Price et al., 1985	2 BP[b] 10 UP[b]	Open; tranylcypromine added to LI	92% responded
Lithium added to antidepressants			
DeMontigny et al., 1981	8 UP	Open; HDR 48 hr after LI addition	100% improved within 48 hr
DeMontigny et al., 1983	34 UP	Open trial of LI added to blind TCA; HDR 48 hr after LI addition	Improvement (>50% drop) in 74% of 42 observations (8 patients had 2 LI trials on 2 different TCAs)
Heninger et al., 1983	1 BP 14 UP	Double-blind LI or placebo added to heterocyclic antidepressant; HDR	LI group significantly improved vs placebo group, which subsequently had similar response to LI; 33% responded within 48 hr; average time to response was 12 days
Louie & Meltzer, 1984	2 BP 7 UP	Open; case method	Both BPs switched into mania; 2 UPs sustained responses; 2 transient; 3 did not respond
DeMontigny et al., 1985	7 UP	Open trial; LI added to iprindole; HDR 48 hr after LI addition	Improvement (>50% drop) in 86%; all patients reported alleviated symptoms
L.H. Price et al., 1985	22 BP & UP	Open; LI added to bupropion in 6 patients; TCA in 5, and adinazolam in 11	45% responded
Kantor et al., 1986	7 UP	Double-blind LI or placebo added to TCA; HDR after 48 hr Response defined as at least 50% drop in HDR	Improvement (transient) in 25% of patients given LI, in none of the placebo patients
Nelson & Mazure, 1986	9 BP 12 UP	Retrospective study of LI added to TCA + neuroleptic; assessment by CGIS	89% of BPs responded to LI augmentation; only 25% of UPs responded
L.S. Cohen et al., 1988	74 UP	Open; LI added to imipramine; assessment by CGIS	67% ultimately improved (majority were markedly improved); 47% responded within 1 wk

All patients were nonresponders to at least 3 weeks of antidepressant treatment, lithium treatment, or combination of both, except Lingjaerde et al., Himmelhoch et al., and Price et al.

LI = lithium, TCA = tricyclic antidepressant, HDR = Hamilton Rating Scale, CGIS = Clinical Global Improvement Scale

[a]"Endogenous depressives"; 13 in one hospital, 32 in 8 others
[b]These 12 patients were those who had not responded to the addition of LI to TCA

their patients who responded did so within the first 3 days. The design employed in the study by Heninger and colleagues (1983) supports the conclusion that the potentiation is not simply due to longer treatment time in the combined group. Although some bipolar patients are included in these studies, lithium potentiation clearly occurs in unipolar patients as well. Whether this effect is more likely to occur among patients with recurrent episodes is not yet clear.

A retrospective analysis showed that the bipolar patients were considerably more responsive than the unipolar patients to lithium potentiation (Nelson and Mazure, 1986). Further, in the study by Louie and Meltzer (1984), two of the nine patients were bipolar, and both switched into mania following lithium potentiation, an observation also made by Price and associates (1984) in two case reports.

Price and colleagues (1985) showed that a large percentage of patients previously unresponsive to a combination of tricyclic and lithium did respond to an MAOI–lithium combination. This observation is consistent with the previously noted clinical observation that nonresponse to tricyclics may predict response to MAOIs, and vice versa.

Second-Generation Antidepressants

The second-generation heterocyclic antidepressants are modifications of the already well-established tricyclics (these agents are listed in Table 22-4). Drugs in this basic class of compounds continue to come to clinical trials, and many are already marketed in some countries. Other classes of drugs reported to have antidepressant properties are discussed later under the heading Experimental Drugs for Depression.

Maprotiline, amoxapine, and *trazodone* have been widely available longer than the other second-generation antidepressants. Studies indicate that as antidepressants they are probably as effective as their predecessors, although recent reviewers dispute claims of a faster onset of action and of reduced side effects. In fact, these drugs may not have an advantage over standard tricyclic drugs, as suggested by the proven neuroleptic activity of amoxapine and possible associated tardive dyskinesia, the propensity for maprotiline to cause seizures, the rare occurrence of priapism with trazodone, and the withdrawal

of nomifensine because of relatively rare but nevertheless severe autoimmune hemolytic anemia.[24]

In contrast, *bupropion* may offer special advantages to bipolar patients with depression. It is especially effective in improving the psychomotor retardation so characteristic of these patients (Fabre et al., 1983), perhaps related to its dopamine agonist properties. It has also been reported to be useful in bipolar patients who are intolerant of other antidepressants (Gardner, 1983), and it may be less likely than other antidepressants to precipitate manic episodes (Gardner, 1983; Shopsin, 1983). Two antidepressant side effects frequently associated with poor compliance—weight gain and decreased sexual function—do not appear to occur with bupropion (Bryant et al., 1983), at least when it is administered alone. As discussed in Chapter 23, this advantage may be especially important for patients also on lithium. Two adverse effects have been reported when the drug is used in doses that are higher than recommended: seizures (Peck et al., 1983; Leber, 1985) and the appearance of psychotic symptoms (Golden et al., 1985, 1988). Another drug with dopamine agonist properties is the dopamine reuptake inhibitor amineptine, now on the market in Europe. To our knowledge, it has not been evaluated in bipolar depression.

The bicyclic antidepressant *fluoxetine,* a serotonin-reuptake inhibitor, has rapidly become widely used and may have a special place in the treatment of bipolar patients. Data from 89 bipolar depressed patients treated for 6 weeks indicate an impressive response rate, 86 percent, compared with 57 percent for those on imipramine (Benfield et al., 1986). Fluoxetine has few if any anticholinergic effects and is not associated with weight gain. Like bupropion, it may be especially useful in patients also on lithium because it does not contribute to compliance problems secondary to additive side effects. It has been suggested that serotonergic antidepressants may be less likely to precipitate mania. Although no such reactions have been reported from the controlled trials (reviewed by Benfield et al., 1986), a few case reports of mania in patients taking fluoxetine have appeared, two involving overdoses.[25] Rickels and colleagues (1985) noted that 3 of 84 unipolar patients treated with fluoxetine for 11 months became manic. Whether this risk is lower than that

Table 22-4. Second-Generation Heterocyclic Antidepressants

On U.S. Market	Marketed Elsewhere	In Clinical Trials
Alprazolam	Amineptine	Adinazolam
Amoxapine	Butriptyline	Alaproclate
Bupropion	Ciclazindol	Citalopram
Fluoxetine	Clomipramine	Clovoxamine
Maprotiline	(Chlorimipramine)	Etoperidone
Trazodone	Dibenzepin	Femoxetine
Trimipramine	Dimet(h)acrine	Fezolamine
	Dothiepin	Idazoxin
	(Dosulepin)	Nefazadone
	Fluvoxamine	Paroxetine
	Iprindole	Pirlindole
	Lofepramine	Salbutamol[a]
	(Clofepramine)	(Albuterol)
	Melitracen	Sertraline
	Mianserin	Tomoxetine
	Noxiptyline	
	Opipramol	
	Viloxazine	

[a] Marketed for other than antidepressant use

associated with other antidepressants remains to be seen. Sertraline and citalopram, both selective serotonin-reuptake inhibitors in vitro, are under development as antidepressants (Lemberger et al., 1985; Dufour et al., 1987). The clinical data to date indicate a low level of anticholinergic and cardiovascular side effects with all three of these serotonergic compounds.

Precipitation of Mania or Hypomania by Antidepressants

Perhaps the most important issue in the prudent clinical management of bipolar depression is the phenomenon of manic reactions to antidepressants. As noted earlier, the initial report of hypomanic-like and manic-like reactions to iproniazid, an antitubercular drug that is also an MAOI, launched the era of antidepressant drug development (Crane, 1956), and manic reactions were noted in one of the earliest studies of the antidepressant effects of imipramine (Ball and Kiloh, 1959). In 1972, Bunney and co-workers, reviewing the largely unsystematic literature on mania following the administration of tricyclic antidepressants and MAOIs, estimated its incidence at about 10 percent for both classes of antidepressants. The manic switches often occurred within a week of initiating treatment. Among the 67 patients who switched and on whom past data

were available, 60 percent had a history of mania, at least three times the expected prevalence of bipolarity among depressed patients. This observation suggests that bipolar-I patients are especially vulnerable to the mania-inducing effect of antidepressants. De la Fuente and colleagues (1986) reported that of 15 patients treated with a combination of amitriptyline and isocarboxazid for refractory depression, the 3 bipolar-I patients but none of the 12 unipolar patients developed manic episodes.

The more systematic studies of bipolar patients bear this out (Table 22-5). In a collaborative study at the Veterans' Administration (VA) and NIMH, Prien and colleagues (1973) compared maintenance lithium with maintenance imipramine in unipolar and bipolar-I patients. They noted that 67 percent of bipolar patients on imipramine had manic episodes, twice the spontaneous rate seen in the placebo group. A subsequent large-scale multicenter study of bipolar-I patients (Prien et al., 1984) compared maintenance treatment using lithium, imipramine, or a combination of the two, but without using a separate placebo group. In that study, mania occurred roughly twice as often in patients treated with imipramine (53 percent) as in those treated with lithium or a combination of the two drugs. Akiskal and associates (1979), in a retrospective

Table 22-5. Manic/Hypomanic Episodes in Bipolar Patients on Tricyclic Antidepressants

Study	Patients N	% with M/HM	Comments
Prien et al., 1973b	9 BPI	67	Does not include those who relapsed during the first 4 months
Akiskal et al., 1977	40 BPI	35	Hypomanic
	25 Cyclothymia	44	Hypomanic
Akiskal et al., 1979b	18 BPI & II	50	Hypomania; episodes determined from retrospective chart review
Wehr & Goodwin, 1979	26 BPI & II	70	Half of the episodes were manic, half hypomanic; average time to mania = 21 days; average time to hypomania = 35 days
Quitkin et al., 1981a	37 BPI	24	Patients on imipramine *plus lithium*
Pickar et al., 1984a	20 BPI & II	30	4 of 13 BPI patients had manic episodes, 2 of 7 BPII patients had hypomanic episodes
Prien et al., 1984	36 BPI	53	Patients on imipramine alone
	36 BPI	28	Patients on imipramine *plus lithium*
Himmelhoch et al., 1986	19 BPI	37	Similar incidence of switches as in patients given tranylcypromine, but qualitatively different; 3 of 7 manic patients required hospitalization
Kupfer et al., 1988a	33 BPII	3	The outpatient study incidence of hypomanic reactions was low in both the UP and BPII groups and was not different. Very strict criteria for hypomania were required

study, reported that one half of their patients with bipolar-I and bipolar-II disorders had hypomanic reactions during antidepressant treatment. These investigators noted parenthetically that the hypomanic syndrome was often misidentified in the charts by such nondescriptive designations as "hysterical acting out" or "flight into health." In a prospective follow-up study of patients with cyclothymia, Akiskal and colleagues (1977) reported that 44 percent developed clear hypomania in the course of treatment with TCAs.

Using daily nurses' ratings under double-blind conditions, Wehr and Goodwin (1979) conducted an intensive longitudinal investigation of a group of 26 bipolar patients (I and II) whose treatment included periods of TCAs. Of the 19 patients who responded to medication, 18 showed manic or hypomanic reactions while on tricyclics (Figure 22-2). Bipolar-I patients had either manic or hypomanic episodes, and the bipolar-II patients experienced only hypomanic episodes. The onset of manic episodes occurred, on average, 21 days after treatment began, whereas the average time of onset of hypomania was longer, 35 days. Similarly, Himmelhoch (personal communication, 1986) observed that in his experience of treating depressed bipolar-I patients with imipramine, more have become manic than have become well. On the other hand, in a careful 5-month prospective study of 24 bipolar-II patients undergoing treatment with imipramine, only one hypomanic episode was registered by strict criteria (mania rating at the time of the follow-up visit and a confirmatory progress note at the same visit) (Kupfer et al., 1988).

The few available prospective studies of bipo-

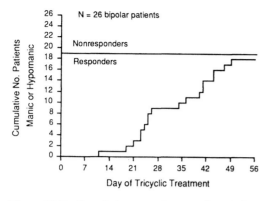

Figure 22-2. Cumulative sum of onsets of mania ($n = 8$) and hypomania ($n = 10$) in 26 depressed bipolar patients treated with tricyclic antidepressants. With few exceptions, manic responses occurred earlier in the course of treatment than hypomanic ones (data from Wehr and Goodwin, 1987a).

lar depressed patients treated with MAOIs appear to indicate a high rate of manic switches—50 percent in a study by Murphy and colleagues (1975), 41 percent in the Himmelhoch study, and 35 percent in a report by Pickar and co-workers (1984). In two of these studies, all of the patients who responded became manic or hypomanic. With MAOIs, the switch seems more likely to be hypomanic, even in bipolar-I patients.

The extent to which the natural course of the illness may contribute to the occurrence of switches on antidepressants needs to be considered (Lewis and Winokur, 1982). For those studies with random assignment to a comparison drug (e.g., the two Prien studies), spontaneous switching cannot be invoked. Patients in the longitudinal study of Wehr and Goodwin were four times as likely to switch into mania when on tricyclics than when they were not. (We return to this question later when we discuss the retrospective study of Lewis and Winokur.) Bipolar patients whose natural course is characterized by the DMI sequence (depression switching directly into a mania or hypomania, followed by a well interval) are apparently more prone to antidepressant-induced switches than are those with the MDI sequence (Kukopulos et al., 1980)

Some investigators suggest that maintenance lithium protects bipolar patients from antidepressant-induced switches, but the results of a 3-year prospective study by Quitkin and co-workers (1981a) indicate that it may not do so

completely (Table 22-6). Seventy-five bipolar-I patients were randomly assigned to maintenance lithium plus placebo (38 patients) and lithium plus imipramine (37 patients), and 24.3 percent of the lithium plus imipramine treatment group experienced manic relapses, compared with only 10.5 percent of the lithium plus placebo group. Women were by far more vulnerable to manic relapses on imipramine, 32 percent compared with 6 percent for the lithium-alone group ($p < 0.05$). The antidepressant did not provide additional protection against depressive relapses, which were, in any case, low in both treatment groups. Since lithium levels did not differ in the two treatment groups, that factor cannot explain the 2.5-fold higher switch rate with combined treatment. The Quitkin group did not consider whether higher lithium levels would have protected the combined treatment group. Jann and colleagues (1982) reported an association between lower lithium levels and increased switching in a group of patients who were also on tricyclics.

There are now several case reports of hypomanic and manic reactions to the addition of lithium to antidepressants (Louie and Meltzer, 1984; Price et al., 1984). Mania following thyroid hormone potentiation of antidepressants has been noted (Evans et al., 1986). Several reports indicate that newer antidepressant treatments, such as trazodone (Warren and Bick, 1984), fluoxetine (Lebegue, 1987), and alprazolam (Arana et al., 1985), can also be associated with hypomania or mania.

Nasrallah and co-workers (1982) found that patients who switch into mania while on tricyclics are likely to be younger than those who do not and to have an earlier onset of illness, higher frequency of hospitalization, and a history of psychiatric illness other than alcoholism among first-degree relatives. On the other hand, age and frequency of episodes were not associated with hypomanic episodes in Kupfer's bipolar-II population.

Angst's 1985 (see also Angst, 1987) analysis of admission records at the Burghölzli Psychiatric Hospital in Zurich, Switzerland, sampled over the six decades from 1920 to 1982, sheds light on the issue of drug-induced mania.[26] His data show that among bipolar and unipolar patients the number of switches into mania and hypomania after admission for an index episode of depression was

Table 22-6. Depressive and Manic Relapses in Bipolar Patients
on Maintenance Medication: A Three-Year Prospective Study

Outcome	Lithium (N = 38)		Lithium + Imipramine (N = 37)		All Patients (N = 75)
	%	Months[a]	%	Months	%
Total Relapses (N = 20)	21		32		27
Depressive Relapses (N = 7)	10	11	8	3	9
Manic Relapses (N = 13)	10	7	24	10	17

65% of all relapses occurred within first 4 months (5 of 7 depressive, 8 of 13 manic)

[a]Months are average time to relapse

Data from Quitkin et al., 1981a

low during the era preceding somatic treatment (1920–1939), and it doubled during the era of electroconvulsive therapy (1940–1949). During the neuroleptic era (1953–1957), it decreased again to levels comparable to the presomatic treatment era, only to increase again in the tricyclic era (1958–1981) (see Figure 23-3).

Despite the apparent agreement between the case report literature and the systematic studies reviewed, some investigators doubt that antidepressants induce mania. Lewis and Winokur (1982) opened the debate when they did not find such a response in bipolar patients receiving acute and continuation treatment with antidepressants chosen by the physician (Table 22-7). In their uncontrolled, retrospective review of hospital charts, they found that bipolar patients who received TCAs switched into mania at a rate not

significantly different from that of unmedicated patients (25 and 41 percent, respectively). The validity of this finding is quite doubtful, however, in view of the very high switch rate among the controls and the variety of uncontrolled factors that could lead to such a higher rate among patients whose physicians chose not to administer antidepressants.[27] The negative conclusion from this study was reinforced by Angst who, when analyzing his data on admission patterns from 1920 to 1982, inexplicably combined the ECT era data (with its expected high switch rates) with the data from the presomatic treatment era and concluded that switch rates did not increase after the introduction of tricyclics.

The current controversy over tricyclic-induced mania was also abetted by ambiguities in the NIMH collaborative study of maintenance drug

Figure 22-3. Switch rates as a function of prevailing treatments for depression (adapted from Angst, 1985).

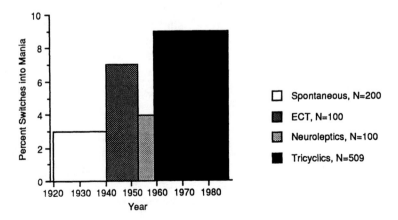

Table 22-7. The Lewis and Winokur Study (1982): The Induction of
Mania: A Natural History Study with Controls

Findings: Incidence of switches into mania in BP patients

Group	Male	Female	Number (%) Switches	
Tricyclic-treated	6	2	2	(25)
No treatment	12	15	11	(41)

Problems with study

1. Small number of subjects

2. Retrospective chart review; patients not randomly assigned to groups
    Women were twice as likely to switch as men, but unfortunately in this study the ratio
    of women to men was twice as high in the control group as in the treated group

3. The majority (55%) of control patients who switched were *not* depressed on
    admission and had other diagnoses that could indicate misdiagnosed impending
    mania (personality disorder 27%) or pharmacological (9%) or organic (9%) factors
    predisposing to mania

4. The remainder (45%) of control patients were depressed but *not* treated. Why not?
    For example, were they beginning to switch before a treatment decision would have
    been made (a selection bias)?

Adapted from Wehr & Goodwin, 1987a

treatment (Prien et al., 1984). Because no placebo controls were included, Prien's group was unable to determine the extent to which mania was induced by imipramine or dampened by lithium. Generalizing from the results of their 1973 VA–NIMH study, which had included a placebo group, Prien and colleagues speculated in the 1984 article that the incidence of mania recorded in the collaborative study reflected the natural switch into mania expected with bipolar-I illness rather than an induction caused by imipramine. A careful analysis of these two studies does not support this conclusion.[28]

Antidepressant Induction of Rapid Cycles

Closely related to the issues just reviewed is the question of the long-term impact of antidepressants on the course of the illness. Although maintenance treatment of bipolar illness is the subject of Chapter 23, we discuss here the effect of antidepressants on the long-term course of the illness, since this is a key consideration in planning the acute treatment of bipolar depression. We consider a phenomenon that is the virtual opposite of prophylaxis: the apparent capacity of antidepressant drugs, in some patients, to accelerate the underlying cyclic process of the illness. In patients with an inherently cyclic illness, both the

onset and recovery from a depressive or manic episode can be viewed as part of the underlying cyclic process. Some treatments that accelerate recovery, if continued too long, may also accelerate the onset of the next episode.

As far back as 1965, the German literature reported that antidepressants may increase the frequency of recurrences after the acute treatment of a depressive episode (Arnold and Kryspin-Exner, 1965; Till and Vuckovic, 1970), sometimes transforming the illness from an episodic course with free intervals to a chronic course with continuous illness (*Chronifizierung*). In some of the case studies, the drugs, rather than producing a true remission, appeared to create a fragile equilibrium near the threshold of depression, where relapses and remissions reflect changes in drug dose. In other cases, the drugs produced a destabilization (*Labilizierung*) in which, for the first time, hypomania was followed by continual cycling between hypomania and depression.

In fact, as noted earlier, the first report of a psychoactive effect of the MAOI iproniazid (which led to the development of the first antidepressants) was of drug-induced rapid cycling between hypomania and depression (Crane, 1956). Today, reports of rapid cycling induced by the continuous (or perhaps even intermittent) administration of antidepressants still appear (Wehr and Goodwin, 1987, 1988). Most of these reports are based on nonblind, uncontrolled studies that relied on observations that were partly or wholly retrospective (Table 22-8). To date, the only prospective, double-blind studies are those of Wehr and Goodwin (1979) and Wehr and colleagues (1988), in which patients served as their own controls. These studies show that tricyclic and MAOI antidepressants could induce rapid cycling between mania and depression in certain bipolar patients. In about one half of 51 patients who had rapid-cycling bipolar illness, the continuation of the rapid cycling appeared to depend on the continued administration of antidepressants. Figure 22-4 illustrates the impact of tricyclics on the cycle length in ten bipolar patients by comparing periods of time on and off the antidepressant while on lithium continuously.

The tricyclic-induced acceleration affected not only the next manic or hypomanic phase but also the next depressive phase, as is seen in the case illustrated in Figure 22-5. Shortly after desipramine treatment began, the patient recovered rapidly from a depressive episode, which before

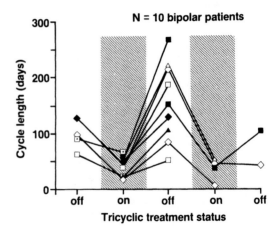

Figure 22-4. Shortening of manic-depressive cycle length (onset of mania to onset of mania) by tricyclic antidepressants in 10 rapid-cycling bipolar patients whose switches from mania to depression and depression to mania were recorded prospectively (adapted from Wehr and Goodwin, 1987a).

this treatment had lasted 2.5 months. However, another depression occurred within two weeks of initiating the tricyclic. During the course of tricyclic treatment, the patient experienced three separate depressive episodes, each lasting about

Table 22-8. Induction of Rapid Cycling by Antidepressants

Study	Patients N (% of total sample)	Cycling %[b]	Drug
Crane, 1956	1		MAOI
Arnold & Kryspin-Exner, 1965	1		Tricyclic
Till and Vuckovic, 1970	7	27	Tricyclic
Coppen et al., 1972a	2	67	Tricyclic
Van Scheyen, 1973	2	2	Tricyclic
Wehr & Goodwin, 1977, 1979	6		Tricyclic, MAOI
Siris et al., 1979	1		Tricyclic
Kukopulos et al., 1980	59	51	Tricyclic, MAOI
Lerer et al., 1980	1		Tricyclic
Ko et al., 1981	1		L-Dopa
Mattsson & Seltzer, 1981	1		MAOI
Extein et al., 1982	1		Tricyclic
Oppenheim, 1982	1		Tricyclic
Wehr et al., 1988	26[a]	51	Tricyclic
Post et al., unpublished data	35	34	Tricyclic
Total	145		

[a]Cumulative total
[b]Where no percent is given, the study involved case report(s)

Adapted from Wehr & Goodwin, 1987a

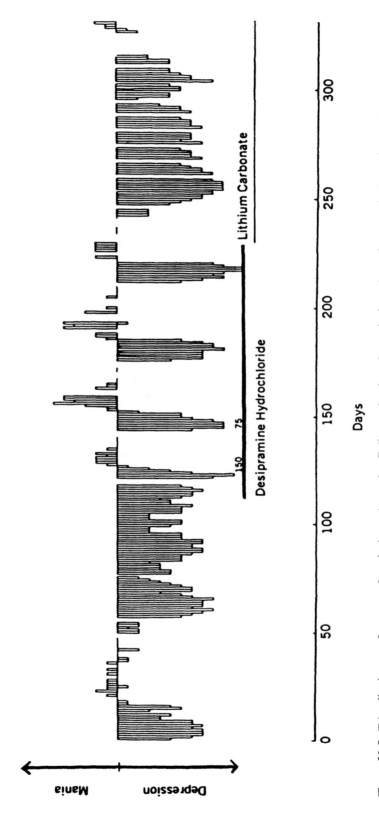

Figure 22-5. Tricyclics increase frequency of manic-depressive cycles. Daily mood ratings for a single patient whose manic-depressive cycling was accelerated by maintenance therapy with desipramine. Desipramine dose indicated above line; lithium carbonate dose was 750 mg. After a brief postrecovery hypomania on lithium, the patient went on to experience continuous mood stability on maintenance lithium, now 3 years in duration (from Wehr and Goodwin, 1979).

649

10 to 12 days. On day 225, a change from desipramine to lithium was associated with a more gradual, but stable, antidepressant response.

Consistent with this study are the nonblind observations of Kukopulos and co-workers (1980), who followed 434 bipolar patients (48 percent bipolar I, 52 percent bipolar II) for an average of 18 years (direct observation averaged 4.5 years, retrospective observation, 13.4 years). In 115 patients, especially the women, the illness changed during the course of observation into a "continuous circular course" unrelieved by a free interval between the depressive and the manic or hypomanic episodes. Fifty-nine of these patients (51 percent) had received nonpharmacological treatments (ECT, psychotherapy) for their several depressive episodes, but the continuous course did not develop until at least one episode had been treated with antidepressants. The investigators concluded that antidepressants probably had precipitated development of a continuous course in this subgroup of patients, 40 of whom developed rapid cycles. The rapid-cycling patients did not respond to prophylactic lithium as long as they were also taking antidepressants, but they improved once the antidepressants were withdrawn. This change suggests that the antidepressant drugs induced resistance to prophylactic lithium. In a later retrospective study of patients with rapid cycles, Kukopulos and colleagues (1983) noted that 32 exhibited the pattern from the outset of the illness. Rapid cycling developed in 86 later in the course, and the change coincided with antidepressant treatment in at least 52. Among these patients, the average number of episodes before treatment was 0.8 per year, a number that increased to 6.5 when they were taking antidepressants. In the majority of these apparently antidepressant-related continuous cycles from the 1980 study, the drugs were given only during the actual depressions. Prospective controlled data on the potential impact of intermittent antidepressants on the course of bipolar illness unfortunately are not available.

A mechanism by which intermittent antidepressants might alter the course of the illness is suggested by the work of Pickar and colleagues (1984), who found that bipolar-I patients who had experienced a manic episode after they began taking an MAOI invariably became manic earlier when they took an MAOI for a subsequent depression. This finding suggests that the initial exposure left the patient more sensitive to subsequent exposure; that is, sensitization may have occurred. It cannot be determined, however, whether the patient is sensitized to the antidepressant or is demonstrating the greater vulnerability to subsequent episodes that follows the manic episode itself (mania sensitizing to further mania).

Which bipolar patients are at greatest risk for antidepressant-induced switches or acceleration of the cycle? As noted, there is some evidence that women have a higher risk than men, and a history of mania proneness (Quitkin et al., 1981b, 1986) or a relatively more cyclic history also may be predictive. Akiskal (1980) and Kukopulos and associates (1980) proposed that bipolar patients with premorbid cyclothymic temperaments (in effect, a continuous low-amplitude cycle) are prone to develop mania or rapid cycling, but as yet no systematic prospective study has been done. Bipolar-II patients may have a lower risk of antidepressant-related acceleration than have bipolar-I patients (Kupfer et al., 1988). Certainly the risk of manic episodes on antidepressant drugs seems largely confined to bipolar-I patients.

An association has been proposed among female gender, hypothyroidism, and drug-induced rapid cycling (Cowdry et al., 1983; Cho et al., 1979). Although findings are equivocal and prospective studies are needed, these potential risk factors are of both practical and theoretical significance. Cowdry and associates (1983), studying patients who had taken lithium for at least 3 months, found overt hypothyroidism in 50 percent of the 24 rapid-cycling patients (83 percent were female) but none of the 19 nonrapid-cycling patients (53 percent were female). Levels of thyroid-stimulating hormone (TSH), a measure of subclinical hypothyroidism, were elevated in 92 percent of the rapid-cycling group and 32 percent of those without rapid cycles. Joffe and colleagues (1988) analyzed the course of illness and thyroid function of 42 bipolar patients and do not replicate these findings. However, direct comparison of the two studies is difficult, since the sex ratio in the study by Joffe's group was reversed: only 41 percent of the rapid-cycling patients were female, compared with 80 percent of the those without rapid cycles.[29]

It is difficult to determine what proportion of bipolar patients on antidepressants develop drug-induced acceleration of the cycle because investigators seldom look for the phenomenon. Further, it cannot be observed if patients who exhibit the response are systematically excluded from studies and if antidepressants are stopped or observations cease as soon as patients become manic.

Descriptions of the clinical course of manic-depressive illness and interpretations of treatment response rarely take into account the possibility that antidepressants can accelerate the underlying cycle. When novel agents or procedures are reported to be effective in maintenance treatment, investigators usually attribute the cessation of frequent recurrences to the new treatment regimens, neglecting the possibility that withdrawal of antidepressants may have been at least partly responsible. Also, as noted in Chapter 6, some studies of the natural course of manic-depressive illness may have been contaminated by this effect of antidepressants.

Tricyclics may also affect the more recurrent forms of unipolar depression. Angst and co-workers (1969) and Van Scheyen (1973) observed an increased frequency of recurrences of unipolar depression among patients on TCAs, but this was not observed by Kupfer and colleagues (1988) in a large-scale prospective study employing very strict criteria for hypomania. As noted in previous chapters, the more recurrent forms of unipolar illness may be related to bipolar illness. The possibility that continuous antidepressants might shorten the cycle length in a subgroup of unipolar patients needs additional study, and that possibility may give new meaning to the prediction of poor response to tricyclics among patients with a history of mania or of recurrent episodes, whether unipolar or bipolar (Deykin and Di-Mascio, 1972; Wittenborn et al., 1973). In addition, these possible effects of antidepressant medications are consistent with the observation that lithium may be superior to imipramine in treating bipolar or unipolar depressed patients with a history of recurrent episodes (Goodwin et al., 1972; Worrall et al., 1979).

The precipitation of hypomanic or manic reactions during antidepressant withdrawal also has been reported.[30] This phenomenon may reflect destabilization in vulnerable individuals.

In summary, absolutely incontrovertible evidence of antidepressant-induced mania and cycle induction is still lacking, and prospective, randomized, double-blind studies are needed. The available evidence strongly suggests, however, that antidepressant drugs can precipitate mania in some bipolar-I patients, especially those who respond to antidepressants, and that some bipolar-II patients appear to be vulnerable to hypomania while taking antidepressants. Although antidepressant-induced rapid cycling does occur in some patients, its frequency is not easy to determine, and, therefore, the generalizability of this observation is unclear.

Experimental Drugs for Depression

In this section, we briefly review studies of experimental antidepressant drugs. Usually these studies did not focus on bipolar patients, since most were designed to explore particular biochemical hypotheses.

Triazolobenzodiazepines

A large, multicenter 1983 study by Feighner documenting the antidepressant effect of *alprazolam* in unipolar depressed patients was followed by a smaller nonblind study by Rush and co-workers (1984), which showed some antidepressant efficacy in five bipolar-I patients. A study by Lenox and colleagues (1984) failed to show antidepressant efficacy in severely depressed patients, however, and the present status of this drug in treating bipolar depressed patients is not clear. Another drug in this class, *adinazolam,* has shown antidepressant efficacy in patients with DSM-III major depression (Smith and Glaudin, 1986; Dunner et al., 1987); 31 percent of the sample in the Dunner study was bipolar II, and no mania or hypomania was noted during this 6-week, double-blind outpatient trial. The mechanism of action of these drugs may involve their effects on γ-aminobutyric acid (GABA) transmission.

Carbamazepine and Clonazepam

A double-blind, placebo-controlled study of 35 depressed patients (29 bipolar) showed that carbamazepine had at least modest antidepressant effects in 57 percent, including substantial effects in 34 percent (Post et al., 1986). Although this latter figure approximates the usual placebo response rate seen in standard studies, it may be more readily accepted because most patients were demonstrably resistant to conventional antidepressant treatments, and all were unaware of the timing of any changes in their medications. The carbamazepine nonresponders were randomly assigned to supplemental lithium or placebo under double-blind conditions, and 53 percent of the lithium plus carbamazepine patients showed a rapid-onset antidepressant response (Kramlinger and Post, 1989b). These findings are supported by two case reports (Schaffer et al., 1985; Nurnberg and Finkel, 1985). The latter demonstrated the efficacy of a lithium–carbamazepine combination in psychotic depression. The onset of the antidepressant effect of carbamazepine appears to be somewhat delayed and similar to that discussed earlier for lithium. Another anticonvulsant, clonazepam, has shown antidepressant effects in an open trial that included bipolar patients (Kishimoto et al., 1988).

Stimulants and Euphoriants

Several stimulant or euphoriant drugs have been the subject of antidepressant trials, including *amphetamine* (Jimerson et al., 1977; Satel and Nelson, 1989), *methylphenidate* (Janowsky et al., 1973), *cocaine* (Post et al., 1974), *morphine* (Extein et al., 1980), and *tetrahydrocannabinol* (Kotin et al., 1973b). All produced varying degrees of nonspecific activation in depressed patients, but so far none has produced a sustained, complete antidepressant effect in a significant proportion of patients. Psychostimulants may be most useful when given to depressed patients who are elderly (Kaplitz, 1975; Katon and Raskind, 1980) or medically ill (Kaufmann et al., 1982) or when used in combination with tricyclics (Drimmer et al., 1983; Feighner et al., 1985) or MAOIs (Feighner et al., 1985).

Renewed interest in morphine, which was used years ago to treat severely depressed patients, followed the discovery of the brain's endogenous opiate systems and their relationship to mood states (see Chapter 15). The NIMH group (Extein et al., 1981) conducted a trial of morphine and methadone in a group of predominantly bipolar patients and found only small, nonsignificant changes in global depression ratings, although the patients appeared less anxious. A preliminary antidepressant trial of FK-33824, a synthetic analog of enkephalin, the endogenous opiate receptor ligand, had little success (Extein et al., 1979). However, buprenorphine, an opiate agonist and antagonist, was reported to have antidepressant effects in a double-blind, placebo-controlled study of depressed patients (Emrich et al., 1982). Des-tyrosine-γ-endorphin, a peptide that is structurally related to endorphins but lacking in opiate activity, was given intramuscularly for 1 week to ten depressed patients in a double-blind placebo study, and it showed highly significant antidepressant activity (Chazot et al., 1985), although an earlier double-blind trial showed none (Fink et al., 1981). Naloxone, an opiate-receptor antagonist, had no effect on depressed mood in moderate doses (Terenius et al., 1977), but in high doses (2 mg/kg) it produced a noticeable worsening of depression (Cohen et al., 1984).

Amine Precursors and Related Agents

As noted in Chapter 17, the use of amino acid precursors of the biogenic amines in the 1970s was a major approach to evaluating the amine hypotheses of depression. L-Dopa, the amino acid precursor of the catecholamines, was evaluated as an antidepressant in several open studies done after Pare and Sandler's initial observation in 1959. In the first double-blind controlled study of this amino acid in depression (Goodwin et al., 1970), results were predominantly negative, but in the small group of responders (5 of 21), all had bipolar-II diagnoses. Similar findings were reported subsequently by Matussek (1971) and by Nähunek and co-workers (1972). In these three studies, the fact that L-dopa had its clearest effect on psychomotor retardation is of interest, since retardation is characteristic of bipolar depressed patients. In the 1970 study by Goodwin and colleagues, hypomania occurred in 55 percent of the bipolar patients after an average of 27 days of treatment. Ko and colleagues (1981) also noted induction of rapid mood cycles with L-dopa. *Tyrosine,* the amino acid precursor of L-dopa, was significantly more effective than placebo in moderately depressed patients of uncertain polarity (Gelenberg et al., 1982-3), whereas *phenylalanine,* tyrosine's precursor, was an effective antidepressant in two open trials, although the patients were primarily unipolar (Fischer et al., 1975; Beckmann et al., 1977).

L-*Tryptophan,* the amino acid precursor of serotonin, has been used with mixed results in ten controlled trials involving 170 depressed patients. Unfortunately, most of the studies that showed positive effects did not distinguish between bipolar and unipolar patients (see, for example, Coppen et al., 1972a). Although the positive results are of considerable interest, these studies failed to use adequate placebo controls (Baldessarini, 1984), and L-tryptophan has yet to achieve recognition in the management of depressive illness. On the other hand, there is agreement that the combination of this amino acid with an MAOI does have clear antidepressant properties (Glassman and Platman, 1969). L-Tryptophan ultimately may be useful as an adjunctive treatment in bipolar patients who are taking lithium (Baldessarini, 1984) if recent serious questions about toxicity can be resolved (see Chapter 21).

The immediate serotonin precursor 5-hydroxy-tryptophan (5-HTP) is reported to be an effective antidepressant (reviewed by Byerley et al., 1987). In his review, Van Praag (1983) noted favorable results in 12 of 14 trials of 5-HTP, with an overall response rate of 53 percent in 547 patients. In one study, it was shown to be equivalent to imipramine (Angst et al., 1977). In studies of medication-resistant bipolar and unipolar depressed patients, 5-HTP showed antidepressant effects in combination with the peripheral decarboxylase inhibitor carbidopa (Van Hiele, 1980), with MAOIs (Mendlewicz and Youdim, 1980), or with tricyclics (Van Hiele, 1980).

In 1963, Pöldinger reported that intramuscular *reserpine* added to standard tricyclic regimens produces a dramatic response in treatment-resistant depressions. Later, better controlled studies (e.g., Price et al., 1987; Amsterdam and Berwish, 1987), however, yielded findings that were predominantly negative, and the use of this treatment must be questioned.

GABA Agonists

γ-Aminobutyric acid is a major inhibitory transmitter in the central nervous system (CNS). As reviewed in Chapter 11, the pathophysiology of depression may involve a reduction in GABA function, and GABA may be involved in the mechanism of action of standard antidepressant treatments. Two compounds that enhance or mimic the function of GABA—progabide and fengabine—have been reported to have antidepressant activity comparable to imipramine, amitriptyline, or clomipramine (Bartholini et al., 1986; Musch and Garreau, 1986) but a low incidence of anticholinergic side effects (Morselli et al., 1987). These interesting reports await further replications. The previously discussed antidepressant effects of carbamazepine (and perhaps clonazepam) are also of interest here, since these anticonvulsants clearly interact with CNS GABA. The putative benzodiazepine-like antidepressants, alprazolam and adinozolam, are also thought to have a primarily GABAergic mechanism of action and can up-regulate GABA receptors when given chronically (Lloyd and Morselli, 1987).

Receptor Agonists and Antagonists

Among the potential antidepressants are several drugs that are agonists (i.e., stimulants) or antagonists to amine receptors.

Dopaminergic Agents. Post and colleagues (1978) administered *piribedil,* a putative central dopamine-receptor agonist, to 11 hospitalized depressed patients (including 5 bipolar-II and 2 bipolar-I patients). They observed mild to moderate antidepressant effects, as well as the precipitation of mania in one individual. The degree of improvement in depression was inversely correlated with pretreatment levels of homovanillic acid (HVA), the dopamine metabolite in the CNS. The emergence of dysphoric effects with prolonged use (Shopsin and Gershon, 1978) may have discouraged further study.

Another dopamine-receptor agonist, *bromocriptine,* used clinically as an adjunctive agent in treating parkinsonism, apparently has some antidepressant activity, particularly in relieving psychomotor retardation (Agnoli et al., 1978). One controlled study found that it was as effective as imipramine and caused fewer side effects (Waehrens and Gerlach, 1981). In addition, an open study found improvement in 60 percent of depressed patients (Nordin et al., 1981), although amelioration of depression correlated with changes in cerebrospinal fluid 3-methoxy-4-hydroxyphenylglycol (MHPG), not HVA, suggesting a noradrenergic rather than a dopaminergic mechanism. Response in bipolar patients was not specified. In the only study that separated bipolar from unipolar patients, Silverstone (1984) reported dramatic and rapid antidepressant effects in five of five bipolar patients (some of whom developed manic symptoms) in contrast to the five unipolar patients who either did not respond or responded very slowly. (For a review of the antidepressant effects of dopamine agonists, see Jimerson, 1987.)

Adrenergic Agents. Clonidine, a drug that stimulates α_2-adrenergic receptors, has been the subject of preliminary antidepressant trials. Jimerson and colleagues (1980) noted that it had beneficial effects in three of five hospitalized depressed patients they studied; two of the three responders were bipolar. One patient became manic during the clonidine withdrawal period.

In related studies, *salbutamol,* a stimulant of β-adrenergic receptors in the CNS, was evaluated for antidepressant properties by Simon and colleagues (1978) and by Lecrubier and co-workers (1980). Simon's study involved a comparison with clomipramine, a recognized antidepressant, each drug being given intravenously to ten hospitalized depressed patients (mixed unipolar and bipolar). Both drugs produced substantial improvement, as reflected in Hamilton depression ratings, but salbutamol was significantly more effective ($p < 0.05$), at least in the first 2 weeks of treatment. In a smaller double-blind, placebo-controlled study of *pirbuterol,* a more selective β agonist, Nurnberger and colleagues (1986) failed to find antidepressant activity in five bipolar depressed women.

The initial positive results with the direct receptor agonists may not be sustained over time. Such tolerance to the antidepressant effects would be expected if direct postsynaptic receptor stimulation produces a gradual down-regulation of the postsynaptic site (as described in Chapter 17). On the other hand, α_2-antagonists, such as yohimbine and idazoxan, might theoretically have sustained antidepressant effects because they accelerate the down-regulation of β-receptors when given chronically to animals (see Chapter 17). Idazoxan was found to be effective in a preliminary study of a small group of bipolar patients (Osman et al., 1989).

Anticholinergic Agents. Early attempts to produce antidepressant effects with atropine and oth-er anticholinergic agents were not successful, and the anticholinergic effects of tricyclics do not correlate with their antidepressant potency. Kasper and co-workers (1981) found in a double-blind, placebo-controlled study that 12 mg of *biperiden* per day was an effective antidepressant in ten severely depressed patients (five bipolar), and Jimerson and colleagues (1982) noted an equally robust effect in a controlled study of two bipolar depressed women receiving up to 20 mg a day of *trihexyphenidyl.* Unfortunately, these findings, which mirror the previously cited efficacy of cholinomimetic drugs in mania, have not been pursued.

S-Adenosylmethionine

S-Adenosylmethionine (S-AMe) is a major donor of methyl groups in the various transmethylation reactions important to central neurotransmitter functioning, such as catechol-*o*-methyl transferase (COMT) (see Chapter 17). Furthermore, methylation reactions have been implicated in the process of postsynaptic receptor activation by monoamine neurotransmitters (Hirata and Axelrod, 1978).

Following a series of uncontrolled studies of an activating antidepressant response to parenterally administered S-AMe, Agnoli and colleagues (1976) conducted a double-blind, placebo-controlled trial in 30 hospitalized depressed patients with mixed diagnoses. Bipolar patients were not specifically identified. Compared with placebo, S-AMe produced substantial improvement in depressed mood, loss of interest, somatic symptoms, and psychomotor retardation. Between 80 and 100 percent of the patients showed some response, and the percentage of improvement averaged between 70 and 80 percent on the Hamilton rating scale. Improvement was rapid—within 4 to 6 days in 80 percent of the patients. It should be noted, however, that most patients in this trial, although hospitalized, were not diagnosed as having endogenous depression. Both the S-AMe group and the placebo group started the trial at an average Hamilton rating of 20 to 21, indicating moderately severe depression. The S-AMe group finished the trial at a 6.5 rating, but the placebo group also showed considerable response, finishing the trial at a 14 rating.

In a subsequent single-blind trial, Del Vecchio and colleagues (1978) compared S-AMe with clomipramine and found no significant difference between the two treatments. S-AMe primarily improved mood, guilt feelings, psychomotor retardation, level of interest, and suicidal tendencies. Miccoli and co-workers (1978) reached a similar conclusion after comparing S-AMe with either intravenous clomipramine or amitriptyline. In a double-blind comparison study, Bell and colleagues (1988) actually found S-AMe to be superior to imipramine in a group of predominantly unipolar patients.

We are aware of only two studies in which bipolar patients have been analyzed separately. In an open trial by Lipinski and colleagues (1984), 7 of 9 depressed patients (5 of 6 bipolar patients) improved with S-AMe, including a few who switched into a euphoric state. Carney and co-workers (1989) administered S-AMe to 29 patients (22 intravenously, 7 orally) in a placebo controlled study. Among the 11 bipolar patients, 9 switched into mania or hypomania within a period ranging from a few hours to 6 days. Among the 18 unipolar patients, 6 improved without switching, and 12 showed no response. These interesting preliminary results suggest that bipolar patients may be especially sensitive to the antidepressant–activating effects of S-AMe. The pharmacology of this interesting compound has been reviewed by Baldessarini (1987). S-AMe may represent a rapidly acting antidepressant with a low incidence of side effects, but the specific role of S-AMe in treating bipolar illness cannot yet be quantified.

Endocrine-Related Substances

Considerable attention has been focused on the role of a wide variety of newly discovered brain peptides. Elaboration of the functional significance of these peptides has stimulated interest in their clinical potential.

Thyroid Hormone. Some, but not all (see, e.g., Gitlin et al., 1987), trials have shown that the thyroid hormone T_3 accelerates the response to tricyclic antidepressants among women with major depression (Prange et al., 1969; Wheatley, 1972) and to potentiate antidepressant response among some tricyclic responders (Goodwin et al., 1982; Targum et al., 1984).[31] One report of two patients found the same potentiation of the MAOI phenelzine (Joffe, 1988). Joffe and Singer

(1988) directly compared supplemental T_3 with T_4 in tricyclic nonresponders and found that 7 of 14 responded to the addition of T_3, compared with only 1 of 15 given T_4. (The prophylactic use of T_4 in rapid-cycling patients is discussed in Chapter 23.) Some of the discrepancy in the results of T_3 potentiation studies may be due to differences in the patient populations. A recent study by Nelson (1988) found that bipolar-II patients were much more likely to respond than were unipolar patients (89 percent vs 25 percent; $p < 0.0003$), and Evans and colleagues (1986) reported on two bipolar-I patients who switched into mania after T_3 was added to their antidepressant regimen. The possibility that bipolar patients are more responsive to T_3 potentiation is interesting but needs further evaluation. The controversies and conceptual issues concerning thyroid potentiation have been nicely reviewed by Bauer and Whybrow (1988), and the comments accompanying their article provide rich and varied perspectives.

Hypothalamic Peptides. Thyrotropin-releasing hormone (TRH), a hypothalamic tripeptide, was evaluated as an antidepressant after the initial positive reports of Prange and his colleagues (1972). Although some of the studies showed a slight, but discernible, improvement (Lipton and Goodwin, 1975), initial hopes for a rapidly acting agent with clinically significant antidepressant action were not borne out by subsequent studies (see, e.g., Takahashi et al., 1973; Hollister et al., 1974; Lipton and Goodwin, 1975).

Following reports of its antidepressant-like activity in several animal tests, MIF-1, the hormone that inhibits the release of the hypothalamic peptide melanocyte-stimulating hormone, was evaluated as an antidepressant in a small trial by Kastin and colleagues (1971). Although four of the five patients showed marked improvement within 2 to 3 days, the relatively high rate of improvement in the placebo group makes this preliminary study difficult to interpret, even though the results are provocative.

Analogs of the opiate peptides, endorphin and synthetic enkephalin, were discussed previously under Stimulants and Euphoriants. Another peptide-related substance with possible mood-elevating properties is *captopril,* an inhibitor of angiotensin-converting enzyme and of enkephalinase. Mood-elevating properties have been reported in a small number of patients (Zubenko and Nixon, 1984; Deicken, 1986; Cohen and Zubenko, 1988).

Vasopressin. As noted in Chapter 17, vasopressin is another important peptide that may be involved in the pathophysiology of some forms of depression (Gold and Goodwin, 1978). When an analog of vasopressin (DDAVP) was administered to five patients hospitalized for major depressive illness, including three with bipolar illness, all five showed statistically significant cognition and memory improvement (Gold et al., 1979). In most cases, these functions returned to normal or exceeded normal, but depressive symptoms did not improve, except in one patient who achieved a remission.

Gonadal Steroid Hormones. Klaiber and co-workers (1979) demonstrated in a double-blind, placebo-controlled trial that high-dose conjugated estrogens (5 to 25 mg of conjugated estrogenic hormone) had modest antidepressant efficacy in 21 premenopausal women. Subsequently, Holsboer and colleagues (1985) reported similar results in an open trial, using ethinyl estradiol 20 mg three times a day along with 40 mg three times a day of vitamin B_6. However, a study of conjugated estrogenic hormone added to imipramine in 11 depressed women patients (Shapira et al., 1985) failed to show any beneficial antidepressant effects. In a complementary study, Vogel and co-workers (1985) showed that 150 mg of mesterolone, a synthetic androgen, was as effective an antidepressant as amitriptyline in a double-blind, parallel-group study of 34 depressed men.

Nonpharmacological Approaches

Several alternatives to medications are now used to treat bipolar depression. With the exception of ECT, these treatments are still considered experimental (psychotherapy is discussed in Chapter 24).

Sleep Deprivation, Phase Advance, and REM Deprivation

Efficacy. Since the initial reports of Schulte (1966) and of Pflug and Tölle (1971), one of the most interesting developments in the treatment of affective disorders is the growing literature documenting dramatic, but transient, improvement in severe depression following one or more nights of sleep deprivation. For most patients, the depressive syndrome reappears after one or two nights of sleep (Post et al., 1976; Roy-Byrne et al., 1984), but in some, the improvement can last longer. In a review of the literature, Wehr and colleagues (1982) found that the overall response rate was about 60 percent, about evenly divided between complete remission and varying degrees of partial improvement. These studies are summarized in Table 22-9.

Schilgen and Tölle (1980) found that even partial sleep deprivation (i.e., during the second half of the night) produced a similar antidepressant response. The patients in this study were put to bed early—at 9 PM—and slept until 1 AM, when they were awakened. Thus, in addition to the reduction of sleep, timing was advanced. As with the earlier reports, sleep deprivation was more effective in patients showing clear endogenous symptoms, particularly sleep disturbance and diurnal variation. (The number of bipolar patients included in these studies was not specified.) In a 1985 study by Dessauer and colleagues, antidepressant-resistant depressed patients (14 unipolar, 4 bipolar), given antidepressants and partially deprived of sleep, recovered as well as did antidepressant-responsive patients given tricyclics alone. Some studies have also suggested that short-term response to sleep deprivation predicts later response to antidepressant drugs (Wirz-Justice et al., 1979; Roy-Byrne et al., 1984).

Table 22-9. Antidepressant Effects of Sleep Deprivation

Technique	Studies N	Patients N	Response[a] %
Total SD	60	1,181	57[b]
Partial SD	10	182	64
Selective REM Deprivation	3	57	56
Totals	73	1,420	59

SD = sleep deprivation
[a]Average response rate (weighted)
[b]BP = 74%, UP = 52%

Adapted from Wehr et al., unpublished

Studies of sleep deprivation are particularly interesting theoretically in relation to disturbed circadian rhythms in affective illness (discussed in Chapter 19). The usefulness of sleep deprivation therapy in the clinical management of depression is limited by the relapse of most patients after sleep is resumed. Among the several attempts to overcome this problem, sleep deprivation has been combined with antidepressant drug therapy in the hope that the rapid antidepressant effect of the former could be sustained by the latter. Evidence concerning the efficacy of this approach is preliminary and partly contradictory. Elsenga and Van dan Hoofdakker (1983) found that antidepressant effects of clomipramine can be accelerated by repeated sleep deprivation treatments during the initial phase of treatment. They were unable to replicate this finding in a later study, however. Baxter and colleagues (1986; Baxter, 1985) reported that the antidepressant effects of sleep deprivation can be sustained by administering lithium, beginning on the day after the sleep-deprived night.

In an interesting elaboration of the sleep deprivation paradigm, Wehr and his NIMH colleagues (1979; Sack et al., 1985) treated hospitalized depressed patients (60 percent of them bipolar) by altering the sleep-wake cycle (phase advance). Following one night of sleep deprivation, these subjects advanced their sleep-wake cycle 6 hours by sleeping from 6 or 7 PM to 1 or 2 AM. They were kept on this schedule for the next 2 weeks. Most experienced rapid relief of their severe depressive symptoms, with remissions persisting for approximately 2 weeks. Souêtre and colleagues (1987) reported similar results.

Some investigators are searching for a way to use sleep interventions over the long term. Patients tolerate repeated partial sleep deprivation in the latter half of the night and phase advance of the sleep-wake cycle more readily than repeated total sleep deprivations. These procedures, the focus of ongoing clinical studies, appear to be effective for some patients (Wehr et al., 1986; Holsboer-Trachsler et al., 1988).

Pursuing another sleep manipulation approach, Vogel and colleagues (1980) reported significant antidepressant effects associated with selective deprivation of REM sleep. Like partial sleep deprivation, the repeated used of this procedure over several weeks is reported to produce a sustained antidepressant response. Although of theoretical interest, the clinical potential of this approach probably is limited by technical complexity.

Induction of Mania. The literature contains several reports of sleep deprivation inducing mania in bipolar patients, but only one study systematically investigated this phenomenon. Wehr and his colleagues (1982) found that a majority of depressed, rapid-cycling, manic-depressive patients switched into hypomania or mania following total sleep deprivation for one night (Figure 22-6). In some cases, patients switched back into depression after recovery sleep. In others, mania persisted for days or weeks. Phase advance of the sleep-wake cycle has been reported to induce switches from depression to hypomania or mania in a few bipolar patients (Wehr et al., 1979, 1982; Wehr and Goodwin, 1983).

Given the experimental evidence that bipolar patients may switch into mania when deprived of sleep, it is possible that this mechanism serves as a final common pathway for diverse factors that have been thought to induce mania (Wehr et al., 1986). Sleep reduction is likely to occur during disruptions of routine due to travel, shift work, social events, and medical and other types of emergencies. Emotional reactions—anxiety, fear, anger, infatuation, or bereavement—can cause insomnia, as can taking such drugs as amphetamines, MAOIs, and excess caffeine, or withdrawing from other drugs (e.g., antidepressants, neuroleptics, and sedatives). Each of these factors reported to induce mania may act through a common mechanism involving sleep reduction (Figure 22-7).

High-Intensity Light

Clinical trials involving more than 243 patients at several centers have shown that some 60 to 80 percent of patients with winter depressions (the most prominent form of SAD) improved significantly with phototherapy (see Chapter 19).[32] These results, reviewed by Rosenthal and colleagues (1989), support several conclusions:

- To be effective, phototherapy requires light several times brighter than that of typical indoor environments. In most studies, patients were exposed to light emitted through a diffus-

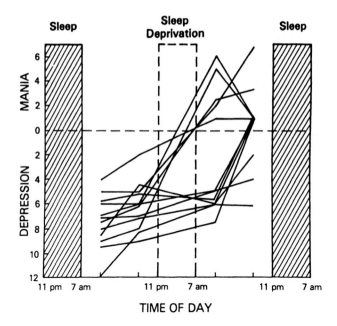

Figure 22-6. Individual patients' response to sleep deprivation, with some showing mania. (Wehr, unpublished data).

ing screen from eight 4-foot fluorescent bulbs at a distance of three feet (2,500 to 3,500 lux).
- Animal models led to the original hypothesis that light treatment would be effective only if it extended the duration of the short winter day. However, light administered in the middle of the day appears to be more or less as effective as light administered at the extremes of the day (Wehr et al., 1986; Jacobsen et al., 1987), although there are some patients for whom phototherapy in the morning appears to be *relatively* more effective than phototherapy in the evening (Lewy et al., 1985; Terman et al., 1987).
- Dosage of light appears to be directly related to response (Terman et al., 1987). Effective treatment seems to require at least 2 hours of exposure per day, and 4 hours are more effective than 2.
- The therapeutic effects of phototherapy are mediated by the eyes and not the skin (Wehr et al., 1987).
- The exact wavelength requirements have not yet been determined.

The relatively quick response to changes in light exposure has practical implications for clinical management. Response to phototherapy is relatively rapid (Rosenthal et al., 1985), and patients sometimes experience slight improvement after 1 or 2 days, attaining the maximum benefit after 4 to 7 days. Relapses after withdrawal of light are similarly rapid. Patients sometimes notice a deterioration in mood after a series of overcast days, even in summertime. Those for whom maintenance phototherapy seems to lose its effectiveness often report neglecting their treatment schedules. In uncontrolled studies, starting phototherapy in late summer appears to prevent winter depression in patients with SAD (Rosenthal and Wehr, 1987).

A major problem in evaluating the clinical trials of phototherapy is the difficulty in establishing blind treatment conditions. It is hard to imagine how patients can be kept blind to a treatment that they literally must see if it is to be effective; thus the response may be engendered by the expectations of the procedure, especially since phototherapy has had a considerable amount of positive publicity.[33] Nevertheless, studies indicate that patients' responses to phototherapy are not primarily due to nonspecific aspects of the intervention (placebo responses). First, patients failed to respond to sham treatments involving yellow light of ordinary intensity, even though they were told that the investigators were interested in the

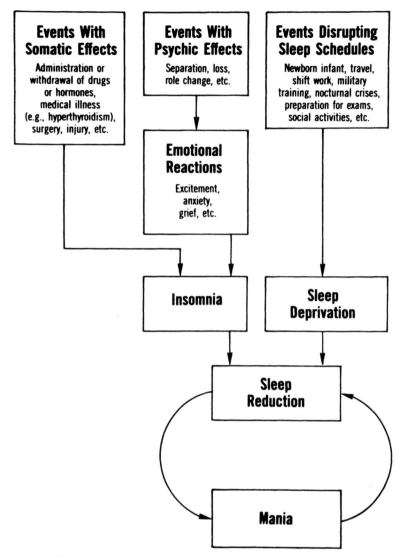

Figure 22-7. Diagram of hypothesis of sleep reduction as final common pathway of diverse factors thought to precipitate mania (from Wehr et al., 1987a).

effects of color on mood (Rosenthal et al., 1984). Second, response and relapse do not follow immediately after initiation and termination of treatment. Third, patients do not appear to develop tolerance to the procedure, as often occurs with placebo. Finally, a study comparing phototherapy administered through the eyes with that administered through the skin found that, although patients expected to benefit from both conditions, they responded only to the eye condition (Wehr et al., 1986). Whether light therapy has any adverse effects is clearly an important issue. In the initial report (Rosenthal et al., 1984), intensive examination of the retina (retinopathy) failed to reveal any adverse effects with short-term use, and no eye problems have yet been reported after several years of accumulated clinical experience. Some patients do report eye strain, headaches, irritability, or difficulty falling asleep. These symptoms usually respond to increasing the distance from the light. In some bipolar patients, excessive light has been noted to be associated with hypomanic symptoms, but there are not controlled data on this point.

The responses of patients with winter SAD to drugs have not been investigated systematically, although clinical impressions strongly suggest that most patients are unresponsive to a wide variety of agents. It has been suggested that artificial light may potentiate antidepressant drugs in patients whose symptoms intensify in winter but who do not experience "pure" winter depression. Definite data are lacking, however. The impact of light therapy on the long-term course of recurrent winter SAD has not been explored. There are some indications that the effective treatment of winter depression may decrease the likelihood or extent of a hypomanic episode in the subsequent summer.

Relationship Between Phototherapy and Sleep Deprivation

Unlike antidepressant drugs, both sleep deprivation therapy and phototherapy act rapidly, and their action stops when the treatment stops. However, the effects of these two treatments are sometimes difficult to differentiate. Early morning light treatments can incidentally deprive patients of sleep, for example, or sleep deprivation may expose patients to light at times when they would ordinarily be asleep in the dark. Further confounding interpretation of results, some patients with SAD respond to sleep deprivation (Wehr et al., 1985). Controlled experiments indicate, however, that the two treatments can operate independently. Patients respond to phototherapy without sleep deprivation (Rosenthal et al., 1985), and they respond to sleep deprivation without exposure to light (Wehr et al., 1985).

Electroconvulsive Therapy

Several studies have compared the efficacy of ECT to that of TCAs in patients with endogenous depressive illness (reviewed by Avery and Mills, 1978; Rudorfer and Linnoila, 1986). Most of these studies (involving more than 3,000 patients) show a higher response rate in the ECT group, especially in the more severely ill patients and in those with delusions. Others show the treatments to be equivalent, and only one found tricyclics superior to ECT.

In 1985, Janicak and colleagues conducted a meta-analysis of studies that used careful methodology and at least single-blind conditions in comparing ECT with simulated ECT, placebo,

tricyclics, or MAOIs. The evidence for the efficacy and superiority of ECT over other treatments is clear-cut and convincing. A report by Davidson and colleagues (1978) also suggests that ECT is superior to combined tricyclic–MAOI treatment.

A substantial proportion of depressed patients who do not respond to a tricyclic do respond to a course of ECT. For example, in a study of 437 patients with endogenous depression, De Carolis and associates (1964) found a 61 percent response rate to imipramine. Those who did not respond to imipramine were given ECT, and 85 percent of them responded. The delusional depressive patients were especially poor imipramine responders (35 percent), but they responded to ECT at the same rate as the overall group (85 percent). Bratfos and Haug reported similar findings in 1965. In a study by Paul and co-workers (1981), bilateral ECT induced remissions in eight of nine severely depressed patients who had been refractory to extensive trials on a variety of antidepressant medication. Although some evidence suggests that bilateral ECT is more effective than unilateral (Abrams et al., 1983), not all reports reach the same conclusion (NIMH/NIH Consensus Conference, 1985). Common clinical experience suggests that the therapeutic effects of ECT begin more rapidly than those of the tricyclics, but we are aware of no controlled study that directly attempts to verify this.

Like studies of antidepressant drugs, most of the literature on the efficacy of ECT does not differentiate bipolar from unipolar depression. Perris (1966) initially reported that bipolar patients respond more favorably to ECT than do unipolar patients. However, subsequent studies by Strömgren (1973) and by Abrams and Taylor (1974) failed to find any bipolar–unipolar difference. When Abrams and Taylor reanalyzed Perris' data, considering only those patients who received ECT alone, they found no significant difference between the groups. Black and colleagues (1987) reported a less favorable response in bipolar than in unipolar patients, although the relatively low overall response rate limits the interpretation of this study. Thus, studies comparing the antidepressant effects of ECT in bipolar and unipolar patients do not suggest a clearly different response pattern.

In the earlier literature on ECT, authors frequently refer to the observation that treatment efficacy tends to be lower in patients with histories of multiple episodes and that in individual patients, ECT is somewhat less effective with each ensuing episode. These observations may be related to what we have already discussed concerning the tendency for antidepressant treatments to work less well in patients with highly recurrent or cyclic illness. As we have suggested, it is in these patients (whether bipolar or unipolar) that lithium may have its most valuable role.

ECT and Long-Term Course. In assessing the potential impact of ECT treatment on the long-term course of bipolar illness, the study by Kukopulos and co-workers (1980) is helpful. Of 434 bipolar patients, 57 were treated for depression with ECT alone. Of this group, 22 (39 percent) experienced mild hypomania following the course of ECT. Unlike the tricyclics, ECT did not seem to be associated with the development of "a continuous circular course" or rapid cycling. In a further attempt to evaluate the relative effect of ECT on the frequency of recurrences, these investigators examined 11 patients who were treated with ECT for their first several episodes and subsequently were treated with tricyclics. The tricyclic treatment was associated with a "remarkable increase in the frequency of recurrences." Of the 11, 6 became continuous cyclers within a few years, 2 having rapid cycles. The possible contribution of the natural course of the illness (with its tendency to increase in frequency) was not discussed. Based on their observations, the investigators suggested that ECT may be preferable to tricyclics in treating bipolar depression, since the risk of shortening the cycle or precipitating mania seems to be lower with ECT. As noted earlier, however, in Angst's historical analysis of admission patterns to the Burghölzli Hospital, admissions increased sharply for mania in the decade after the introduction of ECT, and the rate was not substantially lower than that subsequently observed during the tricyclic era. Additional longitudinal studies are needed, particularly prospective studies of how ECT, tricyclics, or MAOIs, when used intermittently, affect the long-term course of the illness.

ECT and Memory Function: An Update. Many clinicians and patients are reluctant to consider the use of ECT because of concern about its impact on memory (reviewed in Fink, 1979, 1987). This concern persists despite evidence that verbal memory effects are substantially reduced by unilateral placement of electrodes on the nondominant side (Abrams et al., 1972; Squire and Slater, 1978) and that performance on a variety of memory tests returns to normal within 6 to 9 months of treatment (reviewed by Squire, 1986; Abrams, 1988).

These studies show that the capacity to learn, retain, and recall new information is unimpaired 6 to 9 months after ECT. The investigators, however, did not directly consider a question of great clinical relevance: Does ECT permanently disrupt memory for events in the recent past (just before the treatment), as subjective memory complaints following ECT suggest?

A study by Squire and colleagues (1981) provides some reassurance on this point. In 43 patients examined before, 1 week after, and 7 months after a course of bilateral ECT, the investigators found that, although bilateral ECT disrupted recall of public and personal events occurring many years earlier, the recovery of these memories was virtually complete within 7 months of ECT. Squire and colleagues noted some apparently permanent loss of memory for events a few days before ECT. In a few patients, the persistence of a very slight memory loss of events 1 to 2 years before ECT could not be entirely ruled out. In an earlier paper, Squire and Chace (1975) observed that the persistence of subjective memory complaints was correlated with the extent of the acute loss, not with the actual performance at the time. This suggests that some patients were sensitized to expect memory difficulties as a result of their experiences in the immediate post-ECT period.

SUMMARY

Somatic treatments for acute depression have proliferated during the past three decades, as have systematic studies of their effects. Since the bipolar–unipolar distinction often is not made in such studies, however, firm knowledge of the impact of many of these treatments on acute bipolar depression is still lacking.

The pharmacological armamentarium for bipolar depression includes tricyclic and second-generation antidepressants, MAOIs, and lithium—all drugs of proven efficacy singly and in selected combinations. Among the nondrug somatic approaches, carefully administered ECT remains an important option for selected patients, particularly those who are delusional or suicidal. Unfortunately, the controversy surrounding ECT impedes its use. Light therapy and the delay or phase shifting of sleep provide additional supplementary approaches.

Despite the demonstrated ability of many antidepressant drugs to relieve depressive symptoms, increasing evidence suggests that antidepressants, especially tricyclics, can precipitate mania or rapid cycling in bipolar depressed patients. Carbamazepine may, like lithium, prove to have some antidepressant properties.

Pretreatment evaluation is the cornerstone of clinical management of depression, establishing the bipolar or recurrent unipolar diagnosis, the family and treatment history (and prior treatment response), medical constraints on treatment choice, the risk of suicide, and the need for hospitalization. Once a bipolar diagnosis is made, barring contraindications, lithium should be part of the initial treatment. If the depression is severe, an antidepressant should be administered along with lithium. Although the use of tricyclic or heterocyclic drugs is still the most frequent, the role of MAOIs in treating bipolar depression is being recognized. Adjunctive thyroid hormone can aid in potentiating responses to antidepressants. Whatever drug is chosen, frequent monitoring is necessary to ensure that adequate blood levels have been reached and to detect incipient adverse reactions. For patients on lithium alone, treatment should continue for 6 to 12 months, at which point maintenance treatment should be considered. Because of the risk of precipitating mania or rapid cycling, however, continuation antidepressant treatment of bipolar patients should be relatively brief.

Alternate or adjunct somatic treatments are available for patients for whom the standard treatment approaches are contraindicated or ineffective. These include ECT, carbamazepine, sleep deprivation, light therapy, and psychostimulants. Clearly, more effort to develop new medications for bipolar depression should be a high priority. For some bipolar depressed patients, hospitalization may be advisable, particularly to enhance treatment efficacy or avert the risk of suicide. The benefits must, of course, be weighed against the negative consequences of hospitalization.

NOTES

1. Cited in Schumann, 1907.
2. For a discussion of maintenance treatment of bipolar depression, see Chapter 23. Psychotherapy of depression is discussed in Chapters 24 and 25.
3. He did not, however, document this with quantitative rating data.
4. Vojtechovsky, 1957; Andreani et al., 1958; Hartigan, 1963. Reported in Dyson and Mendels, 1968.
5. Management of breakthrough depressions occurring during maintenance treatment are covered in Chapter 23. Several useful reviews of the management of depressive disorders in general are available: Goodwin, 1977; Kupfer and Detre, 1978; Klein et al., 1981; Akiskal, 1985; Baldessarini, 1985.
6. The issue of managing the suicidal patient is discussed separately in Chapter 27.
7. In bipolar depressed patients, the predominance of retardation over agitation may be associated with younger age and with less severe episodes (see Chapter 18).
8. Some recommend that two different drugs from each class be tried before a patient is declared nonresponsive to that class of drug.
9. Schuckit et al., 1971; Spiker and Pugh, 1976; White and Simpson, 1981; Marley and Wozniak, 1983; Razani et al., 1983. However, this combination may be more likely to precipitate mania than either drug alone (De la Fuente, et al., 1986).
10. For more details on the proper use of these combinations, see Baldessarini, 1985, and the articles cited there.
11. Potter and Linnoila, 1984; Amsterdam et al., 1980; Van Brunt 1983; APA Task Force Report, 1985.
12. The role of supplemental thyroid in managing breakthrough depressions in patients on maintenance lithium is discussed in Chapter 23.
13. Reports of seizures with bupropion occurred almost exclusively in patients with anorexia and bulimia syndromes, and they may have been in electrolyte imbalance.
14. Because of the long half-life of fluoxetine (100 hours for one active metabolite), a too rapid dose increase can result in overshooting the optimal blood level because of accumulation. Since at this writing the drug is only available in 20 mg capsules, the long half-life allows for gradual dose buildup by using every other day increments. Special caution should be exercised when combining fluoxetine with a MAOI because of the risk of hyperthermia (the serotonin syndrome).

15. The pure seasonal affective disorder pattern with winter depression responds to light therapy alone in the absence of medication.

16. This caution may not apply to the antidepressant effects of the mood stabilizers, such as lithium and carbamazepine.

17. If the patient is taking carbamazepine or another anticonvulsant, it should probably be discontinued before starting ECT treatment, since these drugs can markedly increase the amount of current necessary to produce a convulsion (Roberts and Attah, 1988).

18. Contemporary experience with the treatment of depression in outpatient settings, particularly clinics with referral populations, probably does not produce response rates this high because of higher rates of axis-II diagnoses, particularly substance abuse, and because the typical tricyclic-responsive patient is not as likely to be referred to specialty clinics.

19. It is our impression that the literature on anti-depressant response in bipolar patients usually refers to bipolar-I patients, although this is rarely spelled out carefully.

20. This qualitative difference is supported and strengthened by an increase in the size of the study group to 55 patients (Himmelhoch, personal communication, 1987).

21. Davidson et al., 1984, 1988; Liebowitz et al., 1984, 1988.

22. Rubidium, an alkali metal element closely related to lithium and potassium, has been evaluated as an antidepressant for theoretical reasons. Although it does, indeed, appear to have antidepressant properties, its very long biological half-life represents a practical barrier to wider evaluation. For a comprehensive review of this interesting substance, see Fieve and Jamison (1982).

23. A more extensive review can be found in Kramlinger and Post (1989).

24. Full discussions of the efficacy, side effects, advantages, and disadvantages of these drugs can be found in several reviews (Kane and Lieberman, 1984; Ostrow, 1985).

25. Settle and Settle, 1984; Turner et al., 1985: Chouinard and Steiner, 1986; Lebegue, 1987.

26. Records were sampled from the era before specific somatic therapies (1920-1939), the electroconvulsive therapy era (1940-1949), and the neuroleptic era (1953-1957). This clinic has enjoyed a remarkable stability in both patients and professional staff.

27. In Lewis and Winokur's 1982 study, few subjects were used (only eight patients were treated with tricyclics alone), and more importantly, the study's patient selection criteria may have introduced powerful distortions. Patients were systematically excluded if their previous manias were induced by drugs. It is this very group that is likely to switch into mania frequently during treatment. Furthermore, instead of being randomly assigned to different treatments, patients received those chosen by their physicians. Selection biases stemming from these treatment decisions may have led to the high number of switches in the unmedicated group. For example, 45 percent of those patients had been depressed. Their physicians may have withheld treatment in some cases because the patients were already beginning to switch from depression into mania. Further, unequal distribution of the sexes in the groups may have skewed the switch rates found in the two groups. Among all the patients, women were twice as likely as men to switch into mania—a finding consistent with the data of Wehr and Goodwin (1979) and of Quitkin and colleagues (1981b)—but the ratio of women to men was twice as high in the no-treatment group as in the tricyclic group. Finally, most of the unmedicated patients who switched into mania had not been depressed on admission. Instead, they had other diagnoses that could indicate misdiagnosed impending mania, such as personality disorder (27 percent) or pharmacological (9 percent) or organic (9 percent) factors predisposing them to mania.

28. In the 1973 study by Prien and colleagues, bipolar patients were treated for 2 years with lithium, imipramine, or placebo. From the 5th to the 24th month, the spontaneous incidence of mania was twice as high in the imipramine-treated group as it was in the placebo group (67 percent vs 33 percent, $p = 0.05$). Every instance of relapse in the imipramine-treated group was a manic episode, whereas both manic and depressive relapses occurred in the lithium-treated and placebo-treated groups. The 1984 interpretation relies on the fact that Prien's team did not find a significantly increased incidence of mania during the first 4 months of the study. The only patients allowed to enter the study were those who were stable on imipramine during the acute treatment phase. This criterion eliminated as many as half of the original patients—precisely the ones at most risk of switching—leaving only those likely to switch slowly, if at all.

In the 1984 study, Prien and colleagues compared the incidence of full mania in bipolar patients maintained on imipramine alone (53 percent), lithium alone (26 percent), or lithium plus imipramine (28 percent). As in the first study, a large number of patients who had an unstable course during the first 2 months of imipramine plus lithium were eliminated (25 percent of the original sample), probably explaining why this study did not, like Quitkin's, reveal significantly more manic relapses in bipolar patients on lithium plus imipramine compared with those on lithium alone. Furthermore, women, who are more likely than men to switch into mania during treatment with antidepressants were underrepresented in the 1973 VA study. Thus, the high switch rate in the imipramine groups was probably less than the actual incidence of mania during imipramine treatment of bipolar patients.

29. Five of the patients in the Joffe et al. study developed lithium-induced clinical hypothyroidism and another three had elevated TSH levels. All were women and had been taking lithium significantly longer than other patients in the study. Although none of the 17 rapid-cycling patients had a thyroid disorder, there were only 7 women in this group. Among the females in the nonrapid-cycling group, 40 percent developed thyroid dysfunction.

30. For tricyclics: Mirin et al., 1981; Nelson et al., 1983; Dilsaver and Greden, 1984. For MAOIs: Pickar et al., 1984; Rothschild, 1985.

31. The possible involvement of thyroid function in mood regulation is discussed in Chapter 17.

32. Rosenthal et al., 1984, 1985, 1989; James et al., 1985; Wirz-Justice et al., 1985; Lewy et al., 1985; Yerevanian et al., 1986; Hellekson et al., 1986; Lewy and Sack, 1986; Bick, 1986; Czeisler et al., 1986, 1987; Kripke et al., 1987; Wehr et al., 1987; Terman et al., 1987, 1989. The syndrome of winter SAD overlaps considerably with that of bipolar-II disorder.

33. This problem, of course, is not unique to phototherapy. Many patients involved in clinical trials of antidepressants are able to determine when they are receiving capsules containing active drugs because of obvious side effects.

23

Maintenance Medical Treatment

He [Robert Lowell] showed me the bottle of lithium capsules. Another medical gift from Copenhagen. Had I heard what his trouble was? "Salt deficiency." This had been the first year in eighteen he hadn't had an [manic] attack. There'd been fourteen or fifteen of them over the past eighteen years. Frightful humiliation and waste. He'd been all set to taxi up to Riverdale five times a week at $50 a session. . . . His face seemed smoother, the weight of distress-attacks and anticipation both gone.
—Richard Stern[1]

Preventing new episodes of manic-depressive illness has been an ambition of clinical investigators since they first recognized the inherently recurrent nature of the illness. In the middle of this century, the pursuit led many clinicians to undertake intensive psychotherapy, without much success. Others tried maintenance electroconvulsive therapy and considered it modestly effective. It was finally pharmacology, however, that provided the realization of that long-standing ambition. The development of lithium as an effective prophylactic treatment for manic-depressive illness, one of the most important advances in modern psychiatry, fundamentally altered both the prognosis for patients and the concepts of the disorder. The widespread clinical acceptance of lithium in treating and preventing manic-depressive illness is indicated by estimates that several years ago in Scandinavia, Great Britain, and the United States 1 of every 750 to 1,000 persons was being treated with this drug (Schou, 1981, 1989).

In the first part of this chapter, we provide practical guidelines for the long-term prophylactic treatment of manic-depressive illness. These guidelines cover the complex issues of patient selection for maintenance treatment, the problem of breakthrough episodes, the question of long-term side effects, and the increasingly important topic of alternative prophylactic strategies, including the use of carbamazepine and other anticonvulsants. Although bipolar illness is our main focus, we also review the prophylaxis of recurrent unipolar depression to emphasize the relationship between these two forms of affective illness. As noted throughout this book, classically the concept of manic-depressive illness included both bipolar and recurrent unipolar forms; in contemporary usage, however, *manic-depressive illness* is too often assumed to represent only the bipolar form.

The second part of the chapter examines the relevant research literature, emphasizing studies of treatment efficacy, predictors of response, and the important issue of the effects of long-term treatments on organ systems. We also discuss more recent efforts to assess the effect of lithium prophylaxis on long-term outcome in bipolar disorder. Some of the studies examining this issue tracked the course of illness in patients maintained on prophylactic lithium for 10 to 15 years, whereas others approached the question indirectly by scrutinizing changes in hospital admissions for mania since lithium was introduced.

Lithium prophylaxis was first described in 1951 by Noack and Trautner, who observed that the drug appeared to prevent additional manic episodes in patients whose acute mania had been alleviated by it. In 1954, Schou and colleagues provided the first case report demonstrating the benefits of lithium for both manic and depressive episodes. The 10 to 12 episodes a year that Schou's patient had experienced before treatment were markedly attenuated in duration and severity after 2 years of taking lithium continuously.[2]

Schou and associates were not encouraged by their early and brief attempts to treat depression with lithium. They continued to explore the drug's potential as an antimanic agent but did not systematically investigate its prophylactic effects. In 1959, Hartigan (the first to refer to lithium treatment as prophylaxis, published in 1963) and, later, Baastrup (1964) independently observed that bipolar patients treated with lithium for mania reported substantially fewer depressive episodes, as well as manic ones, during followup. Reviewing these early reports in 1973, Schou noted that neither Hartigan nor Baastrup had expected lithium to ameliorate depression and were initially reluctant to believe their own observations. Schou concluded that their skepticism made the findings all the more credible.

CLINICAL GUIDELINES

Most bipolar patients are maintained on lithium alone or in combination with other drugs. The following general guidelines, although emphasizing lithium, apply to alternative prophylactic drugs as well.

Selection of Patients for Maintenance Treatment

Before beginning treatment of an acute episode of illness with a drug such as lithium, the clinician should have already weighed the potential for medical complications and tested the patient's ability to tolerate the drug. Often the decision to embark on the maintenance treatment phase comes after the patient has already received the drug for the treatment of an episode. These acute and continuation phases of treatment allow for ongoing evaluation of side effects, functioning between episodes, and psychological reactions.

Even though most bipolar patients eventually experience recurrences frequently enough to justify prophylactic treatment, not all patients should be placed on maintenance treatment at the first sign of the illness. The clinician and the pa-

tient together must weigh the overwhelming likelihood of a relapse, keeping in mind that the natural recurrences of bipolar illness tend to become more frequent as the illness progresses, at least up to the point where the relapse frequency becomes constant or the disease chronic. Restructuring a patient's history into a life chart can be useful in determining the need for prophylactic treatment. One example of such a chart is illustrated in Figure 23-1.

Criteria for patient selection usually involve the type, frequency, total number, and severity of prior episodes. Bipolar or unipolar patients who experience episodes requiring hospitalization every year or two clearly need prophylactic treatment. Studies reviewed later demonstrate that such patients have a very high relapse rate, averaging 73 percent within the first year, when treated only with placebo (Schou, 1979). As discussed in Chapter 6, relapses also may follow catastrophic life events in some patients (Aronson and Shukla, 1987).

The need for prophylaxis is less obvious in patients with lower relapse rates. Naturalistic observation of 95 bipolar patients over many years led Angst (1981) and Grof and colleagues (1979a) to the conclusion that a total of two previous episodes is the best minimum criterion for lithium prophylaxis. If more stringent criteria were set, a substantial number of patients would be deprived of prophylaxis and would relapse. Considering the relative safety of long-term lithium treatment and the devastation caused by bipolar illness, treating some patients during a period when they would not relapse seems preferable to excluding from treatment many patients who would otherwise relapse quickly. If the criteria were more rigid—two episodes in 2 years, for example—two thirds of the patients excluded from lithium maintenance would relapse within 2 years. Zarin and Pass (1987) have proposed a quantitative model for deciding whether to initiate lithium after the first manic episode. Applying their model to the available literature, they estimate that approximately 5 years of maintenance lithium is needed to avoid an additional episode. Waiting to start maintenance lithium until the patient has already had a second episode requires 2 years of lithium to avoid a third episode.[3]

The wisdom of basing selection for prophylaxis on number rather than frequency of epi-

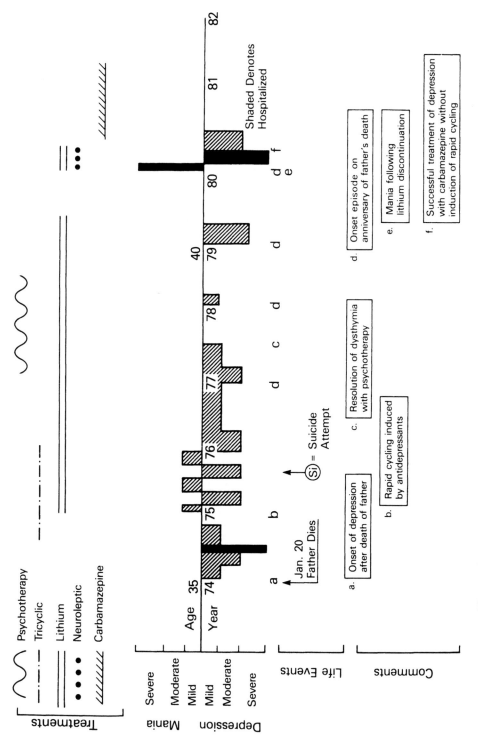

Figure 23-1. Graphing the course of affective illness. Prototype of a life chart (from Post, 1989).

sodes is underscored by the irregularity in the course of the illness, since episodes sometimes occur in bursts. Experienced clinicians do use other selection criteria, however. Many are so wary of the potential danger of future episodes that they initiate maintenance lithium after the first manic episode, even if it is the first episode of illness (NIMH/NIH Consensus Statement, 1985). In one study, for example, 57 percent of first-admission manic patients in Edinburgh were taking lithium at discharge (Mander, 1986).

It is now well established that episodes of bipolar affective illness tend to occur closer together as the illness progresses, particularly through the first several episodes. Some evidence suggests that the latency between the first and second episodes is longer in patients with an early age of onset (see Chapter 6). Women may thus be able to avoid taking lithium during their middle to late 20s, the prime childbearing years—an important advantage, given the drug's potential harm to a fetus in the first trimester.

On the other hand, the kindling models reviewed in Chapters 15 and 20 suggest that early treatment may reduce the long-term morbidity of the illness. Perhaps related to this is recent evidence from bipolar adolescents indicating a very high relapse rate among those who stop lithium prophylaxis after acute treatment for a manic episode (Strober et al., in press).[4]

Lithium prophylaxis is crucial when the patient is more vulnerable to mania than to depression. Since evidence suggests that a manic first episode may predict a course dominated by mania (Perris, 1968), early prophylaxis may be justified when the first episode is mania. Similarly, evidence of a higher ratio of manic to depressive episodes in men than women (see Chapter 6) implies that prophylaxis should start earlier in men (Mander, 1986).[5]

The rapidity of onset of previous episodes should also be considered when deciding whether to initiate maintenance treatment. Sudden onset of the prior manic episode provides a strong indication for prophylaxis, since there may be no warning period of hypomania during which treatment could be started.

A final illness characteristic to be considered is, of course, the severity of episodes. Obviously, when there is a history of psychotic mania, no real question exists. But what about severe cyclo-

thymia? The literature on this question is thin. The effect of lithium on the hypomanic pole seems more clear, although it is more often the depressive phases that bring such patients into treatment (Peselow et al., 1980).

Individual patient characteristics also affect decisions about prophylaxis. Questions the clinician should consider include: How reliable is the patient in noting early signs and seeking early treatment? What is the risk of suicide? Is the patient likely to deny difficulty until it is too late? Does the patient have family help or other support systems available? Since a patient may not consider hypomania a problem requiring treatment, concerned family members may have to detect it early and persuade the patient to seek professional care (Jacobsen, 1965; Molnar et al., 1988).

Some clinicians advise taking into account extenuating circumstances that might have contributed to the first manic episode, such as high levels of psychosocial stress, physical illness, or drugs of abuse. This recommendation is based on the assumption that so-called precipitated manias represent less inherent vulnerability and, therefore, less need for prophylaxis. Although this supposition seems reasonable to us, it is not well documented by research.

In summary, although no set of guidelines can be applied uniformly to all patients, some general principles can be followed. For almost all bipolar patients, lithium maintenance is indicated after the second major episode. Prophylaxis should be considered earlier if the first episode is manic, the patient is male, onset is sudden or later than age 30, the episode(s) has been severe and disruptive and/or involved a high suicide risk, the episode was not precipitated by external factors, the patient has a poor family and social support system, and the patient is an adolescent, especially one with substantial genetic loading.

Pretreatment Evaluation

Pretreatment evaluation should emphasize contraindications that could mitigate against the use of lithium (see discussion in Chapter 21 and Table 21-1). Most, if not all, contraindications are relative rather than absolute and involve the three systems most likely to be adversely affected by lithium: the kidney, the cardiovascular system, and the CNS. The routine pretreatment laboratory evaluation is outlined in Table 23-1. Some con-

Table 23-1. Pretreatment Evaluation
for Lithium Maintenance
(Healthy Individuals Under Age 50)

Laboratory[a]
Minimum Recommendations:
BUN
Creatinine
T_4, Free T_4
TSH
Urinalysis including protein and
microscopic examination

Additional Tests Recommended by
Some Authorities:
24-hour urine volume
Creatinine clearance
Urine osmolality
T_3 resin uptake
Complete blood count
Electrolytes
EKG (over age 50)
Blood pressure (over age 50)

Clinical
Medical History Focusing on Renal, Thyroid,
Cardiac, and Central Nervous Systems

Catalog of Present and Past Drug Use:
Prescription drugs
Over-the-counter preparations
Illicit drugs
Caffeine, nicotine, alcohol

Baseline Weight and History of Recent
Weight Change

Dietary Habits, Including Estimate of Salt
Intake

Exercise and Recreational Habits

[a]From Goodwin & Roy-Byrne, 1987

traindications may justify the use of alternative medications.

Monitoring of Maintenance Lithium

The Appropriate Lithium Level

The optimal blood level for maintenance lithium treatment generally is between 0.5 and 1.0 mEq/liter, the lower range being most appropriate in older patients. In earlier studies of prophylaxis, blood levels were maintained near the high end,[6] but a lower range more recently has become the accepted norm. Several studies indicate that, for patients stabilized on lithium for some time, a drop in prophylactic efficacy is unlikely to occur until blood levels fall below 0.6

mEq/liter (Jerram and McDonald, 1978; Hullin, 1980; Sashidharan et al., 1982; Maj et al., 1986; Goodnick et al., 1987). There are two random-assignment, double-blind prospective study that consider this issue: (1) Coppen and colleagues (1983) observed a significant decrease in affective morbidity among a group of bipolar and recurrent unipolar patients who had their maintenance lithium dose reduced, compared with those who did not.[7] (2) Gelenberg and colleagues (1989) randomly assigned 94 bipolar-I patients to either standard-dose lithium (dose adjusted to give 0.8–1.0 blood level, with group median of 0.83) or to low-dose lithium (dose adjusted to give 0.4–0.6 level, with group median of 0.54). The low-dose group showed a 2.6 times greater risk of relapse. These are group data, however, and individuals vary in their responses. Therefore, the best approach is to start with a blood level near the point at which side effects become troublesome and very gradually reduce it until side effects almost disappear completely or until 0.6 or 0.7 is reached. For older patients, however, a lower limit of 0.5 is not uncommon.

Fine-tuning the lithium dose is very important,

Table 23-2. Achieving 75-mg Increments of
Lithium Using the 300-mg and 450-mg
Dosage Forms

Dosage Level (mg)	Number of 300-mg Tablets[a]		Number of 450-mg Tablets[a]
150	_[a]		
225			1/2
300	1		
375	_[a]	&	1/2
450			1
525	1	&	1/2
600	2		
675			1+1/2
750	1	&	1
825	2	&	1/2
900	3	or	2
975	1	&	1+1/2
1,050	2	&	1
1,125			2+1/2
1,200[b]	4		
1,275	2	&	1+1/2
1,350			3
1,425	4	&	1/2
1,500[c]	5		

[a] 150 mg is available as a capsule or as 1/2 of a scored 300 mg pill
[b] Could also be one 300 mg and two 450 mg
[c] Could also be two 300 mg and two 450 mg

but it can require ingenuity, at least in the United States, where the drug (in tablet or capsule form) is available in only three strengths, 150, 300, and 450 mg of the carbonate salt (the last a sustained-release preparation). Table 23-2 illustrates how these strengths can be combined to provide increments of 75 mg. Lithium citrate in liquid form can be used for even finer tuning (1 ml = 60 mg of the carbonate salt), but many patients find the liquid inconvenient.

When maintenance treatment first begins, the frequency of blood level monitoring varies with the clinical situation. For the first several weeks, levels should be evaluated every week to determine the dose/blood level ratio for that patient. As noted in the discussion of acute treatment, the patient's clinical state, as well as a variety of other factors (sex, age, muscle mass, and diet), contribute to that ratio. Frequent monitoring during the initiation phase of maintenance treatment also helps establish compliance by emphasizing to the patient the importance of the blood level. Once the dose and blood level have been stabilized, most patients can be adequately managed by monitoring every 4 to 8 weeks during the first year or so and less frequently after that. Continuous monitoring remains important because unexpected medical conditions can alter the lithium level. Monitoring is also important for its psychological effects, since it reminds the patient of the illness and the importance of the medication, and it offers the patient an opportunity to participate in pharmacological management of the illness. Poor compliance is the most important factor limiting the prophylactic efficacy of lithium. For example, Baastrup (1969) estimated that 75 percent of his relapsing patients did so because of poor compliance. As discussed in Chapter 25, regular monitoring of blood levels is one important aspect of the psychological enhancement of compliance. Monitoring every 4 to 8 weeks indefinitely is, of course, not necessary for everyone. Some highly reliable patients who self-monitor side effects and who are aware of the factors that can alter lithium blood levels can be managed with less frequent monitoring.

Ever since lithium was introduced for treating manic-depressive illness, investigators have attempted to circumvent the need to draw blood by using alternative methods for monitoring lithium levels. The most promising is salivary monitoring, a method that is far easier to use with children, with adults with needle phobias, and in settings where needles are difficult to obtain. Although salivary monitoring has been widely studied, it has not generally been used in clinical settings (for a review of the subject, see Cooper, 1987). Concentrations of lithium in saliva, roughly twice as great as those in plasma, vary substantially from one individual to the next. Consequently the ratio of salivary levels to plasma levels must be established for each patient. Whether salivary levels more accurately reflect tissue levels is still unclear.

Several studies have suggested strategies by which the plasma level response to a single test dose of lithium might be used to predict the dose levels needed to produce the desired maintenance plasma level.[8] However, these approaches have not yet been applied generally in clinical practice.

Frequency of Other Laboratory Tests

Patients on lithium who do not show clinical indications of developing problems can be monitored according to the routine program summarized in Table 23-3. Authorities differ on the extent of minimum monitoring.

Special Circumstances

Both clinician and patient must be aware of circumstances that can affect lithium levels. Medical illness is probably the most common. The plasma lithium level can be elevated, for example, by even brief episodes of influenza severe enough to substantially reduce food (and therefore, salt) intake and produce changes in fluid balance. Distinguishing the early signs of lithium toxicity from symptoms of the medical illness itself can sometimes be difficult. One helpful clue is the prominence of CNS symptoms associated with lithium toxicity. If the illness persists for more than a few days, plasma lithium should be checked, and if it is accompanied by vomiting or diarrhea, plasma electrolytes should be measured.

Surgical Procedures. Surgical procedures that involve general anesthesia require attention, but there are no absolute contraindications to general anesthesia in patients on lithium. Two or three days before surgery, it is generally advisable to reduce the dose by half, withholding it altogether

Table 23-3. Medical Monitoring of Healthy Patients on Maintenance Lithium

Test	Frequency
Minimum recommendations	
Plasma lithium	4-8 weeks[a]
T4, Free T4, TSH	6 months
Creatinine[b]	6 months
Urinalysis	1 year
Additional recommendations by some authorities	
24-hour urine volume	6-12 months
Creatinine clearance	6-12 months
Urine osmolality	6-12 months
CBC	6-12 months
EKG (over age 50)	6-12 months

Special circumstances that can alter dose/blood level relationships
- Medical illness, especially with diarrhea, vomiting, or anorexia
- Surgery
- Crash dieting
- Strenuous exercise
- Very hot climate
- Advanced age
- Pregnancy and delivery

---

[a] This frequency can be reduced over time, especially with reliable patients

[b] Recently Schou (1989) has expressed his doubt that routine creatinine monitoring is still necessary, in light of the failure to find any decrease in glomerular filtration among his cohort of patients followed over a long period of time.

---

for 24 hours before the procedure. Lithium levels can be brought up to the therapeutic range as soon as the fluid and electrolyte balance is normalized, that is, after the patient is again taking nourishment by mouth. Lithium has been found to potentiate some anesthetics which has also been noted in a few case reports (reviewed in Jefferson et al., 1987), and patients on lithium have been noted to need less pain medication during postoperative recovery.

Diet. Alterations in diet can sometimes be the source of puzzling changes in the lithium level. Crash diets (i.e., severe weight-reducing efforts), undertaken without the physician's knowledge, are most frequently the cause. The bulk of daily salt intake comes from food, and severe dieting can cause sodium depletion, producing increased plasma lithium levels. Patients on diets should pay special attention to salt intake; more frequent plasma monitoring is also advisable.

Physical Activity. Major changes in physical activity can be important. For example, when a program of strenuous exercise, such as long-distance running, is started, care is required to maintain adequate hydration, replace lost electrolytes (especially sodium and potassium), and monitor lithium more closely. Clinical experience suggests that strenuous physical activity in hot climates may increase the risk of lithium intoxication, although not all experienced clinicians observe this effect. Two groups (Jefferson et al., 1982; Norman et al., 1987) report cases in which the selective excretion of lithium (over sodium) in the sweat during exercise actually produced a lower plasma lithium level. Whatever the real physiological effect of increased sweating on plasma lithium, it is probably advisable to monitor the lithium dose more closely.

Clinical State and Age. In some patients on a constant lithium dose, changes in the blood level can occur in association with major shifts in mood state (see Chapter 21 for a review of the literature). A shift into depression can be accompanied by an increase in plasma lithium, and a shift into hypomania can be associated with a decreased level.

Renal lithium clearance gradually decreases with age (Vestergaard and Schou, 1984), indicating that periodic dosage reduction will probably be necessary in the course of long-term lithium administration. One of the few groups that has studied lithium prophylaxis in the elderly (Hardy et al., 1987; Shulman et al., 1987) recommends a 12-hour serum lithium concentration of 0.5 mEq/liter or less, achieved at an average dose of 400 mg/day given in a single dose at bedtime.

Experience with lithium prophylaxis in adolescents and children dates back to its early use in adults, but the research is scattered and unsystematic. As noted in Chapter 21, the faster renal clearance in the young would predict a greater tolerance of the drug. Clinical reports substantiate this prediction. In general, dosages and serum levels should follow adult guidelines. As noted earlier, saliva monitoring may, in some conditions, serve as an alternative to plasma monitoring for children averse to having their blood drawn (see, e.g., Weller et al., 1987). Carbamazepine has also been used in manic-depressive children and adolescents, although systematic studies are lacking (for a review, see Evans et al., 1987).

Pregnancy and Birth. The many issues involved in deciding whether a woman should be off lithium or on an alternative drug during pregnancy are discussed later in this chapter (see Table 23-7). Here we simply note that if lithium is to be used, peaks should be avoided by using divided doses, and plasma levels should be followed closely because the hormonal and physiological changes accompanying pregnancy can alter the dose/plasma level ratio. These changes are particularly profound during delivery and require a temporary dosage reduction of at least 50 percent, which is best accomplished by gradually stepping the dose down during the week before the due date. The full maintenance blood level should be reestablished as soon as possible after the delivery, as normal dietary intake resumes and fluid balance and electrolytes normalize. The prompt reestablishment of prophylactic lithium levels should substantially reduce the likelihood of postpartum mania. Although preventing postpartum depression may require a longer period of restabilization, this is largely offset by the longer lag after parturition before depression develops.

Management of Side Effects

Managing the side effects of lithium is as much a psychotherapeutic as a medical task. Even before lithium is prescribed, the physician should mention the type of side effects that can occur and reassure the patient about their meaning. Patients should regularly be encouraged to voice their concerns about the subject, especially since side effects often lead to poor compliance. (These issues are covered in depth in Chapters 24 and 25.) Here we are concerned with the medical aspects of managing side effects.

Although any side effect that intensifies with the dose should respond to a reduction in dose, such a course of action is not always wise, particularly if prior experience suggests that the risk of relapse is unacceptably high. Some patients may tolerate side effects after simple reassurance, but others may require supplemental treatment. Fine tremor, a common side effect of lithium, is one of the easiest to treat; if left untreated, it can contribute to poor compliance. Although reducing the blood level may help, the tremor often persists even at the minimum level needed for prophylaxis. β-Adrenergic receptor blockers, such as propranolol (10 to 80 mg/day), metoprolol (20 to 80 mg/day) or atenolol (50 mg/day) control lithium-induced tremor very effectively and, at modest dosage, are essentially without other effects. These drugs usually begin to reduce tremor within 30 minutes and continue to do so for 4 to 6 hours.[9] When other drugs with a potential for causing tremors (e.g., tricyclics, caffeine) are used with lithium, propranolol may be less effective.

Excessive polyuria, that is, lithium-induced nephrogenic diabetes insipidus (NDI), can occasionally become so severe that either the patient or the clinician stops the drug. In a patient who clearly needs lithium and whose problem is not alleviated by a reduction in dosage, two alternate strategies are available: The first involves addition of a diuretic, preferably a loop diuretic, such as furosemide, which is considerably safer than a thiazide in combination with lithium.[10] Amiloride, a potassium-conserving diuretic, has also been used to treat lithium-induced polyuria (for review, see Boton et al., 1987). The second strategy for managing polyuria is to substitute (completely or partially) carbamazepine for lithium, since the former does not antagonize the antidiuretic hormone. Carbamazepine will not reverse NDI in the presence of a continued high lithium level, but it may substantially decrease the need for lithium.

The antithyroid effects of lithium can and should be treated with supplemental thyroid when both laboratory and clinical evidence confirms hypothyroidism. Clinical manifestations may be limited to such nonspecific symptoms as lassitude, tiredness, weight gain, and decreased cognitive functioning. The use of adjunctive thyroid hormone as an experimental treatment for breakthrough depressions or for lithium-resistant cycling in the absence of chemical evidence of hypothyroidism is discussed later.

One of the most troublesome of the common side effects of lithium and one frequently associated with poor compliance is weight gain. We are not referring to the small amounts (less than 5 to 7 pounds) gained by most patients when they begin lithium therapy, much of which is probably due to fluid retention and can be expected to recede gradually. Instead, we are considering the approximately 25 percent of patients who gain more than 10 pounds over and above what can be explained by fluid retention. Women, especially those who have had prior difficulty controlling their weight, are particularly likely to experience this weight gain. It must be managed early and vigorously, at first by restricting carbohydrates and encouraging regular exercise. Lithium treatment frequently produces a mild hypoglycemia-like pattern in which the patient will experience carbohydrate craving associated with low plasma glucose 2 to 3 hours after ingesting carbohydrates, especially sugar. Sometimes simply eliminating sugar-containing foods (such as orange juice at breakfast) can alleviate the midmorning or late-morning hunger that might otherwise contribute to the weight problem. Lithium-induced hypothyroidism, also associated with weight gain, can be corrected easily. Patients should also be warned not to increase their caloric intake inadvertently by using high-calorie drinks to quench lithium-induced thirst.

For patients who experience discrete periods of carbohydrate craving, either of two amino acids (L-glutamine or L-tryptophan) may prove to be helpful. L-Glutamine in doses of 500 to 1500 mg can suppress carbohydrate craving in some patients. If the time of the craving can be anticipated, the amino acid can be taken to prevent its onset. L-Tryptophan in similar doses may also suppress carbohydrate craving. Because of its sedative properties, it may be more useful for carbohydrate cravings that occur in the evening or at night. These two amino acids are available over the counter, although some preparations may be too impure to be useful. Two precautionary notes are necessary here. Instances of a switch into mania have been reported following large doses of L-glutamine, and large doses of L-tryptophan have recently been associated with a serious eosinophilia myalgia syndrome, causing its withdrawal from the market. Finally, we should note that although the above strategies can be helpful to some, weight gain remains a difficult problem for patients on lithium.

The management of lithium's effects on memory and cognition first involves reducing the dose to the lowest level consistent with effective prophylaxis. Since there is some evidence that increased CNS symptoms may be related to lower plasma levels of folate (Coppen and Abou-Saleh,

1982),[11] it is advisable to maintain all lithium-treated patients on a high-potency, multivitamin B preparation supplemented with 400 μg of folic acid. In our experience this strategy can attenuate the cognitive and memory side effects of lithium in some patients.

Treatment of Lithium Toxicity

Prevention is the most important principle in managing lithium toxicity or intoxication. By detecting early signs and adjusting dosages, the problem can be averted. The most sensitive indicator of incipient lithium toxicity is the CNS, perhaps particularly the cerebellum. Patients must be alerted in advance to CNS symptoms, and each encounter with the patient should include some assessment of CNS functioning. The agitation and restlessness of early intoxication are similar to symptoms of mixed affective states, and distinguishing between the two phenomena can be difficult. The signs of lithium intoxication are listed in Table 23-4.

If the intoxication is so severe that lithium withdrawal is not sufficient, the patient should be admitted to a hospital and cared for by a specialist in the treatment of poisoning. The first of several methods used to treat lithium poisoning (Table 23-4) is the vigorous application of general supportive measures appropriate in any CNS poisoning. Obviously, kidney function should be preserved by maintaining blood pressure and by replacing fluids and salt, but if it falters, hemodialysis is necessary. Although most patients recover after deliberately or accidentally overdosing on lithium, some are left with a persistent neurological or renal defect, and a few die. Because of these severe complications, the possibility of lithium intoxication should never be taken lightly. Patients with pre-existing vulnerabilities, particularly in kidney or CNS function, plainly require more careful monitoring.

Interaction of Lithium with Other Drugs

Surprisingly few problems are associated with the use of lithium in combination with other drugs. The major interactions are outlined in Table 23-5.

Psychoactive Drugs

Sedative hypnotics, as well as the benzodiazepines and other related minor tranquilizers, have no clinically significant interactions with lithium,

Table 23-4. Lithium Intoxication

Mild

Recurrence and/or intensification of a previously transient or mild side effect
Difficulty concentrating, cognitive impairment
Muscle weakness, heaviness of the limbs
Irritability
Nausea

Moderate

Drowsiness, lassitude
Dullness, disorientation, confusion
Slurred or indistinct speech
Blurred vision
Unsteady gait
Coarse hand tremor
Restlessness
Muscle twitches
Lower jaw tremor
Giddiness
Vomiting

Severe

Intensification of any of the above
Marked apathy, impaired consciousness, may
   progress to coma
Ataxia
Irregular hand tremor
Prominent generalized muscle twitches
Choreiform/parkinsonian movements

Neurotoxicity Treatment Guidelines[a]

Withdraw lithium
Obtain serum lithium, electrolyte, creatinine
   levels
Carry out complete physical examination
Increase lithium clearance by saline infusion
   in mild to moderate toxic reactions
   (plasma lithium < 3 mmol/liter)
Closely monitor and maintain fluid and
   electrolyte balance
Measure plasma lithium level at least every
   12 hours
Start renal hemodialysis (or peritoneal
   dialysis) If:
      patient is comatose, in shock, severely
         dehydrated, **and/or if**
      plasma lithium level ≥ 3 mmol/liter;
      or if patient fails to respond to 24 hours
         of conservative treatment,
      or if patient's condition deteriorates

---

[a]Adapted from G. Johnson, 1984

although the CNS depressant effects can be additive. The most widely studied interaction is that with neuroleptic drugs, particularly haloperidol. Studies discussed in Chapter 21 suggest that lithium and neuroleptics can be administered together safely as long as the clinician is aware of potential additive effects and uses the lowest effective doses of both drugs (Schou, 1989).

Lithium is quite compatible with tricyclic antidepressants (TCAs), monoamine oxidase inhibitors (MAOIs), and carbamazepine and other anticonvulsants, although some side effects may be additive. For example, patients on lithium plus carbamazepine may experience problems with cognition, memory, and alertness if full doses of both are used.[12] Lithium plus a tricyclic could theoretically have additive effects on cardiac conduction in susceptible individuals, and it is probably unwise to use this combination in patients with pre-existing severe or unstable cardiac conduction defects. This combination may exert additive and even synergistic effects on the production of tremors.

Nonpsychoactive Drugs

Some diuretics (especially the thiazides) can elevate serum lithium levels and produce toxicity, but, as discussed subsequently, this lithium–diuretic synergy can be used therapeutically in some patients. The effects of certain drugs (such as quinidine) on cardiac conduction could, at least theoretically, be potentiated by lithium. Some animal data suggest that lithium potentiates digitalis toxicity by lowering intracellular potassium, but whether this occurs in humans is not clear. What is clear is that the combination of lithium with cardiac drugs, although not contraindicated, requires particularly careful monitoring, including periodic electrocardiograms initially.

Any drug that alters renal function should be used cautiously in patients on lithium, especially if there is a history of kidney disease. Some nonsteroidal anti-inflammatory agents can increase lithium levels and, since these are readily available over the counter, patients should be cautioned accordingly.

Lithium is known to prolong the action of neuromuscular agents. Primarily for this reason, some authorities have suggested that lithium be temporarily discontinued during a course of electroconvulsive therapy (ECT). Small and colleagues (1980) have shown that ECT can be neurotoxic when administered to a patient taking lithium.

Although lithium does not generally interfere with alcohol-induced highs, some patients report that they need more alcohol to produce the de-

Table 23-5. Clinically Important Drug Interactions with Lithium

Drug	Interaction
Diuretics	
Thiazides	Reduce lithium clearance by effect on distal tubular function
Loop diuretics (furosemide)	No effect on lithium clearance
Potassium-sparing diuretic (amiloride)	Can be used to treat lithium-induced polyuria
Nonsteroidal Anti-inflammatory drugs	
Indomethacin Phenylbutazone Naproxen Ibuprofen and others	May increase lithium level by interfering with clearance
Sulindac	No effect on serum lithium levels and lithium clearance
Antibiotics[a]	
Metronidazole Erythromycin	Probable renal effect; may increase lithium level; may also induce diarrhea
Antihypertensives	
Methyldopa	May increase lithium level, may cause neurotoxic symtoms; mechanism uncertain
Clonidine	Lithium may decrease antihypertensive effect
Cardiac Medications	
Digitalis	In combination with elevated lithium levels may cause serious prolonged dysrhythmias
Calcium channel blockers (verapamil, etc.)	May increase rate of lithium excretion
Bronchodilators Aminophylline Theophylline	Significantly increased lithium excretion, possibly increased risk of mortality in those with certain cardiovascular abnormalities
Insulin and Oral Hypoglycemics	Careful monitoring of glucose levels is necessary, since lithium can increase glucose tolerance; mechanism unclear
Digoxin Quinidine	Cardiac conduction effects may be potentiated by lithium; digoxin may reduce effect of lithium
Neuroleptics	Increased risk of neurotoxicity (?); tardive dyskinesia
Anticonvulsants	
Carbamazepine	Additive CNS effects can produce neurotoxicity unless doses are modified
Valproate	May decrease lithium level

[a]In 1978, a case report suggested that tetracycline might cause an increase in lithium levels (McGennis, 1978). This report caused some concern, since tetracycline is commonly used to treat skin eruptions secondary to lithium. However, no other such cases have been reported (Jefferson et al., 1987), and in normal volunteers tetracycline has actually been shown to decrease lithium levels (Fankhauser et al., 1988).

sired alteration in mood, and some inadvertently drink more alcoholic beverages in response to the lithium-induced increase in thirst. Alcohol-related complications, such as cirrhosis, could result. Some patients, on the other hand, drink less alcohol on lithium, particularly if their drinking had been strongly linked to extremes of mood. Lithium has been reported to interfere with cocaine- and amphetamine-induced highs.

Lithium may also decrease the need for certain

medications. Some forms of headache respond to lithium (Abou-Saleh and Coppen, 1983), as does labile hypertension, at least partially. The interaction of lithium with other drugs has been extensively reviewed by Himmelhoch and colleagues (1980) and by Jefferson and Greist (1987).

Impact of Lithium on Other Functions

Lithium produces noticeable effects in addition to attenuating bipolar episodes, and these become especially apparent in the periods between episodes. Patients on lithium sometimes report an apparent intensification of smaller cycles. A woman might become aware of the mood changes accompanying her menstrual cycle, or another patient might identify subtle cycles of activity and energy. These observations are of interest in light of the occasional reports of lithium-induced rapid cycling (see Chapter 22). Such experiences could, however, simply reflect the elimination or attenuation of the major cycles of the illness, which allows the more subtle phenomena to manifest themselves.

Lithium alters sleep, as monitored by the electroencephalogram. Overall depth and length are increased, as are the duration of REM sleep and its latency (reviewed by F.N. Johnson, 1984). It is not clear how much these changes represent alterations in the illness or generalized effects of lithium per se, but lithium's clinical effects on sleep are not striking. In most patients, a large dose at bedtime has a mild sedative effect. Occasionally, patients will report feeling activated after their nighttime dose of lithium, a state that may reflect a high blood level.

One interesting but almost unstudied aspect of long-term lithium maintenance is its potential to improve some aspects of general health. Many lithium-treated patients note fewer common colds and flu-like episodes—a phenomenon that, if real, may be traceable to stimulatory effects of the ion on the immune system. Anecdotal reports have suggested that myocardial infarctions occur less frequently than expected in men maintained on lithium. If true, this might be partially due to a general decrease in mood-related stress or perhaps a direct membrane effect of the drug.

Management of Breakthrough Manias and Depressions

Managing breakthrough episodes (Table 23-6) involves strategies similar to those used for acute

Table 23-6. Management of
Breakthrough Episodes

Hypomania/Mania
(including mixed states)

Increase clinical contact; consider interfering factors
  (e.g., alcohol, drugs, stress)
Increase lithium to maximum tolerable level
Benzodiazepine for sleep (e.g., clonazepam)
Add clonazepam, neuroleptic, or carbamazepine for
  rapidly escalating manic symptoms

Moderate Depression

Increase clinical contact; consider interfering factors
Increase lithium to approximately 1.2 mEq/liter level
  (for bipolar patients)
Maximize thyroid function
Add tricyclic (or heterocyclic) antidepressant or MAO
  inhibitor
Consider alternative/adjunctive experimental
  approach:
    Partial sleep deprivation/phase advance
    High-intensity light (if seasonal)
    Carbamazepine
    Valproate

Severe Depression

Increase clinical contact; consider interfering factors
Add antidepressant and optimize lithium and thyroid
  function
Consider alternative or adjunctive approaches,
  including ECT

---

treatment and described in Chapters 21 and 22. When breakthrough symptoms appear, the most important initial consideration should focus on psychological issues (see Chapter 24), alcohol or drug abuse (Chapter 26), and, especially, compliance (see Chapter 25). Enhanced psychotherapeutic support is especially important at this time and may obviate the need for new medications.

Breakthrough Hypomania and Mania

Detecting hypomania early is critical and often can be done by watching for a decreased need for sleep. If correction of interfering factors or compliance problems does not suffice, the symptoms of hypomania should be treated with increased doses of lithium while closely monitoring the blood level. If hypomanic symptoms persist after reaching a maximum tolerable lithium level, clonazepam, a neuroleptic, or carbamazepine may be added, initially in small doses and preferably at bedtime. Clonazepam is perhaps the easiest to use and, if it aborts the episode by enhancing sleep, may be all that is necessary. Because carbamazepine often is prophylactically effective in patients with rapid cycles, it may be the best alternative for breakthrough episodes in such patients, who can then be maintained on it. Schizoaffective symptoms may require neuroleptics. An alternative for breakthrough hypomania is to add 1.5 to 3 g of L-tryptophan, although use of this strategy cannot be resumed until the origins of the serious eosinophilia myalgia syndrome in patients on L-tryptophan can be clarified.

If full manic symptoms appear rapidly, that is, without a warning period of hypomania, the adjunctive agent must be added immediately without waiting to adjust the lithium level. In this circumstance, neuroleptics may be needed. If these agents are used, they should be tapered off and discontinued soon after the symptoms are under control. A few bipolar patients, generally those with schizoaffective symptoms, will have further breakthrough symptoms when the neuroleptics are discontinued, and for such patients, low maintenance doses generally will be sufficient.

Mania (or hypomania) is associated with a profoundly decreased need for sleep, a symptom that in turn reinforces the mania. Once set in motion by other factors, mania and sleep reduction could keep triggering one another in a vicious cycle that might escalate out of control. Clinicians should counsel patients at risk for mania to avoid situations likely to disrupt sleep routine, help them manage emotional crises that might disturb sleep, avoid using drugs known to interfere with sleep, and carefully monitor drug withdrawal that could precipitate insomnia, such as the rapid withdrawal from antidepressants. When sleep disruption cannot be avoided, such as that associated with flying across several time zones (jet lag), short-acting hypnotics should be employed.

Breakthrough Depression

Breakthrough symptoms of depression, which range from mild to severe, are among the most frequent challenges in managing bipolar patients on lithium. The first response to the appearance of depressive symptoms should include a re-evaluation of interfering substances, of compliance, and of the lithium level and thyroid function, as well as a reassessment of the patient's life situation, with particular attention to real or perceived losses. The lithium level should be raised

to at least 1.2 mEq/liter or higher, since some breakthrough depressions will respond to increased lithium, usually within 7 to 10 days.[13]

A diagnosis of hypothyroidism that is supported by chemical indices should be corrected by supplemental thyroid medication. Even indices in the low-normal range can justify the use of thyroid supplements in the presence of breakthrough depressive symptoms. Since thyroid indices have a wide normal range, it is not always clear whether a normal value is really optimal for a given patient. Many patients with affective illness have low-normal thyroid function before starting on lithium (see Chapter 17). Thus, lithium-induced hypothyroidism may not be obvious from the chemical indices.

Among the lithium clinics surveyed,[14] 44 percent indicated that they would place a patient on supplemental thyroid medication if chemical indices were in the low-normal range and the patient was complaining of fatigue, apathy, and possible depression. Thirty-three percent said they use supplemental thyroid medication even when the indices are in the normal range if the patient is suffering from a refractory depression characterized by psychomotor retardation.

In our own practices, we find that rigid adherence to the range of thyroid indices usually considered normal would deprive many patients of the considerable benefits provided by small doses of supplemental thyroid medication. Dosages should start at 10 μg of T_3 or 25 μg of T_4 once a day (but not in the evening or night) and progress in increments of 10 (or 25) μg, with monitoring of blood thyroid indices.[15]

If the response to thyroid optimization and increased lithium is not satisfactory, the clinician and patient must decide whether to add an antidepressant drug. If the depression is only moderately severe, more psychological support is preferable to antidepressants, which could precipitate mania and worsen the course of the illness, particularly among patients who are especially vulnerable to this (see Chapter 22). This conservative approach is especially appropriate for the patient who has been on lithium for only 1 or 2 years, since clinical experience suggests that prophylactic efficacy may improve with time.

Antidepressants are indicated for patients whose depression is severe enough to cause considerable suffering, especially if it significantly impairs normal functioning. Tricyclics and the newer heterocyclics are the most frequently used antidepressants in this situation. Those with less sedative effects, such as bupropion, fluoxetine, desmethylimipramine, or nortriptyline, are preferred, since breakthrough depressions in bipolar patients on lithium are frequently characterized by anergy and lassitude rather than anxiety, sleep disturbance, and intense psychic distress.

The second-generation heterocyclic antidepressants (e.g., fluoxetine or bupropion) may be preferred if side effects associated with the traditional tricyclic drugs are a source of concern. The efficacy of these new drugs is generally less well established than that of traditional tricyclics, especially when the breakthrough depression is quite severe. However, these new drugs are already widely used, and it would not be surprising if they replaced the classic tricyclics for bipolar patients.

Antidepressant dosages generally should be somewhat lower than those used in the absence of lithium, since some side effects, such as tremor and sedation, can be additive. Because of the risk of precipitating mania or hypomania (even in the presence of lithium), these drugs should be withdrawn gradually shortly after the antidepressant response is achieved.

The use of MAOIs has undergone a minor renaissance, and they are increasingly used as an alternative to tricyclic (or heterocyclic) antidepressants to treat breakthrough depressions in patients on lithium. Some authorities now even recommend MAOIs as the treatment of choice in such cases, and a recent study directly comparing imipramine and tranylcypromine in the treatment of bipolar depression (Thase et al., 1988) found significantly better results with the MAOI. (Studies of the combination of MAOIs and lithium are reviewed in Chapter 22.)

The use of ECT to treat breakthrough depressions in patients on lithium has been advocated by some clinicians, such as Kukopulos and colleagues (1980), because ECT is less likely than antidepressant medication to precipitate a postdepression mania. However, ECT has been reported to cause increased memory loss and neurological abnormalities when administered to patients on lithium (Small et al., 1985; El-Mallakh, 1988).[16] Breakthrough depressions occurring in patients on maintenance lithium often do not fall in the very severe range usually associ-ated with ECT treatments. Nevertheless, it remains an important alternative for this indication.

The alternate antidepressant treatments discussed in Chapter 22 (carbamazepine, partial sleep deprivation or phase advance, high-intensity light) also should be considered in dealing with breakthrough symptoms during prophylactic management. As noted earlier, when carbamazepine and lithium are administered together, dosages may need to be reduced because of possible additive effects on the CNS.

Other Issues in Lithium Maintenance

Timing of the Dose

The pharmacokinetics of lithium have been the subject of a great deal of attention in the medical literature, as have the advantages and disadvantages of various lithium preparations and schedules of administration. Clinical investigators have argued extensively about these issues and whether the greater cost of sustained-release preparations is justified.[17]

It has been suggested that renal side effects (secondary to decreased concentrating ability) are somewhat less frequent when a single daily dose is used, the lower rates presumably due to the rest given the kidneys during the trough in plasma lithium levels 18 to 24 hours after the dose (see, e.g., Hetmar et al., 1986). Several clinical investigators in our survey reported that side effects were exacerbated or illness recurred in some patients shifted from standard preparations to a sustained-release preparation, or vice versa.

Patients prefer as few doses a day as possible. Once a day dosing is more convenient, easier to remember (especially when there are few, if any, symptoms to serve as reminders), and less socially embarrassing; as a result, compliance is better. If the entire dose is taken at bedtime, the peak blood level and the worst side effects occur at night, when the patient is unaware of them. There is extensive evidence that the prophylactic results of once a day administration are as satisfactory as those of divided doses. Some patients require relatively high maintenance levels of lithium but are exquisitely sensitive to its cognitive side effects. They may do better on divided doses or sustained-release preparations, which make it possible to avoid the morning carryover of nighttime peak levels from regular lithium.

Plasma Monitoring

Plasma monitoring should be done as closely as possible to 12 hours after the last dose of lithium, that is, the morning after a bedtime dose. Patients who take their entire dose at night have 12-hour blood levels about 15 to 20 percent higher than those on a divided dose of the standard preparation. Patients who cross several time zones while on lithium must be careful to avoid confusion about the timing of the doses. Anecdotal evidence that jet lag can be associated with mood destabilization in some patients (probably secondary to sleep disruption) indicates that an adequate lithium level is important. For our own patients who travel, we suggest splitting the difference between the old and the new time in planning the dosage schedule.[18] Adequate hydration must be scrupulously maintained during travel, since flying across meridians can induce shifts in fluid and electrolyte balance. Because of the risk of precipitating a switch into mania, sleep disruption should be minimized during travel by using hypnotics when necessary.

Lithium Holidays, Including Pregnancy

Lithium holidays, analogous to neuroleptic holidays, have been advocated by Ayd (1981). They are intended to minimize long-term side effects by giving the body's systems an opportunity to recover from sustained exposure to the drug. Ayd reported mixed results; some patients were able to sustain progressively longer holidays (to the point of withdrawal) without relapse, but others relapsed relatively quickly. In fact, the phenomenon of rapid relapse after lithium withdrawal has now been extensively documented by others (see review in the second part of this chapter). Thus, although lithium holidays may deserve further exploration, they certainly cannot be recommended for clinical practice. A brief holiday is equivalent to lowering the lithium level. Using the lowest maintenance levels that preserve effective prophylaxis, a good practice to follow, can be accomplished best by gradually reducing the daily doses, a procedure that does not produce repeated sudden changes in plasma level. When lithium must be discontinued for appropriate medical reasons, it should be reduced gradually to avoid withdrawal symptoms, particularly sleep disruption.

Lithium holidays may subtly encourage poor compliance. Patients who find themselves free of symptoms and side effects while off lithium with the doctor's blessing may mistakenly assume that they no longer need the drug. Every experienced clinician knows that when patients are taken off lithium for medical or surgical reasons, it can be difficult to convince them to go back on it. If the clinician believes that a patient may be receiving more lithium than needed, the preferred approach is to lower the daily dose gradually. If it is necessary to take a patient off lithium, the safest approach is to decrease the dose gradually until the drug is fully withdrawn rather than gradually lengthening the drug-free periods. Some patients can identify a time of the year associated with less vulnerability, the best time to be off lithium. Conversely, it may be advisable to increase the lithium dose during certain times of the year in patients with a history of seasonal exacerbations.

The most common reason for withdrawing lithium is when the patient wishes to become pregnant. Table 23-7 outlines the risks and the clinical considerations involved in this decision. Many, but by no means all, manic-depressive patients can tolerate being off lithium during pregnancy. Because of the high risk of postpartum mania or depression, those who do go off should resume taking lithium at least a few weeks before the birth is expected.[19] As discussed earlier in this chapter, lithium levels should be lowered immediately before parturition and followed carefully during the immediate postpartum period until the fluid and electrolyte balance is normalized again. Carbamazepine had been suggested as an alternative to lithium because fetal anomalies associated with the anticonvulsant were thought to be rare (Elia et al., 1987), but a recent report (Jones et al., 1989) challenges this opinion.

Lithium Withdrawal or Discontinuation

Extending the lithium holiday into total lithium withdrawal raises the question of whether the patient is thereby rendered even more vulnerable to relapse in the near term. Some investigators have found no difference in relapse rates between the period before lithium was started and after it was withdrawn. Others, however, focusing on bipolar patients, have found relapse rates during with-

Table 23-7. Risks of Lithium During Pregnancy

Teratogenic effects – (Primarily a risk during the first trimester)
Animal studies
- Evidence of abnormal fetal development (Szabo, 1970; Smithberg & Dixit, 1982)
- Limitations in extrapolating animal findings to humans
    Species differences in susceptibility
    Harmful in humans; may not be in animals (e.g., thalidomide)

Lithium birth-registry data (Schou & Weinstein, 1980)
- Increased rate of congenital malformations (11.5% vs 1-3% in general population) especially cardiac anomalies (8%), e.g., Ebstein's anomaly
- Limitations to interpretation
    No control groups
    Potential for bias — overreporting of pathology
    Low overall incidence of birth defects
- 5-year follow-up of 50 normal lithium infants (Schou, 1976)
    No significant differences in incidence of developmental anomalies compared with 51 siblings (20% vs 12% in sibs)
    But findings based on subjective report rather than objective examination

Swedish cohort study (Källén & Tandberg, 1983)
- 350 infants born to manic-depressive mothers compared with all infants born during same period
- Higher than expected rates of perinatal death and congenital malformations
- 4/59 infants (7%) born to lithium-treated mothers had heart defects
    3/4 of these infants died (none had Ebstein's anomaly)
    No cardiac defects in 38 infants whose mothers were treated with psychotropic drugs other than lithium
    2/80 infants of mothers treated without drugs had heart defects (1 had Down's syndrome)

International register of lithium babies (Elia et al., 1987)
- Approximately one case of Ebstein's anomaly per 100 exposures (0.1%)
- Substantially lower risk than earlier estimates, but still 20 times the general population rate
- Fetal ultrasound at 18 weeks can help detect major cardiovascular anomalies (Elia et al., 1987)

Absence of evidence for any teratogenic effect of paternal lithium treatment

Risks during later pregnancy — fetal toxicity potential and blood level changes
Increased glomerular filtration rate during pregnancy speeds lithium clearance
Increased lithium dose may be necessary to maintain symptom control
Lithium freely crosses placenta
Toxicity in neonate manifested by hypotonia, cyanosis, lethargy

Risks during and following delivery
Decreased maternal glomerular filtration rate leads to reduced lithium clearance, higher serum level
Lithium concentration in breast milk about one-half maternal serum lithium level

---

drawal to be higher than expected from the natural course of the illness. On the other hand, Molnar and associates (1987) found a 12-month relapse rate lower than expected from the literature after they had gradually terminated lithium in 15 bipolar patients, although these results require confirmation in more rigorous studies.[20] At any rate, it is known that sudden discontinuation of lithium can produce a cluster of disturbing withdrawal symptoms, such as anxiety, irritability, and emotional lability (King and Hullin, 1983), and it may precipitate a new episode.

We wish to emphasize the common clinical belief that the great majority of bipolar patients withdrawn from lithium will eventually relapse. The wisdom of this assumption is reinforced by long-term follow-up studies (Bouman et al., 1986; Abou-Saleh and Coppen, 1986; Page et al.,

Table 23-7a. Lithium During Pregnancy: Considerations

Manic-Depressive illness itself is associated with some risk to fetus:
Cohort study found higher than expected rates of perinatal death and congenital defects
    regardless of maternal treatment, if any
Potential for suicide during an affective episode
Potential for harm or injury to fetus during an affective episode
Extremely high risk of postpartum depression/mania, especially with previous history of such
    an episode, results in potential risk to mother and infant due to interference with bonding.
    While lithium (re)administered after delivery may prevent postpartum mania, it often takes
    longer term administration to achieve prophylaxis against depression

On the other hand
Some patients report a positive effect of pregnancy on mood
A regular pattern of episodes may permit planning a pregnancy during a "safe" period

Lithium treatment during pregnancy is associated with some risks
Early lithium registry data and cohort study each showed similar high rate of cardiac anomalies
    (7-8%), but recent more extensive registry data indicate a substantially lower risk
Maternal and/or fetal toxicity is possible since increased GFR (and therefore faster lithium
    clearance) may necessitate higher dose for control of affective symptoms

On the other hand
Recent technological advances permit:
    A. neonatal echocardiography to screen for cardiac defects
    B. early surgical correction of most cases of Ebstein's anomaly
Careful monitoring of maternal lithium levels:
    A. reduces risk of developing toxicity
    B. facilitates maintaining minimal effective dose
Alternative drugs are available, i.e., carbamazepine

1987). The Page study involved 101 bipolar and recurrent unipolar patients maintained on lithium for a median time of 13 years. Of the 31 who stopped lithium, all but 2 suffered relapses, and those 2 were unipolar patients; that is, all bipolar patients who discontinued lithium relapsed. We return to these issues later in the review of the literature.

Approaches to Lithium Resistance

Management of Contributing Factors
A poor prophylactic response to lithium is associated with three principal conditions, which frequently overlap: rapid cycling, mixed manic-depressive states, and concomitant alcohol or drug abuse. As discussed in Chapter 22, most rapid cycling occurs when patients are taking antidepressant or neuroleptic drugs. In light of the evidence that some rapid cycling will stop when these drugs are withdrawn (Kukopulos et al., 1980; Wehr et al., 1988), we recommend doing so whenever it is possible. Once off these potentially cycle-inducing drugs, bipolar patients may again become responsive to lithium (Reginaldi et al., 1981).

Mixed states are often confounded with rapid cycling. Because of the mixture of manic and depressive symptoms, patients in these states are usually already taking antidepressants, neuroleptics, or both and are also more likely to be abusing drugs or alcohol. Thus, it is difficult to know whether pure mixed states are in fact resistant to lithium. We recommend that substance abuse be treated aggressively before alternative or adjunctive treatments to lithium prophylaxis are begun.

The Anticonvulsants
Carbamazepine. Like lithium, carbamazepine has been shown to have prophylactic effects in manic-depressive illness in addition to its acute antimanic and antidepressant effects. Although the proper role for this drug in maintenance treatment is not yet completely established, the most important indication for it is unsuccessful prior lithium treatment, because of either unacceptable side effects or prophylactic failure (Table 23-8).[21] When used in these circumstances, carbamazepine is usually given in conjunction with lithium. To minimize CNS side effects for such patients, the maintenance lithium blood

Table 23-8. Alternative or Adjunctive Treatments for Poor Responders to Lithium (Often Rapid Cyclers)

- Evaluate possible cycle-inducing effect of adjunctive antidepressant or antimanic medication

- Evaluate contribution of drug or alcohol abuse

- Anticonvulsants (carbamazepine or valproate)

- MAO-A inhibitor (clorgyline)

- Thyroxine (hypermetabolic doses)

- L-tryptophan

- Calcium channel blockers (verapamil and others)

- Maintenance ECT

- Periodic sleep deprivation

- Magnesium aspartate

level may need to be somewhat lower than that previously described for lithium alone.

Some authorities now recommend that patients with rapid cycles be treated initially with lithium–carbamazepine combinations without first establishing failure on lithium alone. In most instances, however, it is probably still wise to first evaluate the prophylactic efficacy of lithium alone. Nevertheless, most rapid-cycling patients will probably end up on the lithium–carbamazepine combination. Patients may have a continuously circular course (i.e., no true symptom-free interval of more than 3 or 4 weeks) yet not meet the criteria for rapid cycling because they have long, low-amplitude episodes. In our experience, some of these patients respond to lithium and others respond like typical rapidly cycling patients to carbamazepine.

Another important candidate for carbamazepine plus lithium maintenance is the patient who cannot tolerate prophylactic levels of lithium, often because of the onset of nephrogenic diabetes insipidus (NDI). Although carbamazepine (a vasopressin agonist) will not reverse lithium-induced NDI, it may sufficiently potentiate the effects of lithium to allow a substantial lowering of maintenance levels and, therefore, of dose-related side effects.

For patients who cannot tolerate any lithium, carbamazepine alone—generally given twice a day—may provide an alternative. In fact, some studies suggest that carbamazepine is as effective prophylactically as lithium in manic-depressive patients without rapid cycles. More studies will be needed before this can be recommended as standard treatment. As an agonist of vasopressin, which is involved in recall mechanisms, carbamazepine may become especially useful as an alternative in patients who experience memory difficulties on lithium. One emerging potential limitation of carbamazepine is that some patients apparently will relapse after several years of successful prophylaxis, a topic we revisit later in the review of the literature.

The side effects of carbamazepine are outlined in Table 23-9, which also contrasts them with side effects associated with lithium. It is best to start with a low dose (100 mg), building it up gradually (100 mg every 4 or 5 days) until the blood level is just within the range reported as therapeutic for its use in convulsive disorders (6 to 10 μg/ml). A too rapid buildup of the dose or a blood level that is too high can produce troublesome CNS side effects, especially if the patient is also on lithium. Although systematic studies are lacking, at least one group (Nolen et al., 1988) recommends using plasma level determinations performed just before the next dose of the drug is administered. These trough levels should be kept between 6 and 8 μg/ml, and peak levels (2 to 4 hours after drug administration) should generally not exceed 10 μg/ml.

The pretreatment laboratory evaluations for carbamazepine are outlined in Table 23-10 and routine monitoring in Table 23-11. During carbamazepine maintenance, a complete blood count, particularly the white count and numbers of platelets, should be monitored regularly (every 2 to 3 weeks initially, then every 1 to 3 months). Although a benign and transient decrease in the white blood count (to the 3,000 to 4,000 range) is not uncommon, true aplastic anemia is rare.[22] Carbamazepine levels should also be monitored, since, over time, the drug can induce the liver to accelerate its metabolism, and blood levels may decrease on a fixed dose. The clinically important interactions between carbamazepine and other drugs are listed in Table 23-11a. Those that increase carbamazepine toxicity, particularly interactions between carbamazepine and verapamil, are especially important and may require a sub-

Table 23-9. Carbamazepine Side Effects Contrasted with Lithium

Side Effect	Carbamazepine %	Lithium %	Comments
Dizziness/Ataxia	19	<1	Transient, associated with rapid increase in carbamazepine dose
Skin problems:			
Acne		1	Essentially absent for carbamazepine
Rash	13	<1	
Psoriasis		1	Not uncommon in lithium-treated patients who have previously had psoriasis or have a family history of it
Gastrointestinal problems:			
Nausea	10	4	G.I. symptoms are generally transient
Diarrhea	<1	9	
Drowsiness, sedation	10	12	Transient and dose-related
Visual problems:			
Blurred vision		0-14	
Diplopia	8		Transient and dose-related for lithium
Slurred speech	4		Transient and dose-related for lithium
Tremor	3	27	
Paresthesia	3		Transient and dose-related
Confusion	2		Memory problems reported by 28% of lithium-treated patients
Excessive thirst		36	
Excessive weight gain		19	
Polyuria	<1	30	

Carbamazepine data from Post, personal communication; lithium effects from Johnson et al., 1984, and Vestergaard et al., 1980

stantial reduction in the carbamazepine dose (Macphee et al., 1986).

Valproic Acid. Valproic acid was initially evaluated primarily as an antimanic agent, but it does appear to have prophylactic efficacy for some patients. Like carbamazepine, it may be most useful in lithium-resistant patients, and it may also benefit patients who have failed to respond to both lithium and carbamazepine. Side effects of valproic acid are generally mild. Coadministration with lithium may not produce the lethargy sometimes associated with lithium–carbamazepine combinations. For prophylaxis, a low dose (300 to 400 mg) is used at first and gradually built up, depending on clinical response, to a blood level in the 50 to 100 $\mu g/ml$ range. This level is usually achieved at a dose around 1,500 mg, but it may require up to 5,000 mg in some patients. Unlike carbamazepine, valproate does not induce its own metabolism and, therefore, ongoing dose increments are not generally needed. When carbamazepine is administered along with valproate, blood levels should be monitored closely and dosages may need to be adjusted, since there are complex metabolic interactions between the two drugs (Bowdle et al., 1979).

Table 23-10. Pretreatment Evaluation for Carbamazepine

- Complete blood count, including platelets, WBC, reticulocyte, and serum iron
- Liver function tests
- Electrolytes
- Thyroid function: T_3, T_4, and TSH
- Complete urinalysis and BUN
- Rule out history of cardiac, hepatic, or renal damage
- Rule out history of adverse hematological response to other drugs

Adapted from Post et al., 1984a, and PDR, 1989

Table 23-11. Clinical Monitoring for Patients on Carbamazepine

Parameter	Finding	Action	Comment
Dose	400-1,800 mg/day	Individualize	Start slowly, decrease if side effects
Blood level	4-12 μg/ml	Individualize	Enzyme induction after 2-3 weeks may necessitate dose increase
WBC	Consistent mild decreases	Monitor, inform; discontinue drug if WBC below 3,000[a]	Very rare, idiosyncratic aplastic anemia
Rash	10-15%	Discontinue	Restart and treat with steroids if carbamazepine requirement continues
Thyroid	$\downarrow T_4$, T_3, little $\uparrow$ in TSH		Larger decreases in responders
Liver	Occasional $\uparrow$ enzymes		Discontinue if persistent; very rare hepatitis
Sodium	Mild hyponatremia		Very rare water intoxication
Calcium	Mild hypocalcemia		No osteoporosis
Cardiac	Slows AV conduction		Avoid use in heart block

[a] Below 4,000 the clinician should become more vigilant, inform the patient and monitor frequently. Carbamazepine might be discontinued earlier, (i.e., between 3,000 and 4,000) if the platelets are also down, in the presence of red cell abnormalities or systemic symptoms. Also, since lithium produces a nonspecific increase in WBC, a drop below 4,000 in a patient on the combination should trigger discontinuation of carbamazepine.

Adapted from Post and Uhde, 1985, 1987

Other Anticonvulsants. Clonazepam, a benzodiazepine derivative, has been used prophylactically without much success so far. In addition to dubious efficacy, the problems of sedation and the development of tolerance would argue against its maintenance use, although periodic use to abort breakthrough hypomania or manic symptoms is quite sensible. There are anecdotal reports of patients occasionally showing a prophylactic response to diphenylhydantoin, but no systematic data are yet available.

Other Adjunctive Approaches. Aside from the anticonvulsants, the principal alternative to lithium in prophylactic treatment is to maintain optimal or even supraoptimal thyroid function using T_4 supplementation. The experimental use of thyroid preparations alone for prophylaxis is described later. Here we simply emphasize that a bipolar patient should not be considered a lithium

prophylactic failure until plasma T_4 levels at least in the high normal range (10 to 12 μg/ml) have been achieved. Other adjunctive approaches are discussed later in this chapter.

REVIEW OF THE LITERATURE

Open Trials of Lithium Prophylaxis

The first major systematic study of lithium's prophylactic efficacy in manic-depressive illness occurred through the collaboration of Baastrup and Schou in 1967. They analyzed the results of a retrospective study initiated at the Psychiatric Hospital in Glostrup, Denmark, involving all patients with recurrent affective disorders admitted from 1960 through 1966. Patients selected for analysis had an episode frequency ranging from two or more episodes in a year to one episode a year for at least 2 years before lithium administra-

Table 23-11a. Clinically Important Interactions
Between Carbamazepine and Other Drugs

**Increased Carbamazepine Levels and Toxicity
Produced by**
      Erythromycin (and analogs)
      Triacetyloleandomycin
      Viloxazine
      Isoniazid
      Verapamil
      Diltiazem

Decreased Carbamazepine Levels Produced by
      Phenobarbital
      Phenytoin
      Primidone

Carbamazepine Decreases Effects of
      Haloperidol (decreases blood level)
      Clonazepam
      Phenytoin
      Valproate
      Ethosuximide
      Theophylline
      Dexamethasone
      Dicumarol
      Warfarin
      Pregnancy Tests

From Post and Uhde, 1987

tion. All had taken lithium for at least 1 year.

The study's results were striking. Compared with the period before lithium was introduced, episodes during the lithium period had become less frequent among 83 of the 88 patients (94 percent) meeting criteria for the study. The magnitude of the effect is suggested by the fact that before lithium, on average, patients were ill 13 weeks a year compared with less than 2 weeks a year while on lithium, a nearly sevenfold reduction. The frequencies of manic and depressive episodes were affected equally. However, lithium's ability to prevent depression, not always evident initially, seemed to improve with time. In this sample, lithium was equally effective in bipolar and recurrent unipolar patients but was less so in schizoaffective patients. The data from this study are illustrated in Figure 24-3.[23]

In 1970, Angst and colleagues undertook a cooperative follow-up study involving 244 patients in Denmark, Czechoslovakia, and Switzerland. The data from all three countries were similar: Most patients on lithium experienced fewer manic and depressive episodes. Regression analysis indicated that the intervals between the episodes were prolonged and the episodes themselves shortened. As in the original Danish study, bipolar and recurrent unipolar depressives showed similar results, with schizoaffectives showing less pronounced lithium-related changes in the course of their illness.

Baastrup and Schou's 1967 report, a medical landmark, stimulated many trials of this sort in the prophylactic management of manic-depressive illness. By 1972, more than 60 clinical studies comparing the prelithium course of the illness with that found while taking the drug had been published. Like the 1970 international collaborative study, these were based on non-blind administration of lithium to patients with a certain minimum frequency of episodes before lithium (generally about one episode per year). Most studies dealt with groups of 30 to 100 patients and 2 to 3 year observation periods. Although a wide range of criteria was used for scoring an episode, these studies consistently showed good to excellent results. Virtually all showed decreases in the frequency, duration, and severity of episodes. Many of the studies did not distinguish between manic and depressive episodes, but of those that did, most reported that lithium reduced both types of episodes. Some, however, reported more impact on mania, others more on depression. These issues are discussed further below.

By this time, most clinicians who had studied lithium's effects on recurrent affective illness were very favorably impressed. However, skeptics, such as Blackwell and Shepherd in England (1968; also see *Lancet* editorial, 1969), noted that, among patients selected for a trial because of a history of relatively frequent episodes, the natural course of the illness might be expected to show a decreased frequency of episodes during the study period; this decrease reflects a regression toward the mean rather than a drug effect. However, the underlying assumption—that the natural course of manic-depressive illness is random—was contradicted by data indicating a strong tendency for the average frequency of manic-depressive episodes to be nonrandom and to increase with time (see Chapter 6). Three independent studies (Laurell and Ottosson, 1968; Isaksson et al., 1969; Angst et al., 1970) examined the natural course of manic-depressive illness in patients with 2-year histories of frequent episodes—that is, the kind of patients selected for the trials just discussed. In all three of these natural course studies, patients remained at high risk for subsequent episodes in the next 2 years if they remained off lithium. Blackwell and Shepherd had also noted that in the absence of double-blind procedures, observer bias or patient expectation might have accounted for the favorable results. Clinicians very familiar with the illness knew, however, that major episodes of mania (and probably also depression) are unlikely to respond fully to subtle psychological suggestion alone.

Placebo-Controlled Studies

The definitive response to the criticism came when the Danish team undertook a study in which female patients given lithium in a clinic setting and stabilized on it for at least a year were then given either lithium or placebo under double-blind conditions (Baastrup et al., 1970). If anything, the results were even better than those of the earlier open studies. Of the 39 bipolar and unipolar patients switched to placebo, 21 relapsed within 5 months, whereas of the 45 given lithium, not one relapsed. This dramatic difference was, of course, highly significant statistically ($p < 0.001$).

A subsequent study by Coppen and colleagues in England (1971) was especially influential in lessening skepticism in Europe, in part because of its more traditional design, in which comparable groups of patients were randomly started on either lithium or placebo. The design permitted psychiatrists who knew the patients' conditions to administer any additional drugs deemed necessary for episodes of mania or depression in both groups. Criteria for selecting bipolar and unipolar patients resembled those of the earlier studies. Only 1 of the 37 placebo-treated patients could be rated as having had "no conspicuous affective disturbance during the trial period" (averaging 1½ years), in contrast to 20 of the 28 lithium-treated patients. Almost all of the placebo-treated patients (35 of 37) received some additional treatment (tricyclics or ECT for depressions and neuroleptics for manias), whereas only half of the lithium-treated patients did (antidepressant drugs and a few instances of neuroleptics for breakthrough hypomania). No lithium-treated patient required ECT for depression, although 16 of the 37 placebo-treated patients did.

The major study influencing the acceptance of lithium prophylaxis in the United States was that of Prien and colleagues (1974), a collaborative effort of the VA and the National Institute of Mental Health (NIMH). This study, which formed the principal basis of the U.S. Food and Drug Administration's 1974 decision to approve the marketing of lithium, was initiated at a time when the drug was poorly accepted in the United States, largely because of unfortunate experiences with toxicity that had occurred before the importance of maintaining sodium was understood.

The data from these studies further document two aspects of lithium maintenance mentioned frequently in the open studies: the common occurrence of mild or moderate depressive breakthroughs, and the unlikelihood of severe episodes (i.e., those that would have required hospitalization and would have been treated with ECT in this setting).

For most observers, the controlled studies of Baastrup and Schou and of Coppen and colleagues essentially laid to rest reservations based on nonblind administration or selection bias. However, the question remained whether patients selected for and maintained on lithium became dependent on it and, therefore, were more likely to relapse when taken off. Two studies examined this question directly. Schou and colleagues (1970a) and Grof and colleagues (1970) both compared patients' relapse rates during lithium withdrawal and before lithium treatment, and both found no difference in either frequency or severity.

There are ten major double-blind studies comparing lithium prophylaxis to placebo in bipolar patients (Table 23-12). Thirty-four percent of those on lithium relapsed during the trial period compared with 81 percent of the patients on placebo. Nine of the ten studies independently established a statistically significant difference between lithium and placebo; the one that did not had only seven patients on lithium (Melia, 1970). Although the placebo and lithium relapse rates differ across studies, probably reflecting differences in patient selection and in criteria for relapse, the percent difference between placebo and lithium is reasonably comparable, as is the power of the statistical significance.

That lithium has profound prophylactic effects

in bipolar illness is now incontrovertible. However, many important clinical questions remain. For example, how does lithium's ability to prevent depression compare with its ability to prevent mania? What is the likelihood of breakthrough episodes not severe enough to require additional treatment or hospitalization? How does lithium affect subclinical mood lability between episodes? How do additional treatments affect patients receiving long-term lithium? Systematic data are available to answer these questions partially, but the information is thin compared with the data proving that lithium is an effective prophylactic agent in manic-depressive illness.

Relative Prophylactic Efficacy in Mania and Depression

Some reviewers, primarily Americans, appear to assume that lithium prevents mania better than it prevents depression, a position that is perhaps influenced by the prevailing biological theories that postulate that mania and depression are opposite states. Conversely, many European investigators apparently expected that both phases would respond equally, since both were viewed as intrinsic aspects of the same illness. Of the important early European studies, most did not distinguish manic from depressive episodes in reporting relapse frequencies.

In their landmark 1967 study, Baastrup and Schou did not specifically analyze the differential effects of lithium on mania and depression. However, inspection of their individual case histories indicates equivalent prevention of depressive and manic episodes (defined as a period in which symptoms were sufficiently pronounced to require hospitalization or supervision in the home). They also noted that "very many of the patients suffered during these nonpsychotic intervals from phases with slight to moderate depressive or, less often, hypomanic symptoms" (p. 168). This comment suggests that there may have been more mild depressions than hypomania, but they do not discuss whether or how this effect might be related to differences in the relative number of manic and depressive episodes before lithium administration.

Among the open studies, some found both phases affected equally, some found mania more affected than depression, and others reported the opposite. Petterson (1977) compared the number and duration of manic and depressive episodes before and during at least 6 months of lithium treatment in a group of 79 bipolar patients. She found that for men, manic episodes on lithium decreased more than depressive episodes did, but for women, both types of episodes were equally reduced. For both men and women, lithium's effect on the duration of episodes was equivalent for mania and depression.

Three studies using balanced mirror-image pretreatment and lithium-treatment periods, careful selection of patients, and quantitative rating instruments directly tried to answer the question of lithium's relative efficacy in preventing depression and mania (Table 23-13). Holinger and Wolpert (1979) reported on 56 bipolar patients followed over at least 5 years on lithium. All had experienced at least one manic or depressive episode yearly for at least 5 years before lithium treatment. On lithium, manic and depressive episodes each showed a similar decrease. This study is of interest because it includes mild episodes defined by well-delineated criteria. Two later studies indicated better prophylaxis against depression than mania. Rybakowski and colleagues (1980) studied a group of 61 bipolar patients on lithium for 1 to 8 years. An episode was defined as at least 2 weeks of symptoms severe enough to require additional drugs or psychiatric hospitalization. The rate of manic episodes on lithium was 28 percent of the prelithium rate, but depressive episodes were reduced to 16 percent of baseline ($p < 0.01$). Poole and co-workers (1978) conducted a retrospective study of 100 randomly selected patients with clearly diagnosed clinical depression or hypomania-mania, who had been ill an average of 10 years before receiving lithium. A comparison of episodes during the 5 years before lithium treatment with those during the first 5 years on the drug indicated a significantly better prophylactic effect against depression than against hypomania-mania ($p < 0.01$). In this study, however, only major episodes were counted, not milder mood swings.

Of the eight double-blind, placebo-controlled studies that tried to answer this question, two found a greater effect in preventing mania or hypomania than depression (Cundall et al., 1972; Dunner et al., 1976a), two were indeterminate (Stallone et al., 1973; Fieve et al., 1976), and

Table 23-12. Lithium Prophylactic Effectiveness in Bipolar

Study	Trial Period (months)	Design	Treatment	N	% Patients Relapsing[a]
Baastrup et al., 1970	5	DD	LI	28	0[d]
			PL	22	55[d]
Melia, 1970	24	DD	LI	7	57
			PL	8	78
Coppen et al., 1971b, 1973	4 to 26	PR	LI	17	18
			PL	21	95
Cundall et al., 1972	12	CD	LI	12	33[b]
			PL	12	83[b]
Stallone et al., 1973	22[e]	PR	LI	25	44[d]
	8[e]		PL	27	93[d]
Prien et al., 1973a	24	PR	LI	101	43[d]
			PL	104	80[d]
Prien et al., 1973b	24	PR	LI	18	28[b]
			PL	13	77[b]
Fieve et al., 1976	40[e]	PR	LI	17	—[a]
	18[e]		PL	18	—[a]
	30[e]		LI	7 BPII	57
	21[e]		PL	11 BPII	73
Dunner et al., 1976e	17[e]	PR	LI	16 BPII	—[a]
	15[e]		PL	24 BPII	—[a]
Quitkin et al., 1978	10[e]	PR	LI	3 BPII	0
	5[e]		PL	3 BPII	67
		Totals	LI	251	34%
			PL	263	81%

CD = Crossover design; patients already stabilized in lithium maintenance assigned randomly to placebo or lithium; switched to other condition after 6 mo.
PR = Prospective design; patients assigned randomly to treatment condition
DD = Double-blind discontinuation design; patients already on lithium maintenance switched to placebo or lithium
LI = Lithium, PL = Placebo

[a] In studies analyzing manic (hypomanic) and depressive episodes separately, the number of patients relapsing may not have been reported; some patients may have had both manic and depressive relapses.
Reported significance of difference in placebo vs. lithium relapse rates:
[b] $p < 0.05$
[c] $p < 0.01$
[d] $p < 0.001$
[e] Mean trial period

four found lithium equally effective against both phases of the illness.[24] As is clear from a detailed analysis of the controlled studies,[25] there is little support for the notion that lithium is prophylactically more effective against mania than against major episodes of depression. However, mild depressive symptoms do seem to be noted more frequently than mild hypomanic symptoms among patients on maintenance lithium. In interpreting this finding, we should remember that

Patients: Double-Blind, Placebo-Controlled Studies

Relapses %		Comments
Manic/Hypomanic	Depressive	
0[c]	0[c]	Relapse defined as episode requiring hospitalization or
27[c]	23[c]	supplemental therapy. 1 relapse was a mixed state
		Relapse defined as episode requiring hospitalization.
		2 patients in each group had history of schizophrenic
		features in addition to bipolar manic-depressive illness
		Relapses in lithium group were significantly shorter than in
		placebo group
8[b]	25	3 patients had more than one relapse on placebo. 1 patient
75[b]	42	remained well throughout trial. High rate of manic or hypo-
		manic relapses on placebo: effect of lithium withdrawal?
20[b]	28	More rapid dropout rate in placebo group; lithium group
56[b]	48	in remission significantly longer
32[d]	16	Relapse defined as episode requiring hospitalization
68[d]	26	(severe) or supplementary drugs (moderate)
11	22	Part of a larger design comparing lithium, imipramine, and
38	62	placebo
59	29	3/17 lithium-treated required hospitalization compared
94	44	with 9/18 placebo-treated
0	57	
9	64	
6	56	BPII and BP "other" patients only. Relapse defined
25	50	as requiring supplemental medication. Lithium reduced
		severity of depressive relapses
	0	BPII patients previously stabilized on imipramine. Part of
	67	a study comparing lithium with and without imipramine
		to placebo with and without imipramine in BPII and
		UP patients
LI 23%	21%	
PL 56%	37%	

Manic relapses appear to be more common than depressive relapses overall (regardless of drug condition). Lithium appears more effective in attenuating the rate of manic relapses, relative to the rates of each in patients on placebo (problem of base-rate of nonresponders)

Potential sources of underestimation of relapses:
- Dropouts were more likely to occur in response to a manic relapse. A patient first suffering a manic relapse might not remain in the study long enough to have a subsequent depressive relapse counted
- Some investigators reported that lithium reduced the *severity* of depressive relapses; in studies with *hospitalization* as the criterion for relapse, the number of depressive relapses may be underestimated
- Hypomanic episodes may not be experienced by the patient as abnormal

patients are probably less likely to report hypomanic symptoms than depressive ones. In a survey of patient and physician attitudes toward lithium, Jamison and colleagues (1979) found physicians more likely than patients to report lithium as less effective against depression than mania. Perhaps some physicians, on theoretical grounds, have more difficulty accepting lithium's antidepressant effects than their patients do. Cul-

tural differences are also likely to influence the reporting of depressive or manic symptoms. Thus, compared with their American counterparts, Scandinavian and British authors generally seem more impressed with lithium's prophylactic effects against depression. This could reflect a relative underreporting of depressive symptoms by Scandinavian and British patients, who are probably more likely than American patients to

Table 23-13. Relative Prophylactic Efficacy of Lithium: Mania vs Depression:
Longitudinal Studies with Mirror-Image Design

Study	BP Patients N	Episode Frequency (% of Prelithium Baseline)	
		Mania	Depression
Holinger & Wolpert, 1979	56	16	18
Rybakowski et al., 1980	61	28 ($p < .01$)	16
Poole et al., 1978	100	Depression prevented more effectively than manias ($p < .01$)	

suffer depressive symptoms quietly and "tough them out." Likewise, tolerance for hypomanic symptoms undoubtedly also differs in various cultural settings, thus affecting the relative impressions of lithium's prophylactic efficacy.

Quality of the Prophylactic Response

Although research demonstrates that 80 to 90 percent of bipolar patients show some prophylactic response to lithium, no systematic studies have been done to clarify how complete and satisfactory that response is. Some tentative conclusions can be reached, however, by drawing on both the available literature and our survey of experienced colleagues.

One would expect large individual differences in the extent of response, for a variety of reasons. First, patients differ considerably in overall severity of illness and in the frequency, type, and pattern of their cycles. In addition, there are wide differences in clinical management of patients, differences that encompass both pharmacological and psychological factors. Finally, patients differ in the adequacy of their psychosocial support systems.

Although acknowledging this considerable variability, we can still draw some general conclusions about the quality of lithium's prophylactic effects. The most consistent finding in the literature is a decrease in intensity of subsequent episodes. This is probably the fundamental effect of lithium on the illness, and it is fair to say that most patients with typical bipolar illness experience some attenuation of episodes on lithium. Baastrup (1980) estimated that no more than 10 percent of manic-depressive patients show abso-

lutely no prophylactic response. It is, of course, the degree of attenuation that determines whether the response is clinically adequate. Lithium's effect in decreasing the duration of subsequent episodes could be viewed, at least in part, as reflecting the fundamental modulation of intensity, so that only the most severe tip of the episode now appears in the pathological range—that is, the episode appears shortened. This is illustrated in Figure 23-2.

By lessening the intensity of episodes, lithium also decreases their frequency, since most, if not all, expressions of the cycle are brought below a threshold necessary to be considered an episode. Thus, in the controlled studies of lithium's prophylactic efficacy, episodes were scored according to strict criteria reflecting major pathology. Any substantial attenuation of episodes was probably recorded as a reduction in frequency.

Lithium also changes the nature of symptoms that characterize breakthrough episodes. Despite the lack of systematic studies in this area, the descriptive literature, along with our own clinical impressions and those of the colleagues we surveyed, suggest that during breakthrough depressions while a patient is taking lithium, anxiety, depressive mood, psychic pain, suicidal ideation, and psychotic features all are attenuated considerably. By contrast, depressive psychomotor slowing and inhibition, which may be less affected by lithium, can become relatively more prominent.[26] However, lithium-altered hypomania or mania has primarily been viewed as an across the board modulation without a noticeable qualitative shift in the nature of the symptoms.

An interesting but as yet unanswered question

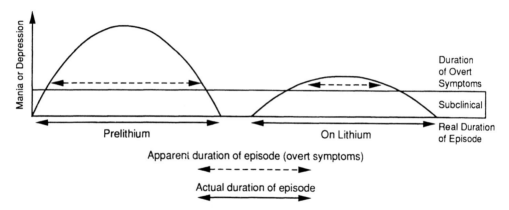

Figure 23-2. Lithium can shorten the apparent duration of episodes by attenuating their severity. By dampening the intensity of an episode, lithium can shorten the duration of overt symptoms. The actual duration of the full episode, including a subclinical phase, need not be shortened. Some episodes will be dampened to a level below the threshold criteria for a clinical episode, contributing to a decrease in frequency as well.

is whether lithium reduces mood lability between episodes. In their classic paper, Baastrup and Schou (1967) noted that patients value this aspect of lithium almost as much as they do the actual prevention of major episodes. Referring to patients' subclinical mood shifts between episodes, these authors noted that:

It was with these patients that some of the most gratifying lithium results were obtained. Hypomanic over-optimism and hyperactivity disappeared, depressive periods with tiredness and lack of initiative were prevented, and capricious phase shifts no longer occurred. (p. 168)

Subsequently, Pons and colleagues (1985) noted an interepisode stabilizing effect of lithium, based on changes in a word-association test. On the other hand, Goodnick and associates (1987) found no difference in interepisode functioning between patients above and below the median lithium level (0.82 and 0.52, respectively). DePaulo and colleagues (1982) noted that when bipolar patients on lithium rated their mood using visual analog scales, they reported less mood variation than normal subjects did. This finding may mean that lithium exerts a general mood-stabilizing effect (i.e., attenuating normal mood fluctuations) or that bipolar patients are accustomed to greater mood variability, which causes them to judge the truly normal range as less variable than normal. The impact of this on medication compliance is discussed in Chapter 25.

In summary, almost all patients have some response to lithium, but reminders of the illness remain while on the medication. Many experienced clinicians have concluded that, in general, the overall quality of the prophylactic response to lithium does appear to improve with time. It is not clear whether this observation primarily reflects progressively improved interepisode mood stability or gradually increased attenuation of the episodes themselves. It is unlikely to be entirely explained as the consequence of poor responders' dropping out of treatment early. Nevertheless, the question of whether one should persist with lithium prophylaxis with patients who fail early in treatment is still unsettled in the literature (Prien et al., 1983).

Prophylaxis in Children, Adolescents, and the Elderly

Although lithium has been used in all age groups since the initial prophylactic trials, studies of treatment efficacy in the very young and the elderly are for the most part uncontrolled. Thus, conclusions about the parameters of lithium administration for these age groups must be more tentative.

DeLong and Aldershof (1987) analyzed the outcome of 59 manic-depressive children and adolescents (mean age, 10.9; range 3.1 to 20) who had been treated with lithium for up to 9 years. For 66 percent of the subjects, lithium prophylaxis was retrospectively judged to be successful. Efficacy in many cases was inferred from the relapses that followed temporary discontinuation of the drug. Those younger than 14 years did as well as those 14 or older. Children who had other conditions without a clear mood component (e.g., attention deficit disorder) did not respond to lithium, although among a group of seven children with unspecified symptoms but with a lithium-responsive parent, five did respond to lithium.

Retrospective parental ratings of the behavior of 21 manic-depressive children were significantly better after successful lithium treatment than before in a study by Younes and colleagues (1986). Posttreatment ratings were still significantly more deviant for the manic-depressive children than those for the control children, however.

In one of the most careful studies done to date on young manic-depressive patients, Strober and colleagues (in press) prospectively followed 37 bipolar-I adolescents stabilized on lithium over 18 months (with serum levels ranging from 0.7 to 1.4 mEq/liter). The relapse rate among the 13 patients who discontinued lithium shortly after being discharged from the hospital was 92.3 percent, nearly three times greater than patients who continued taking the drug. Among those who continued, early relapse was associated with an increased risk of recurrence.

The prophylactic efficacy of lithium among the elderly has rarely been studied, although the sensitivity of these patients to certain side effects and the lower dosages they require have been emphasized.[27] In their prospective study of 166 bipolar and recurrent unipolar outpatients, Murray and colleagues (1983) found no age-related decrease in lithium efficacy. They did note that, with age, manic symptoms grew increasingly prevalent and severe, a trend they interpreted as reflecting the natural course of the illness. The lithium treatment of the elderly has been reviewed by Foster and Rosenthal (1980).

Lithium Prophylaxis of Bipolar-II and Cyclothymic Disorders

As noted in Chapter 4, the subgroups of bipolar-II and cyclothymia probably exist on a continuum with bipolar-I manic-depressive illness. Although most of the prophylactic studies reviewed previously are limited to bipolar-I patients, it is not always clear whether some patients from these subgroups are included. Although bipolar II and cyclothymia are often referred to as "milder

forms" of bipolar illness, this notion can be misleading, especially for the bipolar-II patient with serious depressive episodes. Less obvious is the potential severity of cyclothymia, where the relentless recurrences can produce cumulative damage to the individual's life.

Unfortunately, there are very few studies of lithium prophylaxis in these subgroups. Dunner and colleagues (1976a) compared bipolar patients on lithium ($n = 12$) with those on placebo ($n = 20$) over a long period of study with an average of about 16 months and found a significant prophylactic effect against hypomania and a trend toward less severe depressive episodes (i.e., fewer hospitalizations for depression in the lithium group). Quitkin and colleagues (1978, 1981b), as part of a larger study, found that three of four bipolar-II patients given lithium remained free of depressive symptoms over the 1-year trial. Peselow and associates (1982), using a longitudinal life table analysis of 102 bipolar-II patients on lithium for 2 years, found that the probability of a depressive relapse averaged about 50 percent. It is difficult to know what this means, since there was no placebo comparison group or an estimate of the relapse rate before lithium was started, nor did the authors comment on preventing relapses of hypomania.

There are even fewer data available on lithium prophylaxis among cyclothymic patients, perhaps partly because the issue of diagnostic boundaries is more difficult. Dunner and colleagues (1976a), during a 14-month study period, noted that one of four cyclothymic patients on lithium had a depressive relapse compared with two of the four on placebo. In a life table analysis by Peselow's group (1982), the cyclothymic patients on lithium ($n = 69$) had a 70 percent probability of a depressive relapse over 2 years. However, as with the bipolar-II patients, no placebo or pretreatment comparisons are available, and the impact of a hypomania is not discussed. Akiskal and colleagues (1979) conducted an open study of lithium over 1 year in 15 cyclothymic patients compared with 10 with "nonaffective personality disorder." Focusing on nonadaptive behavior associated with hypomania, they found clinically significant improvement (greater than a 50 percent decrease in the behavior) in 60 percent of the cyclothymic patients vs only 20 percent of those with personality disorders. Prophylaxis against depression, although not specifically commented on, is suggested by the fact that the majority of the cyclothymic patients on lithium opted to remain on it.

Alternative or adjunctive prophylactic approaches (e.g., antidepressants) are capable of inducing mania or shortening the cycle length in bipolar patients (discussed in Chapter 22). Given these potential risks, it is all the more important that there be a credible research base on which to make prophylactic treatment decisions for bipolar-II or cyclothymic patients. Until more data are available, we continue to believe that if prophylactic medication is to be used for these milder cyclic mood disorders, the regimen should include lithium (or another mood stabilizer).

Comparison of Bipolar and Recurrent Unipolar Illness

How does lithium's prophylactic efficacy compare in bipolar and recurrent unipolar illness? As noted earlier, most of the early open studies of lithium prophylaxis included both unipolar and bipolar patients, although generally bipolar patients predominated. Of the studies that make the distinction, four reported equivalent efficacy in both groups,[28] and two noted slightly better prophylactic effects in the recurrent unipolar patients (Misra and Burns, 1977; Hullin et al., 1975). Davis (1976) conducted a critical review of the literature and concluded that unipolar patients had a slightly better response than bipolar patients when differences in numbers of subjects were weighted (Davis, 1976). Interestingly, none of these studies reported a better prophylactic effect in bipolar than in unipolar patients, although the inclusion of a few rapid-cycling patients in some of the bipolar samples could have biased the results somewhat. Overall, the results of the open studies suggest that lithium is as effective in preventing recurrent unipolar illness as it is in preventing bipolar illness. As observed by Baastrup and Schou (1967), "Patients with predominantly depressive phases in the history almost always became ardent devotees of the treatment and attended to the daily intake with great punctuality" (p. 168).

Four controlled studies compared lithium and placebo in unipolar and bipolar groups separately. Three of these (Prien et al., 1973b; Coppen et al., 1971; Baastrup et al., 1970) showed no difference between the two groups. In a crossover study, Cundall and colleagues (1972) reported a strong effect in bipolar patients, but they could draw no conclusions about unipolar patients because of a high dropout rate.

In his review of the literature, Schou (1978), using weighted means of the percentages of patients relapsing within 1 year, calculated that the proportions of unipolar and bipolar patients relapsing on lithium were virtually identical (22 percent vs 20 percent) (Table 23-14).

In a collaborative study, Prien (1984) found maintenance imipramine superior to lithium overall in preventing unipolar depression, a difference primarily due to the superior efficacy of the tricyclic against more severe depressive episodes. On the other hand, several groups have found lithium equivalent or superior to tricyclics in the prophylaxis of unipolar illness.[29]

In his review of prophylaxis in recurrent unipolar illness, Schou (1979b) calculated that the 1-year relapse rate was 35 percent for TCAs among 187 patients vs only 22 percent for lithium among 76 patients (Table 23-14). The difference between these data and the results of Prien and others might be explained by two factors: First, patients with more severe depressions may do better on tricyclics. Second, the unipolar data reviewed by Schou are drawn from patient groups having recurrence rates similar to the bipolar patients, that is, an episode every 12 to 24 months. Many of the patients in the Prien study had less recurrent forms of unipolar illness. Indeed, the median number of prior episodes in Prien's bipolar group was nearly twice that in the unipolar sample.

As pointed out by Baldessarini and Tohen (1988), the literature on pharmacological prevention of recurrences among unipolar patients is dominated by heterogeneous unipolar samples and by relatively short-term trials, with only a few studies going on for 2 years and fewer still for 3 years, probably the minimum time needed to evaluate the true prophylactic effect of a drug. In other words, what is probably the dominant phenomenon assessed in these studies is the ability of a drug to stabilize the recovery from an acute episode, that is, diminish the likelihood of an episode reemerging (continuation treatment as opposed to prophylaxis). In an interesting reanalysis of the 1984 collaborative study of Prien

Table 23-14. Prevention of Manic-Depressive Illness with Lithium and with
Tricyclic Antidepressants: Summary of the Controlled Trials

Diagnostic Group	Medication	Patients[a] N	Relapsing Within a Year[b] %
Lithium vs Placebo			
Bipolar	Lithium	186	20
	Placebo	187	73
Unipolar	Lithium	76	22
	Placebo	77	65
Antidepressants vs Placebo			
Bipolar	Antidepressants[c]	26	65
	Placebo	10	68
Unipolar	Antidepressants[d]	187	35
	Placebo	187	67

[a]Excludes patients who withdrew from trial for reason other than relapse
[b]Includes patients who withdrew from trial because of relapse
[c]10 patients received imipramine; 1 received maprotiline
[d]72 patients received imipramine; 107 received amitriptyline; 8 received maprotiline

Update of Schou, 1979b

and colleagues, Shapiro and colleagues (1989) established the importance of the type of index episode for the prevention of relapse or recurrence in a 2-year follow-up period. For patients whose index episode was manic, lithium provided the greatest stability and imipramine the least, whereas results with the combination were intermediate. For those whose index episode was a depression, the combination was superior to either drug alone (lithium and imipramine results were similar). The importance of the index episode may reflect the fact that much of what is being measured in relatively short-term studies is the impact of postepisode stabilization during the traditional continuation phase of treatment.

After their review of the so-called long-term maintenance studies of recurrent unipolar depression, Baldessarini and Tohen (1988) conclude:

These studies provide strong evidence for a partial protective effect of lithium or of a few imipramine like agents for several months after apparent recovery from an acute episode of major depression. . . . The evidence for a longer-lasting average protective effect against major recurrences . . . and for reduced morbidity . . . over 1–2 years is good for lithium alone or in combination with a TCA [tricyclic], but not as strong for a TCA alone. (pp. 137–138)

We strongly support Baldessarini and Tohen's call for longer-term studies of unipolar patients, starting when they have fully recovered and stabilized, perhaps 6 to 9 months after remission of the acute symptoms. However, as we and others (Prien et al., 1984) have noted elsewhere, it is difficult to recruit such successful patients into long-term, placebo-controlled studies, since they are being asked to run the risk of suffering a relapse by being assigned to the placebo group. Hence, contemporary long-term studies tend to attract patients who have not responded to treatment or are otherwise dissatisfied with it.

Lithium Prophylaxis of Schizoaffective Disorders

The problematic diagnostic category of schizoaffective disorder has undergone various evolutions and transformations (see Chapter 5). After reviewing studies employing RDC or DSM-III criteria, we concluded that the bulk of what has been called schizoaffective disorders (especially schizomania) cannot be distinguished from bipolar illness on the basis of family history, outcome, or response to treatment. Smaller segments of the schizoaffective spectrum appear to represent a variant of schizophrenia or a true coexistence of schizophrenia and affective illness.

Diagnostic heterogeneity confounds the literature on lithium prophylaxis of schizoaffective disorder, especially in early studies that did not use quantifiable criteria of proven reliability. In their comprehensive review of ten studies comparing lithium's prophylactic efficacy among schizoaffective patients ($n = 220$) with that among bipolar patients ($n = 574$), Goodnick and Meltzer (1984) noted that the earlier studies generally reported somewhat better results with bipolar patients, whereas the more recent studies find equivalent efficacy. Perhaps the most important difference between the earlier and the more recent studies is that contemporary diagnostic criteria for schizoaffective disorder require a return to normal functioning between episodes. The study of Bouman and colleagues (1986) is representative of the more recent literature. Using the individual retrospective control method over a 10-year period,[30] they found that lithium was associated with a 92 percent reduction in the number of episodes among schizoaffective patients compared with a 71 percent reduction among the bipolar patients. One of the criteria defining an episode in this study was a preceding symptom-free period of at least 1 month.

Patients with a predominance of schizomanic episodes have a better prophylactic response than those with more schizodepressive episodes (Brockington et al., 1980a, b; Kemali et al., 1985; Maj, 1988). This observation is consistent with the data reviewed in Chapter 5 that links schizomania with bipolar disorder and schizodepressive syndromes with schizophrenic disorders.

Impact of Lithium on Naturalistic Outcome

What is the relevance of the impressive results of the earlier controlled studies of lithium prophylaxis to the ordinary bipolar patient? Although approximately 70 percent of the bipolar patients studied remained free of relapses when maintained on lithium, their experience may not be typical. They were carefully selected, treated in optimal settings, and followed for relatively short periods.

Several attempts have been made to examine the impact of prophylactic lithium from a larger public health perspective. These efforts range from studies of outcome among bipolar patients receiving treatment in the community to analyses of year by year changes in hospital admission rates for mania as a function of when lithium became established as a standard treatment.

In one major outcome study, for example, Harrow and colleagues (in press) followed 73 bipolar patients for 1.7 years after hospitalization for mania and found that overall outcome was not encouraging: 26 percent good, 40 percent intermediate, and 30 percent poor. Poor outcome was similar among those on lithium (36 percent) and not on lithium (32 percent) during the month before follow-up. Similar findings have been reported from the Chestnut Lodge follow-up study (McGlashan et al., 1984). On the other hand, a recent report from a major lithium clinic in the United Kingdom (Coppen and About Saleh, 1988) continues to report very high effectiveness in both bipolar and recurrent unipolar illness, using the same indicators employed in the original double-blind studies.

Length of follow-up cannot be invoked to explain the differences between these recent studies and the earlier controlled trials for two reasons. (1) Like the controlled trials, the follow-up studies also involved relatively brief periods. (2) Long-term studies (10 to 15 years) of lithium prophylaxis have produced results that are at least as good as the short-term controlled studies (see, e.g., Page et al., 1987), as one would expect from other data suggesting that short-term prophylactic outcome is predictive of subsequent long-term outcome (Carroll, 1979; Cazzulo et al., 1980; Page et al., 1987).

Disparities in patient characteristics probably explain some of the discrepancy in findings. Given the widespread use of lithium, it is likely that patients who are referred to university-based research settings may already have failed to respond to lithium when administered as part of the standard treatment available in the community. They also may be diagnostically atypical. For instance, lithium was a much better prophylactic agent for the bipolar patients in the 1973 VA-NIMH collaborative study (Prien et al., 1974) than it was in the 1984 NIMH collaborative study (Prien et al., 1984), conducted after lithium was an established treatment in the community.

Differences in treatment setting also explain some of the discrepancy between recent follow-up studies and the earlier prophylactic trials. The optimal maintenance treatment of bipolar disorder is generally not simple, especially finding the appropriate treatment for breakthrough episodes and dealing with compliance issues. Since lithium's prophylactic efficacy is widely accepted, clinicians may not pay sufficient attention to psychosocial factors that influence the patient.

Dickson and Kendell's report (1986) of a threefold increase of admissions for mania to the Royal Edinburgh Hospital between 1970 and 1981 has generated considerable interest. During that 12-year period, lithium use increased tenfold in that hospital, and the authors assert that the increase in admissions for mania "cast some doubt on the efficacy of lithium prophylaxis in ordinary clinical practice" (p. 521). However, it is questionable whether there has been a real increase in the diagnoses of mania in Edinburgh.[31] Certainly, major diagnostic shifts from schizophrenia to bipolar illness have been demonstrated in the United Kingdom (Horgan, 1981) and elsewhere (Baldessarini, 1970; Parker et al., 1985). Dickson and Kendell dismiss this possibility, citing stability in the proportion of manic, hypomanic, and schizoaffective diagnoses in their hospital over the 12 years. However, since the diagnostic shift in question is from schizophrenia to affective illness, it is difficult to see how the point helps their argument.

It is also quite possible that the actual incidence of bipolar illness could have increased, as it has in the United States (see Chapters 7 and 16).[32] Although the rate of mania in Scotland was apparently stable over those 12 years, the possibility of an increase in Edinburgh, possibly caused by immigration, was not considered. Drug and alcohol abuse increased sharply in Edinburgh during that period, which could increase the baseline rate for mania and also render more bipolar patients resistant to lithium. Also not discussed was the likelihood of increased use of antidepressant drugs during this period, with the attendant greater risk of mania and lithium-resistant mania, as suggested by Kukopulos and Tondo (1980) (see Chapter 22).

Despite its problems,[33] the Dickson and Kendell study is useful because it emphasizes two important points: First, more than two thirds of patients with major affective illness do not seek treatment (Shapiro et al., 1984), and, of those

who do, many comply poorly with medication regimens (see Chapter 25). Second, the treatment available to many manic-depressive patients in the community is unfortunately still not the optimal treatment used in many studies and outlined here.

Clinical Predictors of Prophylactic Response to Lithium

Interpretation of data on response predictors for lithium prophylaxis is clouded by variability in the patient groups studied, in methods of lithium administration, in compliance, and in criteria for response. Some conclusions are nonetheless possible if the interdependence of some presumptive predictors is kept in mind. For example, if typicality of the manic-depressive features predicts lithium response, one might expect that a family history of affective illness would also predict it, since diagnostic features and family history are related. The same predictive power might also be expected from any of the biological measures associated with bipolar illness. Unfortunately, these variables are usually studied individually. The clinical predictors of response are summarized in Table 23-15.

General Demographic Characteristics

There is no association between patients age and response to lithium prophylaxis. The relationship between gender and lithium response is less clear. Only a few studies analyze results for men and women separately. Hofmann and colleagues (1974) reported better prophylactic effects for women. Rybakowski and co-workers (1980) noted that men had a greater preponderance of antidepressant over antimanic prophylactic effect, and Petterson (1977) found that although lithium's prophylactic effect on depressive episodes is the same for both sexes, it is more effective against mania in men than in women. Race, nationality, marital status, and other demographic factors have not been studied sufficiently to permit any conclusions, although Prien and colleagues (1974) found marital status to be unrelated to prophylactic outcome.

Diagnosis

The nature of the illness is probably the single most important predictor of prophylactic lithium response. Baastrup and Schou (1967) reported

Table 23-15. Clinical Predictions of Prophylactic Response to Lithium

Patient Characteristics	Prediction
Demographic	
Age	None
Sex	May differ for prevention of mania and depression
Marital status	None
Clinical	
Diagnosis	"Pure" bipolar may respond better than schizoaffective
Family history	For bipolar, shown predictive in some but not all studies. Some confounding with diagnosis
Age of onset	None
Duration of illness	Later stages may be less responsive; confounded with rapid cycling and with tricyclic use
Presence of mixed states	Somewhat poorer response
Frequency of episodes	Rapid cycling (>3 episodes / year) predicts poor reponse (? role of antidepressant treatment)
BPI vs BPII	Unclear
Episode sequence	MDI course significantly more responsive than DMI (see text)
Quality of symptom-free intervals	Fewer symptoms during intervals predict better episode prevention
Pharmacological	
Acute antimanic and/or antidepressant response	Probably predictive but no systematic data
Initial prophylactic response	4 of 5 studies report significant predictive value
Substance abuse	Interference with prophylactic efficacy

lessened response among patients with the most "atypical" features of manic-depressive illness. Although they do not define atypical precisely, their sample apparently included a number of patients in whom schizophrenia-like symptoms occurred both during manic or depressive episodes and during the interval between episodes. Such patients would probably qualify as schizophrenic by contemporary diagnostic criteria. We have just reviewed the data indicating that lithium's prophylactic efficacy among patients with recurrent schizoaffective disorder is equivalent to that among pure bipolar patients. There we noted that an episodic course with well intervals was more predictive of lithium response than was the symptomatic picture within an episode.

Clinical Features

Rosenthal and colleagues (1979) found that among bipolar patients who functioned well between episodes, those with psychotic symptoms during mania responded better to lithium prophylaxis than those without such symptoms. Several groups of investigators have associated the presence of mixed states with a relatively poor

prophylactic response to lithium, at least in the short term (Keller et al., 1986; Himmelhoch et al., 1976; Prien et al., 1988). Some of the atypical patients included among the poor responders in other studies were, no doubt, patients with such mixed states.[34]

Neither the age of onset of the illness nor its overall duration predicts prophylactic response to lithium (Prien et al., 1974; Dunner et al., 1976a), although as described before, both of these variables may be useful in selecting patients most likely to need long-term prophylaxis. Prien (1984) found that bipolar patients whose first episode was manic experienced better prophylactic effects with lithium than did those whose first episode was a depression.

Frequency of Episodes

Virtually all studies of lithium's prophylactic efficacy have focused on patients with relatively frequent episodes, a practical necessity for outcome-based research. However, clinical experience supports the assumption that patients with less frequent episodes also respond to lithium prophylaxis, and at least two controlled studies provide some support for this conclusion. When Prien and colleagues (1974) and Dunner and associates (1976a) separately compared patients with moderate frequencies (one to two episodes every 2 years) and those with lower frequencies (no episodes in two years preceding the study), no significant difference in lithium prophylaxis was found. Patients with rapid cycles (three to four or more episodes per year) have a significantly reduced prophylactic response to lithium.[35] There is some evidence that depressive episodes of patients with rapid cycles are more resistant to lithium than manic ones. The relationship among antidepressant drugs, rapid cycling, and lithium resistance in patients with rapid cycles, as well as alternate approaches to the management of these patients, are discussed in Chapter 22 and previously in this chapter.

Type and Sequence of Episodes

The differential prophylactic effect of lithium in bipolar-I and bipolar-II patients is difficult to tease out of the original lithium prophylactic studies, which were conducted when the boundaries between bipolar I and bipolar II had not been delineated. Undoubtedly, some of the patients included in earlier bipolar groups would be classified as bipolar II under RDC.

Dunner and colleagues (1976a) initially noted that depressive episodes were more effectively prevented in bipolar-I than in bipolar-II patients, although in an update of their data (Dunner et al., 1979), they did not replicate this finding. Kukopulos and colleagues (1980) and Quitkin and coworkers (1978) found that bipolar-II patients experienced a significant prophylactic effect of lithium against depression. When interpreting any pharmacological differences between bipolar-I and bipolar-II patients, one must consider the possibility that the higher incidence of personality and other axis-II disorders among bipolar-II patients (substance abuse, e.g.) could affect drug response (Abou-Saleh and Coppen, 1986).

How lithium prophylaxis is related to episode sequence has not been considered in the major controlled studies. However, in their systematic observations on 434 bipolar patients in a clinical setting, Kukopulos and colleagues (1980) noted significant differences in lithium prophylaxis as a function of episode sequence. They divided their patients into three groups on the basis of the sequence of their episodes: the classic mania-depression-normal interval (MDI) course, which involves a switch into mania from a normal interval, followed by depression, then back to a normal interval, the depression-mania-interval (DMI) course, in which the most profound change occurs—the switch from depression into mania—and the continuous circular (CC) course, in which there is essentially no normal interval (i.e., any symptom-free period is less than 2 weeks). The differential lithium response rates in the three groups are summarized in Table 23-16. The classic MDI course was associated with the most favorable prophylactic response. The DMI course had significantly more patients with only partial responses. Patients with the CC course and short cycles (analogous to rapid cycles) show essentially no response to lithium, and continuous cycles with long cycle lengths respond reasonably well. The best lithium responders in this study were bipolar-II patients with the classic MDI course; all of them showed at least a partial response. Kukopulos's finding has been replicated by three groups (Haag et al., 1987; Grof et al., 1987; Maj et al., 1989), all of whom noted a significantly more favorable prophylactic response among the MDI patients than among the DMI patients. The study of Maj and colleagues is especially noteworthy, since it is limited to patients not previously treated with lithium and prior course was evaluated independently of lithium efficacy. The relatively poor results in patients with the DMI course may reflect the impact of tricyclics given to treat depression; that is, the mania following a depression may often be drug-induced, and such manias may be relatively resistant to lithium treatment.

The pattern of the onset of manic episodes (abrupt vs gradual) was evaluated by Dunner and colleagues (1976a) and found to be unrelated to prophylactic response to lithium. This important issue merits further study. Finally, Post and associates (1988) have suggested that lithium prophylactic efficacy is reduced in the later stages of the illness, an observation that is confounded by rapid cycling and antidepressant treatment.

Acute Response in Mania or Depression

To our knowledge and surprise, there are no systematic studies on the relationship between acute

Table 23-16. Differential Lithium Response Rates

Type of Course	Patients N	Response to Lithium Prophylaxis %		
		Good	Partial	Poor
MDI	119	61	19	20
DMI	78[a]	33		67
CC-long cycle	56	57	20	23
CC-short cycle (rapid cyclers)	50	16	12	72

MDI = Mania, followed by depression, followed by a well interval
DMI = Depression, followed by mania, followed by a well interval
CC = Continuously circular (no well interval exceeding 2 weeks)

[a]32 of these patients (41%) developed a continuously circular course while on lithium

Adapted from Kukopulos et al.,1980; similar results have been obtained by Haag et al., 1986, and by Maj et al., 1989.

antimanic or antidepressant response to lithium and prophylactic response, although clinical experience suggests that acute response probably does predict prophylactic response. There are reports of a significant association between the initial response (during the continuation phase, i.e., the first 6 to 12 months) and the subsequent response.[36] Likewise, in their follow-up study, Prien and colleagues (1974) found that patients who relapsed during the first 6 months on lithium showed a strong tendency to additional relapses in the ensuing 18 months. We must remember, however, that nonpharmacological factors could influence these results. In the multihospital VA setting with a large number of clinicians using lithium for the first time, early relapses may have resulted in considerable discouragement for both physicians and patients, causing less vigorous continued management and reduced compliance. Further study is needed in this area, since clinical experience suggests that an initial failure does not represent adequate justification for discontinuing lithium. We must recall also the frequently cited observation (based primarily on gradual improvement in subclinical episodes) that lithium's prophylactic efficacy improves with time (Schou et al., 1970a). Whether this also applies to major relapses in patients carefully maintained on optimal levels of lithium with good psychosocial support and compliance has not been systematically studied.

Coexisting Problems

Some conditions that exist along with manic-depressive illness, such as the previously noted schizophrenic-like symptoms, also affect lithium's prophylactic efficacy. Presence of alcohol abuse has been associated with decreased lithium response (see, e.g., Himmelhoch et al., 1976; Prien et al., 1974), although the contribution of poor compliance to these results has not been evaluated. Alcohol abuse may be more likely to occur in association with mixed states, which, as we have seen, are associated with relatively poor prophylactic response to lithium. Himmelhoch and associates (1980) noted a relationship between coexisting neurological difficulties and relatively poor response to lithium. The primary problem was the patients' decreased ability to tolerate adequate prophylactic levels of lithium because unacceptable neurotoxicity developed even at low levels. At least one study (Himmelhoch et al., 1976) has shown that the coexistence of other medical illnesses, although complicating administration of lithium, does not interfere with its prophylactic efficacy.

The coexistence of drug abuse has been associated with poor prophylactic response (Himmelhoch et al., 1980). This area requires further study to evaluate the contributions of diagnostic specificity and of lithium compliance. Regarding this latter point, it is possible that individuals prone to alter their moods by taking drugs might also alter them by stopping a drug such as lithium.

Personality characteristics have been examined as predictors of lithium response (reviewed by F.N. Johnson, 1984 and by Abou-Saleh and Coppen, 1986), most in relation to short-term response. It is difficult to interpret these findings because variations in compliance have not been controlled. Lane (1985) noted that patients who did not respond to lithium evidenced continued psychopathology between episodes as measured by the Minnesota Multiphasic Personality Inventory (MMPI). Similarly, O'Connell and colleagues (1985) found that the quality of the patient's social support system predicted good outcome among 60 bipolar patients, but here too differences in compliance were not controlled. Personality predictors of lithium response are discussed in Chapter 12 (see, especially, Table 12-9).

Family History

Many studies that have examined family history show a significant association between a positive family history of bipolar illness and a good prophylactic response to lithium,[37] but not all agree (Dunner et al., 1976a; Misra and Burns, 1977). In an interesting twin study, Mendlewicz (1979) found that identical twins concordant for affective illness have a significantly higher rate of lithium prophylaxis compared with those whose identical twin did not have the illness.

Patient Compliance

All efforts at prophylaxis with lithium are affected by patient compliance. Some estimates of lithium noncompliance exceed 50 percent (see Chapter 25), making it probably the most important variable contributing to differences in prophylactic efficacy (Baastrup, 1969). It may be an especially important intervening variable in the association between certain personality types or behavioral disorders (e.g., substance abuse) and poor lithium response.

Predictors Among Unipolar Patients

Some of the studies cited previously, principally the European ones, included recurrent unipolar patients in the sample but generally did not analyze them separately. Abou-Saleh and Coppen (1986) found that among their recurrent unipolar patients, good prophylactic response to lithium was predicted by more endogenous features, the presence of pure familial depressive disease (see Chapter 5), less personality disturbance, and a good response to lithium during the first 6 months. It has also been suggested that effective lithium prophylaxis among unipolar patients is predicted by the presence of bipolar features,

such as high episode frequency, early age of onset, and family history of mania (Ramsey and Mendels, 1978). Thus, Schou (1979) concludes that the prophylactic efficacy of lithium among unipolar patients with a cycle length between 12 and 24 months (i.e., an episode every year or two, a typical cycle frequency for bipolar patients) is equivalent to that among bipolar patients. Akiskal cites early age of onset and family history of mania ("pseudounipolar" characteristics) as associated with a good prophylactic response to lithium (Akiskal, 1983; Akiskal and Mallya, 1987). Although this formulation corresponds with our clinical experience, controlled data are lacking.

Conclusion

As in general prophylactic studies, investigations of predictors of response to lithium prophylaxis tend to select patients with relatively serious forms of manic-depressive illness and use relatively narrow episode frequency criteria. These limitations must be kept in mind in applying response predictors to clinical practice. In addition, as noted earlier, since the studies we have reviewed focus on a single variable at a time, the contribution of any individual variable relative to the others is not known.

Grof and associates (1979a) tried to remedy this situation in a very careful longitudinal study of 90 patients followed on lithium for an average of 9 years. Evaluating a wide range of clinical features, they conducted a discriminate function analysis on an initial sample, then replicated it with a separate group of patients. The majority of variance in lithium prophylactic response (i.e., reduction in episode frequency) could be accounted for by the following three factors: (1) the diagnosis, (2) the quality of the symptom-free interval, and (3) the recent frequency of episodes. They noted that a good prophylactic response to lithium became increasingly more likely the closer the patient met the criteria for a true recurrent endogenous disorder (involving not only disturbances in mood but also functional incapacity and other carefully defined diagnostic features of manic-depressive illness). They also observed that the more normal the free interval between episodes, the more likely was a good response to lithium. Patients with a history of very frequent recurrences did not show good prophylactic responses. Using this multivariant discriminant analysis, the investigators predicted prophylactic response (or nonresponse) correctly in 87 percent of the patients.

Side Effects of Lithium

In this section, we review the extensive literature on the side effects of lithium, examining first the subjective complaints of patients, then evidence of the drug's effects on organ systems.[38] Studies reporting rates of individual subjective complaints, which are critical to compliance, are summarized in Chapter 25 (Table 25-8), and the pooled data[39] from these individual studies are displayed in Table 23-17.

Subjective Complaints

Most patients receiving lithium experience some side effects. Some effects are relatively pronounced at the beginning of treatment but generally diminish or disappear rapidly (e.g., gastrointestinal symptoms) or more gradually (e.g., tremor in some patients). Surveys of large numbers of patients in lithium clinics (see Chapter 25) indicate that frequency of subjective complaints of individual side effects ranges from approximately 65 percent to 90 percent, roughly twice the rate recorded in manic-depressive patients not on medication (Cassidy et al., 1957).

Not listed in Table 23-17 are the less frequent side effects, including skin problems, loss of libido, and altered taste sensation. In some of the studies reviewed, certain complaints were elicited by specific questions (e.g., tremor, thirst, weight gain, diarrhea, and edema in the Ves-

tergaard study), whereas others were volunteered by the patients, thereby introducing some bias based on what was expected. Indeed, in an earlier study from the same clinic as Vestergaard's (Schou et al., 1970b), the "big five" were reported far less frequently when only spontaneous reports were counted. The very important issue of memory complaints is discussed subsequently.

Sex differences in the rates of reported side effects have received little study. Although Vestergaard and colleagues (1980) and Johnston and co-workers (1979) did report that men complain of tremor more frequently than do women, Duncavage and associates (1983) and a more recent and extensive study from Schou's group (Vestergaard et al., 1988) found no such sex difference.

Side effects become increasingly problematic as people age. The very young tend to tolerate lithium as well or better than middle-aged adults, even over long periods (DeLong and Aldershof, 1987). The elderly must be carefully monitored for signs of toxicity, primarily because of decreased renal clearance.[40]

Some studies, such as those of Judd and colleagues (1977; Judd, 1979), have used normal subjects to evaluate subjective side effects of lithium in order to isolate them from symptoms of the illness being treated. Interpretation of these studies is somewhat limited, however, because lithium was administered for too short a duration for side effects to begin to attenuate, as they are observed to do in clinical practice.

In Chapter 25, we deal with the relationship between subjective side effects and noncompliance and review the complaints most frequently cited as reasons for discontinuing lithium. Side effects may be the most important reason for discontinuing lithium. In a 10-year follow-up of 74 patients, 9 percent had to permanently discontinue lithium because of side effects (Holinger and Wolpert, 1979). McCreadie and Morrison (1985), in a study of lithium discontinuance patterns in southwest Scotland, found that 40 percent of the lithium patients had discontinued the drug; 28 percent of the total patient population attributed their having stopped to side effects. In a long-term follow-up study of 59 lithium patients treated in Britain, Page and associates (1987) found that 19 percent stopped lithium because of side effects. Interestingly, the

Table 23-17. The Most Frequently Reported Subjective Side Effects of Lithium[a]

Side Effect	Pooled %
Excessive thirst	35.9
Polyuria	30.4
Memory problems	28.2
Tremor	26.6
Weight gain	18.9
Drowsiness/Tiredness	12.4
Diarrhea	8.7
No complaints	26.2

[a] Pooled percentages from 12 individual studies. Refer to Table 25-9 for data on the individual studies

three side effects that contribute most to non-compliance involve the CNS, a system that has received perhaps too little emphasis in the studies summarized in Table 23-17.

The well-established, clear relationship between lithium blood level and side effects in individual patients does not appear in cross-sectional studies (Vestergaard et al., 1980; Johnston et al., 1979), probably because clinicians lower the dose (and blood level) in response to side effects. The relationship between blood levels and side effects may also be obscured by individual differences in tissue sensitivity to lithium. Nevertheless, longitudinal studies do show that the lower doses of lithium currently in use (average blood level of 0.67) are associated with a lower incidence of a broad range of side effects when compared with the earlier practice associated with blood levels that were, on average, 30 percent higher (Coppen and Swade, 1986; Vestergaard and Schou, 1988).

Elizur and colleagues (1977) and Zakowska-Dabrowska and Rybakowski (1973) have suggested that the ratio of red cell lithium to plasma lithium may correlate more closely with certain side effects than the plasma level alone, but not all studies support this hypothesis. The type of lithium preparation appears unimportant. Neither Vestergaard and co-workers (1980) nor Johnston and colleagues (1979) could find any difference in overall subjective side effects when they compared sustained-release lithium with standard preparations. Bone and associates (1980) found that patients complained significantly less frequently of lithium side effects when euthymic than when either depressed or manic, but Lyskowski and colleagues (1982) found the opposite.

Effect of Long-Term Lithium on Organs and Systems

Lithium affects all parts of the body, but three targets are the most important: thyroid, kidney, and the CNS, especially when treatment extends over a long period. These effects are outlined in Table 23-18.

Thyroid. Since the first description of goiter in lithium-treated patients (Schou et al., 1968), the ion's antithyroid effects have been studied extensively and shown to involve several different mechanisms (Berens and Wolff, 1975; Cho et al.,

1979). Although relatively few patients experience actual clinical hypothyroidism when treated with lithium, milder manifestations of lowered thyroid function are frequent. From the literature, Männistö (1980) calculated that definite clinical hypothyroidism occurs among 3.28 percent of lithium-treated patients, with women predominating nine to one. However, goiter was encountered in about 5 percent of patients, primarily in those without clinical hypothyroidism, and slightly more frequently in males (Myers et al., 1985). Using broader criteria for hypothyroidism, Wolff (1974) calculated an overall rate of 14 percent. Even higher figures, with estimates ranging up to 34 percent (Männistö, 1980), were obtained when patients were counted who had at least one abnormal thyroid laboratory test during lithium administration. However, Schou's group found that when T_4 and TSH were studied longitudinally, the initial decrease in T_4 was reversed with time, returning to the prelithium level within 12 months (Maarbjerg et al., 1987). These investigators found a low incidence of patients requiring thyroxine treatment for hypothyroidism and recommended that single low values be reevaluated over time.[41] A substantially higher incidence of hypothyroidism has been noted in three other longitudinal studies—7.8 percent at a mean of 3.4 years on the drug (Yassa et al., 1988), 19 percent at a mean of 6.8 years (Joffe et al., 1988), and 42 percent at a mean of 15 years (Stancer and Forbath, 1989).

One problem in evaluating the effect of lithium on thyroid function is the relatively wide range of normal values; substantial changes can occur in individual patients without their falling outside the normal range. In one study that measured the effect of lithium on thyroid, Transbøl and co-workers (1978) evaluated 86 patients on long-term lithium treatment and compared them with a control population. Elevated TSH levels were found in 23 percent (39 percent of the women) of the lithium-treated patients. Significant reductions in free T_3 and T_4, averaging 25 percent, were associated with the TSH elevations. This reduction within the normal range may have clinical significance. Thus, in a group of patients who had been on lithium for at least 6 months, Hatterer and colleagues (1989) found a significant association between low-normal T_4 and complaints of lethargy and cognitive impairment. Moreover,

Table 23-18. Systemic Effects of Lithium

Thyroid
Hypothyroidism in 5-35% of patients — *apparently dose-related*
Nontoxic goiter in 4-12% of patients

Kidney[a]
Tubular function impairment — *related to dose and duration of treatment*
    Decreased renal concentrating ability in 15-30% of patients
    Polyuria in 50% of patients transiently — *persists in 20-40% of patients on long-term*
        maintenance therapy
Glomerular function preserved
Histological change not lithium specific

Nervous System[a]
Usually transient and dose-related; significant as reasons for noncompliance;
    intensification may be evidence of neurotoxicity
Fine tremor in 33-65% of patients — *more frequent in males; persists in 4-50% of patients in*
    maintenance therapy
Decreased motor coordination — *mild ataxia may signal toxicity*
Muscular weakness
Extrapyramidal
"Cogwheel" rigidity (slight in most) in 48-59% of patients — *associated with longer treatment*
Nonspecific EEG changes
Cognitive and memory function (see Chapter 18)

Metabolic
Weight gain in 11-33% of patients — *some may be secondary to hypothyroidism or to*
    thirst-related increases in caloric intake
Altered glucose metabolism
Hyperparathyroidism — *rare*
Mild decalcification, but without clinical osteoporosis

Dermatological[a]
Maculopapular and acne-like lesions — *occur early; reversible; may not recur on resumption of*
    lithium
Psoriasis — *not uncommon in patients with a past or family history of psoriasis*
Moderate hair loss infrequently reported — *almost all cases female*

Cardiovascular[a]
EKG: T-wave flattening or inversion — *benign; reversible*
Sinus node dysfunction — *rare; reversible*
Cardiac arrythmias — *rare, generally dose-related*

Gastrointestinal
Transient, related to rapid dose increase and timing of dose

Respiratory (see text)

Teratogenic (see discussion of lithium and pregnancy in Table 23-7 & 23-7a)

Many of the systemic effects are reflected in subjective complaints (see Table 25-10).

FN Johnson (1984) has reviewed the literature on the potential effects of lithium on sensory systems.

[a]Effects to these systems constitute the majority of the inquiries received at the Lithium Information Center
(Carroll et al., 1986).

mean T_3 within the normal range was significantly lower in patients who relapsed, and it inversely correlated with affective state.

One of the factors contributing to the relatively high rate of lithium-related thyroid effects is a higher than normal rate of prior thyroid disease in this population (Whybrow et al., 1969), especially among rapid-cycling patients (Cowdry et al.,

1983; Bauer and Whybrow, 1988a). There is also a greater frequency of a family history of thyroid disease, reported as 14 percent in one study (Lazarus et al., 1981). Of the many potentially abnormal thyroid indices in patients on lithium, a relatively high prevalence of thyroid autoantibodies (15 to 30 percent in different studies) is of interest because it suggests a mechanism for antithyroid effects (Lazarus et al., 1981, 1986; Deniker et al., 1978). In fact, two studies (Calabrese et al., 1985; Myers et al., 1985) suggest that the presence of autoantibodies before treatment may be disproportionately associated with the development of hypothyroidism on lithium, since the ion produces a further rise in antibody levels. The effects of lithium on thyroid and other endocrine systems has been extensively reviewed by Lazarus (1986).

Kidney. Since the kidney provides virtually the only excretion route for lithium, good renal function is critical for lithium-treated patients. It has long been known that lithium reduces the kidney's ability to concentrate urine, an effect that is largely reversible.[42] Similarly, although serious renal complications were long known to accompany lithium intoxication, the renal effects seen in normal dose ranges were considered innocuous and reversible. Reports of histological changes in the kidneys of patients on long-term lithium prompted a major reevaluation of the question of renal effects, however.

The initial studies of kidney morphology[43] were conducted in patients already showing signs of lithium toxicity or renal problems, such as severe polyuria. Among the 54 patients examined in these studies, 53 had at least one abnormal biopsy. These alarming initial histological reports stimulated a more careful renal biopsy study in which the patients on lithium were not selected for clinical evidence of renal pathology or intoxication (Rafaelsen et al., 1979). Of the 37 patients who volunteered for biopsy, 6 (15 percent) showed histological abnormalities. As in the earlier report, the histological changes involved interstitial fibrosis, tubular atrophy, and sclerotic glomeruli.

Although there is still some controversy concerning the incidence and specificity of the histological changes, the reports set in motion a useful, comprehensive evaluation of lithium's effect on kidney function. The conclusions are summarized in Table 23-18. There is little evidence of any deleterious lithium effect on filtration, the most important renal function. In the studies reviewed, more than 90 percent of the patients showed glomerular filtration rates (GFR) in the normal range, with very few below 50 ml/minute and none below 20 ml/minute.[44] In an interesting study comparing 101 patients on long-term lithium with a control group of patients with affective disorders but not on lithium, no effect of the ion on glomerular filtration (creatinine clearance) was found, and, in fact, men who had never been exposed to lithium (but who had received other psychotropic drugs) actually had a significantly lower clearance than did men treated with lithium (Coppen et al., 1980). In a similar study comparing 268 patients treated with lithium for an average of 38 months with 59 affectively ill controls not on lithium, Gelenberg and colleagues (1987) found no renal damage associated with lithium and only a slight but not significant decrease in GFR. They did, however, note a modest, statistically significant decrease in GFR in association with concomitant antipsychotic therapy. A study using a sensitive measure of GFR (DePaulo et al., 1986) reported a small negative correlation with duration of lithium therapy in a group of 86 patients, but the correlation could be attributed to just a few subjects apparently predisposed to progressive lithium-induced polyuria. Caution in the long-term use of neuroleptics and lithium together is, however, suggested by the small study of Bucht and colleagues (1980), who found more pronounced histopathological changes and lower concentrating capacity in ten patients on combination therapy than in ten who were taking lithium alone.

Thus, the combined clinical experience of a large number of lithium clinics suggests little or no clinically important effect of lithium on glomerular function. This experience is reinforced by individual studies and reviews[45] indicating that while lithium decreases GFR slightly, by and large the measure remains within the normal range. Furthermore, no association has been found between lithium administration and renal failure or terminal azotemia requiring dialysis, even in patients continually on the drug for 20 years or more. It is important to note, however, that lithium administration under research clinic conditions (careful monitoring, tendency to use lowest effective dose) is not always replicated in practice settings (Masterton et al., 1988). Thus, the possibility of glomerular filtration problems cannot be ignored.

The effects of lithium on renal tubular function are well established. Estimates of lithium-related impairment in renal concentrating ability range from 15 to 30 percent, an effect that appears to be related to dose. Among 788 patients in nine separate studies, persistent lithium-related polyuria (24-hour urine volume greater than 3 liters) was found in 23 percent. More severe cases of polyuria have been described as lithium-induced NDI, sometimes requiring discontinuation of lithium (Schou, 1968). The study by Coppen and colleagues (1980) is again of interest, since these investigators reported only a very modest difference in concentrating ability between lithium-treated patients and manic-depressive patients not treated with lithium. The low incidence of this effect in the British study may be due, in part, to the practice at that time of using lithium doses lower than in the Scandinavian studies, where more polyuria was encountered.

In summary, the continuous use of lithium over many years does not seem to lead to clinically significant alterations in glomerular filtration. However, tubular concentrating ability is impaired in some patients, and the extent of impairment appears to be related to dosage and, to a lesser extent, to the duration of lithium treatment. Initially, Schou suggested that this effect may be greater in patients who have high peak blood levels associated with once a day administration of regular lithium preparations. Plenge and colleagues (1982) and Grof and co-workers (1982) reported lower urine volume with single-dose lithium, and Rafaelsen and colleagues (1979) suggested there may be an advantage to a single-dose regimen. To answer this question, a study directly compared the Schou and the Rafaelsen clinics (Schou et al., 1982). Single daily doses of regular lithium were found to be associated with less effect on distal tubular function, as reflected by urinary volume.[46]

Certainly, renal problems are more extensive in patients who have had episodes of lithium overdose and intoxication. The possibility that these changes could become irreversible provides a strong reason for scrupulously avoiding periods of lithium intoxication. It is now clear, however, that when lithium intoxication occurs it is due to deliberate overdose or an inappropriately high blood level, usually the result of a failure to adjust the dose during periods of physical illness with fever and dehydration (Schou et al., 1989).[47]

Knowledge concerning lithium's effects on the kidney is quite extensive, more so than most long-term drug effects in medicine. The main effect, decreased concentrating ability in some patients, does not portend a functional deficit in the kidney. Rather, it constitutes an inconvenience that only infrequently becomes a reason for discontinuing lithium. Knowledge of this complication of course underlines the need to monitor kidney function carefully and to maintain adequate hydration.

Nervous System. Side effects related to the nervous system are prominent at the initiation of lithium treatment, but as some accommodation develops, they recede to a more subtle place in the hierarchy of symptoms. Neurological and neuromuscular effects are generally sensitive to blood level, the presence of other CNS-active drugs, and individual patient characteristics, such as age and preexisting neurological status. The importance of these effects stems from two considerations. First, the exaggeration of these subtle changes (particularly those affecting the CNS) often provides the first and most reliable clue to impending toxicity. Second, CNS effects seem to be disproportionately important as reasons for noncompliance. Indeed, because of the importance of the cognitive effects of lithium to compliance, we have chosen to review that entire topic separately.

Tremor, one of the most commonly reported side effects, affects from 30 to 70 percent of lithium-treated patients. It is generally a fine tremor of the hands that tends to become exacerbated with intentional fine coordinated movements. Tremor can vary in intensity, perhaps in relation to mood, psychological stress, and drugs, such as caffeine and antidepressants. In some patients, it decreases with time, although not invariably. It can be treated with β-adrenergic receptor blockers, such as propranolol and atenolol.

Decreased motor coordination occurs more frequently than is generally assumed, perhaps because patients do not volunteer complaints. It is most noticeable early in treatment, but gradually becomes attenuated, a process that probably includes elements of true tolerance as well as adaptive learning. This phenomenon is most clear in athletes,[48] who frequently alter the way they play a game (such as tennis or golf) to compensate for their decreased coordination.

Muscular weakness is noted primarily at the

beginning of treatment. Although most patients do not complain of it beyond this point, some experience decreased tolerance for prolonged exercise, such as long-distance running. It is not clear to what extent these subtle effects are neuromuscular in origin or related to other metabolic changes.

Although extrapyramidal side effects are not commonly seen, concern about them increased after Shopsin and Gershon (1975) reported cogwheel rigidity in 16 of 27 patients receiving lithium, with the incidence related to duration of treatment. Of the 20 patients on lithium for a year or more, 15 showed evidence of cogwheeling. However, in a careful study of 100 patients on lithium alone, Asnis and colleagues (1979) found a moderate level of cogwheel rigidity in 7 percent and very slight evidence of it in an additional 26 percent. Among those on lithium plus neuroleptics, the rate jumped to 55 percent, although symptoms were moderate in most of these patients. Since lithium has some modest antidopamine effects, one might expect mild extrapyramidal symptoms and synergism with neuroleptics. In addition to their association with neuroleptics, the cogwheel symptoms were correlated with older age, higher lithium levels, longer duration of treatment, and the presence of a more marked lithium tremor. These side effects do not respond to anticholinergic medications.

Some (Perényi et al., 1984; Mukherjee et al., 1986) but not all (Waddington and Youssef, 1988) studies of tardive dyskinesia in manic-depressive patients[49] show an association between the syndrome and the duration of neuroleptic treatment. The suggestion that lithium might induce tardive dyskinesia, an inference drawn primarily from case reports, has not been supported by most systematic studies (Perényi et al., 1984; Mukherjee et al., 1986; Waddington and Youssef, 1988). One study, however, links a higher incidence of tardive dyskinesia with longer periods of lithium administration (Dinan and Cohen, 1989), and the question remains unresolved.

Changes in the electroencephalograph (EEG), such as increased amplitude and generalized slowing, are clinically benign at usual lithium doses and may not be detectable. As blood levels of lithium increase, so do EEG changes, which then correlate with the emergence of neurotoxic symptoms (Small and Small, 1973). A few seizures have been cited in case reports, but the relationship to lithium is often not clear. At any rate, at routine blood levels and in the absence of neurotoxicity, a seizure would be an extremely rare occurrence. Among bipolar patients with concomitant seizure disorders, Shukla and colleagues (1988) did not find any worsening of seizure frequency on lithium, and it did not induce seizures in those whose seizure disorder was in remission. Benign intracranial hypertension (pseudo-tumor cerebre), that is, increased intracranial pressure of unknown etiology, has been linked to lithium administration by scattered case reports (see, e.g., Saul et al., 1985 and Cermeño, 1989). Since the syndrome typically occurs and remits spontaneously, a link to lithium is not yet established.

Cognitive Effects. The well-known neurotoxic effects of lithium are documented extensively in the literature.[50] Since the drug's primary action is mediated through the central nervous system, it is not surprising that lithium can cause cognitive impairments of varying types and degrees of severity. Indeed, memory problems are among the side effects of lithium treatment that patients report most frequently (see Chapter 25). Although affective illness itself contributes both to cognitive deficits (see Chapter 11) and complaints about such deficits (Coppen et al., 1978; Abou-Saleh and Coppen, 1983; Englesmann et al., 1988), it is important to bear in mind that impairment of intellectual functioning caused by lithium is not uncommon and, in many patients, leads to noncompliance. Creativity can also be affected (see Chapter 14).

The many complex methodological problems involved in studying cognitive changes associated with lithium have led to conflicting results.[51] In their review of the literature, Ananth and colleagues (1987) found that evidence was equivocal for lithium-induced cognitive impairment, partly because of sample heterogeneity and concurrent affective illness. Animal studies reviewed by Ananth and colleagues were inconclusive, since it is difficult to distinguish toxic effects from pharmacological effects of the drug in nonhuman animals. The authors concluded: "There is no convincing proof that lithium causes memory disorders." Jefferson and associates (1987), on the other hand, while acknowledging the major methodological problems in this literature, found "evidence of impaired cognitive and motor functioning" caused by lithium. Judd and colleagues (1987) came to similar conclusions and wrote, in their summary of lithium's effects on normal subjects, that

... lithium often induces subjective feelings of cognitive slowing together with decreased ability to learn, concentrate and memorize. In addition, controlled studies have consistently described small but consistent performance decrements on various cognitive tests, including memory tests. The available data suggest that the slowing of performance is likely to be secondary to a slowing in rate of central information processing. (p. 1468)

Evidence for lithium's detrimental effects on long-term memory, associative processing, semantic reasoning, memory retrieval, and speed of cognitive and psychomotor performance comes, in fact, from many studies.[52] Results from investigations of lithium and intellectual functioning in patients are less consistent, although certainly suggestive.[53]

Evidence to date, although somewhat inconclusive, leads us to believe that cognitive problems from lithium are far from rare. Our clinical experience, along with that of many of our colleagues, suggests the same conclusion. Furthermore, the fact that lithium exerts its ameliorative effects through the CNS and, at high doses, is neurotoxic suggests that cognitive processes also might be affected. Cognitive problems are too often dismissed as being simply secondary to the affective illness rather than to lithium or to some combination of lithium and underlying illness. Because these effects usually vary with the serum level, here is yet another reason for keeping patients at the lowest effective lithium level.

Neurotoxicity. Clinical signs and symptoms of neurotoxicity (see Table 23-4), which are quite similar to those encountered with other CNS poisonings, provide an early indication of generalized lithium toxicity. Early signs, occurring at levels of 1.3 to 2.0 mEq/liter and entirely reversible, include confusion, cognitive impairment, lassitude, disorientation, slurred speech, restlessness, and irritability. The last two symptoms can be difficult to distinguish from the mixed affective states that are part of the illness in many patients. West and Meltzer (1979) reported on

five patients who developed neurotoxicity, some at relatively modest blood levels (0.7 to 1.7 mEq/liter). These patients had marked anxiety and psychosis during mania, symptoms that the investigators suggested might be associated with increased vulnerability to neurotoxic effects. This finding is of interest in light of the naturalistic observation that psychotic mania is frequently associated with organic symptoms, such as delirium (Kraepelin, 1921; Carlson and Goodwin, 1973). Lithium-induced delirium resolves 1 to 2 weeks after levels return to normal (DePaulo et al., 1982). As the neurological syndrome progresses, frank cerebellar symptoms, ataxia, choreiform or parkinsonian movements, and seizures can occur. This stage is not always reversible, and coma and even death may follow.

In his literature review on long-lasting neurological consequences of lithium intoxication, Schou (1984) noted that coexisting physical illness and use of neuroleptics were very frequent in such patients. Fortunately, the early symptoms usually begin over a number of days. Thus, if the clinician, patient, and family are alert to this possibility, early intervention can be effective.

One group noted the benefits of the early use of hemodialysis (Apte and Langston, 1983). After reviewing the charts of 55 patients with lithium intoxication, Gadallah and colleagues (1988) concluded that hemodialysis should be used when symptoms are severe or when serum lithium levels are high in chronically intoxicated patients (who almost always do show severe symptoms). They found that serum lithium concentrations alone were a poor indicator of severity of the intoxication. Toxicity that developed gradually during maintenance therapy, even at serum concentrations in the therapeutic range, was associated with more serious symptoms than the acute intoxication resulting from a suicidal overdose. However, none of the patients in the Gadallah sample died or suffered permanent impairment as a result of the lithium intoxication.

Reports of more frequent lithium-related neurotoxicity in older patients are somewhat misleading. Age per se probably does not substantially increase the risk of neurotoxicity, but since renal clearance in older patients is decreased, they achieve higher lithium levels on standard doses and are more likely to have elevated blood levels unless the clinician is very careful. Older people are also more vulnerable to lithium-induced neurotoxicity because neurological problems that are independent of their psychiatric illness or its treatment become more common with increasing age, as does the likelihood of being on other drugs.

Some investigators have reported a relationship between neurotoxicity and a higher ratio of red cell to plasma lithium (see, e.g., Elizur et al., 1977), although others have disagreed (West and Meltzer, 1979). Evidence from animal and human studies suggests that brain concentration of lithium may be a more significant measure of neurotoxicity than is serum level. Brain concentrations of lithium rise more slowly after initial administration and stay higher than serum levels after a steady state is attained. Lithium uptake in the brain is not uniform. Some parts of the brain may have toxic concentrations even though the serum level is within the therapeutic range (reviewed by Sansone and Ziegler, 1985).

Since the report by Cohen and Cohen (1974) of irreversible brain damage associated with the combined use of lithium and haloperidol (see Chapter 21), there has been considerable interest in this question. However, recent extensive reviews indicate that if any special synergistic neurotoxicity exists at all, it is uncommon. Nonetheless, these two classes of drugs certainly have additive effects, and when high doses of both are used together, some neurological symptoms can be expected.

In summary, we should refer to the experience of Schou and his colleagues (1989), who studied all cases of lithium intoxication that were recorded for their region of Denmark over a 9-year period. During a total exposure time of 4,900 patient years, there were 24 cases of intoxication. Because each case had a probable cause, principally a suicide attempt or obvious mismanagement, the authors concluded that this complication is quite predictable and, therefore, preventable in most cases.

Cardiovascular System. Lithium has a variety of effects on the heart, which are generally benign. Most common is flattening and inversion of the T-wave on the EKG, seen most often when sensitive measures are used. Lithium's ability to affect conduction mechanisms (Tilkian et al., 1976) or to cause sinus node dysfunction (Roose et al.,

1979) or sinoatrial block (Mitchell and MacKensie, 1982) may be particularly relevant for elderly patients, who are generally more prone to develop these dysfunctions than are younger patients.

There are occasional reports of arrhythmias in patients on lithium. After comprehensively reviewing the literature, Albrecht and Müller-Oerlinghausen (1980),[54] concluded that with careful lithium management, arrhythmias are extremely rare. Six of the ten reported cases involved preexisting heart disease or additional psychotropic medication. Shopsin and colleagues (1979) reported that 4 of their 105 patients taking lithium had died suddenly, a rate that is well above the expected mortality rate. The patients, who were 47, 61, 66, and 69 years old, had family histories of severe cardiac pathology. The authors suggested that lithium may unmask an underlying cardiac defect in highly susceptible individuals.

In a follow-up study of 791 Scottish patients treated with lithium for more than 2 months between 1967 and 1976, Norton and Whalley (1984) found that the mortality rate was similar to the (excess) mortality observed among manic-depressive patients in the prelithium era (see Chapter 6).[55] Similarly, Glen and colleagues (1979) found no relationship between death while on lithium and the length of time on the drug.

Metabolic Effects. Studies of the metabolic effects of lithium have focused on alterations in glucose metabolism, partly because of the very common side effect of weight gain (Peselow et al., 1980; Mellerup et al., 1983; Garland et al., 1988). These studies are confusing and conflicting, probably because of lithium's multiple effects on enzymes and receptors involved in these processes. Lithium's inhibition of cyclic AMP formation is well established and would be expected to produce insulin-like effects, particularly increased cellular glucose uptake, decreased lactate formation, and increased glycogen formation and storage. Although lithium has intensified diabetes in some patients (Mellerup et al., 1983), its long-term use is not associated with any increase in blood sugar (Vestergaard and Schou, 1987), and to our knowledge, it has not been associated with the induction of diabetes de novo.

Lithium produces mild to moderate primary hyperparathyroidism, reflected both in increased parathyroid hormone concentrations (Christiansen et al., 1978) and in modest increases of serum calcium and magnesium. Although earlier studies suggested that these changes were rarely of clinical significance, a more recent report by Stancer and Forbath (1989) challenges this conclusion.[56] Also, the association between increased calcium and depression (Carman and Wyatt 1979) suggests that this phenomenon may contribute to breakthrough depressions. The clinical importance of other endocrine effects of lithium (Männistö, 1980) has not been established. The metabolic effects of lithium have been comprehensively reviewed by Lazarus (1986).

Skin Reactions. Skin reactions to lithium are reported infrequently. Fifty cases in the literature have been reviewed by Bakker and Pepplinkhuizen (1980). The most serious dermatological reaction, although not the most common, is the exacerbation of pre-existing psoriasis, or, rarely, its induction de novo (Skoven and Thormann, 1979). A family history of psoriasis has been suggested as a predisposing factor in some cases, and psoriasis frequently responds to the discontinuation of lithium.

The most frequently encountered skin reaction is a nonspecific maculopapular eruption that generally appears early in treatment, disappears with cessation, and frequently does not reappear when lithium is reintroduced. Acneiform eruptions have been reported occasionally, and rarely folliculitis and exfoliative dermatitis. One study (Sarantidis and Waters, 1983) suggested that skin reactions occur far more frequently in women than in men. Most skin reactions, with the exception of some psoriatic cases, can be managed without discontinuing lithium. The mechanism of lithium-induced skin reactions is not clear, although it probably involves an allergic component. Lithium is excreted in the sweat, and some patients may be sensitized to a foreign substance on or in the skin. Reports that lithium may increase immunoglobulin formation (Weetman et al., 1982) and alter antibody function (Presley et al., 1976), as well as a report of a lithium-induced lupus-like syndrome (Shukla and Borison, 1982), may provide some insight into these dermatological effects.

Hair loss attributed to lithium has been the subject of a number of case reports, which have been reviewed by Mortimer and Dawber (1984). The great majority of the patients have been female. In some cases, the hair loss can be attributed to hypothyroidism and responds to hormonal replacement. Generally the loss begins to be noticed about 6 months after the initiation of lithium treatment. From the relatively infrequent case reports, we might assume that this side effect is uncommon. However, in a survey of 99 lithium-treated patients questioned about hair changes (McCreadie and Morrison, 1985), 42 percent answered in the affirmative, about equally divided between complaints of hair thinning and texture change. These effects may correlate with the concentration of lithium in the hair (McCreadie and Farmer, 1985). Total alopecia areata may occur, but it is very rare (Silvestri et al., 1988).

Bone. Since lithium is known to accumulate in bone, there has been some interest in the possibility of its causing bone decalcification. Earlier reports of this phenomenon were apparently in error, however, and subsequent research indicates that lithium has no clinically significant effect on the mineral content of bone (Birch et al., 1982). There are no reports of increased pathological fractures associated with lithium use.

Respiratory System. The effects of lithium on the respiratory system were noted much later than in other body systems. Although one investigator has reported coincidental improvement of asthma in two patients taking lithium, two reports note that lithium can induce a clinically significant opiate-like depression in patients with chronic obstructive pulmonary disease (Weiner et al., 1983; Wolpert et al., 1985).

Teratogenic Effects. The discovery of lithium-induced teratogenic effects in animals led to the establishment in 1968 of registers for babies born to mothers who had been on lithium during the first 3 months of pregnancy. Fetal abnormalities occur more frequently in these "lithium babies" than in the general population. These very important findings and their clinical implications are discussed in the clinical guidance section of this chapter (see especially Table 23-7).

Adjunctive Treatments for Breakthrough Episodes During Lithium Prophylaxis

Lithium alone is not always adequate as a long-term treatment of manic-depressive illness. When asked how many bipolar patients require supplemental drug treatment, respondents to our survey of clinical investigators gave estimates ranging from 10 to 90 percent, with a median of 50 percent. Some of this variance seemed to arise from differences in patient populations. Respondents with hospital experience, especially in large public hospitals, were less optimistic about the efficacy of lithium alone than were those from private outpatient settings. As demonstrated by Dunner and colleagues (1976a), some breakthrough depressive episodes can be treated successfully by increasing the lithium level. Additionally or alternatively, enhancing thyroid function can ameliorate a depressive episode (Hatterer et al., 1988).

The use of supplemental antidepressants and neuroleptics and other drugs for breakthrough depressions and manias is common clinical practice. In a comprehensive survey of 20 major lithium clinics, Gitlin and Jamison (1984) found that 25 percent of bipolar patients on lithium had been given supplemental tricyclics and 16 percent supplemental MAOIs. Although potentiation of antidepressant effects with combined treatments has been reported (see Chapter 22), remarkably few controlled studies have been done on the treatment of breakthrough depression in bipolar patients receiving lithium.

In Chapter 22, we introduced evidence suggesting that in some bipolar patients antidepressants can precipitate manic or hypomanic episodes and can accelerate the underlying cycle. We reintroduce this important topic here to emphasize that it remains an issue even in patients maintained on prophylactic lithium. Few systematic studies have examined the two important parts of this issue. First, how effective are supplemental antidepressants in preventing or reversing breakthrough depressions when administered continuously or intermittently? And, second, what effect do these treatments have on the long-term course of lithium-treated bipolar patients?

At this writing, we are aware of only two prospective, double-blind studies of bipolar patients that have compared the prophylactic efficacy of lithium alone with lithium supplemented by a tricyclic antidepressant (Quitkin et al., 1981a; Shapiro et al., 1989). Although reviewed previously, both of these studies warrant mention here also. In the Quitkin study, combined treatment was associated with 50 percent more total relapses and two and a half times more manic relapses than lithium alone over the 3-year follow-up period. Women were significantly more vulnerable to manic relapses than were men ($p < 0.05$). What is more, the added cost of the additional tricyclic (i.e., the increase in manic relapses) was not offset by any additional protection against depressive relapses—they occurred at virtually the same (low) rate in both treatment groups. Patients who were most vulnerable to tricyclic-related manic relapses were mania prone—that is, their most recent episode had been a manic episode. In the reanalysis of the original 2-year NIMH collaborative study on maintenance drug therapy in recurrent affective illness (Prien et al., 1984) done by Shapiro and colleagues (1989), lithium provided greater stability than lithium combined with imipramine for patients whose index episode was manic, but this difference did not achieve statistical significance. Unlike the Quitkin study, however, the NIMH collaborative study found that for those whose index episode was depressive, the combination of lithium plus imipramine was superior to lithium alone. It is possible that differences in the results of these two studies reflect differences in the length of follow-up or in dropout rates.

In Chapter 22, we focused on the longitudinal observations of Kukopulos and colleagues (Kukopulos et al., 1980; Kukopulos and Tondo, 1980), who followed 434 bipolar patients over an average of 17 years (Figure 23-3). Kukopulos and Tondo, commenting on the resistance to lithium among patients who developed a postdepressive excitement, offered this hypothesis:

> We suspected that the antidepressant drugs given during the depressive phase were responsible. . . . Therefore, whenever possible, we let the depression finish without antidepressant drugs. The subsequent course of the cases was very different: the end of the depression was gradual; in most cases no hypomania followed. . . .
>
> We tried all of the antidepressant drugs: tricyclics, tetracyclics, MAOIs . . . and all had the effect of mak-

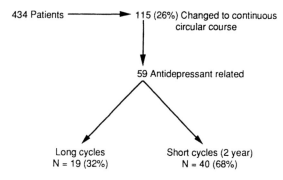

Figure 23-3. An open longitudinal study of 434 bipolar patients (from Kukopulos et al., 1980).

ing the post-depressive mania or hypomania refractory to lithium. Ten non-responders became responders as a result of *not* receiving antidepressants. [emphasis in the original]. . . .

When antidepressants are not given during the depressive phase, the following mania or hypomania disappears [if lithium is maintained]. . . . Only one [continuously cycling patient] kept switching rapidly from depression to mania during lithium treatment, even though he was not given antidepressants. (1980, pp. 146–147)

Kukopulos's experience probably approximates routine treatment approaches with bipolar patients; that is, supplemental antidepressants are used frequently. We recognize, however, that firm conclusions cannot be based on this report alone, since it is not a controlled study, nor does it say how many of the patients who did not develop cycling were treated with tricyclics. Also, it does not indicate how many were continuously on antidepressants. Most problematic is the absence of information on the pretreatment cycle frequency in this group of patients.[57]

In Chapter 22, we discussed the possibility that the impact of antidepressants on the course of the illness in some bipolar patients could be contributing to the higher recurrence rates when the recent (drug) era is compared with the earlier era before drugs were introduced (see Chapter 6). The relative importance of this factor compared to others (e.g., better detection of hypomania, intrinsic change in the illness, greater use of illicit drugs) can only be clarified by further long-term prospective studies, which are sorely needed.

The impact of MAOIs on the long-term course of bipolar illness is even less clear than is the case

with the tricyclics, and we know of no systematic studies on this issue. In his review of the literature, Bunney (1978) noted that MAOIs were apparently as likely to precipitate mania or hypomania as were tricyclics. These data were not derived from patients maintained on prophylactic lithium, however. As noted in Chapter 22, both Himmelhoch's group and Quitkin's group reported that the majority of their lithium-treated bipolar patients whose breakthrough depressions had not responded to TCAs did respond when an MAOI was added to the lithium. The previously discussed study of Kukopulos and colleagues (1980) included an unspecified number of patients whose breakthrough depressions had been treated with an MAOI. These authors imply that the course and outcome were similar to the course and outcome of patients treated with tricyclics. Clearly, further systematic studies are needed.

Two new heterocyclic antidepressants, fluoxetine and bupropion, because of their favorable side effect profiles, are now being used extensively to treat breakthrough depressions in patients on maintenance lithium. Although each of these drugs appears to be less likely to precipitate mania than are the classic tricyclics, this advantage is not yet established. Nor is it yet known what effects these two new drugs will have on the long-term course of the illness.

Even less information is available on how the use of neuroleptics in bipolar patients affects the course of the illness. As will be noted in the section on maintenance neuroleptics, this approach has received little systematic attention. Although the initial study of flupenthixol in bipolar patients suggested that manic episodes might be controlled with the neuroleptic (Ahlfors et al., 1981), a later, better controlled study (Esparon et al., 1986) showed that depot flupenthixol was no better than placebo in preventing breakthrough manias in bipolar patients for whom lithium was inadequate. Nevertheless, experienced clinicians reported in our survey that they continue maintenance neuroleptics in 5 to 30 percent (median 15 percent) of their patients on lithium. The patients most likely to be managed in this way are those who have schizoaffective features while manic, those with rapid cycles, and those with repeated histories of breakthrough manias or mixed states on lithium.

Although the frequency of brief occasional use of neuroleptics to supplement maintenance lithium is not known, this practice is probably more common than the continuous use of these drugs. Several authors have noted the potential for increased incidence and severity of postmania depressions and for tardive dyskinesia when the manic episode has been treated too vigorously and too long with neuroleptics (see Chapter 21).

The effect of acutely administered ECT on the subsequent course of illness has been studied by Small and associates (1986), who reported that patients treated for mania with ECT, then given lithium prophylactically, have lower relapse rates than patients treated with lithium acutely and then maintained on it. This finding may have special relevance for kindling models (see Chapter 15), since ECT has been shown in animals to counteract kindling effects.

MacNeil and co-workers (1975) and Himmelhoch and colleagues (1977) have suggested that some patients with lithium-refractory affective episodes will respond to lithium and thiazide diuretics administered together. This combination should be used with considerable caution, however, since thiazide diuretics produce electrolyte changes and interfere with lithium clearance by the kidney. In Himmelhoch's patients, however, clinical improvement apparently was associated with an increase in plasma lithium to levels that previously could not be achieved without unacceptably severe NDI. These investigators have suggested that, in addition to producing higher lithium levels, thiazide may exert some synergistic action contributing to the improvement, a possibility that requires further study.

Lithium Withdrawal

Several studies document recurrence of illness within a few days to a few weeks in substantial portions of patients withdrawn from lithium (reviewed by Balon et al., 1988).[58] Some authors also report typical withdrawal symptoms, including insomnia. Since sleep loss can precipitate mania, this might explain the unusually high proportion of patients who appear to relapse with sudden lithium withdrawal.

For both theoretical and practical reasons, it would be interesting to know whether long-term lithium treatment produces a rebound effect—that is, a greater likelihood of relapse during withdrawal than would have been the case before lithium was administered. This question has received little attention, and studies that have considered it are difficult to interpret.

The original double-blind study of prophylactic lithium involved its discontinuation (with placebo substitution) for a period of 5 months (Baastrup et al., 1970). The relapse rate during this phase was similar to the prelithium rate and was seen as reflecting simply a recrudescence of the illness. Similar findings were noted by Grof and colleagues (1970). Sashidharan and McGuire (1983) were unable to find any evidence of rebound in their careful retrospective study of 22 patients, and in an open 12-month prospective study of gradual lithium discontinuation, Molnar and colleagues (1987) found no evidence of rebound among 15 bipolar patients.

In contrast, two studies have shown a higher relapse frequency during withdrawal of lithium in bipolar patients. Lapierre and colleagues (1980) compared the frequency of relapse during withdrawal with the pretreatment state, and Mander (1987) compared it with a nonrandomly selected control group of bipolar patients who had not received lithium and who were matched for factors proposed as predictive of outcome. Mander found that 8 of the 29 patients relapsed in the first 3 months, and 7 of the 8 relapses were manic.

The issue is clouded by the heterogeneity of the patient groups. Three of the studies that found no rebound effects involved both unipolar and bipolar patients, and those that did find it involved bipolar patients only. The rate at which lithium is withdrawn may be important, as suggested by Molnar and associates (1987). At this point, the probability of a rebound during lithium withdrawal is still difficult to assess.

Alternate or Adjunctive Approaches to Prophylactic Treatment

Alternatives to lithium in the prophylactic management of bipolar illness have been the subject of a few studies, many of which focus on patients who have failed to respond adequately to lithium. Some alternate treatments are given to supplement rather than to supplant lithium. Some are considered experimental because their efficacy in manic-depressive illness has not been fully demonstrated, whereas others are not truly experimental because major aspects of their clinical use, such as dosage and safety, have already been established. This area has been reviewed by Prien and Gelenberg (1989).

The Anticonvulsants: Carbamazepine and Valproate

Carbamazepine is used to treat a wide range of seizure disorders, especially psychomotor epilepsy or complex partial seizures, and various paroxysmal pain syndromes, such as trigeminal neuralgia. It was tried in manic-depressive patients because it had stabilized the moods of some patients with convulsive disorders, and it counteracted kindling in laboratory animals (see Chapter 17). It was used initially in acute manic states (see Chapter 21), then in prophylactic trials, and the results have continued to be encouraging. So widespread is its use that the practical aspects of prophylactic carbamazepine administration were covered earlier in the clinical guidelines section. Table 23-19 displays the results of the controlled trials, as well as a summary of the open trials.

In a preliminary open study, Okuma and colleagues (1973) reported a prophylactic effect in 14 of their 27 bipolar patients. Ballenger and Post (1978), in the first double-blind trials, noted a prophylactic effect in 13 bipolar patients maintained on carbamazepine for up to 4 months (Figure 23-4). Many of their patients had rapid cycles or had failed to respond to lithium. Okuma and colleagues (1981) conducted a 1-year, placebo-

controlled prophylactic trial in 22 bipolar patients drawn from eight centers. Six of the ten carbamazepine-treated patients, compared with two of the nine placebo-treated patients, had no affective recurrences during the trial, a result that tends to indicate a prophylactic effect ($p < 0.1$). These authors did not indicate how many of their patients had previously responded to lithium. Kishimoto and colleagues (1983) have suggested that responders to carbamazepine prophylaxis are likely to be those with an onset of illness before age 20 and those with frequent illness episodes.

Carbamazepine may be a useful alternative for the prophylactic management of bipolar patients who respond poorly to lithium (see, e.g., Placidi et al., 1986; Watkins et al., 1987), including those with rapid cycles and, perhaps, some with schizoaffective features. Further research is needed to determine whether a carbamazepine–lithium combination is more effective than the anticonvulsant alone. Whether carbamazepine will be as effective as lithium among patients without rapid cycles also requires more investigation, although one study suggests that it is at least as effective prophylactically as lithium in severely ill patients (Lusznat et al., 1988). Kobayashi and colleagues (1988) described a recurrent unipolar patient who was treated successfully with carbamazepine. Among some patients, it appears that the initial prophylactic effect of carbamazepine is not sustained after 3 to 4 years (Frankenburg et al., 1988; Post, 1988a). Post has suggested that this "conditioned tolerance" might be prevented if a symptomatic period off the drug is allowed to ensue.

Although the studies of carbamazepine are encouraging, the number of patients evaluated in double-blind controlled studies is still quite small (less than 50 at this writing), and even these studies suffer from major methodological problems, such as the uncontrolled use of adjunctive medications for breakthrough symptoms. Given the availability of this marketed anticonvulsant, it may never be possible to do the kinds of large studies necessary for its approval by the FDA as a prophylactic agent in manic-depressive illness.

Another anticonvulsant derived from theoretical considerations is *valproate* (or valproic acid), an agent that enhances the action of GABA, an inhibitory neurotransmitter in the CNS hypoth-

Table 23-19. Carbamazepine Prophylaxis in Manic-Depressive Illness

Study	Patients N	Diagnosis	Design	mg / day CBZ (blood level)	Other Drugs	Duration	Results
Controlled Studies							
Ballenger & Post, 1978b	10 CBZ	6 BP 2 UP 2 SA	CBZ vs PBO double-blind controlled on - off	200-1600	Acute treatments added when necessary in 3 patients	Varied	7/10 improved
Okuma et al., 1981	12 CBZ 10 PBO	MDI	CBZ vs PBO double-blind	400-600 ($5.6 \pm 2.0\mu g/ml$)	Acute treatments added during episode breakthroughs	12 mos	6/10 improved on CBZ
Placidi et al., 1986	29 CBZ 27 LI	20 CAD 9 ADSF 19 CAD 8 ADSF	CBZ vs LI random assignment	400 CBZ 300 LI (7-12 mg/L CBZ) (0.6-1.0 mEq/L LI)	Acute treatments added during episode breakthroughs	2-36 mos	At least 2/3 from each group were very much to moderately improved within 3 mo. Diagnostic groups not separated
Watkins et al., 1987	19 CBZ 18 LI	20 BP 17 UP	CBZ vs LI double-blind random assignment	5-12 mg/L CBZ 0.4-0.9 mEq/L LI	Acute treatments added for episode breakthroughs (63% of CBZ patients, 61% of LI patients)	16 mos (CBZ) 20 mos (LI)	Approximately 75% significantly improved on each; but LI associated with a significantly longer remission (16 mo vs 9.4 mo; $p < 0.001$)
Lusznat et al., 1988	20 CBZ 20 LI	Mania or hypomania	12 month follow-up after double blind random assignment	200 CBZ 400 LI (0.6-1.2 mg/ml CBZ) (0.6-1.4 mmol/ml LI)	Acute treatements (antidepressants or neuroleptics) added for episode breakthroughs		9/20 CBZ patients vs 5/20 LI patients were "satisfactory responders"

Summary of open and controlled studies
• Most were LI resistant prior to CBZ administration
• CBZ appears effective in both rapid cyclers and nonrapid cyclers
• Some patients have a better reponse to the combination of CBZ and LI than either drug alone
Overall improvement rate: 271/417 (65%)

CBZ = carbamazepine, PBO = placebo, LI = lithium, CAD = "classic" affective disorder, ADSF = affective disorder with schizophrenic features, SA = schizoaffective

Post and Uhde, 1988, Strömgren and Boller, 1985, and Prien and Gelenberg, 1989, revised and updated

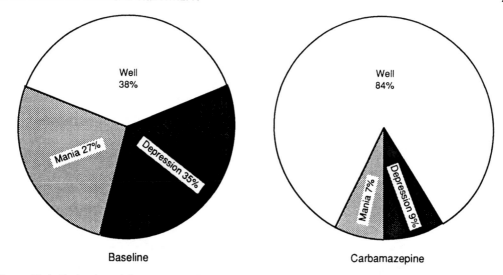

Figure 23-4. Reduction of time spent manic or depressed after treatment with carbamazepine. Thirteen patients with a prior history of rapid cycles or lithium resistance were crossed over to carbamazepine under double-blind conditions. The pie charts illustrate the dramatic reduction in the total time spent ill for the group as a whole (from Post and Uhde, 1987).

esized to be reduced in manic-depressive illness. After a preliminary success in treating acute mania with this drug (see Chapter 21), Emrich and colleagues (1981) conducted a prophylactic trial in seven patients, all of whom remained well during the 18 to 36 month period of observation. This finding suggests an active drug effect, since these patients had histories of relatively frequent relapses. Other studies have confirmed these results.[59] Its prophylactic efficacy may be enhanced when given in combination with lithium (see, e.g., Calabrese and Delucchi, 1989). To date, the prophylactic effect of valproate has been evaluated in nearly 300 bipolar patients, approximately half of whom have been judged as responders. Earlier uncontrolled studies of dipropylacetamide (DPA), which is rapidly metabolized to valproate in the body, showed prophylactic efficacy in bipolar patients when used alone (Lambert et al., 1966) or in combination with lithium (Lambert et al., 1975).

Two other anticonvulsants, diphenylhydantoin and clonazepam (reviewed by Chouinard, 1987), also have been used prophylactically in some bipolar patients,[60] but to our knowledge, controlled studies have not yet been published.

Thyroid Hormone

Thyroid abnormalities have been associated with periodic psychotic states for many years. Gjess-

ing (1976) conducted an extensive series of now classic studies on periodic catatonia, in which he demonstrated major shifts in thyroid function. On the basis of this work, they undertook therapeutic trials with large doses of exogenous thyroid hormone in an attempt to suppress these endogenous fluctuations. Later, Stancer and associates (1970) established the effectiveness of this approach in a controlled trial. Although some therapeutic successes have been achieved, side effects and medical management complications prevented this approach from being pursued in manic-depressive illness. Our survey of clinical investigators revealed anecdotal reports that several lithium-resistant, usually rapid-cycling manic-depressive patients improved when replacement doses of thyroid hormone were used. No further systematic studies have been done, however, and the potential for complications suggests caution in using these hypermetabolic doses of thyroid except under experimental conditions.

A related and more clinically feasible approach has been studied by Bauer and Whybrow (1988b). They found that supplemental T_4, in doses sufficient to produce "supranormal" T_4 levels, successfully converted 10 of 11 lithium-resistant patients with rapid cycles into lithium responders. Of the 4 patients taken off T_4 under double-blind conditions, 3 quickly relapsed. This interesting preliminary finding is consistent with the previously reviewed data (see Chapter 17) indicating an association between low-normal thyroid indices and relapse in bipolar patients on lithium (see, e.g., Extein et al., 1982 and Hatterer et al., 1988).

A Selective Monoamine Oxidase-A Inhibitor

MAOIs appear to be effective antidepressants in some bipolar patients, including some who do not respond to TCAs. The case report literature indicates that MAOIs, like the tricyclics, can precipitate mania and worsen the course of the illness. The clinically available MAOIs are nonspecific. They inhibit both the A and B form of the enzyme (see Chapter 17). Indirect evidence suggests that inhibition of the B form may be associated with some of the deleterious behavioral effects of MAOIs, particularly those associated with the induction of mania and cycles. In a trial of *clorgyline*, an MAOI specific for the A form, the NIMH group noted sustained prophylactic effects in a group of bipolar patients with rapid cycles previously unresponsive to lithium and a variety of other treatments (Table 23-20) (Potter et al., 1982). Despite the small number of patients involved, these dramatic changes are difficult to ignore. Several of the patients have been continued successfully on clorgyline, usually in combination with lithium, for up to 8 years. Preliminary data on two standard (mixed A and B) MAOIs also suggest that there may be a modest lengthening of the cycle among patients with rapid cycles (Table 23-20) (Cowdry, unpublished data). *Moclobemide* is a selective MAO-A inhibitor on the market in several European countries. To our knowledge, it has not yet been evaluated as a treatment for rapid-cycling patients.

Serotonergic Agents

The so-called permissive hypothesis of serotonin was formulated after serotonin metabolites were observed to be low in both mania and depression. Low serotonin function, according to this hypothesis, is associated with decreased modulation of other mood-related neurotransmitter systems, such as norepinephrine, and thus is viewed as part of the predisposition to manic-depressive cycles (see Chapter 17). The hypothesis led to trials of serotonin precursors in the acute treatment of mania and depression (see Chapters 21 and 22).

Table 23-20. Effect of MAO Inhibitors on Average Cycle Length in Days

Patient	Placebo	Lithium	Lithium +TCA	MAOI[a]
		Clorgyline[b]		
1	>220		39	>510
2	32	38		93
3	145	43		90
4	23	10		72
5		35		50
		Tranylcypromine or Phenelzine[c]		
6[d]	>220		39	>58
7[e]	32	38		53
8	25	28	16	>350
9	111			>300
10	75	>72	61	49
11	>106	96	63	42
Adjusted Means	99	45	44	152

TCA = Tricyclic antidepressant
MAOI = Monoamine oxidase inhibitor

[a] Given with conventional treatment in most cases
[b] Adapted from Potter et al., 1982
[c] Adapted from Cowdry, unpublished data
[d] Same as patient 1
[e] Same as patient 2

They have been tried also, but less extensively, for prophylactic management.

Van Praag and DeHaan (1980) conducted interesting preliminary work that integrates the evaluation of drug efficacy with biochemical measures in patients (the biochemical data are discussed in Chapter 17). These investigators reported on a prophylactic trial of the serotonin precursor, 5-hydroxytryptophan (5-HTP) in 20 patients with recurrent major affective disorder, including 6 bipolar patients. Using a drug–placebo crossover paradigm (with patients receiving either a year of 5-HTP followed by a year of placebo, or vice versa), they showed a significant effect of 5-HTP compared with placebo. The prophylactic effect was significantly superior in those patients whose serotonin metabolite levels were relatively low after recovery from the depressive episode.

Use of another precursor of serotonin, L-tryptophan, has, as noted, been suspended pending clarification of its role in the eosinophilia myalgia syndrome. Chouinard and colleagues (1979) reported a case of a rapid-cycling bipolar woman who did not respond to lithium until L-tryptophan was added, a combination that resulted in substantial prophylaxis against both manic and depressive phases. Chouinard later reviewed his clinical experience with this use of tryptophan (1987). Beitman and Dunner (1982) reported a case of a bipolar woman with two episodes a year for 16 years. Although unresponsive to lithium and imipramine, she responded to L-tryptophan (2 gm 4 times daily) alone.

Another approach to evaluating the low serotonin (permissive) hypotheses was taken by Coppen and colleagues (1984), who used a drug presumed to enhance serotonergic neurotransmission by selectively inhibiting the reuptake of the neurotransmitter. They found that this treatment (zimelidine) could not be substituted for lithium in the prophylactic management of bipolar patients, and the drug was later withdrawn from the market because of toxicity.

Fluoxetine is another antidepressant thought to be selective for the inhibition of serotonin uptake. Its antidepressant effects are reviewed in Chapter 22. To our knowledge, no studies have been done of its potential usefulness as an adjunctive agent in the prophylaxis of bipolar disorder, although it has been reported to effectively prevent relapses in recurrent unipolar illness (Montgomery et al., 1988), and, as noted, it is being widely used to treat breakthrough depressions. Its evaluation as an adjunct for the prophylaxis of bipolar illness should be a high priority.

Maintenance Neuroleptic

The prophylactic efficacy of a maintenance neuroleptic (*flupenthixol decanoate*) was evaluated by Ahlfors and colleagues (1981) in 85 bipolar patients, all of whom had been treated with lithium but either responded poorly or had problems with compliance or side effects. When the 2 years before the study were compared with the 18 months on flupenthixol, both the frequency of manic episodes and the percent of time spent ill with mania were significantly reduced. Unfortunately, the frequency of depressive episodes and the percentage of time spent depressed increased significantly. In a later, smaller, but methodologically superior, double-blind study of similar patients, Esparon and colleagues (1986) found no prophylactic effect of supplemental flupenthixol, and, in fact, they found that the patients did worse

than on the placebo. At this juncture it is not clear that this strategy deserves further evaluation, particularly given the risk of tardive dyskinesia (Gardos and Casey, 1984).

Miscellaneous Agents

The new antidepressant drug *bupropion* (see Chapter 22) may also have prophylactic efficacy against both phases of the illness (Shopsin, 1983; Wright et al., 1985). This question clearly deserves further evaluation, particularly in light of the low side effect profile of this agent.

A few case reports and at least one double-blind study (Giannini et al., 1987) suggest that the calcium-channel blocker *verapamil* may have prophylactic effects in rapid-cycling bipolar illness, although not all reports are positive (Barton and Gitlin, 1987). The fact that this drug, unlike other calcium-channel blockers, also blocks dopamine receptors suggests that dopaminergic effects might be mediating its clinical effects. Giannini and colleagues (1987) compared lithium and verapamil in a 1-year, double-blind, crossover study of 20 manic-depressive men already stabilized and maintained on lithium. They found that the patients treated first with verapamil showed clinical improvement after 60 days, whereas the lithium-treated patients improved after 180 days; 60 days after crossover, the group first treated with verapamil and then switched to lithium no longer showed improvement, and the other group was still doing well. The complex interaction of lithium and verapamil suggested by this study warrants further investigation.

Rubidium, an element related to lithium but with physical properties and biological effects opposite to it, has been investigated as an acute antidepressant agent with mixed results in very small numbers of patients. To our knowledge, there is only one report of rubidium as a possible prophylactic agent in manic-depressive illness (Paschalis et al., 1978). Among five bipolar patients with fairly frequent recurrences of episodes, two showed a prolongation of manic episodes and one showed prolongation of both the depressive and manic phases. These changes reversed when the rubidium was withdrawn. Because of the long biological half-life of rubidium and its resulting tendency to accumulate in the body, further trials of this agent probably are not justified.

Magnesium aspartate has been reported to have mood-stabilizing properties in rapid-cycling bipolar patients (Chouinard et al., 1988). To our knowledge, however, no controlled data have been published.

Hypotheses of membrane instability in manic-depressive patients (see Chapter 17) and evidence of abnormal aldosterone fluctuations prompted Hendler (1978) to reason that an *aldosterone antagonist* might stabilize the illness. Of the six patients given spironolactone after demonstrating lithium intolerance, four became stable for 12 to 18 months. Although the follow-up period was short, the fact that the patients had suffered frequent relapses before treatment suggests that there was a medication effect.

Another group of experimental treatments is based on a hypothesized deficiency of membrane ATPase (the sodium pump) in manic-depressive illness and the notion that this deficiency is caused by an endogenous ATPase inhibitor, vanadium. *Methylene blue*, which dampens the effects of vanadium on Na,K-ATPase, was initially reported to be effective in both phases of the illness based on open clinical experience (Narsapur and Naylor, 1983). In a subsequent double-blind, 2-year prophylactic trial in bipolar patients already on lithium, methylene blue was associated with significant additional prophylaxis against depression but not against mania (Naylor et al., 1986). In other studies, this group has noted therapeutic effects of *ascorbic acid* and ethylene diaminetetraacetic acid (*EDTA*), both of which also decrease endogenous vanadium (Kay et al., 1984). Low-vanadium diets (Naylor and Smith, 1981) have been tried with some success as well. Although theoretically interesting, the acceptance of these approaches awaits independent replication.

Sleep Deprivation

As indicated in Chapter 22, sleep deprivation may provide a nonpharmacological alternative or adjunct to psychotropic drugs in some patients. Its prophylactic potential has been explored briefly by one group (Christodoulou et al., 1978; Papadimitriou et al., 1981). Frequency of episodes in the 2 years before initiating weekly sleep deprivation therapy and in the 2 years of follow-up treatment was compared in a mirror-image design. Among the five bipolar patients, two met criteria as responders, one had an equivocal response, and two failed to respond. Further work on this very interesting question is eagerly awaited.

Maintenance ECT

As an approach to prophylaxis, the intermittent use of one or two ECT treatments on an ongoing basis actually predated the use of lithium (Kramer, 1986; Abrams, 1988). Clinical accounts suggest that it is successful in some patients, although to our knowledge, no controlled studies have been done. Clarke and his associates (1988) reported considerable success with the use of maintenance ECT in sustaining ECT-induced remissions among patients with drug-resistant (or drug-intolerant) major depression (whether unipolar or bipolar was not specified). Seventeen of the 24 patients (71 percent) sustained remissions over a minimum follow-up period of 6 months. Almost all of those who relapsed (six of seven) had already dropped out of the maintenance ECT program (described only as "weekly treatments for a few weeks, then biweekly, then monthly for at least four months"). Loo and colleagues (1988) presented case reports of four treatment-resistant patients with affective disorders who also benefited from maintenance ECT. Decina and colleagues (1987) used ECT for continuation treatment of three seriously ill patients over a period of 3 to 6 months and found that it prevented relapses in the two who complied with the treatment schedule.

The use of psychosurgery in patients with severe, treatment-resistant bipolar illness is reviewed in Chapter 18.

SUMMARY

Many years of research were required to convince a skeptical medical community that maintenance lithium can lessen the frequency and severity of episodes in bipolar manic-depressive illness (and in the more recurrent forms of unipolar depression). Substantial clinical research evidence supports the prophylactic power of lithium with striking consistency. Contrary to common belief, among bipolar patients lithium maintenance has been shown to be equally effective against major episodes of mania and of depression, although it may prevent less serious manic episodes more effectively than less serious depressive ones. By lessening the intensity and altering the character of recurrent episodes, lithium reduces their apparent frequency, bringing some below perceptible thresholds. It also alters mood lability between episodes.

For the recurrent unipolar patient who requires maintenance treatment, the clinician must choose between lithium and an antidepressant. Since both have shown prophylactic efficacy in controlled trials, the decision must be based on individual patient characteristics. A maintenance tricyclic (or MAOI)[61] is most appropriate with the more severely depressed patient who required the antidepressant to recover from the acute episode and who has neither a family history of bipolar illness nor bipolar characteristics, that is, a history of cyclothymia, early age of onset, or frequent episodes. For patients with these bipolar characteristics, lithium is the better choice for prophylaxis, even if the severity of the depression required antidepressants for the acute and continuation phases of treatment.

For the bipolar patient, the principal selection criterion for lithium maintenance is a history of at least two major episodes, regardless of frequency. It should be considered earlier when the first episode is manic, the patient is male, onset is sudden or later than age 30, and the patient's family and social network offer little support. For the more recurrent forms of unipolar illness, a minimum of three episodes, usually within 5 years, is generally considered a threshold for prophylaxis, although, compared with bipolar illness, there is less known about the natural course of untreated unipolar illness.

Bipolar patients least likely to respond to lithium prophylaxis include those with atypical, particularly schizophrenic, features, mixed manias, or rapid cycling (perhaps especially when it is related to antidepressants). Patient compliance may well be the most powerful factor of all affecting prophylactic responses.

During lithium maintenance, moderate breakthrough depressive episodes may respond to optimization of lithium and of thyroid supplements, along with additional psychotherapeutic support. More serious episodes generally call for adjunctive antidepressant drugs. Adjunctive tricyclics have received more study than other antidepressants, but recent data suggest that, among bipolar patients, MAOIs, or the newer heterocyclics, fluoxetine and bupropion, may be preferable for this indication. Other alternatives for breakthrough depression include ECT, sleep deprivation, high-intensity light (for winter episodes), and other experimental agents. For breakthrough mania, clonazepam, carbamazepine, or neuroleptics can be added, depending on the type of patient and the severity of the episode.

Promising alternatives to lithium prophylaxis are the anticonvulsants, primarily carbamazepine. In addition to the drug's importance for the patient who cannot tolerate lithium, preliminary data suggest that it is effective for lithium-resistant patients, especially those with rapid cycles. Whether it has a legitimate role in patients who would otherwise be responsive to lithium is not yet clear.

The side effects of lithium have been studied extensively and found to vary considerably in importance and severity. Some, if mismanaged, can be life threatening. Patients most frequently mention such effects as tremor, thirst, weight gain, and gastrointestinal symptoms, most of which subside spontaneously over time. Extensive studies of lithium's bodily effects have revealed three main targets of particular concern—kidney, thyroid, and CNS. Lithium does not impair renal filtration appreciably, but tubular concentrating ability is reduced in some patients, an effect apparently related to dose and duration of administration and one that necessitates monitoring kidney function and ensuring adequate hydration.

Lithium lowers thyroid function (which may already be low or low-normal in some patients). Although most patients compensate for this on their own, many require thyroid supplementation. The effects of lithium on the CNS (initially prominent but then usually subsiding) include decreased motor coordination and cognitive impairment. These effects must be tracked carefully, not only because they can portend impending neurotoxicity but also because they are one of the major reasons for noncompliance.

An additional effect of concern is an elevated rate of a cardiac anomaly (Ebstein's) in infants born to lithium-treated mothers—approximately 1 in 1,000 exposures or 20 times the rate in the general population. Thus, in those cases where it is feasible, lithium should be withheld in anticipation of pregnancy and during at least the first trimester.

The optimal blood level for lithium maintenance treatment of the bipolar patient is generally between 0.6 and 0.9 mEq/liter, somewhat lower than the level recommended for acute treatment of mania. Prophylactic levels for recurrent unipolar illness can be slightly lower. The prophylactic effects of once a day dosing (generally at bedtime to minimize side effects) are as satisfactory as divided doses.

During the first several weeks, blood levels should be monitored weekly to determine the dose/blood level ratio for the individual patient. After stabilization, the frequency of monitoring can be flexible. The patient's clinical state, sex, age, muscle mass, and diet all contribute to the ratio. Special circumstances that require close monitoring and possible adjustment of dosage include the initiation of surgery, weight reduction diets, or unusual physical activity such as long-distance running.

Many of lithium's early side effects can be readily alleviated by altering dosage or giving the appropriate supplemental treatment, such as propranolol (10 to 40 mg/day) for tremor. Loop diuretics can be added to help control lithium-induced NDI. Supplemental thyroid medication can aid in treating hypothyroidism or its clinical manifestations, which can include breakthrough depressions or continued cycling. Weight gain, often associated with noncompliance, requires early and vigorous carbohydrate restriction and attention to the possibility of reactive hypoglycemia and be combined, if necessary, with the use of L-glutamine, which may reduce carbohydrate craving.

Lithium toxicity can be averted by early detection and dose reduction. Patient education and cooperation are essential to aid in monitoring CNS symptoms. Rarely, hospitalization and specialized care may be required for severe intoxication. Lithium has relatively few adverse interactions with psychoactive and nonpsychoactive drugs. The effects of some combinations may be additive, however, requiring dose adjustments of both drugs.

We do not recommend the routine use of lithium holidays, especially when dealing with bipolar patients. Not only is relapse a serious risk,

but such holidays may encourage noncompliance when the medication is resumed.

The fact that lithium maintenance treatment for manic-depressive illness is one of modern medicine's major success stories should not engender complacency. There are still too many patients who do not respond completely. Further pharmacological developments for the treatment of bipolar disorder are urgently needed. We encourage the pharmaceutical industry and the research community to redouble their efforts.

NOTES

1. *Tri-Quarterly* 5, (Winter, 1981) pp. 270–271. Cited in Hamilton, 1982, p. 370.

2. In light of subsequent studies indicating that patients with rapid cycles often do not respond to prophylactic lithium, it is interesting that the initial report of prophylactic efficacy was in a rapidly cycling patient.

3. This complex actuarial study examined increasingly aggressive maintenance strategies. In addition to the most aggressive—starting patients on maintenance lithium after the first episode (an average of 5 years on lithium required to prevent another episode)—the second most aggressive was waiting for the second episode to start maintenance lithium, and the third was to not start maintenance lithium unless the patient experienced a second episode within 2 years. "Patients who do not believe it would be worth 5 years on lithium to avoid one episode but believe it would be worth 2 years should choose one of these two 'wait-and-see' strategies," according to the authors.

4. The majority of patients in this study (21 of 37) were placed on maintenance lithium after their first manic episode. Of those who discontinued the drug during the 18-month follow-up period, 92 percent relapsed, compared with a 37 percent relapse rate among those who stayed on lithium ($p < 0.001$). As noted in Chapter 8, bipolar illness with a very early onset (adolescence) appears to have an unusually high degree of genetic loading, a factor that may predict both greater morbidity and responsiveness to lithium prophylaxis.

5. In assessing the proportion of patients who were maintained on lithium after discharge, Mander (1986) did not differentiate between continuation treatment (up to 1 year) and true prophylaxis (beyond 1 year).

6. The "desirable" lithium level cited in the *Physician's Desk Reference* and package inserts (0.6 to 1.2) is based on earlier literature.

7. In the Coppen et al. (1983) study, the independent variable was the lithium blood level during the trial rather than assignment to one or the other of

the two dose-reduction groups. This leaves open the possibility of an uncontrolled variable. For example, patients who are feeling well over some time may reduce their dose on their own, contributing to the association between lower plasma level and favorable course.

8. Cooper et al., 1973; Perry et al., 1982; Zetin et al., 1986; Lobeck et al., 1987; Rosenberg et al., 1987; Karki et al., 1987.

9. Since some patients may develop tolerance to beta-blockers after prolonged use, Schou and Vestergaard (1987) suggest that their use be on an as needed basis, such as before a social occasion or public appearance. Atenolol, which has a long half-life, can be administered once a day, although its usefulness may thereby be limited for patients who are instructed to take it as needed.

10. Thiazides can be used with caution, however. Himmelhoch and colleagues (1977) offered rough guidelines for the combined use of lithium and thiazide diuretics: 500 mg of chlorothiazide produces approximately a 50 percent increase in lithium levels, and 1 g produces a 70 percent increase. To initiate this combined regimen, the lithium dose should be cut in half, then a low dose (250 mg) of chlorothiazide given. Gradually, both drugs should be increased, with frequent monitoring of the lithium level, electrolytes, and urine output.

11. The association between low folate levels and affective morbidity was not replicated in a later study involving a small number of patients (Stern et al., 1988), and the issue remains unresolved.

12. Compared to carbamazepine, another anticonvulsant, valproic acid, may produce fewer CNS effects when combined with lithium (Calabrese and Delucchi, 1989).

13. A breakthrough depression may result from a drop in the lithium level 10 to 14 days earlier. In other words, the lag in onset of efficacy seems also to be mirrored by a lag in offset of the beneficial clinical effect.

14. Data on the lithium clinics were drawn from the survey conducted by Gitlin and Jamison (1984).

15. Data reviewed in Chapter 22 (Joffe et al., 1988) indicate that T_3 is more effective than T_4 in potentiating antidepressant response to a tricyclic. Whether this also applies to the use of thyroid in patients on lithium is not known. T_3 has the disadvantage of confounding the plasma monitoring of thyroid hormone level.

16. Carbamazepine can complicate ECT treatment by raising the seizure threshold.

17. See reviews by Amdisen and Schou, 1980; Grof et al., 1979b; Coppen et al., 1983; Cooper, 1987.

18. For example, a patient who was flying from the east coast of the United States to Europe would take medications 3 hours earlier on the day before and the day of departure (i.e., the dose schedule would be moved up 3 hours to split the difference between the time in the eastern United States and western Europe). Once in Europe, the dose timing would be according to local time.

19. For a discussion of conflicting opinions on this subject, see Targum et al., 1979; Brockington et al., 1982; Oates, 1986; Stewart, 1988.

20. This was an open prospective study with a sample that was not randomly selected.

21. Among the alternatives to lithium for patients with rapid cycles is magnesium aspartate, a treatment studied as early as 1932 (Mestrallet and Larrivé, 1932).

22. The *Physician's Desk Reference* and package insert warnings about the risk of carbamazepine-induced bone marrow suppression were apparently based on earlier literature, in which carbamazepine was administered in combination with other anticonvulsant drugs.

23. Figure 24-3, from the 1967 Baastrup and Schou study, provides both an excellent illustration of the variability of the natural course of the illness and a dramatic demonstration of lithium's efficacy. It is reproduced in Chapter 24 because we find it useful as part of one important component of psychotherapy in teaching patients about the illness and its treatment.

24. Baastrup et al., 1970; Coppen et al., 1973; Prien et al., 1973a; Prien et al., 1973b.

25. In the first double-blind lithium–placebo discontinuation study, Baastrup and colleagues (1970) reported that 12 of 22 bipolar patients relapsed (6 manic, 5 depressive, 1 mixed state) within 5 months when switched from lithium to placebo. None of the 28 bipolar patients maintained on lithium relapsed within that time. In the double-blind prospective trial by Coppen and co-workers (1973), the mean "affective morbidity" was virtually the same for mania and depression. Cundall and associates (1972) studied lithium prophylaxis in a crossover design with 12 patients already stabilized on lithium. The predominance of manic episodes during placebo treatment, especially in contrast to the low incidence on lithium, suggests a greater antimanic than antidepressive effect for lithium.

Prien and co-workers (1973a) reported a study of 205 patients hospitalized for mania, then randomly assigned to either lithium treatment or a placebo for 2 years after discharge. The overall incidence of severe relapses was reduced by half in the lithium group, compared with no reduction in the placebo group ($p < 0.001$), a difference primarily due to the impact of lithium on manic episodes. The proportion of patients with depressive relapses was reduced from 16 percent before treatment to 8 percent after lithium treatment. For patients on placebo, comparable figures were 13 and 11 percent, but the lithium–placebo difference was not significant given the low numbers involved. The relatively low number of depressive relapses is probably an artifact, resulting from a large number of dropouts in both groups after their first manic relapse. Thus, lithium's relative efficacy in preventing depression and mania cannot be determined. Nonetheless, the study is frequently cited as evidence that lithium more effectively prevents mania than depression, although the investigators themselves made no such claim and, in fact, have pointed out that the large difference in the distribution of manic and depressive relapses makes any such comparisons meaningless. This same group (Prien et al., 1973b) also reported on a somewhat smaller number of patients with bipolar illness hospitalized for depression and randomly assigned at discharge to placebo, lithium, or imipramine. During the 2-year follow-up, the placebo vs lithium difference in manic episodes was 21 (from 33 percent to 12 percent) compared to 43 for depressive episodes (from 55 percent to 12 percent). This indicates that lithium prevented the recurrence of depressive episodes at least as well as it prevented manic ones.

Fieve and colleagues (1976) studied 35 bipolar-I patients randomly assigned to either lithium or placebo and followed for periods ranging from 2 1/2 to 4 1/2 years. The placebo–lithium difference appeared to be greater for manic episodes (from 94 percent to 59 percent) than for depressive episodes (from 44 percent to 29 percent). As with the study by Prien and colleagues, the most interesting aspect of these data is the relatively low number of depressive relapses in both groups, probably reflecting dropouts resulting from manic episodes in both group. The mean number of depressive episodes per year among lithium-treated patients was one fourth that of the placebo-treated patients ($p <$ 0.01), but unfortunately the authors do not present comparable data for manic episodes. Thus, this study does not clarify whether lithium is more effective prophylactically against mania or depression. In a related study from the same group, Dunner and colleagues (1976a) reported on 40 bipolar-II patients followed in an outpatient clinic, 16 of whom received maintenance lithium and 24 placebo. Although lithium did not appear to reduce the total number of depressive episodes, there was a threefold reduction in hospitalization for depression. The depression-related dropout rate was three times higher in the placebo group than in the lithium group, again an indication of considerable lithium protection against the more serious forms of depression.

In a 2-year prospective double-blind study of 38 lithium-treated bipolar patients, Quitkin and co-workers (1981a) found that of the 21 percent who relapsed on lithium, half were depressive and half manic. Prien and associates (1984) also noted a similar rate of depressive and manic relapses in 42 lithium-treated bipolar patients over a 1 to 2 year follow-up period.

26. Some patients experience activation on lithium. The reasons for these individual differences have not been clarified.

27. Hewick et al., 1977; Fann and Wheless, 1977; Roose et al., 1979; Murray et al., 1983.

28. Hartigan, 1963; Baastrup and Schou, 1967; Poole et al., 1978; Angst et al., 1970.

29. Coppen et al., 1976; Kane et al., 1982; Glen et al., 1981, 1984.

30. The literature on the efficacy of lithium prophylaxis in schizoaffective disorder suffers from a dearth of placebo-controlled studies. This is understandable when one considers that the focus on this diagnostic group is relatively recent, coming after the efficacy of lithium is well established. Thus, ethical considerations mitigate against placebo-controlled trials even for a diagnostic group for which baseline rates of relapse (i.e., on placebo) are not established.

31. These points are well-expressed in letters written in response to the *Lancet* editorial of February 21, 1987; note especially Schou's response.

32. The U.S. increase occurred especially among the young. Dickson and Kendell noted that their 1981 patients were younger than those in 1970.

33. Only a minority of Dickson and Kendell's patients were taking lithium before admission (22 percent in 1970 and 1971 vs 35 percent in 1980 and 1981). The median length of stay for the patients previously on lithium was only half as long as that for the patients not treated with it. The authors cite this as "no difference" even though the small numbers preclude meaningful statistical evaluation.

34. As noted earlier, bipolar patients with mixed states are more likely to be on antidepressants and to be abusing illicit drugs or alcohol, all factors that would compromise their response to prophylactic lithium.

35. Stancer et al., 1970; Dunner and Fieve, 1974; Prien et al., 1974; Kukopulos et al., 1980; Misra and Burns, 1977.

36. Prien et al., 1974; Dunner and Fieve, 1974; Abou-Saleh and Coppen, 1986; Page et al., 1987.

37. Stallone et al., 1973; Mendlewicz et al., 1972b, 1973; Grof et al., 1979b; Mendlewicz, 1982; Maj et al., 1984; Smeraldi et al., 1984; Abou-Saleh and Coppen, 1986.

38. Several excellent comprehensive reviews of lithium side effects are available, including those of Reisberg and Gershon, 1979; Johnson, 1980; Vestergaard et al., 1980; Jefferson and Greist, 1977, 1987.

39. These averages include only data from patients on lithium alone. Thus, Bone and co-workers (1980) and Lyskowski and colleagues (1982) report significantly higher rates of various side effects in patients on combinations of lithium and other psychotropic agents than on lithium alone, although this was not confirmed by Duncavage and associates (1983).

40. Roose et al., 1979; Vestergaard and Schou, 1984; Hardy et al., 1987; Shulman et al., 1987.

41. In the Maarbjerg et al. study, the incidence of lithium-induced hypothyroidism was calculated at two per hundred years of lithium exposure, a figure similar to that of Smigan et al., 1984.

42. The reversibility of the effect of lithium on the urine concentrating ability may be explained by the fact that this effect is partly caused by the ion's interference with antidiuretic hormone.

43. Hansen et al., 1977, 1979; Hestbech et al., 1977; Aurell et al., 1981; Thysell et al., 1981.

44. Because the direct measurement of GFR requires a 24-hour urine collection, attempts have been made to estimate changes in GFR by changes in blood levels of creatinine or more recently B_2-microglobulin. Although the former does not correlate with GFR, the latter does (Viberti et al., 1981; Samiy and Rosnick, 1987).

45. Bendz, 1983, 1985; Smigan, et al., 1984; Jørgensen et al., 1984; Johnson et al., 1984; Tyrer et al., 1983; Boton et al., 1987; Mellerup et al., 1987; Gelenberg et al., 1987; Schou et al., 1989; Santella et al., 1988; Conte et al., 1989.

46. As Masterson and colleagues (1988) pointed out, these clinics keep patients maintained at modest blood lithium levels. Once a day dosing may not be as benign when higher blood levels are maintained.

47. The cohort study of Schou and colleagues covered 4,900-patient years. Of the 24 instances of lithium intoxication recorded, 15 were due to deliberate overdose (suicide attempts). The authors note that "in no instance did lithium intoxication develop as a consequence of gradually deteriorating kidney function."

48. In adolescents and young adults, particularly males engaged in competitive sports, the deleterious effects of lithium on muscle coordination can contribute to compliance problems. To prevent this, the lithium dose should be reduced to the minimum necessary to control the illness.

49. The general issue of tardive dyskinesia in manic-depressive illness, its relationship to other signs of CNS dysfunction, and its relevance to course are discussed in Chapter 18.

50. See, for example, Donaldson and Cunningham, 1983; Johnson, 1984; Schou, 1984; Sansone and Ziegler, 1985.

51. These issues have been reviewed by Shaw et al. 1986, 1987; Ananth et al., 1987; Jefferson et al., 1987; and Judd et al., 1987.

52. See, for example, Schou et al., 1968b; Judd et al., 1977b; Karniol et al., 1978; Judd, 1979; Kropf and Müller-Oerlinghausen, 1979; Weingartner et al., 1983a,b, 1985; Glue et al.,1987.

53. Those reporting detrimental effects of lithium on cognitive abilities and speed of performance include, among others, Demers and Heninger, 1971; Reus et al., 1979b; Lund et al., 1982; Pons et al., 1985; Shaw et al., 1986, 1987. Additionally, Aminoff et al., (1974) found that lithium caused a reversible deterioration in cognitive functioning in patients with Huntington's disease. The degree of cognitive impairment was not correlated with the degree of dementia in these patients.

Studies reporting no significant effect of lithium on memory or other cognitive abilities include, for example, Telford and Worrall, 1978; Kjellman et al., 1980; Ghadirian et al., 1983; Engelsmann et al., 1988. A comparison of manic-depressive patients (who were medication free, lithium treated, or carbamazepine treated) with normal controls found no differences among groups on tests of attention, concentration, visuomotor function, or memory (Joffe et al., 1988b).

54. In addition to the review by Albrecht and Müller-Oerlinghausen (1980), other excellent reviews of cardiac effects include those by Jefferson and Greist (1977), Tilkian and colleagues (1976), and Mitchell and MacKenzie (1982).

55. In the Norton and Whalley study (1984) there was a relationship between prelithium signs of physical illness and later death on lithium. Thus, of the 14 patients who died of cardiovascular disease, 9 had clinical abnormalities attributable to cardiovascular disease before they began taking lithium, and 6 had multiple signs or symptoms.

56. Stancer and Forbath (1989) studied 19 patients who had been on lithium for more than 10 years. They found 8 (42 percent) with elevated parathyroid hormone levels, 3 of whom had clinical signs of hyperparathyroidism, including degenerative spine disease, osteoporosis, and hypertension/cardiomegaly.

57. Notwithstanding imperfections in its study, this group's work merits attention, particularly in light of its interesting subclassification of patients by different illness courses. Since the DMI sequence is relatively infrequent, the tendency for tricyclics to worsen the course of illness in such patients may simply have gone unnoticed by others with smaller patient samples. An additional factor is probably relevant to American clinicians in particular. Shorter follow-up periods and higher dropout rates (in part, a product of the mobility of the population) decrease the likelihood of any individual clinician or group detecting the longer-term effects of treatment interventions. As reported by Kukopulos, some of the patients in the depression-mania-interval group went on to become continuously cycling.

58. Bunney et al., 1968; Goodwin et al., 1969; Baastrup et al., 1970; Small et al., 1971; Lapierre et al., 1980; Klein et al., 1981; Margo and McMahon, 1982; Christodoulou and Lykouras, 1982.

59. Puzynski and Klosiewicz, 1984; Vencovsky et al., 1984; Prasad, 1984; Brennan et al., 1984; McElroy et al., 1988; Hayes, 1989; Calabrese and Delucchi, 1989.

60. An open study of clonazepam prophylaxis in five lithium-refractory bipolar patients (Aronson et al., 1989) was quite discouraging. All of the patients relapsed quickly when switched to clonazepam. However, the report of Sacks (1989) is more encouraging.

61. Among the antidepressants, only imipramine and amitriptyline have been evaluated in controlled studies of prophylaxis. However, open studies and clinical experience suggest that the MAOIs also have prophylactic efficacy in recurrent unipolar depression.

24

Psychotherapy

At this point in my life, I cannot imagine leading a normal life without both taking lithium and being in psychotherapy. Lithium prevents my seductive but disastrous highs, diminishes my depressions, clears out the wool and webbing from my disordered thinking, slows me down, gentles me out, keeps me from ruining my career and relationships, keeps me out of a hospital, alive, and makes psychotherapy possible. But, ineffably, psychotherapy *heals*. It makes some sense of the confusion, reins in the terrifying thoughts and feelings, returns some control and hope and possibility of learning from it all. Pills cannot, do not, *ease* one back into reality; they only bring one back headlong, careening, and faster than can be endured at times. Psychotherapy is a sanctuary, it is a battleground, it is a place I have been psychotic, neurotic, elated, confused and despairing beyond belief. But, always, it is where I have believed—or have learned to believe—that I might someday be able to contend with all of this.

No pill can help me deal with the problem of not wanting to take pills; likewise, no amount of analysis alone can prevent my manias and depressions. I need both. It is an odd thing owing life to pills, one's own quirks and tenacities, and this unique, strange and ultimately profound relationship called psychotherapy.

—Patient with manic-depressive illness

INTRODUCTION

Untreated manic-depressive illness is, by any measure, gravely serious—complex in its origins, diverse in its expression, unpredictable in its course, severe in its recurrences, and often fatal in its outcome. Yet in its milder forms, it can enhance productivity, creativity, and sociability. Severe mania and depression are debilitating, but mild hypomania is a state that is often sought. Moods are such an essential part of the substance of life, of individuality and identity, that distinguishing normal moods from mild and moderate expressions of the illness is an exacting task for patients. Given such complexity, it is clearly unrealistic to expect treatment to proceed smoothly simply because effective medications are available—even in the best of circumstances.

Problems that typically accompany manic-depressive illness invite psychotherapeutic intervention. The personal, interpersonal, and social consequences, which are usually severe, can include suicide, violence, alcoholism, drug abuse, and hospitalization. Biological variables predominate in etiology. Nonetheless, the primary manifestations of the illness are behavioral and psychological, with profound changes in perception, attitudes, personality, mood, and cognition. Psychological interventions can be of unique value to patients undergoing such devastating changes in the way they perceive themselves and are perceived by others.

Medication is the central treatment for manic-depressive illness, not an adjunctive one. From time to time, lithium noncompliance becomes a major theme in the therapy of many patients (Jamison et al., 1979; Jamison and Akiskal, 1983). Confusion often arises because the illness itself, as well as its pharmacological treatments, can affect cognition, perception, mood, and behavior. Although the emphasis in this chapter is on psychotherapeutic issues for patients treated with lithium, most of the discussion is applicable to issues that arise for patients maintained on other medications, such as carbamazepine. Psychotherapeutic sessions often involve concerns about being on medication in general and lithium in particular. Lithium's effectiveness in ameliorating the illness is not always welcome, since it deprives some patients of energy and much sought-after highs and, additionally, can burden them with bothersome side effects.

Given the efficacy of lithium, clinicians may minimize the value of psychotherapy and their own role in the treatment of manic-depressive illness. Vasile and colleagues (1987), for example, found that psychiatrists and mental health professionals de-emphasized psychodynamic psychotherapy in the treatment of affectively ill patients. Patients themselves, by contrast, often find psychotherapy a potent adjunct to lithium. In the one study in which patients were actually asked, twice as many patients as therapists thought psychotherapy was helpful to them in remaining compliant to medication (Jamison et al., 1979). There are also times when clinicians encounter manic-depressive patients who are not on medication, and psychotherapy may have to serve as the sole treatment (e.g., patients who refuse medication or women who stop lithium during their pregnancies). In addition, psychotherapy, in conjunction with lithium, may be the treatment of choice for breakthrough depressions in patients prone to antidepressant-induced cycling. There are also theoretical grounds to expect that psychotherapy may help to ameliorate some of the stress-related precipitants of manic and depressive episodes. Such intervention may, one hopes, temper the progression of the natural course of the illness (Post et al., 1986).

Psychological support for the treatment of manic-depressive patients ranges from a few minutes with the prescribing physician to combined use of individual and group psychotherapy. Most commonly, a general psychiatrist or psychopharmacologist is the one who treats lithium patients, usually within a limited time frame of 20 to 30 minutes, every several weeks. Although comprehensive psychotherapeutic work cannot take place in such a context, the doctor can create an emotionally supportive atmosphere, be aware of and focus on the general psychological issues involved in being on lithium and having an affec-

tive illness, and encourage patients to express their concerns. Providing a therapeutic relationship of this kind increases the likelihood of lithium compliance and makes it more probable that the patient will be referred for formal psychotherapy when there is a need for it. Formal, structured psychotherapy—for example, cognitive or interpersonal therapy—best follows control of acute episodes.

Conception of the Chapter

The first section of this chapter emphasizes general psychological issues of importance in treating manic-depressive illness. These issues are relevant to all aspects of clinical management, whether the patient is being seen for medications only (the most common clinical situation) or for medications in conjunction with formal psychotherapy—individual, group, or family—or involvement in a self-help group. Specific psychotherapeutic techniques are not discussed in detail, in part because we assume a basic knowledge of the principles and practice of psychotherapy and in part because no one type of psychotherapy has been demonstrated to be uniquely effective in this patient population.

The lack of psychotherapeutic specificity reflects the reality of clinical practice, namely, the predominance of pharmacological treatments for manic-depressive illness and the relatively recent emphasis on psychological interventions. However, we wish to emphasize our belief that formal psychotherapy is extremely beneficial to many manic-depressive patients and unquestionably essential for many others, especially those who are suicidal or unwilling to take medication in the manner prescribed. The limits of even the most beneficial medications are increasingly apparent to clinicians treating affective illness. Ongoing and future psychotherapy research efforts will determine the specific nature of the most effective psychological interventions.

Specific studies of treatment modalities combining psychotherapy and lithium are reviewed in the second part of this chapter. Strategies useful in increasing medication compliance are discussed in detail in Chapter 25.

Historical Background

Clinical pragmatism, buttressed by biological assumptions about etiology, long ago determined the dominance of organic therapies in the treatment of bipolar illness. Thus, physicians, ancient and modern, have for the most part sought cures not through talking and listening but through direct actions of control: mineral baths, bloodletting, herbs, chains, vapors, bromides, opiates, warm waters, cold waters, and physical and chemical restraints.[1]

Even the pioneers of psychotherapy, the psychoanalysts, tended to perceive patients suffering from manic-depressive illness as not very good candidates for psychoanalytic treatment. Fromm-Reichmann (1949) characterized them as lacking in "complexity and subtlety," Abraham (1911) as "impatient, envious, exploitive, and with dominating possessiveness," and Rado (1928) as continually involved in a "raging orgy of self-torture." Manic-depressive patients generally were compared with schizophrenic patients and found to lack introspection and to be too dependent and "clinging" (Fromm-Reichmann, 1949), disconcertingly able to find vulnerable spots in the therapist (Fromm-Reichmann, 1949; Janowsky et al., 1970), and prone to eliciting strong feelings of countertransference in the analyst (English, 1949; Rosenfeld, 1963). Despite these perceived difficulties, many leading analysts from the prepharmacotherapy era sustained a dedicated commitment to the analytic treatment of manic-depressive illness. Thus Abraham (1911) noted:

Psycho-analysis, which has hitherto enabled us to overcome this obstacle [depression interfering with the development of the transference], seems to me for this reason to be the only rational therapy for manic-depressive psychoses. (pp. 153–154)

Nevertheless, before lithium was available, enthusiasm for treating bipolar illness was limited—understandably so. One can imagine the frustration of attempting to treat a hypomanic or manic patient in psychotherapy. Getting such a patient into the office and keeping him or her there was difficult enough; engaging in a meaningful therapeutic endeavor must have been daunting. Likewise, any clinician can appreciate the different kind of frustration involved in treating a profoundly depressed patient. The exceedingly high spontaneous remission rate characteristic of manic-depressive illness no doubt encouraged therapists in some cases to attribute clinical changes to their therapeutic interventions. Conversely, when no change or a relapse occurred,

therapists tended to assume responsibility as well.

The psychoanalysts and early psychotherapists provide a source of clinically descriptive information, virtually all of it from unmedicated patients. This material is all the more significant because present medical ethics strongly discourage the psychotherapeutic treatment of unmedicated patients with bipolar illness. The psychoanalytic school is also important because it has had a profound effect on clinical thinking about manic-depressive illness. Not only most psychotherapists but also many who contribute to the biological and pharmacological literature have been influenced by psychoanalytic conceptions of the illness.

CLINICAL MANAGEMENT

Psychotherapeutic Issues

Overview

The competent and compassionate psychotherapy of manic-depressive illness is predicated on a solid knowledge of the illness. Kraepelin's injunction to his turn of the century medical students remains compelling: "It is one of the physician's most important duties to make himself, as far as possible, acquainted with the nature and phenomena of insanity" (Kraepelin, 1904). A solid knowledge of bipolar illness encompasses phenomenology, the natural history of the illness (including its recurrent nature, worsening course, and seasonal patterns), biological aspects of the illness (including drug responses in mania and depression), biological theories of etiology, and mechanisms of action of the drugs used in its treatment. Therapists with a good scientific grasp of psychological phenomenology and biology generally are more sure of their own therapeutic competence. They also avoid the biological determinism common in therapists who are well grounded in biological theories but poorly trained in psychological studies such as personality theory and development, perception, motivation, and learning theory.

The psychotherapy of bipolar illness requires considerable flexibility in style and technique. Flexibility is necessary because of the patient's changing mood, cognition, and behavior and the fluctuating levels of dependency intrinsic to the illness. In the therapeutic relationship, a long-lead approach is often useful to maximize the patient's sense of control over his or her behavior. It is important not to control the patient unduly and not to allow lithium or other medications to become the focus of a power struggle. The symbolic value of lithium is enormous, and its role as a protective device also is extremely important. A thin line exists between too much therapeutic control and too little. Too much can lead to increased dependency and acting out or decreased self-esteem and compliance. Too little control occasionally leads to feelings of insecurity, an unnecessarily tenuous hold on reality, and feelings of abandonment. The patient may see signs of caring in the therapist's firm, consistent orders for routine lithium levels or tests of thyroid and kidney functioning but engage in unnecessary power struggles and refuse to comply with medication regimens when the therapist places undue emphasis on precise medication patterns (e.g., not allowing for some degree of self-titration). Collaborative aspects of management through self-ratings, chartings, and patient and family education (using films, lectures, books, or handouts) are integral parts of good clinical care. These issues are discussed later in the chapter. The therapist must also be able to use hospitalization when appropriate as an occasionally necessary adjunct to outpatient care and must not regard hospitalization as an indication of failure in the therapeutic endeavor.

In the next section, we discuss issues that commonly arise in the psychotherapy of manic-depressive illness: anger, denial, and ambivalence surrounding both the illness and its treatment, disappointments and frustrations attendant to less than complete treatment success, losses associated with lithium treatment, fears of recurrence, learning to discriminate normal from abnormal moods, developmental tasks, concerns about family and relationships, and concerns about genetics.

Anger, Denial, and Ambivalence

History bears witness to the tendency of some people to resist with passion when cornered by fate, "to rage against the dying of the light." Others more readily submit to what may or may not have been inevitable. Such different reactions are unmistakable in individuals who face an uncertain future because of manic-depressive illness. Some patients resist for years, irate at their diagnosis, their treatment, and their physicians. Others accept the illness and its treatment with remarkable equanimity. Most fall between the extremes.

Manic-depressive illness can push patients to the limits of their resources. It is a complicated and frustrating illness, seemingly impossible to sort through. It takes a heavy emotional toll on family members and friends, the repercussions of which add further psychological stress to the patient. The illness often seems within the patient's control, yet it is not. It often carries with it a psychotic diagnosis, an uncertain course, and a lifetime sentence of medication. Especially when not treated early and aggressively, it is costly in loss of self-esteem, disrupted relationships, secondary alcoholism and drug abuse, economic chaos, hospitalizations, lost jobs, years consumed by illness, and suicide.

Contending with such a reality understandably rouses patients to anger. A common reaction to acute stress, danger, and uncertainty, anger can be seen as natural and, up a point, highly adaptive. It is useful because it drives patients to question assumptions, summon up motivation, and refuse to accept the unacceptable. Despite its usefulness, the anger often leads patients to reject an effective treatment irrationally or to direct their wrath—at times legitimately—at the clinicians who treat the disease.

Manic-depressive patients also use denial to cope with their illness. Even in the presence of severe and obvious pathology, they deny its severity, the odds of its recurring, its consequences, and at times its very existence. Like anger, denial is a normal response to the unpleasant, the painful, the unpredictable, and the destructive in life. Not to deny some aspects of a serious disease, such as manic-depressive illness, would be unusual, even troubling. Denial clearly is an essential part of healing, allowing slow assimilation of otherwise overwhelming thoughts and feelings.

Symptoms of manic-depressive illness contribute to the process of denial. They may also be mistaken for it. Thus, cognitive and memory impairments in depression often are pronounced and, even without denial, would produce problems in recollection. Repression, psychological distance, and the necessity to adapt to the realities of life frequently cause memories of the depression to pale over time. The severity and nature of the manic episodes are also frequently minimized or forgotten. This can be due to the relatively clearer perception of earlier, milder, and more enjoyable stages of mania, amnesia from the organic features of manic psychosis, repression, and the sheer volume of thoughts, perceptions, behaviors, and feelings that occur during mania and make good recall unlikely. Many clinical investigators believe that denial is critical to lithium noncompliance, an issue discussed further in Chapter 25.

The treatment of denial, although not always successful, frequently becomes easier as time passes and the illness reappears too often to disown, even unconsciously. Denial can be weakened also by exploring in psychotherapy the meaning of the illness for the patient. Ongoing education about the natural history of the illness, with emphasis on its high relapse rate, also undercuts the process of denial, as do discussions of the risks and benefits of medication.

Ambivalence is another common reaction, especially ambivalence caused by the incongruence between the behavioral expression of manic-depressive illness and its biological treatment. Occurring as a disorder of mood and behavior, the symptoms and consequences of the illness are largely psychological and interpersonal in nature. Lithium, on the other hand, is a highly effective biological treatment that results in relatively rapid improvement. The treatment response is obvious and gratifying to the clinician, if not the patient, and lends credence to a strongly biological treatment program. This view is further encouraged by the demonstrated inability of psychotherapy alone to relieve or prevent manic-depressive episodes. Adding to the biological emphasis is the fact that lithium therapy is imbued with a medical ambience and embedded in a highly structured medical regimen: The physician orders laboratory tests of serum lithium levels and kidney and thyroid functioning and asks specific medical questions about side effects, usually focusing on the somatic, not the cognitive, effects. A psychiatric review of systems is done to determine the presence or absence of the signs and symptoms of mania and depression. The understandable focus of physicians on medical aspects of manic-depressive illness is thus placed in a point-

counterpoint position with patients, who are often more focused on psychological aspects of their illness and its treatment. These disparate perspectives can easily lead to a quite arbitrary split of the biological from the psychological.

Conceptualizing manic-depressive illness as fundamentally a medical disorder has many advantages for the patient. It can decrease stigma, provide effective and specific treatment, and minimize family and individual responsibility for the origin of the illness. It can also, however, discourage discussion of significant life issues and problems involved in adjusting to the illness and its consequences. An overly medical approach can also mean that psychological concerns about taking lithium, carbamazepine, or other medications may be ignored. Furthermore, taking lithium may create its own stigma, since society and patients themselves disparage the continuing need for psychiatric medication.

Biological assumptions about the illness can also rob patients of a sense of personal control. Many, for example, maintain the belief that if only they changed their work or dietary habits, if only they conducted their love affairs in a different way, if only they more stringently heeded the counsel of their priests, therapists, and consciences—in other words, if only they behaved as they think they should—they would be able to prevent recurrences of manic and depressive episodes. Biological treatments, the major real control a person can exert over his illness, threaten these beliefs. When lithium is beneficial, some patients continue to believe that they ought to have been able to handle things without medication. Some may attribute their improvement to a combination of their own efforts and the efficacy of the medication. Others believe the medication alone made the difference and they had little or no control over the illness. Psychotherapy can help to clarify the ambivalence that inevitably results from such beliefs, underscore the patient's role in the medication regimen, and identify psychological issues that are important and amenable to the patient's control.

Disappointments Attendant to Less Than Complete Treatment Success

Expecting the treatment of manic-depressive illness to proceed in a straightforward manner is likely to create secondary problems. For many patients, lithium is an uncertain treatment imposed on an uncertain illness, a problematic treatment for a problematic disease. For many, life before lithium can be likened to a kite on a string in exceedingly unpredictable winds. Lithium gives some control over the winds, but often it is not complete. And therein lies much of the disappointment and frustration. Clinicians frequently define successful control very differently than patients do. The clinician looks at certain types of evidence—fewer or no hospitalizations or little or no need for adjunctive neuroleptics and antidepressants—and finds lithium effective. The patient who continues to experience disruptive and upsetting mood swings is likely to interpret the same evidence in much more equivocal terms. In essence, physicians more often focus on the successes of lithium, that is, the contrasts with untreated illness. Patients, while living with the successes, live with the failures and disappointments as well. Patients also see the contrast, but they find themselves comparing the dramatic improvements with day to day discontents. The improvements tend to be forgotten, and with time, the seriousness of the illness is denied. Day to day discontents then emerge as the compelling factor in feelings about lithium. In the words of one P.G. Wodehouse character, ". . . I could see that, if not actually disgruntled, he was far from being gruntled."[2] Lithium patients are often far from being gruntled.

The resentment patients feel at their partial cure is, in some respects, proportional to the severity of illness and concomitant hope. Unrealistic expectations of lithium and of physicians not only derive from the fragile hopes of patients but also are rooted in the hyperbole of journalists and in the exaggerated claims of some physicians. Paradoxically, the very existence of lithium as an effective treatment has given rise to a new generation of patients with a new set of expectations. When lithium was first used in the Scandinavian clinical trials, there was no alternative, and the patients were grateful for a treatment that revolutionized their lives (Schou, personal communication). Even though alternative medications are showing clear promise, the availability and efficacy of lithium have made it a part of the pharmaceutical establishment, which creates an inevitable groundswell of expanded expectations, disappointments, and criticism.

Losses Associated with Lithium Treatment

The subtle and powerful clinician–patient alliance possible in lithium therapy is predicated on a thorough understanding of not only the benefits of lithium to the patient but also the realistic and unrealistic fantasies of loss that many patients experience during lithium treatment. These fantasies often focus on missing the highs and cannot effectively be understood through the simplistic formulation that the patient is shortsighted, regressive, or escapist. Effective therapy with manic-depressive patients, whether it involves using drugs alone or combines drugs with psychotherapy, must address the reality of the patient's positive perceptions of the illness, as well as the altered states of perception induced by phases of the illness.

Patients may experience many different kinds of losses, realistic and otherwise, as a result of taking lithium. These losses and their relationship to medication noncompliance are discussed in detail in Chapter 25. Here we present an overview of the psychotherapeutic issues involved.

Realistic losses are those changes brought about by lithium that the patient does not desire. They can include decreases in energy level, loss of euphoric states, increased need for sleep, possible decreases in productivity and creativity, and decreased sexuality.[3] One patient described a few of these subtle lithium effects:

> People expect that you will welcome being "normal," be appreciative of lithium, doctors, and modern science, and take in stride having normal energy and sleep. But if you are used to sleeping only five hours a night and now sleep eight, are used to staying up all night for days and weeks in a row and now cannot, it is a very real adjustment to blend into a three-piece-suit schedule which, while comfortable to many, is new, restrictive, seemingly less productive, and for sure less fun. People say, when I complain of being less lively, less energetic, "Well, now you're just like the rest of us," meaning, among other things, to be reassuring. What they don't realize is that I compare myself with my former self, not with others. Not only that, I always compare my current self with the best I have been, which is when I have been hypomanic. When I am my present "normal" self, I am far removed from when I have been my liveliest, most productive, most intense, most outgoing and effervescent. In short, for myself, I am a hard act to follow.

The side effects of lithium can be difficult to separate from the medication's effect on hypomanic symptoms. They are also sometimes indistinguishable from symptoms of inadequately treated depressive episodes. A study of manic-depressive patients in remission suggests that many patients feel that their illness makes positive contributions to their lives in one or more important ways (Jamison et al., 1980).

A substantial majority of the patients perceived pronounced short-term and long-term positive effects from their manic-depressive illness in addition to whatever disabling and dysphoric symptoms they might also have experienced. Most patients reported increased sensitivity, sexual intensity, productivity, creativity, and outgoingness (social ease). Men and women varied enormously in what they regarded as the most enjoyable and important changes when hypomanic. Men found increased social ease the most positive attribute, and women rated increases in sexual intensity, productivity, and social ease equally important.

Such attributions are important for several reasons. From a clinical perspective, it is important to realize the meaning, nature, and value of positive behavior and mood changes (as well as negative ones) for an individual patient. From a learning theory point of view, such euphoric states can be powerful reinforcers that create in some patients a potentially strong, variable reinforcement schedule with significant benefits on the one hand and the risk of severe emotional and pragmatic problems on the other.

Treatment management under such circumstances is not altogether straightforward. For example, compliance with a therapeutic lithium regimen, which, at best, has a tenuous and delayed relationship with the alleviation of the dysphoric features of manic-depressive illness, competes with behavior maintained by a highly positive and intermittent reinforcement schedule, an exceedingly difficult behavior pattern to modify. It is in some ways analogous to a drug self-administration paradigm in which a highly pleasurable and relatively rapid state can be obtained. For some patients, the illness may represent, in effect, an endogenous stimulant addiction. Clinical experience suggests that patients may attempt to induce mania by discontinuing lithium, not just at times when they are depressed but also when they have to face problematic decisions and life events. Because the negative consequences accrue only later, it is not always clear to the patient that the benefits of lithium outweigh its costs.

For these reasons, the clinician must be aware of the positive features of mood swings in order to better understand and thereby treat affective disorders.

Other realistic losses include alterations in the patient's cognitive, perceptual, physical, emotional, or social spheres that result from the side effects of lithium and social sequelae, such as self-labeling or social stigma. The most significant side effects from a psychotherapeutic point of view, described further in Chapter 25, are those detailed by Schou and Baastrup (1973) and Schou (1980): decreased energy, enthusiasm, and sexuality (all of which can be a factor in increased marital problems), curbing of activities, and the common perception that life is flatter and less colorful. Again, of course, it may be difficult to separate lithium's side effects from its impact on symptoms of the illness.

Unrealistic losses include circumstances where lithium and psychotherapy come to symbolize the patient's personal failures. In addition to experiencing the normal difficulties in adjusting to the need for treatment, patients occasionally project all of their other life failures, thwarted ambitions, and inadequacies onto lithium. Lithium can become the psychological scapegoat and represent a rationalization for other failures that predate the onset of an affective disorder.

Therapeutic issues of general concern involve many areas of patients' adjustment to having manic-depressive illness: fears of recurrence, denial of the illness, discrimination of normal from pathological moods, effects of the illness on normal developmental tasks, and others.

Fears of Recurrence

The worst fear for most manic-depressive patients is recurrence of the illness. Many patients maintain a deep and fatalistic pessimism, however entwined with denial and optimism, about again becoming manic or depressed. Robert Lowell, in a poem from *Day by Day,* wrote, "If we see the light at the end of the tunnel,/ it's the light of an oncoming train" (p. 31). Some patients become preoccupied with such fears of recurrence and are almost illness-phobic. They become unduly self-protective and hyperalert for signs of an impending episode. These concerns are often reflected in the process of learning to differentiate normal from abnormal moods and states. A perceived decreasing tolerance for affective episodes is a concern that is usually secondary to the stress of the illness and to the large amount of psychological energy consumed by earlier bouts. Patients, often with good cause, fear that their families and friends will grow ever more intolerant with each new recurrence. Manic-depressive illness also takes a severe toll on other relationships, professional activities, and the individual's ability to handle the emotional stress of the affective episodes. Thus, Lowell wrote, "but the breakage can go on repeating once too often" (Lowell, 1977, p. 113). And Joshua Logan described in his autobiography a certain weariness: "I was only forty-five years old, but I felt exhausted by this last experience, hollowed out, as though I were a live fish disemboweled" (Logan, 1976, p. 388).

Learning to Discriminate Moods

Problems in learning to discriminate normal from abnormal moods are common throughout the psychotherapy of bipolar patients. Because of the intensity of their emotional responses, many manic-depressive patients fear that a normal depressive reaction will deepen into a major episode and that a state of well-being will escalate into hypomania or mania. Many common emotions range across several mood states, spanning euthymia, depression, and hypomania. For example, irritability and anger can be a part of normal human existence or alternately can be symptoms of both depression and hypomania. Tiredness, sadness, and lethargy can be due to normal circumstances, medical causes, or clinical depression. Feeling good, being productive and enthusiastic, and working hard can be either normal or pathognomonic of hypomania. These overlapping emotions can be confusing and arouse anxiety in many patients, who may then question their own judgment and become unduly concerned about recurrences of their affective illness. Occasionally, patients become conservative or excessively conforming. Benson (1976) noted that bipolar patients "tend to be more conservative and more conforming to others' attitudes because they are afraid that their ideas are the result of their misperception."

Helping the patient discriminate normal from abnormal affect is common in psychotherapy. The patient must learn to live within a narrower range of emotions yet master the skill of using those emotions with greater subtlety and discretion. Closely related to the discrimination of moods is the slow, steady process involved in patients' learning to unravel what is normal personality from what the illness has superimposed upon it—turbulence, impulsiveness, lack of predictability, and depression.

Developmental Tasks

Developmental tasks, previously overshadowed by the manic-depressive illness, often become issues for patients in remission. Ironically, manic-depressive illness can act as a protection against many of the slings and arrows of fortune encountered in normal life. Because late adolescence and early adulthood are the highest risk periods for the onset of the illness, many of the developmental tasks of these periods—separation from parents and family, development of close personal relationships, romantic involvements, hurts and rejections, child-bearing and child-rearing, and career development—are impaired or temporarily halted. (Conversely, these developmental transitions or crises can also precipitate the onset or occurrence of subsequent episodes.) Once the illness is under control, patients often have to deal with these problems, as well as those of a more general, existential nature, within the therapeutic relationship.

Concerns About Family and Relationships

Concerns about the effects of manic-depressive illness on a family system can be profound. Patients report feeling guilty about things done while manic and those left undone while depressed. The most frequently voiced concerns center on the interpersonal consequences of the illness, effects strongly felt by spouses, family members, and friends as well. Unmarried patients are often unclear about when and what to tell people they are dating about their illness. Similar concerns are involved in relationships with employers and co-workers. Interpersonal aspects of manic-depressive illness are covered more fully in Chapter 12.

Concerns About Genetics

Concerned about the genetic component of manic-depressive illness, many patients worry about possible transmission of the disorder to children.

They tend to overidentify with any close family member who has the illness, particularly if it is a parent. Occasionally, they feel guilt over receiving effective treatments—lithium or carbamazepine—that were not available to an afflicted parent. This latter phenomenon, although not common, is particularly striking in those patients whose parents committed suicide or were hospitalized for a long time. A similar guilt is sometimes seen in patients successfully treated with lithium whose siblings or parents refuse treatment. Recent advances in locating specific genetic deficits involved in manic-depressive illness (Baron et al., 1987; Egeland et al., 1987) are likely to increase concerns and desire for information. Genetic counseling issues are discussed in Chapter 16.

Countertransference Issues

As noted earlier, many psychoanalysts who worked in the prelithium era found it frustrating to treat manic-depressive patients. The psychoanalytic literature discussed countertransference issues extensively and described in some detail the anger analysts felt at such patients for their seeming inconstancy and lack of insight (or desire for insight):

The extraverted, apparently unsubtle, manic depressive is a threat . . . in several ways: In the first place, communicative efforts are a strain because of the lack of response. Secondly, the so-called healthy extraverted approach to reality is likely to fill the more sensitive, introspective person [the psychoanalyst] with self-doubts as to the possibility that he makes mountains out of molehills, reads meanings in where none were meant, and so forth . . . Thirdly, the therapist tends to dislike this sort of person and to think of him as "shallow." And, finally, the patient's difficulty in recognizing or discussing his or another's feelings or meanings throws the therapist into a situation of helplessness, since these things are the coin in which he deals. (Cohen et al., 1954, p. 131).

English (1949) said succinctly what others have said at great length: "The manic-depressive rejects you because he seems to be unsure that he needs you at all" (p. 126).

Although many aspects of therapeutic work with manic-depressive patients have radically changed as a result of lithium, such patients continue to elicit strong feelings from some therapists. One contemporary clinical team wrote:

. . . bipolar patients, with their alienating behavior, incessant demands, opaqueness, and difficulty in adhering to medication regimes, are generally viewed as difficult to treat, providing a therapist with a sense of unease and minimal gratification (Davenport et al., 1979, p. 33)

Other therapists who work with bipolar patients are frustrated by the inconsistencies that patients show during different mood states in their behavior and attitudes toward self, therapist, therapy, and lithium. Their various moods can result in fluctuating levels of intimacy and trust within the therapeutic relationship, both from patient to therapist and from therapist to patient. The patient who appears at a session angry and irritable might produce a reaction in the therapist, whose feelings may then persist longer than the patient's fleeting mood. Or the therapist may make an interpretation at one session, find the patient feeling better at the next, and attribute the improved mood to the interpretation—only to discover the patient is depressed again at the next session. Without understanding that fluctuating mood is not a reliable signal but is rather intrinsic to the illness, such situations could lead to a misperception of the role of therapy.

Anger and frustration can also be engendered in the therapist when the patient rejects an effective treatment. Such encounters may arise when the therapist fails to comprehend what the illness means to the patient or the patient fails to understand, usually through processes of denial, consequences of rejecting such a treatment regimen. Greenson (1967) emphasized that the therapist should have a broad and rich background for empathy. A breadth of fantasy is particularly relevant and useful to the therapist who deals with psychotic patients, whose emotions and ideas are often not from the same experiential base as that of the therapist (see Chapter 12). In addition to having the kind of personal background advocated by Greenson, a therapist can reduce the feelings of being excluded from and not understanding the patient's experience by having a solid grounding in phenomenology.

A therapist often experiences anger and feelings of impotence when the patient's denial leads to lithium noncompliance and results in rehospitalization for manic or depressive episodes, suicide attempts, or exacerbations in hostile and aggressive behaviors. Feelings of inadequacy and failure when illness recurs can develop even when the patient is compliant. Such feelings may be commonplace when therapists treat patients who are depressed, suicidal, or hypomanic (Fromm-Reichmann, 1949; Janowsky et al., 1970). Hypomanic patients regularly show special sensitivity to vulnerabilities in the therapist, and this tuning-in to the therapist's "jugular" is the core of many therapists' acute and intense feelings of anger. Although such a pattern of interaction is most likely to occur during hypomania and mania, it is not uncommon during the depressive phase when the patient's defenses are down and levels of paranoia, irritability, and hopelessness have increased. Patients under such circumstances are often exquisitely tuned in to feelings of frustration, annoyance, and impotence in the therapist. The anger and hopelessness a patient expresses at such times often have a significant impact on the already vulnerable therapist. Therapists, of course, must recognize countertransference feelings and cope effectively with them so that repercussions for the patient will be minimal.

Yet another problem with countertransference potential centers on misinterpretation of resistance in bipolar patients. We have already discussed their difficulties in differentiating normal from pathological mood states and their fears of recurrence. Therapists occasionally assume that a patient's depression is a reaction to a particular environmental, interpersonal, or therapeutic event. They, therefore, attribute problems in discussing and handling the depression to resistance, when often such depression actually represents mild breakthrough cycling in the illness, something which the patient senses but cannot articulate. The therapist's tendency to link such feelings with external events can be problematic. Even when the depressions are not really endogenous, patients are often frightened by the similarity between such thoughts and feelings and those experienced in earlier severe major depressive episodes. Therapists need a delicate approach to help the patient differentiate types of feelings while at the same time recognizing when they themselves need to deny recurrence or to see psychological causality when little exists.

Another area of potential countertransference problems can develop when the therapist acts out through the patient. The therapist is in an unusual position for influencing the patient by unconsciously encouraging both lithium noncompliance and the behaviors linked to affective states. The special appeal of hypomania in particular is also relevant. The potential exists for envy, projective identification, and psychological seduction. Guilt over depriving the patient of a special state, another possible reaction, is heightened when a patient resists lithium and proclaims that he misses the highs. Unconscious collusion in medication resistance is not uncommon. Likewise, the seductive aspects of hypomania are often impossible to ignore. Moods are obviously contagious, and occasionally the loss of a patient's hypomania results in a corresponding, albeit lesser, loss reaction in the therapist. Some psychotherapists espouse a set of attitudes about psychosis that we term the Equus-Laingian view, which refers to a romanticization of madness. It can range from a tendency toward overvaluing the positive aspects of bipolar illness while minimizing the negative, painful ones to a conviction that psychopharmacological interventions in manic-depressive patients are oppressive and contraindicated.

Mood Charting

Mood charting by patients can provide invaluable information about seasonal and premenstrual patterns of moods, psychological and biological correlates of mood swings, and responsiveness to treatment, including possible worsening of the illness due to treatment (e.g., increased cycling induced by antidepressant therapy). Speaking to this last point, Post and colleagues (1986) stressed the utility of identifying "critical psychosocial stresses and areas of sensitivity in a given patient, which appear to be temporally related to repeated episodes of affective illness" (p. 198). The administration of the Visual Analogue Scale is straightforward, requiring little time on the part of the patient. The patient is given sheets of paper, each with a 100-mm line, anchored by a 1 ("worst I've ever felt") on the left (or the bottom) and 100 ("best I've ever felt") on the right (or the top). The patient is then asked to put a mark across the line at the point most representative of his or her overall mood (or whatever other variable, e.g., energy or anxiety level, is being assessed) for the day. To control for diurnal variations in mood and behavior, ratings should be done at approximately the same time of day or evening. Significant life events and additional medications required should be noted on the rating sheet. After completion, the dated form should be placed aside to avoid contamination from earlier ratings. A 100-mm ruler is used to score the patient's mood ratings. The results can then be graphed, with time plotted along the horizontal axis and mood ratings, from 1 to 100, plotted along the vertical axis. In some instances, patients can do their own graphing.

We have found that graphing these mood ratings is useful not only in noticing patterns of mood and treatment response but also in giving patients a sense of control, instilling a feeling of collaborative effort, and underscoring the importance of systematic observation. It also provides a relatively objective basis for persuading patients when their treatment regimens require modification. At the beginning of treatment, we frequently use other patients' charts as examples of different patterns of mood fluctuation to illustrate the use of daily mood ratings in diagnostic and treatment decisions. Figure 24-1 portrays one such pattern, in which the time course and efficacy of antidepressant medications are demonstrated in a woman with bipolar-II disorder. The essential teaching point is that there is an uneven, sawtooth nature to the recovery pattern. Predicting occasional serious relapses on the way to remission is important in minimizing serious, potentially lethal discouragement in a high-risk (i.e., transitional) period.

Patient Education

"Am I manic-depressive?" "We don't use that term, but I would guess from the record that you are bipolar." "Which is a nice way of saying that yes, I'm manic-depressive? . . . that I'm lucky as all get-out to be a complete nut because we real bats get much more help from lithium than simple neurotics can—" "I've never heard it put just that way, but there is some truth in it."   —Sloan Wilson, 1976

Patients often express resentment at how little information they receive about manic-depressive illness and its treatment. Most affective disorders clinics and some practitioners routinely provide formal and informal education to patients and families through lectures, books, articles, pamphlets, discussion groups, videotapes, and ongoing communication between clinicians and patients. This is the ideal scenario, however, not the prevailing one. Clinicians, in whatever setting, have a clinical and legal obligation to engage patients in a continuing process of education and informed consent. Patients vary considerably in their ability to assimilate information about their medications and illness, and they need to participate actively in the treatment process. Too often a physician becomes a unilateral advocate of lithium and other maintenance medications, and this frequently leads to an adversarial rather than

Figure 24-1. The course of recovery in a bipolar-II female treated with antidepressant medications.

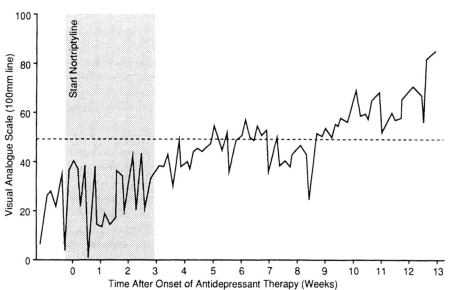

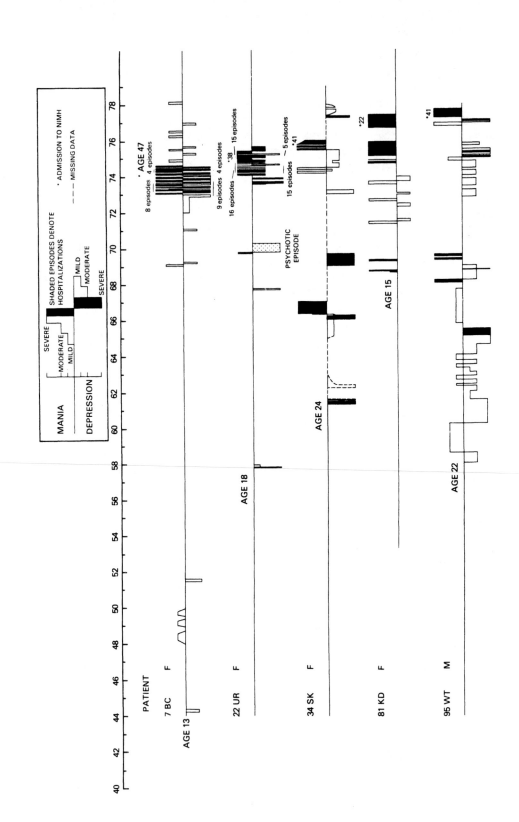

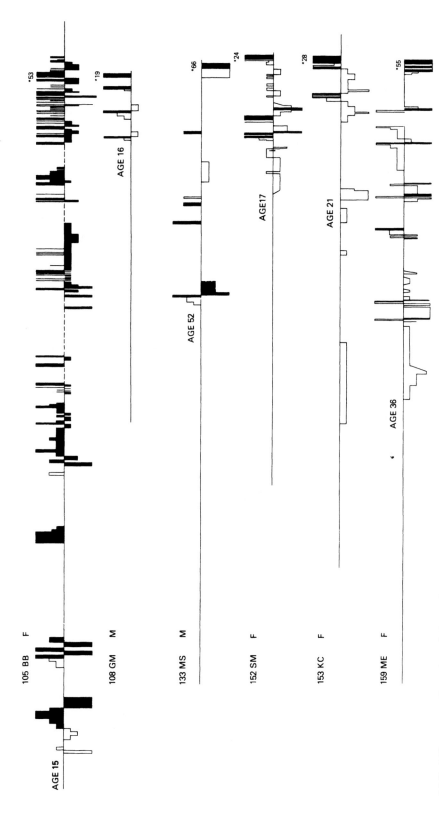

Figure 24-2. Life course of manic and depressive episodes in bipolar affective illness. Patterns of recurrent affective illness are illustrated in individual bipolar-I patients (those hospitalized for a manic episode). Manias are plotted above the line and depression below. Hospitalizations are *shaded*, and *dotted* lines indicate uncertain or missing data. Note that most patients show a course of increased severity or frequency of affective episodes over time (from Squillace et al., 1984).

collaborative effort. Patients should be encouraged to question their clinicians about diagnosis and treatment, to discuss their concerns about undue delays in getting the desired results, and to seek second opinions where appropriate. If the treating physician or psychotherapist disparages second opinions or consultations, patients should be encouraged to challenge this opinion and obtain the consultation anyway.

Patient education and informed consent, integrally bound, require an informed clinician. The chronic and highly recurrent nature of manic-depressive illness should be emphasized and re-emphasized to the patient. In our own practices, we frequently use charts illustrating the relapse rate and worsening course in the untreated illness (Figure 24-2). The dramatic effect of lithium on the course of manic-depressive illness is highlighted to patients and their families (Figure 24-3). Patients are encouraged to read about the illness and its treatment (suggested reading materials are listed in Appendix I). They also are given very specific information about their medications and potential risks and side effects. One such highly detailed information sheet about lithium can be found in Wyatt (in press). Informed consent and education do not end at a discussion of risks and benefits and distribution of fact sheets, however. Ongoing discussions with the clinician are essential. Lectures and videotapes can be useful in supplementing patient–physician talks. As with any form of treatment, safety and efficacy and the risks of no treatment should be outlined. Special attention should be paid to the discussion of potential dangers of antidepressant use in manic-depressive patients (such as induction of mania and worsening of the natural course of the illness, i.e, shortening of the cycle length).

Patients need to be alerted to the symptoms of impending episodes. Changes in sleep patterns are particularly important, since they precede mania, and sleep loss may precipitate it. As discussed in Chapter 19, environmental changes leading to insomnia (e.g., anxiety, excitement, grief) or others (such as hormonal changes, travel, drugs) can lead to mania through sleep deprivation. Wehr and colleagues (1987) advise that manic-depressive patients should be warned that a single night of unexplainable sleep loss should be taken as an early warning of possible impending mania. They further suggest counsel-

ing patients to avoid situations likely to disrupt sleep and advise clinicians to consider prescribing clonazepam to prevent significant sleep loss. Factors leading to sleep reduction and their relationship to the precipitation of mania are illustrated in Figure 22-7. This illustration can be used in educating patients about the necessity for maintaining adequate levels of sleep. The regularization of circadian rhythms through the regularization of meals, exercise, and other activities should also be stressed to patients.

The collaborative nature of the patient–clinician relationship is central to effective treatment. Not only must patients be taught about the natural course and symptoms of manic-depressive illness, they should be actively encouraged to express to their doctors concerns about their illness and treatment. Patients who when rational and in a normal mood wish to have electroconvulsive therapy when depressed (or manic) but know that they are unlikely to consent in the midst of an episode can in some states draw up Odysseus arrangements. Derived from the same principle as that used by Odysseus when he required protection from seduction by the Sirens, the Odysseus agreement allows patients to agree in advance to certain treatments.[4]

Family Education and Family Therapy

Family members and close friends often find that the educational information given to patients is useful to them as well. Families are, of course, in a unique position to observe the behavior and moods of bipolar patients. Education about the illness can increase the awareness and acceptance of patients and underscore the family's role in encouraging the patient to take prescribed medications and to live sensibly. Waiting for symptom-free intervals between episodes to discuss the meaning and nature of manic-depressive illness allows for education and collaborative decision making in a less emotionally charged atmosphere. Family members, in addition to being educated about medications and the illness, should be informed about the importance of recognizing the early signs and symptoms of hypomanic, manic, and depressive episodes. Changes in sleep patterns, sexual and financial behavior, mood (expansiveness or undue enthusiasm, pessimism and hopelessness), involvements in excessive numbers of projects, and changes in judg-

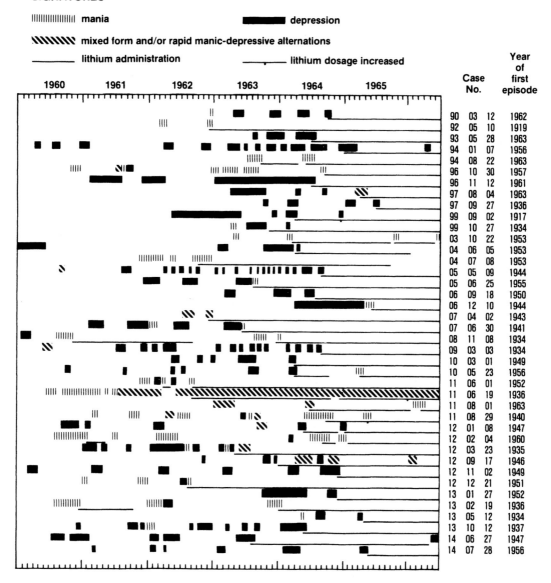

SIGNATURES

|||||||||||||||||| mania   ██████ depression

\\\\\\\\ mixed form and/or rapid manic-depressive alternations

————— lithium administration   ————•— lithium dosage increased

Diagrammatic presentation of the case histories. The patients are arranged according to age; the first two digits of each case number indicate the year of birth. In the second column is shown the year when the first manic or depressive episode appeared. The diagram shows, for each patient, all psychotic episodes that occurred between January 1, 1960, and July 1, 1966.

Figure 24-3. Effect of lithium in decreasing frequency and duration of subsequent manic and depressive episodes (from Baastrup and Schou, 1967).

ment are all highly characteristic of impending affective episodes. Often these changes are first noted by family members and can be crucially important to the patient in early intervention. Strategies for contacting the clinician should be determined, if possible, during times when the patient is normal. To the extent feasible, general contingency plans and agreements should be made in advance to cover possible emergencies (e.g., suicidal thinking and behavior; see Chapter 27), hospitalization plans for mania, and financial protection for the patient and family during hypomanic and manic episodes.

The potential problems of violation of confidentiality are substantial and need to be discussed openly with patients and their families.

Family therapy, when indicated, can be a useful adjunct to treatment. Many issues arise in treating families with one or more members who suffer from manic-depressive illness. These are covered extensively in Chapter 12. Specific studies using family interventions are covered later in this chapter and are summarized in Table 24-1. Interpersonal aspects of manic-depressive illness are discussed in Chapter 12.

National and Local Support Associations

Both manic-depressive patients and their families can participate in excellent self-help programs, many conducted under the auspices of the National Depressive and Manic-Depressive Association (NDMDA). Nationally organized in 1986, the association has its roots in a local support group set up in Chicago in 1978. There are now more than 100 groups in existence, with approximately two or three new ones forming each month. The stated purpose of the NDMDA is "to provide personal support and direct service to persons with clinical depression or manic depression and their families; to educate the public concerning the nature and management of these treatable medical disorders; and to promote related research."

Services provided by chapters of the NDMDA and other support organizations such as the National Alliance for the Mentally Ill (NAMI) include educational programs for patients, their family members, and the general public, self-help support groups for patients and families, determination of lithium levels, Alcoholics Anonymous meetings, telephone hotlines for emergencies, newsletters, summaries of relevant research findings, employment counseling, and referrals to clinicians with expertise in treating manic-depressive and depressive illness. The NDMDA works in collaboration, not in competition, with clinicians.

Most major cities now have a branch of the NDMDA or similar groups, and we feel strongly that patients and their families should be encouraged to seek support from their local group. This in no way takes away from the primary care of the patient by physicians and psychotherapists. Rather, it offers supplementary support that in addition to other benefits, frequently enhances compliance with the medical regimen. If there is no local branch of the NDMDA or NAMI, the national office can be contacted for information about the nearest group.

REVIEW OF THE LITERATURE

The potential advantages of combining psychotherapy with pharmacotherapy in bipolar illness must be inferred from the related but very different field of drug–psychotherapy interactions in the treatment of unipolar depression.[5] No comparable controlled studies exist for bipolar illness. Klerman (1975) has outlined several potential negative and positive drug–psychotherapy interactions. Particularly relevant to the treatment of bipolar patients are the hypothesized positive effects of drug treatment on psychotherapy. These include the patient's increased accessibility and such psychotherapeutically useful symptomatic changes as increased memory, improved sleep, enhanced verbal skills, and decreased distractibility. Also relevant are the positive effects of psychotherapy on drug treatment, which include more reliable patient attendance and increased compliance with the drug regimen. Weissman (1978) reviewed the controlled studies of antidepressants alone and in combination with psychotherapy and came to two pertinent conclusions. First, in ambulatory, unipolar depressed outpatients, the combination of antidepressant medications with psychotherapy (group, individual, or conjoint) was more efficacious than either treatment alone. Second, there were no negative drug–psychotherapy interactions (findings further documented by Rounsaville et al., 1981).

Analogous studies of the treatment of bipolar illness do not exist. Thus, the discussions that follow are limited to hypothetical issues, supplemented by a few uncontrolled clinical investigations. Several modalities of psychotherapy are available to the clinician wishing to work with patients on lithium. Informal psychological treatments include the supportive role of the physician in medication management, educational models that convey medical information about manic-depressive illness and lithium through lectures, handouts, films, or information-giving groups, and self-help groups run by patients for themselves. A wide range of theoretical orientations governs more formal psychological treatments, such as individual, group, family, and conjoint psychotherapy or some combination of these.

Little is known about the appropriateness of any of these modalities or orientations for a particular patient or type of problem. For example, we do not know if cognitive behavior therapy is more effective for lithium compliance problems or if psychodynamic therapy is more appropriate for the interpersonal sequelae of manic-depressive illness. We also do not know if group therapy is more useful for problems of illness denial and self-esteem or if individual therapy is more appropriate for short-term crisis intervention in such problems as suicidal behavior or for the long-term treatment of idiosyncratic, intrapsychic problems. Several studies involving couples and family therapy have been done,[6] and most are summarized in Table 24-1.

Post (1986) suggests using the life charting method to help identify specific, repeated psychosocial stresses that have special meaning to a patient and that become linked in time to repeated episodes of affective illness. This hierarchy of events and ideas likely to evoke dysphoric feelings can become a focus for psychotherapy using systematic desensitization. For patients who have been conditioned to high states of emotional reactivity or sensitized to stress, modified behavioral techniques can serve as an adjunct to drugs and psychotherapy. Cognitive psychotherapy has been demonstrated to be useful in treatment with manic-depressive patients (Cochran, 1984). Interpersonal therapy, although not formally evaluated in bipolar illness, has been found useful in depressive illness (Klerman et al., 1984).

The available clinical reports on combined lithium treatment and psychotherapy are summarized here and in Table 24-1. Few of the studies used comparison groups for the analysis of treatment outcomes or pretest and posttest measures. The substantial methodological shortcomings in most of these investigations make meaningful interpretation virtually impossible, but the clinical observations made by the therapists conducting the studies (noted in Table 24-1) are conceptually very useful.

Better controlled studies (Cochran, 1984; Glick et al., 1985) indicate that both individual and family psychotherapy, when combined with lithium, seem to result in a better clinical outcome and increased lithium compliance. The Cochran

study and specific strategies for coping with noncompliance are further discussed in Chapter 25. A specific strategy for cognitive–behavioral intervention for bipolar patients taking lithium is given in Appendix II. Jacobs (1982) also described specific cognitive therapy techniques to help patients overcome postmanic and postdepressive dysphoria. Wulsin and colleagues (1988) reviewed the literature on group therapy in manic-depressive illness and argue for its efficacy, stressing that several aspects of the illness make group therapy a likely intervention: (1) the patient's need for information about the illness, (2) the patient's need for lithium and other medical management, and (3) the interpersonal difficulties that develop during the course of manic-depressive illness.

SUMMARY

Manic-depressive illness is treated most effectively with a combination of lithium or other medications and adjunctive psychotherapy. Drug treatment, which is primary, frees most patients from the severe disruptions of manic and depressive episodes. Psychotherapy can help them to come to terms with the repercussions of past episodes and to comprehend the practical and existential implications of having manic-depressive illness.

Although not all patients need psychotherapy, most can benefit from one of its many forms—individual, group, or family. Participation in a self-help group can supplement or supplant formal psychotherapy. Which option is most appropriate can often be determined by the psychiatrist or psychopharmacologist who supervises the patient's medications. When drugs are administered in an emotionally supportive atmosphere, patients are more likely to express their concerns and physicians are better able to assess the need for psychological interventions, and lithium compliance is enhanced.

Psychotherapeutic issues are dictated by the character of the illness: Manifested by profound changes in perception, attitudes, personality, mood, and cognition, manic-depressive illness can lead to suicide, violence, alcoholism, drug abuse, and hospitalization. Although reactions vary widely, patients typically feel angry and ambivalent about both the illness and its treatment.

Table 24-1. Clinical Reports on Combined Lithium Treatment and Psychotherapy

Study	Therapy/Design/ Patients N	Results	Clinical Observations
Fitzgerald, 1972	Family therapy and lithium, eclectic: educational, emphasis on communications. Clinical study: no comparison, 25 BP, index hospitalization for mania	No systematic follow-up	Family therapy can help manic patients: (1) take lithium, (2) prevent relapses, and (3) improve verbal communication within the family (i.e., replace the role of mania in the expressions of anger and frustration)
Davenport et al., 1977	Group I – psychodynamic couples' group + lithium, 4 times wk; 12 BP	No rehospital-izations; no marital failures	At follow-up, Group I patients significantly improved on social functioning and family interactions vs Group III; better on family interaction vs Group II; no significant differences beween Groups II and III. Strong recommendation for co-therapist model. Marital dynamics: (1) fear by both spouses of recurrence, (2) sense of help-lessness, (3) need to control all affect and defend against closeness, (4) use of massive denial, and (5) themes related to early parental loss and failure to grieve
	Group II – NIMH outpatient dept. lithium maintenance 4 times monthly; crisis treat-ment as needed; 11 BP	2 rehospital-ized; 5 marital failures	
	Group III – Referral to com-munity clinic or private care; Note: Marriages intact at time of discharge from index hospitalization for all; follow-up period variable for all (2-10 yr posthospitalization) 42 BP	16 rehospital-ized; 10 marital failures; 3 suicides	
Shakir et al., 1979	Group therapy + lithium; interpersonal, interactional Clinical study; compared group means of patients' pre- and posthospitalization records. 75 min 4 times wk; lithium dispensed during last 30 min of group; 15 BP - 13 M, 2 F; Mean age: 43; Range: 19-63; Months on lithium prior to group: 21	Pregroup: 16 wk/yr in hospital Postgroup: 3 wk/ yr in hospital. Two-yr follow-up	Group themes: (1) initial skepticism about lithium and group therapy, (2) complaints about loss of well-being due to lithium, (3) denial of problems, (4) projection of responsibility for lithium deficiency onto psychiatrists, (5) concerns: recurrence, illness chronicity, social adjustment, and social acceptance
Rosen, 1980	Group therapy + lithium, directive. Clinical study; no comparison, pre- or posttest; 90 min 4 times wk for 4 wk 25 mixed patients, 12 M, 13 F, mean age: 36; range: 25-27	No systematic follow-up; over 2.5 yr 8 patients remained in group	Group themes: (1) lithium, (2) concerns about manic-depressive illness, (3) lowered morale when member hospi-talized. Described lively atmosphere where "therapist works not so much to stimulate interaction as to moderate it"
Volkmar et al., 1981	Group therapy + lithium; Interpersonal, interactional (Continuation of group therapy outlined in Shakir et al.)		Group themes as reported in Shakir et al. Also: Cessation of lithium use from denial of illness, lack of information, lack of support. "It is not clear whether the high rate of compliance is secondary to the effects of group therapy per se or to the close follow-up the patients received or to the interaction between the two"

Continued

Cochran, 1984	Individual therapy + lithium, 6 sessions cognitive-behavioral therapy vs standard clinic care; 26 BP, 13 in each condition	Significantly more lithium compliance & fewer hospital-izations in psychotherapy group	Although two groups did not differ significantly in number of affective episodes, psychotherapy patients were less likely to be hospitalized
Glick et al., 1985	Inpatient family intervention. Compared with a standard multi-model inpatient treatment; 12 BP families in therapy group, 8 in comparison	At 18 mo follow-up, sig-nificantly fewer rehospitalized and better work/social role functioning in family therapy group	Clinical outcome was best. Family intervention was the most effective when the patient's family was assessed as low on "patient rejection" and patient was compliant with medication
Kripke & Robinson, 1985	Group outpatient, problem solving. Blood levels and prescriptions monitored. VA setting. Started with 13 M, 1 F; 8 remained at 12th year of group. 90 min every 2 weeks	Decreased hospitalization rates, improved socioeconomic functioning	Leader's attempts at a psychodynamic and introspective focus worked less well than problem-solving
Haas et al., 1988, and Spencer et al., 1988	Inpatient family intervention, psychoeducational, 169 psychiatric patients (50 affective disorder) randomly assigned to family intervention or none (with an increase in individual psychotherapy for the latter). Six 45-60 min sessions average	At discharge, improved hospital treat-ment outcome for the family intervention group, especially in females with affective disorders. At 6 and 18 mo follow-up, a better outcome was also seen among the schizophrenics in this group	Attitudes of families toward treatment improved in the study group. Later follow-ups showed greater openness to social support, less patient rejection and family burden
Miklowitz et al., 1988 and Goldstein & Miklowitz, unpublished data	Behavioral family treatment (including education, com-munication training, problem-solving) + lithium. 8 BPs treated for 9 mo with natu-ralistic follow-up. Compared with 23 BP families receiving lithium only	13% of behavioral + lithium group relapsed, 70% of lithium-alone group relapsed	

Update and adaptation of Jamison & Goodwin, 1983

They may deny its existence, its severity, or its consequences. Such denial may cause them to stop taking their medication. When treatment is not completely successful, they are understandably disappointed and frustrated. They are disturbed by losing the energy and vitality that accompanies mania. They fear recurrences. They have difficulty discriminating normal from abnormal moods. They are concerned about relationships and the possibility of genetically transmitting the illness to their children.

No one technique has been shown to be superior in the psychotherapy of manic-depressive patients. The therapist must be guided by knowledge of the illness itself and its manifestation in the individual patient. In style and technique, the therapist must remain flexible to adjust to the patient's fluctuating levels of dependency and ever changing mood, cognition, and behavior. The therapist must be especially alert to the countertransference issues that commonly occur when working with manic-depressive patients.

Charting moods is useful to provide an objective record of patterns of mood and treatment response. It gives patients a sense of control and collaboration in their treatment. Educating patients and their families is essential because it encourages compliance and helps them to recognize new episodes. Informed consent for treatment is imperative for both clinical and legal reasons. Patients should be encouraged, when appropriate, to participate in self-help groups.

APPENDIX I: READING LIST FOR PATIENTS AND FAMILIES

Custance J: *Wisdom, Madness, and Folly: The Philosophy of a Lunatic.* London: Victor Gollancz Ltd., 1951.

DePaulo R, Ablow KR: *How to Cope with Depression: A Complete Guide for You and Your Family.* New York: McGraw Hill, 1989.

Fieve RR: *Moodswing: The Third Revolution in Psychiatry.* 2nd ed. New York: William Morrow, 1989.

Fitzgerald FS: "The Crack-Up." In: *The Crack-Up With Other Pieces and Stories.* Middlesex: Penguin, 1965 (first published 1936).

Goodwin FK: *Depression and Manic-Depressive Illness.* NIH Publication No. 82-1940, February 1982.

Hamilton I: *Robert Lowell: A Biography.* New York: Random House, 1982.

Jamison KR, Winter R: *Moods and Music.* Program notes for a concert performed by the National Symphony Orchestra at the John F. Kennedy Center for

the Performing Arts, Washington, DC, November 1988.

Lobel B, Hirschfeld RMA: *Depression: What We Know.* DHHS Publication No (ADM) 85-1318, Rockville, Md, 1985.

Logan J: *Josh: My Up and Down, In and Out Life.* New York: Delacorte Press, 1976.

Mondimore F: *Mood Disease: The Biological Basis and Medical Treatment for Depression, Mood Swings, and Other Affective Disorders.* Baltimore: Johns Hopkins University Press, 1989.

Rosenberg JD: *The Darkening Glass: A Portrait of Ruskin's Genius.* New York: Columbia University Press, 1986.

Rosenthal NE: *Seasons of the Mind: Why You Get the Winter Blues & What You Can Do About It.* New York: Bantam Books, 1989.

Schou M: *Lithium Treatment of Manic-Depressive Illness: A Practical Guide.* Basel: Karger, 1986.

APPENDIX II: COGNITIVE–BEHAVIORAL INTERVENTION STRATEGY FOR BIPOLAR PATIENTS ON LITHIUM*

These are outlines of psychotherapy sessions that might take place with bipolar patients. The therapy is highly structured, and patients are encouraged to think about and express their thoughts and reactions to the medication they have been prescribed.

First Session Topic: Introduction
1. Introduce purpose of meeting together
   a. Acknowledge that there may be difficulties with taking medication.
   b. Working together to plan strategies may be helpful.
   c. Work outside of the session may be necessary and important to provide information.
2. Elicit patient's thoughts and reactions to taking lithium and medication in general. Keep a record of these.
3. Educate patient about lithium and manic-depressive illness.
4. Introduce notion that thoughts and beliefs about things affect behavior.
5. Introduce notion that situations can be altered to affect behavior, such as medication compliance.

Second Session Topic: Identifying Negative Thoughts
1. Note any difficulties and together generate some solutions to behavioral aspects of noncompliance. Pay attention to location of pills and filling of prescriptions, and suggest changes where appropriate.
2. Indicate that people have many feelings about tak-

* From Goldstein et al., 1986, p. 299, in which it was adapted from Cochran SD: "Strategies for Preventing Lithium Noncompliance in Bipolar Affective Illness." Unpublished doctoral dissertation. University of California at Los Angeles, 1982.

ing medication. Bring in and discuss last session's responses.

3. Use thought-tracking form (keeping a systematic record) to work to identify negative thoughts.

Homework: Have patient track thoughts at time of taking pills at least once during the week.

Third Session Topic: Countering Negative Thoughts
1. Discuss homework and any difficulties related to the medication regimen that have occurred in the previous week.
2. Teach technique of countering negative thoughts using homework.

Homework: Have patient track thoughts and attempt to counter them.

Fourth Session Topic: Further Countering Negative Thoughts
1. Discuss homework and any difficulties with medication regimen.
2. Again attempt to counter negative thoughts. Elicit patient's degree of belief in counterthoughts and discuss as necessary.
3. Further develop skills at generating coping thoughts.

Homework: Have patient track thoughts, counter, and generate coping thoughts.

Fifth Session Topic: Planning for the Future
1. Discuss homework and any difficulties with the medication regimen.
2. Attempt to anticipate and problem-solve future difficulties likely to arise. Problem areas may include visits from relatives, trips, feeling OK, just not wanting to take pills any more, anger at physicians.

Homework: Have patient contemplate potential future difficulties and generate solutions to have available.

Sixth Session Topic: Wrap-up
1. Discuss homework.
2. Get feedback from patient about what was most and least valuable.
3. Have patient complete forms.
4. Remind patient that he or she will be contacted for follow-up.

NOTES

1. For obvious reasons, psychotherapy has never been as integral or comfortable a part of the treatment of bipolar illness as it has been of unipolar illness. Clearly, the psychotic disorders and their empirically derived remedies long predate psychological treatments. Both history and necessity have embedded bipolar illness in medicine, much more so than other psychiatric disorders. Unipolar depressions, on the other hand, have had an easier alliance with psychotherapy, partly because they generally constitute a wider spectrum of psychopathology that shows a range of milder syndromes with prominent psychological factors. Because the concept of *depression* encompasses a relatively normal spectrum of emotions and feelings, it has traditionally stimulated counsel from priests, physicians, and friends.

2. From *The Code of the Woosters*, 1975.

3. Polatin and Fieve, 1971; Schou and Baastrup, 1973; Van Putten, 1975; Jamison et al., 1979; Schou, 1980.

4. These arrangements are covered under the legal mechanism of *advanced instruction directives*, one of two such mechanisms in general medicine by which a person can make arrangements for treatment should he or she become incapacitated. The other, *advanced proxy directive*, allows a person to appoint another person to act for him or her. This durable power-of-attorney, unlike a regular power-of-attorney, does not become invalid if the person is incapacitated. In fact, it sometimes only takes effect then. The advanced proxy directive has been tested in the courts, and there is a trend to accept its validity.

Psychiatric patients do not necessarily come under the same precedents, statutes, and regulations as general medicine patients. Neither of the mechanisms applies directly, especially for psychiatric hospitalization, ECT, and, increasingly, the use of neuroleptics. Many states have rules that prevent a guardian from giving consent for these treatments without going through an additional procedure. Unless a person otherwise meets the standards for incompetence, these mechanisms have questionable enforceability. Then, of course, there are additional statutory restrictions on the use of ECT.

Nevertheless, these mechanisms could still carry weight, adding evidence when judges make their decisions, whether they are making a substituted judgment, trying to reflect what the person would want, or if they are trying to act in the best interest of the patient (Appelbaum, 1987; Appelbaum et al., 1987).

5. Covi et al., 1974; Klerman et al., 1974; Friedman, 1975; Klerman and Schechter, 1979; Weissman, 1979; Weissman et al., 1979, 1987; Janowsky and Neborsky, 1980; Neborsky et al., 1980; Blackburn et al., 1981; Murphy et al., 1984; Simons et al., 1984; Frank and Kupfer, 1984.

6. Fitzgerald, 1972; Davenport et al., 1977; Glick et al., 1985; Haas et al., 1988; Spencer et al., 1988; Weber et al., 1988.

25

Medication Compliance

The endless questioning finally ended. My psychiatrist looked at me, there was no
uncertainty in his voice. "Manic-depressive illness." I admired his bluntness. I
wished him locusts on his lands and a pox upon his house. Silent, unbelievable
rage. I smiled pleasantly. He smiled back. The war had just begun.
—Patient with manic-depressive illness

Many patients with affective illness seem to have
little or no difficulty in taking potent daily medications for an indeterminate period. They do not
appear to be unduly concerned about potential or
actual side effects, nor do they seem to struggle
with the existential issues that might reasonably
be raised when a person is required to take powerful mind- and mood-altering drugs. Because of
temperament or past experience, they do not protest or disobey their physicians' orders but often
are grateful for the medications and thank the
doctors who prescribe them. Often such patients
state that lithium or antidepressants have rescued
them from chaos, despair, debilitating hospitalization, or suicide. Compliant patients are an interesting, although inadequately studied, group.
Certainly they are a source of gratification to their
physicians.

For every patient who follows the treatment
course, however, there is at least one who does
not—one who resists, protests, objects, takes too
little, takes too much, or takes none at all.
Clearly, the patient who refuses to take lithium or
takes it incorrectly negates its therapeutic
efficacy. One of these noncompliant patients is
quoted in Table 25-1.

We focus on lithium for several reasons. (1)
The consequences of lithium noncompliance[1] are
profound and can be life-threatening. (2) Lithium
often is prescribed on an exceptionally long-term
or lifelong basis. (3) Lithium noncompliance is a
frustrating, common, and perplexing clinical

problem. (4) Poor lithium compliance is almost
certainly the single most important factor in poor
treatment response. (5) Essentially no compliance research has been carried out on carbamazepine (Lenzi et al., 1989).

The consequences of noncompliance are
clinically equivalent to those of untreated or inadequately treated manic-depressive illness: recurrence and intensification of affective episodes
that are often accompanied by interpersonal
chaos, alcohol and drug abuse, personal anguish
and family disruption, financial crises, conjugal
failure, psychiatric hospitalization, suicide, and
violence. This point may be obvious, but it is frequently ignored. Unlike unresponsiveness, however, noncompliance is reversible and can be
changed through experience, education, learning, and psychotherapy.

In addition to the costs in human suffering
brought about by noncompliance, the potential
economic costs to society are staggering. Reifman and Wyatt (1980) estimated that the use of
lithium in the decade between 1969 and 1979
saved the United States $4 billion through reduc-
tions in medical costs and restoration of productivity. A recent updating of these figures, in 1989
dollars, suggests a saving of more than $40 bil-
lion from 1969 to 1989 (Wyatt, personal communication). Noncompliance substantially un-
dermines potential economic gains. From a
practical point of view, the development of effective techniques to deal with lithium non-

Table 25-1. Rules for the Gracious Acceptance of Lithium into Your Life

1. Clear out the medicine cabinet before guests arrive for dinner or new lovers stay the night.

2. Remember to put the lithium back into the cabinet the next day.

3. Don't be too embarrassed by your lack of co-ordination or your inability to do well the sports you once did with ease.

4 Learn to laugh about spilling coffee, having the palsied signature of an eighty year old, and being unable to put on cufflinks in less than ten minutes.

5. Smile when people joke about how they think they "need to be on lithium."

6. Nod intelligently, and with conviction, when your physician explains to you the many advantages of lithium in leveling out the chaos in your life.

7. Be patient when waiting for this leveling off. Very patient. Re-read the Book of Job. Continue being patient. Contemplate the similarity between the phrases "being patient" and "being a patient."

8. Try not to let the fact that you can't read without effort annoy you. Be philosophical. Even if you could read, you probably wouldn't remember most of it anyway.

9. Accommodate to a certain lack of enthusiasm and bounce which you once had. Try not to think about all the wild nights you once had. Probably best not to have had those nights anyway.

10. Always keep in perspective how much better you are. Everyone else certainly points it out often enough and, annoyingly enough, it's probably true.

11. Be appreciative. Don't even consider stopping your lithium.

12. When you do stop, get manic, get depressed, expect to hear two basic themes from your family, friends, and healers:
    • But you were doing so much better, I just don't understand it.
    • I told you this would happen.

13. Restock your medicine cabinet.

From a patient with manic-depressive illness

compliance has major implications for insurance companies and health maintenance organizations.

Another consequence of lithium noncompliance is the probable bias of research findings in clinical studies related to lithium. Frank and colleagues (1985) stressed that investigators "have an obligation to account for nonadherent patients in their analyses" (p. 42) by specifying how many and which patients fail to comply (patient, history of illness, and therapist variables). Data should be analyzed with and without end-point analysis techniques.

In this chapter, we approach the discussion from the perspective of the clinician, by first detailing strategies for dealing with lithium noncompliance. In the second section, we review research findings from anecdotal and systematic observations (rates, correlates, and results of interventions). Some of the issues discussed here were covered, in less detail, by earlier reviews.[2] There is also overlap with our discussions of noncompliance and psychotherapy (see Chapter 24) and maintenance medication (see Chapter 23).

CLINICAL MANAGEMENT

Patient Factors

Risk factors for lithium noncompliance, summarized from studies reviewed later, are presented in Table 25-2. Generally, compliance appears to increase with age, which coincides with a period of increasing risk of episodes recurring. The first year after the initiation of lithium treatment is a particularly high-risk period for stopping lithium against medical advice. A constellation of related mood variables seems to predict noncompliance: missing the highs, elevated mood in its own right, and a history of grandiose delusions. There is some evidence that patients experiencing proportionately more manic than depressive episodes are more likely to be noncompliant.

Table 25-2. Risk Factors for Lithium Noncompliance[a]

- First year of lithium treatment
- History of noncompliance
- Younger
- Male
- Fewer episodes
- History of grandiose, euphoric manias
- Elevated mood
- Complaints of "missing highs"

[a]Summary based on studies of both bipolar and unipolar patients

Medication Factors

Patients report that weight gain, cognitive impairment, tremor, increased thirst, and lethargy are their major reasons for stopping lithium. They mention gastric irritation, nausea, vomiting, and diarrhea less often. The frequency of these side effects and their importance in noncompliance are reviewed later in the chapter. (See Chapter 23 for the clinical management of specific side effects.) The effects of lithium on personality are also relevant to compliance, since some patients become less sociable, outgoing, active, and elated while taking the drug.

Conceivably, some of the lethargy and memory difficulties attributed to lithium actually may be symptoms of the unrecognized, atypical, retarded depressive relapses that lithium sometimes fails to prevent.[3] Along with cognitive problems and hopelessness secondary to the depression, lethargy and cognitive difficulties caused by lithium can increase the likelihood of medication noncompliance. As reviewed in Chapter 22, concomitant chronic use of antidepressants sometimes increases episode frequency. Discouraged by the episodes, patients may stop taking lithium, or they may fail to recognize these mini-episodes and ascribe the accompanying emotional blunting to lithium.

The similarity of lithium-induced changes in cognitive functioning and energy levels to the symptoms of affective illness may cause the opposite problem as well. Some complaints from patients are mistakenly attributed entirely to breakthrough depressions or other manifestations of illness. Although difficult to differentiate clinically, in research settings cognitive side effects of lithium have been observed in normal subjects, as well as in patients with affective disorders (See Chapter 23).

Misunderstandings about lithium can arise between patients and physicians because psychiatrists tend to stress the medical side effects of lithium (e.g., thyroid and renal effects, polyuria, tremor). This emphasis may stem from early studies when clinical investigators were very concerned about the long-term somatic effects of lithium but paid relatively little attention to side effects that many patients find more distressing, such as weight gain, decreased energy, slowing of cognition, decreased memory and concentration, and lessened enthusiasms.

Even though some cognitive effects may be unavoidable and as yet untreatable, and not all patients on lithium experience them, they must be taken seriously and corrected to the extent possible. In some instances, lithium-induced hypothyroidism may be responsible for decreased energy and slowed intellectual functioning. This condition can be treated easily. In other cases, when too little lithium leads to breakthrough depressions or too much lithium leads to mild neurotoxicities, subtle titration of the dosage can improve the problem substantially. Strategies for minimizing the long-term side effects of lithium are outlined in Chapter 23.

Special reinforcement schedules intrinsic to lithium treatment force clinicians to contend with a singularly difficult set of problems:

- Lithium (unlike analgesics, neuroleptics, or benzodiazepines) has delayed therapeutic actions: 5 to 7 days for an antimanic effect, usually 3 to 5 weeks for an antidepressant effect.
- Lithium has no known intrinsic reinforcing qualities, either immediate or delayed.
- Patients are expected to stay on the drug for an indeterminate time, much of it in a more or less normal state, with no immediate felt need for the drug.
- If a patient stops the medication, the negative consequences of noncompliance (recurrences of the affective illness) are often long-delayed (there is no immediate negative reinforcer).
- The onset of lithium treatment often is paired with unpleasant events (psychosis, hospitalization, family problems).
- If lithium is first prescribed for a manic episode, the natural history of the illness predicts that the patient is at significant risk for a postmanic depression, which further pairs the onset of lithium treatment with unpleasant psychological and physical experiences.
- The cessation of lithium is often accompanied by relatively immediate positive experiences, either because of the disappearance of side effects or because of breakthrough hypomania (often a contributing factor in lithium noncompliance in the first place).

Treatment Issues

Guidelines for maximizing lithium compliance are summarized in Table 25-3. Sackett and associates (1985) emphasize the "uniformly dismal performance of clinicians" in predicting and assessing compliance in their patients. They found that detecting which patients are noncompliant could be done more quickly, less expensively, and about as well simply by asking patients about taking their medications as by using drug levels. To increase the reliability of patients' responses, they suggest an interview format that makes the admission of noncompliance socially acceptable; for example, "Most people have trouble taking all of their pills. Do you have any trouble taking all of yours?" The physician should order lithium level determinations regularly and inquire frequently about possible problems with compliance and concerns about the medication.

Also critical are the attitudes toward lithium of all physicians and psychotherapists involved in patient care. In general, clinicians who are ambivalent about the role of biological factors in the

Table 25-3. Guidelines for Maximizing
Lithium Compliance

Monitor compliance
Regular lithium levels
Inquire frequently
Encourage queries and concerns from patients and
families

Side effects
Forewarn
Treat aggressively (especially hypothyroidism and
tremor)
Minimize lithium level

Education
Early symptoms of mania and depression
Unremitting and worsening course of (untreated)
manic-depressive illness

Medication
Minimize number of daily doses
Pillboxes (7 day), especially if on two or more
medications
Involve family members in administering, if
appropriate
Written information about lithium and side effects
(Limited) patient-titration of lithium level

Adjunctive psychotherapy

Self-help groups

causation and treatment of affective disorders tend to convey their ambivalence to their patients and possibly contribute to unsatisfactory compliance. Findings from a study by Cochran and Gitlin (1988) underscore the importance of the role of the patient's psychiatrist in ensuring compliance. The results of their study suggest that the more strongly the psychiatrist believes in the treatment regimen, the more likely the patient is to comply. The problem is further compounded by the antagonism toward lithium and other psychoactive medications on the part of some mental health workers, who may subtly or overtly sabotage drug compliance. In contrast, clinicians with an extreme biological bias may oversell lithium and thereby pave the way to patient disillusionment when minor relapses occur, or they may underestimate the role of psychological factors in the illness and its treatment and overlook subjective symptoms, like emotional dulling or memory disturbance, that many patients find extremely troublesome. The evidence from studies in general medical settings and lithium clinics suggests that physicians may inadvertently contribute to lithium noncompliance by failing to educate the patient and family. A clear understanding of manic-depressive disease, its course without treatment, and the role of lithium in attenuating this course (Frank et al., 1985) can enhance compliance.

As emphasized in Chapter 24, psychotherapy is important in the treatment of manic-depressive illness, specifically in encouraging lithium compliance. Lithium patients tend to place a far greater value on adjunctive psychotherapy than do clinicians, and noncompliant patients have been shown to regard psychotherapy as highly useful in helping them adhere to a regimen of lithium treatment (Jamison et al., 1979). Consistent with these observations are findings that show that patients treated with cognitive therapy more often took their lithium as prescribed than did patients who did not receive psychotherapy (Cochran, 1982). Because of their compliance, the psychotherapy patients also had fewer affective episodes and fewer hospitalizations. Self-help groups, such as those organized by the National Depressive and Manic-Depressive Association, are beneficial to many patients and their families (see Chapter 24).

Many clinicians, having once diagnosed the illness and prescribed an effective drug, tend to assume that the difficult part is over. On the contrary. In the words of the patient quoted at the beginning of the chapter, "the war has just begun."

REVIEW OF THE LITERATURE

General Issues in Medication Compliance

Noncompliance to medication regimens, a major clinical problem, has been reported to range from 15 to 85 percent in medical illnesses.[4] It is especially common in outpatients and those with chronic relapsing disorders, such as diabetes and hypertension. Despite the immensity of the problem, there is no single concept or definition of compliance that is satisfactory for most clinical situations. Questions quickly arise: What does it mean to comply or not to comply? How does one measure compliance? Can it be predicted? Can its course be altered? Is it inevitable? Are there compliers and noncompliers, or can circumstances significantly change behavior patterns? Clinical experience teaches about compliance what it teaches about all complicated and meaningful behavior: the many patterns are not bound into discrete categories. People change, illnesses change, and environments change.

Investigations in general medicine provide information relevant for determining the meaning of compliance to lithium and other psychoactive medications. According to Boyd and colleagues (1974a), medication noncompliance, or drug defaulting, is "the failure to comply (intentional or accidental) with the physician's directions (expressed or implied) in the self-administration of any medication" (p. 326). Blackwell (1976, 1980, 1982) specified how drug defaulting can occur through four types of errors: (1) omission, where the patient either fails to fill the prescription at all or, once having filled it, fails to take the drug, (2) dosage, (3) timing, and (4) purpose or commission (taking drugs for the wrong reason). One study of nonpsychiatric patients (Boyd et al., 1974a,b) found that the most common medication errors were mistimed dosages (56 percent of prescriptions), premature termination of the drug (45 percent), and deliberate skipping of dosages (35 percent). Mazzullo and Lasagna (1972) con-

sidered physician factors in drug noncompliance, including failure to inquire about eating and sleeping habits that relate to prescribed medication schedules, failure to give warning about the time course of expected benefits and side effects, and too little time spent in educating patients about the illness and the prescription. They noted:

Too often, this most important part of the patient's visit is handled in a most superfluous manner, as the doctor rushes on to his next patient. But the process of educating the patient is really crucial to establishing the close working relationship between physician and patient that is the *sine qua non* of optimal care. (p. 15)

Other factors related to adherence to treatment regimens include chronicity of illness and the duration of treatment.

Insight into lithium compliance can be gained from compliance studies conducted in nonpsychiatric settings (Blackwell, 1976, 1982; Haynes et al., 1979). Disease, patient, and treatment factors associated with general medical compliance are summarized in Table 25-4. Factors that seem to predict medical compliance include chronicity of illness, amount of time asymptomatic, number of symptoms experienced, extent of disability, health beliefs of the patient (perceived seriousness of illness and perceived efficacy of treatment), and social supports. Aspects of the treatment regimen are also predictive, such as its complexity, number of medications and their cost, and route and ease of administration, as are aspects of the health care delivery system (convenience of the clinical setting, continuity of care, and extent of supervision by others) and physician attitudes. Demographic variables, such as age (except in its extremes), sex, intelligence, and educational level, are not predictive of compliance. The relationship of personality variables and medication side effects to medical compliance is uncertain, although they appear more relevant to lithium noncompliance.

Noncompliance in psychiatric settings is at least as high as it is in nonpsychiatric settings. In one study of psychiatric outpatients (Willcox et al., 1965), as many as 50 percent of depressive and schizophrenic patients were not taking their medication (imipramine or chlorpromazine), and those treated with the wrong drug (e.g., depressed patients treated with chlorpromazine) or unsupervised patients (e.g., single males) were more likely to default. In a study of schizophrenic

Table 25-4. Factors Associated with Medical Compliance

Factor	Predictive of Compliance	Predictive of Noncompliance	Not Predictive	Unclear
Disease				
Chronicity of illness	X			
Amount of time asymptomatic		X		
Severity of disease:				
As a general factor			X	
Number of symptoms experienced	X			
Extent of disability	X			
Type of illness: psychiatric		X		
Patient				
Demographics:				
Age (except extremes)			X	
Sex			X	
Intelligence			X	
Education level			X	
Attitudes and personality				
Personality				X
Health beliefs:				
Seriousness of illness	X			
Perceived efficacy of treatment	X			
Social supports				
Living alone		X		
Unstable / nonsupportive families		X		
Treatment				
Treatment regimen:				
Complexity of regimen		X		
Number and costs of medication		X		
Oral administration	X			
Safety caps		X		
Frequency of dosage				X
Side effects of medication				X
Health care delivery:				
Convenience of clinical setting	X			
Continuity of care	X			
Extent of supervision by others	X			

Based on data in Haynes et al., 1979; Blackwell, 1980; Cochran, unpublished data

patients, Van Putten and colleagues (1976) reported that drug defaulting occurred because of unpleasant extrapyramidal effects, such as akathisia. Studies of lithium noncompliance, undertaken only in the past several years, have examined many factors in addition to side effects.

Patterns of lithium compliance also vary over time and from patient to patient. Some patients refuse to take medication at all, some adhere to a given medication but titrate their own dose (instead of following the physician-prescribed schedule), and some alternate between total and partial adherence. *Full compliance* refers to the practice of patients who take lithium in the manner prescribed and for the period of time specified by their physicians. This pattern is relatively un-

common; most patients who are considered compliant only approximate full compliance. *Late compliance* is a pattern of initial resistance to medication, followed by recurrences of affective illness and subsequent hospitalizations. There may then be a sudden switch toward compliance as patients begin to recognize the relationship between stopping lithium and recurrences of their illness. In *intermittent compliance*, probably the most common pattern, patients comply for a period of time (usually ranging from days to months) and then stop taking lithium (or start taking it in a manner not prescribed) against medical advice. After a recurrence of their illness, they begin taking lithium again. Before more consistent compliance is achieved, patients stop and start lithium, take it in subtherapeutic dosages, and experience recurrences of illness repeatedly. This pattern, however, varies tremendously from patient to patient. The most extreme pattern is, of course, *total noncompliance,* which every physician encounters at some time.

The most commonly employed methods for measuring compliance include review of chart notes, patient self-reports, records of unkept appointments and unfilled prescriptions, blood and urine levels of the drug in question, spouse estimates of the patient's drug-taking behavior, physician assessments of such behavior, pill counts, and measures of illness outcome (which assumes a direct relationship between medication compliance and exacerbations or recurrences of illness). All of these measures of medication compliance have substantial problems in reliability and validity.

Rates of Lithium Noncompliance

Of the more than 10,000 articles written about lithium, fewer than 50 deal in a substantive way with the primary clinical problem associated with it, that is, noncompliance. This lack of research is extraordinary, given the extent of the clinical problem presented by patients who refuse to take lithium as prescribed. There is little information about how many patients stop taking lithium against medical advice, for what reasons they stop, for how long, at what point in their therapeutic regimen or mood cycles, and whether there are sex and age differences in reasons for noncompliance or incomplete compliance. Little systematic research has been done on patients' perceptions of the positive and negative consequences of taking the drug regularly and the effect of these perceptions on actual patterns of lithium use.

Rates of lithium noncompliance, summarized in Table 25-5, range from 18 to 53 percent. These rates, although high and of concern, are lower than those cited for patients given tricyclics alone, 32 to 76 percent, although tricyclic noncompliance rates are considerably lower, ranging from 10 to 47 percent, when the medications are used in combination with psychotherapy (Frank et al., 1985).

Clinical Reports of Lithium Noncompliance

The first reported instance of lithium noncompliance in a manic-depressive patient was the

Table 25-5. Rates of Lithium Noncompliance

Study	%
Angst et al., 1970	18[a]
Van Putten, 1975	20–30
Bech et al., 1976	24
Jamison et al., 1979	47[b]
Connelly et al., 1982	25
Cochran, 1982	52
Vestergaard & Amdisen, 1983	23[a]
Jamison et al., 1984	28[b]
Frank et al., 1985	
Danion et al., 1987	53
Maarbjerg et al., 1988	23[a]
Lenzi et al., 1989	51[c]

[a] Within the first 6 months of treatment
[b] Differences in the socioeconomic status (SES) of the patients probably account for the differences in the two Jamison et al. studies (more noncompliance among lower SES patients)
[c] Compared with 38% of those patients taking carbamazepine

first patient treated with the drug. After recounting the initial dramatic success of lithium, Cade, years later, described the subsequent course:

> It was with a sense of the most abject disappointment that I readmitted him to hospital 6 months later as manic as ever but took some consolation from his brother who informed me that Bill had become overconfident about having been well for so many months, had become lackadaisical about taking his medication and finally ceased taking it about 6 weeks before. (1978, p. 13)

Several anecdotal reports of lithium noncompliance have been published, along with proposed explanations for the phenomenon. Polatin and Fieve (1971) emphasized that a patient often attributes decreases in creativity and productivity to lithium. They also stressed the role of denial in chronic, serious illnesses. Fitzgerald (1972) speculated that refusal to take lithium stemmed from intolerance of reality-based depressions, preference for a hypomanic way of life, or provocation from a spouse or other family member who also missed the patient's hypomanic episodes. Van Putten (1975), in addition to stressing the preference for hypomania, saw the importance of side effects and lithium-induced dysphoria, characterized by a driveless, anhedonic condition. Like Schou and colleagues (1970), he suggested that depressive relapses, as well as a tendency to feel well and to see no further need for medication, were significant variables in lithium refusal. Grof and associates (1970) found that the majority of their patients who stopped lithium of their own accord had been free of relapse and felt no need to continue. Schou and Baastrup (1973) cited several reasons for lithium noncompliance: decreased energy, enthusiasm, or sexuality, increased marital difficulties, and a common perception that life was flatter and less colorful than before lithium treatment began. Some of these complaints no doubt result from direct effects of lithium on the illness, and some are due to side effects. Kerry (1978) suggested that the social stigma associated with manic-depressive psychosis may lead to rejection of lithium, the most concrete symbol of the illness.

Cochran (1982) found that patient concerns clustered around the following issues:

- Personal control: frustrations with the "medical model," which they perceived as more focused on symptoms than personal gains, and insufficient emphasis on the establishment of alternative means of control, such as changes in diet or reduction in stress
- Changes in life brought about by successful lithium treatment: missing of highs, impact of stabilization on relationships
- Lack of predictability in the course of the illness, possible breakthrough episodes, and length of time on lithium and discomfort about having to be passive in light of possible impending episodes
- Issues concerning lithium, such as safety, mechanism of action, side effects, and efficacy

Cochran noted that, during treatment of noncompliance, patients often followed a pattern in their ability and willingness to articulate their attitudes toward lithium. Initially, they discussed their appreciation of lithium and expressed little ambivalence. By the third session, however, patients frequently spoke of massive ambivalence about lithium and considerable concern about future compliance. Miklowitz and colleagues (1986) found that:

Medication compliance was not by itself significantly associated with illness course in this sample, but did tend to mediate the relations between family factors and 9-month clinical outcome. Specifically, when the family environment to which the patient returned following hospitalization was negative, patients were at high risk for a poor clinical outcome regardless of whether they were medically compliant. However, a neutral or benign family environment was associated

with a good clinical outcome only when the patient consistently adhered to his/her medication regimen. (p. 631)

Data-Based Studies of Lithium Noncompliance

UCLA Studies

In a more systematic exploration of the earlier clinical reports described previously, Jamison and colleagues (1979) pursued two obvious sources of information and experience: the attitudes of patients themselves (47 lithium patients from the Affective Disorders Clinic at the University of California at Los Angeles) and, independently, the attitudes of clinicians well experienced in the use of lithium (50 physicians, each of whom had treated at least 50 patients with lithium). Nearly one half of the patients reported having stopped taking lithium at some time against medical advice, and 34 percent of those said that they stopped more than once. Of those who reported that they had not stopped, more than 90 percent stated that they had never considered doing so. These findings raised the possibility that patient practices in medication compliance tend to divide into two distinct subgroups, a distribution perhaps more bimodal than continuous in nature. (The pattern of full compliance may be fundamentally different from the three other patterns of late compliance, intermittent compliance, and complete noncompliance.)

Demographic Findings. In the UCLA study, no significant differences were found in sex, age, education, or income between the group of 22 patients who reported that they discontinued lithium treatment against medical advice and the group of 25 who continued. Patients with a prior history of mania (bipolar I) tended to be less compliant than those with a prior history of hypomania (bipolar II). The number of months on lithium was the only variable that differentiated significantly between the groups. More patients reported discontinuing lithium during long-term treatment. This finding may simply reflect the effect of increasing the period at risk for noncompliance.

Perceived Effectiveness of Lithium. Both groups of patients reported lithium to be highly effective in preventing recurrences of mania and effective, although somewhat less so, in preventing recurrent depressions. Ninety-six percent of the clinicians and 73 percent of the patients found lithium an extremely or very effective treatment for mania. More patients (40 percent) than clinicians (24 percent), however, regarded lithium as an effective treatment for depression. No significant relationship existed between perceived effectiveness and reported compliance.

Motivation for Continuing Lithium Treatment. Both the compliant and noncompliant patient groups indicated that fear of depression was a stronger reason for staying on lithium than fear of mania. The clinicians concurred in this perception.

Perceived Importance of Psychotherapy. Fifty percent of the patients considered psychotherapy to be "very important" in lithium compliance, but only 27 percent of the clinicians, most of whom were practicing psychotherapists, thought that psychotherapy was that important. This finding suggests a tendency among clinicians to value the potency of an effective medication so highly that they underestimate the psychological aspects of the illness and their impact on medication compliance. Nevertheless, over half the clinicians indicated that they almost always encouraged patients to seek adjunctive psychotherapy.

Side Effects of Lithium. Clinicians rated side effects as more important in noncompliance than did patients who reported discontinuing lithium therapy. Both patients and clinicians viewed lethargy, impairment in coordination, and lithium-induced tremor as important side effects in noncompliance. Patients regarded dulling of senses as equally important, whereas clinicians emphasized weight gain. Three of the four side effects most important to clinicians (tremor, weight gain, and nausea and vomiting) are all relatively somatic in nature, perhaps reflecting a tendency for patients to mention physical rather than cognitive changes. Conversely, clinicians may be reluctant to acknowledge substantial cognitive changes, or perhaps they view such changes as manifestations of affective episodes (as indeed they can be) rather than of medication. Female patients regarded lethargy and dulling of senses as significantly more problematic, which may reflect the often unrecognized lithium-induced hypothyroidism more often present in women than in men.

Psychodynamic Issues. Nearly two thirds of physicians thought that lithium noncompliance was "somewhat" or "very" related to patients acting out their denial of a serious lifelong illness. Other physicians believed that noncomplying patients were acting out psychodynamic factors in therapy. A few thought that anger at the therapist or at a significant other was also an important reason for a patient stopping lithium against medical advice.

General Reasons for Noncompliance. Table 25-6 lists in order of importance the reasons for noncompliance cited by the entire patient sample, by the group that had reported noncompliance, and by the clinicians. (When patients reported that they had always complied, they were asked to give reasons that might cause them not to comply.) From the patients' perspective, the four most important reasons for noncompliance were:

- A dislike of medication controlling their moods
- A dislike of the idea of having a chronic illness, symbolized by the necessity for lithium therapy
- Feeling depressed
- Side effects, particularly lethargy, decreased coordination, and dulling of senses

Patient and clinician perceptions seldom disagreed, but when they did, they were significant. Patients were much more bothered than clinicians believed them to be by their moods being controlled by medication. Those patients who reported discontinuing lithium were more likely to report missing highs and the hassle of taking medications as reasons for noncompliance. On the other hand, patients generally perceived that a decrease in productivity, creativity, and attractiveness to spouse or friends was not that important in deciding to discontinue lithium. This finding contrasts with prevailing notions about reasons for noncompliance, and it suggests that many patients do not necessarily equate highs with creativity or productivity. From the clinicians' point of view, the three most important reasons for lithium noncompliance were:

- The patient felt well and saw no need to continue the medication

Table 25-6. Rank Orders of General Reasons for Noncompliance: UCLA Study

Rank Order	Total Patient Sample (N = 47)	Patients Who Reported Discontinuing Lithium Treatment (N = 22)	Independent Clinician Sample (N = 50)
1	Bothered by idea that moods are controlled by medication	Bothered by idea that moods are controlled by medication	Felt well, saw no need for lithium
2	Felt depressed	Missed highs[a]	Missed highs
3	Bothered by idea of chronic illness	Felt depressed	Bothered by idea of chronic illness
4	Felt less attractive to spouse	Bothered by idea of chronic illness	Felt less creative
5	Felt well, saw no need for lithium	Felt well, saw no need for lithium	Felt less productive
6	Hassle to take medications[a]	Hassle to take medications[a]	Bothered by idea that moods are controlled by medication
7	Missed highs	Felt less attractive to friends	Hassle to take medication
8	Felt less creative	Felt less creative	Felt less attractive to friends
9	Felt less productive	Felt less productive	Felt depressed
10	Felt less attractive to friends	Felt less attractive to spouse	Felt less attractive to spouse

[a] $p < 0.05$. Patients who actually discontinued lithium rated these reasons significantly more important than did patients who did not stop lithium.

From Jamison et al., 1979

- The patient missed the highs of hypomania
- The patient was bothered by the idea of having a chronic illness

Although men and women in this sample showed no overall significant differences in reasons for noncompliance, the women were more likely to stress "missing highs" and "bothered by the idea of moods being controlled by medication." It may be that women perceive more desirable benefits from their highs because they show more extensive changes from baseline experience in such areas as sexuality, energy, and productivity. Some corroborating evidence for this hypothesis has been presented (Jamison et al., 1980). Furthermore, women may be accustomed to accepting extremes of moods and emotions as within the bounds of normal feminine and culturally sanctioned experience; consequently, they may

be upset by the idea of external control. As a result of the natural history of bipolar illness, women may also experience more frequent miniepisodes, leading to further accommodation of mood swings, if not actual acceptance and learned modulation.

Men, on the other hand, may regard fluctuating moods as aberrant and, therefore, legitimately subject to external or medical control. Although not systematically studied, the legal and financial sequelae of affective episodes may be more extensive for men than for women. Differences in cultural expectations and the actual phenomenology of the illness may partially account for this attitude among men, as may their higher ratio of mania/depressive episodes, more aggressive and destructive behavior when manic, and greater physical strength.

UCLA-Columbia Study

Jamison and colleagues, in an unpublished study, extensively examined 71 manic-depressive patients from two very different geographic, social, and economic settings. One group of 31 patients came from Dr. Ronald Fieve's private practice, located in the highly affluent upper east side of Manhattan, and the other group of 40 came from a public university clinic in Los Angeles, the UCLA Affective Disorders Clinic.[5]

Despite significant geographic and socioeconomic differences in the results, overall the two groups were impressively similar. In the discussion that follows, data from patients in both samples were combined.

Overview of Findings. Two patient variables were significantly related to lithium compliance. Older patients were more compliant ($p < 0.05$), and women were far more compliant than men ($p < 0.007$). There was no significant relationship between compliance and IQ, ethnicity, marital status, income, or religious background.

The 1979 UCLA study did not examine the relationship between illness variables and lithium compliance. The UCLA-Columbia study found that the number of both depressive ($p < 0.05$) and manic ($p < 0.05$) episodes was significantly related to compliance. The more affective episodes a patient had, the more likely he or she was to report compliance, even though more episodes also meant more time had passed in which the patient could have been noncompliant. Almost certainly, this finding reflects an early high-risk period for noncompliance and a tendency to have to experience one or more recurrences of illness before the initial denial alters appreciably. The study showed no relationship between compliance and polarity of the first episode, type of mania or hypomania (euphoric, dysphoric, mixed), or the extent of perceived positive aspects of hypomania. Unlike the earlier study, there were no differences in the rates of compliance between bipolar-I and bipolar-II patients.

Attitudes toward treatment also differed. Compared with compliant patients, those who were not more often reported feeling that psychotherapy was important to them in complying with a lithium treatment schedule ($p < 0.02$). Noncompliant patients were more likely to say they

stopped lithium because they felt well and saw no further need for it ($p < 0.01$). Far more than compliant patients, they perceived taking lithium as a hassle to remember ($p < 0.02$). On a semantic differential test of attitudes toward lithium, antidepressants, and psychotherapy, there were no significant differences. There also were no differences in the experience of lithium side effects.

The following psychological measures revealed no significant differences between the compliant and noncompliant groups: Beck Depression Inventory, Manic-Depressive Scale, Eysenck Personality Inventory, Breskin Rigidity Test Aesthetic Preference Scale, Sensation-Seeking Scale, Internal-External Locus of Control, and the Jenkins Activity Survey, a measure of Type A or cardiac-prone behavior. The Semantic-Differential was used to assess attitudes toward different kinds of treatment. Figure 25-1 shows the relatively strong, positive feelings patients held about lithium compared with those for psychotherapy (evaluated as the next most positive treatment) and antidepressants.

Side Effects. The earlier UCLA study neglected to include memory problems in the listing of lithium side effects, reflecting the fact that cognitive effects were seldom mentioned in the lithium literature at that time. Because patients complained of memory problems, however, the UCLA-Columbia study included them. When asked, patients said these problems were the most important reason for stopping lithium against medical advice. Fully one third found memory problems very important in noncompliance, compared with only 18 percent who believed polyuria to be a significant contributor. Ironically, polyuria is probably the most studied of the lithium side effects and changes in memory functioning the least. Weight gain and problems with coordination and tremor were also cited as very important in noncompliance.[6]

General Reasons for Noncompliance. Table 25-7 outlines several reasons for lithium noncompliance in the UCLA-Columbia study. Patients who had stopped taking lithium were asked why they had, and those who had not stopped were asked what might make them do so. The results vary somewhat from the earlier UCLA

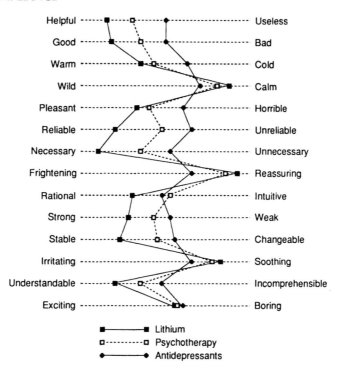

Figure 25-1. Semantic Differential. Lithium, antidepressants, and psychotherapy (from Jamison et al., unpublished data).

study, which did not frame questions about side effects in the same way as did the UCLA-Columbia study (where they were given as the most important reason for stopping lithium against medical advice). The perception of de-

Table 25-7. Rank Orders of Reasons for Lithium Noncompliance: UCLA-Columbia Study[a]

Rank Order	Reasons for Noncompliance (N = 71)
1	Side effects[a]
2	Indefinite intake / chronicity of illness
3	Less creative
4[b,c]	Felt well, saw no need to take lithium
5	Less productive
6	Missed highs
7	Less interesting to spouse
8	Disliked idea of moods being controlled by medication
9[d]	Hassle to remember to take medication
10	Felt depressed, thought mood would improve

a See Table 25-10 for rank ordering of the importance of individual side effects in noncompliance
b Males > females, $p < .05$
c Those who stopped lithium > those who did not, $p < .01$
d Those who stopped lithium > those who did not, $p < .02$

From Jamison et al., unpublished

creased creativity ranked as a more important side effect in the UCLA-Columbia study, perhaps reflecting a greater proportion of professional and creative individuals in the New York private practice group. Dislike of being on medication ranked as less important than in the earlier investigation, again perhaps because of the different nature of the patient populations. Differences in social attitudes toward mood disorders over the past several years also may have had an effect.

Other Studies

Several other studies that have examined correlates of lithium compliance are summarized in Table 25-8.

Demographic Variables. A variety of compliance measures has been used across a range of clinical settings and predictive variables. Few demographic variables (age, sex, income, education) seem to predict lithium compliance consistently, an observation consistent with results of medication compliance studies in general. Among the exceptions to this rule are the findings that being married was associated with better

Table 25-8. Correlates of Lithium Compliance: Data-Based Studies

Study	Patients N	Measures of Compliance	Correlates of Lithium Compliance	Factors Unrelated to Compliance
Jamison et al., 1979	47 (38 BP)	Patient self-report	Noncompliant patients significantly more likely to miss "highs" ($p < .05$) or regard medication as a "hassle" ($p < .05$)	Age, sex, education, income, BPI vs BPII[a], side effects
Cochran, 1982	26 BP	Blind judge examining self-report data, physician ratings, reports from significant others, lab values, chart notations	None	Age, sex, education. Found compliance was a better predictor of attitudes than attitudes were of compliance
Connelly et al., 1982	48 (40 BP)	Lithium level 0.5-1.5 mEq/l; Attendance at 75% or more clinic appointments for 9 months	Noncompliance associated with elevated mood ($p < .01$). Compliance associated with men ($p < .01$) and a perception of the continuity of care ($p < .05$)	Education, age, diagnostic sub-categories, side effects, Health Belief Model Score
Frank et al., 1985	216 BP	Not specified	Compliance associated with increasing age ($p < .05$), being married ($p < .05$), higher education ($p < .05$), history of good compliance ($p < .002$)	Previous interepisode functioning, duration of previous episodes, age at first onset, number of previous episodes
Danion et al., 1987	73 (36 BP)	Lithium level below 0.5 and above 1.0; psychiatrist estimate of compliance	Noncompliance associated with low intellectual level, cognitive deficit, affective relapses, personality disorders	Age, sex, polarity, severity, duration, side effects
Maarbjerg et al., 1988	133 (61 BP)	Patient considered noncompliant if not taking lithium six months after start of treatment	Noncompliance associated with early onset of illness, large number of previous hospital admissions, personality disorder, substance abuse	Diagnostic subgroup

Continued

compliance (Connelly et al., 1982), that women were much more likely than men to be compliant (Jamison et al., unpublished data), and that compliance increases with age (Rosen and Mukherjee, in press; Frank et al., 1985; Jamison et al., unpublished data). The last factor coincides with a greater risk period of affective recurrences. The UCLA-Columbia study also found that better compliance was associated with a larger number of affective episodes requiring treatment. Thus, increasing compliance may be secondary to de-

creasing denial as the illness continues to recur. A related possibility is that it reflects the fact that the severity of consequences ultimately leads to better compliance.

Relative Proportion of Manic to Depressive Episodes and Other Illness Factors. A pattern evolves for the one consistent illness predictor, a constellation of elevated mood variables. Jamison and colleagues (1979) found that "missing of highs" was one of the few factors significantly

Table 25-8 Continued. Correlates of Lithium Compliance: Data-Based Studies

Study	Patients N	Measures of Compliance	Correlates of Lithium Compliance	Factors Unrelated to Compliance
Lenzi et al., 1989	67[b] (53 BP)	Lithium and carbamazepine plasma levels	Compliance associated with social support, unpleasant psychotic experiences, treatment for depressive episode. Noncompliance associated with treatment for mania, grandiosity and hypochondriacal concerns	Diagnostic subgroup, nature of medication side-effects
Rosen & Mukherjee, unpublished	56	Number of months on lithium	Noncompliance associated with history of grandiose delusions ($p <.001$). Compliance associated with increasing age ($p <.05$), history of ECT ($p <.001$), history of state hospitalization ($p <.05$), symptomatic decreased need for sleep ($p <.05$)	Family history, diagnosis, frequency of previous episodes
Jamison et al., unpublished	71 BP	Patient self-reports, physician ratings	Compliance associated with increasing age ($p <.05$), females ($p <.01$), number of depressive episodes requiring treatment ($p <.05$), number of manic episodes ($p <.05$), higher occupational status ($p <.02$) Noncompliance associated with more positive experiences when manic (for women, $p <.05$)	Ethnicity, marital status, income, religious background, polarity of first episode, type of mania or hypomania, degree of positive experience associated with hypomania, BPI vs BPII, side effects, attitudes toward treatments, Beck Depression Inventory, Eysenck Personality Inventory, BRT, Aesthetic Preferences, Sensation Seeking, Internal-External Locus of Control, Jenkins Activity Survey

[a] Although there was a tendency for BPI patients to be less compliant.
[b] 35 patients on lithium, 32 patients on carbamazepine, all female.

differentiating compliant from noncompliant patients. Connelly and colleagues (1982) reported that noncompliance was associated with elevated mood, although the direction of causality was not specified, and Lenzi and associates (1989) found that grandiosity was significantly associated with noncompliance. Rosen and Mukherjee (unpublished data) found that noncompliance was associated with a history of grandiose delusions. Although grandiosity predicts a good acute response to lithium, they hypothesized that:

The presence of grandiose delusions increases the probability of both an acute response to lithium carbonate in the manic phase and rapid drop-out from lithium prophylaxis thereafter . . . personality factors (denial of dependency, etc.) which are expressed as grandiosity in the acute manic phase of the illness also operate to promote discontinuance of medication in the prophylactic period of treatment.

This condition is borne out by a study in bipolar-I disorder that showed lithium compliance to be less likely in those who experienced recurrent manic episodes (without evidence for clinical depression) than in those who experienced both disabling depressive and manic episodes (Lenzi et al., 1989). Other illness factors, such as polarity of episodes, severity, family history, diagnostic subtype, and frequency of affective episodes are not clearly related to compliance.[7]

Subjective Complaints and Lithium Compliance

The subjective experience was primarily one of indifference and slight general malaise. This led to a certain passivity. The subjects often had a feeling of being at a distance from their environment, as if separated from it by a glass wall. The subjective feeling of having been altered by the treatment was disproportionately strong in relation to objective behavioral changes. The subjects could engage in discussions and social activities but found it difficult to comprehend and integrate more than a few elements of a situation. Intellectual initiative was diminished and there was a feeling of lowered ability to concentrate and memorize; but thought processes were un-affected, and the subjects could think logically and produce ideas.   —Mogens Schou[8]

Medical aspects of the side effects of lithium and clinical strategies for treating them are presented in Chapter 23. Psychotherapeutic aspects of lithium side effects, as well as the drug's impact on the course and symptoms of manic-depressive illness, are discussed in Chapter 24. In this sec-tion, available data on frequently reported subjec-tive complaints associated with lithium treatment are presented. Conceptual and methodological problems are common in the literature of lithium side effects, where important variables are often unspecified, unclear, or uncontrolled, for exam-ple, serum lithium level, duration of lithium treat-ment, use of other medications or nonprescription drugs, diagnosis, age, and gender. The degree and type of inquiry into side effects (spontaneous report, checklists, scaled measures of frequency and severity) vary enormously from study to study, and control subjects rarely are included in the design of the investigation. Prelithium pro-files of side effects (a baseline of functioning be-fore lithium) are seldom obtained from patients, making the subsequent interpretations of lithium side effects difficult. Differentiating the simple presence or absence of a side effect from its sever-ity or relationship to noncompliance is even less common.

Several authors stress the worrisome meth-odological problem of distinguishing lithium side effects from the symptomatic manifestations of the underlying affective disorder.[9] Abou-Saleh and Coppen (1983) found, for example, that drug-free depressed patients reported more side effects than both control subjects and lithium-treated patients and that subjective side effects reported by lithium-treated patients were related to their affective symptoms and personality vari-ables. Lyskowski and colleagues (1982), on the

other hand, found that the presence of non-euthymic mood was not associated with changes in the incidence of side effects.

The rates of the most frequently reported lithium side effects are presented in Table 25-9. In the 12 reviewed studies, 35 to 93 percent of the lithium-treated patients reported subjective com-plaints from their medication. The pooled per-centage, based on a total of 1,035 patients, is 74 percent. Lyskowski and co-workers (1982), in a longitudinal study of 67 patients, found that 7 percent were free from all side effects, 63 percent had only mild complaints, and 30 percent re-ported persistent moderate or severe side effects (especially polyuria and thirst). The persistent side effects were not related to age, age at onset of illness, severity of illness, or duration of lithium treatment.

Somatic Effects of Lithium

In our review, slightly more than a third of pa-tients (36 percent) complained of excessive thirst, the most commonly reported lithium side effect. Polyuria (30 percent) and tremor (27 percent) were the next most frequent somatic complaints, followed by weight gain (19 percent), drowsi-ness/lethargy (12 percent), and diarrhea (9 per-cent). When asked the importance of a given side effect in actually stopping lithium against medi-cal advice, however, patients showed a different pattern (Table 25-10). Of the somatic side effects, they perceived weight gain and problems with coordination and tremor as the most likely to lead to noncompliance, followed by polyuria, tiredness/lethargy, dulling of senses, blurred vi-sion, and nausea and vomiting.

The difference between acknowledging the presence of a side effect and perceiving it as trou-bling and likely to lead to noncompliance is fur-ther underscored by the findings of Gitlin and Cochran (unpublished data). They asked 49 bipo-lar patients to indicate whether they had experi-enced various side effects while on lithium. The five most frequently cited side effects were thirst, excessive urination, weight gain, dry mouth, and fatigue. When asked which side effects were most bothersome to them, however, a signifi-cantly different list emerged: weight gain, mental confusion, poor concentration, mental slowness, and memory problems. Four of the five most

Table 25-9. Lithium Side Effects: Percentage of Patients with Subjective Complaints

Study	Patients N	Excessive Thirst	Polyuria	Memory Problems	Tremor	Weight Gain	Drowsiness	Diarrhea	None
Schou et al., 1970a									
Initial treatment (<1 wk)	30	18[a]	18[a]		16	0			4
Extended (1-2 yr)	100	23[a]	23[a]		4	11			65
Bech et al., 1976	39	62		38	51				
Ghose, 1977	50	42	38	52	34	18	24	8	
Bech et al., 1979b[b]	26	62		46	65				
Johnston et al., 1979	49	45[a]	45[a]		31				37
Bone et al., 1980	69	23	38		25		13	10	18
Vestergaard et al., 1980[c]	237	70			45	20		20	10
Lyskowski et al., 1982									
Cross-sectional analysis	142[d]	32	25	3[e]	7	7	6	3	10
Longitudinal analysis	67[f]	13	15	0	10	3	1	0	7
Abou-Saleh & Coppen, 1983									
Males	30	36		57	39		36		
Females	64	49		44	51	34			
Duncavage et al., 1983	21	48	57		14	43		10	19
McCreadie & Morrison, 1985	40	38	30	45	28	43	23	30	35
Page et al., 1987	59	36[a]	36[a]	39	39	36		17	
Jamison et al., unpublished	71		18[g]	33[g]	32[g]	30	24[g]		
Total N	1,094								
Pooled Percentages[h]		35.9	30.4	28.2	26.6	18.9	12.4	8.7	26.2

[a] Polyuria and excessive thirst combined as a single symptom
[b] Patients with Ménière's disease; no history of psychiatric illness
[c] Two-thirds of patients on other medications in addition to lithium
[d] One rating only
[e] Mental confusion
[f] ≥3 ratings
[g] Percent rated as "very important" in lithium noncompliance
[h] Pooled percentages based on patients taking lithium only

Table 25-10. Importance of Side Effects in Lithium Noncompliance

Rank Order[a]	Side Effect	Very Important %	Unimportant %
1	Memory problems	33	22
2	Weight gain	30	28
3	Coordination / tremor	32	31
4	Polyuria	18	17
5	Tiredness / lethargy	24	25
6	Dulling of senses	29	32
7	Blurred vision	26	40
8	Nausea / vomiting	23	40

On the mean scores, there were no significant differences by sex or intelligence
[a] For means of scale scores, ranging from 1 (unimportant) to 5 (very important)

Data from Jamison et al., unpublished

bothersome lithium side effects were cognitive in nature.

Cognitive Effects of Lithium

Disturbance of memory was the most important "late" side effect observed in our patients, not on account of its frequency but because it was very troublesome. Contrary to the other side-effects of lithium which were usually not reported by the patients unless the therapists asked specifically about them, memory dysfunction was an inconvenience patients did complain about. This symptom was not associated with a mild depressive phase, as one might hypothesize, since all patients who complained of memory reduction were clearly normothymic and were only receiving lithium prophylactically. (p. 263)   —Christodoulou et al., 1977

The objective effects of lithium on memory, acquisition of new learning, and other aspects of cognition are reviewed in Chapter 23. It is significant to the discussion of lithium noncompliance that, in the review of studies summarized in Table 25-9, memory problems were the third most frequently cited side effect (28 percent of patients). In one study, fully one third of patients reported that memory problems were very important in their decisions to stop lithium against medical advice (Jamison et al., unpublished data). Memory problems were more important than any other side effects in noncompliance (Table 25-10).

SUMMARY

Noncompliance to lithium among manic-depressive patients is costly to themselves, those who know them, and society as a whole. Patients who fail to comply are usually young, early in their illness, reluctant to give up their highs, or prone to frequent elevated moods and grandiose delusions. Patients themselves cite medication side effects (e.g., weight gain, cognitive impairment) and several psychological factors as their major reasons for stopping lithium.

Clinicians wishing to increase lithium com-

pliance can take several steps: minimize, whenever possible, the lithium level, minimize and treat aggressively the drug's side effects, track the patient's compliance, examine their own ambivalence about lithium maintenance, educate patients and their families about manic-depressive illness and the role of lithium in attenuating its course, and encourage adjunctive psychotherapy.

NOTES

1. Parts of this chapter were published originally in Jamison and Goodwin (1983a,b) and Jamison and Akiskal (1983).
2. Jamison et al., 1979; Jamison and Akiskal, 1983; Jamison and Goodwin, 1983a,b.
3. Treatment for these relapses is outlined in Chapter 23.
4. Mazzullo and Lasagna, 1972; Haynes et al., 1979; Becker and Maiman, 1980; Docherty and Fiester, 1985.
5. All patients were bipolar, but a significantly higher proportion of the Los Angeles sample was bipolar I ($p < 0.05$). There was no significant difference in mean age for the samples or in number of months on lithium treatment. The combined samples had a mean age of 37.7 years and a mean length of treatment of 36.0 months. Mean incomes, not surprisingly, were strikingly different: among the New York patients $64,000, among the Los Angeles patients $16,000.
6. In this study, in contrast to others, questions were tied to a behavioral base (e.g., "How important is the side effect in question to your decision making about continuing to take lithium?") rather than to a presence or absence of the symptom format, probably resulting in some of the differences in findings across studies.
7. Frank et al., 1985; Danion et al., 1987; Maarbjerg et al., 1988; Rosen and Mukherjee, in press.
8. From Schou's description of lithium's effects on himself and other researchers during an early experimental trial (Schou, 1968, p. 78).
9. Bech et al., 1979; Abou-Saleh and Coppen, 1983; Vestergaard, 1983; Jefferson and Greist, 1987.

26

Treatment of Alcohol and Drug Abuse in Manic-Depressive Patients

Dylan was now having blackouts at frequent intervals. On more than one occasion he had been warned by his doctor that he must go on a regime of complete abstinence from alcohol if he was to survive . . . Dylan seemed exhausted, self-preoccupied, and morbidly depressed. He went out alone, and an hour and a half later returned to announce, "I've had eighteen straight whiskeys. I think that's the record." On November 9 he died.   —W. Read, *The Days of Dylan Thomas*

Clinicians often have difficulty recognizing and treating manic-depressive illness, even when it is uncomplicated by other conditions. Alcoholism or drug abuse added to the clinical picture radically compounds treatment issues. Symptoms frequently overlap, and resistance to treatment of one disorder can undermine the treatment of both. Few clinicians are adequately trained to treat the complicated common ground of simultaneous presentation. The study of each condition tends to proceed independently, and advances go unnoticed by those whose primary focus is elsewhere. Traditionally, clinicians who work with affective disorders have only a basic knowledge of alcohol and drug abuse, and vice versa, although recently this tendency has been changing.

As long as clinicians fail to recognize the presence of substance abuse, patients are at risk of suffering lethal consequences. In spite of these dangers and notwithstanding the increasing attention being paid to comorbidity and the dual diagnosis patient, little research has been done on issues specific to assessing and treating manic-depressive patients who suffer concurrent alcoholism and/or drug abuse problems. Examples of such issues include:

• Clinical differentiation of the coexisting disor-

ders and their separate but necessarily related treatments
• The high suicide risk attendant to both illnesses and, suggestively, yet higher rates when affective illness and substance abuse exist together in the same individual
• The importance of early identification and treatment of substance abuse in manic-depressive illness, and vice versa

ASSESSMENT

The difference between mood changes brought about by affective illness and those brought about by alcohol and drug abuse is subtle and complex, as discussed in Chapter 9. Distinguishing transitory drug-induced or alcohol-induced symptoms from those intrinsic to manic-depressive illness is sometimes difficult. In some cases, chance alone accounts for the coexistence of the two disorders in the same individual, whereas in others, the alcohol and drug abuse can be genetically determined or attributed to attempts at self-treatment of manic-depressive illness. Affective illness can mask substance abuse just as substance abuse often masks affective illness. The accurate diagnosis of both disorders is vital because treatment decisions depend on it. It is, for example, unnecessary and unwise to prescribe lithium or anti-depressants for transient mood and cognitive symptoms that will spontaneously remit with abstinence. Many investigators (e.g., Schuckit 1984, 1986; Akiskal et al., 1979b) have noted that with primary alcoholism and an apparent secondary affective disorder, affective symptoms usually remit within 2 to 4 weeks after cessation of alcohol use. Treating substance abuse and not affective illness, on the other hand, risks compounding the problems associated with mood disorders.

Adequate assessment of a patient with possible diagnoses of manic-depressive illness and substance abuse requires systematic inquiry, using standardized diagnostic criteria, about the signs and symptoms of both. Family histories of affective and substance abuse problems, as well as a detailed chronicling of symptom onset, also are important. Such histories help in teasing out the more probable or primary diagnosis, and they help to identify and counsel the manic-depressive patient who has a family history of alcoholism, a history that makes the patient more liable to become alcoholic. Morrison (1975) has described the usefulness of this strategy in preventing problematic drinking. It is important to differentiate between adolescent affective disorders and type II alcoholism, a form that, like manic-depressive illness, has an early age of onset and is associated with aggressive and impulsive behavior. Famularo and colleagues (1985), for example, diagnosed bipolar illness in seven of ten cases of alcohol abuse developing before the age of 13. Ascertaining medical complications secondary to alcohol and drug abuse also is needed. In addition to a general medical evaluation, a urine screen for drugs often is crucial. Estroff and colleagues (1985) found "little relationship between patients' self-reported patterns of drug abuse . . . and the results of the urine analysis" (p. 38).

Probably most important to the discussion of manic-depressive illness, alcoholism, and drug abuse is the simple but pivotal recognition of the importance and extent of the coexistence of these disorders. Manic-depressive patients should always be asked about their patterns of alcohol and drug abuse. Although in what follows we discuss alcohol abuse and drug abuse separately, in reality they often coexist.

TREATMENT

Alcoholism and Alcohol Abuse

The treatment of alcoholism, especially when it coexists with manic-depressive illness (i.e., the dual diagnosis patient), often requires more than one type of intervention. In-depth discussion of the treatment of alcoholism is beyond the purpose of this chapter, and several excellent reviews already exist.[1] Here we outline a few of the treatment issues specific to alcoholism in manic-depressive patients.

Mayfield (in Liskow et al., 1982) made the important point that each disorder, alcoholism and affective illness, needs treatment in its own right:

It is appealing to our sense of parsimony to consider the excessive drinking as merely a ramification of affective disorder, and we prefer to believe that alcoholism will cease to be a problem when the affective disorder is under control. In practice, this is usually not the case. These patients need the same commitment to sobriety, the same understanding of their drinking behavior, the same organized approach to the appropriate selection of the same array of treatment resources as do alcoholics without affective disorder. (p. 146)

Specific studies of pharmacological agents used in the treatment of primary alcoholism (e.g., disulfiram) have not been carried out in manic-depressive patients. The use of lithium and antidepressants as treatments for alcoholism and alcohol abuse, described and reviewed elsewhere,[2] clearly has less relevance for patients with affective illness—generally already taking one or more of these medications—than it does for other alcoholic populations. Himmelhoch and colleagues (1983) summarized much of the literature:

Many drinkers will eschew anything which interferes with their drinking. . . . If they have successfully defied the impressive effects of disulfiram and the unmodulated ferocity of the WCTU [Women's Christian Temperance Union], they will easily survive the modest biological effects of lithium salts. At best lithium salts represent "an opportunity" for the well motivated alcoholic. (p. 87)

Akiskal and colleagues describe a woman who tried to treat her own episodes of irritability and hypomania with alcohol but was successfully treated with lithium:

This 31 year old divorced female teacher. . . . complained of "inability to maintain an even keel." Since the age of 19, she had been in psychotherapy intermittently because of verbal explosive outbursts towards loved ones. Sometimes they occurred under the influence of alcohol, but repeated electroencephalographic studies had revealed no abnormalities. [Her] verbally abusive behavior . . . typically lasted from a few hours to a few days [and] had cost her two marriages and a succession of lovers; she had alienated her parents and friends; and had come under disciplinary action in her current school job. Furthermore, she had had numerous DWI arrests. . . . the patient had periods when she felt "great pressure to be involved," was full of energy—"wired"—and inexhaustible. . . . like "a speed trip without amphetamines." During these times, she was "nervous and dissatisfied about many things" and could not go to bed until she had rearranged her entire household, only to rearrange it again. Impulsive shopping sprees were not uncommon. These "wired" periods extended over 2 to 6 days and occurred more frequently than her "explosive" periods, but they were considered "normal" by her and her acquaintances (as she was "aware, intense, loving and involved" at such times). She often drank to bring herself down from these "hyperwired states." It emerged that the explosive periods tended to come after these "wired states" and were sometimes followed by periods of self-reproach, guilt, and fleeting suicidal ideation. She suffered from chronic insomnia, usually averaging 3 to 4 hours sleep per night. . . . she had a tendency to be involved in various activities and withdrawing in midstream.

[The] patient's father suffered from chronic alcoholism, and a paternal aunt had been treated for manic-depressive illness . . . while one paternal uncle had committed suicide. . . .

. . . [she] was noticeably accelerated in her movements and speech. . . . Thought progression was logical with no evidence for associative slippage. Hallucinations and delusions were not elicited. Cognitive functions were intact. . . . Within one year [of lithium treatment]. . . . Sleep was virtually normalized to a 7 to 8 hour pattern, while dipsomania, shopping sprees, and explosive outbursts were all reduced by more than 75 percent. . . . "I can now sleep. Therefore I don't crave alcohol . . . anymore". . . . The patient could now make constructive use of psychotherapy to structure her life. (Akiskal et al., 1979a, pp. 545–547)

Little, if anything, is written about specific psychosocial treatments for manic-depressive patients with concurrent alcoholism. The psychotherapeutic interventions for bipolar illness in general are reviewed in Chapter 24. Psychological treatments for alcoholism per se are reviewed elsewhere.[3] Our own view is that both disorders, manic-depressive illness and alcoholism, should be treated aggressively and separately. O'Sullivan and colleagues (1988) believe that even if alcoholism is secondary to the affective disorder, alcoholism is the most clinically important illness because of its effects on social behavior and treatment compliance. A dual diagnosis probably increases the need for inpatient treatment. The recently established hospital programs that have parallel treatment components—one for affective illness and one for alcohol and drug abuse—provide one example of a sophisticated appreciation of the interactions between the two disorders.

Woodruff and colleagues (1973) and Murray and associates (1984) observed a much higher prevalence of depression among alcoholics in psychiatric treatment than among untreated alcoholics. This suggests that depressive symptoms may prompt alcoholics to seek treatment and that patients diagnosed as both alcoholic and manic-depressive may have a better chance for recovery from alcoholism. On the other hand, O'Sullivan and associates (1988) also found that the alcoholics with a coexisting affective disorder received more treatment for both illnesses than those who were alcoholic alone, although there were no significant differences for follow-up relapse rates between the groups. These findings are based on inpatients, whose addiction to alcohol has presumably advanced, and may not represent the experience of less seriously addicted patients.

Specific psychotherapeutic and counseling issues overlap both disorders. First, all bipolar patients, whether or not they have drinking problems, should be educated about certain aspects of alcohol:

- Alcohol has additive, occasionally synergistic, effects with lithium. These effects are especially important for judgment and driving.
- Lithium can alter the nature of alcohol intoxication. For example, it may attenuate the euphoria usually associated with drinking (Judd et al., 1979), which can lead to increased drinking in an attempt to recapture earlier, prelithium, alcohol-induced states.
- Alcohol may alter an individual's ability or desire to comply with a prescribed medication regimen.
- Alcohol can alter sleep patterns, which can, in

turn, exacerbate or precipitate manic and mixed states.

- Increased thirst secondary to lithium or a decreased psychological effect from alcohol can lead to an increase in alcohol consumption. We have seen patients with liver damage resulting from insidious, often unnoticed, increases in drinking behavior.
- Alcohol can induce pathological mood changes in susceptible individuals (see Chapter 9). Therefore, patients with manic-depressive illness should be cautioned either to abstain or to be especially careful to keep their use at a very moderate level.
- A patient with a history of mixed states is especially vulnerable to a compromised treatment response when abusing alcohol or sedatives (Himmelhoch and Garfinkel, 1986) and should be strongly advised to limit or eliminate alcohol intake.
- All patients should be educated about the possible deleterious effect of alcohol on the efficacy of pharmacological treatments for manic-depressive illness (Himmelhoch et al., 1976).[4]

The second overlapping issue is that a manic-depressive patient with a family history of alcoholism should be advised about the increased risk for alcoholism, even though he or she may not have developed a drinking problem by the time of clinical examination (see Chapter 9). Patients may or may not choose to alter their drinking behavior, but they will at least have been informed.

Third, a patient with a personal or family history of both alcoholism and bipolar illness is at an increased risk for suicide (Morrison, 1975; Berglund, 1984) and should be followed with particular care (see Chapter 27). The danger is particularly great during detoxification. As Himmelhoch (1987) points out, "Sedativism (alcohol and sedative tolerance and/or addiction) can be at the same time the most obvious and the most subtly insidious clinical factor leading to suicide" (p. 50). It greatly increases the risk of suicide after loss, and the majority of such suicides occur within 6 weeks of the loss. From these facts, Himmelhoch suggests a plan for treatment:

The clinical lesson is obvious; sedative tolerance drastically lowers stress tolerance. Addicted individuals, therefore, must be frequently seen and carefully inter-

rogated. Brief hospitalizations under intensive observation often form the most important part of treatment. Family therapy, group therapy, and other strategies aimed at mobilizing a social network are a sine qua non, as is forced attendance at an Alcoholics Anonymous-type therapy. Finally, associated depressive symptomatology can present management problems. Often, detoxification and reconstruction of social networks obviate the need for antidepressant medications. However, when core depressive symptomatology lingers after full-fledged treatment of sedative addiction, the proper drug must be administered, even if the patient's drug therapist offers the primary clinician resistance to initiating pharmacologic treatment. Primary depressed patients with secondary sedativism tend to respond very slowly to treatment and are particularly dangerous to manage. Ironically, patients suffering primary sedativism with secondary depressions experience rapid relief of depressed mood and are less acutely dangerous, although eventually more likely to relapse because of their primary sedativism. (p. 50)

Manic-depressive patients and their families should be counseled about adjunctive treatments for alcoholism—individual and group psychotherapy, pharmacotherapy—and, when appropriate, they should be vigorously encouraged to use them. We focus here on the adjunctive use of the most clinically significant of these programs, Alcoholics Anonymous (AA).

The most widely known and used treatment program for alcoholism, AA has more than one million members and more than 30,000 groups in at least 70 different countries. Determining efficacy rates and delineating types of individuals for whom AA is most beneficial are difficult in such an anonymous, self-help group setting. As Ogborne and Glaser (1985) point out:

It remains unclear (1) what proportion of any population of problem drinkers would either accept or benefit from a referral to A.A.; (2) whether or not benefits to be derived from involvement with A.A. are greater than those to be gained from other programs; and (3) whether or not involvement with A.A. has any detrimental effects on those concerned. (p. 187)

On the positive side, AA clearly benefits many individuals at little or no cost to themselves or society. Alcoholics Anonymous apparently derives much of its success from acceptance of the belief that only an alcoholic can help and understand another alcoholic, from the continuous support, hope, and help provided by peers, from exposure to successfully abstinent alcoholics, from substitutions of other AA members for former drinking companions, and from increased self-esteem gained through helping other people in like circumstances (Vaillant, 1978).

On the other hand, not all alcoholics are attracted to or are able to tolerate AA's self-examining approach or religious underpinnings. Of particular relevance to manic-depressive patients with drinking problems is the opposition expressed by some AA members to other treatments (e.g., tranquilizers and mood-altering medications), a stance that has jeopardized the complete rehabilitation of many of its members and discouraged others from joining. In the past, this type of influence presented potentially life-threatening problems for the individual involved and was particularly frustrating to the clinician who, having finally persuaded a reluctant or ambivalent patient to take lithium, found the patient under strong group pressure to stop taking the drug. Many lithium patients find it difficult enough under the best of circumstances to take lithium (see Chapter 25) and may find it a relief to be with others who encourage their resistance. The consequences of discontinuing lithium can be catastrophic. We have seen some manic-depressive patients, who were referred to AA for their drinking problems, discontinue their lithium and become manic, requiring hospitalization, or become suicidally depressed. This phenomenon is described by a recovering alcoholic psychiatrist who detailed his experiences in AA (R.S., AA Grapevine, December 1981):

During the past four years, I have seen two women commit suicide and two others have to be hospitalized because they were encouraged by well-meaning AA members to stop all medication. Some mentally ill people do not seem normal even when on medication, and some AA members attribute the problem to the medication rather than to the illness, from which the medication is giving some relief. (p. 16)

Evidence from a large survey (Maxwell, 1984) suggests that antiprofessional attitudes in AA are changing, however. Nearly one third of the sample reported that they had obtained important professional help from some non-AA professional source after being in AA. Likewise, attitudes of professionals toward AA appear to be more positive than they were at one time. The same survey found that nearly 38 percent of AA members reported that professional help played an important role in their coming to AA. Indeed, there are now some AA groups specifically for dual diagnosis patients. Instrumental to these shifts in attitude has been a very important pamphlet, *AA: Medications and Other Drugs*, published by the AA General Service Conference, which is recognized as the sole official policy voice of the AA movement. This pamphlet, which is available through local AA offices, clearly distinguishes necessary and important prescription medications from self-administered drugs. It can provide important support for a lithium-treated manic-depressive patient encountering antimedication pressures from individual AA members, who are trying to discredit lithium as a crutch and to persuade the patient to stop taking it.

We believe that AA is potentially invaluable to some manic-depressive patients. There are, however, no systematic research data to support our strong clinical impressions. Patients should be advised that they may encounter intense pressure to stop taking their medications. For some, knowing about this possibility and being prepared for it may be all that is necessary. Others, especially those reasonably new to their illness or medication and those with compliance problems, may be well advised not to mention that they are taking medication for a psychiatric condition.

Drug Abuse

There are no treatment guidelines specific for intervention with manic-depressive patients who abuse drugs, such as cocaine or the opiates. Pharmacological and psychological treatments for cocaine abusers in general have been outlined by several clinical researchers.[5] Similarly, several authors have reviewed the treatment of affective symptoms in opiate addicts.[6] There appears to be no clinical indication that treatment for drug abuse in bipolar patients substantially differs from the aggressive treatment of both the affective illness and the drug abuse. As in the case of alcohol abuse, however, the dual diagnosis increases the need for inpatient treatment. The hospital-based programs that have been set up recently to deal with both problems are a good choice for such treatment. Narcotics Anonymous, a self-help organization modeled on AA, can provide essential social support to the patient. Because it is newer than AA, it has bypassed the era when all medications were seen as objectionable.

We wish to reemphasize, as Liskow and colleagues (1982) did in discussing the concurrent treatment of affective illness and alcoholism, that the disorders should be evaluated and treated separately:

The greatest error in treating these patients is to consider one illness a consequence of the other and, therefore, to focus all therapeutic attention on one to the exclusion of the other. There is no good evidence that such an approach is beneficial in the total care of the patient. Until more data are available on the best way to treat such patients, it would appear sensible to apply our best treatment techniques for each of these illnesses to any individual who exhibits both of them. (p. 147)

The principal responsibility of professionals and paraprofessionals is to be knowledgeable about the treatment of both manic-depressive illness and substance abuse. The necessary cross-fertilization of separate fields is now being enhanced through such organizations as the American Academy of Psychiatrists in Alcoholism and Addictions and the American Medical Society on Alcoholism and Other Drug Dependencies, Inc., and through educational programs sponsored by the U.S. federal government through the National Institute on Alcohol Abuse and Alcoholism.[7]

SUMMARY

Patients with a dual diagnosis of manic-depressive illness and substance abuse are at high risk of exacerbated mood symptoms, toxic reactions, and suicide. The coexistence of these diagnoses is, however, difficult for many clinicians to recognize, partly because one condition can mask the other.

Manic-depressive patients should always be asked about their patterns of alcohol and drug abuse. Although some manic-depressive patients undoubtedly abuse drugs and alcohol in an attempt to medicate themselves, especially to come down from manic highs, not all abuse fits this pattern. Routine diagnostic workups should include questions about the signs and symptoms of both conditions, family histories of both, and details about onset.

When a dual diagnosis is made, each disorder should be treated separated and aggressively. Inpatient treatment is likely to be needed. Manic-depressive patients should always be educated about the interactions of lithium with alcohol and other commonly abused drugs. They should be encouraged to participate in Alcoholics Anonymous, Narcotics Anonymous, or other groups that can provide psychological and social support and be made aware of the official AA pamphlet supporting the appropriate use of prescription drugs.

NOTES

1. See, for example, Goodwin and Erickson, 1979; Mendelson and Mello, 1979; Kleber and Gawin, 1984; Schuckit, 1984; Bratter and Forrest, 1985; Russell, 1986.
2. See Ditman, 1967; Coppen et al., 1971, 1976; Viamontes, 1972; Cooper et al., 1974; Kline et al., 1974; Merry et al., 1976; Schuckit, 1986.
3. See, for example, Berenson, 1979; Forrest, 1985; Freudenberger, 1985; Kaufman, 1985.
4. For example, Ciraulo and colleagues (1982) found that recently detoxified alcoholics clear imipramine so rapidly that plasma levels achieved at the usual therapeutic dose may be inadequate.
5. Anker and Crowley, 1982; Siegel, 1982; Cohen, 1984; Gawin and Kleber, 1984; Kleber and Gawin, 1984; Estroff and Gold, 1986.
6. Woody et al., 1975, 1982; Spensley, 1976; Dorus and Senay, 1980; Steer and Kotzker, 1980; Rounsaville et al., 1982; Kleber et al., 1983; Dackis and Gold, 1984; Mirin et al., 1988.
7. Through organizations such as these the clinician can learn about the quality of local substance abuse treatment facilities, including guidance on those AA or NA groups that are most appropriate for the dual diagnosis patient. The addresses are:

American Medical Society on Alcoholism & Other Drug Dependencies, Inc.
12 West 21st Street
New York, NY 10010

The American Academy of Psychiatrists in Alcoholism & Addictions
Post Office Box 376
Greenbelt, MD 20770

The National Institute on Alcohol Abuse and Alcoholism
5600 Fishers Lane
Rockville, MD 20857

27

Clinical Management of Suicidal Patients

I remember sitting in your office a hundred times during those grim months and each time thinking, what on earth can he say that will make me feel better or keep me alive? Well, there never was anything you could say, that's the funny thing. It was all the stupid, desperately optimistic, condescending things you didn't *say that kept me alive; all the compassion and warmth I felt from you that could not have been said; all the intelligence, competence, and time you put into it; and your granite belief that mine was a life worth living. You were terribly direct which was terribly important, and you were willing to admit the limits of your understanding and treatments and when you were wrong. Most difficult to put into words but in many ways the essence of everything: You taught me that the road from suicide to life is cold and colder and colder still, but—with steely effort, the grace of God, and an inevitable break in the weather—that I could make it.*
—Patient with manic-depressive illness

The most reliable method of preventing suicide in manic-depressive patients is to treat the underlying illness effectively. Most manic-depressive patients are at high risk for suicide, but some are at even higher risk because of a family history of suicide or because of their clinical state. Early and accurate diagnosis is critical to the identification of these especially vulnerable patients. It is also important because the danger of suicide appears to be greatest in the initial phases of the illness (see Chapter 10), a pattern of risk that also influences treatment decisions, such as the timing of lithium maintenance therapy and the timing and frequency of supportive psychotherapy.

In this chapter, we examine issues of central importance to clinicians dealing with actually or potentially suicidal manic-depressive patients: clinical assessment, risk factors, and psychological and pharmacological treatment. Like Chapter 26 and unlike others in the treatment section, this chapter does not include a formal review of the literature, which can be found in Chapter 10. Instead, a few of the most pertinent studies are interwoven in the discussion of clinical issues. The first part emphasizes the all important clinical task of assessing suicidal risk. The second part

discusses treatment decisions that follow from this evaluation.

CLINICAL EVALUATION

Predicting and managing suicidal behavior in manic-depressive patients begin with an assessment of the patient's personal and family history. The evaluation should also cover the patient's present psychiatric status, psychological assets and liabilities, and treatment history.

Family History
Patients and, if possible, their families should be asked in detail about any history of suicide, suicide attempts, or violence in a first-degree relative. Also important are relatives' responses to different treatments—to different classes of the tricyclics, for example, or to MAO inhibitors, electroconvulsive therapy, lithium, or the anticonvulsants. In their study of manic-depressive patients at the Salzburg (Austria) Psychiatric Clinic, Mitterauer and colleagues (1988) found striking differences in patients who had a family history of suicide and those who did not. Pro-

bands who had a relative (within three generations) who had committed suicide showed more suicidal "tendencies" and suicide attempts. This is consistent with the genetic findings reviewed in Chapter 15.

Patient History

In ascertaining suicidal risk, a clinician must obtain a thorough history of suicidal ideation, suicide attempts, and grossly morbid thought patterns. Such a history should be reviewed with the patient or the patient's family (Table 27-1). Patients who report a history of suicidal ideation or attempts should be asked what the clinician and the family did in the past that was particularly helpful. Frequent reassurances and short but frequent contacts may have been helpful, for example, or brief telephone calls initiated at planned times by the therapist.

Diagnostic studies indicate that within the general population of bipolar patients, suicide risk may be somewhat greater in those experiencing only hypomanic, rather than manic, episodes (see Chapter 10). This difference is neither sufficiently documented nor predictive to be useful in current clinical practice, however. The literature reviewed in Chapter 10 also suggests that, although patients are unlikely to kill themselves during a manic episode, they are at risk of doing so during the depressions and transitional states that follow mania. Those with mixed states are at highest risk. The presence of delusions also appears to be associated with a higher risk for suicide. The prominence of other symptoms may predict suicide as well. Anhedonia, severe psychic anxiety, and moderate alcohol abuse were associated with suicide within the first year of assessment in the National Institute of Mental Health (NIMH) collaborative study (Fawcett et

al., in press). Late suicides, those after the first year, were most associated with severe hopelessness, somatic anxiety, suicidal ideation, and a history of suicide attempts.

Research findings consistently underscore the importance of a history of attempted suicide in determining suicide risk, especially for manic-depressive patients. Clinicians clearly acknowledge this association, but they may not give enough attention to a history of suicidal ideation, perhaps because suicidal thinking is commonplace among depressed patients. Information pertaining to suicidal ideation should be gathered from all sources (see Chapter 10).

History of Violence

It is difficult, but extremely important, to elicit an accurate history of violent feelings, thoughts, and behaviors. Patients are not always questioned in sufficient detail. Many women are reluctant to disclose thoughts and actions at variance with socially accepted behavior and traditional notions of femininity (those who do reveal such histories are often diagnosed as borderline or hysteric). Patients for whom violent feelings and relationships are an integral part of life may not realize their lives are unusual, or they may have no realistic idea of what constitutes an abnormal level of violence. Possibilities to be explored are shown in Table 27-2.

Patients also should be asked about cyclicity in their violent feelings and behaviors. Women should be asked if there are variations related to the menstrual cycle. Both sexes should be questioned about diurnal or seasonal patterns and about whether violence is particularly pronounced in a given mood state (e.g., mixed states, depression, hypomania, or mania).

Course of Illness

Suicide may be a greater risk during certain periods in the course of both the illness and individual episodes. Although the evidence is equivocal, the danger of suicide may be greatest in the first years of an illness. During any one episode, the patient may be particularly concerned with sleep, which in fact appears to be more disrupted just before suicide. Diagnostic considerations include the rare incidence of suicide in manic states and the high suicide rate found in mixed states. There is, in addition, a striking peak incidence of suicide in

---

Table 27-1. Clinical Evaluation of Suicidal
Potential: General Risk Factors

- Patient's stated plans
- Delusions and/or hallucinations
- Mixed and transitional states
- Family history of suicide
- Previous suicide attempts
- Close proximity to onset of illness
- Poor medication response or compliance
- Alcohol & drug abuse
- Violence & impulsivity

Table 27-2. Clinical Assessment: Determining History of Violence / Impulsivity

- Bad or violent temper
- Frequent physical violence or fighting with others
- Child, spouse, or animal abuse
- Frequent provocation of violence in others
- Frequent and pronounced irritability, or a "quick fuse"
- Feeling wired; sense of pent-up energy (usually dysphoric)
- Frequent sense of wanting to put a fist through the wall or a pane of glass, to lash out physically, or actually doing so
- Frequent vitriolic scenes of verbal abuse
- Pattern of tempestuous relationships
- Violent sexual behaviors (not intended to stimulate a response but from a sense of feeling overstimulated)
- Impulsive behaviors, such as throwing things, attempting to jump out of moving cars, bolting in restaurants, impetuousness in social situations
- Impulsivity manifested by sociopathic behavior, e.g., shoplifting and frequent conflicts with authority figures

From Jamison, 1987

May and a second one in October. (See Chapter 10 for further discussion.) Prediction of suicide must rely heavily on the patient's own history, however, and for this reason, a thorough history should include the following points:

- When in the *overall course of the illness* did past suicide attempts or severe suicidal ideation take place, especially latency from onset of illness and latency from onset of diagnosis and treatment
- When in the *sequence of episodes* did attempts or ideation take place (Did the patient attempt suicide in a depressive episode preceding or following a manic episode?)
- When in the *individual episode* the patient appeared to be most vulnerable to suicide
  - In the transition from manic to depressive, depressive to manic, manic to euthymic state
  - Relatively soon after the beginning of a depressive episode, well into it, or during the recovery period
- When the patient, on the basis of past episodes (if any), might reasonably be expected to begin recovery, and to be recovered
- When in the menstrual cycle, in combination with an episode, the patient might be in special

jeopardy (e.g., in the premenstrual phase during a depressive episode)
- When, in general, the patient might be at increased risk for suicide—for example, postpartum, seasonally, or at important anniversaries.

The life-charting approach to recording data relevant to course described in Chapter 6 is useful in tracking this information.

Assets and Liabilities

Minimum pathology in a suicidal person bereft of strengths may be lethal, while severe pathology in a person with unusual strengths may constitute only a moderate risk. (p. 239) —Motto, 1975

The severity of manic-depressive illness and the associated constitutional and biological factors underlying suicide probably account for most, but by no means all, of the variance between those who kill themselves and those who do not. In addition, various personal assets and liabilities combine with the strength of the suicidal state to form a frighteningly delicate balance between the decision to live or die. To some extent, assets and liabilities become relative terms, since serious mood disorders, ironically, can convert characteristics that would be strengths under normal circumstances into liabilities when an individual is depressed or suicidal. Individuals who are used to being independent, confident, and self-determined may kill themselves, yet those for whom seeking help or lacking self-confidence is neither new nor particularly demoralizing may not. Suicide in otherwise normal, even extremely successful people is not uncommon. Among professional and accomplished individuals, especially men, the inability to accept help has been described often. As Motto (1975) wrote:

A person whose self-esteem rests on meeting high standards of performance, in a society which reveres rugged individualism, tends to avoid any situation that can be interpreted as reflecting weakness, dependence, or inability to cope with the stresses of living. Especially threatening is any suggestion of a "mental" disorder, with its implication of diminished control over one's behavior and intellectual functions. (p. 238)

Among the specific factors involved in the ability to survive suicidal inclinations, Motto noted the following:

- Capacity to control behavior—that is, the ability to stand the pain or impulse
- Capacity to relate readily and in a meaningful

way to someone else; presence of family members and friends who are supportive

- Motivation for help and willingness to work actively on the problem
- Variety of resources that facilitate the therapeutic process and the transition back to a stable life pattern—for example, job skills, intelligence, physical health, communication skills, a capacity to trust, close ties to a church, or freedom from severe personality disturbance or addictive problems

To this list might be added financial resources—a factor that is particularly important in gaining access to good medical treatment, covering financial excesses from manic episodes, and meeting expenses during time lost from work—a strong marriage or close relationship, willingness and ability to follow a prescribed treatment regimen, and the kind of personality during normal times that will accumulate a backlog of goodwill. Depression strains and depletes relationships, and there is little restocking during such a state. The support of family and friends—always crucial for depressed and suicidal individuals, particularly if they are to stay out of the hospital—depends largely on how well relationships were maintained before the depression began. The importance of distributing responsibilities and anxieties over several friends and family members is discussed later.

Some depressed people are better than others at garnering support. The hostile, paranoid, and irritable person is unlikely to elicit support, whereas the person who is passive and sad when depressed usually will be offered help, especially if he is normally outgoing and filled with joie de vivre. Unfortunately, the patient with the most dangerous depression—that is, the most perturbed, volatile, irritable, and delusional—is often the most likely to put off potential sources of support.

Present Psychiatric Status

The clinician should use both the history and clinical findings obtained during a psychiatric examination to judge the risk of suicide, weighing past evidence of impulsivity along with the current severity of suicidal ideation and the precision of the patient's planning for suicide. Asking the patient directly about plans for committing sui-

cide is one of the most reliable ways to make such an assessment. If the patient denies immediate plans, the clinician should ask about any possible plans to commit suicide within the next week or month, assuming the current level of distress persists, and about any recent changes in mood, whether better or worse. Severe depression, marked hopelessness, and limited insight into the nature of the depression all augur poorly for outcome. Finally, specific symptoms and combinations of symptoms increase the probability of suicide and require close examination and monitoring. These include mixed states, delusions, psychomotor agitation, severe sleep disorders or excessive concern about the quality and quantity of sleep, panic attacks, severe anxiety (especially somatic anxiety), alcohol abuse, and anhedonia. Other typical signs of suicidal behavior—for example, patients making wills, buying guns, or giving things away—should also alert the clinician to potential risk.

Substance abuse is a particularly strong predictor of lethality in suicide, especially in males. Alcohol and illicit drugs diminish impulse control, impair judgment, and worsen the course of affective illness. Patients often use these substances to lessen the severe anxiety and pain associated with suicidal depression. Since the combination greatly increases the risk of suicide, recognition and treatment of substance abuse must be a priority (see Chapter 26).

From our review of the scientific literature and our clinical experience, we believe that the risk factors summarized in Table 27-1 are primary in the clinical evaluation of a suicidal, or potentially suicidal, manic-depressive patient.

TREATMENT

General Issues

The seriously suicidal person, whether inpatient or outpatient, requires intensive care. The clinician must commit more time and psychological energy than usual, prescribe more or different medications, change psychotherapy practices, and increase involvement with the patient's family members and friends. A suicidal crisis while a patient is already under psychiatric care often provides the opportunity and impetus to reappraise previous assumptions about diagnosis, psychiatric history, treatment response, and relationships with family and others.

The first and foremost clinical priority is, of course, keeping the patient alive. It is also vital to develop a systematic plan to prevent future episodes of depression, mania, and suicidal behavior.

Once the immediate danger of suicide is past, the patient should almost always continue in psychotherapy, which is particularly important when the patient and those close to the patient experience the emotional repercussions of the suicidal behavior. Psychotherapy can help the patient deal with the anger and resentment previously withheld by other people, as well as with the personal emotional consequences of having been depressed and suicidal. Second, the patient must have continuity of care for the basic psychiatric problem underlying the suicidal thoughts and behaviors.

General clinical management of acutely suicidal manic-depressive patients is presented in this section, and more specific psychotherapeutic and medical aspects in the next. The recommendations are based on both our clinical experience and that of others.

Psychotherapy

In general, treating acutely suicidal manic-depressive patients, especially those who are not hospitalized, requires psychotherapy or an intensification of the existing clinical care. Acute and dangerous perturbations in the clinical state are best monitored by close contact with someone trained to recognize and, it is hoped, ameliorate them. As Himmelhoch (1987) has observed:

. . . suicide is the ultimate expression of disconnection (anomie) and uninvolvement (aberration). The clinician must construct with the patient a new, safe, and rewarding social network. In the beginning the clinician is the center of this network, but in the end the patient is at the center and back in control. Psychotherapy becomes a process of reconnection. (p. 51)

Medication noncompliance can become a life-threatening problem, and interpersonal and intrapsychic stresses of the illness require therapeutic support.[1] The specifics of psychotherapy are detailed later in this chapter.

Frequency of Clinician–Patient Contact

When patients are suicidal, they should be seen and contacted more frequently than usual. If financial or scheduling problems exist, the clinician should attempt to see the patient for shorter periods of time but more often. It may help to establish a time each day, or each few days, for a brief telephone conversation (Winokur et al., 1969; Motto, 1975). Because the slowed anergic quality of bipolar depression often makes telephoning a difficult task for the patient, we find it helpful to instigate these contacts, asking the patient frequently and regularly to give his or her own assessment of suicidal intent.

Availability of Clinician

The patient must be told clearly how to reach the clinician in an emergency or during an acute exacerbation of suicidal thoughts and feelings. Directions for dealing with answering services, on-call systems, and coverage by other clinicians should be explicit and conveyed both verbally and in writing. Depressive confusional states, as well as guilt or fear about overburdening and alienating clinicians, often prevent patients from indicating that they do not fully understand practical details about access. Putting this in writing on an appointment card (e.g., "Please do not hesitate to call") can be both concrete and reassuring. The clinician needs a clear contract with all suicidal patients stipulating that they will call if they are in danger of losing control of their feelings or actions, become acutely suicidal, or feel the need for immediate care. It generally is also prudent to share this information with the closest family member or friend.

Consultations with Colleagues

Suicidal manic-depressive patients can challenge and frustrate the clinician because of the need for complicated diagnostic judgments, sophisticated psychopharmacological decisions, unusual conflicts arising from countertransference (particularly in dealing with anger, frustration, and demands on time and emotional reserves), and other problems in managing suicidal behavior. Consultation with specialists in the psychological and pharmacological treatment of affective illness can be helpful clinically, personally, and legally.

Medication Monitoring

The importance of prescribing only limited amounts of lethal medications, especially antidepressants, cannot be overstated. Murphy (1975) concluded that half of the patients who killed themselves through overdose had obtained their lethal dose in a single prescription. Instructions about medications—dosages, timing, potential side effects, dangerous adverse reactions, and potentiation by alcohol and other drugs—should be explicit and in writing. If possible, another concerned individual (family member or friend) should become involved in monitoring medications because confusion, subconscious suicidal wishes, and ambivalence about taking drugs make depressed patients particularly susceptible to errors in taking prescribed medications. Plastic pill boxes with separate sections for each day of the week are helpful to many, particularly those who are confused or taking more than one medication.

Family Members and Friends

The involvement of family members and friends can lessen the need for hospitalization and increase the family's and patient's sense of control over a potentially catastrophic situation. By participating during a patient's acute risk period, families can be actively involved in much of the decision making and learn ways to avert future crises. The clinician can alleviate family members' understandable sense of hopelessness and helplessness by providing information and reassurance, by giving them realistic expectations about likely difficulties in the acute and recovery phases, and by establishing clear contingency plans for serious problems that might arise. Families, like patients, should be given direct, preferably written, information about the patient's illness, medications, suicide risk, and ways of contacting the clinician.

A clinician can set up a suicide alert system by meeting with the patient, relevant family members, and a few close friends (if advisable) to coordinate an effective and direct method for noting particularly dangerous changes in the patient's mental condition and mood. At that meeting the clinician should clarify the limits of confidentiality in situations of potential suicide and should stress that the ultimate responsibility for assessing lethality and making decisions about hospitalization rests with the clinician. This avoids confusion about responsibility and lessens guilt should suicide occur. The clinician must maintain an ongoing surveillance of the system to assess the stress on all participants as well as the patient's need for inpatient care.

Hospitalization

The decision to admit a suicidal patient to a psychiatric hospital is often straightforward and reassuring to all concerned. On the other hand, when a patient equates hospitalization with total failure or symbolic defeat or when the stigma of hospitalization might severely and negatively affect work or personal relationships, the decision becomes more complicated. The psychological, social, and clinical disadvantages to the patient must be weighed not only against the risk of suicide but also against the pragmatic and emotional costs to the family and the clinician if the patient remains out of the hospital.

Hospitalization, while decreasing the risk of suicide, does not eliminate it. Robins and co-workers (1959) found that 7 percent of the patients in their sample had committed suicide while in a psychiatric hospital. Weeke (1979) reported an even higher rate: 27 percent of manic-depressive patients killed themselves while under hospital care, and half of them were on pass from a hospital or had absconded. Like Winokur and co-workers (1969) and Roose and colleagues (1983), Weeke emphasized the necessity of special suicide precautions to supplement hospitalization and the clear observation of patients even when they appear substantially improved or recovered.

Motto (1975) and Hawton and Catalan (1982) provided specific examples of ways to document evidence and to improve communication among hospital staff members in order to prevent suicide:

- The degree of suicide risk should be carefully assessed, and the risk should be stated explicitly, for example, low, moderate, or high.
- The measures to be taken to deal with the acutely suicidal patient should be stated in clear, specific terms. Most hospitals have devised suicide observation procedures that give detailed instructions to nursing and physician staffs.

- The nursing staff should be required to document on the chart that the suicide prevention measures have been carried out.

Other factors important in preventing suicide in hospitalized patients are a high staff/patient ratio, a reduced number of exits on the ward or a locked ward, and an awareness that increased risk periods exist when one nursing shift changes over to another and when a crisis on one part of the ward distracts staff attention from the suicidal patient (Hawton and Catalan, 1982).

Follow-up Care

The chronic, recurrent, and serious nature of manic-depressive illness makes follow-up care a necessary part of treatment. Already in the early 19th century, Benjamin Rush called attention to the danger of this period:

We should be careful to distinguish between a return of reason and a certain cunning, which enables mad people to talk and behave correctly for a short time, and thereby to deceive their attendants, so as to obtain a premature discharge from their place of confinement. To prevent the evils that might arise from a mistake of this kind, they should be narrowly watched during their convalescence, nor should they be discharged until their recovery had been confirmed by weeks of correct conversation and conduct. Three instances of suicide have occurred in patients soon after they left the Pennsylvania Hospital, and while they were receiving the congratulations of their friends upon their recovery. (1812, p. 239)

Hankoff (1982) has noted the advantages of specialty affective disorder clinics in providing continuity of care. Because of their biological associations, these clinics are also relatively free of the "stigmatization handicap of other psychiatric programs." Gitlin and Jamison (1984) and Fieve (1975) have pointed out the ability of such specialty clinics to make rigorous diagnoses, provide highly specialized and up to date treatment, and treat a large number of patients with similar types of problems. Although affective disorders clinics can provide such services, most patients with manic-depressive illness are not, in fact, treated in such facilities, and other settings, such as solo practice, can provide these advantages as well. On the whole, continuity of care and expertise in diagnosis and treatment (via consultation when necessary) are the important points in treating these patients. Several studies (e.g., Roy, 1982; Fawcett et al., 1987) have found that the first 6 to 12 months after hospital discharge comprise a period of very high risk of suicide. Fawcett's group concludes:

Programs designed to reduce suicide rates might use clinical resources most effectively by developing more intensive follow-up and support systems for patients showing features of high risk over the first year after hospital discharge. Clinicians treating patients with depression who have recently been discharged from the hospital should be especially alert to a greater danger of suicide during the first posthospital year. (p. 38)

Psychological Aspects

The psychological treatment of suicidal manic-depressive patients, although often emotionally draining and time consuming, is critical. The suicidal manic-depressive patient has many problems that need psychological support or therapy, reassurance, or general informational counseling. Ongoing professional assessment of suicide potential is essential if the person is to be treated as an outpatient. Often a suicidal depression will follow a manic episode. This clinical depression is confounded by circumstances—financial and employment chaos, marital problems, legal difficulties—that intensify the postmanic depression and require adjunctive management. Other psychological problems rise from reactions to the illness itself; these have been discussed in Chapters 24 and 25.

Important general psychotherapeutic issues include the patient's need for reassurance, the countertransference issues engendered by the suicidal patient, and, especially, a direct and involved therapeutic approach. As Himmelhoch (1987) has noted:

Psychotherapeutic style should always be designed to obtain information and protect the patient. The amount of information necessary for effective suicide management is immense, and the nature is often subtle. (p. 51)

Therapeutic Style

Most clinicians agree that in-depth psychotherapy is contraindicated for suicidal patients, especially those who are manic-depressive (Winokur et al., 1969; Hankoff, 1982). Shneidman (1975) recommends a direct and active approach and the National Institute of Mental Health Task Force on Suicide agreed when it suggested that the therapist maintain an "active relatedness" to the suicidal patient rather than a "reflective approach." The therapist should be willing to take more initiative with severely depressed patients than might be appropriate with others. Directness with a suicidal patient is imperative because the gravity of the situation demands immediate action, and the patient's paralysis of will demands active intervention. Also, most suicidal manic-depressive patients are hyperalert and hypersensitive, as well as guarded and suspicious, and often possess an uncanny ability to sense fear, cautiousness, and evasiveness in their therapists. Directness on the part of the clinician can help allay unnecessary anxiety and unwarranted fantasies, decrease a rather pervasive sense of negative omnipotence, and establish a basis for trust that can extend into other aspects of clinical care.

Along with directness, the therapist must demonstrate an ability to understand complicated and painful feelings. As described by Cassem (1978):

Despite his status as an ally for life, the therapist must also have the capacity to hear out carefully and to tolerate the feelings of despair, desperation, anguish, rage, loneliness, emptiness, and meaninglessness articulated by the suicidal person. The patient needs to know that the therapist takes him seriously and understands. (p. 595)

Because manic-depressive illness by and large is regarded as a biological disorder, psychotherapeutically oriented clinicians often refer suicidal bipolar patients to psychopharmacologists, some of whom may not have the time, interest, or skill to provide psychotherapy. Clinicians who are biologically oriented may tend toward too much reliance on medication while slighting psychotherapy, just as those who are primarily psychotherapists may tend toward too little emphasis on psychopharmacology. This point, made earlier in Chapters 24 and 25, takes on particular significance with suicidal patients, who need both psychological and medical care.

Providing Reassurance

The liberal and intelligent use of reassurance, which is an integral part of the treatment of manic-depressive illness, is especially important when the patient is suicidal. It is reasonable to offer hope when dealing with a treatable and spontaneously remitting illness. Winokur and colleagues (1969) suggest frequent reassurance to patients and families that, first, manic-depressive illness is an illness, second, it is time-limited, and

third, the clinician is familiar with this kind of problem. While depressed, suicidal patients are unlikely to acknowledge that the reassurance is helpful (West, 1975). Since they are likely to reject any reassurance, the clinician needs considerable skill and perseverance to maintain credibility while reassuring them. For example, it is helpful to acknowledge negativistic skepticism, with an understanding of the patient's current depression. After the acute suicidal crisis, however, most patients spontaneously mention the importance of such reassurances.

Communicating Information

Explicit information about manic-depressive illness, its treatment, and suicide is particularly important when dealing with suicidal patients, who may feel profound hopelessness and be cognitively impaired. Whenever feasible, information should be provided to them in both oral and written form. One of the first messages needing clear communication concerns the limits on confidentiality between suicidal patients and their therapists. This message becomes very significant for patients who are paranoid, irritable, and hostile or are experiencing mixed states and rapidly fluctuating moods. Other explanations and predictions for the patient and, where appropriate, the family are listed in Table 27-3.

It is important to communicate consistently that, although manic-depressive illness is serious, it can be treated successfully in the vast majority of cases. Left untreated, however, particularly early in the illness, it often results in suicide. The clinician must explain to the patient and family that denial of recurrence is common, but it can also be dangerous. Such an explanation predicts feelings and thereby lends credence to the clinician's recommendations.

The patient must take lithium and other medications as prescribed and be assured that the drug can often work as effectively against depression as it does against mania but that there is usually more time delay before it has an effect in the prevention or treatment of depression. The patient (and clinician) should not be discouraged by this delay nor assume that depression and suicidal feelings are inevitable.

It is important to communicate explicitly that many side effects occurring with medications can

Table 27-3. Communication to Patients and Families

General Issues
- Written information whenever possible
- Ways of contacting clinician
- Limits on confidentiality
- Postpone major life decisions
- Treatable nature of affective illness

Medication Issues
- Many effective medications available
- Imperative to take medications as prescribed
- Instructions should be in writing
- Side effects usually transient and/or treatable

When to Contact Physician
- Worsening of suicidal ideation
- Worsening of symptoms, especially:
  - sleep loss
  - agitation, severe restlessness
  - delusions
  - feelings of violence, impulsivity
- Problems with medication compliance

Alcohol and Drugs
- Worsen sleep and judgment
- Potentiate prescribed medications
- Undermine efficacy of medication
- Increase likelihood of mixed states

Recovery Issues
- High-risk nature of recovery period
- Recovery likely to be frustrating and tumultuous
- Sawtooth curve pattern
- Time course and recovery pattern with antidepressants

From Jamison, 1988

be ameliorated; others cannot. The clinician should be specific about possible side effects and about how transitory or permanent they are likely to be. (See Chapters 23 and 25 for further discussion of side effects.)

Patients who are on antidepressant medications should be warned that the time course for a drug response may lead to a discrepancy between what their physician sees as improvement and what they themselves are experiencing. For example, the physician and family may see improvement because the patient has more energy and is sleeping better, and the face and body are more animated. These changes generally occur before improvements in mood and thinking, changes that are likely to be more important to the patient. Predicting this discrepancy in perceptions can lessen some of the patient's discouragement, which is particularly important because at this stage in the illness, the patient is at high risk for suicide.

As the patient's condition begins to improve, the clinician may find it necessary to explain that a particularly frustrating and difficult period lies ahead and that temporary setbacks are common. The clinician should inform the patient and family that recovery from a suicidal depression is exceptionally difficult and likely to be filled with ups and downs, successes and setbacks (see Figure 24-1).

The patient should be aware that alcohol generally worsens depression, interferes with sleep, impairs judgment, and potentiates the effects of other medications. The patient should be advised also to avoid significant social or personal changes when depressed and to obtain a leave of absence from school or work rather than quit (Winokur et al., 1969).

Countertransference

Therapists should always be sensitive to the feelings, thoughts, and actions a patient engenders in them, but when the patient is suicidal, countertransference feelings must be examined even more closely. The therapist's reactions often reflect the added stress, responsibility, and time commitments involved in treating a suicidal patient, combined with the psychodynamics of the individual clinician. Problems can surface, such as overt or covert hostility toward patients (e.g., impatience, brusqueness on the telephone) or a tendency to avoid treating suicidal patients (thereby eliminating many manic-depressive patients from private practice).

The tendency for some therapists to overidentify with patients, particularly with professionally successful ones, can increase their own psychological distress and can lead to denial or overprotectiveness. The serious possibility of suicide reminds most therapists of their own vulnerabilities and limits. This is well stated by Cassem (1978):

The need to balance consideration for the patient's safety with the goal that he live his life independently . . . reminds us how limited the therapist's powers are—that is, they are no stronger than the patient's desire to make use of help. The therapist who appreciates his ultimate inability to stop the person who really wants to kill himself is far more likely to be effective in restoring the person's sense of self-esteem and wholeness. . . . Clarifying these limitations with the patient helps convey respect for his autonomy and reminds the therapist that a completed suicide can occur despite complete fulfillment of his responsibility. Both are thereby better enabled to see that the risks of their mutual encounter are worth taking. (pp. 595–596)

Medical Aspects

Effective suicide prevention depends in large measure on good medical management (acute and prophylactic). The sophisticated use of medications in treating manic-depressive illness is the single best protection against suicide, although it is by no means sufficient. In choosing a pharmacologic treatment, the most important aspect is efficacy.[2] Accordingly, some of the recommendations made here summarize what has been covered in detail in the drug treatment chapters.

Symptomatic Relief

Severe sleep disorders, delusions, mixed states, and severe anxiety in manic-depressive illness are not only disruptive and upsetting but also dangerous, since their presence can increase the risk of suicide. In addition to managing the depression itself, the clinician must treat these symptoms aggressively in a suicidal patient. Hypnotics, antipsychotics, or anxiolytics may be appropriate for short-term use.

Antidepressants

As detailed in Chapters 22 and 23, the management of depression of moderate severity, including breakthrough episodes in patients on maintenance treatment, should emphasize lithium initially. When the greater severity of symptoms requires adjunctive antidepressants, those with a less activating profile are preferred for the suicidal patient. If delusions or mixed states are present, an adjunctive neuroleptic or clonazepam may be temporarily necessary. Carbamazepine may be beneficial because of its antiaggressive properties, especially if the suicidal behavior is part of a mixed state. Along with a more anxiolytic antidepressant, benzodiazepines can be helpful in the management of anxiety.

Electroconvulsive Therapy

One of the most compelling indications for the use of electroconvulsive therapy (ECT) is acute suicidal depression in a manic-depressive patient. Even the most up to date and creatively used pharmacological interventions will fail in 20 to 30 percent of suicidal patients (Himmelhoch, 1987).

Yet ECT continues to be underused, particularly in the United States, because of the presence of obstructive legal and bureaucratic pressures that make it difficult and cumbersome, the risks of litigation by a small minority within patient advocacy groups, the availability of alternative treatments, such as tricyclics and MAO inhibitors, the influence of a bad press from outside the medical field, and, within the psychiatric field, a relative lack of awareness of ECT's advantages in treating the acutely suicidal patient. Himmelhoch (1987) has stated it bluntly:

The narcissistic ponderings of psychiatrists whose political agenda supersedes their clinical experience must not be allowed to keep patients who are suffering the most severe form of pain from relief. (p. 53)

Because tricyclics may worsen the course of illness in some bipolar patients (see Chapter 22), ECT becomes an important option for treating suicidal depression in these patients. Compared with tricyclics, ECT has several advantages. The antidepressant response is more rapid, thereby decreasing the immediate risk of suicide, there may be less potential for worsening the course of the illness, and the interruption of the depressive episode allows the prophylactic effect of lithium to become established (Rose et al., 1985).

SUMMARY

Treatment of the underlying illness is the most powerful method for preventing suicide in manic-depressive patients, who are at high risk for attempting suicide. Treatment should be pursued most aggressively in the early stages of the illness, when suicide is most likely to occur.

Predicting who is particularly at risk for suicide involves assessment of personal and family history and the patient's present psychiatric status, psychological assets and liabilities, and treatment history. A history of attempts is an important predictor, but so too is past and present suicidal ideation. The patient's tendency to act violently also should be assessed, along with past phases in the course of illness most often associated with suicidal, impulsive, or violent behavior. Patients should be monitored carefully in the period following hospitalization.

Treatment entails, first, keeping the patient safe—by hospitalization if necessary. Different medications or increased dosages of those already being taken may be necessary, and in some cases, a course of ECT is required. Anxiolytics or other additional treatments may be needed for symptoms associated with high risk of suicide—delusions, severe anxiety, sleep disorders—and special caution should be paid to patients with mixed states. Psychotherapy should accompany these treatments and continue after the initial threat has abated.

NOTES

1. Motto, 1975; Shneidman, 1975; West, 1975; Cassem, 1978; Hankoff, 1982; Jamison and Akiskal, 1983; Jamison, 1986; Schou and Weeke, 1988.

2. Obviously, other things being equal, it makes sense to use a drug with the lowest lethal dose when dealing with the suicidal patient.

Epilogue

Man is a harp whose chords elude the sight,
Each yielding harmony dispos'd aright;
The screws revers'd (a task which if he please,
God in a moment executes with ease)
Ten thousand thousand strings at once go loose,
Lost till he tune them, all their power and use.

—William Cowper

William Cowper was an 18th century poet whose manic-depressive illness caused him to spend much of his life in an insane asylum. Over the years that it has taken us to write this book, we have been impressed with the aptness of Cowper's image of "ten thousand thousand" strings—the numerous, finely tuned, complicated, and interwoven strings of the mind. As if mirroring this complexity, the study of manic-depressive illness and its related temperaments has itself become vast and various. It ranges across the fields of human knowledge and experience, from the arts to the neurosciences. In some of these specialties, research has developed so rapidly that its output threatens to overwhelm those who might learn and profit from it.

Throughout this book, we have tried to emphasize aspects of manic-depressive illness that are essential to its understanding: its recurrent nature and its similarities with the recurrent unipolar illnesses; its awesome lethality, often underemphasized because suicide appears more volitional than, for example, melanoma or renal failure; its distribution of symptoms and severities across a wide variety of dimensions; the frequent, clinically and theoretically pivotal, yet often overlooked existence of simultaneously expressed manic and depressive symptoms (i.e., mixed states); the importance of psychological features in a biologically based but psychologically expressed illness; the fascinating role of environment (e.g., psychological, light, and temperature) in a genetic disorder of incomplete penetrance; gender differences; kindling models; biological rhythms; and the close kinship between manic-depressive illness and certain epilepsies.

This book has discussed at length the clinical, psychological, and pathophysiological studies of manic-depressive illness. Rather than summarize them again (already done at the end of each chapter) we prefer to focus our attention here on a few general remarks about diagnosis and treatment.

Diagnostic issues remain an important part of the clinical practice and scientific understanding of manic-depressive illness. The very fact that an illness can be expressed in various ways—as temperament, seasonal swings of mood, morbid melancholia, mixtures of mania and depression, or unmanageable psychosis—speaks to the complexity of the manic-depressive spectrum. The tendency of clinicians to underdiagnose bipolar disorder in favor of schizophrenia or borderline personality disorders is now being replaced by an opposite tendency to diffuse the core concept of manic-depressive illness by including mild seasonal affective disorders and often unclearly defined bipolar-II conditions. Clearly, under-inclusiveness results in an unacceptably large number of patients being denied effective treatment. Overinclusion, on the other hand, risks trivialization of a serious disease, inappropiate treatment, blurring of meaningful diagnostic and genetic borders, and the labeling as pathological that which is in many people simply a variant of normal temperament. These diagnostic subtleties will, no doubt, be clarified by increasingly sophisticated diagnostic criteria using combined measures of biological markers, family history, subtypings on the basis of natural course and treatment response, and, eventually, neuropsychological profiles, brain-imaging patterns, laboratory techniques, and chromosome specification.

Treatment of manic-depressive illness remains one of the true successes of modern medicine. That very success has led to the complacent assumption that available treatments are adequate and that new ones are being developed at a sufficiently rapid rate. Both assumptions are wrong. Development of new medications for manic-depressive illness is a clear public health priority, since some patients respond only partially or not at all to available treatments. Patients who find the side effects of lithium and other mood-stabilizing drugs distressing or unacceptable may feel that they must choose between a compromised life-style and a high risk of recurrence. The basics of lithium therapy are now widespread in clinical practice. Far less widespread are the use of adjunctive medications, the subtle use of medication titration, mood charting, adjunctive psychotherapy, systematic patient and family education, and referral to patient and family support groups. The development of specific approaches for psychotherapy with manic-depressive patients is essential.

The variety of alternative medical interventions now available is promising, but many questions remain about the long-term efficacy of anti-convulsants and calcium channel blockers. While recognizing the tremendous impact these drugs have had on many patients with otherwise intractable illness, we remain concerned by the tendency to switch too readily from a well-established medication, such as lithium, often without an adequate trial, to newer, less proven drugs. The clinical research literature may be partly responsible for this tendency. The research commonly is done in facilities that treat patients who are unresponsive to standard treatments and who were referred for that very reason. Not surprisingly lithium is found to be less effective in such patients, and alternative medications are prescribed. The overall impression is created that lithium is less effective than it, in fact, is.

Finally, we wish to stress the clinical importance of early and aggressive treatment. It can prevent the psychological damage caused by affective episodes, lessen the chance of suicide, and decrease the probability of triggering a kindling phenomenon, which can render the system more vulnerable to subsequent attacks. These mechanisms may make patients less responsive to otherwise effective treatments and more likely to develop a worsening form of the illness.

Manic-depressive illness spans the range of human nature in its changes in mood, thinking, energies, and actions. Many positive features can accompany the basic destructiveness of the disease, a paradox that raises fascinating and profound issues of philosophy and ethics. It also raises the question of what role such a volatile, extreme, environmentally responsive, and fluctuating disorder plays in the societies and evolution of man. We have considered some of these issues, although we recognize that they are, in many ways, as elusive and complex as the chords of man described by William Cowper.

References

Abdulla YH, Hamadah K: Effect of ADP on PGE1 formation in blood platelets from patients with depression, mania and schizophrenia. *Br J Psychiatry* 127:591–595, 1975.

Ablon SL, Davenport YB, Gershon ES, Adland ML: The married manic. *Am J Orthopsychiatry* 45:854–866, 1975.

Abou-Saleh MT: Platelet MAO, personality and response to lithium prophylaxis. *J Affective Disord* 5:55–65, 1983.

Abou-Saleh MT, Coppen A: Subjective side-effects of amitriptyline and lithium in affective disorders. *Br J Psychiatry* 142:391–397, 1983.

Abou-Saleh MT, Coppen A: Classification of depressive illnesses: Clinico-psychological correlates. *J Affective Disord* 6:53–66, 1984.

Abou-Saleh MT, Coppen A: Who responds to prophylactic lithium? *J Affective Disord* 10:115–125, 1986.

Abou-Saleh MT, Coppen A: Serum and red blood cell folate in depression. *Acta Psychiatr Scand* 80:78–82, 1989.

Abraham K: Notes on the psycho-analytical investigation and treatment of manic-depressive insanity and allied conditions. (1911). In: *Selected Papers of Karl Abraham, M.D.* Translated by D Bryan and A Strachey. London: Hogarth Press, 1927. pp 137–156.

Abraham K: A short study of the development of the libido, viewed in the light of mental disorders. (1924). In: *Selected Papers of Karl Abraham, M.D.* Translated by D Bryan and A Strachey. London: Hogarth Press, 1927. pp 418–480.

Abrams R: *Electroconvulsive Therapy*. New York: Oxford University Press, 1988.

Abrams R, Taylor MA: Unipolar and bipolar depressive illness: Phenomenology and response to electroconvulsive therapy. *Arch Gen Psychiatry* 30:320–321, 1974a.

Abrams R, Taylor MA: Unipolar mania: A preliminary report. *Arch Gen Psychiatry* 30:441–443, 1974b.

Abrams R, Taylor MA: Mania and schizoaffective disorder, manic type: A comparison. *Am J Psychiatry* 133:1445–1447, 1976.

Abrams R, Taylor MA: Differential EEG patterns in affective disorder and schizophrenia. *Arch Gen Psychiatry* 36:1355–1358, 1979.

Abrams R, Taylor MA: A comparison of unipolar and bipolar depressive illness. *Am J Psychiatry* 137:1084–1087, 1980.

Abrams R, Taylor MA: Importance of schizophrenic symptoms in the diagnosis of mania. *Am J Psychiatry* 138:658–661, 1981.

Abrams R, Fink M, Dornbush RL, Feldstein S, Volavka J, Roubicek J: Unilateral and bilateral electroconvulsive therapy: Effects on depression, memory, and electroencephalogram. *Arch Gen Psychiatry* 27:88–91, 1972.

Abrams R, Taylor MA, Hayman MA, Krishna NR: Unipolar mania revisited. *J Affective Disord* 1:59–68, 1979.

Abrams R, Redfield J, Taylor MA: Cognitive dysfunction in schizophrenia, affective disorder and organic brain disease. *Br J Psychiatry* 139:190–194, 1981.

Abrams R, Taylor MA, Faber R, Ts'o TO, Williams RA, Almy G: Bilateral versus unilateral electroconvulsive therapy: Efficacy in melancholia. *Am J Psychiatry* 140:463–465, 1983.

Abse J: *John Ruskin: The Passionate Moralist*. London: Quartet Books, 1980.

Ackerknecht EH: *A Short History of Psychiatry*. New York: Hafner Publishing Co, 1959.

Ackerknecht EH: *A Short History of Medicine*. Revised Ed. Baltimore: The Johns Hopkins University Press, 1982.

Ader R, Cohen N: Behaviorally conditioned immunosuppression. *Psychosom Med* 37:333–340, 1975.

Adler D, Harrow M: Idiosyncratic thinking and personally overinvolved thinking in schizophrenic patients during partial recovery. *Compr Psychiatry* 15:57–67, 1974.

Agnoli A, Andreoli V, Casacchia M, Cerbo R: Effect of s-adenosyl-l-methionine (SAMe) upon depressive symptoms. *J Psychiatr Res* 13:43–54, 1976.

Agnoli A, Ruggieri S, Cerone G, Aloisi P, Baldassarre M, Stramentinoli G: The dopamine hypothesis of depression: Results of treatment with dopaminergic drugs. In: S Garattini, ed: *Symposium Medica Hoechst*. Stuttgart: Schattauer-Verlag, 1978. pp 447–458.

Ågren H: Symptom patterns in unipolar and bipolar depression correlating with monoamine metabolites in the cerebrospinal fluid: I. General patterns. *Psychiatry Res* 3:211–224, 1980.

Ågren H: Depressive symptom patterns and urinary MHPG excretion. *Psychiatry Res* 6:185–196, 1982.

Ågren H: Life at risk: Markers of suicidality in depression. *Psychiatr Dev* 1:87–103, 1983.

Ågren H, Niklasson F: Creatinine and creatine in CSF: Indices of brain energy metabolism in depression. *J Neural Transm* 74:55–59, 1988.

Ågren H, Potter WZ: Effects of drug washout on CSF monoamine and psychoendocrine variables. *Psychopharmacol Bull* 22:937–941, 1986.

Ågren H, Mefford IN, Rudorfer MV, Linnoila M, Potter WZ: Interacting neurotransmitter systems: A non-experimental approach to the 5HIAA-HVA correlation in human CSF. *J Psychiatr Res* 20:175–193, 1986.

Ahlfors UG, Baastrup PC, Dencker SJ, Elgen K, Lingjaerde O, Pedersen V, Schou M, Aaskoven O: Flupenthixol decanoate in recurrent manic depressive illness: A comparison with lithium. *Acta Psychiatr Scand* 64:226–237, 1981.

Ahlström CH: Mortality in mental hospitals with special regard to tuberculosis. *Acta Psychiatr Neurol Scand* (Suppl 24): 1942.

Akagawa K, Watanabe M, Tsukada Y: Activity of erythrocyte NaK-ATPase in manic patients. *J Neurochem* 38:258–260, 1980.

Akimoto H, Nakakuki M, Honda Y, Takahashi Y, Toyoda J, Sasaki K, Machiyama Y: Clinical evaluation of the effect of central stimulants, MAO inhibitors, and imipramine in the treatment of affective disorders. In: *Proceedings of the 3rd World Congress of Psychiatry, 1961*. Toronto: University of Toronto Press, 1962–1963. pp 958–963.

Akiskal HS: External validating criteria for psychiatric diagnosis: Their application in affective disorders. *J Clin Psychiatry* 41:6–15, 1980.

Akiskal HS: Subaffective disorders: Dysthymic, cyclothymic and bipolar II disorders in the "borderline" realm. *Psychiatr Clin North Am* 4:25–46, 1981.

Akiskal HS: The bipolar spectrum: New concepts in classification and diagnosis. In: L Grinspoon, ed: *Psychiatry Update*. Vol. II. Washington, DC: American Psychiatric Press, 1983a. pp 271–292.

Akiskal HS: Diagnosis and classification of affective disorders: New insights from clinical and laboratory approaches. *Psychiatr Dev* 2:123–160, 1983b.

Akiskal HS: Dysthymic and cyclothymic disorders: A paradigm for high-risk research in psychiatry. In: JM Davis, JW Maas, eds: *The Affective Disorders*. Washington DC: The American Psychiatric Press, 1983c. pp 211–231.

Akiskal HS: Characterologic manifestations of affective disorders: Toward a new conceptualization. *Integr Psychiatry* May-June:83–88, 1984.

Akiskal HS: The clinical management of affective disorders. In: R Michels, JO Cavenar, HKH Brodie, AM Cooper, SB Guze, LL Judd, GL Klerman, AJ Solnit, eds: *Psychiatry* Vol 1. Philadelphia: JB Lippincott, 1985. Ch. 61, pp 1–25.

Akiskal HS, Akiskal K: Reassessing the prevalence of bipolar disorders: Clinical significance and artistic creativity. *Psychiatr Psychobiol* 3:29s–36s, 1988.

Akiskal HS, Mallya G: Criteria for the "soft" bipolar spectrum: Treatment implications. *Psychopharmacol Bull* 23:68–73, 1987.

Akiskal HS, Puzantian VR: Psychotic forms of depression and mania. *Psychiatr Clin North Am* 2:419–439, 1979.

Akiskal HS, Djenderedjian AH, Rosenthal RH, Khani MK: Cyclothymic disorder: Validating criteria for inclusion in the bipolar affective group. *Am J Psychiatry* 134:1227–1233, 1977.

Akiskal HS, Bitar AH, Puzantian VR, Rosenthal TL, Walker PW: The nosological status of neurotic depression: A prospective three- to four-year follow-up examination in light of the primary-secondary and unipolar-bipolar dichotomies. *Arch Gen Psychiatry* 35:756–766, 1978a.

Akiskal HS, Djenderedjian AH, Bolinger JM, Bitar AH, Khani MK, Haykal RF: The joint use of clinical and biological criteria for psychiatric diagnosis: II. Their application in identifying subaffective forms of bipolar illness. In: HS Akiskal, WL Webb, eds: *Psychiatric Diagnosis: Exploration of Biological Predictors*. New York: SP Medical and Scientific Books, 1978b. pp. 133–146.

Akiskal HS, Khani MK, Scott-Strauss A: Cyclothymic temperamental disorders. *Psychiatr Clin North Am* 2:527–554, 1979a.

Akiskal HS, Rosenthal RH, Rosenthal TL, Kashgarian M, Khani MK, Puzantian VR: Differentiation of primary affective illness from situational, symptomatic, and secondary depressions. *Arch Gen Psychiatry* 36:635–643, 1979b.

Akiskal HS, Hirschfeld RMA, Yerevanian BI: The relationship of personality to affective disorders: A critical review. *Arch Gen Psychiatry* 40:801–810, 1983a.

Akiskal HS, Walker P, Puzantian VR, King D, Rosenthal TL, Dranon M: Bipolar outcome in the course of depressive illness: Phenomenologic, familial, and pharmacologic predictors. *J Affective Disord* 5:115–128, 1983b.

Akiskal HS, Chen SE, Davis GC, Puzantian VR, Kashgarian M, Bolinger JM: Borderline: An adjective in search of a noun. *J Clin Psychiatry* 46:41–48, 1985a.

Akiskal HS, Downs J, Jordan P, Watson S, Daugherty D, Pruitt DB: Affective disorders in referred children and younger siblings of manic-depressives: Mode of onset and prospective course. *Arch Gen Psychiatry* 42:996–1003, 1985b.

Akiskal HS, Yerevanian BI, Davis GC, King D, Lemmi H: The nosologic status of borderline personality: Clinical and polysomnographic study. *Am J Psychiatry* 142:192–198, 1985c.

Alarcon RD: Rapid cycling affective disorders: A clinical review. *Compr Psychiatry* 26:522–540, 1985.

Albers HE, Ferris CF: Neuropeptide Y: Role in the light-dark cycle entrainment of hamster circadian rhythms. *Neurosci Lett* 50:163–168, 1984.

Albers HE, Ferris CF, Leeman SE, Goldman BD: Avian pancreatic polypeptide phase shifts hamster circadian rhythms when microinjected into the suprachiasmatic region. *Science* 223:833–835, 1984.

Albrecht J, Müller-Oerlinghausen B: Zur klinischen bedeutung der intraerythrozytaren lithium konzentration: Ergebnisse einer katamnestischen studie. *Arzneim Forsch* 26:1145–1147, 1976.

Albrecht J, Müller-Oerlinghausen B: [Cardiovascular side effects of lithium]. *Dtsch Med Wochenschr* 105:651–655, 1980.

Albrecht J, Helderman JH, Schlesser MA, Rush AJ: A controlled study of cellular immune function in affective disorders before and during somatic therapy. *Psychiatry Res* 15:185–193, 1985.

Alexander DR, Deeb M, Bitar F, Antun F: Sodium-potassium, magnesium, and calcium ATPase activities in erythrocyte membranes from manic-depressive patients responding to lithium. *Biol Psychiatry* 21:997–1007, 1986.

Alexander F: *Fundamentals of Psychoanalysis*. New York: WW Norton, 1948.

Alexander FG, Selesnick ST: *The History of Psychiatry: An Evaluation of Psychiatric Thought and Practice From Prehistoric Times to the Present*. New York: Harper & Row, 1966.

Ali SA, Peet M, Ward NI: Blood levels of vanadium, caesium, and other elements in depressive patients. *J Affective Disord* 9:187–191, 1985.

Allen AD, Tilkian SM: Depression correlated with cellular immunity in systemic immunodeficient Epstein-Barr virus syndrome (SIDES). *J Clin Psychiatry* 47:133–135, 1986.

Allen AD, Fudenberg HH, Allen RE: Affective disorder and viral infections. Letter. *Arch Gen Psychiatry* 44:760, 1987.

Allison JB, Wilson WP: Sexual behaviors of manic patients: A preliminary report. *South Med J* 53:870–874, 1960.

Allport GW: *Pattern and Growth in Personality*. New York: Holt, Rinehart and Winston, 1961.

Almy GL, Taylor MA: Lithium retention in mania. *Arch Gen Psychiatry* 29:232–234, 1973.

Alvarez A: *The Savage God: A Study of Suicide*. New York: Random House, 1973.

Alvarez-Cermeño JC, Fernández JM, O'Neill A, Moral L, Saiz-Ruiz J: Lithium-induced headache. *Headache* 29:245–246, 1989.

Amark C: A study in alcoholism. *Acta Psychiatria et Neurologia* (Suppl 70):1–283, 1951.

Ambelas A: Psychologically stressful events in the precipitation of manic episodes. *Br J Psychiatry* 135:15–21, 1979.

Amdisen A, Schou M: Lithium. In: MNG Dukes, ed: *Side Effects of Drugs Annual 4*. Amsterdam: Excerpta Medica, 1980. pp 22–25.

American Psychiatric Association. *Diagnostic and Statistical Manual of Mental Disorders*. 1st ed. Washington, DC: The Association, 1952.

American Psychiatric Association. *Diagnostic and Statistical Manual of Mental Disorders*. 2nd ed. Washington, DC: The Association, 1968.

American Psychiatric Association. *Diagnostic and Statistical Manual of Mental Disorders*. 3rd ed. Washington, DC: The Association, 1980.

American Psychiatric Association. *Diagnostic and Statistical Manual of Mental Disorders*. 3rd ed.-revised. Washington, DC: The Association, 1987.

American Psychiatric Association (APA) Task Force on the use of laboratory tests in psychiatry: Tricyclic antidepressants, blood level measurements and clinical outcome. *Am J Psychiatry* 142:155–162, 1985.

American Psychiatric Association (APA) Task Force on the use Laboratory Tests in Psychiatry: The dexamethasone suppression test: An overview of its current status in psychiatry. *Am J Psychiatry* 144:1253–1262, 1987.

Aminoff MJ, Marshall J, Smith E, Wyke M: Cognitive function in patients on lithium therapy. *Br J Psychiatry* 125:109–110, 1974.

Amsel A: Partial reinforcement effects on vigor and persistance: Advances in frustration theory derived from a variety of within-subject experiments. In: KW Spence, JT Spence, eds: *The Psychology of Learning and Motivation: Advances in Research and Theory. Vol. 1*. New York: Academic Press, 1967. pp 1–65.

Amsterdam JD, Berwish N: Treatment of refractory depression with combination reserpine and tricyclic antidepressant therapy. *J Clin Psychopharmacol* 7:238–242, 1987.

Amsterdam J, Brunswick D, Mendels J: The clinical application of tricyclic antidepressant pharmacokinetics and plasma levels. *Am J Psychiatry* 137:653–662, 1980.

Amsterdam JD, Winokur A, Abelman E, Lucki I,

Rickels K: Cosyntropin (ACTH alpha 1-24) stimulation test in depressed patients and healthy subjects. *Am J Psychiatry* 140:907–909, 1983a.

Amsterdam JD, Winokur A, Lucki I, Caroff S, Snyder P, Rickels K: A neuroendocrine test battery in bipolar patients and healthy subjects. *Arch Gen Psychiatry* 40:515–521, 1983b.

Amsterdam JD, Winokur A, Dyson W, Herzog S, Gonzalez F, Rott R, Koprowski H: Borna disease virus: A possible etiologic factor in human affective disorders? *Arch Gen Psychiatry* 42:1093–1096, 1985.

Amsterdam JD, Henle W, Winokur A, Wolkowitz OM, Pickar D, Paul SM: Serum antibodies to Epstein-Barr virus in patients with major depressive disorder. *Am J Psychiatry* 143:1593–1596, 1986.

Amsterdam JD, Schweizer E, Winokur A: Multiple hormonal responses to insulin-induced hypoglycemia in depressed patients and normal volunteers. *Am J Psychiatry* 144:170–175, 1987.

Amsterdam JD, Maislin G, Winokur A, Berwish N, Kling M, Gold P: The oCRH stimulation test before and after clinical recovery from depression. *J Affective Disord* 14:213–222, 1988a.

Amsterdam JD, Rybakowski J, Gottlieb J, Frazer A: Kinetics of erythrocyte lithium-sodium countertransport in patients with affective illness before and during lithium therapy. *J Affective Disord* 14:75–81, 1988b.

Amsterdam JD, Maislin G, Skolnick B, Berwish N, Winokur A: Multiple hormone responses to clonidine administration in depressed patients and healthy volunteers. *Biol Psychiatry* 26:265–278, 1989.

Ananth J, Engelsmann NF, Kiriakos R, Kolivakis T: Prediction of lithium response. *Acta Psychiatr Scand* 60:279–286, 1979.

Ananth J, Ghadirian AM, Engelsmann F: Lithium and memory: A review. *Can J Psychiatry* 32:312–316, 1987.

Anderson GM, Bowers MB, Roth RH, Young JG, Hrbek CC, Cohen DJ: Comparison of high-performance liquid chromatographic, gas chromatographic—mass spectrometric, and fluorometric methods for the determination of homovanillic acid and 5-hydroxyindoleacetic acid in human cerebrospinal fluid. *J Chromatogr* 277:282–286, 1983.

Anderson LE, Phillips RD: Biological effects of electric fields: An overview. In: M Grandolfo, SM Michaelson, A Rindi, eds: *Biological Effects and Dosimetry of Static and ELF Electromagnetic Fields*. New York: Plenum Press, 1985. pp 345–378.

Andreani G, Caselli G, Martelli G: Relievi clinici ed elettroencefalografici duranti il trattamento consali di litio in malati psichiatrici. *G Psichiat Neuropat* 86:273–328, 1958.

Andreasen NC: Thought, language, and communication disorders: I. Clinical assessment, definition of terms, and evaluation of their reliability. *Arch Gen Psychiatry* 36:1315–1321, 1979a.

Andreasen NC: Thought, language, and communication disorders: II. Diagnostic significance. *Arch Gen Psychiatry* 36:1325–1330, 1979b.

Andreasen NC: Mania and creativity. In: RH Belmaker, HM van Praag, eds: *Mania: An Evolving Concept*. New York: Spectrum, 1980. pp 377–386.

Andreasen NC: Concepts, diagnosis and classification. In: Paykel ES, ed. *Handbook of Affective Disorders*. Edinburgh: Churchill Livingstone, 1982a. pp 24–44.

Andreasen NC: Negative symptoms in schizophrenia: Definition and reliability. *Arch Gen Psychiatry* 39:784–788, 1982b.

Andreasen NC: The clinical differentiation of affective and schizophrenic disorders. In: MR Zales, ed: *Affective and Schizophrenic Disorders: New Approaches to Diagnosis and Treatment*. New York: Brunner/Mazel Pub, 1983. pp 29–52.

Andreasen NC: The clinical significance of "thought disorder." Hibbs Award Lecture, 137th annual meeting of the American Psychiatric Association, May, 1984.

Andreasen NC: Creativity and mental illness: Prevalence rates in writers and their first-degree relatives. *Am J Psychiatry* 144:1288–1292, 1987a.

Andreasen NC: The diagnosis of schizophrenia. *Schizophr Bull* 13:9–22, 1987b.

Andreasen NC: The phenomenology of bipolar depression. Abstract of paper presented at the American Psychiatric Association, May, 1988.

Andreasen NC: Schizophrenia and bipolar disorder: CAT scan and MRI. Abstract of paper presented at the 142nd annual meeting of the American Psychiatric Association, 1989.

Andreasen NJC, Canter A: The creative writer: Psychiatric symptoms and family history. *Compr Psychiatry* 15:123–131, 1974.

Andreasen NC, Grove WM: The classification of depression: Traditional versus mathematical approaches. *Am J Psychiatry* 139:45–52, 1982.

Andreasen NJC, Pfohl B: Linguistic analysis of speech in affective disorders. *Arch Gen Psychiatry* 33:1361–1367, 1976.

Andreasen NJC, Powers PS: Creativity and psychosis: An examination of conceptual style. *Arch Gen Psychiatry* 32:70–73, 1975.

Andreasen NC, Winokur G: Secondary depression: Familial, clinical, and research perspectives. *Am J Psychiatry* 136:62–66, 1979.

Andreasen NC, Grove WM, Shapiro RW, Keller MB, Hirschfeld RMA, McDonald-Scott P: Reliability of lifetime diagnosis: A multicenter collaborative perspective. *Arch Gen Psychiatry* 38:400–405, 1981.

Andreasen NC, Hoffman RE, Grove WM: Mapping abnormalities in language and cognition. In: M Alpert, ed: *Controversies in Schizophrenia: Changes and Constancies*. New York: Guilford Press, 1985. pp 199–227.

Andreasen NC, Scheftner W, Reich T, Hirschfeld RMA, Endicott J, Keller MB: The validation of the concept of endogenous depression. *Arch Gen Psychiatry* 43:246–251, 1986.

Andreasen NC, Grove WM, Coryell WH, Endicott J,

Clayton PJ: Bipolar versus unipolar and primary versus secondary affective disoder: Which diagnosis takes precedence? *J Affective Disord* 15:69–80, 1988.

Angold A: Childhood and adolescent depression: I. Epidemiological and aetiological aspects. *Br J Psychiatry* 152:601–607, 1988.

Angst J: *Zur Ätiologie und Nosologie endogener depressiver Psychosen.* Berlin: Springer, 1966.

Angst J: The course of affective disorders: II. Typology of bipolar manic-depressive illness. *Arch Psychiat Nervenkr* 226:65–73, 1978.

Angst J: Verlauf unipolar depressiver, bipolar manisch-depressiver und schizo-affektiver Erkrankungen und Psychosen: Ergebnisse einer prospektiven Studie. *Fortschr Neurol Psychiatr* 48:3–30, 1980.

Angst J: Clinical indications for a prophylactic treatment of depression. *Adv Biol Psychiatry* 7:218–229, 1981a.

Angst J: Course of affective disorders. In: HM Van Praag, MH Lader, OJ Rafaelsen, EJ Sachar, eds: *Handbook of Biological Psychiatry.* New York: Marcel Dekker, Inc, 1981b. pp 225–242

Angst J, ed: *The Origins of Depression: Current Concepts and Approaches.* Berlin: Springer-Verlag, 1983.

Angst J: The course of affective disorders. In: *Mood Disorders: Pharmacologic Prevention of Recurrences.* Consensus Development Conference. National Institutes of Health/National Institute of Mental Health, 1984.

Angst J: Switch from depression to mania: A record study over decades between 1920 and 1982. *Psychopathology* 18:140–154, 1985.

Angst J: The course of major depression, atypical bipolar disorder, and bipolar disorder. In: H Hippius, GL Klerman, N Matussek, eds: *New Results in Depression Research.* Berlin: Springer-Verlag, 1986a. pp 26–35.

Angst J: Zurich genetic study findings. Presented at the NIMH affective disorders workshop, September, 1986b.

Angst J: The course of schizoaffective disorders. In: A Marneros, MT Tsuang, eds: *Schizoaffective Psychoses.* Berlin-Heidelberg: Springer-Verlag, 1986c. pp 63–93.

Angst J: The course of affective disorders. *Psychopath* 19(Suppl 2): 47–52, 1986d.

Angst J: Switch from depression to mania, or from mania to depression: Role of psychotropic drugs. *Psychopharmacol Bull* 23:66–67, 1987.

Angst J: Suicides among depressive and bipolar patients. Abstract of paper presented at the 141st annual meeting of the American Psychiatric Association, 1988.

Angst J: "A Genetic Validation of Diagnostic Concepts for Schizo-Affective Psychoses." Unpublished paper.

Angst J, Clayton P: Premorbid personality of depressive, bipolar, and schizophrenic patients with special reference to suicidal issues. *Compr Psychiatry* 27:511–532, 1986.

Angst J, Weis P: Periodicity of depressive psychoses. In: H Brill, JO Cole, P Deniker, eds: *Neuropsychopharmacology: Proceedings of the Fifth International Congress of the Collegium Internationale Neuro-psycho-pharmalogicum.* Amsterdam: Excerpta Medica, 1967. pp 703–710.

Angst J, Grof P, Hippius H, Pöldinger W, Weis P: La psychose maniaco-dépressive est-elle périodique ou intermittente? In: J de Ajuriaguerra, ed: *Cycles Biologiques et Psychiatrie.* Geneva: George & Cie, SA, 1968. pp 339–351.

Angst J, Dittrich A, Grof P: Course of endogenous affective psychoses and its modification by prophylactic administration of imipramine and lithium. *Int Pharmacopsychiatry* 2:1–11, 1969.

Angst J, Weis P, Grof P, Baastrup PC, Schou M: Lithium prophylaxis in recurrent affective disorders. *Br J Psychiatry* 116:604–614, 1970.

Angst J, Woggon B, Schoepf J: The treatment of depression with L-5-hydroxytryptophan versus imipramine: Results of two open and one double-blind study. *Arch Psychiatr Nervenkr* 224:175–186, 1977.

Angst J, Felder W, Frey R, Stassen HH: The course of affective disorders: I. Change of diagnosis of monopolar, unipolar, and bipolar illness. *Arch Psychiat Nervenkr* 226:57–64, 1978.

Angst J, Autenreith V, Brem F, Koukkou M, Meyer H, Stassen HH, Storck U: Preliminary results of treatment with β-endorphin in depression. In: E Usdin, WE Bunney, NS Kline, eds: *Endorphins in Mental Health Research.* New York: Oxford University Press, 1979a. pp 518–528.

Angst J, Felder W, Frey R: The course of unipolar and bipolar affective disorders. In: M Schou, E Strömgren, eds: *Origin, Prevention and Treatment of Affective Disorders.* New York: Academic Press, 1979b. pp 215–226.

Angst J, Felder W, Lohmeyer B: Schizoaffective disorders: Results of a genetic investigation. I. *J Affective Disord* 1:139–153, 1979c.

Angst J, Felder W, Lohmeyer B: Are schizoaffective psychoses heterogeneous? Results of a genetic investigation, II. *J Affective Disord* 1:155–165, 1979d.

Angst J, Frey R, Lohmeyer B, Zerbin-Rüdin E: Bipolar manic-depressive psychoses: Results of a genetic investigation. *Hum Genet* 55:237–254, 1980a.

Angst J, Felder W, Lohmeyer B: Course of schizoaffective psychoses: Results of a followup study. *Schizophr Bull* 6:579–585, 1980b.

Anker AL, Crowley TJ: Use of contingency contracts in specialty clinics for cocaine abuse. In: LS Harris, ed: *Problems of Drug Dependence 1981.* National Institute on Drug Abuse research monograph 41, 1982. pp 452–459.

Anonymous: Manic-depressive illness. *Lancet* 8414: 1268, 1984.

Ansseau M, Kupfer DJ, Reynolds CF III, McEachran AB: REM latency distribution in major depression: Clinical characteristics associated with sleep onset

REM periods. *Biol Psychiatry* 19:1651–1666, 1984.

Ansseau M, Kupfer DJ, Reynolds CF III: Internight variability of REM latency in major depression: Implications for the use of REM latency as a biological correlate. *Biol Psychiatry* 20:489–505, 1985a.

Ansseau M, Machowski R, Franck G, Timsit-Berthier M: REM sleep latency and contingent negative variation in endogenous depression: Suggestion for a common cholinergic mechanism. *Biol Psychiatry* 20:1303–1307, 1985b.

Ansseau M, Von Frenckell R, Cerfontaine JL, Papart P, Franck G, Timsit-Berthier M, Geenen V, Legros JJ: Blunted response of growth hormone to clonidine and apomorphine in endogenous depression. *Br J Psychiatry* 153:65–71, 1988.

Antel JP, Richman DP, Medof ME, Arnason BG: Lymphocyte function and the role of regulator cells in multiple sclerosis. *Neurology* 28:106–110, 1978.

Antelman SM, Caggiula AR: Norepinephrine-dopamine interactions and behavior. *Science* 195:646–653, 1977.

Anthony EJ: Childhood depression. In: EJ Anthony, T Benedek, ed: *Depression and Human Existence*. Boston: Little, Brown, 1975a.

Anthony EJ: The influence of a manic-depressive environment on the developing child. In: EJ Anthony, T Benedek, eds. *Depression and Human Existence*. Boston: Little, Brown, 1975b. pp 279–315.

Anthony EJ, Scott P: Manic-depressive psychosis in childhood. *J Child Psychol Psychiatry* 1:53–72, 1960.

Anthony JC, Folstein M, Romanoski AJ, Von Korff MR, Nestadt GN, Chahal R, Merchant A, Brown CH, Shapiro S, Kramer M, Gruenberg EM: Comparison of lay Diagnostic Interview Schedule and a standardized psychiatric diagnosis: Experience in eastern Baltimore. *Arch Gen Psychiatry* 42:667–675, 1985.

Appelbaum PS, Lidz CW, Meisel A: *Informed Consent: Legal Theory and Clinical Practice*. New York: Oxford University Press, 1987.

Apte SN, Langston JW: Permanent neurological deficits due to lithium toxicity. *Ann Neurol* 13:453–455, 1983.

Apter A, Borengasser M, Hamovit J, Bartko J, Cytryn L, McKnew DH Jr: A four-year follow-up of depressed children. Paper presented at the American Psychiatric Association, New Orleans, 1981.

Arana GW, Barreira PJ, Cohen BM, Lipinski JF, Fogelson D: The dexamethasone suppression test in psychotic disorders. *Am J Psychiatry* 140:1521–1523, 1983.

Arana GW, Pearlman C, Shader RI: Alprazolam-induced mania: Two clinical cases. *Am J Psychiatry* 142:368–369, 1985.

Arató M, Rihmer Z, Banki CM, Grof P: The relationships of neuroendocrine tests in endogenous depression. *Prog Neuropsychopharmacol Biol Psychiatry* 7:715–718, 1983.

Arató M, Rihmer Z, Szádöczky E: Seasonal influence on the dexamethasone suppression test results in unipolar depression. *Arch Gen Psychiatry* 43:813, 1986.

Arce AA, Vergare MJ: Identifying and characterizing the mentally ill among the homeless. In: HR Lamb, ed: *The Homeless Mentally Ill: A Task Force Report of the American Psychiatric Association*. Washington, DC: The American Psychiatric Association, 1984. pp 75–89.

Arce AA, Tadlock M, Vergare MJ, Shapiro SH: A psychiatric profile of street people admitted to an emergency shelter. *Hosp Community Psychiatry* 34:812–817, 1983.

Archer T, Fredriksson A, Jonsson G, Lewander T, Mohammed AK, Ross SB, Söderberg U: Central noradrenaline depletion antagonizes aspects of d-amphetamine-induced hyperactivity in the rat. *Psychopharmacology (Berlin)* 88:141–146, 1986.

Arieti S: Manic-depressive psychoses. In: S Arieti, ed: *American Handbook of Psychiatry*. Vol. 1. New York: Basic Books, 1959. pp 419–454.

Arieti S: *Creativity: The Magic Synthesis*. New York: Basic Books, 1976.

Arieti S: The manifest symptomatology of depression in adults. In: Arieti S, Bemporad J: *Severe and Mild Depression: The Psychotherapeutic Approach*. New York: Basic Books, 1978. pp 57–86.

Aristotle: *Problems II: Books XXII-XXXVIII*. Translated by WS Hett. Cambridge, Mass: Harvard University Press, 1936.

Arkowitz H, Buck F, Shanfield F: Interpersonal factors in depression: The reactions of family and friends to the depressed patient. Paper presented at the Annual Meeting of the Western Psychological Association, San Diego, 1979.

Arnold OH, Kryspin-Exner K: Zur Frage der Beeinflussung des Verlaufes des manisch-depressiven Krankheitsgeschehens durch Antidepressiva. [The problem of control of manic-depressive processes by antidepressants]. *Wien Med Wochenschr* 115:929–934, 1965.

Aronoff MS, Epstein RS: Factors associated with poor response to lithium carbonate: A clinical study. *Am J Psychiatry* 127:472–480, 1970.

Aronson TA, Shukla S: Life events and relapse in bipolar disorder: The impact of a catastrophic event. *Acta Psychiatr Scand* 75:571–576, 1987.

Aronson TA, Shukla S, Hoff A, Cook B: Proposed delusional depression subtypes: Preliminary evidence from a retrospective study of phenomenology and treatment course. *J Affective Disord* 14:69–74, 1988.

Aronson TA, Shukla S, Hirschowitz J: Clonazepam treatment of five lithium-refractory patients with bipolar disorder. *Am J Psychiatry* 146:77–80, 1989.

Arora RC, Meltzer HY: Serotonergic measures in the brains of suicide victims: 5-HT$_2$ binding sites in the frontal cortex of suicide victims and control subjects. *Arch Gen Psychiatry* 146:730–736, 1989.

Asano N: Clinicogenetic study of manic-depressive

psychoses. In: H Mitsuda, ed: *Clinical Genetics in Psychiatry*. Tokyo: Igaku Shoin, 1967.

Asarch KB, Shih JC, Kulsar A: Decreased ^{3}H-imipramine binding in depressed males and females. *Commun Psychopharmacol* 4:425–432, 1980.

Åsberg M, Bertilsson L, Tuck D, Cronholm B, Sjöqvist F: Indoleamine metabolites in the cerebrospinal fluid of depressed patients before and during treatment with nortriptyline. *Clin Pharmacol Ther* 14:277–286, 1973.

Åsberg M, Montgomery SA, Perris C, Schalling D, Sedvall G: A comprehensive psychopathological rating scale. *Acta Psychiatr Scand* (Suppl 271): 5–27, 1978.

Åsberg M, Bertilsson L, Mårtensson B, Scalia-Tomba GP, Thorén P, Träskman-Bendz L: CSF monoamine metabolites in melancholia. *Acta Psychiatr Scand* 69:201–219, 1984.

Aschoff J: Annual rhythms in man. In: J Aschoff, ed: *Handbook of Behavioral Neurobiology, Vol 4 Biological Rhythms*. New York: Plenum Press, 1981a. pp 475–487.

Aschoff J: Circadian rhythms: Interference with and dependence on work-rest schedules. In: LC Johnson, DI Tepas, WP Colquhoun, MJ Colligan, eds: *The 24-Hour Workday: A Symposium on Variations in Work-Sleep Schedules*. National Institute for Occupational Safety and Health. Washington, DC, 1981b. pp. 13–50.

Aschoff J: Freerunning and entrained circadian rhythms. In: J Aschoff, ed: *Handbook of Behavioral Neurobiology, Vol 4 Biological Rhythms*. New York: Plenum Press, 1981c. pp 81–93.

Aschoff J, ed: *Handbook of Behavioral Neurobiology, Vol 4 Biological Rhythms*. New York: Plenum Press, 1981d. pp 547–548.

Aschoff J: Disorders of the circadian system as discussed in psychiatric research. In: TA Wehr, FK Goodwin, eds: *Circadian Rhythms in Psychiatry*. Pacific Grove, CA: The Boxwood Press, 1983. pp 33–39.

Aschoff J, Wever R: The circadian system of man. In: J Aschoff, ed: *Handbook of Behavioral Neurobiology, Vol 4 Biological Rhythms*. New York: Plenum Press, 1981. pp 311–331.

Ashcroft GW, Glen AIM: Mood and neuronal functions: A modified amine hypothesis for the etiology of affective illness. *Adv Biochem Psychopharmacology* 11:335–339, 1974.

Ashcroft GW, Sharman DF: 5-hydroxyindoles in human cerebrospinal fluids. *Nature* 186:1050–1051, 1960.

Ashcroft GW, Crawford TBB, Eccleston D, Sharman DF, MacDougall EJ, Stanton JB, Binns JK: 5-hydroxyindole compounds in the cerebrospinal fluid of patients with psychiatric or neurological diseases. *Lancet* 2:1049–1052, 1966.

Ashcroft GW, Blackburn IM, Eccleston D, Glen AI, Hartley W, Kinloch NE, Lonergan M, Murray LG, Pullar IA: Changes on recovery in the concentrations of tryptophan and the biogenic amine metabolites in the cerebrospinal fluid of patients with affective illness. *Psychol Med* 3:319–325, 1973.

Ashcroft G, Dow R, Yates C: Significance of lumbar CSF metabolite measurements in affective illness. In: J Tuomisto, M Paasonen, eds: *CNS and Behavioral Pharmacology*. Helsinki: University of Helsinki, 1976. pp 277–284.

Ashworth CM, Blackburn IM, McPherson FM: The performance of depressed and manic patients on some repertory grid measures: A cross-sectional study. *Br J Med Psychol* 55:247–255, 1982.

Ashworth CM, Blackburn IM, McPherson FM: The performance of depressed and manic patients on some repertory grid measure: A longitudinal study. *Br J Med Psychol* 58:337–342, 1985.

Asnis GM, Asnis D, Dunner DL, Fieve RR: Cogwheel rigidity during chronic lithium therapy. *Am J Psychiatry* 136:1225–1226, 1979.

Asnis GM, Sachar EJ, Halbreich U, Nathan RS, Ostrow L, Halpern FS: Cortisol secretion and dexamethasone response in depression. *Am J Psychiatry* 138:1218–1221, 1981.

Assal G, Zander E, Hadjiantoniou J: Les troubles mentaux au cours des tumeurs de la fosse posterieure. *Schweizer Archiv fur Neurologie, Neurochirurgie un Psychiarie* 116:17–127, 1957.

Astrup C, Fossum A, Holmboe R: A follow-up study of 270 patients with acute affective psychoses. *Acta Psychiat Neurol Scand* 34(Suppl 135):11–65, 1959.

Astrup C, Fossum A, Holmboe R: *Prognosis in Functional Psychoses: Clinical Social and Genetic Aspects*. Springfield, IL: Charles C Thomas, 1962.

Atkinson JH, Kremer EF, Risch SC, Janowsky DS: Basal and post-dexamethasone cortisol and prolactin concentrations in depressed and non-depressed patients with chronic pain syndromes. *Pain* 25:23–34, 1986.

Aurell M, Svalander C, Wallin L, Alling C: Renal function and biopsy findings in patients on long-term lithium treatment. *Kidney Int* 20:663–670, 1981.

Avery D, Casey D: Resynchronization of the temperature rhythm in a catatonic patient treated with ECT. Paper presented at the 42nd Annual convention of the Society of Biological Psychiatry. Chicago, 1987.

Avery D, Mills M: Electroconvulsive therapy and antidepressants in the treatment of depression. In: F Ayd, IJ Taylor, eds: *Mood Disorders: The World's Major Public Health Problem*. Baltimore: Ayd Medical Research Publication, 1978. pp 139–153.

Avery D, Winokur G: Mortality in depressed patients treated with electroconvulsive therapy and antidepressants. *Arch Gen Psychiatry* 33:1029–1037, 1976.

Avery D, Winokur G: The efficacy of electroconvulsive therapy and antidepressants in depression. *Biol Psychiatry* 12:507–523, 1977.

Avery D, Wildschiødtz G, Rafaelsen O: REM latency and temperature in affective disorder before and after treatment. *Biol Psychiatry* 17:463–470, 1982.

Avery DH, Wildschiødtz G, Smallwood RG, Martin

D, Rafaelsen OJ: REM latency and core temperature relationships in primary depression. *Acta Psychiatr Scand* 74:269–280, 1986.

Avery DH, Khan A, Dager S, Dunner DL: Winter depression and response to a.m. and p.m. light. Abstract of paper presented at the 141st annual meeting of the American Psychiatric Association, May, 1988.

Axelrod J: The pineal gland: A neurochemical transducer. *Science* 184:1341–1348, 1974.

Axelrod J, Reisine TD: Stress hormones: Their interaction and regulation. *Science* 224:452–459, 1984.

Ayd FJ: Lithium holidays. *Intl Drug Ther Newsletter* 16:17–20, 1981.

Baasher T, Elhakim ASED, ElFawal K, Geil R, Harding TW, Wankiiri VB: On vagrancy and psychosis. *Community Ment Health J* 19:27–41, 1983.

Baastrup PC: The use of lithium in manic-depressive psychosis. *Compr Psychiatry* 5:396–408, 1964.

Baastrup PC: Practical clinical viewpoints regarding treatment with lithium. *Acta Psychiatr Scand* 207:12–16, 1969.

Baastrup PC: Lithium in the prophylactic treatment of recurrent affective disorders. In: FN Johnson, ed: *Handbook of Lithium Therapy.* Baltimore: University Park Press, 1980. pp 26–38.

Baastrup PC, Schou M: Lithium as a prophylactic agent: Its effect against recurrent depression and manic-depressive psychosis. *Arch Gen Psychiatry* 16:162–172, 1967.

Baastrup PC, Poulsen JC, Schou M, Thomsen K, Amdisen A: Prophylactic lithium: Double-blind discontinuation in manic-depressive and recurrent-depressive disorders. *Lancet* 2:326–330, 1970.

Baastrup PC, Hollnagel P, Sorensen R, Schou M: Adverse reactions in treatment with lithium carbonate and haloperidol. *JAMA* 236:2645–2646, 1976.

Baastrup PC, Christiansen C, Transbøl I: Calcium metabolism in lithium-treated patients: Relation to unibipolar dichotomy. *Acta Psychiatr Scand* 57:124–128, 1978.

Babcock JW: The colored insane. *Alienist and Neurologist* 16:423–447, 1895.

Babor TF, Mirin SM, Meyer RE: Behavioral and social effects. In: Babor TF, Mirin SM, Meyer RE, eds: *The Heroin Stimulus: Implications for a Theory of Addiction.* New York: Plenum Press, 1979. pp 119–135.

Bacher NM, Lewis HA: Lithium plus reserpine in refractory manic patients. *Am J Psychiatry* 136:811–814, 1979.

Bacopoulos NG, Hattox SE, Roth RH: 3,4-Dihydroxyphenylacetic acid and homovanillic acid in rat plasma: Possible indicators of central dopaminergic activity. *Eur J Pharmacol* 56:225–236, 1979.

Baer L, Durell J, Bunney WE Jr, Levy BS, Murphy DL, Greenspan K, Cardon PV: Sodium balance and distribution in lithium carbonate therapy. *Arch Gen Psychiatry* 22:40–44, 1970.

Baer L, Glassman AH, Kassir S: Negative sodium bal-

ance in lithium carbonate toxicity: Evidence of mineralocorticoid blockade. *Arch Gen Psychiatry* 29:823–827, 1973.

Bagehot, W: *The English Constitution.* London: Chapman & Hall, 1867.

Bagley C: Occupational status and symptoms of depression. *Soc Sci Med* 7:327–339, 1973.

Bagshaw MH, Kimble DP, Pribram KH: The GSR of monkeys during orienting and habituation after ablation of the amygdala, hippocampus and inferotemporal cortex. *Neuropsychologia* 3:111–119, 1965.

Bailey J, Coppen A: A comparison between the Hamilton Rating Scale and the Beck Inventory in the measurement of depression. *Br J Psychiatry* 128:486–489, 1976.

Baillarger J: De la folie à double forme. *Ann Med Psychol* 6:367–391, 1854a.

Baillarger J: Note sur un genre de folie dont les accès sont caractérisés par deux périodes régulières, l'une de dépression et l'autre d'excitation. *Gazette Hebdomadaire de Medecine et Chirurgie* 132:263–265, 1854b.

Baker EF: Sodium transfer to cerebrospinal fluid in functional psychiatric illness. *Can Psychiatr Assoc J* 16:167–170, 1971.

Baker M, Dorzab J, Winokur G, Cadoret RJ: Depressive disease: Classification and clinical characteristics. *Compr Psychiatry* 12:354–365, 1971.

Bakker JB, Pepplinkhuizen L: Cutaneous side-effects of lithium. In: FN Johnson, ed: *Handbook of Lithium Therapy.* Baltimore: University Park Press, 1980. pp 372–377.

Baldessarini RJ: Frequency of diagnoses of schizophrenia versus affective disorders from 1944 to 1968. *Am J Psychiatry* 127:757–763, 1970.

Baldessarini RJ: The basis for the amine hypotheses in affective disorders. *Arch Gen Psychiatry* 32:14–35, 1975.

Baldessarini RJ: Treatment of depression by altering monoamine metabolism: Precursors and metabolic inhibitors. *Psychopharmacol Bull* 20:224–239, 1984.

Baldessarini RJ: *Chemotherapy in Psychiatry.* Cambridge: Harvard University Press, 1985.

Baldessarini RJ: Neuropharmacology of s-adenosyl-l-methionine. *Am J Med* 83(Suppl 5A):95–103, 1987.

Baldessarini RJ, Arana GW: Does the dexamethasone suppression test have clinical utility in psychiatry? *J Clin Psychiatry* 46:25–29, 1985.

Baldessarini RJ, Tohen M: Is there a long-term protective effect of mood-altering agents in unipolar depressive disorder? In: DE Casey, AV Christensen, eds: *Psychopharmacology: Current Trends.* Berlin: Springer-Verlag, 1988. pp 130–139.

Baldwin JA: Schizophrenia and physical disease. *Psychol Med* 9:611–618, 1979.

Ball JRB, Kiloh LG: A controlled trial of imipramine in treatment of depressive states. *Br Med J* 2:1052–2055, 1959.

Ballantine HT, Giriunas IE: Advances in psychiatric surgery. In: T Rasmussen, R Marino, eds: *Functional Neurosurgery*. New York: Raven Press, 1979. pp 155–164.

Ballantine HT, Levy BS, Dagi TF, Giriunas IE: Cingulotomy for psychiatric illness: Report of 13 years' experience. In: WH Sweet, S Obrador, JG Martin-Rodríguez, eds: *Neurosurgical Treatment in Psychiatry, Pain, and Epilepsy*. Baltimore: University Park Press, 1977. pp 333–353.

Balldin J, Berggren U, Rybo E, Kjellbo H, Lindstedt G: Treatment resistant mania with primary hypothyroidism: A case of recovery after levothyroxine. *J Clin Psychiatry* 48:490–491, 1987.

Ballenger JC, Post RM: Kindling as a model for alcohol withdrawal syndromes. *Br J Psychiatry* 133:1–14, 1978a.

Ballenger JC, Post RM: Therapeutic effects of carbamazepine in affective illness: A preliminary report. *Commun Psychopharmacol* 2:159–175, 1978b.

Ballenger JC, Post RM: Carbamazepine in manic-depressive illness: A new treatment. *Am J Psychiatry* 137:782–790, 1980.

Ballenger JC, Goodwin FK, Major FL, Brown GL: Alcohol and central serotonin metabolism in man. *Arch Gen Psychiatry* 36:224–227, 1979.

Ballenger JC, Post RM, Gold PW, Goodwin FK, Bunney WE, Robertson G: Endocrine correlates of personality and cognition in normals. Abstract of paper presented at the 133rd Annual Meeting of the American Psychiatric Association, 1980. pp 144–145.

Ballenger JC, Reus VI, Post RM: The "atypical" clinical picture of adolescent mania. *Am J Psychiatry* 139:602–606, 1982.

Balon R, Yeragani VK, Pohl RB, Gershon S: Lithium discontinuation: Withdrawal or relapse? *Compr Psychiatry* 29:330–334, 1988.

Banay-Schwartz M, Wajda IJ, Manigault I, DeGuzman T, Lajtha A: Lithium: Effect on [³H]spiperone binding, ionic content, and amino acid levels in the brain of rats. *Neurochem Res* 7:179–189, 1982.

Banki CM: Correlation between cerebrospinal fluid amine metabolites and psychomotor activity in affective disorders. *J Neurochem* 28:255–257, 1977.

Banki CM, Vojnik M, Molnar G: Cerebrospinal fluid amine metabolites, tryptophane and clinical parameters in depression. *J Affective Disord* 3:91–99, 1981.

Banki CM, Vojnik M, Papp Z, Balla KZ, Arató M: Cerebrospinal fluid magnesium and calcium related to amine metabolites, diagnosis, and suicide attempts. *Biol Psychiatry* 20:163–171, 1985.

Banki CM, Bissette G, Arato M, O'Connor L, Nemeroff CB: CSF corticotropin-releasing factor-like immunoreactivity in depression and schizophrenia. *Am J Psychiatry* 144:873–877, 1987.

Banki CM, Bissette G, Arato M, Nemeroff CB: Elevation of immunoreactive CSF TRH in depressed patients. *Am J Psychiatry* 145:1526–1531, 1988.

Barczak P, Edmunds E, Betts T: Hypomania following complex partial seizures. *Br J Psychiatry* 152:137–139, 1988.

Baron M: Linkage between an X-chromosome marker (deutan color blindness) and bipolar affective illness: Occurrence in the family of a lithium carbonate-responsive schizo-affective proband. *Arch Gen Psychiatry* 34:721–725, 1977.

Baron M, Gershon ES, Rudy V, Jonas WZ, Buchsbaum M: Lithium carbonate response in depression: Prediction by unipolar/bipolar illness, average-evoked response, catechol-O-methyl transferase, and family history. *Arch Gen Psychiatry* 32:1107–1111, 1975.

Baron M, Mendlewicz J, Gruen R, Gruen R, Asnis L, Fieve RR: Assortative mating in affective disorders. *J Affective Disord* 3:167–171, 1981a.

Baron M, Mendlewicz J, Klotz J: Age-of-onset and genetic transmission in affective disorders. *Acta Psychiatr Scand* 64:373–380, 1981b.

Baron M, Gruen R, Asnis L, Kane J: Schizoaffective illness, schizophrenia and affective disorders: Morbidity risk and genetic transmission. *Acta Psychiatr Scand* 65:253–262, 1982.

Baron M, Barkai A, Gruen R, Kowalik S, Quitkin F: ³H-imipramine platelet binding sites in unipolar depression. *Biol Psychiatry* 18:1403–1409, 1983a.

Baron M, Risch N, Mendlewicz J: Age at onset in bipolar-related major affective illness: Clinical and genetic implications. *J Psychiatric Res* 17:5–18, 1983b.

Baron M, Barkai A, Gruen R, Peselow E, Fieve R, Quitkin F: Platelet ³H-imipramine binding in affective disorders: Trait versus state characteristics. *Am J Psychiatry* 143:711–717, 1986.

Baron M, Risch N, Hamburger R, Mandel B, Kushner S, Newman M, Drumer D, Belmaker RH: Genetic linkage between X-chromosome markers and bipolar affective illness. *Nature* 326:289–292, 1987.

Barraclough B: The diagnostic classification and psychiatric treatment of 100 suicides. In: R Fox, ed: *Proceedings of the Fifth International Conference for Suicide Prevention*. Vienna: IASP, 1970. pp 129–132.

Barraclough B: Suicide prevention, recurrent affective disorder and lithium. *Br J Psychiatry* 121:391–392, 1972.

Barraclough B, Bunch J, Nelson B, Sainsbury P: A hundred cases of suicide: Clinical aspects. *Br J Psychiatry* 125:355–373, 1974.

Bartholini G, Lloyd KG, Morselli PL, eds: *GABA and Mood Disorders: Experimental and Clinical Research*. New York: Raven Press, 1986.

Barton BM, Gitlin MJ: Verapamil in treatment-resistant mania: An open trial. *J Clin Psychopharmacol* 7:101–103, 1987.

Bashir M, Russell J, Johnson G: Bipolar affective disorder in adolescence: A 10-year study. *Aust NZ J Psychiatry* 21:36–43, 1987.

Baskow J, Gottfries CG, Roos BE, Winblad B: Determination of monoamine and monoamine metabolites in the human brain: Post mortem studies in a group of suicides and in a control group. *Acta Psychiatr Scand* 53:7–20, 1976.

Bassuk EL, Rubin L, Lauriat A: Is homelessness a mental health problem? *Am J Psychiatry* 141:1546–1550, 1984.

Bassuk EL, Rubin L, Lauriat A: Characteristics of sheltered homeless families. *Am J Public Health* 76:1097–1101, 1986.

Bauer MS, Whybrow PC: Thyroid hormones and the central nervous system in affective illness: Interactions that may have clinical significance. *Integ Psychiatry* 6:75- 100, 1988a.

Bauer MS, Whybrow PC: Rapid cycling bipolar affective disorder: Thyroid function and response to adjuvant treatment with high-dose thyroxine. Abstract of paper presented at the 43rd annual meeting of the Society for Biological Psychiatry, May, 1988b.

Baumann U: Methodische Untersuchungen zur Hamilton-Depression-Skala. *Arch Psychiat Nervenkr* 222:359–375, 1976.

Baumann U: Recent development of the AMDP system. In: P Pichot, P Berner, R Wolf, K Thau, eds: *Psychiatry: The State of the Art. Vol 1: Clinical Psychopathology, Nomenclature and Classification.* New York: Plenum Press, 1985. pp 155–160.

Baumann U, Angst J: Methodological development of the AMP system. In: JR Boissier, H Hippius, P Pichot, eds: *Neuropsychopharmacology: Proceedings of the IX Congress of the Collegium Internationale Neuropsychopharmacologicum.* Amsterdam: Excerpta Medica, 1975. pp 72–78.

Baumgartner A, Gräf KJ, Kürten I, Meinhold H: The hypothalamic-pituitary-thyroid axis in psychiatric patients and healthy subjects: Parts 1–4. *Psychiatry Res* 24:271–332, 1988.

Baxter LR Jr: Can lithium carbonate prolong the antidepressant effect of sleep deprivation? *Arch Gen Psychiatry* 42:635, 1985.

Baxter L, Edell W, Gerner R, Fairbanks L, Gwirtsman H: Dexamethasone suppression test and axis I diagnoses of inpatients with DSM-III borderline personality disorder. *J Clin Psychiatry* 45:150–153, 1984.

Baxter LR Jr, Phelps ME, Mazziotta JC, Schwartz JM, Gerner RH, Selin CE, Sumida RM: Cerebral metabolic rates for glucose in mood disorders: Studies with positron emission tomography and fluorodeoxyglucose F 18. *Arch Gen Psychiatry* 42:441–447, 1985.

Baxter LR Jr, Liston EH, Schwartz JM, Altshuler LL, Wilkins JN, Richeimer S, Guze BH: Prolongation of the antidepressant response to partial sleep deprivation by lithium. *Psychiatry Res* 19:17–23, 1986.

Baxter LR Jr, Phelps ME, Mazziotta JC, Guze BH, Schwartz JM, Selin CE: Local cerebral glucose metabolic rates in obsessive-compulsive disorder: A comparison with rates in unipolar depression and in normal controls. *Arch Gen Psychiatry* 44:211–218, 1987.

Baxter LR Jr, Schwartz JM, Phelps ME, Mazziotta JC, Guze BH, Selin CE, Gerner RH, Sumida RM: Reduction of prefrontal cortex glucose metabolism common to three types of depression. *Arch Gen Psychiatry* 46:243–250, 1989.

Bazzoui W: Affective disorders in Iraq. *Br J Psychiatry* 117:195–203, 1970.

Bear DM, Fedio P: Quantitative analysis of interictal behavior in temporal lobe epilepsy. *Arch Neurol* 34:454–467, 1977.

Beardslee WR, Bemporad J, Keller MB, Klerman GL: Children of parents with major affective disorder: A review. *Am J Psychiatry* 140:825–832, 1983.

Bech P: Rating scales for affective disorders: Their validity and consistency. *Acta Psychiatr Scand* (Suppl 295):11–101, 1981.

Bech P, Rafaelsen OJ: The use of rating scales exemplified by a comparison of the Hamilton and the Bech-Rafaelsen Melancholia Scale. *Acta Psychiatr Scand* (Suppl 285):128–132, 1980.

Bech P, Gram E, Dein E, Jacobsen O, Vitger J, Bolwig TG: Quantitative rating of depressive states: Correlation between clinical assessment, Beck's Self-Rating Scale and Hamilton's Objective Rating Scale. *Acta Psychiatr Scand* 51:161–170, 1975.

Bech P, Vendsborg PB, Rafaelsen OJ: Lithium maintenance treatment of manic-melancholic patients: Its role in the daily routine. *Acta Psychiatr Scand* 53:70–81, 1976.

Bech P, Kirkegaard C, Bock E, Johannesen M, Rafaelsen OJ: Hormones, electrolytes, and cerebrospinal fluid proteins in manic-melancholic patients. *Neuropsychobiology* 4:99–112, 1978.

Bech P, Bolwig TG, Kramp P, Rafaelsen OJ: The Bech-Rafaelsen Mania Scale and the Hamilton Depression Scale: Evaluation of homogeneity and inter-observer reliability. *Acta Psychiatr Scand* 59:420–430, 1979a.

Bech P, Thomsen J, Prytz S, Vendsborg PB, Zilstorff K, Rafaelsen OJ: The profile and severity of lithium-induced side effects in mentally healthy subjects. *Neuropsychobiology* 5:160–166, 1979b.

Bech P, Shapiro RW, Sihm F, Nielsen BM, Sørensen B, Rafaelsen OJ: Personality in unipolar and bipolar manic-melancholic patients. *Acta Psychiatr Scand* 62:245–257, 1980.

Bech P, Kastrup M, Rafaelsen OJ: Mini-compendium of rating scales for states of anxiety, depression, mania and schizophrenia with corresponding DSM-III syndromes. *Acta Psychiatr Scand* (Suppl 326):1–37, 1986.

Beck AT: *Depression: Causes and Treatment.* Philadelphia: University of Pennsylvania Press, 1967.

Beck AT, Beamesderfer A: Assessment of depression: The Depression Inventory. *Mod Probl Pharmacopsychiat* 7:151–169, 1974.

Beck AT, Ward CH, Mendelson M, Mock J, Erbaugh J: An inventory for measuring depression. *Arch Gen Psychiatry* 4:561–571, 1961.

Beck AT, Kovacs M, Weisman A: Hopelessness and suicidal behavior. *JAMA* 234:1146–1149, 1975.

Beck-Friis J, Von Rosen D, Kjellman BF, Ljunggren JG, Wetterberg L: Melatonin in relation to body measures, sex, age, season and the use of drugs in patients with major affective disorders and healthy subjects. *Psychoneuroendocrinology* 9:261–277, 1984.

Becker G: *The Mad Genius Controversy: A Study in the Sociology of Deviance.* Beverly Hills: Sage, 1978.

Becker J: Achievement related characteristics of manic-depressives. *J Abnorm and Soc Psychol* 60:334–339, 1960.

Becker J, Altrocchi J: Peer conformity and achievement in female manic-depressives. *J Abnorm Psychol* 73:585–589, 1968.

Becker MH, Maiman LA: Strategies for enhancing compliance. *J Community Health* 6:113–135, 1980.

Beckman L, Cedergren B, Perris C, Strandman E: Blood groups and affective disorders. *Hum Hered* 28:48–55, 1978.

Beckmann H, Goodwin FK: Urinary MHPG in subgroups of depressed patients and normal controls. *Neuropsychobiology* 6:91–100, 1980.

Beckmann H, Heinemann H: [Proceedings: D-Amphetamine in manic syndrome (author's transl)]. *Arzneimittelforschung* 26:1185–1186, 1976.

Beckmann H, Strauss MA, Ludolph E: Dl-phenylalanine in depressed patients: An open study. *J Neural Transm* 41:123–134, 1977.

Bedi AR, Halikas JA: Alcoholism and affective disorder. *Alcoholism: Clinical and Experimental Research* 9:133–134, 1985.

Behar D, Winokur G: Research in alcoholism and depression: A two-way street under construction. In: RW Pickens, LL Heston, eds: *Psychiatric Factors in Drug Abuse.* New York: Grune and Stratton, 1979. pp 125–152.

Beigel A, Murphy DL: Assessing clinical characteristics of the manic state. *Am J Psychiatry* 128:688–694, 1971a.

Beigel A, Murphy DL: Unipolar and bipolar affective illness: Differences in clinical characteristics accompanying depression. *Arch Gen Psychiatry* 24:215–220, 1971b.

Beigel A, Murphy DL, Bunney WE: The Manic-State Rating Scale: Scale construction, reliability, and validity. *Arch Gen Psychiatry* 25:256–262, 1971.

Beitman BD, Dunner DL: L-Tryptophan in the maintenance treatment of bipolar II manic-depressive illness. *Am J Psychiatry* 139:1498–1499, 1982.

Bell CC, Mehta H: The misdiagnosis of black patients with manic depressive illness. *J Natl Med Assoc* 72:141–145, 1980.

Bell KM, Plon L, Bunney WE, Potkin SG: S-adenosylmethionine in the treatment of depression: A controlled clinical trial. *Am J Psychiatry* 145:1110–1114, 1988.

Bell L: On a form of disease resembling some advanced stages of mania and fever, but so contradistinguished from any ordinarily observed or described combination of symptoms as to render it probable that it may be an overlooked and hith-erto unrecorded malady. *Am J Insanity* 6:97–127, 1849.

Bell Q: *Virginia Woolf: A Biography.* London: Hogarth Press, 1972. New York: Harcourt Brace Jovanovich, 1972.

Belloc H: *Cromwell.* London: Cassell and Company, 1934.

Belmaker RH: Receptors, adenylate cyclase, depression, and lithium. *Biol Psychiatry* 16:333–350, 1981.

Belmaker RH, Van Praag HM, eds: *Mania: An Evolving Concept.* New York: Spectrum Publications, 1980a.

Belmaker RH, Van Praag HM: Mania: Disease entity or symptom cluster. In: RH Belmaker, HM van Praag, eds: *Mania: An Evolving Concept.* Jamaica, NY: Spectrum Publications, 1980b. pp 1–5.

Belmaker RH, Wyatt RJ: Possible X-linkage in a family with varied psychoses. *Isr Ann Psychiatry* 14:345–353, 1976.

Belmaker RH, Lehrer R, Ebstein RP, Lettik H, Kugelmass S: A possible cardiovascular effect of lithium. *Am J Psychiatry* 136:577–579, 1979.

Belmaker RH, Zohar J, Levy A: Unidirectionality of lithium stabilization of adrenergic and cholinergic receptors. In: HM Emrich, JB Aldenhoff, HD Lux, eds: *Basic Mechanisms in the Action of Lithium.* Amsterdam: Excerpta Medica, 1982. pp 146–153.

Bendz H: Kidney function in lithium-treated patients. A literature survey. *Acta Psychiatr Scand* 68:303–324, 1983.

Bendz H: Kidney function in a selected lithium population. A prospective, controlled, lithium withdrawal study. *Acta Psychiatr Scand* 72:451–463, 1985.

Benfield P, Heel RC, Lewis SP: Fluoxetine: A review of its pharmacodynamic and pharmacokinetic properties, and therapeutic efficacy in depressive illness. *Drugs* 32:481–508, 1986.

Berens SC, Wolff J: The endocrine effects of lithium. In: FN Johnson, ed: *Lithium Therapy and Research.* Baltimore: Academic Press, 1975. pp 445–464.

Berenson D: The therapist's relationship with couples with an alcoholic member. In: E Kaufman, P Kaufman, eds: *Family Therapy of Drug and Alcohol Abuse.* New York: Plenum Press, 1979. pp 233–242.

Berger PA, Faull KF, Kilkowski J, Anderson PJ, Kraemer H, Davis KL, Barchas JD: CSF monoamine metabolites in depression and schizophrenia. *Am J Psychiatry* 137:174–180, 1980.

Berglund M: Suicide in alcoholism: A prospective study of 88 suicides: I. The multidimensional diagnosis at first admission. *Arch Gen Psychiatry* 41:888–891, 1984.

Berglund M, Nilsson K: Mortality in severe depression: A prospective study including 103 suicides. *Acta Psychiatr Scand* 76:372–380, 1987.

Berlioz H: *Memoirs.* Translated by D Cairns. London: Granada, 1969.

Berlioz HL: *Memoirs of Hector Berlioz from 1803 to*

1865. Paris: Michel Lévy Bros, 1870. Annotated and translated by E Newman. New York: Dover, 1966.

Berman KF: Prefrontal activation during cognition in depression. Abstract of paper presented at the 142nd annual meeting of the American Psychiatric Association, 1989.

Bernad PG, Ballantine HT, Giriunas IE: Neuropathological study of bilateral cingulotomy for mood disturbance. In: ER Hitchcock, HT Ballantine Jr, BA Meyerson, eds: *Modern Concepts in Psychiatric Surgery*. Amsterdam: Elsevier, 1979. pp 283–302.

Bernadt MW, Murray RM: Psychiatric disorder, drinking and alcoholism. *Br J Psychiat* 148:393–400, 1986.

Bernasconi R: The GABA hypothesis of affective illness: Influence of clinically effective antimanic drugs on GABA turnover. In: HM Emrich, JB Aldenhoff, HD Lux, eds: *Basic Mechanisms in the Action of Lithium*. Amsterdam: Excerpta Medica, 1982. pp 183–192.

Berner P, Gabriel E, Katschnig H, Kieffer W, Koehler K, Lenz G, Simhandl C: *Diagnostic Criteria for Schizophrenia and Affective Psychoses* (World Psychiatric Association). Washington, DC: American Psychiatric Association, 1983.

Berner P, Lesch OM, Walter H: Alcohol and depression. *Psychopathology* 19(Suppl 2):177–183, 1986.

Berrettini WH: A case of erythromycin-induced carbamazepine toxicity. *J Clin Psychiatry* 47:147, 1986.

Berrettini WH, Post RM: GABA in affective illness. In: RM Post, JC Ballenger, eds: *Neurobiology of Mood Disorders*. Baltimore: Williams & Wilkins, 1984. pp 673–685.

Berrettini WH, Nurnberger JI Jr, Post RM, Gershon ES: Platelet ^{3}H-imipramine binding in euthymic bipolar patients. *Psychiatry Res* 7:215–219, 1982a.

Berrettini WH, Nurnberger JI Jr, Worthington EK, Simmons-Alling S, Gershon ES: Platelet vasopressin receptors in bipolar affective illness. *Psychiatry Res* 7:83–86, 1982b.

Berrettini WH, Umberkoman-Wiita B, Nurnberger JI Jr, Vogel WH, Gershon ES, Post RM: Platelet GABA-transaminase in affective illness. *Psychiatry Res* 7:255–260, 1982c.

Berrettini WH, Nurnberger JI Jr, Hare TA, Simmons-Alling S, Gershon ES, Post RM: Reduced plasma and CSF gamma-aminobutyric acid in affective illness: Effect of lithium carbonate. *Biol Psychiatry* 18:185–194, 1983.

Berrettini WH, Goldin LR, Nurnberger JI Jr, Gershon ES: Genetic factors in affective illness. *J Psychiatr Res* 18:329–350, 1984.

Berrettini WH, Nurnberger JI Jr, Gold PW, Chretien M, Chrousos GP, Chan JS, Goldin LR, Gershon ES: Neuropeptides in human cerebrospinal fluid. *Life Sci* 37:1265–1270, 1985a.

Berrettini WH, Nurnberger JI Jr, Scheinin M, Seppala T, Linnoila M, Narrow W, Simmons-Alling S, Gershon ES: Cerebrospinal fluid and plasma monoamines and their metabolites in euthymic bipolar patients. *Biol Psychiatry* 20:257–269, 1985b.

Berrettini WH, Rubinow DR, Nurnberger JI Jr, Simmons-Alling S, Post RM, Gershon ES: CSF substance P immunoreactivity in affective disorders. *Biol Psychiatry* 20:965–970, 1985c.

Berrettini WH, Nurnberger JI Jr, Hare TA, Simmons-Alling S, Gershon ES: CSF GABA in euthymic manic-depressive patients and controls. *Biol Psychiatry* 21:844–846, 1986.

Berrettini WH, Bardakjian J, Cappellari CB, Barnett AL, Jr, Albright A, Nurnberger JI Jr, Gershon ES: Skin fibroblast beta-adrenergic receptor function in manic-depressive illness. *Biol Psychiatry* 22:1439–1443, 1987a.

Berrettini WH, Cappellari CB, Nurnberger JI Jr, Gershon ES: Beta-adrenergic receptors on lymphoblasts: A study of manic-depressive illness. *Neuropsychobiology* 17:15–18, 1987b.

Berrettini WH, Nurnberger JI, Simmons-Alling S: Growth hormone releasing factor in human cerebrospinal fluid. *Psychiatry Res* 22:141–147, 1987c.

Berrettini WH, Nurnberger JI Jr, Zerbe RL, Gold PW, Chrousos GP, Tomai T: CSF neuropeptides in euthymic bipolar patients and controls. *Br J Psychiatry* 150:208–212, 1987d.

Berrettini WH, Hoehe M, Lentes KU: Molecular genetic studies of beta-adrenergic receptor genes in manic-depressive illness. Abstract of paper presented at the 43rd Annual Meting of the Society of Biological Psychiatry, 1988.

Berrettini WH, Goldin LR, Gelernter J, Gejman PV, Gershon ES, Detera-Wadleigh S: X-chromosome markers and manic-depressive illness: Rejection of linkage to Xq28 in nine bipolar pedigrees. *Arch Gen Psychiatry* in press.

Berridge MJ, Downes CP, Hanley MR: Lithium amplifies agonist-dependent phosphatidylinositol responses in brain and salivary glands. *Biochem J* 206:587–595, 1982.

Berrios GE, Hauser R: The early development of Kraepelin's ideas on classification: A conceptual history. *Psychol Med* 18:813–821, 1988.

Bertelsen A: A Danish twin study of manic-depressive disorders. In: M Schou, E Strömgren, eds: *Origin, Prevention and Treatment of Affective Disorders*. London: Academic Press, 1979. pp 227–239.

Bertelsen A, Harvald B, Hauge M: A Danish twin study of manic-depressive disorders. *Br J Psychiatry* 130:330–351, 1977.

Besedovsky HO, del Rey AE, Sorkin E: What do the immune system and the brain know about each other? *Immunol Today* 4:342–346, 1983a.

Besedovsky H, del Rey A, Sorkin E, Da Prada M, Burri R, Honegger C: The immune response evokes changes in brain noradrenergic neurons. *Science* 221:564–566, 1983b.

Bevis W: Psychological traits of the southern Negro, with observations as to some of his psychoses. *Am J Psychiatry* 1:69–78, 1921.

Bick PA: Seasonal major affective disorder. *Am J Psychiatry* 143:90–91, 1986.

Bidzinska EJ: Stress factors in affective diseases. *Br J Psychiatry* 144:161–166, 1984.

Biederman J, Lerner Y, Belmaker RH: Combination of lithium carbonate and haloperidol in schizoaffective disorder: A controlled study. *Arch Gen Psychiatry* 36:327–333, 1979.

Bielski RJ, Friedel RO: Prediction of tricyclic antidepressant response: A critical review. *Arch Gen Psychiatry* 33:1479–1489, 1976.

Binder RL: Three case reports of behavioral disinhibition with clonazepam. *Gen Hosp Psychiatry* 9:151–153, 1987.

Binite A: A factor analytic study of depression across cultures (African and European). *Br J Psychiatry* 117:559–563, 1975.

Birch NJ, Horsman A, Hullin RP: Lithium, bone and body weight studies in long-term lithium-treated patients and in the rat. *Neuropsychobiology* 8:86–92, 1982.

Birkmayer W, Riederer P: Biochemical post-mortem findings in depressed patients. *J Neural Transm* 37:95–109, 1975.

Birtchnell J: Social class, parental social class, and social mobility in psychiatric patients and general population controls. *Psychol Med* 1:209–221, 1971.

Bissette G, Widerlöv E, Walléus H, Karlsson I, Eklund K, Forsman A, Nemeroff CB: Alterations in cerebrospinal fluid concentrations of somatostatinlike immunoreactivity in neuropsychiatric disorders. *Arch Gen Psychiatry* 43:1148–1151, 1986.

Bitensky MW, Miki N, Keirns JJ, Keirns M, Baraban JM, Freeman J, Wheeler MA, Lacy J, Marcus FR: Activation of photoreceptor disk membrane phosphodiesterase by light and ATP. *Adv Cyclic Nucleotide Res* 5:213–240, 1975.

Björum N, Plenge P, Rafaelsen OJ: Electrolytes in CSF in endogenous depression. *Acta Psychiatr Scand* 48:533–539, 1972.

Black DW, Nasrallah A: Hallucinations and delusions in 1,715 patients with unipolar and bipolar affective disorders. *Psychopathology* 22:28–34, 1989.

Black DW, Warrack G, Winokur G: The Iowa record-linkage study: I. Suicides and accidental death among psychiatric patients. *Arch Gen Psychiatry* 42:71–75, 1985.

Black DW, Winokur G, Nasrallah A: Is death from natural causes still excessive in psychiatric patients? A follow-up of 1593 patients with major affective disorder. *J Nerv Ment Dis* 175:674–680, 1987a.

Black DW, Winokur G, Nasrallah MA: Suicide in subtypes of major affective disorder: A comparison with general population suicide mortality. *Arch Gen Psychiatry* 44:878–880, 1987b.

Black DW, Winokur G, Nasrallah A: The treatment of depression: Electroconvulsive therapy v. antidepressants: A naturalistic evaluation of 1,495 patients. *Compr Psychiatry* 28:169–182, 1987c.

Black DW, Winokur G, Nasrallah A: Treatment of mania: A naturalistic study of electroconvulsive therapy versus lithium in 438 patients. *J Clin Psychiatry* 48:132–139, 1987d.

Black DW, Winokur G, Hulbert J, Nasrallah A: Predictors of immediate response in the treatment of mania: The importance of comorbidity. *Biol Psychiatry* 24:191–198, 1988a.

Black DW, Winokur G, Nasrallah A: Effect of psychosis on suicide risk in 1,593 patients with unipolar and bipolar affective disorders. *Am J Psychiatry* 145:849–852, 1988b.

Black DW, Winokur G, Nasrallah A, Emmanuel M, Woolson R: Does treatment influence mortality in depressives? Abstract of paper presented at the 141st annual meeting of the American Psychiatric Association, 1988c.

Black DW, Hulbert J, Nasrallah A: The effect of somatic treatment and comorbidity on immediate outcome in manic patients. *Compr Psychiatry* 30:74–79, 1989.

Black PM, Ballantine HT, Carr DB, Beal MF, Martin JB: Beta-endorphin and somatostatin concentrations in the ventricular cerebrospinal fluid of patients with affective disorder. *Biol Psychiatry* 21:1075–1077, 1986.

Black S, Walter WG: Effects on anterior brain responses of variation in the probability of association between stimuli. *J Psychosom Res* 9:33–43, 1965.

Blackard WG, Heidingsfelder SA: Adrenergic receptor control mechanism for growth hormone secretion. *J Clin Invest* 47:1407–1414, 1968.

Blackburn IM: The pattern of hostility in affective illness. *Br J Psychiatry* 125:141–145, 1974.

Blackburn IM: Mental and psychomotor speed in depression and mania. *Br J Psychiatry* 132:329–335, 1975.

Blackburn IM, Loudon JB, Ashworth CM: A new scale for measuring mania. *Psychol Med* 7:453–458, 1977.

Blackburn IM, Bishop S, Glen AIM, Whalley LJ, Christie JE: The efficacy of cognitive therapy in depression: A treatment using cognitive therapy and pharmacotherapy, each alone and in combination. *Br J Psychiatry* 139:181–189, 1981.

Blackenmore CB, Ettlinger G, Falconer MA: Cognitive abilities in relation to frequency of seizures and neuropathology of the temporal lobes in man. *J Neurol Neurosurg Psychiatry* 29:268–272, 1966.

Blackwell B: Treatment adherence. *Br J Psychiatry* 129:513–531, 1976.

Blackwell B: Why don't patients take their medicines? Presented at the annual meeting of the American Association for the Advancement of Science. Toronto, Canada, January, 1980.

Blackwell B: Treatment compliance. In: JH Greist, JW Jefferson, RL Spitzer, eds: *Treatment of Mental Disorders*. New York: Oxford University Press, 1982. pp 501–516.

Blackwell B, Shepherd M: Prophylactic lithium: Another therapeutic myth? *Lancet* 1:968–971, 1968.

Blair JA, Barford PA, Morar C, Pheasant AE, Hamon CG, Whitburn SB, Leeming RJ, Reynolds GP, Coppen A: Tetrahydrobiopterin metabolism in depression. Letter. *Lancet* 2:163, 1984.

Blalock JR: Psychology of the manic phase of the manic-depressive psychoses. *Psychiatr Q* 10:263–344, 1936.

Bland RC, Newman SC, Orn H: Recurrent and non-recurrent depression: A family study. *Arch Gen Psychiatry* 43:1085–1089, 1986.

Blaney PH: Affect and memory: A review. *Psychol Bull* 99:229–246, 1986.

Blazer D, George LK, Landerman R, Pennybacker M, Melville ML, Woodbury M, Manton K, Jordan K, Locke B: Psychiatric disorders: A rural/urban comparison. *Arch Gen Psychiatry* 42:651–656, 1985.

Blehar MC, Rosenthal NE: Seasonal affective disorders and phototherapy. *Arch Gen Psychiatry* 46:469–474, 1989.

Bleuler E: *Dementia Praecox or the Group of Schizophrenias*. Translated by J Zinkin. New York: International Universities Press, 1950. [Originally published in German as a volume of *Aschaffenburg's Handbuch, Dementia Praecox oder die Gruppe der Schizophrenien*, 1911.]

Bleuler E: *Textbook of Psychiatry*. English ed by AA Brill. New York: The Macmillan Co, 1924. (4th German ed)

Bloom FE: Future directions and goals in basic pharmacology and neurobiology. In: HY Meltzer, ed: *Psychopharmacology: The Third Generation of Progress*. New York: Raven Press, 1987. pp 1685–1689.

Bluemel CS: *War, Politics, and Insanity*. Denver: World Press, 1948.

Blumenthal RL, Egeland JA, Sharpe L, Nee J, Endicott J: Age of onset in bipolar and unipolar illness with and without delusions or hallucinations. *Compr Psychiatry* 28:547–554, 1987.

Board F, Wadeson R, Persky H: Depressive affect and endocrine functions. *Arch Neurol Psychiatry* 78:612–620, 1957.

Bodmer WF: Human genetics: The molecular challenge. *Cold Spring Harbor Symp Quant Biol* 51:1–13, 1986.

Bohus B, Kovács GL, De Wied D: Oxytocin, vasopressin and memory: Opposite effects on consolidation and retrieval processes. *Brain Res* 157:414–417, 1978.

Bolander AM: Nordic suicide statistics. In: J Waldenström, T Larsson, N Ljungstedt N, eds: *Suicide and Attempted Suicide*. Stockholm: Nordiska Bokhandelns Förlag, 1972.

Bond ED, Braceland FJ: Prognosis in mental disease. *Am J Psychiatry* 94:263–274, 1937.

Bond PA, Howlett DR: Measurement of the two conjugates of 3-methoxy-4-hydroxyphenyglycol in urine. *Biochem Med* 10:219–228, 1974.

Bond TC: Recognition of acute delirious mania. *Arch Gen Psychiatry* 37:553–554, 1954.

Bone S, Roose SP, Dunner DL, Fieve RR: Incidence of side effects in patients on long-term lithium therapy. *Am J Psychiatry* 137:103–104, 1980.

Bonetti U, Johansson F, Von Knorring L, Perris C, Strandman E: Prophylactic lithium and personality variables: An international collaborative study. *Int Pharmacopsychiatry* 12:14–19, 1977.

Bonham-Carter S, Sandler M, Sepping P, Bridges PK: Decreased conjugated tyramine outputs in depression: Gastrointestinal factors. *Br J Clin Pharmacol* 5:269–272, 1978.

Bonney GE: Regressive logistic models for familial disease and other binary traits. *Biometrics* 42:611–625, 1986.

Borbély AA: A two-process model of sleep regulation. *Hum Neurobiol* 1:195–204, 1982.

Borbély AA, Wirz-Justice A: Sleep, sleep deprivation and depression: A hypothesis derived from a model of sleep regulation. *Hum Neurobiol* 1:205–210, 1982.

Borbély AA, Tobler I, Loepfe M, Kupfer DJ, Ulrich RF, Grochocinski V, Doman J, Matthews G: All-night spectral analysis of the sleep EEG in untreated depressives and normal controls. *Psychiatry Res* 12:27–33, 1984.

Borge GF, Buchsbaum M, Goodwin F, Murphy D, Silverman J: Neuropsychological correlates of affective disorders. *Arch Gen Psychiatry* 24:501–504, 1971.

Born GV, Grignani G, Martin K: Long-term effect of lithium on the uptake of 5-hydroxytryptamine by human platelets. *Br J Clin Pharmacol* 9:321–325, 1980.

Boswell PC, Murray EJ: Depression, schizophrenia, and social attraction. *J Consult Clin Psychol* 49:641–647, 1981.

Bothwell S, Weissman MM: Social impairments four years after an acute depressive episode. *Am J Orthopsychiatry* 47:231–237, 1977.

Boton R, Gaviria M, Batlle C: Prevalence, pathogenesis, and treatment of renal dysfunction associated with chronic lithium therapy. *Am J Kidney Dis* 10:329–345, 1987.

Botstein D, White RL, Skolnick M, Davis RW: Construction of a genetic linkage map in man using restriction fragment length polymorphism. *Am J Hum Genet* 32:314–331, 1980.

Boulton AA, Baker GB, Dewhurst WG, Sandler M, eds: *Neurobiology of the Trace Amines*. Clifton, NJ: Humana Press, 1984.

Bouman TK, Niemantsverdriet JG, Ormel J, Slooff CJ: The effectiveness of lithium prophylaxis in bipolar and unipolar depressions and schizo-affective disorders. *J Affective Disord* 11:275–280, 1986.

Bourgeois M, Campagne A: Maniaco-depressive et syndrome de Garcin. *Ann Med Psychol* 125(Suppl 2):451–460, 1967.

Bourne HR, Bunney WE, Colburn RW, Davis JM, Shaw DM, Coppen AJ: Noradrenaline, 5-hydroxytryptamine and 5-hydroxy-indoleacetic acid in hindbrains of suicidal patients. *Lancet* 2:805–808, 1968.

Bovier P, Widmer J, Gaillard J-M, Tissot R: Evolution of red blood cell membrane transport and plasma level of L-tyrosine and L-tryptophan in depressed treated patients according to clinical improvement. *Neuropsychobiol* 19:125–134, 1988.

Bowden CL, Sarabia F: Diagnosing manic-depressive illness in adolescents. *Compr Psychiatry* 21:263–269, 1980.

Bowden CL, Koslow S, Maas JW, Davis J, Garver DL, Hanin I: Changes in urinary catecholamines and their metabolites in depressed patients treated with amitriptyline or imipramine. *J Psychiatr Res* 21:111–128, 1987.

Bowden CL, Huang LG, Javors MA, Johnson JM, Seleshi E, McIntyre K, Contreras S, Maas JW: Calcium function in affective disorders and healthy controls. *Biol Psychiatry* 23:367–376, 1988.

Bowdle TA, Levi RH, Cutler RE: Effects of carbamazepine on valproic acid kinetics in normal subjects. *Clin Pharmacol Ther* 26:629–634, 1979.

Bowen RC, Cipywnyk D, D'Arcy C, Keegan DL: Types of depression in alcoholic patients. *Can Med Assoc J* 130:869–874, 1984.

Bower GH: Affect and cognition. *Phil Trans R Soc Lond* 302:387–402, 1983.

Bower GH, Cohen PR: Emotional influences in memory and thinking: Data and theory. In: Clark MS, ST Fiske, eds: *Affect and Cognition: The Seventeenth Annual Carnegie Symposium on Cognition.* Lawrence Erlbaum Associates: Hillsdale, New Jersey, 1982. pp 291–331.

Bower GH, Gilligan SG, Monteiro KP: Selectivity of learning caused by affective states. *J Exp Psychol [Gen]* 110:451–473, 1981.

Bowers MB: Psychoses precipitated by psychotomimetic drugs. *Arch Gen Psychiatry* 34:832–835, 1977.

Bowers MB, Freedman DX: Psychoses associated with drug use. In: S Arieti, ed: *American Handbook of Psychiatry.* Vol 4. New York: Basic Books, 1975. pp 356–370.

Bowers MB, Heninger GR: Lithium: Clinical effects and cerebrospinal fluid acid monoamine metabolites. *Communications in Psychopharmacology.* 1:135–145, 1977.

Bowers MB, Heninger GR, Gerbode FA: Cerebrospinal fluid 5-HIAA and HVA in psychiatric patients. *Int J Neuropharmacol* 8:255–162, 1969.

Bowman KM, Raymond AF: A statistical study of delusions in the manic-depressive psychoses. *Am J Psychiatry* 88:111–121, 1931–1932a.

Bowman KM, Raymond AF: A statistical study of hallucinations in the manic-depressive psychoses. *Am J Psychiatry* 88:299–309, 1931–1932b.

Boyce P, Parker G: Seasonal affective disorder in the southern hemisphere. *Am J Psychiatry* 145:96–99, 1988.

Boyd JH, Weissman MM: Epidemiology of affective disorders: A reexamination and future directions. *Arch Gen Psychiatry* 38:1039–1046, 1981.

Boyd JH, Weissman MM: Epidemiology of major affective disorders. In: R Michels, JO Cavenar, HKH Brodie, AM Cooper, SB Guze, LL Judd, GL Klerman, AJ Solnit, eds: *Psychiatry, Vol. 3.* Philadelphia: JB Lippincott, 1985. Ch 13. pp 1–16.

Boyd JH, Weissman MM, Thompson WD, Myers JK: Different definitions of alcoholism I. Impact of seven definitions on prevalence rates in a community survey. *Am J Psychiatry* 140:1309–1313, 1983.

Boyd JH, Burke JD, Gruenberg E, Holzer CE, Rae DS, George LK, Karno M, Stoltzman R, McEvoy L, Nestadt G: Exclusion criteria of DSM-III: A study of co-occurrence of hierarchy-free syndromes. *Arch Gen Psychiatry* 41:983–989, 1984.

Boyd JH, Pulver AE, Stewart W: Season of birth: Schizophrenia and bipolar disorder. *Schizophr Bull* 12:173–186, 1986.

Boyd JR, Covington TR, Stanaszek WF, Coussons RT: Drug defaulting part i: Determinants of compliance. *Am J Hosp Pharm* 31:362–367, 1974a.

Boyd JR, Covington TR, Stanaszek WF, Coussons RT: Drug defaulting part ii: Analysis of noncompliance patterns. *Am J Hosp Pharm* 31:485–491, 1974b.

Boyle GJ: Self-report measures of depression: Some psychometric considerations. *Br J Clin Psychol* 24:45–59, 1985.

Braden W, Ho CK: Racing thoughts in psychiatric inpatients. *Arch Gen Psychiatry* 38:71–75, 1981.

Braden W, Qualls CB: Racing thoughts in depressed patients. *J Clin Psychiatry* 40:336–339, 1979.

Bradford E: *Nelson: The Essential Hero.* London: Granada, 1979.

Bragman LJ: The case of John Ruskin: A study in cyclothymia. *Am J Psychiatry* 91:1137–1159, 1935.

Brainard GC, Morgan WW: Light-induced stimulation of retinal dopamine: A dose-response relationship. *Brain Res* 424:199–203, 1987.

Brand N, Jolles J: Information processing in depression and anxiety. *Psychol Med* 17:145–153, 1987.

Bratfos O, Haug JO: Electroconvulsive therapy and antidepressant drugs in manic-depressive disease Treatment results at discharge and 3 months later. *Acta Psychiatr Scand* 41:588–596, 1965.

Bratfos O, Haug JO: The course of manic-depressive psychosis: A follow-up investigation of 215 patients. *Acta Psychiatr Scand* 44:89–112, 1968.

Bratter TE, Forrest GG, eds: *Alcoholism and Substance Abuse.* New York: Free Press, 1985.

Brazier MAB: The human amygdala: Electrophysiological studies. In: BE Eleftheriou, ed: *The Neurobiology of the Amygdala.* New York: Plenum Press, 1972. pp 397–420.

Breakey WR, Goodell H: Thought disorder in mania and schizophrenia evaluated by Bannister's Grid Test for schizophrenic thought disorder. *Br J Psychiatry* 120:391–395, 1972.

Breakey WR, Goodell H, Lorenz PC, McHugh PR: Hallucinogenic drugs as precipitants of schizophrenia. 4:255–261, 1974.

Breier A: AE Bennett award paper: Experimental approaches to human stress research: Assessment of neurobiological mechanisms of stress in volunteers and psychiatric patients. *Biol Psychiatry* 26:438–462, 1989.

Breier A, Albus M, Pickar D, Zahn TP, Wolkowitz OM, Paul SM: Controllable and uncontrollable stress in humans: Alterations in mood and neuroendocrine and psychophysiological function. *Am J Psychiatry* 144:1419–1425, 1987.

Brennan M, Sandyk R, Borsook D: Use of sodium valproate in the management of affective disorders: Basic and clinical aspects. In: HM Emrich, T Okuma, AA Muller, eds: *Anticonvulsants in Affective Disorders.* Amsterdam: Elsevier, 1984. pp 56–65.

Brent DA, Perper JA, Goldstein CE, Kolko DJ, Allan MJ, Allman CJ, Zelenak JP: Risk factors for adolescent suicide: A comparison of adolescent suicide victims with suicidal inpatients. *Arch Gen Psychiatry* 45:581–588, 1988.

Breslau N, Meltzer HY: Validity of subtyping psychotic depression: Examination of phenomenology and demographic characteristics. *Am J Psychiatry* 145:35–40, 1988.

Breslow R, Kocsis J, Belkin B: Memory deficits in depression: Evidence utilizing the Wechsler Memory Scale. *Percept Mot Skills* 51:541–542, 1980.

Breslow RE, DeMuth GW, Weiss C: Lithium incorporation in the fibroblasts of manic-depressives. *Biol Psychiatry* 20:58–65, 1985.

Brewerton TD: Lithium counteracts carbamazepine-induced leukopenia while increasing its therapeutic effect. *Biol Psychiatry* 21:667–685, 1986.

Brewerton TD, Reus VI: Lithium carbonate and L-tryptophan in the treatment of bipolar and schizoaffective disorders. *Am J Psychiatry* 140:757–760, 1983.

Breyer U, Quadbeck G: [The cerebrospinal fluid content of magnesium and other cations in central nervous system diseases]. *Dtsch Z Nervenheilkd* 187:595–607, 1965.

Bridge TP, Mirsky AF, Goodwin FK, eds: *Psychological, Neuropsychiatric and Substance Abuse Aspects of AIDS: Advances in Biochemical Psychopharmacology.* Vol 44. New York: Raven press, 1988.

Brierly CE, Szabadi E, Rix KJB, Bradshaw CM: The Manchester Nurse Rating Scales for daily simultaneous assessment of depressive and manic ward behaviours. *J Affective Disord* 15:45–54, 1988.

Briley MS, Raisman R, Langer SZ: Human platelets possess high-affinity binding sites for ^{3}H-imipramine. *Eur J Pharmacol* 58:347–348, 1979.

Briley MS, Langer SZ, Raisman R, Sechter D, Zarifian E: Tritiated imipramine binding sites are decreased in platelets of untreated depressed patients. *Science* 209:303–305, 1980.

Briley MS, Raisman R, Arbilla S, Casasamonte M, Langer SZ: Concomitant decrease in ^{3}H-imipramine binding in cat brain and platelets after chronic treatment with imipramine. *Eur J Pharmacol* 81:309–314, 1982.

Briscoe CW, Smith JB: Depression and marital turmoil. *Arch Gen Psychiatry* 29:811–817, 1973.

Brochet DM, Martin P, Soubrié P, Simon P: Triiodothyronine potentiation of antidepressant-induced reversal of learned helplessness in rats. *Psychiatry Res* 21:267–275, 1987.

Brockington IF, Leff JP: Schizo-affective psychoses: Definitions and incidence. *Psychol Med* 9:91–99, 1979.

Brockington IF, Wainwright S, Kendell RE: Manic patients with schizophrenic or paranoid symptoms. *Psychol Med* 10:73–83, 1980a.

Brockington IF, Kendell RE, Wainwright S: Depressed patients with schizophrenic or paranoid symptoms. *Psychol Med* 10:665–675, 1980b.

Brockington IF, Altman E, Hillier V, Meltzer HY, Nand S: The clinical picture of bipolar affective disorder in its depressed phase: A report from London and Chicago. *Br J Psychiatry* 141:558–562, 1982a.

Brockington IF, Perris C, Kendell RE, Hillier VE, Wainwright S: The course and outcome of cycloid psychosis. *Psychol Med* 12:97–105, 1982b.

Brockington IF, Winokur G, Dean C: Puerperal psychosis. In: IF Brockington, R Kumar, eds: *Motherhood and Mental Illness.* London: Academic Press, 1982c. pp 37–69.

Brockington IF, Hillier VF, Francis AF, Helzer JE, Wainwright S: Definitions of mania: Concordance and prediction of outcome. *Am J Psychiatry* 140:435–439, 1983.

Brodie HK: Affective changes associated with L-dopa therapy. In C Eisdorfer, WE Fann, eds: *Psychopharmacology and Aging.* New York: Plenum Press, 1973. pp 97–104.

Brodie HKH, Leff MJ: Bipolar depression—A comparative study of patient characteristics. *Am J Psychiatry* 127:1086–1090, 1971.

Brodie HK, Murphy DL, Goodwin FK, Bunney WE Jr: Catecholamines and mania: The effect of alpha-methyl-para-tyrosine on manic behavior and catecholamine metabolism. *Clin Pharmacol Ther* 12:218–224, 1971.

Brodie H, Sach R, Siever L: Clinical studies of L-5-hydroxytryptophan. In: J Barchas, E Usdin: *Serotonin and Behavior.* New York: Academic Press, 1973. pp 549–559.

Brody EB: *The Lost Ones.* New York: International Universities Press, 1973.

Bromet EJ, Dunn LO, Connell MM, Dew MA, Schulberg HC: Long-term reliability of diagnosing lifetime major depression in a community sample. *Arch Gen Psychiatry* 43:435–440, 1986.

Brooke EM: National statistics in the epidemiology of mental illness. *J Ment Sci* 105:893–908, 1959.

Brower D, Oppenheim S: The effects of electroshock therapy on mental functions as revealed by psychological tests. *J Gen Psychol* 45:171–188, 1951.

Brown D, Silverstone T, Cookson J: Carbamazepine vs. haloperidol in acute mania. Abstract of paper presented at the 41nd Annual Meeting of the Society of Biological Psychiatry. May, 1986.

Brown GL, Goodwin FK: Cerebrospinal fluid correlates of suicide attempts and aggression. *Ann NY Acad Sci* 487:175–188, 1986.

Brown GL, Goodwin FK, Bunney WE: Human aggression and suicide: Their relationship to neuro-psychiatric diagnoses and serotonin metabolism. *Adv Biochem Psychopharmacol* 34:287–307, 1982.

Brown JH: Suicide in Britain: More attempts, fewer deaths, lessons for public policy. *Arch Gen Psychiatry* 36:1119–1124, 1979.

Brown O: Relation of WAIS verbal and performance IQs for four psychiatric conditions. *Psychol Rep* 20:1015–1020, 1967.

Brown R: U.S. experience with valproate in manic depressive illness: A multicenter trial. *J Clin Psychiatry* 50(Suppl):13–16, 1989.

Brown R, Kocsis JH, Caroff S, Amsterdam J, Winokur A, Stokes PE, Frazer A: Differences in nocturnal melatonin secretion between melancholic depressed patients and control subjects. *Am J Psychiatry* 142:811–816, 1985.

Brown RM, Crane AM, Goldman PS: Regional distribution of monoamines in the cerebral cortex and subcortical structures of the rhesus monkey: Concentrations and in vivo synthesis rates. *Brain Res* 168:133–150, 1979.

Brown WA, Mueller B: Alleviation of manic symptoms with catecholamine agonists. *Am J Psychiatry* 136:230–231, 1979.

Brown WA, Johnston R, Mayfield D: The 24-hour dexamethasone suppression test in a clinical setting: Relationship to diagnosis, symptoms, and response to treatment. *Am J Psychiatry* 136:543–547, 1979.

Bruce LC: Notes of a case of dual brain action. *Brain* 18:54–65, 1895.

Bruder G, Spring B, Yozawitz A, Sutton S: Auditory sensitivity in psychiatric patients and non-patients: Monotic click detection. *Psychol Med* 10:133–138, 1980.

Bruder G, Sutton S, Berger-Gross P, Quitkin F, Davies S: Lateralized auditory processing in depression: Dichotic click detection. *Psychiatry Res* 4:253–266, 1981.

Bruder GE, Quitkin FM, Stewart JW, Martin C, Voglmaier MM, Harrison WM: Cerebral laterality and depression: Differences in perceptual asymmetry among diagnostic subtypes. *J Abnorm Psychol* 98:177–186, 1989.

Brumback RA: Wechsler performance IQ deficit in depressed children. *Percept Mot Skills* 61:331–335, 1985.

Brunello N, Barbaccia ML, Chuang DM, Costa E: Down-regulation of β-adrenergic receptors following repeated injections of desmethylimipramine: Permissive role of serotonergic axons. *Neuropharmacology* 21:1145–1149, 1982.

Brunswick DJ, Frazer A, Koslow SH, Casper R, Stokes PE, Robins E, Davis JM: Insulin-induced hypoglycaemic response and release of growth hormone in depressed patients and healthy controls. *Psychol Med* 18:79–91, 1988.

Brusov OS, Beliaev BS, Katasonov AB, Zlobina GP, Factor MI, Lideman RR: Does platelet serotonin receptor supersensitivity accompany endogenous depression? *Biol Psychiatry* 26:375–381, 1989.

Bryant SG, Guernsey BG, Ingrim NB: Review of bupropion. *Clin Pharm* 2:525–537, 1983.

Bucher KD, Elston RC: The transmission of manic depressive illness: I: Theory, description of the model and summary of results. *J Psychiat Res* 16:53–63, 1981.

Buchsbaum MS: Average evoked response augmenting/reducing in schizophrenia and affective disorders. In: DX Freedman, ed: *Biology of the Major Psychoses: A Comparative Analysis.* Research Publications: Association for Research in Nervous and Mental Disease. Vol 54. New York: Raven Press, 1975. pp 129–142.

Buchsbaum M, Goodwin F, Murphy D, Borge G: AER in affective disorders. *Am J Psychiatry* 128:19–25, 1971.

Buchsbaum M, Landau S, Murphy D, Goodwin F: Average evoked response in bipolar and unipolar affective disorders: Relationship to sex, age of onset, and monoamine oxidase. *Biol Psychiatry* 7:199–212, 1973.

Buchsbaum MS, Haier RJ, Murphy DL: Suicide attempts, platelet monoamine oxidase and the average evoked response. *Acta Psychiatr Scand* 56:69–79, 1977.

Buchsbaum MS, Muscettola G, Goodwin FK: Urinary MHPG, stress response, personality factors and somatosensory evoked potentials in normal subjects and patients with major affective disorders. *Neuropsychobiology* 7:212–224, 1981.

Buchsbaum MS, DeLisi LE, Holcomb HH, Cappelletti J, King AC, Johnson J, Hazlett E, Dowling-Zimmerman S, Post RM, Morihisa J, Carpenter W, Cohen R, Pickar D, Weinberger DR, Margolin R, Kessler RM: Anteroposterior gradients in cerebral glucose use in schizophrenia and affective disorders. *Arch Gen Psychiatry* 41:1159–1166, 1984.

Buchsbaum MS, Wu J, DeLisi LE, Holcomb H, Kessler R, Johnson J, King AC, Hazlett E, Langston K, Post RM: Frontal cortex and basal ganglia metabolic rates assessed by positron emission tomography with [18F]2-deoxyglucose in affective illness. *J Affective Disord* 10:137–152, 1986.

Bucht G, Wahlin A, Wentzel T, Winblad B: Renal function and morphology in long-term lithium and combined lithium-neuroleptic treatment. *Acta Med Scand* 208:381–385, 1980.

Buchwald AM, Neale JM: Editorial. *J Abnorm Psychol* 93:131–132, 1984.

Buckholtz NS, Davies AO, Rudorfer MV, Golden RN, Potter WZ: Lymphocyte beta adrenergic receptor function versus catecholamines in depression. *Biol Psychiatry* 24:451–457, 1988.

Buhrich N, Cooper DA, Freed E: HIV infection associated with symptoms indistinguishable from functional psychosis. *Br J Psychiatry* 152:649–653, 1988.

Bukstein OG, Brent DA, Kaminer Y: Comorbidity of substance abuse and other psychiatric disorders in adolescents. *Am J Psychiatry* 146:1131–1141, 1989.

Bunney WE Jr: Psychopharmacology of the switch process in affective illness. In: M Lipton, A DiMascio, K Killam, eds: *Psychopharmacology—A Generation of Progress*. New York: Raven Press, 1978. pp 1249–1259.

Bunney WE Jr, Davis J: Norepinephrine in depressive reactions. *Arch Gen Psychiatry* 13:483–494, 1965.

Bunney WE Jr, Garland-Bunney BL: Mechanisms of action of lithium in affective illness: Basic and clinical implications. In: HY Meltzer, ed: *Psychopharmacology: The Third Generation of Progress*. New York: Raven Press, 1987. pp 553–565.

Bunney WE, Hamburg DA: Methods for reliable longitudinal observation of behavior. *Arch Gen Psychiatry* 9:280–294, 1963.

Bunney WE Jr, Hartman EL, Mason JW: Study of a patient with 48-hour manic-depressive cycles. *Arch Gen Psychiatry* 12:619–625, 1965.

Bunney WE Jr, Goodwin FK, Davis JM, Fawcett JA: A behavioral-biochemical study of lithium treatment. *Am J Psychiatry* 125:499–512, 1968.

Bunney WE Jr, Brodie HKH, Murphy DL, Goodwin FK: Psychopharmacological differentiation between two subgroups of depressed patients. Abstract of a paper presented at the 125th Annual Meeting of the American Psychiatric Association. May, 1970.

Bunney WE Jr, Murphy D, Goodwin FK, Borge GF: The "switch process" in manic-depressive illness: I. A systematic study of sequential behavior change. *Arch of Gen Psychiatry* 27:295–302, 1972a.

Bunney WE Jr, Goodwin FK, Murphy DL, House KM, Gordon EK: The "switch process" in manic-depressive illness: II: Relationship to catecholamines, REM sleep, and drugs. *Arch Gen Psychiatry* 27:304–309, 1972b.

Bunney WE Jr, Goodwin FK, Murphy DL: The "switch process" in manic-depressive illness: III: Theoretical implications. *Arch Gen Psychiatry* 27:312–317, 1972c.

Bunney WE Jr, Post RM, Andersen AE, Kopanda RT: A neuronal receptor sensitivity mechanism in affective illness (a review of evidence). *Commun Psychopharmacol* 1:393–405, 1977.

Burdick BM, Holmes CB: The use of the lithium response scale with an outpatient psychiatric sample. *Psychol Rep* 47:69–70, 1980.

Burke JD Jr: Diagnostic categorization by the Diagnostic Interview Schedule (DIS): A comparison with other methods of assessment. In: JE Barrett, RM Rose, eds: *Mental Disorders in the Community*. New York: The Guilford Press, 1986. pp 255–285.

Burnam MA, Karno M, Hough RL, Escobar JI, Forsythe AB: The Spanish Diagnostic Interview Schedule: Reliability and comparison with clinical diagnoses. *Arch Gen Psychiatry* 40: 1189–1196, 1983.

Burnam MA, Hough RL, Escobar JI, Karno M, Timbers DM, Telles CA, Locke BZ: Six-month prevalence of specific psychiatric disorders among Mexican Americans and non-Hispanic whites in Los Angeles. *Arch Gen Psychiatry* 44:687–694, 1987.

Burton R: *The Anatomy of Melancholy*. Edited by F Dell, P Jordan-Smith. New York: Tudor Publishing Company, 1927.

Butterfield DA, Markesbery WR: Specificity of biophysical and biochemical alterations in erythrocyte membranes in neurological disorders—Huntington's disease, Friedreich's ataxia, Alzheimer's disease, amyotrophic lateral sclerosis, and myotonic and duchenne muscular dystrophy. *J Neurol Sci* 47:261–271, 1980.

Buydens-Branchey L, Branchey MH, Noumair D: Age of alcoholism onset: I: Relationship to psychopathology. *Arch Gen Psychiatry* 46:225–230, 1989.

Byerley WF, Judd LL, Reimherr FW, Grosser BI: 5-hydroxytryptophan: A review of its antidepressant efficacy and adverse effects. *J Clin Psychopharmacol* 7:127–137, 1987.

Cade JFJ: Lithium salts in the treatment of psychotic excitement. *Med J Aust* 36:349–352, 1949.

Cade JFJ: Lithium—Past, present and future. FN Johnson, S Johnson, eds: *Lithium in Medical Practice*. Baltimore: University Park Press, 1978. pp 5–16.

Cadoret R, Winokur G: Depression in alcoholism. *Ann NY Acad Sci* 233:34–38, 1974.

Caillard V: Treatment of mania using a calcium antagonist—preliminary trial. *Neuropsychobiology* 14:23–26, 1985.

Cairns J, Waldron J, MacLean AW, Knowles JB: Sleep and depression: A case study of EEG sleep prior to relapse. *Can J Psychiatry* 25:259–263, 1980.

Calabrese JR, Delucchi GA: Phenomenology of rapid cycling manic depression and its treatment with valproate. *J Clin Psychiatry* 50(Suppl):30–34, 1989.

Calabrese JR, Gulledge AD, Hahn K, Skwerer R, Kotz M, Schumacher OP, Gupta MK, Krupp N, Gold PW: Autoimmune thyroiditis in manic-depressive patients treated with lithium. *Am J Psychiatry* 142:1318–1321, 1985.

Calabrese JR, Skwerer RG, Barna B, Gulledge AD, Valenzuela R, Butkus A, Subichin S, Krupp NE: Depression, immunocompetence, and prostaglandins of the E series. *Psychiatry Res* 17:41–47, 1986.

Calev A, Erwin PG: Recall and recognition in depressives: Use of matched tasks. *Br J Clin Psychol* 24:127–128, 1985.

Calev A, Nigal D, Chazan S: Retrieval from semantic memory using meaningful and meaningless constructs by depressed, stable bipolar and manic patients. *Br J Clin Psychol* 28:67–73, 1989.

Calogero AE, Gallucci WT, Chrousos GP, Gold PW: Interaction between GABAergic neurotransmission and rat hypothalamic corticotropin-releasing hormone in vitro *Brain Res* 463:28–36, 1988a.

Calogero AE, Gallucci WT, Chrousos GP, Gold PW: Catecholamine effects upon rat hypothalamic corticotropin-releasing hormone secretion in vitro. *J Clin Invest* 82:839–846, 1988b.

Calogero AE, Gallucci WT, Bernardini R, Saoutis C, Gold PW, Chrousos GP: Effect of cholinergic agonists and antagonists on rat hypothalamic corticotropin-releasing hormone secretion in vitro. *Neuroendocrinology* 47:303–308, 1988c.

Calogero AE, Bernardini R, Margioris AN, Bagdy G, Gallucci WT, Munson PJ, Tamarkin L, Tomai TP, Brady L, Gold PW, Chrousos GP: Effects of serotonergic agonists and antagonists on corticotropin-releasing hormone secretion by explanted rat hypothalami. *Peptides* 10:189–200, 1989.

Campbell CA, Peet M, Ward NI: Vanadium and other trace elements in patients taking lithium. *Biol Psychiatry* 24:775–781, 1988.

Campbell DR, Kimball RR: Replication of "prediction of antidepressant response to lithium": Problems in generalizing to a clinical setting. *Am J Psychiatry* 141:706–707, 1984.

Campbell J: *The Hero With a Thousand Faces*. (1949) Princeton, NJ: Princeton University Press, Bollingen, 1972.

Campbell JD: *Manic-Depressive Disease: Clinical and Psychiatric Significance*. Philadelphia: JB Lippincott, 1953.

Campbell M, Perry R, Green WH: Use of lithium in children and adolescents. *Psychosomatics* 25:95–106, 1984.

Cancro R: Clinical prediction of outcome in schizophrenia. *Compr Psychiatry* 10:349–354, 1969.

Canino GL, Bird HR, Shrout PE, Rubio-Stipec M, Bravo M, Martinez R, Sesman M, Guevara LM: The prevalence of specific psychiatric disorders in Puerto Rico. *Arch Gen Psychiatry* 44:727–735, 1987.

Cantley LC Jr, Josephson L, Warner R, Yanagisawa M, Lechene C, Guidotti G: Vanadate is a potent (Na,K)-ATPase inhibitor found in ATP derived from muscle. *J Biol Chem* 252:7421–7423, 1977.

Cantoni GL, Mudd SH, Andreoli V: Affective disorders and s-adenosylmethionine: A new hypothesis. *Trends in Neurosci* 12:319–324, 1989.

Cantor N, Genero N: Psychiatric diagnosis and natural categorization: A close analogy. In: T Millon, GL Klerman, eds. *Contemporary Directions in Psychopathology: Toward the DSM-IV*. New York: The Guilford Press, 1986. pp 233–256.

Cantwell DP, Sturzenberger S, Burroughs J, Salkin B, Green JK: Anorexia nervosa: An affective disorder? *Arch Gen Psychiatry* 34:1087–1093, 1977.

Cappel R, Sprecher S: Are herpes viruses responsible for neuropsychiatric diseases? *Adv Biol Psychiatry* 12:168–173, 1983.

Caramagno T: *Virginia Woolf: A Neurobiography*. Berkeley: University of California Press, in press.

Carlson GA: Manic-depressive illness and cognitive immaturity. In: RH Belmaker, HM van Praag, eds: *Mania: An Evolving Concept*. New York: Spectrum Books, 1980. pp 281–289.

Carlson GA: Bipolar affective disorders in childhood and adolescence. In: DP Cantwell, GA Carlson, eds: *Affective Disorders in Childhood and Adolescence: An Update*. New York: Spectrum Publications, 1983. pp 61–83.

Carlson GA, Goodwin FK: The stages of mania: A longitudinal analysis of the manic episode. *Arch Gen Psychiatry* 28:221–228, 1973.

Carlson GA, Kashani JH: Phenomenology of major depression from childhood through adulthood: Analysis of three studies. *Am J Psychiatry* 145:1222–1225, 1988a.

Carlson GA, Kashani JH: Manic symptoms in a non-referred adolescent population. *J Affective Disord* 15:219–226, 1988b.

Carlson GA, Strober M: Affective disorder in adolescence: Issues in misdiagnosis. *J Clin Psychiatry* 39:59–66, 1978.

Carlson G, Strober M: Affective disorders in adolescence. *Psychiatr Clin North Am* 2:511–526, 1979.

Carlson GA, Kotin JL, Davenport YB, Adland M: Follow-up of 53 bipolar manic-depressive patients. *Br J Psychiatry* 124:134–139, 1974.

Carlson GA, Davenport YB, Jamison K: A comparison of outcome in adolescent- and late-onset bipolar manic-depressive illness. *Am J Psychiatry* 134:919–922, 1977.

Carlsson A, Lindqvist M: Effects of antidepressant agents on the synthesis of brain monoamines. *J Neural Transm* 43:73–91, 1978.

Carman JS, Wyatt RJ: Calcium: Bivalent cation in the bivalent psychoses. *Biol Psychiatry* 14:295–336, 1979a.

Carman JS, Wyatt RJ: Calcium: Pacesetting the periodic psychoses. *Am J Psychiatry* 136:1035–1039, 1979b.

Carman JS, Wyatt RJ: Use of calcitonin in psychotic agitation or mania. *Arch Gen Psychiatry* 36:72–75, 1979c.

Carman JS, Post RM, Teplitz TA, Goodwin FK: Divalent cations in predicting antidepressant response to lithium. Letter. *Lancet* 2:1454, 1974.

Carman JS, Post RM, Goodwin FK, Bunney WE Jr: Calcium and electroconvulsive therapy of severe depressive illness. *Biol Psychiatry* 12:5–17, 1977.

Carman JS, Post RM, Runkle DC, Bunney WE Jr, Wyatt RJ: Increased serum calcium and phosphorus with the "switch" into manic or excited psychotic state. *Br J Psychiatry* 135:55–61, 1979.

Carman JS, Bigelow LB, Wyatt RJ: Lithium combined with neuroleptics in chronic schizophrenic and schizoaffective patients. *J Clin Psychiatry* 42:124–128, 1981.

Carman JS, Wyatt ES, Smith W, Post RM, Ballenger JC: Calcium and calcitonin in bipolar affective disorder. In: RM Post, JC Ballenger, eds: *Neurobiology of Mood Disorders*. Baltimore: Williams & Wilkins, 1984. pp 340–355.

Carney MWP, Roth M, Garside RF: The diagnosis of depresssive syndromes and the prediction of E.C.T. response. *Br J Psychiatry* 111:659–674, 1965.

Carney MWP, Chary TKN, Bottiglieri T, Reynolds EH: The switch mechanism and the bipolar/unipolar dichotomy. *Br J Psychiatry* 154:48–51, 1989a.

Carney MWP, Chary TKN, Bottiglieri T, Reynolds EH: Switch and s-adenosylmethionine. *Ala J Med Sci* 25:316–319, 1989b.

Carney PA, Fitzgerald CT, Monaghan CE: Influence of climate on the prevalence of mania. *Br J Psychiatry* 152:820–823, 1988.

Carney RM, Hong BA, O'Connell MF, Amano H: Facial electromyography as a predictor of treatment outcome in depression. *Br J Psychiatry* 138:485–489, 1981.

Carothers JC: *The African Mind in Health and Disease.* Geneva: World Health Organization, 1953.

Carpenter WT, Strauss JS, Mulch S: Are there pathognomonic symptoms in schizophrenia? An empiric investigation of Schneider's first rank symptoms. *Arch Gen Psychiatry* 28:847–852, 1973.

Carpenter WT, Bartko JJ, Strauss JS, Hawk AB: Signs and symptoms as predictors of outcome: A report from the International Pilot Study of Schizophrenia. *Am J Psychiatry* 135:940–945, 1978.

Carr V, Dorrington C, Schrader G, Wale J: The use of ECT for mania in childhood bipolar disorder. *Br J Psychiatry* 143:411–415, 1983.

Carroll BJ: Hypothalamic-pituitary function in depressive illness: insensitivity to hylycaemia. *Br Med J* 3:27–28, 1969.

Carroll BJ: Sodium and potassium transfer to cerebrospinal fluid in sever depression. In: B Davies, BJ Carroll, RM Mowbray, eds: *Depressive Illness: Some Research Studies.* Springfield, Il: Charles C Thomas, 1972. pp 247–257.

Carroll BJ: Prediction of treatment outcome with lithium. *Arch Gen Psychiatry* 36:870–878, 1979.

Carroll BJ: The dexamethasone suppression test for melancholia. *Br J Psychiatry* 140:292–304, 1982.

Carroll BJ: Neurobiologic dimensions of depression and mania. In: J Angst, ed: *The Origins of Depression: Current Concepts and Approaches.* Berlin: Springer-Verlag, 1983. pp 163–186.

Carroll BJ, Feinberg MP: Intracellular lithium. *Neuropharmacology* 16:527, 1977.

Carroll BJ, Sharp PT: Rubidium and lithium: Opposite effects on amine-mediated excitement. *Science* 172:1355–1357, 1971.

Carroll BJ, Martin FI, Davies B: Resistance to suppression by dexamethasone of plasma 11-O.H.C.S. levels in severe depressive illness. *Br Med J* 3:285–287, 1968.

Carroll BJ, Fielding JM, Blashki TG: Depression rating scales: A critical review. *Arch Gen Psychiatry* 28:361–366, 1973.

Carroll BJ, Curtis GC, Mendels J: Neuroendocrine regulation in depression. II. Discrimination of depressed from nondepressed patients. *Arch Gen Psychiatry* 33:1051–1058, 1976a.

Carroll BJ, Curtis GC, Mendels J: Cerebrospinal fluid and plasma free cortisol concentrations in depression. *Psychol Med* 6:235–244, 1976b.

Carroll BJ, Feinberg M, Greden JF, Haskett RF, James NM, Steiner M, Tarika J: Diagnosis of endogenous depression: Comparison of clinical, research and neuroendocrine criteria. *J Affective Disord* 2:177–194, 1980.

Carroll BJ, Feinberg M, Smouse PE, Rawson SG,

Greden JF: The Carroll Rating Scale for Depression: I. Development, reliability and validation. *Br J Psychiatry* 138:194–200, 1981.

Carroll JA, Greist JH, Jefferson JW, Baudhuin MG, Hartley BL, Erdman HP, Ackerman DL: Lithium information center: One model of a computer-based psychiatric information center. *Arch Gen Psychiatry* 43:483–485, 1986.

Carstens M, Engelbrecht A, Russell V, Aalbers C, Gagiano C, Chalton D, Taljaard J: Imipramine binding sites on platelets of patients with major depressive disorder. *Psychiatry Res* 18:333–342, 1986.

Casat CD, Powell K: The dexamethasone suppression test in children and adolescents with major depressive disorder: A review. *J Clin Psychiatry* 49:390–393, 1988.

Casey DE: Tardive dyskinesia and affective disorders. In: G Gardos, DE Casey, eds: *Tardive Dyskinesia and Affective Disorders.* Washington, DC: American Psychiatric Press, 1984. pp 2–19.

Casper RC, Davis JM, Pandey GN, Garver DL, Dekirmenjian H: Neuroendocrine and amine studies in affective illness. *Psychoneuroendocrinology* 2:105–113, 1977.

Casper RC, Redmond E Jr, Katz MM, Schaffer CB, Davis JM, Koslow SH: Somatic symptoms in primary affective disorder: Presence and relationship to the classification of depression. *Arch Gen Psychiatry* 42:1098–1104, 1985.

Cassano GB, Musetti L, Perugi G, Soriani A, Mignani V, McNair DM, Akiskal HS: A proposed new approach to the clinical subclassification of depressive illness. *Pharmacopsychiat* 21:19–23, 1988.

Cassem NH: Treating the person confronting death. In: AM Nicholi, ed: *Harvard Guide to Modern Psychiatry.* Cambridge, Mass: Belknap Press of Harvard University Press, 1978. pp 579–606.

Cassidy WL, Flanagan NB, Spellman M, Cohen ME: Clinical observations in manic-depressive disease. *JAMA* 164:1535–1546, 1957.

Castaneda R, Galanter M, Franco H: Self-medication among addicts with primary psychiatric disorders. *Compr Psychiatry* 30:80–83, 1989.

Castellani S, Petrie WM, Ellinwood E: Drug induced psychosis: Neurobiological mechanisms. In: Alterman AI, ed: *Substance Abuse and Psychopathology.* New York: Plenum Press, 1985. pp 173–210.

Cattell RB: *Personality and Mood by Questionnaire.* San Francisco: Jossey-Bass Publishers, 1973.

Caudrey DJ, Kirk K, Thomas PC, Ng KO: Perceptual deficit in schizophrenia: A defect in redundancy utilization, filtering or scanning? *Br J Psychiatry* 137:352–60, 1980.

Causemann B, Müller-Oerlinghausen B: Does lithium prevent suicides and suicidal attempts? In: NJ Birch, ed: *Lithium: Inorganic Pharmacology and Psychiatric Use.* Oxford: IRL Press, 1988. pp 23–24.

Cazzullo CL, Smeraldi E, Sacchetti E, Bottinelli S: Intracellular lithium concentration and clinical response. *Br J Psychiatry* 126:298–300, 1975.

Cazzullo CL, Sacchetti E, Smeraldi E: New trends on

long-term lithium treatment in affective disorders. *Prevention in Psychiatry* 1:115–130, 1980.

Chabanier MJ, Pelisser H, Minivielle MJ: Electroclinical correlations in 100 patients in a psychiatric clinic. *Electroencephalogr Clin Neurophysiol* 17:722, 1964.

Chambers CA, Naylor GJ: A controlled trial of L-tryptophan in mania. *Br J Psychiatry* 132:555–559, 1978.

Chambers CA, Smith AH, Naylor GJ: The effect of digoxin on the response to lithium therapy in mania. *Psychol Med* 12:57–60, 1982.

Chambers WJ, Puig-Antich J, Tabrizi MA, Davies M: Psychotic symptoms in prepubertal major depressive disorder. *Arch Gen Psychiatry* 39:921–927, 1982.

Chambers WJ, Puig-Antich J, Hirsch M, Paez P, Ambrosini PJ, Tabrizi MA, Davies M: The assessment of affective disorders in children and adolescents by semistructured interview. *Arch Gen Psychiatry* 42:696–702, 1985.

Chapman LJ, Chapman JP: *Disordered thought in schizophrenia.* New York: Appleton-Century-Crofts, 1973.

Charlton BG, Ferrier IN: Hypothalamo-pituitary-adrenal axis abnormalities in depression: A review and a model. *Psychol Med* 19:331–336, 1989.

Charney DS, Nelson JC: Delusional and nondelusional unipolar depression: Further evidence for distinct subtypes. *Am J Psychiatry* 138:328–333, 1981.

Charney DS, Nelson JC, Quinlan DM: Personality traits and disorder in depression. *Am J Psychiatry* 138:1601–1604, 1981a.

Charney DS, Menkes DB, Heninger GR: Receptor sensitivity and the mechanism of action of antidepressant treatment: Implications for the etiology and therapy of depression. *Arch Gen Psychiatry* 38:1160–1180, 1981b.

Chaturvedi SK, Upadhyaya M: Secondary mania in a patient receiving isonicotinic acid hydrazide and pyridoxine: Case report. *Can J Psychiatry* 33:675–676, 1988.

Chaugule VB, Master RS: Impaired cerebral dominance and schizophrenia. *Br J Psychiatry* 139:23–24, 1981.

Chazot G, Fournis Y, Robert JM, Aimard G, Devic M: [Modifications of serum creatine phosphokinase activity under the influence of lithium gluconate in Duchenne's myopathy]. *Lyon Med* 228:421–425, 1972.

Chazot G, Chalumeau A, Mornex R, Schott B, Girard PF: [Thyrotropin releasing factoor and depressive state: Acroagonines of TRH.] *Probl Actuels Endocrinol Nutr* 18:261–271, 1974.

Chazot G, Claustrat B, Brun J, Olivier M: Rapid antidepressant activity of destyr gamma endorphin: Correlation with urinary melatonin. *Biol Psychiatry* 20:1026–1030, 1985.

Checkley SA: Corticosteroid and growth hormone responses to methylamphetamine in depressive illness. *Psychol Med* 9:107–115, 1979.

Checkley SA, Slade AP, Shur E: Growth hormone and other responses to clonidine in patients with endogenous depression. *Br J Psychiatry* 138:51–55, 1981.

Cheung WY: Calmodulin plays a pivotal role in cellular regulation. *Science* 207:19–27, 1980.

Chiodo LA, Antelman SM: Tricyclic antidepressants induce subsensitivity of presynaptic dopamine autoreceptors. *Eur J Pharmacol* 64:203–204, 1980.

Cho JT, Bone S, Dunner DL, Colt E, Fieve RR: The effect of lithium treatment on thyroid function in patients with primary affective disorder. *Am J Psychiatry* 136:115–116, 1979.

Chodoff P: The depressive personality: A critical review. *Arch Gen Psychiatry* 27:666–673, 1972.

Choi SJ, Taylor MA, Abrams R: Depression, ECT, and erythrocyte adenosinetriphosphatase activity. *Biol Psychiatry* 12:75–81, 1977.

Choi SJ, Derman RM, Lee KS: Bipolar affective disorder, lithium carbonate and Ca^{++} ATPase. *J Affective Disord* 3:77–79, 1981.

Chouinard G: Clonazepam in acute and maintenance treatment of bipolar affective disorder. *J Clin Psychiatry* 48(Suppl):29–36, 1987.

Chouinard G, Steiner W: A case of mania induced by high-dose fluoxetine treatment. *Am J Psychiatry* 143:686, 1986.

Chouinard G, Jones BD, Young SN, Annable L: Potentiation of lithium by tryptophan in a patient with bipolar illness. *Am J Psychiatry* 136:719–720, 1979.

Chouinard G, Young SN, Annable L: Antimanic effect of clonazepam. *Biol Psychiatry* 18:451–466, 1983.

Chouinard G, Young SN, Annable L: A controlled clinical trial of L-tryptophan in acute mania. *Biol Psychiatry* 20:546–557, 1985.

Chouinard G, Beauclair L, Etienne P: Magnesium aspartate hydrochloride (magnesiocard) as a mood stabilizer for rapid cyclers. Abstract of paper presented at the 27th annual meeting of the American College of Neuro-Psychopharmacology, 1988.

Chouvet G, Mouret J, Coindet J, Siffre M, Jouvet M: Periodicite bicircadienne du cycle veille-sommeil dans de conditions hors du temps: Etude polygraphique. *Electroencephalogr Clin Neurophysiol* 37:367–380, 1974.

Christiansen C, Baastrup PC, Lindgren P, Transbøl I: Endocrine effects of lithium: II. "Primary" hyperparathyroidism. *Acta Endocrinol (Copenh)* 88:528–534, 1978.

Christensen NJ, Vestergaard P, Sørensen T, Rafaelsen OJ: Cerebrospinal fluid adrenaline and noradrenaline in depressed patients. *Acta Psychiatr Scand* 61:178–182, 1980.

Christie KA, Burke JD, Regier DA, Rae DS, Boyd JH, Locke BZ: Epidemiologic evidence for early onset of mental disorders and higher risk of drug abuse in young adults. *Am J Psychiatry* 145:971–975, 1988.

Christie MJ, Little BC, Gordon AM: Peripheral indices of depressive states. In: HM Van Praag, MH Lader, OJ Rafaelsen, EJ Sachar, eds: *Handbook of Biological Psychiatry Part II: Brain Mechanisms and Ab-*

normal Behavior Psychophysiology. New York: Marcel Dekker, Inc, 1980. pp 145–182.

Christodoulou GN, Lykouras EP: Abrupt lithium discontinuation in manic-depressive patients. *Acta Psychiatr Scand* 65:310–314, 1982.

Christodoulou GN, Siafakas A, Rinieris PM: Side-effects of lithium. *Acta Psychiatr Belg* 77:260–266, 1977.

Christodoulou GN, Malliaras DE, Lykouras EP, Papadimitriou GN, Stefanis CN: Possible prophylactic effect of sleep deprivation. *Am J Psychiatry* 135:375–376, 1978.

Chuang DM, Kinnier WJ, Farber L, Costa E: A biochemical study of receptor internalization during beta-adrenergic receptor desensitization in frog erythrocytes. *Mol Pharmacol* 18:348–55, 1980.

Ciraulo DA, Alderson LM, Chapron DJ, Jaffe JH, Subbarao B, Kramer PA: Imipramine disposition in alcoholics. *J Clin Psychopharmacol* 2:2–7, 1982.

Clancy J, Crowe R, Winokur G, Morrison J: The Iowa 500: Precipitating factors in schizophrenia and primary affective disorder. *Compr Psychiatry* 14:197–202, 1973.

Clark DC, Clayton PJ, Andreasen NC, Lewis C, Fawcett J, Scheftner WA: Intellectual functioning and abstraction ability in major affective disorders. *Compr Psychiatry* 26:313–325, 1985.

Clark DM, Teasdale JD: Diurnal variation in clinical depression and accessibility of memories of positive and negative experiences. *J Abnorm Psychol* 91:87–95, 1982.

Clark RE: Psychoses, income, and occupational prestige. *Am J Sociology* 54:433–440, 1949.

Clarke T, Coffey CE, Figiel GS, Weiner RD: Continuation therapy of depression with outpatient ECT. Abstract of paper presented at the 43rd annual meeting of the Society for Biological Psychiatry, May, 1988.

Claustrat B, Chazot G, Brun J, Jordan D, Sassolas G: A chronobiological study of melatonin and cortisol secretion in depressed subjects: Plasma melatonin, a biochemical marker in major depression. *Biol Psychiatry* 19:1215–1228, 1984.

Clayton PJ: The epidemiology of bipolar affective disorder. *Compr Psychiatry* 22:31–43, 1981.

Clayton P, Pitts FN Jr, Winokur G: Affective disorder: IV. Mania. *Compr Psychiatry* 6:313–322, 1965.

Cleary P, Guy W: Factor analysis of the Hamilton Depression Scale. *Drugs Exp Clin Res* 1:115–120, 1977.

Clerget-Darpoux F, Goldin LR, Gershon ES: Clinical methods in psychiatric genetics: III: Environmental stratification may simulate a genetic effect in adoption studies. *Acta Psychiatr Scand* 74:305–311, 1986.

Cloninger CR, Reich T, Wetzel R: Alcoholism and affective disorders: Familial associations and genetic models. In: DW Goodwin, CK Erickson, eds: *Alcoholism and Affective Disorders: Clinical, Genetic, and Biochemical Studies.* New York: SP Medical and Scientific Books, 1979. pp 57–86.

Coate M: *Beyond All Reason.* London: Constable & Co, 1964.

Coccaro EF, Siever LJ, Klar HM, Maurer G, Cochrane K, Cooper TB, Mohs RC, Davis KL: Serotonergic studies in patients with affective and personality disorders. *Arch Gen Psychiatry* 46:587–599, 1989.

Cochran E, Robins E, Grote S: Regional serotonin levels in brain: A comparison of depressive suicides and alcoholic suicides with controls. *Biol Psychiatry* 11:283–294, 1976.

Cochran SD: Strategies for preventing lithium noncompliance in bipolar affective illness. Doctoral dissertation, University of California, Los Angeles, 1982.

Cochran SD: Preventing medical noncompliance in the outpatient treatment of bipolar affective disorders. *J Consult Clin Psychol* 52:873–878, 1984.

Cochran SD, Gitlin MJ: Attitudinal correlates of lithium compliance in bipolar affective disorders. *J Nerv Ment Dis* 176:457–464, 1988.

Coffey CE: Cerebral laterality and emotion: The neurology of depression. *Compr Psychiatry* 28:197–219, 1987.

Coffey CE, Figiel GS, Djang WT, Cress M, Saunders WB, Weiner RD: Leukoencephalopathy in elderly depressed patients referred for ECT. *Biol Psychiatry* 24:143–161, 1988.

Coffman JA, Petty F: Plasma GABA: A potential indicator of altered GABAergic function in psychiatric illness. In: G Bartholini, KG Lloyd, PL Morselli, eds: *GABA and Mood Disorders: Experimental and Clinical Research.* New York: Raven Press, 1986. pp 179–185.

Cohen BM, Zubenko GS: Captopril in the treatment of recurrent major depression. *J Clin Psychopharmacol* 8:143–144, 1988.

Cohen BM, Miller AL, Lipinski JF, Pope HG: Lecithin in mania: A preliminary report. *Am J Psychiatry* 137:242–243, 1980.

Cohen BM, Lipinski JF, Altesman RI: Lecithin in the treatment of mania: Double-blind, placebo-controlled trials. *Am J Psychiatry* 139:1162–1164, 1982.

Cohen LS, Rosenbaum JF: Clonazepam: New uses and potential problems. *J Clin Psychiatry* 48:50–56, 1987.

Cohen LS, Heller VL, Rosenbaum JF, Goldstein S, Hirshfeld D: Adjuvant lithium carbonate in refractory depression. Abstract of paper presented at the 141st annual meeting of the American Psychiatric Association, May, 1988.

Cohen MB, Baker G, Cohen RA, Fromm-Reichmann F, Weigert EV: An intensive study of twelve cases of manic-depressive psychosis. *Psychiatry* 17:103–137, 1954.

Cohen MR, Niska RW: Localized right cerebral hemisphere dysfunction and recurrent mania. *Am J Psychiatry* 137:847–848, 1980.

Cohen MR, Cohen RM, Pickar D, Sunderland T, Mueller EA III, Murphy DL: High dose naloxone in depression. *Biol Psychiatry* 19:825–832, 1984.

Cohen RM, Nordahl T: Brain imaging techniques. In: JG Howells, ed: *Modern Perspectives in Clinical Psychiatry*. New York: Brunner/Mazel, 1988. pp 102–129.

Cohen RM, Weingartner H, Smallberg SA, Pickar D, Murphy DL: Effort and cognition in depression. *Arch Gen Psychiatry* 39:593–597, 1982.

Cohen RM, Semple WE, Gross M, Nordahl TE, King AC, Pickar D, Post RM: Evidence for common alterations in cerebral glucose metabolism in major affective disorders and schizophrenia. *Neuropsychopharmacology*, 2:241–254, 1989.

Cohen S: Recent developments in the abuse of cocaine. *Bull Narcotics* 36:3–14, 1984.

Cohen S, Khan A, Robison J: Significance of mixed features in acute mania. *Compr Psychiatry* 29:421–426, 1988.

Cohen WJ, Cohen NH: Lithium carbonate, haloperidol, and irreversible brain damage. *JAMA* 230:1283–1287, 1974.

Cohn CK, Dunner DL, Axelrod J: Reduced catechol-O-methyltransferase activity in red blood cells of women with primary affective disorder. *Science* 170:1323–1324, 1970.

Colbert J, Harrow M: Psychomotor retardation in depressive syndromes. *J Nerv Ment Dis* 145:405–419, 1967.

Cole BJ, Robbins TW: Amphetamine impairs the discriminative performance of rats with dorsal noradrenergic bundle lesions on a 5-choice serial reaction time task: New evidence for central dopaminergic-noradrenergic interactions. *Psychopharmacology (Berlin)* 91:458–466, 1987.

Coleridge ST: *Coleridge: Poems and Prose Selected.* K Raine, ed. Middlesex: Penguin Books, 1957.

Coll PG, Bland R: Manic-depressive illness in adolescence and childhood: Review and case report. *Can J Psychiatry* 24:255–263, 1979.

Colt EW, Dunner DL, Wang J, Ross DC, Pierson RN, Fieve RR: Body composition in affective disorder before, during, and after lithium carbonate therapy. *Arch Gen Psychiatry* 39:577–581, 1982.

Comings DE: Pc 1 Duarte, a common polymorphism of a human brain protein, and its relationship to depressive disease and multiple sclerosis. *Nature* 277:28–32, 1979.

Connelly CE, Davenport YB, Nurnberger JI Jr.: Adherence to treatment regimen in a lithium carbonate clinic. *Arch Gen Psychiatry* 39:585–588, 1982.

Connelly TL: *The Marble Man: Robert E. Lee and Image in American Society.* New York: Knopf, 1977.

Conners CK, Himmelhoch J, Goyette CH, Ulrich R, Neil JF: Children of parents with affective illness. *J Am Acad Child Psychiatry* 18:600–607, 1979.

Conte G, Vazzola A, Sacchetti E: Renal function in chronic lithium-treated patients. *Acta Psychiatr Scand* 79:503–504, 1989.

Cook BL, Shukla S, Hoff AL: EEG abnormalities in bipolar affective disorder. *J Affective Disord* 11:147–149, 1986.

Cook BL, Shukla S, Hoff AL, Aronson TA: Mania with associated organic factors. *Acta Psychiatr Scand* 76:674–677, 1987.

Cook FA: Gynecology and obstetrics among the Eskimos. *Brooklyn Med J* 8:154–169, 1894.

Cooke RG, Langlet F, McLaughlin BJM: Age-specific prevalence of Epstein-Barr virus antibodies in adult patients with affective disorders. *J Clin Psychiatry* 49:361–363, 1988.

Cooklin RS, Ravindran A, Carney MWP: The patterns of mental disorder in Jewish and non-Jewish admissions to a district general hospital psychiatric unit: Is manic-depressive illness a typically Jewish disorder? *Psychol Med* 13:209–212, 1983.

Cookson JC: The neuroendocrinology of mania. *J Affective Disord* 8:233–241, 1985.

Cookson JC, Silverstone T, Wells B: A double-blind controlled study of pimozide versus chlorpromazine in mania. *Psychopharmacol Bull* 16:38–41, 1980.

Cooper AJ: Hypomanic psychosis precipitated by hemodialysis. *Compr Psychiatry* 8:168–172, 1967.

Cooper JE, Kendell RE, Gurland BJ, Sharpe L, Copeland JRM, Simon R: *Psychiatric Diagnosis in New York and London: A Comparative Study of Mental Hospital Admissions.* Maudsley Monograph No. 20. London: Oxford University Press, 1972.

Cooper SD, Sellers EM, Khouw V, Zilm DH, Israel Y: Lithium treatment during ethanol ingestion and withdrawal. *Pharmacologist* 16:304, 1974.

Cooper SJ, Kelly JG, King DJ: Adrenergic receptors in depression: Effects of electroconvulsive therapy. *Br J Psychiatry* 147:23–29, 1985.

Cooper TB: Pharmacokinetics of lithium. In: HY Meltzer, ed: *Psychopharmacology: The Third Generation of Progress.* New York: Raven Press, 1987. pp 1365–1375.

Cooper TB, Simpson GM: The 24-hour lithium level as a prognosticator of dosage requirements: A 2-year follow-up study. *Am J Psychiatry* 133:440–443, 1976.

Cooper TB, Berner PE, Simpson GM: The 24-hour serum lithium level as a prognosticator of dosage requirements. *Am J Psychiatry* 130:601–603, 1973.

Coppen A: Abnormality in the blood-cerebrospinal fluid barrier of patients suffering from a depressive illness. *J Neurol Neurosurg Psychiatry* 23:156–161, 1960.

Coppen A, Abou-Saleh MT: Plasma folate and affective morbidity during long-term lithium therapy. *Br J Psychiatry* 141:87–89, 1982.

Coppen A, Abou-Saleh MT: Lithium therapy: From clinical trials to practical management. *Acta Psychiatr Scand* 78:754–762, 1988.

Coppen A, Ghose K: Peripheral alpha-adrenoreceptor and central dopamine receptor activity in depressive patients. *Psychopharmacology (Berlin)* 59:171–177, 1978.

Coppen A, Metcalfe H: Effect of a depressive illness on M.P.I. scores. *Br J Psychiatry* 111:236–239, 1965.

Coppen A, Shaw DM: Mineral metabolism in melancholia. *Br Med J* 2:1439–1444, 1963.

Coppen A, Swade C: Reduced lithium dosage improves prophylaxis: A possible mechanism. In: H Hippius, GL Klerman, N Matussek, eds: *New Results in Depression Research*. Berlin: Springer-Verlag, 1986. pp 126–130.

Coppen A, Shaw DM, Malleson A, Costain R: Mineral metabolism in mania. *Br Med J* 1:71–75, 1966.

Coppen A, Shaw DM, Herzberg B, Maggs R: Tryptophan in the treatment of depression. *Lancet* 2:1178–1180, 1967.

Coppen A, Prange AJ Jr, Whybrow PC, Noguera R, Paez JM: Methysergide in mania: A controlled trial. *Lancet* 2:338–340, 1969.

Coppen A, Brooksbank BW, Noguera R, Wilson DA: Cortisol in the cerebrospinal fluid of patients suffering from affective disorders. *J Neurol Neurosurg Psychiatry* 34:432–435, 1971a.

Coppen A, Noguera R, Bailey J, Burns BH, Swani MS, Hare EH, Gardner R, Maggs R: Prophylactic lithium in affective disorders: Controlled trial. *Lancet* 2:275–279, 1971b.

Coppen A, Whybrow PC, Noguera R, Maggs R, Prange AJ: The comparative antidepressant value of l-tryptophan and imipramine with and without attempted potentiation by liothyonine. *Arch Gen Psychiatry* 26:234–245, 1972a.

Coppen A, Prange AJ Jr, Whybrow PC, Noguera R: Abnormalities of indoleamines in affective disorders. *Arch Gen Psychiatry* 26:474–478, 1972b.

Coppen A, Peet M, Bailey J, Noguera R, Burns B, Swani M, Maggs R, Gardner R: Double-blind and open prospective studies of lithium prophylaxis in affective disorders. *Psychiatr Neurol Neurochir* 76:500–510, 1973.

Coppen A, Montgomery SA, Gupta RK, Bailey J: A double-blind comparison of lithium carbonate and maprotiline in the prophylaxis of the affective disorders. *Br J Psychiatry* 128:479–485, 1976.

Coppen A, Swade C, Wood K: Platelet 5-hydroxytryptamine accumulation in depressive illness. *Clin Chim Acta* 87:165–168, 1978.

Coppen A, Rama Rao VA, Ruthven CRJ, Goodwin BL, Sandler M: Urinary 4-hydroxy-3-methoxyphenylglycol is not a predictor for clinical response to amitriptyline in depressive illness. *Psychopharmacology (Berlin)* 64:95–97, 1979.

Coppen A, Bishop ME, Bailey JE, Cattell, Price RG: Renal function in lithium and non-lithium treated patients with affective disorders. *Acta Psychiatr Scand* 62:343–355, 1980a.

Coppen A, Swade C, Wood K: Lithium restores abnormal platelet 5-HT transport in patients with affective disorders. *Br J Psychiatry* 136:235–238, 1980b.

Coppen A, Abou-Saleh M, Milln P, Bailey J, Wood K: Decreasing lithium dosage reduces morbidity and side-effects during prophylaxis. *J Affective Disord* 5:353–362, 1983.

Coppen A, Abou-Saleh MT, Wood KM, Mitchell MJ: Treatment of bipolar affective illness with zimeldine, a 5-HT uptake inhibitor. *J Affective Disord* 7:339–342, 1984.

Coppen A, Swade C, Jones SA, Armstrong RA, Blair JA, Leeming RJ: Depression and tetrahydrobiopterin: The folate connection. *J Affective Disord* 16:103–107, 1989.

Corkin S, Twitchell TE, Sullivan EV: Safety and efficacy of cingulotomy for pain and psychiatric disorder. In: ER Hitchcock, HT Ballantine, BA Meyerson, eds: *Modern Concepts in Psychiatric Surgery*. Amsterdam: Elsevier, 1979. pp 253–272.

Corn TH, Checkley SA: A case of recurrent mania with recurrent hyperthyroidism. *Br J Psychiatry* 143:74–76, 1983.

Coryell W, Norten SG: Mania during adolescence: The pathoplastic significance of age. *J Nerv Ment Dis* 168:611–613, 1980.

Coryell W, Tsuang MT: Primary unipolar depression and the prognostic importance of delusions. *Arch Gen Psychiatry* 39:1181–1184, 1982.

Coryell W, Endicott J, Reich T, Andreasen N, Keller M: A family study of bipolar II disorder. *Br J Psychiatry* 145:49–54, 1984.

Coryell W, Endicott J, Andreasen N, Keller M: Bipolar I, bipolar II, and nonbipolar major depression among the relatives of affectively ill probands. *Am J Psychiatry* 142:817–821, 1985.

Coryell W, Grove W, VanEerdewegh M, Keller M, Endicott J: Outcome in RDC schizo-affective depression: The importance of diagnostic subtyping. *J Affective Disord* 12:47–56, 1987a.

Coryell W, Andreasen NC, Endicott J, Keller M: The significance of past mania or hypomania in the course and outcome of major depression. *Am J Psychiatry* 144:309–315, 1987b.

Coryell W, Endicott J, Keller M, Andreasen N, Grove W, Hirschfeld RMA, Scheftner W: Bipolar affective disorder and high achievement: A familial association. *Am J Psychiatry* 146:983–988, 1989a.

Coryell W, Keller M, Endicott J, Andreasen N, Clayton P, Hirschfeld R: Bipolar II illness: Course and outcome over a five-year period. *Psychol Med* 19:129–141, 1989b.

Costello EJ, Edelbrock CS: Detection of psychiatric disorders in pediatric primary care: A preliminary report. *J Am Acad Child Psychiatry* 24:771–774, 1985.

Couch FH, Fox JC: Photographic study of ocular movements in mental disease. *Arch Neurol Psychiatry* 34:556–578, 1934.

Court JH: Manic-depressive psychosis: An alternative conceptual model. *Br J Psychiatry* 114:1523–1530, 1968.

Court JH: The continuum model as a resolution of paradoxes in manic-depressive psychosis. *Br J Psychiatry* 120:133–141, 1972.

Covi L, Lipman RS, Derogatis LR, Smith JE, Pattison JH: Drugs and group psychotherapy in neurotic depression. *Am J Psychiatry* 131:191–198, 1974.

Cowdry RW, Goodwin FK: Amine neurotransmitter

studies and psychiatric illness: Toward more meaningful diagnostic concepts. In R Spitzer, DF Klein, eds: *Critical Issues in Psychiatric Diagnosis*. New York: Raven Press, 1978. pp 281–304.

Cowdry RW, Goodwin FK: Biological and physiological predictors of drug response. In: HM Van Praag, MH Lader, OJ Rafaelsen, EJ Sachar, eds: *Handbook of Biological Psychiatry, Part VI: Practical Applications of Psychotropic Drugs and Other Biological Treatments*. New York: Marcel Dekker, Inc, 1981a. pp 263–308.

Cowdry RW, Goodwin FK: Dementia of bipolar illness: Diagnosis and response to lithium. *Am J Psychiatry* 138:1118–1119, 1981b.

Cowdry RW, Ebert MH, Van Kammen DP, Post RM, Goodwin FK: Cerebrospinal fluid probenecid studies: A reinterpretation. *Biol Psychiatry* 18:1287–1299, 1983a.

Cowdry RW, Wehr TA, Zis AP, Goodwin FK: Thyroid abnormalities associated with rapid-cycling bipolar illness. *Arch Gen Psychiatry* 40:414–420, 1983b.

Cowen PJ, Grahame-Smith DC, Green AR, Heal DJ: β-adrenoceptor agonists enhance 5-hydroxytryptamine mediated behavioural responses. *Br J Pharmacol* 76:265–270, 1982.

Cowen PJ, Parry-Billings M, Newsholme EA: Decreased plasma tryptophan levels in major depression. *J Affective Disord* 16:27–31, 1989.

Cowper W: *Letters of William Cowper*. Edited by W Benham. London: MacMillan, 1884.

Cox SM, Ludwig AM: Neurological soft signs and psychopathology: I. Findings in schizophrenia. *J Nerv Ment Dis* 167:161–165, 1979.

Coyne JC: Depression and the response of others. *J Abnorm Psychol* 85:186–193, 1976.

Coyne JC, Kessler RC, Tal M, Turnbull J, Wortman CB, Greden JF: Living with a depressed person. *J Consult Clin Psychol* 55:347–352, 1987.

Crammer JL: Review of ES Paykel, ed: *Handbook of Affective Disorders*. *Br J Psychiatry* 140:643–644, 1982.

Crane GE: The psychiatric side effects of iproniazid. *Am J Psychiatry* 112:494–501, 1956.

Crawley JN: Evaluation of a proposed hamster separation model of depression. *Psychiatry Res* 11:35–47, 1984.

Crawley JN: A monoamine oxidase inhibitor reverses the "separation syndrome" in a new hamster separation model of depression. *Eur J Pharmacol* 112:129–133, 1985.

Crawley JN, Hattox SE, Maas JW, Roth RH: 3-Methoxy-4- hydroxyphenethyleneglycol increase in plasma after stimulation of the nucleus locus coeruleus. *Brain Res* 141:380–384, 1978.

Crawley JN, Sutton ME, Pickar D: Animal models of self-destructive behavior and suicide. *Psychiatr Clin North Am* 8:299–310, 1985.

Creese I, Iversen SD: The pharmacological and anatomical substrates of the amphetamine response in the rat. *Brain Res* 83:419–436, 1975.

Crick FHC: Thinking about the brain. *Sci Amer* 241:219–232, 1979.

Cronholm B, Ottosson JO: Experimental studies of the therapeutic action of electroconvulsive therapy in endogenous depression: The role of the electrical stimulation and of the seizure studied by variation of stimulus intensity and modification by lidocaine of seizure discharge. *Acta Psychiatr Neurol Scand* (Suppl 145):69–101, 1960.

Cronholm B, Ottosson JO: Memory functions in endogenous depression: Before and after electroconvulsive therapy. *Arch Gen Psychiatry* 5:193–199, 1961.

Crookes TG, Hutt SJ: Scores of psychotic patients on the Maudsley Personality Inventory. *J Consult Psychol* 27:243–247, 1963.

Cross RJ, Markesbery WR, Brooks WH, Roszman TL: Hypothalamic-immune interactions: I. The acute effect of anterior hypothalamic lesions on the immune response. *Brain Res* 196:79–87, 1980.

Crow TJ: A re-evaluation of the viral hypothesis: Is psychosis the result of retroviral integration at a site close to the cerebral dominance gene? *Br J Psychiatry* 145:243–253, 1984.

Crow TJ: The continuum of psychosis and its implication for the structure of the gene. *Br J Psychiatry* 149:419–429, 1986.

Crow TJ: Commentary on EF Torrey: Functional psychoses and viral encephalitis. *Integr Psychiatry* 5:59–60, 1987.

Crow TJ, Deakin JFW: Affective change and the mechanisms of reward and punishment: A neurochemical hypothesis. In: C. Perris, G Struwe, B Jansson, eds: *Biological Psychiatry 1981*. Amsterdam: Elsevier, 1981. pp 536–541.

Crow TJ, Cross AJ, Cooper SJ, Deakin JFW, Ferrier IN, Johnson JA, Joseph MH, Owen F, Poulter M, Lofthouse R, Corsellis JAN, Chambers DR, Blessed G, Perry EK, Perry RH, Tomlinson BE: Neurotransmitter receptors and monoamine metabolites in the brains of patients with Alzheimer-type dementia and depression, and suicides. *Neuropharmacology* 23:1561–1569, 1984.

Culliton BJ: Genetic screening: NAS recommends proceeding with caution. *Science* 189:119–120, 1975.

Cummings JL: Organic psychoses: Delusional disorders and secondary mania. *Psychiatr Clin North Am* 9:293–311, 1986.

Cummings JL, Mendez MF: Secondary mania with focal cerebrovascular lesions. *Am J Psychiatry* 141:1084–1087, 1984.

Cundall RL, Brooks PW, Murray LG: A controlled evaluation of lithium prophylaxis in affective disorders. *Psychol Med* 2:308–311, 1972.

Curtius H-Ch, Muldner H, Niederweiser A: Tetrahydrobiopterin: Efficacy in endogenous depression and Parkinson's disease. *J Neural Transm* 55:301–318, 1982.

Curtius H-Ch, Niederwieser A, Levine RA, Lovenberg W, Woggon B, Angst J: Successful treatment of depression with tetrahydrobiopterin. Letter. *Lancet* 1:657–658, 1983.

Curzon G, Kantamaneni BD, Van Boxel P, Gillman PK, Bartlett JF, Bridges PK: Substances related to 5-hydroxytryptamine in plasma and in lumbar and ventricular fluid of psychiatric patients. *Acta Psychiatr Scand* (Suppl 280):13–17, 1980.

Custance J: *Wisdom, Madness, and Folly: The Philosophy of a Lunatic.* New York: Farrar, Straus & Cudahy, 1952.

Cutler NR, Post RM: Life course of illness in untreated manic-depressive patients. *Compr Psychiatry* 23: 101–115, 1982a.

Cutler NR, Post RM: State-related cyclical dyskinesias in manic-depressive illness. *J Clin Psychopharmacol* 2:350–354, 1982b.

Cytryn L, Gershon ES, McKnew DH: Childhood depression: Genetic or environmental influences? *Integr Psychiatry* 2:17–27, 1984.

Czeisler CA, Zimmerman JC, Ronda JM, Moore-Ede MC, Weitzman ED: Timing of REM sleep is coupled to the circadian rhythm of body temperature in man. *Sleep* 2:329–346, 1980.

Czeisler CA, Allan JS, Strogatz SH, Ronda JM, Sanchez R, Rios CD, Freitag WO, Richardson WO, Kronauer RE: Bright light resets the human circadian pacemaker independent of the timing of the sleep-wake cycle. *Science* 233:667–671, 1986.

Czeisler CA, Kronauer RE, Mooney JJ, Anderson JL, Allan JS: Biologic rhythm disorders, depression, and phototherapy: A new hypothesis. *Psychiatr Clin North Am* 10:687–709, 1987.

Dackis CA, Gold MS: Depression in opiate addicts. In: SM Mirin, ed: *Substance Abuse and Psychopathology.* Washington: American Psychiatric Press, 1984. pp 19–40.

Dackis CA, Gold MS, Pottash AL, Sweeney DR: Evaluating depression in alcoholics. *Psychiatry Res* 17:105–109, 1986.

Dahlgren KG: Entstehung undd Bedeutung der 2: Schutzzone bei der Salzäurekollargolreaktion. *Monatschr Psychiatr Neurol* 109:74–92, 1944.

Dahlström A, Fuxe K: Evidence for the existencce of monoamine-containing neurons in the central nervous system: I. Demonstration of monoamines in the cell bodies of brain stem neurons. *Acta Physiol Scand* 62(Suppl 232):1–55, 1964.

Daiguji M, Meltzer HY, U'Prichard DC: Human platelet alpha 2-adrenergic receptors: Labeling with ^{3}H-yohimbine, a selective antagonist ligand. *Life Sci* 28:2705–2717, 1981a.

Daiguji M, Meltzer HY, Tong C, U'Prichard DC, Young M, Kravitz H: Alpha-2-adrenergic receptors in platelet membranes of depressed patients: No change in number or ^{3}H-yohimbine affinity. *Life Sci* 29:2059–2064, 1981b.

Dalby JT, Williams R: Preserved reading and spelling ability in psychotic disorders. *Psychol Med* 16:171–175, 1986.

Dalby MA: Behavioral effects of carbamazepine. In: JK Penry, DD Daly, eds: *Complex Partial Seizures*

and Their Treatment, Vol 11: Advances in Neurology.* New York: Raven Press, 1975. pp 331–344.

Dalén P: Family history, the electroencephalogram and perinatal factors in manic conditions. *Acta Psychiatr Scand* 41:527–563, 1965.

Daniels EK, Shenton ME, Holzman PS, Benowitz LI, Levin S, Levine D: Patterns of thought disorder associated with right cortical damage, schizophrenia, and mania. *Am J Psychiatry* 145:944–949, 1988.

Danion JM, Neunreuther C, Krieger-Finance F, Imbs JL, Singer L: Compliance with long-term lithium treatment in major affective disorders. *Pharmacopsychiatry* 20:230–231, 1987.

Darko DF, Gillin JC, Risch SG, Golshan S, Bulloch K, Baird SM: Peripheral white blood cells and HPA axis neurohormones in major depression. *Int J Neurosci* 45:153–159, 1989.

Dauncey K: Mania in the early stages of AIDS. *Br J Psychiatry* 152:716–717, 1988.

Davenport YB, Adland ML: Postpartum psychoses in female and male bipolar manic-depressive patients. *Am J Orthopsychiatry* 52:288–297, 1982.

Davenport YB, Ebert MH, Adland ML, Goodwin FK: Couples group therapy as an adjunct to lithium maintenance of the manic patient. *Am J Orthopsychiatry* 47:495–502, 1977.

Davenport YB, Adland ML, Gold PW, Goodwin FK: Manic-depressive illness: Psychodynamic features of multigenerational families. *Am J Orthopsychiatry* 49:24–35, 1979.

Davenport YB, Zahn-Waxler C, Adland ML, Mayfield A: Early child-rearing practices in families with a manic-depressive parent. *Am J Psychiatry* 141: 230–235, 1984.

Davidson J, McLeod M, Law-Yone B, Linnoila M: A comparison of electroconvulsive therapy and combined phenelzine- amitriptyline in refractory depression. *Arch Gen Psychiatry* 35:639–642, 1978.

Davidson JRT, Miller RD, Turnbull CD, Sullivan JL: Atypical depression. *Arch Gen Psychiatry* 39:527–534, 1982.

Davidson J, Miller R, Turnbull CD, Belyea M, Strickland R: An evaluation of two doses of isocarboxazid in depression. *J Affective Disord* 6:201–207, 1984.

Davidson J, Turnbull CD, Strickland R, Miller R, Graves K: The Montgomery-Åsberg Depression Scale: Reliability and validity. *Acta Psychiatr Scand* 73:544–548, 1986.

Davidson JRT, Giller EL, Zisook S, Overall JE: An efficacy study of isocarboxazid and placebo in depression, and its relationship to depressive nosology. *Arch Gen Psychiatry* 45:120–127, 1988.

Davidson M: Studies in the application of mental tests to psychotic patients. *Br J Med Psychol* 18:44–52, 1939.

Davis BM, Pfefferbaum A, Krutzik S, Davis KL: Lithium's effect of parathyroid hormone. *Am J Psychiatry* 138:489–492, 1981.

Davis D: Mood changes in alcoholic subjects with programmed and free choice drinking. In: Mello NK, Mendelson J, eds: *Recent Advances in Studies of*

Alcoholism. Washington, DC: US Government Printing Office, 1971. pp 596–618.

Davis GC, Buchsbaum MS: Pain sensitivity and endorphins in functional psychoses. *Mod Prob Pharmacopsychiat* 17:97–108, 1981.

Davis GC, Bunney WE, Buchsbaum MS, DeFraites EG, Duncan W, Gillin JC, Van Kammen DP, Kleinman J, Murphy DL, Post RM, Reus V, Wyatt RJ: Use of narcotic antagonists to study the role of endorphins in normals and psychiatric patients. In: E Usdin, WE Bunney, NS Kline, eds: *Endorphins in Mental Health Research.* New York: Oxford University Press, 1979. pp 393–406.

Davis GC, Extein I, Reus VI, Hamilton W, Post RM, Goodwin FK, Bunney WE Jr: Failure of naloxone to reduce manic symptoms. *Am J Psychiatry* 137:1583–1585, 1980.

Davis H: Self-reference and the encoding of personal information in depression. *Cog Ther Res* 3:97–110, 1979a.

Davis H: The self-schema and subjective organization of personal information in depression. *Cog Ther Res* 3:415–425, 1979b.

Davis H, Unruh WR: Word memory in non-psychotic depression. *Percept Mot Skills* 51:699–705, 1980.

Davis JM: Overview: Maintenance therapy in psychiatry: II. Affective disorders. *Am J Psychiatry* 133:1–13, 1976.

Davis JM, Maas JW, eds: *The Affective Disorders.* Washington, DC: American Psychiatric Press, Inc, 1983.

Davis KL, Berger PA, Hollister LE, Defraites E: Physostigmine in mania. *Arch Gen Psychiatry* 35:119–122, 1978.

Davis KL, Davis BM, Mohs RC, Mathe AA, Vale W, Krieger D: CSF corticotropin releasing factor in neuropsychiatric disease. Abstract of paper presented at the 137th Annual Meeting of the American Psychiatric Association, May 1984.

Davis PA: Electroencephalograms in manic-depressive patients. *Am J Psychiatry* 98:430–433, 1941.

Davis RE: Manic-depressive variant syndrome of childhood: A preliminary report. *Am J Psychiatry* 136:702–705, 1979.

Dax EC: *Experimental Studies in Psychiatric Art.* London: Faber & Faber, 1953.

Deakin JF, Baker HF, Frith CD, Joseph MH, Johnstone EC: Arousal related to excretion of noradrenaline metabolites and clinical aspects of unmedicated chronic schizophrenic patients. *J Psychiatry Res* 15:57–65, 1979.

Deakin JFW, Owen F, Cross AJ, Dashwood MJ: Studies on possible mechanisms of action of electroconvulsive therapy: Effects of repeated electrically induced seizures on rat brain receptors for monoamines and other neurotransmitters. *Psychopharmacology (Berlin)* 73:345–349, 1981.

De Carolis V, Gilberti F, Roccatagliata G, Rossi R, Venutti G: Imipramine and electroshock in the treatment of depression: A clinical statistical analysis of 437 cases. *Sist Nerv* 16:29–42, 1964.

Decina P, Kestenbaum CJ, Farber S, Kron L, Gargan M, Sackeim HA, Fieve RR: Clinical and psychological assessment of children of bipolar probands. *Am J Psychiatry* 140:548–553, 1983.

Decina P, Guthrie EB, Sackeim HA, Kahn D, Malitz S: Continuation ECT in the management of relapses of major affective episodes. *Acta Psychiatr Scand* 75:559–562, 1987.

Deglin VL, Nikolaenko NN: Role of the dominant hemisphere in the regulation of emotional states. *Human Physiol* 1:394–402, 1975.

Deicken RF: Captopril treatment of depression. *Biol Psychiatry* 21:1425–1428, 1986.

De la Fuente JR, Berlanga C, León-Andrade C: Mania induced by tricyclic-MAOI combination therapy in bipolar treatment-resistant disorder: Case reports. *J Clin Psychiatry* 47:40–41, 1986.

Delay J, Deniker P: Drug-induced extrapyramidal syndromes. In: Vinken PJ, Bruyn GW, eds: *Handbook of Clinical Neurology: Diseases of the Basal Ganglia.* Amsterdam: North Holland, 1968. pp 248–266.

Deleon-Jones F, Maas JW, Dekirmenjian H, Sanchez J: Diagnostic subgroups of affective disorders and their urinary excretion of catecholamine metabolites. *Am J Psychiatry* 132:1141–1148, 1975.

d'Elia G, Perris C: Selbstmordversuche im Laufe unipolarer und bipolarer Depressionen [Attempted suicide during depressive (unipolar) and manic depressive (bipolar) psychoses.] *Acta Psychiatr Nervenkr* 212:339–356, 1969.

d'Elia G, Perris C: Cerebral functional dominance and depression: An analysis of EEG amplitude in depressed patients. *Acta Psychiatr Scand* 49:191–197, 1973.

DeLisi LE, King AC, Targum S: Serum immunoglobulin concentrations in patients admitted to an acute psychiatric in-patient service. *Br J Psychiatry* 145:661–665, 1984.

DeLisi LE, Goldin, Hamovit JR, Maxwell ME, Kurtz D, Gershon ES: A family study of the association of increased ventricular size with schizophrenia. *Arch Gen Psychiatry* 43:148–153, 1986a.

DeLisi LE, Nurnberger JS, Goldin LR, Simmons-Alling S, Gershon ES: Epstein-Barr virus and depression. Letter. *Arch Gen Psychiatry* 43:815–816, 1986b.

DeLong GR, Aldershof A: Associations of special abilities with juvenile manic-depressive illness. *Ann Neurol* 14:362, 1983.

DeLong GR, Aldershof AL: Long-term experience with lithium treatment in childhood: Correlation with clinical diagnosis. *J Am Acad Child Adolesc Psychiatry* 26:389–394, 1987.

DeLong GR, Nieman GW: Lithium-induced behavior changes in children with symptoms suggesting manic-depressive illness. *Psychopharmacol Bull* 19:258–265, 1983.

Del Vecchio M, Iorio G, Cocorullo M, Vacca L, Amati A: Has SAMe (Ado-Met) an antidepressant effect? A preliminary trial versus chlorimipramine. *Revista Sperimentale di Freniatria* 102:343–358, 1978.

Del Zompo M, Bocchetta A, Goldin LR, Corsini GU: Linkage between X-chromosome markers and manic-depressive illness: Two Sardinian pedigrees. *Acta Psychiatr Scand* 70:282–287, 1984.

Demeester-Mirkine N, Dumont JE: The hypothalamo-pituitary thyroid axis. In: M de Visscher, ed: *The Thyroid Gland*. New York: Raven Press, 1980. pp 145–152.

Dement W, Kleitman N: Cyclic variations in EEG during sleep and their relation to eye movements, body motility, and dreaming. *Electroencephalogr Clin Neurophysiol* 9:673–690, 1957.

Demers RG, Davis LS: The influence of prophylactic lithium treatment on the marital adjustment of manic-depressives and their spouses. *Compr Psychiatry* 12:348–353, 1971.

Demers RG, Heninger GR: Visual-motor performance during lithium treatment: A preliminary report. *J Clin Pharmacol* 11:247–279, 1971.

Demitrack MA, Gold PW: Oxytocin: Neurobiologic considerations and their implications for affective illness. *Prog Neuropsychopharmacol Biol Psychiatry* 12(Suppl):S23-S51, 1988.

dé Montigny C, Grunberg F, Mayer A, Deschenes JP: Lithium induces rapid relief of depression in tricyclic antidepressant drug non-responders. *Br J Psychiatry* 138:252–256, 1981.

dé Montigny C, Cournoyer G, Morissette R, Langlois R, Caillé G: Lithium carbonate addition in tricyclic antidepressant-resistant unipolar depression: Correlations with the neurobiologic actions of tricyclic antidepressant drugs and lithium ion on the serotonin system. *Arch Gen Psychiatry* 40:1327–1334, 1983.

dé Montigny C, Elie R, Caillé G: Rapid response to the addition of lithium in iprindole-resistant unipolar depression: A pilot study. *Am J Psychiatry* 142:220–223, 1985.

Deniker P, Eygiem A, Bernheim R, Lôo H, Delarue P: Thyroid antibody levels during lithium therapy. *Neuropsychobiology* 4:270–275, 1978.

DePaulo JR, Folstein MF, Correa EI: The course of delirium due to lithium toxicity. *J Clin Psychiatry* 43:447–449, 1982.

DePaulo JR, Correa EI, Folstein MF: Does lithium stabilize mood? *Biol Psychiatry* 18:1093–1097, 1983.

DePaulo JR, Correa EI, Sapir DG: Renal function and lithium: A longitudinal study. *Am J Psychiatry* 143:892–895, 1986.

Deptula D, Yozawitz A: Lateralized brain dysfunction in depression: Analysis of memory. *Int J Neurosci* 24:319, 1984.

Depue RA: Criteria for a hyperthymic period. Presented at the NIMH Seasonal Affective Disorder Workshop. Bethesda, May, 1987.

Depue RA, Iacono WG: Neurobehavioral aspects of affective disorders. *Annu Rev Psychol* 40:457–492, 1989.

Depue RA, Klein DN: Identification of unipolar and bipolar affective conditions in nonclinical and clinical populations by the General Behavior Inventory.

In: DL Dunner, ES Gershon, JE Barrett, eds: *Relatives at Risk for Mental Disorder*. New York: Raven Press, 1988. pp 179–204.

Depue RA, Monroe SM: The unipolar-bipolar distinction in the depressive disorders. *Psychol Bull* 85:1001–1029, 1978.

Depue RA, Spoont MR: Conceptualizing a serotonin trait: A behavioral dimension of constraint. *Ann NY Acad Sci* 487:47–62, 1986.

Depue RA, Slater JF, Wolfstetter-Kausch H, Klein D, Goplerud E, Farr D: A behavioral paradigm for identifying persons at risk for bipolar depressive disorder: A conceptual framework and five validation studies. *J Abnorm Psychol Monograph* 90:381–437, 1981.

Depue RA, Kleiman RM, Davis P, Hutchinson M, Krauss SP: The behavioral high-risk paradigm and bipolar affective disorder, VIII: Serum free cortisol in nonpatient cyclothymic subjects selected by the General Behavior Inventory. *Am J Psychiatry* 142:175–181, 1985.

Depue RA, Krauss SP, Spoont MR: A two-dimensional threshold model of seasonal bipolar affective disorder. In: D Magnusson, A Öhman: *Psychopathology: An Interactional Perspective*. Orlando: Academic Press, 1987. pp 95–123.

Depue RA, Iacono WG, Muir R, Arbisi P: Effect of phototherapy on spontaneous eye blink rate in subjects with seasonal affective disorder. *Am J Psychiatry* 145:1457–1459, 1988.

Depue RA, Krauss S, Spoont MR, Arbisi: General Behavior Inventory identification of unipolar and bipolar affective conditions in a nonclinical university population. *J Abnorm Psychol* 98:117–126, 1989a.

Depue RA, Arbisi P, Spoont MR, Krauss S, Leon A, Ainsworth B: Seasonal and mood independence of low basal prolactin secretion in premenopausal women with seasonal affective disorder. *Am J Psychiatry* 146:989–995, 1989b.

Derby IM: Manic-depressive "exhaustion" deaths: An analysis of "exhaustion" case histories. *Psychiatr Q* 7:435–449, 1933.

Derogatis LR, Lipman RS, Rickels K, Uhlenhuth EH, Covi L: The Hopkins Symptom Checklist (HSCL): A measure of primary symptom dimensions. *Mod Probl Pharmacopsychiat* 7:79–110, 1974.

Desai NG, Gangadhas BN, Channabasavanna SM, Shetty KT: Carbamazepine hastens therapeutic action of lithium in mania. *Proc Intl Conf on New Directions in Affective Disorders*. April, 1987. p 47.

Dessauer M, Goetze U, Tölle R: Periodic sleep deprivation in drug-refractory depression. *Neuropsychobiology* 13:111–116, 1985.

Detera-Wadleigh SD, Berrettini WH, Goldin LR, Boorman D, Anderson S, Gershon ES: Close linkage of c-Harvey-ras-1 and the insulin gene to affective disorder is ruled out in three North American pedigrees. *Nature* 325:806–808, 1987.

Detre T, Himmelhoch J, Swartzburg M, Anderson CM, Byck R, Kupfer DJ: Hypersomnia and manic-depressive disease. *Am J Psychiatry* 128:1303–1305, 1972.

Deutsch SI, Campbell M: Status of cholinesterase activities in blood in neuropsychiatric disorders. *Neurochem Res* 9:863–869, 1984.

Deutsch SI, Peselow ED, Banay-Schwartz M, Gershon S, Virgilio J, Fieve RR, Rotrosen J: Effect of lithium on glycine levels in patients with affective disorders. *Am J Psychiatry* 138:683–684, 1981.

Deutsch SI, Stanley M, Peselow ED, Banay-Schwartz M: Glycine: A possible role in lithium's action and affective illness. *Neuropsychobiology* 9:215–218, 1983.

Devanand DP, Bowers MB, Hoffman FJ, Nelson JC: Elevated plasma homovanillic acid in depressed females with melancholia and psychosis. *Psychiatry Res* 15:1–4, 1985.

Devanand DP, Lo I, Sackeim HA, Halbreich U, Ross F, Cooper T: Acute and subacute effects of electroconvulsive therapy on plasma oxytocin and vasopressin in depressed patients. Abstract of paper presented at the 42nd Annual Meeting of the Society of Biological Psychiatry, May 1987. p 284.

Devanand DP, Bowers MB Jr, Hoffman FJ Jr, Sackeim HA: Acute and subacute effects of ECT on plasma HVA, MHPG, and prolactin. *Biol Psychiatry* 26:408–412, 1989.

Dewan MJ, Haldipur CV, Lane E, Donnelly MP, Boucher M, Major LF: Normal cerebral asymmetry in bipolar patients. *Biol Psychiatry* 22:1058–1066, 1987.

Dewan MJ, Haldipur CV, Lane EE, Ispahani A, Boucher MF, Major LF: Bipolar affective disorder I: Comprehensive quantitative computed tomography. *Acta Psychiatr Scand* 77:670–676, 1988a.

Dewan MJ, Haldipur CV, Boucher MF, Ramachandran T, Major LF: Bipolar affective disorder II: EEG, neuropsychological, and clinical correlates of CT abnormality. *Acta Psychiatr Scand* 77:677–682, 1988b.

Dewhurst K: A seventeenth-century symposium on manic-depressive psychosis. *Br J Med Psychology* 35:113–125, 1962.

Dewhurst WG: Methysergide in mania. *Nature* 219:506–507, 1968.

De Wied D: Peptides and adaptive behaviour. In: D de Wied, PA Van Keep, eds: *Hormones and the Brain*. Baltimore: University Park Press, 1980. pp 103–113.

Deykin EY, DiMascio A: Relationship of patient background characteristics to efficacy of pharmacotherapy in depression. *J Nerv Ment Dis* 155:209–215, 1972.

Deykin EY, Levy JC, Wells V: Adolescent depression, alcohol and drug abuse. *Am J Public Health* 77:178–182, 1987.

Diaz J, Ellison G, Masuoka D: Opposed behavioral syndromes in rats with partial and more complete central serotonergic lesions made wiith 5,6-dihyroxytrytamine. *Psychopharmacology* 37:67–79, 1974.

Dick DAT, Naylor GJ, Dick EG: Effects of lithium on sodium transport across membranes. In: FN Johnson, S Johnson, eds: *Lithium in Medical Practice*. Baltimore: University Park Press, 1978. pp 173–182.

Dick DAT, Naylor GJ, Dick EG: Plasma vanadium concentration in manic-depressive illness. *Psychol Med* 12:533–537, 1982.

Dick G, Gay D: Multiple sclerosis—autoimmune or microbial? A critical review with additional observations. *J Infect* 16:25–35, 1988.

Dickson WE, Kendell RE: Does maintenance lithium therapy prevent recurrences of mania under ordinary clinical conditions? *Psychol Med* 16:521–530, 1986.

Diefendorf AR, Dodge R: An experimental study of the ocular reactions of the insane from photographic records. *Brain* 31:451–489, 1908.

Dietzel M, Saletu B, Lesch OM, Sieghart W, Schjerve M: Light treatment in depressive illness: Polysomnographic, psychometric and neuroendocrinological findings. *Eur Neurol* 25 (Suppl 2):93–106, 1986.

Dilsaver SC: The pathophysiologies of substance abuse and affective disorders: An integrative model? *J Clin Psychopharm* 7:1–10, 1987.

Dilsaver SC, Flemmer DD: Bright light blocks the capacity of forced swim stress to supersensitize a muscarinic mechanism. ACNP abstract, 1988.

Dilsaver SC, Greden JF: Antidepressant withdrawal-induced activation (hypomania and mania): Is withdrawal-induced cholinergic overdrive causally significant? *J Clin Psychopharmacol* 4:174–175, 1984.

Dinan TG, Kohen D: Tardive dyskinesia in bipolar affective disorder: Relationship to lithium therapy. *Br J Psychiatry* 155:557–57, 1989.

Dion GL, Tohen M, Anthony WA, Waternaux CS: Symptoms and functioning of patients with bipolar disorder six months after hospitalization. *Hosp Community Psychiatry* 39:652–657, 1988.

Direkze M, Baylias SG, Cutting J: Primary tumours of the frontal lobe. *Br J Clin Practice* 25:207–213, 1971.

Ditman KS: Review and evaluation of current drug therapies in alcoholism. *Int J Psychiatry* 3:248–258, 1967.

Dix J: *The Life of Thomas Chatterton*. London: Hamilton, Adams & Co, 1837.

Docherty JP, Fiester SJ: The therapeutic alliance and compliance with psychopharmacology. In: RE Hales, AJ Frances, eds: *American Psychiatric Association Annual Review, vol 4*. American Psychiatric Press Inc, 1985. pp 607–632.

Docherty JP, Fiester SJ, Shea T: Syndrome diagnosis and personality disorder. In: RE Hales, AJ Frances, eds: *Psychiatry Update: Annual Review, Vol 5*. Washington, DC: American Psychiatric Press, 1986. pp 315–355.

Dohrenwend BP, Dohrenwend BS: Social and cultural influences on psychopathology. *Ann Rev Psychol* 25:417–452, 1974.

Dolan RJ, Calloway SP, Mann AH: Cerebral ventricular size in depressed subjects. *Psychol Med* 15:873–878, 1985.

Dolan RJ, Calloway SP, Thacker PF, Mann AH: The cerebral cortical appearance in depressed subjects. *Psychol Med* 16:775–779, 1986.

Domino EF, Riaz A, Rodin E, Demetriou S, Mathews B, Tait S: Effect of duration of lithium therapy of various psychiatric patients on red blood cell/plasma choline ratio. *Psychopharmacol Bull* 17:174–175, 1981.

Donaldson IM, Cunningham J: Persisting neurologic sequelae of lithium carbonate therapy. *Arch Neurol* 40:747–751, 1983.

Donis-Keller H, Green P, Helms C, Cartinhaur S, Weiffenbach B, Stephens K, Keith TP, Bowden DW, Smith DR, Lander ES, Botstein D, Akots G, Rediker KS, Gravius T, Brown VA, Rising MB, Parker C, Powers JA, Watt DE, Kauffman ER, Bricker A, Phipps P, Muller-Kahle H, Fulton TR, Ng S, Schumm JW, Braman JC, Knowlton RG, Barker DF, Crooks SM, Lincoln SE, Daly MJ, Abrahamson J: A genetic linkage map of the human genome. *Cell* 51:319–337, 1987.

Donnelly EF, Murphy DL: Social desirability and bipolar affective disorder. *J Consult Clin Psychol* 41:469, 1973.

Donnelly EF, Murphy DL: Primary affective disorder: Bender-Gestalt sequence of placement as an indicator of impulse control. *Percept Mot Skills* 38:1079–1082, 1974.

Donnelly EF, Dent JK, Murphy DL, Mignone RJ: Comparison of temporal lobe epileptics and affective disorders on the Halstead-Reitan Test Battery. *J Clin Psychol* 28:61–62, 1972.

Donnelly EF, Murphy DL, Scott WH: Perception and cognition in patients with bipolar and unipolar depressive disorders: A study in Rorschach responding. *Arch Gen Psychiatry* 32:1128–1131, 1975.

Donnelly EF, Murphy DL, Goodwin FK: Cross-sectional and longitudinal comparisons of bipolar and unipolar depressed groups on the MMPI. *J Consult Clin Psychol* 44:233–237, 1976.

Donnelly EF, Goodwin FK, Waldman IN, Murphy DL: Prediction of antidepressant responses to lithium. *Am J Psychiatry* 135:552–556, 1978a.

Donnelly EF, Murphy DL, Goodwin FK: Primary affective disorder: Anxiety in unipolar and bipolar depressed groups. *J Clin Psychol* 34:621–623, 1978b.

Donnelly EF, Waldman IN, Murphy DL, Wyatt RJ, Goodwin FK: Primary affective disorder: Thought disorder in depression. *J Abnorm Psychol* 89:315–319, 1980.

Donnelly EF, Murphy DL, Goodwin FK, Waldman IN: Intellectual function in primary affective disorder. *Br J Psychiatry* 140:633–636, 1982.

Donovan DM, O'Leary MR: Relationship between distortions in self-perception of depression and psychopathology. *J Clin Psychol* 32:16–19, 1976.

Dooley L: A psychoanalytic study of manic depressive psychoses. *Psychoanal Rev* 8:38–72 and 144–167, 1921.

Doran AR, Rubinow DR, Roy A, Pickar D: CSF somatostatin and abnormal response to dexamethasone administration in schizophrenic and depressed patients. *Arch Gen Psychiatry* 43:365–369, 1986.

Dorpat TL, Ripley HS: A study of suicide in the Seattle area. *Compr Psychiatry* 1:349–359, 1960.

Dorus E, Pandey GN, Davis JM: Genetic determinant of lithium ion distribution: An in vitro and in vivo monozygotic-dizygotic twin study. *Arch Gen Psychiatry* 32:1097–1102, 1975.

Dorus E, Pandey GN, Shaughnessy R, Davis JM: Low platelet monoamine oxidase activity, high red blood cell lithium ratio, and affective disorders: A multivariate assessment of genetic vulnerability to affective disorders. *Biol Psychiatry* 14:989–993, 1979a.

Dorus E, Pandey GN, Shaughnessy R, Gaviria M, Val E, Ericksen S, Davis JM: Lithium transport across red cell membrane: A cell membrane abnormality in manic-depressive illness. *Science* 205:932–934, 1979b.

Dorus E, Pandey GN, Shaughnessy R, Davis JM: Lithium transport across the RBC membrane: A study of genetic factors. *Arch Gen Psychiatry* 37:80–81, 1980.

Dorus E, Cox NJ, Gibbons RD, Shaughnessy R, Pandey GN, Cloninger CR: Lithium ion transport and affective disorders within families of bipolar patients: Identification of a major gene locus. *Arch Gen Psychiatry* 40:545–552, 1983.

Dorus W, Senay EC: Depression, demographic dimensions and drug abuse. *Am J Psychiatry* 137:699–704, 1980.

Drake ME: Episodic depression and hypomania with temporal EEG paroxysms. *Psychosomatics* 29:354–357, 1988.

Dratman MB, Crutchfield FL, Gordon JT, Jennings AS: Iodothyronine homeostasis in rat brain during hypo- and hyperthyroidism. *Am J Physiol* 245:E185–E193, 1983.

Drimmer EJ, Gitlin MJ, Gwirtsman HE: Desipramine and methylphenidate combination treatment for depression: Case report. *Am J Psychiatry* 140:241–242, 1983.

Drugan RC, Skolnick P, Paul SM, Crawley JN: A pretest procedure reliably predicts performance in two animal models of inescapable stress. *Pharmacol Biochem Behav* 33:649–654, 1989.

Duarte-Escalante O, Ellinwood EH: Effects of chronic amphetamine intoxication on adrenergic and cholinergic structures in the central nervous system: Histochemical observations in cats and monkeys. In: E Ellinwood, S Cohen, eds: *Current Concepts on Amphetamine Abuse*. Washington, DC: National Institute of Mental Health, United States Government Printing Office, 1972. pp 97–106.

Dubé S, Kumar N, Ettedgui E, Pohl R, Jones D, Sitaram N: Cholinergic REM induction response: Separation of anxiety and depression. *Biol Psychiatry* 20:408–418, 1985.

Dubé S, Jones D, Bush C, Muskiewsky C, Sitaram N: Presence of ACh supersensitivity increases familial risk of MDD and panic in MDD probands. *Int J Neurs* 32:1–2, 1987.

Dubovsky SL, Franks RD: Intracellular calcium ions in affective disorders: A review and an hypothesis. *Biol Psychiatry* 18:781–797, 1983.

Dubovsky SL, Franks RD, Lifschitz M, Coen P: Effectiveness of verapamil in the treatment of a manic patient. *Am J Psychiatry* 139:502–504, 1982.

Dubovsky SL, Franks RD, Schrier D: Phenelzine-induced hypomania: Effect of verapamil. *Biol Psychiatry* 20:1009–1014, 1985.

Dubovsky SL, Christiano J, Daniell LC, Franks RD, Murphy J, Adler L, Baker N, Harris RA: Increased platelet intracellular calcium concentration in patients with bipolar affective disorders. *Arch Gen Psychiatry* 46:632–638, 1989.

Duch DS, Woolf JH, Nichol CA, Davidson JR, Garbutt JC: Urinary excretion of biopterin and neopterin in psychiatric disorders. *Psychiatry Res* 11:83–89, 1984.

Dufour H, Bouchacourt M, Thermoz P, Viala A, Rop PP, Gouezo F, Durand A, Petersen HEH: Citalopram: A highly selective 5-HT uptake inhibitor in the treatment of depressed patients. *Int Clin Psychopharmacol* 2:225–237, 1987.

Duncan WC, Wehr TA: Pharmacological and non-pharmacological chronotherapies of depression. In: A Reinberg, M Smolensky, G Labrecque, eds: *Annual Review of Chronopharmacology*. Vol. 4, New York: Pergamon Press, 1988. pp 137–170.

Duncan WC Jr, Pettigrew KD, Gillen JC: REM architecture changes in bipolar and unipolar depression. *Am J Psychiatry* 136:1424–1427, 1979.

Duncavage MB, Nasr SJ, Altman EG: Subjective side effects of lithium carbonate: A longitudinal study. *J Clin Psychopharmacol* 3:100–102, 1983.

Dunner DL: Unipolar and bipolar depression: Recent findings from clinical and biologic studies. In: *The Psychobiology of Affective Disorders*. Pfizer Symp. Depression. Basel: Karger, 1980. pp 11–24.

Dunner DL: Stability of bipolar II affective disorder as a diagnostic entity. *Psychiatr Ann* 17:18–20, 1987.

Dunner DL, Fieve RR: Clinical factors in lithium prophylaxis failure. *Arch Gen Psychiatry* 30:229–233, 1974.

Dunner DL, Goodwin FK: Effect of L-tryptophan on brain serotonin metabolism in depressed patients. *Arch Gen Psychiatry* 26:364–366, 1972.

Dunner DL, Dwyer T, Fieve R: Depressive symptoms in patients with unipolar and bipolar affective disorder. *Compr Psychiatry* 17:447–451, 1976a.

Dunner DL, Fleiss JL, Fieve RR: The course of development of mania in patients with recurrent depression. *Am J Psychiatry* 133:905–908, 1976b.

Dunner DL, Fleiss JL, Fieve RR: Lithium carbonate prophylaxis failure. *Br J Psychiatry* 129:40–44, 1976c.

Dunner DL, Gershon ES, Goodwin FK: Heritable factors in the severity of affective illness. *Biol Psychiatry* 11:31–42, 1976d.

Dunner DL, Stallone F, Fieve RR: Lithium carbonate and affective disorders: V. A double-blind study of

prophylaxis of depression in bipolar illness. *Arch Gen Psychiatry* 33:117–120, 1976e.

Dunner DL, Levitt M, Kumbaraci T, Fieve RR: Erythrocyte catechol-o-methyltransferase activity in primary affective disorder. *Biol Psychiatry* 12:237–244, 1977a.

Dunner DL, Patrick V, Fieve RR: Rapid cycling manic depressive patients. *Compr Psychiatry* 18:561–566, 1977b.

Dunner DL, Meltzer HL, Fieve RR: Clinical correlates of the lithium pump. *Am J Psychiatry* 135:1062–1064, 1978.

Dunner DL, Hensel BM, Fieve RR: Bipolar illness: Factors in drinking behavior. *Am J Psychiatry* 136:583–585, 1979a.

Dunner DL, Murphy D, Stallone F, Fieve RR: Episode frequency prior to lithium treatment in bipolar manic-depressive patients. *Compr Psychiatry* 20:511–515, 1979b.

Dunner DL, Murphy D, Stallone F, Fieve RR: Affective episode frequency and lithium therapy. *Psychopharmacol Bull* 16:49–50, 1980.

Dunner DL, Russek FD, Russek B, Fieve RR: Classification of bipolar affective disorder subtypes. *Compr Psychiatry* 23:186–189, 1982.

Dunner DL, Jie SQ, Ping ZY, Dunner PZ: A study of primary affective disorder in the People's Republic of China. *Biol Psychiatry* 19:353–359, 1984.

Dunner DL, Myers J, Khan A, Avery D, Ishiki D, Pyke R: Adinazolam: A new antidepressant: Findings of a placebo-controlled, double-blind study in outpatients with major depression. *J Clin Psychopharmacol* 7:170–172, 1987.

Dupont RM, Jernigan TL, Gillin JC, Butters N, Delis DC, Hesselink JR: Subcortical signal hyperintensities in bipolar patients detected by MRI. *Psychiatry Res* 21:357–358, 1987.

Dupont RM, Cullum CM, Jeste DV: Poststroke depression and psychosis. *Psychiatr Clin North Am* 11:133–149, 1988.

Dupont RM, Jernigan TL, Butters N, Delis DC, Hesselink JR, Heindel W, Gillin JC: Subcortical abnormalities detected in bipolar affective disorder using magnetic resonance imaging: Clinical and neuropsychological significance. *Arch Gen Psychiatry* 47:55–59, 1990.

Dvoredsky AE, Stewart MA: Hyperactivity followed by manic-depressive disorder: Two case reports. *J Clin Psychiatry* 42:212–214, 1981.

Dwyer JT, DeLong GR: A family history study of twenty probands with childhood manic-depressive illness. *J Am Acad Child Adol Psychiatry* 26:176–180, 1987.

Dyson WL, Mendels J: Lithium and depression. *Curr Ther Res* 10:601–608, 1968.

Eagles JM, Whalley LJ: Decline in the diagnosis of schizophrenia among first admissions to Scottish mental hospitals from 1969–78. *Br J Psychiatry* 146:151–154, 1985.

Eastwood MR, Peacocke J: Seasonal patterns of suicide, depression and electroconvulsive therapy. *Br J Psychiatry* 129:472–475, 1976.

Eastwood MR, Peter AM: Editorial: Epidemiology and seasonal affective disorder. *Psychol Med* 18:799–806, 1988.

Eastwood MR, Stiasny S: Psychiatric disorder, hospital admission, and season. *Arch Gen Psychiatry* 35:769–771, 1978.

Eastwood MR, Stiasny S, Meier HMR, Woogh CM: Mental illness and mortality. *Compr Psychiatry* 23:377–385, 1982.

Eastwood MR, Whitton JL, Kramer PM, Peter AM: Infradian rhythms: A comparison of affective disorders and normal persons. *Arch Gen Psychiatry* 42:295–299, 1985.

Eaton JW, Weil RJ: *Culture and Mental Disorders: A Comparative Study of the Hutterites and Other Populations.* New York: Free Press, 1955.

Eaton WW, Kessler LG, eds: *Epidemiologic Field Methods in Psychiatry: The NIMH Epidemiologic Catchment Area Program.* New York: Academic Press, 1985.

Eaton WW, Regier DA, Locke BZ, Taube CA: The Epidemiologic Catchment Area Program of the National Institute of Mental Health. *Public Health Rep* 96:319–325, 1981.

Eaton WW, Kramer M, Anthony JC, Dryman A, Shapiro S, Locke BZ: The incidence of specific DIS/DSM-III mental disorders: Data from the NIMH Epidemiologic Catchment Area Program. *Acta Psychiatr Scand* 79:163–178, 1989.

Ebstein RP, Oppenheim G, Ebstein BS, Amiri Z, Stessman J: The cyclic AMP second messenger system in man: The effects of heredity, hormones, drugs, aluminum, age and disease on signal amplification. *Prog Neuropsychopharmacol Biol Psychiatry* 10:323–353, 1986.

Ebstein RP, Moscovich D, Zeevi S, Amiri Z, Lerer B: Effect of lithium in vitro and after chronic treatment on human platelet adenylate cyclase activity: Postreceptor modification of second messenger signal amplification. *Psychiatry Res* 21:221–228, 1987.

Ebstein RP, Lerer B, Shapira B, Shemesh Z, Moscovich DG, Kindler S: Cyclic AMP second-messenger signal amplification in depression. *Br J Psychiatry* 152:665–669, 1988.

Economou SG, Stefanis CN: Changes of electrooculogram (EOG) in Parkinson's disease. *Acta Neurol Scand* 58:44–52, 1978.

Economou SG, Stefanis CN: Electrooculographic (EOG) findings in manic-depressive illness. *Acta Psychiatr Scand* 60:155–162, 1979.

Edman G, Åsberg M, Levander S, Schalling D: Skin conductance habituation and cerebrospinal fluid 5-hydroxyindoleacetic acid in suicidal patients. 43:586–592, 1986.

Edmunds LN Jr: *Cellular and Molecular Bases of Biological Clocks: Models and Mechanisms for Circadian Timekeeping.* New York: Springer-Verlag, 1988.

Edwards DJ, Spiker DG, Neil JF, Kupfer DJ, Rizk M: MHPG excretion in depression. *Psychiatry Res* 2:295–305, 1980.

Egeland JA: Bipolarity: The iceberg of affective disorders? *Compr Psychiatry* 24:337–344, 1983.

Egeland JA, Hostetter AM: Amish Study, I: Affective disorders among the Amish, 1976–1980. *Am J Psychiatry* 140:56–61, 1983.

Egeland JA, Sussex JN: Suicide and family loading for affective disorders. *JAMA* 254:915–918, 1985.

Egeland JA, Hostetter AM, Eshleman SK III: Amish Study, III: The impact of cultural factors on diagnosis of bipolar illness. *Am J Psychiatry* 140:67–71, 1983.

Egeland JA, Kidd JR, Frazer A, Kidd KK, Neuhauser VI: Amish study, V: Lithium-sodium countertransport and catechol *O*-methyltransferase in pedigrees of bipolar probands. *Am J Psychiatry* 141:1049–1054, 1984.

Egeland JA, Blumenthal RL, Nee J, Sharpe L, Endicott J: Reliability and relationship of various ages of onset criteria for major affective disorder. *J Affective Disord* 12:159–165, 1987a.

Egeland JA, Gerhard DS, Pauls DL, Sussex JN, Kidd KK, Allen CR, Hostetter AM, Housman DE: Bipolar affective disorders linked to DNA markers on chromosome 11. *Nature* 325:783–787, 1987b.

Ehlers CL, Frank E, Kupfer DJ: Social zeitgebers and biological rhythms: A unified approach to understanding the etiology of depression. *Arch Gen Psychiatry* 45:948–952, 1988.

Ehrensing RH, Kastin AJ: Melanocyte-stimulating hormone-release inhibiting hormone as a antidepressant: A pilot study. *Arch Gen Psychiatry* 30:63–65, 1974.

Ehrlich BE, Diamond JM: Lithium fluxes in human erythrocytes. *Am J Physiol* 237:C102-C110, 1979.

Ehrlich BE, Diamond JM: Lithium, membranes, and manic-depressive illness. *J Membr Biol* 52:187–200, 1980.

Ehsanullah RS: Uptake of 5-hydroxytryptamine and dopamine into platelets from depressed patients and normal subjects—influence of clomipramine, desmethylclomipramine and maprotiline. *Postgrad Med J* 56 (Suppl 1):31–35, 1980.

Eisemann M: Social class and social mobility in depressed patients. *Acta Psychiatr Scand* 73:399–402, 1986.

Eisenbruch M: Affective disorders in parents: Impact upon children. In: DP Cantwell, GA Carlson, eds: *Affective Disorders in Childhood and Adolescence: An Update.* Jamaica, NY: Spectrum Publications, 1983. pp 279–333.

Eissler KR: Psychopathology and creativity. *Am Imago* 24:35–81, 1967.

Eitinger L: The incidence of mental disease among refugees in Norway. *J Ment Sci* 105:326–338, 1959.

Ekman P, Friesen WV: Nonverbal behavior in psychopathology. In: KJ Friedman, MM Katz, eds: *The Psychology of Depression: Contemporary Theory and Research.* Washington, DC: VH Winston & Sons, 1974. pp. 203–224.

El-Guebaly N: Manic-depressive psychosis and drug abuse. *Can Psychiatr Assoc J* 20:595–598, 1975.

El-Mallakh RS: The Na,K-ATPase hypothesis for manic-depression: II. The mechanism of action of lithium. *Med Hypotheses* 12:269–282, 1983.

El-Mallakh RS: Complications of concurrent lithium and electroconvulsive therapy: A review of clinical material and theoretical considerations. *Biol Psychiatry* 23:595–601, 1988.

Elia J, Katz IR, Simpson GM: Teratogenicity of psychotherapeutic medications. *Psychopharmacol Bull* 23:531–586, 1987.

Elizur A, Shopsin B, Gershon S, Ehlenberger A: Intra:extracellular lithium ratios and clinical course in affective states. *Clin Pharmacol Ther* 13:947–953, 1972.

Elizur A, Groff E, Steiner, Davidson S: Intra/extra red blood cell lithium and electrolyte distributions as correlates of neurotoxic reactions during lithium therapy. In: ES Gershon, RH Belmaker, SS Kety, Rosenbaum M, eds: *The Impact of Biology on Modern Psychiatry*. New York: Plenum Press, 1977. pp 55–64.

Ellicott AG: A prospective study of stressful life events and bipolar illness. Unpublished doctoral dissertation, University of California, Los Angeles, 1988.

Ellinwood EH, Petrie WM: Drug-induced psychoses. In: RW Pickens, LL Heston, eds: *Psychiatric Factors in Drug Abuse*. New York: Grune and Stratton, 1979. pp 301–336.

Ellis H: *A Study of British Genius*. London: Hurst & Blackett, 1904.

Elsenga S, Van den Hoofdakker RH: Clinical effects of sleep deprivation and clomipramine in endogenous depression. *J Psychiatr Res* 17:361–74, 1983.

Elsenga S, Van den Hoofdakker RH: Body core temperature and depression during total sleep deprivation in depressives. *Biol Psychiatry* 24:531–540, 1988.

Elston RC: Ascertainment and age of onset in pedigree analysis. *Hum Hered* 23:105–112, 1973.

Elston RC, Lange K: The prior probability of autosomal linkage. *Ann Hum Genet* 38:341–350, 1975.

Elston RC, Sobel E: Sampling considerations in the gathering and analysis of pedigree data. *Am J Hum Gen* 31:62–69, 1979.

Elston RC, Stewart J: A general model for the genetic analysis of pedigree data. *Hum Hered* 21:523–542, 1971.

Elston RC, Yelverton KC: General models for segregation analysis. *Am J Hum Genet* 27:31–45, 1975.

Emerson RW: Experience. In: RW Emerson: *Selected Essays*. New York: Viking Penguin, 1982.

Emery R, Weintraub S, Neale JM: Effects of marital discord on the school behavior of children of schizophrenic, affectively disordered, and normal parents. *J Abnorm Child Psychol* 10:215–228, 1982.

Emrich HM, Eilert P: Evaluation of speech and language in neuropsychiatric disorders. *Arch Psychiat Nervenkr* 225:209–221, 1978.

Emrich HM, Cording C, Piree S, Kölling A, Möller HJ, Von Zerssen D, Herz A: Actions of naloxone in

different types of psychoses. In: E Usdin, WE Bunney, NS Kline, eds: *Endorphins in Mental Health Research*. New York: Oxford University Press, 1979. pp 452–460.

Emrich HM, Von Zerssen D, Kissling W, Möller HJ, Windorfer A: Effect of sodium valproate on mania: The GABA-hypothesis of affective disorders. *Arch Psychiatr Nervenkr* 229:1–16, 1980.

Emrich HM, Von Zerssen D, Kissling W, Möller HJ: On a possible role of GABA in mania: Therapeutic efficacy of sodium valproate. *Adv Biochem Psychopharmacol* 26:287–296, 1981.

Emrich HM, Aldenhoff JB, Lux HD, eds: *Basic Mechanisms in the Action of Lithium*. Amsterdam: Excerpta Medica, 1982a.

Emrich HM, Vogt P, Herz A: Possible antidepressive effects of opioids: Action of buprenorphine. *Ann NY Acad Sci* 398:108–112, 1982b.

Emrich HM, Vogt P, Herz A, Kissling W: Antidepressant effects of buprenorphine. Letter. *Lancet* 2:709, 1982c.

Emrich HM, Altmann H, Dose M, von Zerssen D: Therapeutic effects of GABA-ergic drugs in affective disorders: A preliminary report. *Pharmacol Biochem Behav* 19:369–372, 1983.

Emrich HM, Dose M, Günther R, Von Zerssen D: The use of valproate and oxcarbamazepine in affective disorders. In: P Pichot, P Berner, R Wolf, K Thau, eds: *Psychiatry: The State of the Art*. New York: Plenum Press, 1985. pp 455–458.

Enâchescu C: Aspects of pictorial creation in manic-depressive psychosis. *Confin Psychiat* 14:133–142, 1971.

Endicott J, Spitzer RL, Fleiss JL, Cohen J: The global assessment scale: A procedure for measuring overall severity of psychiatric disturbance. *Arch Gen Psychiatry* 33:766–771, 1976.

Endicott J, Nee J, Andreasen N, Clayton P, Keller M, Coryell W: Bipolar II: Combine or keep separate? *J Affective Disord* 8:17–28, 1985.

Endicott J, Nee J, Coryell W, Keller M, Andreasen N, Croughan J: Schizoaffective, psychotic, and nonpsychotic depression: Differential familial association. *Compr Psychiatry* 27:1–13, 1986.

Endicott NA: Psychophysiological correlates of "bipolarity." *J Affective Disord* 17:47–56, 1989.

Endler NS: *Holiday of Darkness: A Psychologist's Personal Journey Out of His Depression*. (1982). Toronto: Wall & Thompson, 1990.

Engelsmann F, Katz J, Ghadirian AM, Schachter D: Lithium and memory: A long-term follow-up study. *J Clin Psychopharmacology* 8:207–212, 1988.

English OS: Observation of trends in manic-depressive psychosis. *Psychiatry* 12:125–133, 1949.

Engstrom FW, Robbins DR, May JG: Manic-depressive illness in adolescence: A case report. *J Am Acad Child Psychiatry* 17:514–520, 1978.

Entwistle C, Taylor RM, MacDonald IA: Treatment of mania with haloperidol (serenace). *J Ment Sci* 108:373–375, 1962.

Erard R, Luisada PV, Peale R: The PCP psychosis:

Prolonged intoxication or drug-induced functional illness? *J Psychedelic Drugs* 12:235–251, 1980.

Erikson EH: *Young Man Luther: A Study in Psychoanalysis and History*. New York: WW Norton, 1962.

Esche I, Joffe RT, Blank DW: Erythrocyte electrolytes in psychiatric illness. *Acta Psychiatr Scand* 78:695–697, 1988.

Escobar JI, Gomez J, Tuason VB: Depressive phenomenology in North and South American patients. *Am J Psychiatry* 140:47–51, 1983.

Esler M, Turbott J, Schwarz R, Leonard P, Bobik A, Skewa H, Jackman G: The peripheral kinetics of norepinephrine in depressive illness. *Arch Gen Psychiatry* 39:295–300, 1982.

Esparon J, Kolloori J, Naylor GJ, McHarg AM, Smith AHW, Hopwood SE: Comparison of the prophylactic action of flupenthixol with placebo in lithium treated manic-depressive patients. *Br J Psychiatry* 148:723–725, 1986.

Esquirol JED: *Des Maladies Mentales* Paris: Balliére, 1838. Translated by EK Hunt as *Mental Maladies: A Treatise on Insanity*. Philadelphia: Lea and Blanchard, 1845 (facsimile edition by Hafner, London, 1966).

Estroff TW, Gold MS: Medical and psychiatric complications of cocaine abuse with possible points of pharmacological treatment. *Adv Alcohol Subst Abuse* 5:61–76, 1986.

Estroff TW, Dackis CA, Gold MS, Pottash ALC: Drug abuse and bipolar disorders. *Int J Psychiatry Med* 15:37–40, 1985.

Ettlinger RW: Suicides in a group of patients who had previously attempted suicide. *Acta Psychiatr Scand* 40:363–378, 1964.

Evans DL, Nemeroff CB: The dexamethasone suppression test in mixed bipolar disorder. *Am J Psychiatry* 140:615–617, 1983.

Evans DL, Strawn SK, Haggerty JJ Jr, Garbutt JC, Burnett GB, Pedersen CA: Appearance of mania in drug-resistant bipolar depressed patients after treatment with L-triiodothyronine. *J Clin Psychiatry* 47:521–522, 1986.

Evans RW, Clay TH, Gualtieri CT: Carbamazepine in pediatric psychiatry. *J Am Acad Child Adolesc Psychiatry* 26:2–8, 1987.

Extein I, Goodwin FK, Lewy AJ, Schoenfeld RI, Fakhur LR: Behavioral and biochemical effects of FK 33–824, a parenterally and orally active enkephalin analog. In: E Usdin, WE Bunney, NS Kline, eds: *Endorphins in Mental Health Research*. New York: Oxford University Press, 1979a. pp 279–292.

Extein I, Lo C, Goodwin FK, Schoenfeld RI: Dopamine-mediated behavior produced by the enkephalin analogue FK 33–824. *Psychiatry Res* 1:333–339, 1979b.

Extein I, Tallman J, Smith CC, Goodwin FK: Changes in lymphocyte beta-adrenergic receptors in depression and mania. *Psychiatry Res* 1:191–197, 1979c.

Extein I, Pottash AL, Gold MS, Sweeney DR, Martin DM, Goodwin FK: Deficient prolactin response to morphine in depressed patients. *Am J Psychiatry* 137:845–846, 1980a.

Extein I, Pottash AL, Gold MS, Martin DM: Differentiating mania from schizophrenia by the TRH test. *Am J Psychiatry* 137:981–982, 1980b.

Extein I, Pickar D, Gold MS, Gold PW, Pottash AL, Sweeney DR, Ross RJ, Rebard R, Martin D, Goodwin FK: Methadone and morphine in depression. *Psychopharmacol Bull* 17:29–33, 1981a.

Extein I, Pottash AL, Gold MS: Relationship of thyrotropin-releasing hormone test and dexamethasone suppression test abnormalities in unipolar depression. *Psychiatry Res* 4:49–53, 1981b.

Extein I, Pottash ALC, Gold MS: Does subclinical hypothyroidism predispose to tricyclic-induced rapid mood cycles? *J Clin Psychiatry* 43:290–291, 1982.

Extein I, Pottash AL, Gold MS: The TRH test in affective disorders: Experience in a private clinical setting. *Psychosomatics* 25:379–80, 383, 385–6 passim, 1984a.

Extein I, Pottash ALC, Gold MS, Cowdry RW: Changes in TSH response to TRH in affective illness. In: RM Post, JC Ballenger, eds: *Neurobiology of Mood Disorders*. Baltimore: Williams & Wilkins, 1984b. pp 297–310.

Eysenck HJ: The questionnaire measurement of neuroticism and extraversion. *Revista di Psicologia* 50:113–140, 1956.

Eysenck HJ: *The Maudsley Personality Inventory: Manual*. London: University of London Press, 1959.

Eysenck HJ: *The Structure of Human Personality*. 3rd ed. (1st ed 1953) London: Methuen and New York: Wiley, 1970.

Eysenck HJ, Eysenck SBG: *Eysenck Personality Inventory*. San Diego: Educational and Industrial Testing Service, 1963a.

Eysenck HJ, Eysenck SBG: *Manual of the Eysenck Personality Inventory*. San Diego: Educational and Industrial Testing Service, 1963b.

Eysenck HJ, Eysenck SBG: *Manual of the Eysenck Personality Inventory*. 4th ed. (1st ed. 1964). London: University, 1971.

Fabian AA, Donohue JF: Maternal depression: A challenging child guidance problem. *Am J Orthopsychiatry* 26:400–405, 1956.

Fabre LF, Brodie HKH, Garver D, Zung WWK: A multicenter evaluation of bupropion versus placebo in hospitalized depressed patients. *J Clin Psychiatry* 44:88–94, 1983.

Fabrega H Jr, Mezzich JE, Mezzich AC, Coffman GA: Descriptive validity of DSM-III depressions. *J Nerv Ment Dis* 174:573–584, 1986.

Fähndrich E, Coper H, Christ W, Helmchen H, Müller-Oerlinghausen B, Pietzcker A: Erythrocyte COMT-activity in patients with affective disorders. *Acta Psychiatr Scand* 61:427–437, 1980.

Falconer DS: The inheritance of liability to certain diseases, estimated from the incidence among relatives. *Ann Hum Genet* 29:51–71, 1965.

Falret JP: Mémoire sur la folie circulaire, forme de maladie mentale caractérisée par la reproduction successive et régulière de l'état maniaque, de l'état mélancolique, et d'un intervalle lucide plus ou moins prolongé. *Bulletin de l'Académie de Médecine* 19:382–415, 1854.

Falret J: La folie circulaire ou folie a formes alternes. In: *Etudes Cliniques sur les Maladies Mentales et Nerveuses*. Paris: Librairie JB Bailliere et Fils, 1890.

Famularo R, Stone K, Popper C: Preadolescent alcohol abuse and dependence. *Am J Psychiatry* 1442:1187–1189, 1985.

Fankhauser MP, Lindon JL, Connolly B, Healey WJ: Evaluation of lithium-tetracycline interaction. *Clin Pharm* 7:314–317, 1988.

Fann WE, Wheless JC: Effects of psychotherapeutic drugs on geriatric patients. In: C Usdin, I Forrest, eds: *Psychotherapeutic Drugs*. Part I. New York: Marcel Dekker, 1977. pp 545–565.

Fann WE, Asher H, Luton FH: Use of lithium in mania (with comment on underlying personality types). *Dis Nerv Syst* 30:605–610, 1969.

Faragalla FF, Flach FF: Studies of mineral metabolism in mental depression: I. The effects of imipramine and electric convulsive therapy on calcium balance and kinetics. *J Nerv Ment Dis* 151:120–129, 1970.

Faravelli C, Pole E: Stability of the diagnosis of primary affective disorder: A four-year follow-up study. *J Aff Disord* 4:35–39, 1982.

Faris REL, Dunham HW: *Mental Disorders in Urban Areas: An Ecological Study of Schizophrenia and Other Psychoses*. Chicago: University of Chicago Press, 1939.

Fauman MA: The central nervous system and the immune system. *Biol Psychiatry* 17:1459–1482, 1982.

Fava GA, Molnar G, Block B, Lee JS, Perini GI: The lithium loading dose method in a clinical setting. *Am J Psychiatry* 141:812–813, 1984.

Fawcett J: Valproate use in acute mania and bipolar disorder: An international perspective. *J Clin Psychiatry* 50(Suppl):10–12, 1989.

Fawcett J, Scheftner W, Clark D, Hedeker D, Gibbons R, Coryell W: Clinical predictors of suicide in patients with major affective disorders: A controlled prospective study. *Am J Psychiatry* 144:35–40, 1987.

Fawcett J, Scheftner W, Fogg L, Clark DC, Young MA, Hedeker D, Gibbons R: Suicide: Time-related predictors of suicide in major affective disorder. *Am J Psychiatry* 147:1189–1194, 1990.

Feder L: *Madness in Literature*. Princeton: Princeton University Press, 1980.

Feighner JP, Robins E, Guze SB, Woodruff RA, Winokur G, Munoz R: Diagnostic criteria for use in psychiatric research. *Arch Gen Psychiatry* 26: 57–63, 1972.

Feighner JP, Meredith CH, Frost NR, Chaimas S, Hendrickson G: A double-blind comparison of alprazolam vs. imipramine and placebo in the treatment of major depressive disorder. *Acta Psychiatr Scand* 68:223–233, 1983.

Feighner JP, Meredith CH, Stern WC, Hendrickson G, Miller LL: A double-blind study of bupropion and placebo in depression. *Am J Psychiatry* 141:525–529, 1984.

Feighner JP, Herbstein J, Damlouji N: Combined MAOI, TCA, and direct stimulant therapy of treatment-resistant depression. *J Clin Psychiatry* 46:206–209, 1985.

Feinberg M, Carroll BJ: Separation of subtypes of depression using discriminate analysis: Separation of bipolar endogenous depression from nonendogenous ("neurotic") depression. *J Affective Disord* 5:129–139, 1983.

Feinberg M, Carroll BJ: Biological "markers" for endogenous depression: Effect of age, severity of illness, weight loss, and polarity. *Arch Gen Psychiatry* 41:1080–1085, 1984.

Feinberg M, Carroll BJ, Smouse PE, Rawson SG: The Carroll Rating Scale for Depression: III. Comparison with other rating instruments. *Br J Psychiatry* 138:205–209, 1981a.

Feinberg M, Greden JF, Carroll BJ: The effect of amphetamine on plasma-cortisol in patients with endogenous and non-endogenous depression. *Psychoneuroendocrinology* 6:355–357, 1981b.

Fenichel O: *The Psychoanalytic Theory of Neuroses*. New York: WW Norton, 1945.

Fernstrom JD: Food-induced changes in brain serotonin synthesis: Is there a relationship to appetite for specific macronutrients? *Appetite* 8:163–182, 1987.

Ferrari E, Bossolo PA, Vailati A, Martinelli I, Rea A, Nosari I: [Effects of a vagolytic substance on the circadian rhythm of the ACTH-secreting system in man]. *Ann Endocrinol (Paris)* 38:203–213, 1977.

Feuchtwanger E: Die funktionen des stirnhirns. *Gesamtgebiete der Neurologie und Psychiatrie Heft* 38:1–194, 1923.

Fibiger HC, Phillips AG: Increased intracranial self-stimulation in rats after long-term administration of desipramine. *Science* 214:683–685, 1981.

Fieve RR: The lithium clinic: A new model for the delivery of psychiatric services. *Am J Psychiatry* 132:1018–1022, 1975a.

Fieve RR: *Moodswing: The Third Revolution in Psychiatry*. New York: William Morrow, 1975b.

Fieve RR, Jamison KR: Rubidium: Overview and clinical perspectives. *Mod Probl Pharmacopsychiatry* 18:145–163, 1982.

Fieve RR, Platman SR, Plutchik RR: The use of lithium in affective disorders I: Acute endogenous depression. *Am J Psychiatry* 125:487–491, 1968.

Fieve RR, Platman SR, Fleiss JL: A clinical trial of methysergide and lithium in mania. *Psychopharmacologia* 15:425–429, 1969.

Fieve RR, Kumbaraci T, Dunner DL: Lithium prophylaxis of depression in bipolar I, bipolar II, and unipolar patients. *Am J Psychiatry* 133:925–930, 1976.

Fieve RR, Go R, Dunner DL, Elston R: Search for biological/genetic markers in a long-term epidemiological and morbid risk study of affective disorders. *J Psychiatr Res* 18:425–445, 1984.

Fink M: *Convulsive Therapy—Theory and Practice.* New York: Raven Press, 1979a.

Fink M: Efficacy of ECT. *Lancet* 2:1303–1304, 1979b.

Fink M: Convulsive therapy in affective disorders: A decade of understanding and acceptance. In: HY Meltzer, ed: *Psychopharmacology: The Third Generation of Progress.* New York: Raven Press, 1987. pp 1071–1076.

Fink M, Simeon J, Itil TM, Freedman AM: Clinical antidepressant activity of cyclazocine—a narcotic antagonist. *Clin Pharmacol Ther* 11:41–48, 1970.

Fink M, Papakostas Y, Lee J, Meehan T, Johnson L: Clinical trials with des-tyr-gamma-endorphin (GK-78). In: C. Perris, G Struwe, B Jansson, eds: *Biological Psychiatry 1981.* Amsterdam: Elsevier, 1981. pp 398–401.

Finley CB, Wilson DC: The relation of the family to manic-depressive psychosis. *Dis Nerv Sys* 12:39–43, 1951.

Fischer E, Spatz H, Heller B, Reggiani H: Phenylethylamine content of human urine and rat brain: Its alteration in pathological conditions and after drug administration. *Experientia* 28:307–311, 1972.

Fischer E, Heller B, Nachon M, Spatz H: Therapy of depression by phenylalanine: Preliminary note. *Arzneimittelforschung* 25:132, 1975.

Fischer KA: Changes in test performance of ambulatory depressed patients undergoing electro-shock therapy. *J Gen Psychol* 41:195–232, 1949.

Fischer PJ, Shapiro S, Breakey WR, Anthony JC, Kramer M: Mental health and social characteristics of the homeless: A survey of mission users. *Am J Public Health* 76:519–524, 1986.

Fitzgerald FS: *The Crack-up.* New York: New Directions, 1956.

Fitzgerald RG: Mania as a message: Treatment with family therapy and lithium carbonate. *Am J Psychother* 26:547–553, 1972.

Flach FF, Faragalla FF: The effects of imipramine and electric convulsive therapy on the excretion of various minerals in depressed patients. *Br J Psychiatry* 116:437–438, 1970.

Flemenbaum A, Larson JW: ABO-RH blood groups and psychiatric diagnosis: A critical review. *Dis Nerv Syst* 37:581–583, 1976.

Fleminger JJ, Dalton R, Standage KF: Handedness in psychiatric patients. *Br J Psychiatry* 131:448–452, 1977.

Flor-Henry P: Psychosis and temporal lobe epilepsy: A controlled investigation. *Epilepsia* 10:363–395, 1969.

Flor-Henry P: Laterality, shifts of cerebral dominance, sinistrality and psychosis. In: J Gruzelier, P Flor-Henry, eds: *Hemispheric Asymmetries of Function in Psychopathology.* New York: Elsevier, 1979. pp 3–19.

Flor-Henry P: *The Cerebral Basis of Psychopathology.* Boston: John Wright, 1983.

Flor-Henry P, Gruzelier J: *Laterality and Psychopathology.* Amsterdam: Elsevier, 1983.

Flor-Henry P, Koles ZJ: Statistical quantitative EEG studies of depression, mania, schizophrenia and normals. *Biol Psychol* 19:257–279, 1984.

Flor-Henry P, Yeudall LT: Neuropsychological investigation of schizophrenia and manic-depressive psychoses. In: Gruzelier J, Flor-Henry P, eds: *Hemisphere Asymmetries of Function in Psychopathology.* Amsterdam: Elsevier, 1979. pp 341–362.

Fogarty SJ, Hemsley DR: Depression and accessibility of memories: A longitudinal study. *Br J Psychiatry* 142:232–237, 1983.

Foley KM, Kourides IA, Inturrisi CE, Kaiko RF, Zaroulis CG, Posner JB, Houde RW, Li CH: Beta-endorphin: Analgesic and hormonal effects in humans. *Proc Natl Acad Sci USA* 76:5377–5381, 1979.

Folstein MF, Luria R: Reliability, validity, and clinical application of the visual analogue mood scale. *Psychol Med* 3:479–486, 1973.

Folstein MF, Maiberger R, McHugh PR: Mood disorder as a specific complication of stroke. *J Neurol Neurosurg Psychiatry* 40:1018–1020, 1971.

Folstein MF, DePaulo JR Jr, Trepp K: Unusual mood stability in patients taking lithium. *Br J Psychiatry* 140:188–191, 1982.

Folstein SE, Abbott MH, Chase GA, Jensen BA, Folstein MF: The association of affective disorder with Huntington's Disease in a case series and in families. *Psychol Med* 13:537–542, 1983.

Ford J, Hillard JR, Giesler LJ, Lassen KL, Thomas H: Substance abuse/mental illness: Diagnostic issues. *Am J Drug Alcohol Abuse* 15:297–307, 1989.

Forrest GG: Psychodynamically oriented treatment of alcoholism and substance abuse. In: Bratter TE, Forrest GG, eds: *Alcoholism and Substance Abuse.* New York: Free Press, 1985. pp 307–336.

Foster JR, Rosenthal JS: Lithium treatment of the elderly. Inn: FN Johnson, ed: *Handbook of Lithium Therapy.* Baltimore: University Park Press, 1980. pp 414–420.

Foulds GA: Temperamental differences in maze performance: Part II: The effect of distraction and of electroconvulsive therapy on psychomotor retardation. *Br J Psychol* 43:33–41, 1952.

Fox HA: Convalescent phase of bipolar disorder. *J Clin Psychiatry* 49:452–454, 1988.

France RD, Krishnan KRR: Alprazolam-induced manic reaction. *Am J Psychiatry* 1127–1128, 1984.

Frances A, Brown RP, Kocsis JH, Mann JJ: Psychotic depression: A separate entity? *Am J Psychiatry* 138:831–833, 1981.

Frangos E, Athanassenas G, Tsitourides S, Psilolignos P, Robos A, Katsanou N, Bulgaris Ch: Seasonality of the episode of recurrent affective psychoses: Possible prophylactic interventions. *J Affective Disord* 2:239–247, 1980.

Frangos E, Athanassenas G, Tsitourides S, Psilolignos P, Katsanou N: Psychotic depressive disorder: A separate entity? *J Affective Disord* 5:259–265, 1983.

Frank E, Kupfer DJ: Maintenance treatment of recurrent unipolar depression: Pharmacology and psychotherapy. In: D Demali, G Racagni, eds: *Chronic Treatments in Neuropsychiatry*. New York: Raven Press, 1985. pp 139–151.

Frank E, Targum SD, Gershon ES, Anderson C, Stewart BD, Davenport Y, Ketchum KL, Kupfer DJ: A comparison of nonpatient with bipolar patient-well spouse couples. *Am J Psychiatry* 138:764–768, 1981.

Frank E, Prien RF, Kupfer DJ, Alberts L: Implications of noncompliance on research in affective disorders. *Psychopharmacol Bull* 21:37–42, 1985.

Frankenburg FR, Tohen M, Cohen BM, Lipinski JF: Long-term response to carbamazepine: A retrospective study. *J Clin Psychopharmacol* 8:130–132, 1988.

Franks RD, Adler LE, Waldo MC, Alpert J, Freedman R: Neurophysiological studies of sensory gating in mania: Comparison with schizophrenia. *Biol Psychiatry* 18:989–1005, 1983.

Franz SI: The time of some mental processes in the retardation and excitement of insanity. *Am J Psychol* 17:38–68, 1906.

Fraser A: *Cromwell: The Lord Protector*. New York: Alfred A Knopf, 1973.

Fraser WI, King KM, Thomas P, Kendell RE: The diagnosis of schizophrenia by language analysis. *Br J Psychiatry* 148:275–278, 1986.

Frazer A, Mendels J: Sodium ion retention and red blood cell lithium ion concentrations in affective disorders. In E Usdin, DA Hamburg, JD Barchas: *Neuroregulators and Psychiatric Disorders*. New York: Oxford University Press, 1977. pp 478–487.

Frazer A, Mendels J, Brunswick D, London J, Pring M, Ramset TA, Rybakowski J: Erythrocyte concentrations of the lithium ion: Clinical correlates and mechanisms of action. *Am J Psychiatry* 135:1065–1069, 1978.

Frazer A, Ramsey TA, Swann A, Bowden C, Brunswick D, Garver D, Secunda S: Plasma and erythrocyte electrolytes in affective disorders. *J Affective Disord* 5:103–113, 1983.

Freed EX: Alcohol abuse by manic patients. *Psychol Rep* 25:280, 1969.

Freed EX: Alcoholism and manic-depressive disorders: Some perspectives. *Q J Stud Alcohol* 31:62–89, 1970.

Freedman DX: Preface. In: DX Freedman, ed: *Biology of the Major Psychoses: A Comparative Analysis*. Research Publications: Association for Research in Nervous and Mental Disease. Vol 54. New York: Raven Press, 1975. pp vii–viii.

Freeman D:. *Margaret Mead and Samoa: The Making and Unmaking of an Anthropological Myth*. Cambridge, Mass: Harvard University Press, 1983.

Freeman DS: *R.E. Lee*. New York: Charles Scribners, 1961.

Freeman RL, Galaburda AM, Cabal RD, Geschwind N: The neurology of depression: Cognitive and behavioral deficits with focal findings in depression and resolution after electroconvulsive therapy. *Arch Neurol* 42:289–291, 1985.

Freinhar JP, Alvarez WH: Use of clonazepam in two cases of acute mania. *J Clin Psychiatry* 46:29–30, 1985a.

Freinhar JP, Alvarez WH: Androgen-induced hypomania. Letter. *J Clin Psychiatry* 46:354–355, 1985b.

Fremming KH: *The Expectation of Mental Infirmity in a Sample of the Danish Population*. No 7. Occasional Papers in Eugenics. London: Cassell & Co, Ltd., 1951.

Freud S: Mourning and melancholia. (1917). In: W Gaylin, ed: *The Meaning of Despair: Psychoanalytic Contributions to the Understanding of Depression*. New York: Science House, 1968.

Freud S: Uber coca. 1884. In: R Byck, ed: *Cocaine Papers: Sigmund Freud*. New York: Stonehill Publishing Co, 1974. pp 49–73.

Freudenberger HJ: Individual treatment of substance abusers in independent practice. In: Bratter TE, Forrest GG, eds: *Alcoholism and Substance Abuse*. New York: Free Press, 1985. pp 337–348.

Frey R: Die prämorbide Persönlichkeit von monopolar und bipolar Depressiven: Ein Vergleich aufgrund von Persönlichkeitstests. *Archiv Psychiatr Nervenkr* 224:161–173, 1977.

Frézal J, Klinger HP, eds: Human Gene Mapping 9: Paris Conference (1987). Ninth International Workshop on Human Gene Mapping. *Cytogenet Cell Genet* 46, 1987.

Friedl W, Propping P: ^{3}H-imipramine binding in human platelets: A study in normal twins. *Psychiatry Res* 11:279–285, 1984.

Friedl W, Propping P, Weck B: ^{3}H-imipramine binding in platelets: Influence of varying proportions of intact platelets in membrane preparations on binding. *Psychopharmacology (Berlin)* 80:96–99, 1983.

Friedman AS: Minimal effects of severe depression on cognitive functioning. *J Abnorm Soc Psychol* 69:237–243, 1964.

Friedman AS: Interaction of drug therapy with martial therapy in depressed patients. *Arch Gen Psychiatry* 32:619–637, 1975.

Friedman MJ: Does receptor supersensitivity accompany depressive illness? *Am J Psychiatry* 135:107–109, 1978.

Friedman RC, Clarkin JF, Corn R, Aronoff MS, Hurt SW, Murphy MC: DSM-III and affective pathology in hospitalized adolescents. *J Nerv Ment Dis* 170:511–521, 1982.

Friedman RC, Aronoff MS, Clarkin JF, Corn R, Hurt SW: History of suicidal behavior in depressed borderline inpatients. *Am J Psychiatry* 140:1023–1026, 1983a.

Friedman RC, Hurt SW, Clarkin JF, Corn R, Aronoff MS: Symptoms of depression among adolescents and young adults. *J Affective Disord* 5:37–43, 1983b.

Friis ML: Antiepileptic drugs and teratogenesis: How should patients, doctors and health authorities be counselled? *Acta Neurol Scand* (Suppl 94):39–43, 1983.

Frith CD, Stevens M, Johnstone EC, Deakin JFW, Lawler P, Crow TJ: Effects of ECT and depression on various aspects of memory. *Br J Psychiatry* 142:610–617, 1983.

Fritze J, Beckmann H: Erythrocyte acetylcholinesterase in psychiatric disorders and controls. *Biol Psychiatry* 22:1097–1106, 1987.

Fromm D, Schopflocher D: Neuropsychological test performance in depressed patients before and after drug therapy. *Biol Psychiatry* 19:55–72, 1984.

Fromm-Auch D: Comparison of unilateral and bilateral ECT: Evidence for selective memory impairment. *Br J Psychiatry* 141:608–613, 1982.

Fromm-Reichmann F: Intensive psychotherapy of manic-depressives: A preliminary report. *Confina Neurologica* 9:158–165, 1949.

Frosch WA: Moods, madness, and music: I. Major affective disease and musical creativity. *Compr Psychiatry* 28:315–322, 1987.

Frosch WA: The "case" of George Frideric Handel. *N Engl J Med* 321:765–769, 1989.

Fukuda K, Etoh T, Iwadate T, Ishii A: The course and prognosis of manic-depressive psychosis: A quantitative analysis of episodes and intervals. *Tohoku J Exp Med* 139:299–307, 1983.

Fuller RW: Serotonergic stimulation of pituitary-adrenocortical function in rats. *Neuroendocrinology* 32:118–127, 1981.

Fyer MR, Frances AJ, Sullivan T, Hurt SW, Clarkin J: Comorbidity of borderline personality disorder. *Arch Gen Psychiatry* 45:348–352, 1988.

Gabel RH, Barnard N, Norko M, O'Connell RA: AIDS presenting as mania. *Compr Psychiatry* 27:251–254, 1986.

Gadallah MF, Feinstein EI, Massry SG: Lithium intoxication: Clinical course and therapeutic considerations. *Mineral Electrolyte Metab* 14:146–149, 1988.

Gaekwad RS, Niyogi AK, Jagtiani R: ABO blood group genes in schizophrenia and manic depressive psychosis. *Ind J Med Sci* 26:493–495, 1972.

Gaensbauer TJ, Harmon RJ, Cytryn L, McKnew DH: Social and affective development in infants with a manic-depressive parent. *Am J Psychiatry* 141:223–229, 1984.

Gagrat DD, Spiro HR: Social, cultural, and epidemiological aspects of mania. In: RH Belmaker, HM van Praag, eds: *Mania: An Evolving Concept.* Jamaica, NY: Spectrum Publications, 1980. pp 291–307.

Gainotti G: Emotional behavior and hemispheric side of the lesion. *Cortex* 8:41–55, 1972.

Gajdusek DC: Unconventional viruses and the origin and disappearance of Kuru. *Science* 197:943–960, 1977.

Gammon GD, John K, Rothblum ED, Mullen K, Tischler GL, Weissman MM: Use of a structured diagnostic interview to identify bipolar disorder in adolescent inpatients: Frequency and manifestations of the disorder. *Am J Psychiatry* 140:543–547, 1983.

García-Sevilla JA, Zis AP, Hollingsworth MA, Greden JF, Smith CB: Platelet α_2-adrenergic receptors in major depressive disorder: Binding of tritiated clonidine before and after tricyclic antidepressant drug treatment. *Arch Gen Psychiatry* 38:1327–1333, 1981.

García-Sevilla JA, Guimón J, García-Vallejo P, Fuster MJ: Biochemical and functional evidence of supersensitive platelet alpha-2-adrenoceptors in major affective disorder: Effect of long-term lithium carbonate treatment. *Arch Gen Psychiatry* 43:51–57, 1986.

Gardner EA: Long-term preventive care in depression: The use of bupropion in patients intolerant of other antidepressants. *J Clin Psychiatry* 44:157–162, 1983.

Gardos G, Casey DE, eds: *Tardive Dyskinesia and Affective Disorders.* Washington, DC: American Psychiatric Press, 1984.

Garety P: Delusions: Problems in definition and measurement. *Br J Med Psychol* 58:25–34, 1985.

Garfinkel PE, Warsh JJ, Stancer HC, Sibony D: Total and free plasma tryptophan levels in patients with affective disorders: Effects of a peripheral decarboxylase inhibitor. *Arch Gen Psychiatry* 33:1462–1466, 1976.

Garfinkel PE, Warsh JJ, Stancer HC, Godse DD: CNS monoamine metabolism in bipolar affective disorder. *Arch Gen Psychiatry* 34:735–739, 1977.

Garfinkel PE, Brown GM, Warsh JJ, Stancer HC: Neuroendocrine responses to carbidopa in primary affective disorders. *Psychoneuroendocrinology* 4:13–20, 1979.

Garfinkel PE, Stancer HC, Persad E: A comparison of haloperidol, lithium carbonate and their combination in the treatment of mania. *J Affective Disord* 2:279–288, 1980.

Garland EJ, Remick RA, Zis AP: Weight gain with antidepressants and lithium. *J Clin Psychopharmacol* 8:323–330, 1988.

Garma A: The deceiving superego and the masochistic ego in mania. *Psychoanal Q* 37:63–79, 1968.

Garver DL, Hutchinson LJ: Psychosis, lithium-induced antipsychotic response, and seasonality. *Psychiatry Res* 26:279–286, 1988.

Garvey MJ, Johnson RA, Valentine RH, Schuster V: Use of an MMPI scale to predict antidepressant response to lithium. *Psychiatry Res* 10:17–20, 1983.

Garvey MJ, Mungas D, Tollefson GD: Hypersomnia

in major depressive disorders. *J Affective Disord* 6:283–286, 1984.

Garvey MJ, Hwang S, Teubner-Rhodes D, Zander J, Rhem C: Dextroamphetamine treatment in mania. *J Clin Psychiatry* 48:412–413, 1987.

Garvey MJ, Wesner R, Godes M: Comparison of seasonal and nonseasonal affective disorders. *Am J Psychiatry* 145:100–102, 1988.

Gasparrini WG, Satz P, Heilman KM, Coolidge FL: Hemisphere asymmetries of affective processing as determined by the Minnesota Multiphasic Personality Inventory. *J Neurol Neurosurg Psychiatry* 41:470–473, 1978.

Gass CS, Russell EW: Differential impact of brain damage and depression on memory test performance. *J Consult Clin Psychology* 54:261–263, 1986.

Gaviria M, Flaherty J, Val E: A comparison of bipolar patients with and without a borderline personality disorder. *Psychiatric J Univ Ottawa* 7:190–195, 1982.

Gawin FH, Kleber HD: Cocaine abuse treatment: Open pilot trial with desipramine and lithium carbonate. *Arch Gen Psychiatry* 41:903–909, 1984.

Gawin FH, Kleber HD: Abstinence symptomatology and psychiatric diagnosis in cocaine abusers. *Arch Gen Psychiatry* 43:107–113, 1986.

Gaylord JJ, Parker AL, Phillips EM, Rowsell AR: Whole blood 5-hydroxytryptamine during treatment of endogenous depressive illness. *Br J Psychiatry* 122:597–598, 1973.

Gelenberg AJ: Lithium: Dealing with difficult treatment issues. Abstract of paper presented at the 142nd annual meeting of the American Psychiatric Association, 1989.

Gelenberg AJ, Wojcik JD, Gibson CJ, Wurtman RJ: Tyrosine for depression. *J Psychiatr Res* 17:175–180, 1982–83.

Gelenberg AJ, Wojcik JD, Falk WE, Coggins CH, Brotman AW, Rosenbaum JF, LaBrie RA, Kerman BJ: Effects of lithium on the kidney. *Acta Psychiatr Scand* 75:29–34, 1987.

Gelernter J, Berrettini W, Nurnberger JI, Simmons-Alling S: Growth hormone response to clonidine in euthymic bipolar patients. Abstract of paper presented at the 42nd Annual meeting of the Society of Biological Psychiatry, May, 1987.

Gentsch C, Lichtsteiner M, Gastpar M, Gastpar G, Feer H: ³H-imipramine binding sites in platelets of hospitalized psychiatric patients. *Psychiatry Res* 14:177–187, 1985.

Geoghegan JJ, Stevenson GH: Prophylactic electroshock. *Am J Psychiatry* 105:494–496, 1949.

Georgi F: Psychophysische Korrelationen: III. Psychiatrische Probleme im Licte der Rhythmusforschung. *Schweiz Med Wochenschr* 49:1276–1280, 1947.

Gerner RH, Hare TA: CSF GABA in normal subjects and patients with depression, schizophrenia, mania, and anorexia nervosa. *Am J Psychiatry* 138:1098–1101, 1981.

Gerner RH, Sharp B: CSF beta-endorphin-immunoreactivity in normal, schizophrenic, depressed, manic and anorexic subjects. *Brain Res* 237:244–247, 1982.

Gerner RH, Wilkins JN: CSF cortisol in patients with depression, mania, or anorexia nervosa and in normal subjects. *Am J Psychiatry* 140:92–94, 1983.

Gerner RH, Yamada T: Altered neuropeptide concentrations in cerebrospinal fluid of psychiatric patients. *Brain Res* 238:298–302, 1982.

Gerner RH, Post RM, Bunney WE Jr: A dopaminergic mechanism in mania. *Am J Psychiatry* 133:1177–1180, 1976.

Gerner RH, Post RM, Gillin JC, Bunney WE Jr: Biological and behavioral effects of one night's sleep deprivation in depressed patients and normals. *J Psychiat Res* 15:21–40, 1979.

Gerner RH, Catlin DH, Gorelick DA, Hui KK, Li CH: Beta-endorphin: Intravenous infusion causes behavioral change in psychiatric inpatients. *Arch Gen Psychiatry* 37:642–647, 1980.

Gerner RH, Fairbanks L, Anderson GM, Young JG, Scheinin M, Linnoila M, Hare TA, Shaywitz BA, Cohen DJ: CSF neurochemistry in depressed, manic, and schizophrenic patients compared with that of normal controls. *Am J Psychiatry* 141:1533–1540, 1984.

Gerö G: Construction of depression. *Int J Psychoanal* 17:423–461, 1936.

Gershon ES: Should science be stopped? The case of recombinant DNA research. *The Public Interest* 71:3–16, Spring, 1983a.

Gershon ES: The genetics of affective disorders. In: L Grinspoon, ed: *Psychiatry Update*. Vol. 2. Washington, DC: American Psychiatric Press, 1983b. pp 434–538.

Gershon ES, Goldin LR: Clinical methods in psychiatric genetics: I. Robustness of genetic marker investigative strategies. *Acta Psychiatr Scand* 74:113–118, 1986.

Gershon ES, Guroff JJ: Information from relatives: Diagnosis of affective disorders. *Arch Gen Psychiatry* 41:173–180, 1984.

Gershon ES, Hamovit J: Genetic methods and preventive psychiatry. *Prog Neuropsychopharmacol Biol Psychiatry* 3:565–573, 1979.

Gershon ES, Jonas WZ: Erythrocyte soluble catechol-O-methyl transferase activity in primary affective disorder: A clinical and genetic study. *Arch Gen Psychiatry* 32:1351–1356, 1975.

Gershon ES, Liebowitz JH: Sociocultural and demographic correlates of affective disorders in Jerusalem. *J Psychiatr Res* 12:37–50, 1975.

Gershon ES, Matthysse S: X-linkage: Ascertainment through doubly ill probands. *J Psychiatr Res* 13:161–168, 1977.

Gershon ES, Dunner DL, Sturt L, Goodwin FK: Assortative mating in the affective disorders. *Biol Psychiatry* 7:63–74, 1973.

Gershon ES, Mark A, Cohen N, Belizon N, Baron M,

Knobe KE: Transmitted factors in the morbid risk of affective disorders: A controlled study. *J Psychiat Res* 12:283–299, 1975.

Gershon ES, Bunney WE, Jr, Leckman JF, Van Eerdewegh M, Debauche BA: The inheritance of affective disorders: A review of data and of hypotheses. *Behav Genet* 6:227–261, 1976.

Gershon ES, Targum SD, Kessler LR, Mazure CM, Bunney WE Jr: Genetic studies and biological strategies in the affective disorders. In: AG Steinberg, AG Bearn, AG Motulsky, B Childs, eds: *Progress in Medical Genetics, Vol. 2.* Philadelphia: WB Saunders Co, 1977. pp 101–164.

Gershon ES, Targum S, Matthysse S, Bunney WE Jr: Color blindness not closely linked to bipolar illness: Report of a new pedigree series. *Arch Gen Psychiatry* 36:1423–1430, 1979.

Gershon ES, Goldin LR, Lake CR, Murphy DL, Guroff JJ: Genetics of plasma dopamine-β-hydroxylase (DBH), erythrocyte catechol-O-methyltransferase (COMT), and platelet monoamine oxidase (MAO) in pedigrees of patients with affective disorders. In: E Usdin, TL Sourkes, MBH Youdim, eds: *Enzymes and Neurotransmitters in Mental Disease.* Chichester: John Wiley & Sons, 1980a. pp 281–299.

Gershon ES, Mendlewicz J, Gastpar M, Bech P, Goldin LR, Kielholz P, Rafaelsen OJ, Vartanian F, Bunney WE, Jr: A collaborative study of genetic linkage of bipolar manic-depressive illness and red/green colorblindness. *Acta Psychiatr Scand* 61:319–338, 1980b.

Gershon ES, Hamovit J, Guroff JJ, Dibble E, Leckman JF, Sceery W, Targum SD, Nurnberger JI Jr, Goldin LR, Bunney WE Jr: A family study of schizoaffective, bipolar I, bipolar II, unipolar, and normal control probands. *Arch Gen Psychiatry* 39:1157–1167, 1982a.

Gershon ES, Hamovit J, Schreiber JL, Dibble ED, Kaye W, Nurnberger JI Jr, Andersen A, Ebert M: Anorexia nervosa and major affective disorders associated in families: a preliminary report. *Proceedings of the Annual Meeting of the American Psychopathological Association.* 1982b.

Gershon ES, Schreiber JL, Hamovit JR, Dibble ED, Kaye W, Nurnberger JI Jr, Andersen AE, Ebert M: Clinical findings in patients with anorexia nervosa and affective illness in their relatives. *Am J Psychiatry* 141:1419–1422, 1984.

Gershon ES, McKnew D, Cytryn L, Hamovit J, Schreiber J, Hibbs E, Pellegrini D: Diagnosis in school-age children of bipolar affective disorder patients and normal controls. *J Affective Disord* 8:283–291, 1985a.

Gershon ES, Nadi NS, Nurnberger JI Jr, Berrettini WH: Failure to confirm muscarinic receptors on skin fibroblasts. Letter. *N Engl J Med* 312:862, 1985b.

Gershon ES, Weissman MM, Guroff JJ, Prusoff BA, Leckman JF: Validation of criteria for major depression through controlled family study. *J Affective Disord* 11:125–131, 1986.

Gershon ES, Berrettini W, Nurnberger J Jr, Goldin LR: Genetics of affective illness. In: HY Meltzer, ed: *Psychopharmacology: The Third Generation of Progress.* New York: Raven Press, 1987a. pp 481–491.

Gershon ES, Hamovit JH, Guroff JJ, Nurnberger JI: Birth-cohort changes in manic and depressive disorders in relatives of bipolar and schizoaffective patients. *Arch Gen Psychiatry* 44:314–319, 1987b.

Gershon ES, DeLisi LE, Hamovit J, Nurnberger JI Jr, Maxwell ME, Schreiber J, Dauphinais D, Dingman CW 2d, Guroff JJ: A controlled family study of chronic psychoses: Schizophrenia and schizoaffective disorder. *Arch Gen Psychiatry* 45:328–336, 1988.

Ghadirian AM, Nair NP, Schwartz G: Transmembrane lithium distribution and hypertension in manic depressive patients. *Prog Neuropsychopharmacol Biol Psychiatry* 13:525–530, 1989.

Ghadirian AM, Lehmann HE: Neurological side effects of lithium: Organic brain syndrome, seizures, extrapyramidal side effects, and EEG changes. *Compr Psychiatry* 21:327–335, 1980.

Ghadirian AM, Engelsmann F, Ananth J: Memory functions during lithium therapy. *J Clin Psychopharmacology* 3:313–315, 1983.

Ghose K: Lithium salts: Therapeutic and unwanted effects. *Br J Hosp Med* 18:578–583, 1977.

Ghose K, Turner P: Intravenous tyramine pressor response in depression. *Lancet* 1:1317–1318, 1975.

Giannini AJ, Extein I, Gold MS, Pottash ALC, Castellani S: Clonidine in mania. *Drug Dev Res* 3:101–103, 1983.

Giannini AJ, Pascarzi GA, Loiselle RH, Price WA, Giannini MC: Comparison of clonidine and lithium in the treatment of mania. *Am J Psychiatry* 143:1608–1609, 1986.

Giannini AJ, Taraszewski R, Loiselle RH: Verapamil and lithium in maintenance therapy of manic patients. *J Clin Pharmacol* 27:980–982, 1987.

Gibbons JL: Total body sodium and potassium in depressive illness. *Clin Sci* 19:133–138, 1960.

Gibbons JL: Electrolytes and depressive illness. *Postgrad Med J* 39:19–25, 1963.

Gibbons JL: Cortisol secretion rates in depressive illness. *Arch Gen Psychiatry* 10:572–575, 1964.

Gibbons RD, Davis JM: Consistent evidence for a biological subtype of depression characterized by low CSF monoamine levels. *Acta Psychiatr Scand* 74:8–12, 1986.

Gibbons RD, Dorus E, Ostrow DG, Pandey GN, Davis JM, Levy DL: Mixture distributions in psychiatric research. *Biol Psychiatry* 19:935–961, 1984.

Gibbs FA, Gibbs EL: *Atlas of Electroencephalography.* Vol. 2, *Epilepsy.* Cambridge, Mass: Addison-Wesley Press, Inc, 1952.

Gibson RW: Psychotherapy of manic-depressive states. *Psychiatr Res Rep* 17:91–102, 1963.

Gibson RW, Cohen MB, Cohen RA. On the dynamics of the manic-depressive personality. *Am J Psychiatry* 115:1101–1107, 1959.

Giles DE, Rush AJ, Roffwarg HP: Sleep parameters in bipolar I, bipolar II, and unipolar depressions. *Biol Psychiatry* 21:1340–1343, 1986.

Giles DE, Jarrett RB, Biggs MM, Guzick DS, Rush AJ: Clinical predictors of recurrence in depression. *Am J Psychiatry* 146:764–767, 1989a.

Giles DE, Roffwarg HP, Kupfer DJ, Rush AJ, Biggs MM, Etzel BA: Secular trends in unipolar depression: A hypothesis. *J Affective Disord* 16:71–75, 1989b.

Gill J, Horne DJ: Psychological testing in depressive illness: 1. Psychomotor performance. *Psychol Med* 4:470–473, 1974.

Gilliland AR, Wittman P, Goldman M: Patterns and scatter of mental abilities in various psychoses. *J Gen Psychology* 29:251–260, 1943.

Gillin JC: The sleep therapies of depression. *Prog Neuropsychopharmacol Biol Psychiatry* 7:351–364, 1983.

Gillin JC, Borbély AA: Sleep: A neurobiological window on affective disorders. *Trends in Neuroscience* 8:537–542, 1985.

Gillin JC, Sitaram N: Rapid eye movement (REM) sleep: Cholinergic mechanisms. *Psychol Med* 14:501–506, 1984.

Gillin JC, Mazure C, Post RM, Jimerson D, Bunney WE Jr: An EEG sleep study of a bipolar (manic-depressive) patient with a nocturnal switch process. *Biol Psychiatry* 12:711–718, 1977.

Gillin JC, Sitaram N, Wehr T, Duncan W, Post R, Murphy DL, Mendelson WB, Wyatt RJ, Bunney WE: Sleep and affective illness. In: RM Post, JC Ballenger, eds: *Neurobiology of Mood Disorders*. Baltimore: Williams & Wilkins, 1984. pp 157–189.

Gillin JC, Kelsoe J, Risch C, Darko D, Kalir H, Janowsky D: Cholinergic supersensitivity in depression. *Int J Neurs* 32:471, 1987.

Giroux R, ed: *Robert Lowell: Collected Prose*. New York: Farrar, Straus, Giroux, 1987.

Gitlin MJ, Jamison KR: Lithium clinics: Theory and practice. *Hosp Community Psychiatry* 35:363–368, 1984.

Gitlin MJ, Weiner H, Fairbanks L, Hershman JM, Friedfeld N: Failure of T_3 to potentiate tricyclic antidepressant response. *J Affective Disord* 13:267–272, 1987.

Gjerris A, Fahrenkrug J, Bøjholm S, Rafaelsen OJ: Vasoactive intestinal polypeptide in cerebrospinal fluid in psychiatric disorder. In: C Perris, G Struwe, B Jansson, eds: *Biological Psychiatry 1981*. Amsterdam: Elsevier, 1981a. pp 359–362.

Gjerris A, Jensen E, Christensen NJ, Rafaelsen OJ: Adrenaline and noradrenaline in psychiatric disorders. In: C. Perris, G Struwe, B Jansson, eds: *Biological Psychiatry 1981*. Amsterdam: Elsevier, 1981b. pp 565–568.

Gjerris A, Rafaelsen OJ, Vendsborg P, Fahrenkrug J, Rehfeld JF: Vasoactive intestinal polypeptide decreased in cerebrospinal fluid (CSF) in atypical depression: Vasoactive intestinal polypeptide, cho-

lecystokinin and gastrin in CSF in psychiatric disorders. *J Affective Disord* 7:325–337, 1984.

Gjerris A, Hammer M, Vendsborg P, Christensen NJ, Rafaelsen OJ: Cerebrospinal fluid vasopressin—changes in depression. *Br J Psychiatry* 147:696–701, 1985.

Gjerris A, Sørenson AS, Rafaelsen OJ, Werdelin L, Alling C, Linnoila M: 5-HT and 5-HIAA in cerebrospinal fluid in depression. *J Affective Disord* 12:13–22, 1987.

Gjessing R: Disturbances of somatic functions in catatonia with periodic course, and their compensation. *J Ment Sci* 84:608–621, 1938.

Gjessing RR: *Contributions to the Somatology of Periodic Catatonia*. Edited by LR Gjessing, FA Jenner. Oxford: Pergamon Press, 1976.

Glaser GH: Psychotic reactions induced by corticotropin (ACTH) and cortisone. *Psychosom Med* 15:280–291, 1953.

Glass L, Mackey MC: *From Clocks to Chaos: The Rhythms of Life*. Princeton, NJ: Princeton University Press, 1988.

Glassman AH, Platman SR: Potentiation of a monoamine oxidase inhibitor by tryptophan. *J Psychiatr Res* 7:83–88, 1969.

Glassman AH, Roose SP: Delusional depression: A distinct clinical entity? *Arch Gen Psychiatry* 38:424–427, 1981.

Glassner B, Haldipur CV: Life events and early and late onset of bipolar disorder. *Am J Psychiatry* 140:215–217, 1983.

Glassner B, Haldipur CV, Dessauersmith J: Role loss and working-class manic depression. *J Nerv Ment Dis* 167:530–541, 1979.

Gleick J: *Chaos: Making a New Science*. New York: Viking, 1987.

Glen AIM: Lithium regulation of membrane ATPases. In: FN Johnson, S Johnson, eds: *Lithium in Medical Practice*. Baltimore: University Park Press, 1978. pp 183–192.

Glen AIM, Ongley GC, Robinson K: Diminished membrane transport in manic-depressive psychosis and recurrent depression. *Lancet* 2:241–243, 1968.

Glen AIM, Dodd M, Hulme EB, Kreitman N: Mortality on lithium. *Neuropsychobiology* 5:167–173, 1979.

Glen AIM, Johnson AL, Shepherd M: Continuation therapy with lithium and amitriptyline in unipolar depressive illness: A controlled clinical trial. *Psychol Med* 11:409–416, 1981.

Glen AIM, Johnson AL, Shepherd M: Continuation therapy with lithium and amitriptyline in unipolar depressive illness: A randomized, double-blind, controlled study. *Psychol Med* 14:37–50, 1984.

Glick ID, Clarkin JF, Spencer JH, Maas GL, Lewis AB, Peyser J, DeMane N, Good-Ellis M, Harris E, Lestelle V: A controlled evaluation of inpatient family intervention: Preliminary results of the six-month follow-up. *Arch Gen Psychiatry* 42:882–886, 1985.

Glover EG: On the etiology of drug addiction. *Int J Psychoanal* 13:298–328, 1932.

Glue P: Rapid cycling affective disorders in the mentally retarded. *Biol Psychiatry* 26:250–256, 1989.

Glue PW, Nutt DJ, Cowen PJ, Broadbent D: Selective effect of lithium on cognitive performance in man. *Psychopharmacology (Berlin)* 91:109–111, 1987.

Godwin CD: The dexamethasone suppression test in acute mania. *J Affective Disord* 7:281–286, 1984.

Godwin CD, Greenberg LB, Shukla S: Consistent dexamethasone suppression test results with mania and depression in bipolar illness. *Am J Psychiatry* 141:1263–1265, 1984.

Goertzel V, Goertzel M: *Cradles of Eminence.* Boston: Little, Brown, 1962.

Goffman E. The insanity of place. *Psychiatry* 32:357–388, 1969.

Goggans FC: A case of mania secondary to vitamin B12 deficiency. *Am J Psychiatry* 141:300–301, 1984.

Gold BI, Bowers MB, Roth RH, Sweeney DW: GABA levels in CSF of patients with psychiatric disorders. *Am J Psychiatry* 137:362–364, 1980.

Gold MS, Pottash AL, Extein I: Hypothyroidism and depression. Evidence from complete thyroid function evaluation. *JAMA* 245:1919–1922, 1981.

Gold MS, Pottash AL, Extein I: "Symptomless" autoimmune thyroiditis in depression. *Psychiatry Res* 6:261–269, 1982.

Gold PW, Chrousos G: Clinical studies with corticotropin releasing factor: Implications for the diagnosis and pathophysiology of depression, Cushing's disease, and adrenal insufficiency. *Psychoneuroendocrinology* 10:401–419, 1985.

Gold PW, Goodwin FK: Vasopressin in affective illness. *Lancet* 1:1233–1236, 1978.

Gold PW, Goodwin FK, Wehr T, Rebar R, Sack R: Growth-hormone and prolactin response to levodopa in affective illness. Letter. *Lancet* 2:1308–1309, 1976.

Gold PW, Goodwin FK, Wehr T, Rebar R: Pituitary thyrotropin response to thyrotropin-releasing hormone in affective illness: Relationship to spinal fluid amine metabolites. *Am J Psychiatry* 134:1028–1031, 1977.

Gold PW, Weingartner H, Ballenger JC, Goodwin FK, Post RM: Effects of 1-desamo-8-D-arginine vasopressin on behaviour and cognition in primary affective disorder. *Lancet* 2:992–994, 1979.

Gold PW, Goodwin FK, Post RM, Robertson GL: Vasopressin function in depression and mania [proceedings]. *Psychopharmacol Bull* 17:7–9, 1981.

Gold PW, Ballenger JC, Robertson GL, Weingartner H, Rubinow DR, Hoban MC, Goodwin FK, Post RM: Vasopressin in affective illness: Direct measurement, clinical trials, and response to hypertonic saline. In: RM Post, JC Ballenger, eds: *Neurobiology of Mood Disorders.* Baltimore: Williams & Wilkins, 1984a. pp 323–339.

Gold PW, Chrousos G, Kellner C, Post R, Roy A, Augerinos P, Schulte H, Oldfield E, Loriaux DL: Psychiatric implications of basic and clinical studies with corticotropin-releasing factor. *Am J Psychiatry* 141:619–627, 1984b.

Gold PW, Loriaux DL, Roy A, Kling MA, Calbrese JR, Kellner CH, Nieman LK, Post RM, Pickar D, Gallucci W, Avgerinos P, Paul S, Oldfield EH, Cutler GB, Chrousos GP: Responses to corticotropin-releasing hormone in the hypercortisolism of depression and Cushing's disease: Pathophysiologic and diagnostic implications. *N Engl J Med* 314:1329–1335, 1986a.

Gold PW, Gwirtsman H, Avgerinos PC, Nieman LK, Gallucci WT, Kaye W, Jimerson D, Ebert M, Rittmaster R, Loriaux DL, Chrousos GP: Abnormal hypothalamic-pituitary-adrenal function in anorexia nervosa: Pathophysiologic mechanisms in underweight and weight-corrected patients. *N Engl J Med* 314:1335–1342, 1986b.

Gold PW, Goodwin FK, Chrousos GP: Clinical and biochemical manifestations of depression: Relation to the neurobiology of stress. *N Engl J Med* 319:348–353, 1988.

Gold PW, Kellner CH, Loriaux DL, Roy A, Post RM, Pickar D, Avgerinos P, Paul S, Schulte H, Oldfield EH, Cutler GB, Chrousos GP: The CRF stimulation test: Implications for the diagnosis and pathophysiology of primary affective disorder and Cushing's disease. *N Engl J Med* in press.

Golden RN, James SP, Sherer MA, Rudorfer MV, Sack DA, Potter WZ: Psychoses associated with bupropion treatment. *Am J Psychiatry* 142:1459–1462, 1985.

Golden RN, Rudorpher MV, Sherer MA, Linnoila M, Potter WZ: Bupropion in depression I: Biochemical effects and clinical response. *Arch Gen Psychiatry* 45:139–143, 1988.

Goldin LR, Gershon ES: Association and linkage studies of genetic marker loci in major psychiatric disorders. *Psychiatr Develop* 4:387–418, 1983.

Goldin LR, Kidd KK, Matthysse S, Gershon ES: The power of pedigree segregation analysis for traits with incomplete penetrance. In: ES Gershon, S Matthysse, XO Breakefield, RD Ciaranello, eds: *Genetic Research Strategies in Psychobiology and Psychiatry.* Pacific Grove, CA: Boxwood Press, 1981. pp 305–317.

Goldin LR, Clerget-Darpoux F, Gershon ES: Relationship of HLA to major affective disorder not supported. *Psychiat Res* 7:29–45, 1982.

Goldin LR, Gershon ES, Targum SD, Sparkes RS, McGinniss M: Segregation and linkage analyses in families of patients with bipolar, unipolar and schizoaffective mood disorders. *Am J Hum Genet* 35:274–287, 1983.

Goldin LR, Cox NJ, Pauls DL, Gershon ES, Kidd KK: The detection of major loci by segregation and linkage analysis: A simulation study. *Gen Epidem* 1:285–296, 1984.

Goldin LR, Nurnberger JI Jr, Gershon ES: Clinical methods in psychiatric genetics: II: The high risk approach. *Acta Psychiatr Scand* 74:119–128, 1986.

Goldney RD, Spence ND: Safety of the combination of lithium and neuroleptic drugs. *Am J Psychiatry* 143:882–884, 1986.

Goldring N, Fieve RR: Attempted suicide in manic-depressive disorder. *Am J Psychother* 38:373–383, 1984.

Goldschmidt TJ, Burch EA, Gutnisky GG: Secondary mania from cerebral embolization with nonfocal neurologic findings. *South Med J* 81:1309–1311, 1988.

Goldstein ET, Preskorn SH: Mania triggered by a steroid nasal spray in a patient with stable bipolar disorder. *Am J Psychiatry* 146:1076–1077, 1989.

Goldstein MJ, Miklowitz DJ: Lithium and family management of bipolar disorder. NIMH Grant Application, 1988.

Goldstein MJ, Baker BL, Jamison KR: *Abnormal Psychology: Experiences, Origins, and Interventions.* Boston: Little, Brown, 1986.

Goldstein PC, Brown GG, Welch KMA, Marcus A, Ewing JR, Rosenbaum G: Age-related decline of rCBF in schizophrenia and major affective disorder. *J Cereb Blood Flow Metab* 5(Suppl): 203–204, 1985.

Golinkoff M, Sweeney JA: Cognitive impairments in depression. *J Affective Disord* 17:105–112, 1989.

Golstein J, Van Cauter E, Linkowski P, Vanhaelst L, Mendlewicz J: Thyrotropin nyctohemeral pattern in primary depression: Differences between unipolar and bipolar women. *Life Sci* 27:1695–1703, 1980.

Goodall E: The exciting cause of certain states of disease, at present classified under "schizophrenia" by psychiatrists, may be infection: The pathogenesis of these states does not, in this country, receive the close, prolonged and co-ordinated clinical and pathological study which it demands. *J Ment Sci* 78:746–755, 1932.

Goodnick PJ, Meltzer HY: Treatment of schizoaffective disorders. *Schizophr Bull* 10:30–48, 1984.

Goodnick PJ, Meltzer HY, Dunner DL, Fieve RR: Repression and reactivation of lithium efflux from erythrocytes. *Psychiatry Res* 1:147–152, 1979.

Goodnick PJ, Fieve RR, Peselow E, Schlegel A, Filippi A: General behavior inventory: Measurement of subclinical changes during depression and lithium prophylaxis. *Acta Psychiatr Scand* 73:529–532, 1986.

Goodnick PJ, Fieve RR, Schlegel A, Kaufman K: Lithium level and inter-episode symptoms in affective disorder. *Acta Psychiatr Scand* 75:601–603, 1987.

Goodwin DW, Erickson CK, eds: *Alcoholism and Affective Disorders: Clinical, Genetic, and Biochemical Studies.* New York: Spectrum, 1979.

Goodwin DW, Alderson P, Rosenthal R: Clinical significance of hallucinations in psychiatric disorders: A study of 116 hallucinatory patients. *Arch Gen Psychiatry* 24:76–80, 1971.

Goodwin DW, Schulsinger F, Knop J, Mednick S, Guze SB: Psychopathology in adopted and non-adopted daughters of alcoholics. In: DW Goodwin, CK Erickson, eds: *Alcoholism and Affective Disorders: Clinical, Genetic, and Biochemical Studies.* New York: SP Medical and Scientific Books, 1979. pp 87–98.

Goodwin FK: Diagnosis of affective disorders. In: ME Jarvik, ed: *Psychopharmacology in the Practice of Medicine.* New York: Appleton-Century-Crofts, 1977a. pp 219–228.

Goodwin FK: Drug treatment of affective disorders: General principles. In: M Jarvik, ed: *Psychopharmacology in the Practice of Medicine.* New York: Appelton-Century-Crofts, 1977b. pp 241–253.

Goodwin FK: Commentary on RG Robinson: Investigating mood disorders following brain injury: An integrative approach using clinical and laboratory studies. *Integr Psychiatry* 1: 41–42, 1983.

Goodwin FK: The biology of depression: Conceptual issues. *Adv Biochem Psychopharmacol* 39:11–26, 1984.

Goodwin FK: Pharmacological consultation in major depressive disorders. In: DC Jimerson, JP Docherty, eds: *Psychopharmacology Consultation.* Washington, DC: American Psychiatric Press, 1986. pp 2–17.

Goodwin FK, Bunney WE Jr: Depressions following reserpine: A reevaluation. *Semin Psychiatry* 3:435–448, 1971.

Goodwin FK, Ebert M: Lithium in mania: Clinical trials and controlled studies. In: S Gershon, B Shopsin, eds: *Lithium: Its Role in Psychiatric Research and Treatment.* New York: Plenum Press, 1973. pp 237–252.

Goodwin FK, Jamison KR: The natural course of manic-depressive illness. In: RM Post, JC Ballenger, eds: *Neurobiology of Mood Disorders.* Baltimore: Williams & Wilkins, 1984. pp 20–37.

Goodwin FK, Post RM: The use of probenicid in high doses for the estimation of central serotonin turnover in affective illness and addicts on methadone. In: J Barchas, E Usdin, eds: *Serotonin and Behavior.* New York: Academic Press, 1972. pp 469–480.

Goodwin FK, Post RM: Studies of amine metabolites in affective illness and in schizophrenia: A comparative analysis. In: DX Freedman, ed: *Biology of the Major Psychoses: A Comparative Analysis.* Research Publications: Association for Research in Nervous and Mental Disease. Vol 54. New York: Raven Press, 1975. pp 299–332.

Goodwin FK, Post RM: 5-hydroxytryptamine and depression: A model for the interaction of normal variance with pathology. *Br J Clin Pharmacol* 15 (Suppl 3):393S–405S, 1983.

Goodwin FK, Roy-Byrne P: Treatment of bipolar disorders. In: RE Hales, AJ Frances, eds: *Psychiatry Update. American Psychiatric Association Annual Review. Vol 6.* Washington, DC: American Psychiatric Press, 1987. pp. 81–107.

Goodwin FK, Sack RL: Affective disorders: The catecholamine hypotheses revisited. In: E Usdin, S Snyder, eds: *Frontiers in Catecholamine Research.* New York: Pergamon Press, 1973. pp 1157–1164.

Goodwin FK, Sack RL: Behavioral effects of a new dopamine-beta-hydroxylase inhibitor (fusaric acid) in man. *J Psychiatr Res* 11:211–217, 1974a.

Goodwin FK, Sack RL: Central dopamine function in

affective illness: Evidence from precursors, enzyme inhibitors, and studies of central dopamine turnover. In: E Usdin: *The Neuropsychopharmacology of Monoamines and Their Regulatory Enzymes.* New York: Raven Press, 1974b. pp 261–279.

Goodwin FK, Zis AP: Lithium in the treatment of mania: Comparisons with neuroleptics. *Arch Gen Psychiatry* 36:840–844, 1979.

Goodwin FK, Murphy DL, Bunney WF Jr: Lithium carbonate treatment in depression and mania: A longitudinal double-blind study. *Arch Gen Psychiatry* 21:486–496, 1969.

Goodwin FK, Murphy DL, Brodie HK, Bunney WE Jr: L-dopa, catecholamines, and behavior: A clinical and biochemical study in depressed patients. *Biol Psychiatry* 2:341–366, 1970.

Goodwin FK, Murphy DL, Dunner DL, Bunney WE Jr: Lithium response in unipolar versus bipolar depression. *Am J Psychiatry* 129:44–47, 1972.

Goodwin FK, Post RM, Dunner DL, Gordon EK: Cerebrospinal fluid amine metabolites in affective illness: The probenecid technique. *Am J Psychiatry* 130:73–79, 1973.

Goodwin FK, Post RM, Wehr TA: Clinical approaches to the evaluation of brain amine function in mental illness: Some conceptual issues. In: MBH Youdim, W Lovenberg, DF Sharman, JR Lagnado, eds: *Essays in Neurochemistry and Neuropharmacology.* Vol. 2. London: John Wiley and Sons, 1977. pp 71–104.

Goodwin FK, Cowdry RW, Webster MH: Predictors of drug response in the affective disorders: Toward an integrated approach. In: MA Lipton, A DiMascio, KF Killam, eds: *Psychopharmacology: A Generation of Progress.* New York: Raven Press, 1978a. pp 1277–1288.

Goodwin FK, Muscettola G, Gold PW, Wehr T: Biochemical and pharmacological differentiation of affective disorders: An overview. In: HS Akiskal, WL Webb, eds: *Psychiatric Diagnoses: Exploration of Biological Predictors.* New York: SP Medical and Scientific Books, 1978b. pp. 313–336.

Goodwin FK, Prange AJ Jr, Post RM, Muscettola G, Lipton MA: Potentiation of antidepressant effects by L-triiodothyronine in tricyclic nonresponders. *Am J Psychiatry* 139:34–38, 1982.

Goodwin JS, Webb DR: Regulation of the immune response by prostaglandins. *Clin Immunol Immunopathol* 15:106–122, 1980.

Goolker P, Schein J: Psychic effects of ACTH and cortisone. *Psychosom Med* 15:589–597, 1953.

Goplerud E, Depue RA: Behavioral response to naturally occurring stress in cyclothymia and dysthymia. *J Abnorm Psychol* 94:128–139, 1985.

Gotlib IH, Robinson LA: Responses to depressed individuals: Discrepancies between self-report and observer-rated behavior. *J Abnorm Psychol* 91:231–240, 1982.

Gottesman IL, Shields J: *Schizophrenia: The Epigenetic Puzzle.* New York: Cambridge University Press, 1982.

Gould SJ: *The Mismeasure of Man.* New York: WW Norton Co, 1981.

Graham PM, Booth J, Boranga G, Galhenage S, Myers CM, Teoh CL, Cox LS: The dexamethasone suppression test in mania. *J Affective Disord* 4:201–211, 1982.

Graves A: *The Eclipse of a Mind.* New York: The Medical Journal Press, 1942.

Graves R: *Clinical Lectures on the Practice of Medicine.* Dublin: Fannin & Co., 1864.

Gray JA: *The Neuropsychology of Anxiety.* Reprinted, 1987. Oxford: Clarenden, Oxford University Press, 1982.

Grayson DA: Can categorical and dimensional views of psychiatric illness be distinguished? *Br J Psychiatry* 151:355–361, 1987.

Greden JF, Carroll BJ: Decrease in speech pause times with treatment of endogenous depression. *Biol Psychiatry* 15:575–587, 1980.

Greden JF, Carroll BJ: Psychomotor function in affective disorders: An overview of new monitory techniques. *Am J Psychiatry* 138:1441–1448, 1981.

Greden JF, Albala AA, Carroll BJ: Speech pause times among endogenous depressives: An objective measure of diurnal variation. Proceedings of the Fifth World Congress of the International College of Psychosomatic Medicine. Jerusalem Psychosomatic Society, 1979.

Greden JF, Albala AA, Smokler IA, Gardner R, Carroll BJ: Speech pause time: A marker of psychomotor retardation among endogenous depressives. *Biol Psychiatry* 16:851–859, 1981.

Greden JF, DeVigne JP, Albala AA, Tarika J, Buttenheim M, Eiser A, Carroll BJ: Serial dexamethasone suppression tests among rapidly cycling bipolar patients. *Biol Psychiatry* 17:455–462, 1982.

Greden JF, Genero N, Price HL, Feinberg M, Levine S: Facial electromyography in depression: Subgroup differences. *Arch Gen Psychiatry* 43:269–274, 1986.

Green AR, Deakin JF: Brain noradrenaline depletion prevents ECS-induced enhancement of serotonin- and dopamine-mediated behaviour. *Nature* 285:232–233, 1980.

Green E: Psychoses among Negroes: A comparative study. *J Nerv Ment Dis* 41:697–708, 1914.

Greenberg DB, Brown GL: Mania resulting from brainstem tumor. *J Nerv Ment Dis* 173434–436, 1985.

Greenhill LL, Shopsin B: Survey of mental disorders in the children of patients with affective disorders. In: J Mendlewicz, B Shopsin, eds: *Genetic Aspects of Affective Illness.* New York: SP Medical and Scientific Books, 1979. pp 75–92.

Greenhouse SW, Geisser S: On methods in the analysis of profile data. *Psychometrika* 24:95–112, 1959.

Greenson RR: *The Technique and Practice of Psychoanalysis.* New York: International Universities Press, 1967.

Greenspan K, Green R, Durell J: Retention and distribution patterns of lithium, a pharmacological tool in studying the pathophysiology of manic-depressive psychosis. *Am J Psychiatry* 125:512–519, 1968.

Greenspan K, Schildkraut JJ, Gordon EK, Baer L, Aronoff MS, Durell J: Catecholamine metabolism in affective disorders: 3. MHPG and other catecholamine metabolites in patients treated with lithium carbonate. *J Psychiatr Res* 7:171–183, 1970.

Gresham SC, Agnew HW, Williams RL: The sleep of depressed patients: An EEG and eye movement study. *Arch Gen Psychiatry* 13:503–507, 1965.

Grewel F: Psychiatric differences in Ashkenazim and Sephardim. *Psychiatria, Neurologia, Neurochirurgia* 70:330–347, 1967.

Griesinger W: *Mental Pathology and Therapeutics.* Translated by CL Robertson and J Rutherford. London: New Sydenhem Society, 1867.

Griffith JD, Fann EW, Tapp J: Drug-seeking behavior of hospitalized drug addicts. Presented at the 121st Annual Meeting of the American Psychiatric Association, Boston, 1968.

Grigoroiu-Serbânescu M, Christodorescu D, Jipescu I, Totoescu A, Marinescu E, Ardelean V: Psychopathology in children aged 10–17 of bipolar parents: Psychopathology rate and correlates of the severity of the psychopathology. *J Affective Disord* 16:167–179, 1989.

Grof E, Haag M, Grof P, Haag H: Lithium response and the sequence of episode polarities: Preliminary report on a Hamilton sample. *Prog Neuropsychopharmacol Biol Psychiatry* 11:199–203, 1987.

Grof P, Cakulis P, Dostal T: Lithium dropouts: A follow-up study of patients who discontinued prophylactic treatment. *Int Pharmacopsychiatry* 5:162–169, 1970.

Grof P, Angst J, Karasek M, Keitner G: Patient selection for long-term lithium treatment in clinical practice. *Arch Gen Psychiatry* 36:894–897, 1979a.

Grof P, Angst J, Karasek M, Keitner G: Selection of an individual patient for long-term lithium treatment in clinical practice. In: TB Cooper, S Gershon, NS Kline, M Schou, eds: *Lithium: Controversies and Unresolved Issues.* Amsterdam: Excerpta Medica, 1979b. pp 370–380.

Grof P, Lane J, MacCrimmon D, Werstiuk E, Blajchman M, Daigle L, Varma R: Clinical and laboratory correlates of the responses to long-term lithium treatment. In: M Schou, E Strömgren, eds: *Origin, Prevention and Treatment of Affective Disorders.* London: Academic Press, 1979c. pp 27–40.

Grof P, Hux, Dressler B, O'Sullivan K: Kidney function and response to lithium treatment. *Prog Neuropsychopharmacol Biol Psychiatry* 6:491–494, 1982.

Grossi E, Sacchetti E, Vita A, Conte G, Faravelli C, Hautman G, Zerbi D, Mesina AM, Drago F, Motta A: Carbamazepine vs. chlorpromazine in mania: A double-blind trial. In: HM Emrich, T Okuma, AA Muller, eds: *Anticonvulsants in Affective Disorders.* Amsterdam: Excerpta Media, 1984. pp 177–187.

Grossman LS, Harrow M, Lazar B, Kettering R,

Meltzer HY, Lechert J: Do thought disorders persist in manic patients? Abstract of paper presented at the 134th Annual Meeting of the American Psychiatric Association, May, 1981.

Grossman LS, Harrow M, Sands JR: Features associated with thought disorder in manic patients at 2–4 year follow-up. *Am J Psychiatry* 143:306–311, 1986.

Grotstein JS: The psychology of powerlessness: Disorders of self-regulation and interactional regulation as a newer paradigm for psychopathology. *Psychoanal Inq* 6:93–118, 1986.

Grove W, Clayton PJ, Endicott J, Hirschfeld RMA, Andreasen NC, Klerman GL: Immigration and major affective disorder. *Acta Psychiatr Scand* 74:548–552, 1986.

Grove W, Andreasen NC, Clayton PJ, Winokur G, Coryell WH: Primary and secondary affective disorders: Baseline characterisics of unipolar patients. *J Affective Disord* 13:249–257, 1987.

Gruzelier J, Venables P: Bimodality and lateral asymmetry of skin conductance orienting activity in schizophrenics: Replication and evidence of lateral asymmetry in patients with depression and disorders of personality. *Biol Psychiatry* 8:55–73, 1974.

Gruzelier J, Seymour K, Wilson L, Jolley A, Hirsch S: Impairments on neuropsychiatric tests of temporohippocampal and frontohippocampal functions and word fluency in remitting schizophrenia and affective disorders. *Arch Gen Psychiatry* 45:623–629, 1988.

Guenther W, Moser E, Mueller-Spahn F, von Oefele K, Buell U, Hippius H: Pathological cerebral blood flow during motor function in schizophrenic and endogenous depressed patients. *Biol Psychiatry* 21:889–899, 1986.

Guilford JP: *Psychometric Methods.* New York: McGraw-Hill, 1954.

Guilford JP: A revised structure of intellect. *Report of the Psychological Laboratory, University of Southern California.* no. 19, 1957.

Guilford JP: *Personality.* New York: McGraw-Hill, 1959a.

Guilford JP: Traits of creativity. In: HH Anderson, ed: *Creativity and its Cultivation.* New York: Harper, 1959b. pp 142–161.

Guillaume V, Conte-Devolx B, Szafarczyk A, Malaval F, Pares-Herbute N, Grino M, Alonso G, Assenmacher I, Oliver C: The corticotropin-releasing factor release in rat hypophysial portal blood is mediated by brain catecholamines. *Neuroendocrinology* 46:143–146, 1987.

Gunderson JG, Elliott GR: The interface between borderline personality disorder and affective disorder. *Am J Psychiatry* 142:277–288, 1985.

Gur RE, Skolnick BE, Gur RC, Caroff S, Rieger W, Obrist WD, Younkin D, Reivich M: Brain function in psychiatric disorders: II. Regional cerebral blood flow in medicated unipolar depressives. *Arch Gen Psychiatry* 41:695–699, 1984.

Gurtman MB: Depression and the response of others:

Reevaluating the reevaluation. *J Abnorm Psychol* 95:99–101, 1986.

Gusella JF, Wexler NS, Conneally PM, Naylor SL, Anderson M, Tanzi RE, Watkins PC, Ottina K, Wallace MR, Sakaguchi AY, Young AB, Shoulson I Bonilla E, Martin JB: A polymorphic DNA marker genetically linked to Huntington's Disease. *Nature* 306:234–238, 1983.

Guttman E, Hermann K: Ueber psychische Storungen bei Hirnstammerkrankungen und das Automatose-syndrom. *Z Ges Neurol Psychiatr* 140:439–472, 1932.

Guy W, Ban TA, eds: *The AMDP-System: Manual for the Assessment and Documentation of Psychopathology.* Berlin: Springer-Verlag, 1982.

Guze SB, Robins E: Suicide and primary affective disorders. *Br J Psychiatry* 117:437–438, 1970.

Guze SB, Woodruff RA Jr, Clayton PJ: The significance of psychotic affective disorders. *Arch Gen Psychiatry* 32:1147–1150, 1975.

Haag H, Heidorn A, Haag M, Greil W: Sequence of affective polarity and lithium response: Preliminary report on the Munich sample. *Prog Neuropsychopharmacol Biol Psychiatry* 11:205–208, 1987.

Haag M, Haag H, Eisenried F, Greil W: RBC-choline: Changes by lithium and relation to prophylactic response. *Acta Psychiatr Scand* 70:389–399, 1984.

Haas GL, Glick ID, Clarkin JF, Spencer JH, Lewis AB, Peyser J, DeMane N, Good-Ellis M, Harris E, Lestelle V: Inpatient family intervention: A randomized clinical trial: II: Results at hospital discharge. *Arch Gen Psychiatry* 45:217–224, 1988.

Hadjiconstantinou M, Neff NH: Catecholamine systems of retina: A model for studying synaptic mechanisms. *Life Sci* 35:1135–1147, 1984.

Haertzen CH, Hooks NT: Changes in personality and subjective experience associated with chronic administration and withdrawal of opiates. *J Nerv Ment Dis* 148:606–613, 1969.

Hagnell O, Lanke J, Rorsman B: Suicide rates in the Lundby study: Mental illness as a risk factor for suicide. *Neuropsychobiology* 7:248–253, 1981.

Hagnell O, Lanke J, Rorsman B, Öjesjö L: Are we entering an age of melancholy? Depressive illnesses in a prospective epidemiological study over 25 years: The Lundby study, Sweden. *Psychol Med* 12:279–289, 1982.

Haile HG: *Luther: An Experiment in Biography.* Princeton: Princeton University Press, 1980.

Hakim AH, Bomb BS, Pandey SK, Singh SV: A study of cerebrospinal fluid calcium and magnesium in depression. *J Assoc Physicians India* 23:311–315, 1975.

Halaris AE: Plasma 3-methoxy-4-hydroxyphenylglycol in manic psychosis. *Am J Psychiatry* 135:493–494, 1978.

Halberg G: Physiologic considerations underlying rhythmometry, with special reference to emotional illness. In: J DeAjuriaguerra, ed: *Cycles Biologiques et Psychiatrie.* Symposium Bel-Air III. Geneva, Masson et Cie, 1968. pp 73–126.

Hall CS, Lindzey G: *Theories of Personality.* 2nd ed. New York: John Wiley & Sons, 1970.

Hall KRL, Stride E: Some factors affecting reaction times to auditory stimuli in mental patients. *J Ment Sci* 100:462–477, 1954.

Hall KS, Dunner DL, Zeller G, Fieve RR: Bipolar illness: A prospective study of life events. *Compr Psychiatry* 18:497–502, 1977.

Hall NR, McGillis JP, Spangelo BL, Healy BL, Goldstein AL: Immunomodulatory peptides and the central nervous system. *Springer Semin Immunopathol* 8:153–164, 1985.

Hallberg H, Almgren O, Svensson TH: Reduced brain serotonergic activity after repeated treatment with β-adrenoceptor antagonists. *Psychopharmacology (Berlin)* 76:114–117, 1982.

Hallonquist JD, Mrosovsky N: Ironies of animal modelling. *Nature* 329:18–19, 1987.

Hallstrom CO, Rees WL, Pare CM, Trenchard A, Turner P: Platelet uptake of 5-hydroxytryptamine and dopamine in depression. *Postgrad Med J* 52:40–46, 1976.

Halper JP, Brown RP, Sweeney JA, Kocsis JH, Peters A, Mann JJ: Blunted β-adrenergic responsivity of peripheral blood mononuclear cells in endogenous depression: Isoproterenol dose-response studies. *Arch Gen Psychiatry* 45:241–244, 1988.

Halpern L: Some data of the psychic morbidity of Jews and Arabs in Palestine. *Am J Psychiatry* 94:1215–1222, 1938.

Hamilton A: *The Papers of Alexander Hamilton.* Edited by HC Syrett. New York: Columbia University Press, 1961–62.

Hamilton I: *Robert Lowell: A Biography.* New York: Random House, 1982.

Hamilton M: A rating scale for depression. *J Neurol Neurosurg Psychiatry* 23:56–62, 1960.

Hamilton M: Development of a rating scale for primary depressive illness. *Br J Soc Clin Psychol* 6: 278–296, 1967.

Hamilton M: Clinical evaluation of depressions: Clinical criteria and rating scales, including a Guttman Scale. In: DM Gallant, GM Simpson, eds: *Depression: Behavioral, Biochemical, Diagnostic and Treatment Concepts.* New York: Spectrum Publications, 1976. pp 155–179.

Hamilton M: Symptoms and assessment of depression. In: ES Paykel, ed: *Handbook of Affective Disorders.* Edinburgh: Churchill Livingstone, 1982. pp 3–11.

Hamilton M: Assessment of depression and mania. In: A Georgotas, R Cancro, eds: *Depression and Mania.* New York: Elsevier, 1988. pp 625–637.

Hammen CL, Peters SD: Differential responses to male and female depressive reactions. *J Consult Clin Psychol* 45:994–1001, 1977.

Hammen CL, Peters SD: Interpersonal consequences of depression: Responses to men and women enacting a depressed role. *J Abnorm Psychol* 87:322–332, 1978.

Hammen C, Gordon D, Burge D, Adrian C, Jaenicke C, Hiroto D: Maternal affective disorders, illness, and stress: Risk for children's psychopathology. *Am J Psychiatry* 144:736–741, 1987.

Hammen C, Ellicott A, Gitlin M, Jamison KR: Sociotropy/autonomy and vulnerability to specific life events in patients with unipolar depression and bipolar disorders. *J Abnorm Psychol* 98:154–160, 1989.

Hanin I, Kopp U, Spiker DG, Neil JF, Shaw DH, Kupfer DJ: RBC and plasma choline levels in control and depressed individuals: A critical evaluation. *Psychiatr Res* 3:345–355, 1980.

Hanin I, Cohen BM, Kopp U, Lipinski JF: Erythrocyte and plasma choline in bipolar psychiatric patients: A follow up study. *Psychopharmacol Bull* 18:186–190, 1982.

Hankoff LD: Suicide and attempted suicide. In: ES Paykel, ed: *Handbook of Affective Disorders*. New York: Guilford Press, 1982. pp 416–428.

Hanna SM, Jenner FA, Souster LP: Electro-oculogram changes at the switch in a manic-depressive patient. *Br J Psychiatry* 149:229–232, 1986.

Hansen HE, Hestbech J, Olsen S, Amdisen A: Renal function and renal pathology in patients with lithium-induced impairment of renal concentrating ability. *Proc Eur Dial Transplant Assoc* 14:518–527, 1977.

Hansen HE, Hestbech J, Sørensen JL, Nørgaard K, Heilskov J, Amdisen A: Chronic interstitial nephropathy in patients on long-term lithium treatment. *Q J Med* 48:577–591, 1979.

Hanus H, Zapletalek M: Sebevrazedna aktivita nemocnych afektivnimi poruchami v prubehu lithioprofylaxe. *Ceskoslovenska Psychiatrie* 80:97–100, 1984.

Haracz JL, Minor TR, Wilkins JN, Zimmerman EG: Learned helplessness: An experimental model of the DST in rats. *Biol Psychiatry* 23:388–396, 1988.

Harding T, Knight F: Marijuana-modified mania. *Arch Gen Psychiatry* 29:635–637, 1973.

Harding TW, DeArango MV, Baltasar J, Climent CE, Ibrahim HHA, Ladrido-Ignacio L, Srinivasa Murthy R, Wig NN: Mental disorders in primary health care: A study of their frequency and diagnosis in four developing countries. *Psychol Med* 10:231–241, 1980.

Hardy A: *The Spiritual Nature of Man: A Study of Contemporary Religious Experience*. Oxford: Clarendon Press, 1979.

Hardy BG, Shulman KI, Mackenzie SE, Kutcher SP, Silverberg JD: Pharmacokinetics of lithium in the elderly. *J Clin Psychopharmacol* 7:153–158, 1987.

Hardy MC, Lecrubier Y, Widlöcher D: Efficacy of clonidine in 24 patients with acute mania. *Am J Psychiatry* 143:1450–1453, 1986.

Hare EH: Mental illness and social class in Bristol. *Br J Prev Soc Med* 9:191–195, 1955.

Hare EH: *Bethlem Royal Hospital and the Maudsley Hospital Triennial Statistical Report: 1964–1966.* 1968.

Hare E: The two manias: A study of the evolution of the modern concept of mania. *Br J Psychiat* 138: 89–99, 1981.

Hare EH: Epidemiological evidence for a viral factor in the aetiology of the functional psychoses. *Adv Biol Psychiatry* 12:52–75, 1983.

Hare EH, Price JS, Slater E: Parental social class in psychiatric patients. *Br J Psychiatry* 121:515–524, 1972.

Harlow HF, Harlow MK: Social deprivation in monkeys. *Sci Am* 207:136–146, 1962.

Harris WH, Beauchemin JA: CSF Ca, Mg, and their ratio in psychoses of organic and functional origin. *Yale J Biol Med* 29:117–124, 1956.

Harrison WM, Cooper TB, Stewart JW, Quitkin FM, McGrath PJ, Liebowitz MR, Rabkin JR, Markowitz JS, Klein DF: The tyramine challenge test as a marker for melancholia. *Arch Gen Psychiatry* 41:681–685, 1984.

Harrow M, Prosen M: Intermingling and disordered logic as influences on schizophrenic thought disorders. *Arch Gen Psychiatry* 35:1213–1218, 1978.

Harrow M, Quinlan D: Is disordered thinking unique to schizophrenia? *Arch Gen Psychiatry* 34:15–21, 1977.

Harrow M, Himmelhoch J, Tucker G, Hersh J, Quinlan D: Overinclusive thinking in acute schizophrenic patients. *J Abnorm Psychol* 79:161–168, 1972a.

Harrow M, Tucker GJ, Adler D: Concrete and idiosyncratic thinking in acute schizophrenic patients. *Arch Gen Psychiatry* 26:433–439, 1972b.

Harrow M, Grossman LS, Silverstein ML, Meltzer HY: Thought pathology in manic and schizophrenic patients: Its occurrence at hospital admission and seven weeks later. *Arch Gen Psychiatry* 39:665–671, 1982.

Harrow M, Lanin-Kettering I, Prosen M, Miller JG: Disordered thinking in schizophrenia: Intermingling and loss of set. *Schizophr Bull* 9:354–367, 1983.

Harrow M, Grossman LS, Silverstein ML, Meltzer HY, Kettering RL: A longitudinal study of thought disorder in manic patients. *Arch Gen Psychiatry* 43:781–785, 1986.

Harrow M, Goldberg JF, Grossman LS, Meltzer HY: Outcome in manic disorders: A naturalistic follow-up study. *Arch Gen Psychiatry*, 47:665–671, 1990.

Hart RG, Easton JD: Carbamazepine and hematological monitoring. *Ann Neurol* 11:309–312, 1982.

Hartigan GP: Experiences with treatment with lithium salts. Paper read to the Southeastern Branch of the Royal Medicopsychological Society, 1959.

Hartigan GP: The use of lithium salts in affective disorders. *Br J Psychiatry* 109:810–814, 1963.

Hartmann E: Longitudinal studies of sleep and dream patterns in manic-depressive patients. *Arch Gen Psychiatry* 19:312–329, 1968.

Harvey PD: Speech competence in manic and schizophrenic psychoses: The association between clinically rated thought disorder and cohesion and reference performance. *J Abnorm Psychol* 92:368–377, 1983.

Harvey PD, Weintraub S, Neale JM: Speech competence of children vulnerable to psychopathology. *J Abnorm Child Psychol* 10:373–388, 1982.

Hashimoto R, Ozaki N, Ohta T, Kasahara Y, Kaneda N, Nagatsu T: Plasma biopterin levels of patients with affective disorders. *Neuropsychobiology* 19:61–63, 1988.

Hashimoto R, Ozaki N, Ohta T, Kasahara Y, Kaneda N, Nagatsu T: The plasma tetrahydrobiopterin levels in patients with affective disorders. *Biol Psychiatry*, 28:526–528, 1990.

Hasin D, Endicott J, Lewis C: Alcohol and drug abuse in patients with affective syndromes. *Compr Psychiatry* 26:283–295, 1985.

Hasin DS, Endicott J, Keller MB: RDC alcoholism in patients with major affective syndromes: Two-year course. *Am J Psychiatry* 146:318–323, 1989.

Häskovec L, Soucek K: Trial of methysergide in mania. *Nature* 219:507–508, 1968.

Hastings DW: Follow-up results in psychiatric illness. *Am J Psychiatry* 114:1057–1066, 1958.

Hathaway SR, McKinley JC: *Minnesota Multiphasic Personality Inventory*. New York: The Psychological Corporation, 1951.

Hatterer JA, Kocsis JH, Stokes PE: Thyroid function in patients maintained on lithium. *Psychiatry Res* 26:249–258, 1989.

Hauge M, Harvald B, Fischer M, Gotlieb-Jensen K, Juel-Nielsen N, Raeblid I, Shapiro R, Videbest T: The Danish twin register. *Acta Geneticae Medicae et Gemellologiae* 17:315–332, 1968.

Hauger R, Luu HM, Goodwin FK, Paul SM: Characterization of [³H]ouabain binding sites in human brain, platelet, and erythrocyte. *J Neurochem* 44:1704–1708, 1985.

Hauser P, Altshuler L, Post RM, Berrettini W, Dauphinais ID, Gelernter J: Temporal lobe size by MRI in affective disorder. Abstract of paper presented at the 141st annual meeting of the American Psychiatric Association, May, 1988.

Hautzinger M, Linden M, Hoffman N: Distressed couples with and without a depressed partner: An analysis of their verbal interaction. *J Behav Ther Exp Psychiatry* 13:307–314. 1982.

Hawton K, Catalan J: *Attempted Suicide: A Practical Guide to its Nature and Management*. New York: Oxford University Press, 1982.

Hayes MHS, Patterson DG: Experimental development of the graphic rating method. *Psychol Bull* 18:98–99, 1921.

Hayes SG: Long-term use of valproate in primary psychiatric disorders. *J Clin Psychiatry* 50(Suppl):35–39, 1989.

Haynes RB, Taylor DW, Sackett DL, eds: *Compliance in Health Care*. Baltimore: The Johns Hopkins University Press, 1979.

Hays P: Modes of onset of psychotic depression. *Br Med J* 2:779–784, 1964.

Healy D: Rhythm and blues: Neurochemical, neuropharmacological and neuropsychological implications of a hypothesis of circadian rhythm dysfunction in the affective disorders. *Psychopharmacology* 93:271–285, 1987.

Healy D, Carney PA, Leonard BE: Monoamine-

related markers of depression: Changes following treatment. *J Psychiat Res* 17:251–260, 1983.

Heath RG, Franklin DE, Shraberg: Gross pathology of the cerebellum in patients diagnosed and treated as functional psychiatric disorders. *J Nerv Ment Dis* 167:585–592, 1979.

Heath RG, Franklin DE, Walker CG, Keating JW: Cerebellar vermal atrophy in psychiatric patients. *Biol Psychiatry* 17:569–583, 1982.

Heathfield KW: Huntington's chorea. Investigation into the prevalence of this disease in the area covered by the North East Metropolitan Regional Hospital Board. *Brain* 90:203–232, 1967.

Hecaen H: *Manie et Inspiration Musicale: Le Cas Hugo Wolf*. Bordeaux: These, 1934.

Hedge GA, de Wied D: Corticotropin and vasopressin secretion after hypothalamic implantation of atropine. *Endocrinology* 88:1257–1259, 1971.

Hedge GA, Smelik PG: Corticotropin release: Inhibition by intrahypothalamic implantation of atropine. *Science* 159:891–892, 1968.

Hedlund B, Abens J, Bartfai T: Vasoactive intestinal polypeptide and muscarinic receptors: Supersensitivity induced by long-term atropine treatment. *Science* 220:519–521, 1983.

Hekimian LJ, Gershon S: Characteristics of drug abusers admitted to a psychiatric hospital. *JAMA* 205:125–130, 1968.

Helgason T: Frequency of depressive states in Iceland as compared with other Scandinavian countries. *Acta Psychiatr Scand* (Suppl 162):37–81, 1961.

Helgason T: Epidemiology of mental disorders in Iceland: A psychiatric and demographic investigation of 5395 Icelanders. *Acta Psychiatr Scand* 40(Suppl 173), 1964.

Helgason T: Epidemiological investigations concerning affective disorders. In: M Schou, E Strömgren, eds: *Origin, Prevention and Treatment of Affective Disorders*. London: Academic Press, 1979. pp 241–255.

Hellekson C: Phenomenology of seasonal affective disorder: An Alaskan perspective. In: NE Rosenthal, M Blehar, eds: *Seasonal Affective Disorders and Phototherapy*. New York: Guilford, 1989. pp. 33–45.

Hellekson CJ, Kline JA, Rosenthal NE: Phototherapy for seasonal affective disorder in Alaska. *Am J Psychiatry* 143:1035–1037, 1986.

Hellhammer D: Learned helplessness: An animal model revisited. In: J Angst, ed: *The Origins of Depression: Current Concepts and Approaches*. Berlin: Springer-Verlag, 1983. pp 147–161.

Helmchen H: The AMP System as a method in clinical pharmacopsychiatry. In: H Hippius, ed: *Assessment of Pharmacodynamic Effects in Human Pharmacology, Part I: Psychopharmacological Screening Tests*. Stuttgart: F.K. Schattauer Verlag, 1975. pp 87–134.

Helmchen H: The AMDP. In: P Pichot, P Berner, R Wolf, K Thau, eds: *Psychiatry: The State of the Art. Vol 1: Clinical Psychopathology, Nomenclature and*

Classification. New York: Plenum Press, 1985. pp 141–146.

Helms PM, Smith RE: Recurrent psychotic depression: Evidence of diagnostic stability. *J Affective Disord* 5:51–54, 1983.

Helzer JE: Bipolar affective disorder in black and white men: A comparison of symptoms and familial illness. *Arch Gen Psychiatry* 32:1140–1143, 1975.

Helzer JE, Pryzbeck TR: The co-occurrence of alcoholism with other psychiatric disorders in the general population and its impact on treatment. *J Stud Alcohol* 49:219–224, 1988.

Helzer JE, Winokur G: A family interview study of male manic-depressives. *Arch Gen Psychiatry* 31:73–77, 1974.

Hemsi LK: Psychiatric morbidity of West Indian immigrants. *Soc Psychiatry* 2:95–100, 1967.

Hemsley DR, Philips HC: Models of mania: An individual case study. *Br J Psychiatry* 127:78–85, 1975.

Henderson D, Gillespie RD: *A Text-book of Psychiatry for Students and Practitioners.* 8th ed. London: Oxford University Press, 1956.

Hendler NH: Spironolactone prophylaxis in manic-depressive disease. *J Nerv Ment Dis* 166:517–520, 1978.

Hendrie HC: Organic brain disorders: Classification, the "symptomatic" psychoses, misdiagnosis. *Psychiatr Clin North Am* 1:3–19, 1978.

Heninger GR, Mueller PS: Carbohydrate metabolism in mania before and after lithium carbonate treatment. *Arch Gen Psychiatry* 23:310–319, 1970.

Heninger GR, Charney DS, Sternberg DE: Lithium carbonate augmentation of antidepressant treatment: An effective prescription for treatment-refractory depression. *Arch Gen Psychiatry* 40:1335–1342, 1983.

Heninger GR, Charney DS, Sternberg DE: Serotonergic function in depression: Prolactin response to intravenous tryptophan in depressed patients and healthy subjects. *Arch Gen Psychiatry* 41:398–402, 1984.

Heninger GR, Charney DS, Price LH: α_2-adrenergic receptor sensitivity in depression: The plasma MHPG, behavioral, and cardiovascular responses to yohimbine. *Arch Gen Psychiatry* 45:718–726, 1988.

Henry GM, Weingartner H, Murphy DL: Idiosyncratic patterns of learning and word association during mania. *Am J Psychiatry* 128:564–574, 1971.

Henry GM, Weingartner H, Murphy DL: Influence of affective states and psychoactive drugs on verbal learning and memory. *Am J Psychiatry* 130:966–971, 1973.

Henry WD: The personality of Oliver Cromwell. *Practitioner* 215:102–110, 1975.

Hensel B, Dunner DL, Fieve RR: The relationship of family history of alcoholism to primary affective disorder. *J Affect Disord* 1:105–113, 1979.

Herrman H, McGorry P, Bennett P, van Riel R, Singh B: Prevalence of severe mental disorders in disaffiliated and homeless people in inner Melbourne. *Am J Psychiatry* 146:1179–1184, 1989.

Hertz M: On rhythmic phenomena in thyroidectomized patients. *Acta Psychiatr Scand* 40(Suppl 180):449–456, 1964.

Hes J Ph: Manic-depressive illness in Israel. *Am J Psychiatry* 116:1082–1086, 1960.

Hesketh JE: Effects of potassium and lithium on sodium transport from blood to cerebrospinal fluid. *J Neurochem* 28:597–603, 1977.

Hesselbrock MN, Meyer RE, Keener JJ: Psychopathology in hospitalized alcoholics. *Arch Gen Psychiatry* 42:1050–1055, 1985.

Hesselbrock V, Stabenau J, Hesselbrock M, Mirkin P, Meyer R: A comparison of two interview schedules: The Schedule for Affective Disorders and Schizophrenia-Lifetime and the NIMH Diagnostic Interview Schedule. *Arch Gen Psychiatry* 39:674–677, 1982.

Hestbech J, Hansen HE, Amdisen A, Olsen S: Chronic renal lesions following long-term treatment with lithium. *Kidney Int* 12:205–213, 1977.

Heston LL: Psychiatric disorders in foster home reared children of schizophrenic mothers. *Br J Psychiatry* 112:819–825, 1966.

Hetmar O, Bolwig TG, Brun C, Ladefoged J, Larsen S, Rafaelsen OJ: Lithium: Long-term effects on the kidney: I. Renal function in retrospect. *Acta Psychiatr Scand* 73:574–581, 1986.

Hewick DS, Newbury P, Hopwood S, Naylor G, Moody J: Age as a factor affecting lithium therapy. *Br J Clin Pharmacol* 4:201–205, 1977.

Hill C: *God's Englishman.* London: Weidenfeld & Nicolson, 1970.

Himmelhoch JM: Mixed states, manic-depressive illness, and the nature of mood. *Psychiatr Clin North Am* 2:449–459, 1979.

Himmelhoch JM: Major mood disorders related to epileptic changes. In: D Blumer, ed: *Psychiatric Aspects of Epilepsy.* Washington, DC: American Psychiatric Press, 1984. pp 271–294.

Himmelhoch JM: Lest treatment abet suicide. *J Clin Psychiatry* 48(Suppl):44–54, 1987.

Himmelhoch JM, Garfinkel ME: Sources of lithium resistance in mixed mania. *Psychopharmacol Bull* 22:613–620, 1986.

Himmelhoch JM, Detre T, Kupfer DJ, Swartzburg M, Byck R: Treatment of previously intractable depressions with tranylcypromine and lithium. *J Nerv Ment Dis* 155:216–220, 1972.

Himmelhoch J, Harrow M, Hersh J, Tucker GJ: *Manual for Assessment of Selected Aspects of Thinking: Object Sorting Test.* ASIS/NAPS #02206, New York: Microfiche Publications, 1973.

Himmelhoch JM, Mulla D, Neil JF, Detre TP, Kupfer DJ: Incidence and significance of mixed affective states in a bipolar population. *Arch Gen Psychiatry* 33:1062–1066, 1976a.

Himmelhoch JM, Coble P, Kupfer DJ, Ingenito J: Agitated psychotic depression associated with severe hypomanic episodes: A rare syndrome. *Am J Psychiatry* 133:765–771, 1976b.

Himmelhoch JM, Forrest J, Neil JF, Detre TP:

Thiazide-lithium synergy in refractory mood swings. *Am J Psychiatry* 134:149–152, 1977.

Himmelhoch JM, Neil JF, May SJ, Fuchs CZ, Licata SM: Age, dementia, dyskinesias, and lithium response. *Am J Psychiatry* 137:941–945, 1980.

Himmelhoch JM, Fuchs CZ, Symons BJ: A double-blind study of tranylcypomine treatment of major anergic depression. *J Nerv Ment Dis* 170:628–634, 1982.

Himmelhoch JM, Hill S, Steinberg B, May S: Lithium, alcoholism and psychiatric diagnosis. *J Psychiatr Treat Eval* 5:83–88, 1983.

Himmelhoch JM, Thase ME, Mallinger AG, Fuchs CZ: Tranylcypromine versus imipramine in manic depression. Abstract of paper presented at the 139th Annual Meeting of the American Psychiatric Association, May, 1986.

Hinchliffe MK, Lancashire M, Roberts FJ: Depression: Defense mechanisms in speech. *Br J Psychiatry* 118:471–472, 1971.

Hinchliffe M, Hooper D, Roberts FJ, Vaughan PW: A study of the interaction between depressed patients and their spouses. *Br J Psychiatry* 126:164–172, 1975.

Hirata F, Axelrod J: Enzymatic methylation of phosphatidylethanolamine increases erythrocyte membrane fluidity. *Nature* 275:219–220, 1978.

Hirschfeld RMA: Personality and bipolar disorder. Paper presented at the Symposium on New Results in Depression Research. Munich, March, 1985.

Hirschfeld RMA, Klerman GL: Personality attributes and affective disorders. *Am J Psychiatry* 136:67–70, 1979.

Hirschfeld RMA, Klerman GL, Clayton PJ, Keller MB, McDonald-Scott P, Larkin BH: Assessing personality: Effects of the depressive state on trait measurement. *Am J Psychiatry* 140:695–699, 1983.

Hirschfeld RMA, Klerman GL, Keller MB, Andreasen NC, Clayton PJ: Personality of recovered patients with bipolar affective disorder. *J Affective Disord* 11:81–89, 1986.

Hitzemann R, Hirschowitz J, Garver D: Membrane abnormalities in the psychoses and affective disorders. *J Psychiatr Res* 18:319–326, 1984.

Hitzemann RJ, Hirschowitz J, Garver DL: On the physical properties of red cell ghost membranes in the affective disorders and psychoses: A fluorescence polarization study. *J Affective Disord* 10:227–232, 1986.

Hobson JA, Steriade M: Neuronal basis of behavioral state control. In: VB Mountcastle, F Blum, SR Geiger, eds: *Handbook of Physiology: A Critical, Comprehensive Presentation of Physiological Knowledge and Concepts*. Volume IV, Section 1, The Nervous System. Bethesda, MD: American Physiological Society, 1986. pp 701–823.

Hodgkinson S, Sherrington R, Gurling H, Marchbanks R, Reeders S, Mallet J, McInnis M, Petursson H, Brynjolfsson J: Molecular genetic evidence for heterogeneity in manic depression. *Nature* 325:805–806, 1987.

Hoehe MR, Berrettini WH, Lentes KU: Dra I identifies a two allele DNA polymorphism in the human alpha 2-adrenergic receptor gene (ADRAR), using a 5.5 kb probe (p ADRAR). *Nucleic Acids Res* 16:9070, 1988.

Hoff AL, Shukla S, Cook BL, Aronson TA, Ollo CL, Pass HL: Cognitive function in manics with associated neurologic factors. *J Affective Disord* 14:251–255, 1988.

Hoffman RE: Computer simulations of neural information processing and the schizophrenia-mania dichotomy. *Arch Gen Psychiatry* 44:178–188, 1987.

Hoffman RE, Stopek S, Andreasen NC: A comparative study of manic vs schizophrenic speech disorganization. *Arch Gen Psychiatry* 43:831–835, 1986.

Hofmann G: Vergleichende untersuchungen zur pramorbiden personlichkeit von patienten mit bipolaren (manisch-depressiven) und solchen mit monopolar depressiven psychosen. *Med Diss* Univ Munchen, 1973.

Hofmann G, Grünberger J, König P, Presslich O, Wolf R: Die mehrjährige lithium therapie affektiver störungen. Langzeiteffekte und begleiterscheinungen. *Psychiatr Clin* 7:129–148, 1974.

Hokin-Neaverson M, Spiegel DA, Lewis WC: Deficiency of erythrocyte sodium pump activity in bipolar manic-depressive psychosis. *Life Sci* 15:1739–1748, 1974.

Holinger PC, Wolpert EA: A ten year follow-up of lithium use *IMJ* 156:99–104, 1979.

Hollingshead AB: *Two-Factor Index of Social Position*. New Haven: Yale University Press, 1957.

Hollingshead AB, Redlich FC: *Social Class and Mental Illness: A Community Study*. New York: Wiley, 1958.

Hollister LE, Berger P, Ogle FL, Arnold RC, Johnson A: Protirelin (TRH) in depression. *Arch Gen Psychiatry* 31:468–470, 1974.

Holmes R: *Shelley: The Pursuit*. New York: Weidenfeld & Nicolson, 1974.

Holmes T, Rahe R: The social adjustment rating scale. *J Psychosom Res* 4:213–218, 1967.

Holsboer F: The dexamethasone suppression test in depressed patients: Clinical and biochemical aspects. *J Steroid Biochem* 19:251–257, 1983.

Holsboer F: Implications of altered limbic-hypothalamic-pituitary-adrenocortical (LHPA)-function for neurobiology of depression. *Acta Psychiatr Scand* (Suppl 341):72–111, 1988.

Holsboer F, Benkert O, Meier L, Kreuz-Kersting A: Combined estradiol and vitamin B6 treatment in women with major depression. *Am J Psychiatry* 142:658, 1985.

Holsboer-Trachsler E, Wiedemann K, Holsboer F: Serial partial sleep deprivation in depression—Clinical effects and dexamethasone suppression test results. *Neuropsychobiology* 19:73–78, 1988.

Holzman PS, Kringlen E, Levy DL, Proctor LR, Haberman SJ, Yasillo NJ: Abnormal-pursuit eye movements in schizophrenia. Evidence for a genetic indicator. *Arch Gen Psychiatry* 34:802–805, 1977.

Holzman PS, Solovay MR, Shenton ME: Thought disorder specificity in functional psychoses. In M Alpert, ed: *Controversies in Schizophrenia: Changes and constancies*. New York: Guilford Press, 1985. pp 228–252.

Hommes OR, Panhuysen LH: Depression and cerebral dominance: A study of bilateral intracarotid amytal in eleven depressed patients. *Psychiatr Neurol Neurochir* 74:259–270, 1971.

Hooley JM, Richters JE, Weintraub S, Neale JM: Psychopathology and marital distress: The positive side of positive symptoms. *J Abnorm Psychol* 96:27–33, 1987.

Hoover CF, Fitzgerald RG: Marital conflict of manic-depressive patients. *Arch Gen Psychiatry* 38:65–67, 1981.

Hopkins GM: *Poems of Gerard Manley Hopkins*. WH Gardner, NH Mackenzie, eds. 4th ed. London: Oxford University Press, 1967.

Horgan D: Change of diagnosis to manic-depressive illness. *Psychol Med* 11:517–523, 1981.

Horn E, Lach B, Lapierre Y, Hrdina P: Hypothalamic pathology in the neuroleptic malignant syndrome. *Am J Psychiatry* 145:617–620, 1988.

Horne JA, Moore VJ: Sleep EEG effects of exercise with and without additional body cooling. *Electroencephalogr Clin Neurophysiol* 60:33–38, 1985.

Horowitz HA: The use of lithium in the treatment of the drug-induced psychotic reaction. *Dis Nerv Sys* 36:159–163, 1975.

Horrobin DF, Lieb J: A biochemical basis for the actions of lithium on behaviour and on immunity: Relapsing and remitting disorders of inflammation and immunity such as multiple sclerosis or recurrent herpes as manic-depression of the immune system. *Med Hypotheses* 7:891–905, 1981.

Höschl C, Koženy J: Verapamil in affective disorders: A controlled, double-blind study. *Biol Psychiatry* 25:128–140, 1989.

Hostetter AM, Egeland JA, Endicott J: Amish study, II: Consensus diagnosis and reliability results. *Am J Psychiatry* 140:62–66, 1983.

House KM, Martin RL: MMPI delineation of a subgroup of depressed patients refractory to lithium carbonate therapy. *Am J Psychiatry* 132:644–646, 1975.

Hsia Z, Zhang M: A follow-up study of 704 cases of affective psychosis and a discussion of the classification of its monophasia and biphasias. *Chung Hua Shen Ching Ching Shen Ko Tsa Chih* 133:151–153, 1980.

Hsu LKG, Starzynski JM: Mania in adolescence. *J Clin Psychiatry* 47:596–599, 1986.

Hubain PP, Sobolski J, Mendlewicz J: Cimetidine-induced mania. *Neuropsychobiology* 8:223–224, 1982.

Hudgens RW: Mental health of political candidates: Notes on Abraham Lincoln. *Am J Psychiatry* 130:110, 1973.

Hudgens RW: *Psychiatric Disorders in Adolescents*. Baltimore: Williams & Wilkins, 1974.

Hudson JI, Lipinski JF, Frankenburg FR, Grochocinski VJ, Kupfer DJ: Electroencephalographic sleep in mania. *Arch Gen Psychiatry* 45:267–273, 1988.

Hudson JI, Lipinski JF, Frankenburg FR, Tohen M, Kupfer DJ: Effects of lithium on sleep in mania. *Biol Psychiatry* 25:665–668, 1989.

Hudson L: *Contrary Imaginations: A Psychological Study of the English Schoolboy*. Middlesex: Penguin Books, 1966.

Hughes CC, Tremblay M, Rapoport RN, Leighton AH: *People of Cove and Woodlot*. New York: Basic Books, 1960.

Hullin RP: Minimum serum lithium levels for effective prophylaxis. In: FN Johnson, ed: *Handbook of Lithium Therapy*. Baltimore: University Park Press, 1980. pp 243–247.

Hullin RP, McDonald R, Allsopp MNE: Further report on prophylactic lithium in recurrent affective disorders. *Br J Psychiatry* 126:281–284, 1975.

Hullin RP, Goodwin JC, Birch NJ: The determination of sodium, potassium, and lithium concentrations in erythrocytes. *Biochem Soc Transactions* 4:331–333, 1976.

Humpheries SR, Dickinson PS: Hypomania following complex partial seizures. Letter. *Br J Psychiatry* 152:571–572, 1988.

Hunt DD, Adamson R, Egan K, Carr JE: Opioids: Mediators of fear or mania. *Biol Psychiatry* 23:426–428, 1988.

Hunt GE, Beilharz GR, Storlien LH, Kuchel PW, Johnson GF: The effect of lithium on rat erythrocyte choline, glycine and glutathione levels. *Biochem Pharmacol* 32:2981–2983, 1983.

Hurst LA, Mundy-Castle AC, Beerstecher DM: The electroencephalogram in manic-depressive psychosis. *J Ment Sci* 100:220–240, 1954.

Huston PE, Locher LM: Involutional psychosis: Course when untreated and when treated with electric shock. *Arch Neurol Psychiatry* 59:385–394, 1948a.

Huston PE, Locher LM: Manic-depressive psychosis: Course when untreated and when treated with electric shock. *Arch Neurol Psychiatry* 60:37–48, 1948b.

Huston PE, Senf R: Psychopathology of schizophrenia and depression: I. Effect of amytal and amphetamine sulfate on level and maintenance of attention. *Am J Psychiatry* 109:131–138, 1952.

Hutt C, Coxon MW: Systematic observation in clinical psychology. *Arch Gen Psychiatry* 12:374–378, 1965.

Iacono WG, Tuason VB: Bilateral electrodermal asymmetry in euthymic patients with unipolar and bipolar affective disorders. *Biol Psychiatry* 18:303–315, 1983.

Iacono WG, Peloquin LJ, Lumry AE, Valentine RH, Tuason VB: Eye tracking in patients with unipolar and bipolar affective disorders in remission. *J Abnorm Psychol* 91:35–44, 1982.

Iacono WG, Lykken DT, Peloquin LJ, Lumry AE, Valentine RH, Tuason VB: Electrodermal activity in euthymic unipolar and bipolar affective disorders: A possible marker for depression. *Arch Gen Psychiatry* 40:557–565, 1983.

Iacono WG, Lykken DT, Haroian KP, Peloquin LJ,

Valentine RH, Tuason VB: Electrodermal activity in euthymic patients with affective disorders: One-year retest stability and the effects of stimulus intensity and significance. *J Abnorm Psychol* 93:304–311, 1984.

Iacono WG, Smith GN, Moreau M, Beiser M, Fleming JAE, Lin T, Flak B: Ventricular and sulcal size at the onset of psychosis. *Am J Psychiatry* 145:820–824, 1988.

Ianzito BM, Cadoret RJ, Pugh DD: Thought disorder in depression. *Am J Psychiatry* 131:703–707, 1974.

Ikeda Y, Ijima M, Nomura S: Serum dopamine-beta-hydroxylase in manic-depressive psychosis. Letter. *Br J Psychiatry* 140:209–210, 1982.

Ingbar SH, Braverman LE, eds: *Werner's, The Thyroid: A Fundamental and Clinical Text*. 5th ed. New York: Lippincott, 1986.

Ingham JG: Changes in M.P.I. scores in neurotic patients: A three year follow-up. *Br J Psychiatry* 112:931–939, 1966.

Ingram RE: Toward an information-processing analysis of depression. *Cog Ther Res* 8:443–478, 1984.

Ingvar DH: Patterns of brain activity revealed by measurements of regional cerebral blood flow. In DH Ingvar, NA Lassen, eds: *Brain Work*. Copenhagen: Munksgaard, 1975. pp 397–413.

Ingvar DH, Franzén G: Abnormalities of cerebral blood flow distribution in patients with chronic schizophrenia. *Acta Psychiatr Scand* 50:425–462, 1974.

Ingvar DH, Lassen NA: Quantitative determination of regional cerebral blood-flow in man. *Lancet* 2:806–807, 1961.

Innis RB, Charney DS, Heninger GR: Differential ^{3}H-imipramine platelet binding in patients with panic disorder and depression. *Psychiatry Res* 21:33–41, 1987.

Insel TR, Goodwin FK: The dexamethasone suppression test: promises and problems of diagnostic laboratory tests in psychiatry. *Hosp Community Psychiatry* 34:1131–1138, 1983.

Insel TR, Donnelly EF, Lalakea ML, Alterman IS, Murphy DL: Neurological and neuropsychological studies of patients with obsessive-compulsive disorder. *Biol Psychiatry* 18:741–751, 1983.

Irvine DG, Miyashita H: Blood types in relation to depressions and schizophrenia: A preliminary report. *Can Med Assoc J* 92:551–554, 1965.

Isaacs G, Stainer DS, Sensky TE, Moor S, Thompson C: Phototherapy and its mechanisms of action in seasonal affective disorder. *J Affective Disord* 14:13–19, 1988.

Isaksson A, Ottosson JO, Perris C: Methologische aspekte der forschung über prophylaktische behandlund bei affektiven psychosen. In: H Hippius, H Selbach, eds: *Das Depressive Syndrom*. Munich: Urban and Schwarzenberg, 1969. pp 561–574.

Itil TM, Polvan N, Holden JM: Clinical and electroencephalographic effects of cinanserin in schizophrenic and manic patients. *Dis Nerv Syst* 32:193–200, 1971.

Iversen SD: Brain dopamine systems and behavior. In: L Iversen, S Iversen, S Snyder, eds: *Handbook of Psychopharmacology*. Vol 8. New York: Liss, 1978. pp 333–384.

Jablensky A: Symptoms, patterns of course and predictors of outcome in the functional psychoses: Some nosological implications. In: G Tognoni, C Bellantuono, M Lader, eds: *Epidemiological Impact of Psychotropic Drugs*. Amsterdam: Elsevier, 1981. pp 71–97.

Jacklet JW: Neural organization and cellular mechanisms of circadian pacemakers. *Int Rev Cytol* 89:251–294, 1984.

Jackson SL: Psychosis due to isoniazid. *Br Med J* 2:743–746, 1957.

Jackson SW: *Melancholia and Depression: From Hippocratic Times to Modern Times*. New Haven: Yale University Press, 1986.

Jaco E: *The Social Epidemiology of Mental Disorders*. New York: Russell Sage, 1960.

Jacobs D, Silverstone T: Dextroamphetamine-induced arousal in human subjects as a model for mania. *Psychol Med* 16:323–329, 1986.

Jacobs LI: Cognitive therapy of postmanic and postdepressive dysphoria in bipolar illness. *Am J Psychotherapy* 36:450–458, 1982.

Jacobsen FM, Sack DA, Wehr TA, Rogers S, Rosenthal NE: Neuroendocrine response to 5-hydroxytryptophan in seasonal affective disorder. *Arch Gen Psychiatry* 44:1086–1091, 1987a.

Jacobsen FM, Wehr TA, Skwerer RA, Sack DA, Rosenthal NE: Morning versus midday phototherapy of seasonal affective disorder. *Am J Psychiatry* 144:1301–1305, 1987b.

Jacobson E: Contribution to the metapsychology of cyclothymic depression. In: P Greenacre, ed. *Affective Disorders: Psychoanalytic Contribution to Their Study*. New York: International Universities Press, Inc, 1953. pp 49–83.

Jacobson JE: The hypomanic alert: A program designed for greater therapeutic control. *Am J Psychiatry* 122:295–299, 1965.

Jacoby RJ, Levy R: Computed tomography in the elderly. 3. Affective disorder. *Br J Psychiatry* 136:270–275, 1980.

Jacoby RJ, Levy R, Dawson JM: Computed tomography in the elderly: I: The normal population. *Br J Psychiatry* 136:249–255, 1980.

Jacoby RJ, Levy R, Bird JM: Computed tomography and the outcome of affective disorder: A follow-up study of elderly patients. *Br J Psychiatry* 139:288–292, 1981.

Jacoby RJ, Dolan RJ, Levy R, Baldy R: Quantitative computed tomography in elderly depressed patients. *Br J Psychiatry* 143:124–127, 1983.

Jaeckle RS, Kathol RG, Lopez JF, Meller WH, Krummel SJ: Enhanced adrenal sensitivity to exogenous cosyntropin (ACTH alpha 1-24) stimulation in major depression: Relationship to dexamethasone suppression test results. *Arch Gen Psychiatry* 44:233–240, 1987.

Jameison GR: Suicide and mental disease: A clinical

analysis of one hundred cases. *Arch Neurol Psychiatry* 36:1–12, 1936.

Jameison GR, Wall JH: Some psychiatric aspects of suicide. *Psychiatr Q* 7:211–229, 1933.

James NM: Early- and late-onset bipolar affective disorder: A genetic study. *Am J Psychiatry* 34:715–717, 1977.

James NM, Chapman CJ: A genetic study of bipolar affective disorder. *Br J Psychiatry* 126:449–456, 1975.

James SP, Wehr TA, Sack DA, Parry BL, Rosenthal NE: Treatment of seasonal affective disorder with light in the evening. *Br J Psychiatry* 147:424–428, 1985.

James SP, Wehr TA, Sack DA, Parry BL, Rogers S, Rosenthal NE: The dexamethasone suppression test in seasonal affective disorder. *Compr Psychiatry* 27(3):224–226, 1986.

James W: *The Varieties of Religious Experience: A Study in Human Nature.* (1902) Middlesex, England: Penguin, 1982.

Jamison KR: Atypical cycloid psychoses. In: CTH Friedmann, RA Faguet, eds: *Extraordinary Disorders of Human Behavior.* New York: Plenum Press, 1982. pp 259–291.

Jamison KR: "Psychological Management of Bipolar Disorders." Presented at Mood Disorders: Pharmacologic Prevention of Recurrences, Consensus Development Conference on Mood Disorders, Bethesda, MD, April, 1984.

Jamison KR: Suicide and bipolar disorders. *Ann NY Acad Sci* 487:301–315, 1986.

Jamison KR: Psychotherapeutic issues and suicide prevention in the treatment of bipolar disorders. In: RE Hales, AJ Frances, eds: *American Psychiatric Association Annual Review, Vol 6.* Washington, DC: American Psychiatric Press, 1987. pp. 108–124.

Jamison KR: Suicide prevention in depressed women. *J Clin Psychiatry* 49:42–45, 1988.

Jamison KR: Mood disorders and seasonal patterns in British writers and artists. *Psychiatry* 52:125–134, 1989.

Jamison KR, Akiskal HS: Medication compliance in patients with bipolar disorders. *Psychiatr Clin North Am* 6:175–192, 1983.

Jamison KR, Goodwin FK: Psychotherapeutic treatment of manic-depressive patients on lithium. In: M Greenhill, A Gralnick, eds: *The Interrelationship of Psychopharmacology and Psychotherapy.* New York: Macmillan, 1983a. pp 53–74.

Jamison KR, Goodwin FK: Psychotherapeutic issues in bipolar illness. In: L Grinspoon, ed: *Psychiatry Update: The American Psychiatric Association Annual Review.* Vol II, Washington, DC: American Psychiatric Press, 1983b. pp 319–345.

Jamison KR, Winter R: *Moods and Music.* Program notes for a concert performed by the National Symphony Orchestra at the John F. Kennedy Center for the Performing Arts. Washington, DC, 1988.

Jamison KR, Gerner RH, Goodwin FK: Patient and physician attitudes toward lithium: Relationship to compliance. *Arch Gen Psychiatry* 36:866–869, 1979.

Jamison KR, Gerner RH, Hammen C, Padesky C: Clouds and silver linings: Positive experiences associated with primary affective disorders. *Am J Psychiatry* 137:198–202, 1980.

Jamison KR, Hammen C, Gong-Guy E, Padesky C, Gerner RH: Self-perceptions of interpersonal functioning in unipolar and bipolar men and women. Unpublished data.

Jamison KR, Litman-Adizes T, Gitlin MJ, Fieve RR: Personality and attitudinal patterns in affective illness. Unpublished data.

Jampala VC, Abrams R: Mania secondary to left and right hemisphere damage. *Am J Psychiatry* 140:1197–1199, 1983.

Jampala VC, Abrams R, Taylor MA: Mania with emotional blunting: Affective disorder or schizophrenia? *Am J Psychiatry* 142:608–612, 1985.

Jampala VC, Taylor MA, Abrams R: The diagnostic implications of formal thought disorder in mania and schizophrenia: A reassessment. *Am J Psychiatry* 146:459–463, 1989.

Janicak PG, Davis JM, Gibbons RD, Ericksen S, Chang S, Gallagher P: Efficacy of ECT: A meta-analysis. *Am J Psychiatry* 142:297–302, 1985.

Janicak PG, Bresnahan DB, Sharma R, Davis JM, Comaty JE, Malinick: A comparison of thiothixine with chlorpromazine in the treatment of mania. *J Clin Psychopharmacol* 8:33–37, 1988a.

Janicak PG, Sharma RP, Altman E, Javaid JI, Kumar PM, Davis JM: Clonidine for mania: Placebo controlled trial. Abstract of paper presented at the 141st annual meeting of the American Psychiatric Association, May, 1988b.

Jann MW, Bitar AH, Rao A: Lithium prophylaxis of tricyclic-antidepressant-induced mania in bipolar patients. *Am J Psychiatry* 139:683–684, 1982.

Janowsky A, Steranka LR, Gillespie DD, Sulser F: Role of neuronal signal input in the down-regulation of central noradrenergic receptor function by antidepressant drugs. *J Neurochem* 39:290–292, 1982.

Janowsky DS, Neborsky RJ: Hypothesized common mechanism in the psychotherapy and psychopharmacology of depression *Psychiatr Ann* 10:356–361, 1980.

Janowsky DS, Risch SC: Cholinomimetic and anticholinergic drugs used to investigate an acetylcholine hypothesis of affective disorders and stress. *Drug Dev Res* 4:125–142, 1984.

Janowsky DS, Leff M, Epstein RS: Playing the manic game: Interpersonal maneuvers of the acutely manic patient. *Arch Gen Psychiatry* 22:252–261, 1970.

Janowsky DS, El-Yousef MK, Davis JM, Sekerke HJ: A cholinergic-adrenergic hypothesis of mania and depression. *Lancet* 2:632–635, 1972.

Janowsky DS, El-Yousef MK, Davis JM, Sekerke HJ: Antagonistic effects of physostigmine and methylphenidate in man. *Am J Psychiatry* 130:1370–1376, 1973a.

Janowsky DS, El-Yousef MK, Davis JM, Sekerke HJ:

Provocation of schizophrenic symptoms by intravenous administration of methylphenidate. *Arch Gen Psychiatry* 28:185–191, 1973b.

Janowsky DS, El-Yousef MK, Davis JM, Sekerke HJ: Parasympathetic suppression of manic symptoms by physostigmine. *Arch Gen Psychiatry* 28:542–547, 1973c.

Janowsky DS, El-Yousef MK, Davis JM: Interpersonal maneuvers of manic patients. *Am J Psychiatry* 131:250–255, 1974.

Janowsky D, Judd L, Huey L, Roitman N, Parker D, Segal D: Naloxone effects on manic symptoms and growth-hormone levels [Letter]. *Lancet* 2:320, 1978.

Janowsky DS, Judd LL, Huey L, Segal D: Effects of naloxone in normal, manic, and schizophrenic patients: Evidence for alleviation of manic symptoms. In: E Usdin, WE Bunney, NS Kline, eds: *Endorphins in Mental Health Research*. New York: Oxford University Press, 1979. pp 435–447.

Janowsky DS, Risch SC, Parker DC, Huey LY, Judd LL: Behavioral-neuroendocrine effects of physostigmine effect. *Proc of the 13th Collegium Internationale Neuropsychopharmacologicum*, 1982.

Jarrett DB, Miewald JM, Kupfer DJ: Recurrent depression is associated with a persistent reduction in sleep-related growth hormone secretion. *Arch Gen Psychiatry* 47:113–118, 1990.

Jaspers K: *General Psychopathology*. Translated by J Hoenig, MW Hamilton, Chicago: University of Chicago Press, 1963. (Originally published in 1913).

Jauch DA, Carpenter WT: Reactive psychosis I: Does the pre-DSM-III concept define a third psychosis? *J Nerv Ment Dis* 176:72–81, 1988a.

Jauch DA, Carpenter WT: Reactive psychosis II: Does DSM-III-R define a third psychosis? *J Nerv Ment Dis* 176:82–86, 1988b.

Jefferson JW: The use of lithium in childhood and adolescence: An overview. *J Clin Psychiatry* 43:174–177, 1982.

Jefferson JW, Greist JH: *Primer of Lithium Therapy*. Baltimore: Williams & Wilkins, 1977.

Jefferson JW, Greist JH: Lithium carbonate and carbamazepine side effects. In: RE Hales, AJ Frances, eds: *Psychiatry Update: American Psychiatric Association Annual Review. Vol 6*. Washington, DC: American Psychiatric Press, 1987. pp 746–780.

Jefferson JW, Greist JH, Clagnaz PJ, Eischens RR, Marten WC, Evenson MA: Effect of strenuous exercise on serum lithium level in man. *Am J Psychiatry* 139:1593–1595, 1982.

Jefferson JW, Greist JH, Ackerman DL, Carroll JA: *Lithium Encyclopedia for Clinical Practice*. 2nd ed. Washington DC: American Psychiatric Press, 1987.

Jelliffe SE: Some historical phases of the manic-depressive synthesis. *Research Publications Association for Research in Nervous and Mental Diseases* 11:3–47, 1931.

Jenner FA, Gjessing LR, Cox JR, Davies-Jones A, Hullin RP, Hanna SM: A manic depressive psychotic with a persistent forty-eight hour cycle. *Br J Psychiatry* 113:895–910, 1967.

Jensen AR: The Maudsley Personality Inventory. *Acta Psychologica* 14:314–325, 1958.

Jernajczyk W: Latency of eye movement and other REM sleep parameters in bipolar depression. *Biol Psychiatry* 21:465–472, 1986.

Jerram TC, McDonald R: Plasma lithium control with particular reference to minimum effective levels. In: FN Johnson, S Johnson, eds: *Lithium in Medical Practice*. Baltimore: University Park Press, 1978. pp 407–413.

Jesberger JA, Richardson JS: Animal models of depression: Parallels and correlates to severe depression in humans. *Biol Psychiatry* 20:764–784, 1985a.

Jesberger JA, Richardson JS: Neurochemical aspects of depression: The past and the future? *Int J Neurosci* 27:19–47, 1985b.

Jesberger JA, Richardson JS: Brain output dysregulation induced by olfactory bulbectomy: An approximation in the rat of major depressive disorder in humans? *Int J Neurosci* 38:241–265, 1988.

Jeste DV, Lohr JB, Goodwin FK: Neuroanatomical studies of major affective disorders: A review and suggestions for further research. *Br J Psychiatry* 153:444–459, 1988.

Jimerson DC: Role of dopamine mechanisms in the affective disorders. In: HY Meltzer, ed: *Psychopharmacology: The Third Generation of Progress*. New York: Raven Press, 1987. pp 505–511.

Jimerson DC, Berrettini W: Cerebrospinal fluid amine metabolite studies in depression: Research update. In: H Beckmann, P Riederer, eds: *Pathochemical Markers in Major Psychoses*. Berlin: Springer-Verlag, 1985. pp 129–143.

Jimerson DC, Gordon EK, Post RM, Goodwin FK: Central noradrenergic function in man: Vanillylmandelic acid in CSF. *Brain Res* 99:434–439, 1975.

Jimerson DC, Post RM, Van Kammen DL, Docherty J, Gillin JC, Buchsbaum M, Ebert M, Bunney WE: Predictors of amphetamine response in depression. Abstract of paper presented at the 130th meeting of the American Psychiatric Association, 1977. pp 100–101.

Jimerson DC, Post RM, Carman JS, Van Kammen DP, Wood JH, Goodwin FK, Bunney WE Jr: CSF calcium: Clinical correlates in affective illness and schizophrenia. *Biol Psychiatry* 14:37–51, 1979.

Jimerson DC, Post RM, Stoddard FJ, Gillin JC, Bunney WE Jr: Preliminary trial of the noradrenergic agonist clonidine in psychiatric patients. *Biol Psychiatry* 15:45–57, 1980a.

Jimerson DC, Post RM, Van Kammen DP, Skyler JS, Brown GL, Bunney WE Jr: Cerebrospinal fluid cortisol levels in depression and schizophrenia. *Am J Psychiatry* 137:979–980, 1980b.

Jimerson DC, Nurnberger JI Jr, Post RM, Gershon ES, Kopin IJ: Plasma MHPG in rapid cyclers and healthy twins. *Arch Gen Psychiatry* 38:1287–1290, 1981.

Jimerson DC, Nurnberger JI Jr, Simmons S, Gershon ES: Anticholinergic treatment for depression. Abstract of paper presented at the 135th meeting of the American Psychiatric Association, 1982. pp 218–219.

Jimerson DC, Insel TR, Reus VI, Kopin IJ: Increased plasma MHPG in dexamethasone-resistant depressed patients. *Arch Gen Psychiatry* 40:173–176, 1983.

Jimerson DC, Cutler NR, Post RM, Rey A, Gold PW, Brown GM, Bunney WE Jr: Neuroendocrine responses to apomorphine in depressed patients and healthy control subjects. *Psychiatry Res* 13:1–12, 1984a.

Jimerson DC, Rubinow DR, Ballenger JC, Post RM, Kopin IJ: Cerebrospinal fluid norepinephrine metabolites in depressed patients: New methodologies. In: Usdin E, Carlsson A, Dahlström A, Engel J, eds: *Catecholamines: Part C: Neuropharmacology and Central Nervous System—Therapeutic Aspects.* New York: Alan R. Liss, 1984b. pp. 123–129.

Joffe RT: Antithyroid antibodies in major depression. *Acta Psychiatr Scand* 76:598–599, 1987.

Joffe RT: Triiodothyronine potentiation of the antidepressant effect of phenelzine. *J Clin Psychiatry* 49:409–410, 1988.

Joffe RT, Brown P: Clinical and biological correlates of sleep deprivation in depression. *Can J Psychiatry* 29:530–536, 1984.

Joffe RT, Singer W: Thyroid hormone potentiation of antidepressants. Abstract of paper presented at the 141st annual meeting of the American Psychiatric Association, May, 1988.

Joffe RT, Roy-Byrne PP, Uhde TW, Post RM: Thyroid function and affective illness: A reappraisal. *Biol Psychiatry* 19:1685–1691, 1984.

Joffe RT, Blank DW, Berrettini WH, Post RM: Erythrocyte sodium and potassium in affective illness. *Acta Psychiatr Scand* 73:416–419, 1986a.

Joffe RT, Post RM, Rubinow DR, Berrettini WH, Hare TA, Ballenger JC, Roy-Byrne PP: Cerebrospinal fluid GABA in manic-depressive illness. In: G Bartholini, KG Lloyd, PL Morselli, eds: *GABA and Mood Disorders: Experimental and Clinical Research.* New York: Raven Press, 1986b. pp 187–193.

Joffe RT, Post RM, Uhde TW: Effects of carbamazepine on serum electrolytes in affectively ill patients. *Psychol Med* 16:331–335, 1986c.

Joffe RT, Lippert GP, Gray TA, Sawa G, Horvath Z: Personal and family history of affective illness in patients with multiple sclerosis. *J Affective Disord* 12:63–65, 1987a.

Joffe RT, Lippert GP, Gray TA, Sawa G, Horvath Z: Mood disorder and multiple sclerosis. *Arch Neurol* 44:376–378, 1987b.

Joffe RT, Kutcher S, MacDonald C: Thyroid function and bipolar affective disorder. *Psychiatry Res* 25:117–121, 1988a.

Joffe RT, MacDonald C, Kutcher SP: Lack of differential cognitive effects of lithium and carbamazepine in bipolar affective disorder. *J Clin Psychopharmacology* 8:425–428, 1988b.

John ER, Karmel BZ, Corning WC, Easton P, Brown D, Ahn H, John M, Harmony T, Prichep L, Toro A, Gerson I, Bartlett F, Thatcher F, Kaye H, Valdes P, Schwartz E: Neurometrics. *Science* 196:1393–1410, 1977.

John ER, Prichep L, Ahn H, Easton P, Fridman J, Kaye H: Neurometric evaluation of cognitive dysfunctions and neurological disorders in children. *Prog Neurobiol* 21:239–290, 1983.

John ER, Prichep L, Fridman J, Easton P: Neurometrics: Computer-assisted differential diagnosis of brain dysfunctions. *Science* 239:162–169, 1988.

Johnson FN: *Handbook of Lithium Therapy.* Baltimore: University Park Press, 1980.

Johnson FN: *The Psychopharmacology of Lithium.* London: Macmillan Press, 1984.

Johnson FS, Hunt GE, Duggin GG, Horvath JS, Tiller DJ: Renal function and lithium treatment: Initial and follow-up tests in manic-depressive patients. *J Affective Disord* 6:249–263, 1984.

Johnson G: Antidepressant effect of lithium. *Compr Psychiatry* 15:43–47, 1974.

Johnson G: Lithium. *Med J Aust* 141: 595–601, 1984.

Johnson G, Gershon S, Hekimian LJ: Controlled evaluation of lithium and chlorpromazine in the treatment of manic states: An interim report. *Compr Psychiatry* 9:563–573, 1968.

Johnson G, Gershon S, Burdock EI, Floyd A, Hekimian L: Comparative effects of lithium and chlorpromazine in the treatment of acute manic states. *Br J Psychiatry* 119:267–276, 1971.

Johnson GF, Hunt G: Suicidal behavior in bipolar manic-depressive patients and their families. *Compr Psychiatry* 20:159–164, 1979.

Johnson LC: Psychophysiological research: Aims and methods. *Int J Psychiatry Med* 5:565–573, 1974.

Johnson MH, Magaro PA: Effects of mood and severity on memory processes in depression and mania. *Psychol Bull* 101:28–40, 1987.

Johnson O, Crockett D: Changes in perceptual asymmetries with clinical improvement of depression and schizophrenia. *J Abnorm Psychol* 91:45–54, 1982.

Johnson RF, Smale L, Moore RY, Morin LP: Lateral geniculate lesions block circadian phase-shift responses to a benzodiazepine. *Proc Natl Acad Sci USA* 85:5301–5304, 1988.

Johnston BB, Dick EG, Naylor GJ, Dick DAT: Lithium side effects in a routine lithium clinic. *Br J Psychiatry* 134:482–487, 1979.

Johnston BB, Naylor GJ, Dick EG, Hopwood SE, Dick DA: Prediction of clinical course of bipolar manic depressive illness treated with lithium. *Psychol Med* 10:329–334, 1980.

Johnston MH, Holzman PS: *Assessing Schizophrenic Thinking.* San Francisco: Josey-Bass, 1979.

Johnstone EC, Owens DG, Crow TJ, Colter N, Lawton CA, Jagoe R, Kreel L: Hypothyroidism as a correlate of lateral ventricular enlargement in manic-depressive and neurotic illness. *Br J Psychiatry* 148:317–321, 1986.

Johnstone EC, Owens DG, Crow TJ, Frith CD, Alexandropolis K, Bydder G, Colter N: Temporal lobe structure as determined by nuclear magnetic resonance in schizophrenia and bipolar affective disorder. *J Neurol Neurosurg Psychiatry* 52:736–741, 1989.

Jones BE, Gray BA, Parson EB: Manic-depressive illness among poor urban blacks. *Am J Psychiatry* 138:654–657, 1981.

Jones BE, Gray BA, Parson EB: Manic-depressive illness among poor urban Hispanics. *Am J Psychiatry* 140:1208–1210, 1983.

Jones BE, Gray BA, Parson EB: Major affective disorders in blacks: A preliminary report. *Integr Psychiatry* 6:131–140, 1988.

Jones D, Kelwala S, Bell J, Dubé S, Jackson E, Sitaram N: Cholinergic REM sleep induction response correlation with endogenous major depressive subtype. *Psychiatry Res* 14:99–110, 1985.

Jones FD, Maas JW, Dekirmenjian H, Fawcett JA: Urinary catecholamine metabolites during behavioral changes in a patient with manic-depressive cycles. *Science* 179:300–302, 1973.

Jones JF, Wilson IC: Lithium therapy in manic states: Prediction of therapeutic effect. *Activ Nerv* 14:52–58, 1972.

Jones KL, Lacro RV, Johnson KA, Adams J: Pattern of malformations in the children of women treated with carbamazepine during pregnancy. *N Engl J Med* 320:1661–1666, 1989.

Jones PM, Berney TP: Early onset rapid cycling bipolar affective disorder. *J Child Psychol Psychiatry* 28:731–738, 1987.

Jope RS, Jenden DJ, Ehrlich BE, Diamond JM, Gosenfeld LF: Erythrocyte choline concentrations are elevated in manic patients. *Proc Natl Acad Sci USA* 77:6144–6146, 1980.

Jørgensen F, Larsen S, Spanager B, Clausen E, Tangø M, Brinch E, Brun C: Kidney function and quantitative histological changes in patients on long-term lithium therapy. *Acta Psychiatr Scand* 70:455–462, 1984.

Joseph RJ: John Ruskin: Radical and psychotic genius. *Psychoanal Rev* 56:425–441, 1969.

Josephson AM, Mackenzie TB: Appearance of manic psychosis following rapid normalization of thyroid status. *Am J Psychiatry* 136:846–847, 1979.

Jouvent R, Lecrubier Y, Puech AJ, Simon P, Widlöcher D: Antimanic effect of clonidine. *Am J Psychiatry* 137:1275–1276, 1980.

Joyce PR: Age of onset in bipolar affective disorder and misdiagnosis as schizophrenia. *Psychol Med* 14:145–149, 1984a.

Joyce PR: Parental bonding in bipolar affective disorder. *J Affective Disord* 7:319–324, 1984b.

Joyce PR, Paykel ES: Predictors of drug response in depression. *Arch Gen Psychiatry* 46:89–99, 1989.

Joyce PR, Sellman JD, Donald RA, Livesey JH, Elder PA: The unipolar-bipolar depressive dichotomy and the relationship between afternoon prolactin and cortisol levels. *J Affective Disord* 14:189–193, 1988.

Judd LL: The effect of lithium on mood, cognition, and personality function in normal subjects. *Arch Gen Psychiatry* 36:860–865, 1979.

Judd LL, Hubbard B, Janowsky DS, Huey LY, Attewell PA: The effect of lithium carbonate on affect, mood, and personality of normal subjects. *Arch Gen Psychiatry* 34:346–351, 1977a.

Judd LL, Hubbard B, Janowsky DS, Huey LY, Takahashi KI: The effect of lithium carbonate on the cognitive functions of normal subjects. *Arch Gen Psychiatry* 34:355–357, 1977b.

Judd LL, Hubbard B, Janowsky DS, Huey LY, Abrams AA, Riney WB, Pendery MM: Ethanol-lithium interaction in alcoholics. In: DW Goodwin, CK Erickson, eds: *Alcoholism and Affective Disorders: Clinical, Genetic, and Biochemical Studies.* New York: Spectrum, 1979. pp 109–135.

Judd LL, Janowsky DS, Segal DS, Huey LY: Naloxone-induced behavioral and physiological effects in normal and manic subjects. *Arch Gen Psychiatry* 37:583–586, 1980.

Judd LL, Squire LR, Butters N, Salmon DP, Paller KA: Effects of psychotropic drugs on cognition and memory in normal humans and animals. In: HY Meltzer, ed: *Psychopharmacology: The Third Generation of Progress.* New York: Raven Press, 1987. pp 1467–1475.

Juhl RP, Tsuang MT, Perry PJ: Concomitant administration of haloperidol and lithium carbonate in acute mania. *Dis Nerv Syst* 38:675–677, 1977.

Jura A: The relationship between high mental capacity and psychic abnormalities. *Am J Psychiatry* 106:296–307, 1949.

Kadrmas A, Winokur G: Manic depressive illness and EEG abnormalities. *J Clin Psychiatry* 40:306–307, 1979.

Kadrmas A, Winokur G, Crowe R: Postpartum mania. *Br J Psychiatry* 135:551–554, 1979.

Kafka MS, Paul SM: Platelet alpha 2-adrenergic receptors in depression. *Arch Gen Psychiatry* 43:91–95, 1986.

Kafka MS, Tallman JF, Smith CC, Costa JL: Alpha-adrenergic receptors on human platelets. *Life Sci* 21:1429–1438, 1977.

Kafka MS, Van Kammen DP, Kleinman JE, Nurnberger JI JR, Siever LJ, Uhde TW, Polinsky RJ: Alpha-adrenergic receptor function in schizophrenia, affective disorders and some neurological diseases. *Commun Psychopharmacol* 4:477–486, 1980.

Kagan DL, Oltmanns TF: Matched tasks for measuring single-word, referent communication: The performance of patients with schizophrenic and affective disorders. *J Abnorm Psychol* 90:204–212, 1981.

Kahlbaum KL: Über cyclisches Irresein. *Der Irrenfreund* 10: 145–157, 1882.

Kahn EM, Weiner RD, Brenner RP, Coppola R: Topographic maps of brain electrical activity—pitfalls and precautions. *Biol Psychiatry* 23:628–636, 1988.

Kahn J, Coyne JC, Margolin G: Depression and marital disagreement: The social construction of despair. *J Soc Pers Rel* 2:447–462, 1985.

Kalin NH, Gibbs DM, Barksdale CM, Shelton SE, Carnes M: Behavioral stress decreases plasma oxytocin concentrations in primates. *Life Sci* 36:1275–1280, 1985.

Källén B, Tandberg A: Lithium and pregnancy: A cohort study on manic-depressive women. *Acta Psychiatr Scand* 68:134–139, 1983.

Kametani H, Nomura S, Shimizu J: The reversal effect of antidepressants on the escape deficit induced by inescapable shock in rats. *Psychopharmacology* 80:206–208, 1983.

Kan YW, Dozy AM: Polymorphism of DNA sequence adjacent to human beta-globin structural gene: Relationship to sickle mutation. *Proc Natl Acad Sci* 75:5631–5635, 1978.

Kanakaratnam G, Direkze M: Aspects of primary tumours of the frontal lobe. *Br J Clin Practice* 30:220–221, 1976.

Kandel ER: Psychotherapy and the single synapse: The impact of psychiatric thought on neurobiologic research. *N Engl J Med* 301:1028–1037, 1979.

Kane FJ Jr: Treatment of mania with cinanserin, an antiserotonin agent. *Am J Psychiatry* 126:1020–1023, 1970.

Kane FJ, Taylor TW: Mania associated with the use of INH and cocaine. *Am J Psychiatry* 119:1098–1099, 1963.

Kane JM, Lieberman J: The efficacy of amoxapine, maprotiline, and trazodone in comparison to imipramine and amitriptyline: A review of the literature. *Psychopharmacol Bull* 20:240–249, 1984.

Kane JM, Quitkin FM, Rifkin A, Ramos-Lorenzi JR, Nayak DD, Howard A: Lithium carbonate and imipramine in the prophylaxis of unipolar and bipolar II illness: A prospective, placebo-controlled comparison. *Arch Gen Psychiatry* 39:1065–1069, 1982.

Kane J, Honigfeld G, Singer J, Meltzer H: Clozapine for the treatment-resistant schizophrenic. *Arch Gen Psychiatry* 45:789–796, 1988.

Kaneko M, Hayashi A, Unno Y, Watanabe K, Takahashi Y: Serum 5-hydroxytryptamine level in manic-depressive illness. *Fukushima J Med Sci* 21:1–9, 1975.

Kanof PD, Coccaro EF, Johns CA, Siever LJ, Davis KL: Platelet [3H] imipramine binding in psychiatric disorders. *Biol Psychiatry* 22:278–286, 1987.

Kansal PC, Buse J, Talbert OR, Buse MG: The effect of L-dopa on plasma growth hormone, insulin, and thyroxine. *J Clin Endocrinol Metab* 34:99–105, 1972.

Kantor D, McNevin S, Leichner P, Harper D, Krenn M: The benfit of lithium carbonate adjunct in refractory depression: Fact or fiction? *Can J Psychiatry* 31:416–418, 1986.

Kaplan RD, Mann JJ: Altered platelet serotonin uptake kinetics in schizophrenia and depression. *Life Sci* 31:583–588, 1982.

Kaplitz SE: Withdrawn, apathetic geriatric patients responsive to methylphenidate. *J Am Geriatr Soc* 23:271–276, 1975.

Kapp FT: Ezra Pound's creativity and treason: Clues from his life and work. *Compr Psychiatry* 9:414–427, 1968.

Karczmar AG, Longo VG, Scotti de Carolis A: A pharmacological model of paradoxical sleep: The role of cholinergic and monoamine systems. *Physiol Behav* 5:175–182, 1970.

Karege F, Bovier P, Gaillard JM, Tissot R: The decrease of erythrocyte catechol-O-methyltransferase activity in depressed patients and its diagnostic significance. *Acta Psychiatr Scand* 76:303–308, 1987.

Karki SD, Carson SW, Holden JM, Nanavati D: Evaluation of a two-point method for prediction of lithium maintenace dosage. *Int Clin Psychopharmacol* 2:343–351, 1987.

Karliner W, Wehrheim HK: Maintenance convulsive treatments. *Am J Psychiatry* 121:1113–1115, 1965.

Karlsson JL: Genetic association of giftedness and creativity with schizophrenia. *Hereditas* 66:177–82, 1970.

Karniol IGG, Dalton J, Lader MH: Acute and chronic effects of lithium chloride on physiological and psychological measures in normals. *Psychopharmacology (Berlin)* 57:289–294, 1978.

Karno M, Hough RL, Burnam MA, Escobar JI, Timbers DM, Santana F, Boyd JH: Lifetime prevalence of specific psychiatric disorders among Mexican Americans and non-Hispanic whites in Los Angeles. *Arch Gen Psychiatry* 44:695–701, 1987.

Karoum F, Linnoila M, Potter WZ, Chuang LW, Goodwin FK, Wyatt RJ: Fluctuating high urinary phenylethylamine excretion rates in some bipolar affective disorder patients. *Psychiatry Res* 6:215–222, 1982.

Karoum F, Korpi ER, Linnoila M, Chuang LW, Wyatt RJ: Reduced metabolism and turnover rates of rat brain dopamine, norepinephrine and serotonin by chronic desipramine and zimelidine treatments. *Eur J Pharmacol* 100:137–144, 1984a.

Karoum F, Potkin S, Chuang LW, Murphy DL, Liebowitz MR, Wyatt RJ: Phenylacetic acid excretion in schizophrenia and depression: The origins of PAA in man. *Biol Psychiatry* 19:165–178, 1984b.

Kasa K, Otsuki S, Yamamoto M, Sato M, Kuroda H, Ogawa N: Cerebrospinal fluid γ-aminobutyric acid and homovanillic acid in depressive disorders. *Biol Psychiatry* 17:877–883, 1982.

Kasanin J: The acute schizoaffective psychoses. *Am J Psychiatry* 90:97–126, 1933.

Kasanin J: The affective psychoses in children. *J Nerv Ment Dis* 116:424–429, 1952.

Kashani JH, Carlson GA: Seriously depressed preschoolers. *Am J Psychiatry* 144:348–350, 1987.

Kashani JH, Husain A, Shekim WO, Hodges KK, Cytryn L, McKnew DH: Current perspectives on childhood depression: An overview. *Am J Psychiatry* 138:143–152, 1981.

Kashani JH, Orvaschel H, Burk JP, Reid JC: Informant

variance: The issue of parent-child disagreement. *J Am Acad Child Psychiatry* 24:437–441, 1985.

Kaskey GB, Salzman LF, Ciccone JR, Klorman R: Effects of lithium on evoked potentials and performance during sustained attention. *Psychiatry Res* 3:281–289, 1980.

Kasper S, Moises HW, Beckmann H: The anticholinergic biperiden in depressive disorders. *Pharmacopsychiatria* 14:195–198, 1981.

Kasper S, Sack DA, Wehr TA, Kick H, Voll G, Vieira A: Nocturnal TSH and prolactin secretion during sleep deprivation and prediction of antidepressant response in patients with major depression. *Biol Psychiatry* 24:631–641, 1988.

Kasper S, Rogers SLB, Yancey A, Skwerer RG, Schulz PM, Rosenthal NE: Psychological effects of light therapy in normals. In: NE Rosenthal, MC Blehar, eds: *Seasonal Affective Disorders and Phototherapy*. New York: Guilford, 1989a. pp. 260–270.

Kasper S, Wehr TA, Bartko JJ, Gaist PA, Rosenthal NE: Epidemiological findings of seasonal changes in mood and behavior: A telephone survey of Montgomery County, Maryland. *Arch Gen Psychiatry* 46:823–833, 1989b.

Kastin AJ, Miller LH, Gonzalez-Barcena D, Hawley WD, Dyster-Aas K, Schally AV, Velasco de Parra ML, Velasco M: Psycho-physiologic correlates of MSH activity in man. *Physiol Behav* 7:893–896, 1971.

Kastin AJ, Ehrensing RH, Schalch DS, Anderson MS: Improvement in mental depression with decreased thyrotropin response after administration of thyrotropin-releasing hormone. *Lancet* 2:740–742, 1972.

Kathol RG: Persistent elevation of urinary free cortisol and loss of circannual periodicity in recovered depressive patients: A trait finding. *J Affective Disord* 8:137–145, 1985.

Katon W, Raskind M: Treatment of depression in the medically ill elderly with methylphenidate. *Am J Psychiatry* 137:963–965, 1980.

Katz MM, Itil TM: Video methodology for research in psychopathology and psychopharmacology: Rationale and application. *Arch Gen Psychiatry* 31:204–210, 1974.

Katz MM, Robins E, Croughan J, Secunda S, Swann A: Behavioural measurement and drug response characteristics of unipolar and bipolar depression. *Psychol Med* 12:25–36, 1982.

Katz MM, Koslow SH, Maas JW, Frazer A, Bowden CL, Casper R, Croughan J, Kocsis J, Redmond E: The timing, specificity and clinical prediction of tricyclic drug effects in depression. *Psychol Med* 17:297–309, 1987.

Katz RJ: Animal models and human depressive disorders. *Neuroscience and Biobehavioral Reviews* 5:231–246, 1981.

Katz RJ: Stress, conflict, and depression. In: J Angst, ed: *The Origins of Depression: Current Concepts and Approaches*. Berlin: Springer-Verlag, 1983. pp 121–132.

Katzenelbogen S, Brody MW, Hayman M, Margolin E: Metrazol convulsions in man: Clinical and biochemical studies. *Am J Psychiatry* 95:1343–1348, 1939.

Katzman R, Pappius HM: *Brain Electrolytes and Fluid Metabolism*. Baltimore: Williams & Wilkins, 1973.

Kaufman E: Family adaptation to substance abuse. In: AI Alterman, ed: *Substance Abuse and Psychopathology*. New York: Plenum Press, 1985. pp 343–366.

Kaufmann MW, Murray GB, Cassem NH: Use of psychostimulants in medically ill depressed patients. *Psychosomatics* 23:817–819, 1982.

Kay DS, Naylor GJ, Smith AH, Greenwood C: The therapeutic effect of ascorbic acid and EDTA in manic-depressive psychosis: Double-blind comparisons with standard treatments. *Psychol Med* 14:533–539, 1984.

Kay DWK: Observations on the natural history and genetics of old age psychoses: A Stockholm material 1931–1937. *Proc Roy Soc Med* 52:29–32, 1959.

Kay DWK, Petterson U: VI. Mortality. In: U Petterson: Manic-depressive illness: A clinical, social and genetic study. *Acta Psychiatr Scand* (Suppl 269):55–60, 1977.

Keeler MH, Taylor CI, Miller WC: Are all recently detoxified alcoholics depressed? *Am J Psychiatry* 136:586–588, 1979.

Keith-Spiegel P, Spiegel DE: Affective states of patients immediately preceding suicide. *J Psychiatr Res* 5:89– 93, 1967.

Keller MB, Lavori PW, McDonald-Scott P, Scheftner WA, Andreasen NC, Shapiro RW, Croughan J: Reliability of lifetime diagnoses and symptoms in patients with a current psychiatric disorder. *J Psychiatr Res* 4:229–240, 1981.

Keller MB, Shapiro RW, Lavori PW, Wolfe N: Relapse in major depressive disorder: Analysis with the life table. *Arch Gen Psychiatry* 39:911–915, 1982.

Keller MB, Lavori PW, Endicott J, Coryell W, Klerman GL: "Double-depression": Two-year follow-up. *Am J Psychiatry* 140:689–694, 1983.

Keller MB, Lavori PW, Coryell W, Andreasen NC, Endicott J, Clayton PJ, Klerman GL, Hirschfeld RMA: Differential outcome of pure manic, mixed/cycling, and pure depressive episodes in patients with bipolar illness. *JAMA* 255:3138–3142, 1986a.

Keller MB, Lavori PW, Rice J, Coryell W, Hirschfeld RMA: The persistent risk of chronicity in recurrent episodes of nonbipolar major depressive disorder: A prospective follow-up. *Am J Psychiatry* 143:24–28, 1986b.

Keller MB, Lavori PW, Friedman B, Nielsen E, Endicott J, McDonald-Scott P, Andreasen NC: The Longitudinal Interval Follow-up Evaluation (LIFE): A comprehensive method for assessing outcome in prospective longitudinal studies. *Arch Gen Psychiatry* 44:540–548, 1987.

Keller MB, Beardslee W, Lavori PW, Wunder J, Drs DL, Samuelson H: Course of major depression in non-referred adolescents: A retrospective study. *J Affective Disord* 15:235–243, 1988.

Keller SE, Stein M, Camerino MS, Schleifer SJ, Sherman J: Suppression of lymphocyte stimulation by anterior hypothalamic lesions in the guinea pig. *Cell Immunol* 52:334–340, 1980.

Keller SE, Weiss JM, Schleifer SJ, Miller NE, Stein M: Suppression of immunity by stress: Effect of a graded series of stressors on lymphocyte stimulation in the rat. *Science* 213:1397–1400, 1981.

Kellner CH, Rakita RM, Rubinow DA, Gold PW, Ballenger JC, Post RM: Tetrahydrobiopterin levels in cerebrospinal fluid of affectively ill patients. Letter. *Lancet* 2:55–56, 1983a.

Kellner CH, Rubinow DR, Gold PW, Post RM: Relationship of cortisol hypersecretion to brain CT scan alterations in depressed patients. *Psychiatry Res* 8:191–197, 1983b.

Kelly JP: Principles of the functional and anatomical organization of the nervous system. In: ER Kandel, JH Schwartz, eds: *Principles of Neural Science*. 2nd Ed. New York: Elsevier, 1985. pp. 211–221.

Kelsoe JR, Gillin C, Janowsky DS, Brown JH, Risch SC, Lumkin B: Failure to confirm muscarinic receptors on skin fibroblasts. Letter. *N Engl J Med* 312:861–862, 1985.

Kelsoe JR, Ginns EI, Egeland JA, Gerhard DS, Goldstein AM, Bale SJ, Pauls DJ, Long RT, Kidd KK, Conte G, Housman DE, Paul SM: Re-evaluation of the linkage relationship between chromosome 11p loci and the gene for bipolar affective disorder in the Old Order Amish. *Nature* 342:238–243, 1989.

Kemali D, Maj M, Ariano MG, Fabrazzo M, Amati A: Response to lithium prophylaxis in schizoaffective psychoses. In: D Kemali, G Racagni, eds: *Chronic Treatments in Neuropsychiatry*. New York: Raven Press, 1985. pp 153–158.

Kemp K, Lion JR, Magram G: Lithium in the treatment of a manic patient with multiple sclerosis: A case report. *Dis Nerv Syst* 38:210–211, 1977.

Kendell RE: *The Classification of Depressive Illness*. London: Oxford University Press, 1968.

Kendell RE: *The Role of Diagnosis in Psychiatry*. Oxford: Blackwell Scientific Publications, 1975.

Kendell RE: The classification of depressions: A review of contemporary confusion. *Br J Psychiatry* 129:15–28, 1976.

Kendell RE, Pichot P, Von Cranach M: Diagnostic criteria of English, French, and German psychiatrists. *Psychol Med* 4:187–195, 1974.

Kendell RE, Wainwright S, Hailey A, Shannon B: Influence of childbirth on psychiatric morbidity. *Psychol Med* 6:297–302, 1976.

Kendell RE, Brockington IF, Leff JP: Prognostic implications of six alternative definitions of schizophrenia. *Arch Gen Psychiatry* 36:25–31, 1979.

Kendell RE, Chalmers JC, Platz C: Epidemiology of puerperal psychoses. *Br J Psychiatry* 150:662–673, 1987.

Kendler KS: Kraepelin and the differential diagnosis of dementia praecox and manic-depressive insanity. *Compr Psychiatry* 27:549–558, 1986.

Kendler KS, Hays P: Schizophrenia subdivided by the family history of affective disorder: A comparison of symptomatology and course of illness. *Arch Gen Psychiatry* 40:951–955,1983.

Kendler KS, Glazer WM, Morgenstern H: Dimensions of delusional experience. *Am J Psychiatry* 140:466–469, 1983.

Kendler KS, Gruenberg AM, Tsuang MT: Psychiatric illness in first-degree relatives of schizophrenic and surgical control patients: A family study using DSM-III criteria. *Arch Gen Psychiatry* 42:770–779, 1985.

Kendler KS, Gruenberg AM, Tsuang MT: A DSM-III family study of nonschizophrenic psychotic disorders. *Am J Psychiatry* 143:1098–1105, 1986.

Kennedy S, Thompson R, Stancer HC, Roy A, Persad E: Life events precipitating mania. *Br J Psychiatry* 142:398–403, 1983.

Kennedy SH, Tighe S, McVey G, Brown GM: Melatonin and cortisol "switches" during mania, depression, and euthymia in a drug-free bipolar patient. *J Nerv Ment Dis* 177:300-303, 1989.

Kermani EJ, Borod JC, Brown PH, Tunnell G: New psychopathologic findings in AIDS: Case report. *J Clin Psychiatry* 46:240–241, 1985.

Kerry RJ: Recent developments in patient management. In FN Johnson, S Johnson, eds: *Lithium in Medical Practice*. Baltimore: University Park Press, 1978. pp 337–353.

Kerry RJ, Orme JE: Lithium, manic-depressive illness and psychological test performance. *Br Med J* 1:230, 1979.

Kerry RJ, McDermott CM, Orme JE: Affective disorders and cognitive performance: A clinical report. *J Affective Disord* 5:349–352, 1983.

Keschner M, Bender MB, Strauss I: Mental symptoms in cases of tumours in the temporal lobe. *Arch Neurol Psychiatry* 35:572–596, 1936.

Keschner M, Bender MB, Strauss I: Mental symptoms associated with brain tumours. *JAMA* 110:714–718, 1938.

Keshavan MS, Goswamy U: Tardive dyskinesia less severe in depression. *Br J Psychiatry* 142:207–208, 1983.

Kestenbaum CJ: Children at risk for manic-depressive illness: Possible predictors. *Am J Psychiatry* 136:1206–1208, 1979.

Kety SS: Brain amines and affective disorders. In: BT Ho, WM McIsaac, eds: *Brain Chemistry and Mental Disease*. New York: Plenum Press, 1971. pp 237–263.

Kety SS: Overall review: Brain amines and affective disorders. In: BT Ho, WM McIsaac, eds: *Brain Chemistry and Mental Disease*. New York: Plenum Press, 1971. pp 237–244.

Kety SS: Disorders of the human brain. *Sci Am* 241:202–214, 1979.

Kety SS, Schmidt CF: The determination of cerebral blood flow in man by the use of nitrous oxide in low concentrations. *Am J Physiol* 143:53–66, 1945.

Kety SS, Rosenthal D, Wender PH, Schulsinger F, Jacobsen B: Mental illness in the biological and adoptive families of adopted individuals who have become schizophrenic: A preliminary report based on psychiatric interviews. In: RR Fieve, D Rosenthal, H Brill, eds: *Genetic Research in Psychiatry*. Baltimore: Johns Hopkins University Press, 1975. pp 147–165.

Keup W: Psychiatric symptoms due to cannabis abuse. *Dis Nerv Sys* 31:119–126, 1970.

Keynes M: Handel's illnesses. *Lancet* 2:1354–1355, 1980.

Khan I, Kling MA, Whitfield H, Gallucci WT, Calabrese JR, Gold PW, Merriam GR: Blunted growth hormone (GH) responses to GH releasing hormone (GHRH) in depressive illness. Abstract of paper presented at 42nd Annual Meeting of the Society of Biological Psychiatry, May 1987. p 303.

Khan MC: Lithium carbonate in the treatment of acute depressive illness. *Bibl Psychiatr* 161:244–248, 1981.

Khantzian EJ: Opiate addiction: A critique of theory and some implications for treatment. *Am J Psychother* 28:59–70, 1974.

Khantzian EJ: The self-medication hypothesis of addictive disorders: Focus on heroin and cocaine dependence. *Am J Psychiatry* 142:1259–1264, 1985.

Kidd KK: Searching for major genes for psychiatric disorders. *Ciba Found Symp* 130:184–196, 1987.

Kielholz P: *Klinik, Differentialdiagnostik und Therapie der Depressiven Zustandsbilder*. Basel: Geigy, 1959.

Kiloh LG, Garside RF: The independence of neurotic depression and endogenous depression. *Br J Psychiatry* 109:451–463, 1963.

Kim YB, Dunner DL, Meltzer HL, Fieve RR: Lithium erythrocyte: Plasma ratio in primary affective disorder. *Compr Psychiatry* 19:129–134, 1978.

Kimura B: Vergleichende Untersuchungen über depressive Erkrankungen in Japan und in Deutschland. *Fortschr Neurol Psychiatr* 33:202–215, 1965.

King DJ, Cooper SJ, Earle JAP, Martin SJ, McFerran NV, Rima BK, Wisdom GB: A survey of serum antibodies to eight common viruses in psychiatric patients. *Br J Psychiatry* 147:137–144, 1985.

King JR, Hullin RP: Withdrawal symptoms from lithium: Four case reports and a questionnaire study. *Br J Psychiatry* 143:30–35, 1983.

King LJ, Pittman GD: A six-year follow-up study of sixty-five adolescent patients: Predictive value of presenting clinical picture. *Br J Psychiatry* 115:1437–1441, 1969.

Kinkelin M: Verlauf und Prognose des manisch-depressiven Irreseins. *Schweiz Arch Neurol Neurochir Psychiatr* 73:100–146, 1954.

Kiriike N, Izumiya Y, Nishiwaki S, Maeda Y, Nagata T, Kawakita Y: TRH test and DST in schizoaffective mania, mania, and schizophrenia. *Biol Psychiatry* 24:415–422, 1988.

Kirkegaard C, Bjørum N, Cohn D, Faber J, Lauridsen UB, Nekup J: Studies on the influence of biogenic amines and psychoactive drugs on the prognostic value of the TRH stimulation test in endogenous depression. *Psychoneuroendocrinology* 2:131–136, 1977.

Kirkegaard C, Bjørum N, Cohn D, Lauridsen UB: Thyrotrophin-releasing hormone (TRH) stimulation test in manic-depressive illness. *Arch Gen Psychiatry* 35:1017–1021, 1978.

Kishimoto A, Ogura C, Hazama H, Inoue K: Long-term prophylactic effects of carbamazepine in affective disorder. *Br J Psychiatry* 143:327–331, 1983.

Kishimoto A, Kamata K, Sugihara T, Ishiguro S, Hazama H, Mizukawa R, Kunimoto N: Treatment of depression with clonazepam. *Acta Psychiatr Scand* 77:81–86, 1988.

Kishimoto H, Takazu O, Ohno S, Yamaguchi T, Fujita H, Kuwahara H, Ishii T, Matsushita M, Yokoi S, Iio M: ^{11}C-glucose metabolism in manic and depressed patients. *Psychiatry Res* 22:81–88, 1987.

Kjellman BF, Karlberg BE, Thorell LH: Cognitive and affective functions in patients with affective disorders treated with lithium. *Acta Psychiatr Scand* 62:32–46, 1980.

Kjellman BF, Beck-Friis J, Ljunggren J-G, Wetterberg L: Twenty-four-hour serum levels of TSH in affective disorders. *Acta Psychiatr Scand* 69:491–502, 1984.

Kjellman BF, Beck-Friis J, Ljunggren JG, Ross SB, Undén F, Wetterberg L: Serum dopamine-beta-hydroxylase activity in patients with major depressive disorders. *Acta Psychiatr Scand* 73:266–270, 1986.

Klaiber EL, Broverman DM, Vogel W, Kobayashi Y: Estrogen therapy for severe persistent depressions in women. *Arch Gen Psychiatry* 36:550–554, 1979.

Kleber HD, Gawin FH: Cocaine abuse: A review of current and experimental treatments. *National Institute on Drug Abuse Research Monograph* 50:111–129, 1984.

Kleber HD, Weissman MM, Rounsaville BJ: Imipramine as treatment for depression in addicts. *Arch Gen Psychiatry* 40:649–653, 1983.

Klein DF: Behavioral effects of imipramine and phenothiazines: Implications for a psychiatric pathogenetic theory and theory of drug action. *Recent Advances Biol Psychiatry* 7:273–287, 1965.

Klein DF: Importance of psychiatric diagnosis in prediction of clinical drug effects. *Arch Gen Psychiatry* 16:118–126, 1967.

Klein DF: Endogenomorphic depression: A conceptual and terminological revision. *Arch Gen Psychiatry* 31:447–454, 1974.

Klein DF, Davis JM: *Diagnosis and Treatment of Psychiatric Disorders*. Baltimore: Williams & Wilkins, 1969.

Klein DF, Gittelman R, Quitkin F, Rifkin A: *Diagnosis and Drug Treatment of Psychiatric Disorders: Adults and Children*. ed. 2. Baltimore: Williams & Wilkins, 1981.

Klein DN: Activity-withdrawal in the differential diagnosis of schizophrenia and mania. *J Abnorm Psychol* 91:157–164, 1982.

Klein DN, Depue RA: Obsessional personality traits and risk for bipolar affective disorder: An offspring study. *J Abnorm Psychol* 94:291–297, 1985.

Klein DN, Depue RA, Slater JF: Cyclothymia in the adolescent offspring of parents with bipolar affective disorder. *J Abnorm Psychol* 94:115–127, 1985.

Klein DN, Depue RA, Krauss SP: Social adjustment in the offspring of parents with bipolar affective disorder. *J Psychopath Behav Assess* 8:355–366, 1986a.

Klein DN, Depue RA, Slater JF: Inventory identification of cyclothymia: IX. Validation in offspring of bipolar I patients. *Arch Gen Psychiatry* 43:441–445, 1986b.

Klein DN, Taylor EB, Harding K, Dickstein S: Double depression and episodic major depression: Demographic, clinical, familial, personality, and socioenvironmental characteristics and short-term outcome. *Am J Psychiatry* 145:1226–1231, 1988.

Klein E, Bental E, Lerer B, Belmaker RH: Carbamazepine and haloperidol *v* placebo and haloperidol in excited psychoses: A controlled study. *Arch Gen Psychiatry* 41:165–170, 1984.

Klein HE, Broucek B, Greil W: Lithium withdrawal triggers psychotic states. *Br J Psychiatry* 139:255–256, 1981.

Klein HE, Seibold B, Bender W, Nedopil N, Albus M, Schmauss M: Postdexamethasone prolactin and cortisol: A biological state variable in depression. *Acta Psychiatr Scand* 70:239–247, 1984.

Kleinman JE, Hong J, Iadarola M, Govoni S, Gillin CJ: Neuropeptides in human brain—Postmortem studies. *Prog Neuropsychopharmacol Biol Psychiatry* 9:91–95, 1985.

Kleist K: Gehirnpathologische und lokalisatorische ergebnisse: Die störungen der ichleistungen und ihre localsation in orbital, iinnenund zwischenhirn. *Monatsschrift für Psychiatrie und Neurologie* 79:338, 1931.

Kleist K: *Fortschritte der Psychiatrie*. Frankfurt-am-Main: W. Kramer, 1947.

Klerman GL: The relationship between personality and clinical depressions: Overcoming the obstacles to verifying psychodynamic theories. *Int J Psychiatry* 11:227–233, 1973.

Klerman GL: Unipolar and bipolar depressions: Theoretical and empirical issues in establishing the validity of nosological concepts in the classification of affective disorders. In: FK Schattauer, ed: *Classification and Prediction of Outcome of Depression*. Symposia Medica Hoechst, No. 8. Stuttgart-New York: Verlag, 1974. pp 49–73.

Klerman GL: Combining drugs and psychotherapy in the treatment of depression. In: M Greenblatt, ed: *Drugs in Combination With Other Therapies*. New York: Grune & Stratton, 1975. pp 67–81.

Klerman GL: The spectrum of mania. *Compr Psychiatry* 22:11–20, 1981.

Klerman GL: History and development of modern concepts of affective illness. In: RM Post, JC Ballenger,

eds.: *Neurobiology of Affective Disorders*. Baltimore: William & Wilkins, 1984. pp 1–19.

Klerman GL: The current age of youthful melancholia: Evidence for increase in depression among adolescents and young adults. *Br J Psychiatry* 152:4–14, 1988.

Klerman GL, Schechter G: Drugs and psychotherapy. In: ES Paykel, ed: *Handbook of Affective Disorders*. New York: Churchill Livingstone, 1982. pp 329–337.

Klerman GL, DeMascio A, Weissman MM, Prusoff BA, Paykel ES: Treatment of depression by drugs and psychotherapy. *Am J Psychiatry* 131:186–191, 1974.

Klerman GL, Weissman MM, Rounsaville BJ, Chevron ES: *Interpersonal Psychotherapy of Depression*. New York: Basic Books, 1984.

Klerman, GL, Lavori PW, Rice J, Reich T, Endicott J, Andreasen NC, Keller MB, Hirschfeld RMA: Birth-cohort trends in rates of major depressive disorder among relatives of patients with affective disorder. *Arch Gen Psychiatry* 42: 689–693, 1985.

Kline NS, Lehmann HE: β-endorphin therapy in psychiatric patients. In: E Usdin, WE Bunney, NS Kline, eds: *Endorphins in Mental Health Research*. New York: Oxford University Press, 1979. pp 500–517.

Kline NS, Wren JC, Cooper TB, Varga E, Canal A: Evaluation of lithium therapy in chronic and periodic alcoholism. *Am J Med Sci* 268:15–22, 1974.

Kling MA, Chrousos GP, Rubinow DR, Doran A, Calabrese JR, Loriaux DL, Gold PW: Reduced cerebrospinal fluid somatostatin in Cushing's syndrome. Serano Symposium Series, Washington, DC, 1986.

Kling MA, Kellner CH, Post RM, Cowdry RW, Gardner DL, Coppola R, Putnam FW, Gold PW: Neuroendocrine effects of limbic activation by electrical, spontaneous, and pharmacological modes: Relevance to the pathophysiology of affective dysregulation in psychiatric disorders. *Prog Neuro-Psychopharmacol Biol Psychiat* 11:459–481, 1987.

Klinger E, Barta SG, Kemble ED: Cyclic activity changes during extinction in rats: A potential model of depression. *Anim Learn Behav* 2:313–316, 1974.

Knapp S, Mandell AJ: Short- and long-term lithium administration: Effects on brain's serotonergic biosynthetic systems. *Science* 180:645–647, 1973.

Knott V, Lapierre YD: Electrophysiological and behavioral correlates of psychomotor responsivity in depression. *Biol Psychiatry* 22:313–324, 1987.

Knott V, Waters B, Lapierre Y, Gray R: Neurophysiological correlates of sibling pairs discordant for bipolar affective disorder. *Am J Psychiatry* 142:248–250, 1985.

Knowles JB, Cairns J, MacLean AW, Delva N, Prowse A, Waldron J, Letemendia FJ: The sleep of remitted bipolar depressives: Comparison with sex and age-matched controls. *Can J Psychiatry* 31:295–298, 1986.

Ko GN, Leckman JF, Heninger GR: Induction of rapid mood cycling during L-dopa treatment in a bipolar patient. *Am J Psychiatry* 138:1624–1625, 1981.

Kobayashi T, Kishimoto A, Inagaki T: Treatment of periodic depression with carbamazepine. *Acta Psychiatr Scand* 77:364–367, 1988.

Koe BK, Weissman A: p-Chlorophenylalanine: A specific depletor of brain serotonin. *J Pharmacol Exp Ther* 154:499–516, 1966.

Koegel P, Burnam MA, Farr RK: The prevalence of specific psychiatric disorders among homeless individual in the inner city of Los Angeles. *Arch Gen Psychiatry* 45:1085–1092, 1988.

Koehler-Troy C, Strober M, Malenbaum R: Methylphenidate-induced mania in a prepubertal child. *J Clin Psychiatry* 47:566–567, 1986.

Koestler A: *The Act of Creation.* (1964) New York: Dell, 1975.

Koh SD, Wolpert EA: Memory scanning and retrieval in affective disorders. *Psychiatry Res* 8:289–297, 1983.

Kolb L: *Modern Clinical Psychiatry.* 7th ed. Philadelphia: WB Saunders, 1968.

Kolodny A: The symptomatology of tumour in the temporal lobe. *Brain* 52:385–417, 1928.

Kontaxakis V, Markianos M, Markidis M, Stefanis C: Clonidine in the treatment of mixed bipolar disorder. *Acta Psychiatr Scand* 79:108–110, 1989.

Kopell BS, Wittner WK, Lunde D, Warrick G, Edwards D: Cortisol effects on averaged evoked potential, alpha-rhythm, time estimation, and two-flash fusion threshold. *Psychosom Med* 32:39–49, 1970.

Kopin IJ, Gordon EK, Jimerson DC, Polinsky RJ: Relation between plasma and cerebrospinal fluid levels of 3-methoxy-4-hydroxyphenylglycol. *Science* 219: 73–75, 1983.

Kopin IJ, Jimerson DC, Markey SP, Ebert MH, Polinsky RJ: Disposition and metabolism of MHPG in humans: Application to studies in depression. *Pharmacopsychiatry* 17:3–8, 1984.

Korf J, Van den Burg W, Van den Hoofdakker RH: Acid metabolites and precursor amino acids of 5-hydroxytryptamine and dopamine in affective and other psychiatric disorders. *Psychiatr Clinica* 16:1–16, 1983.

Koslow SH, Stokes PE, Mendels J, Ramsey A, Casper R: Insulin Tolerance Test: Human growth hormone response and insulin resistance in primary unipolar depressed, bipolar depressed and control subjects. *Psychol Med* 12:45–55, 1982.

Koslow SH, Maas JW, Bowden CL, Davis JM, Hanin I, Javaid J: CSF and urinary biogenic amines and metabolites in depression and mania: A controlled, univariate analysis. *Arch Gen Psychiatry* 40:999–1010, 1983.

Kosten TR, Rounsaville BJ: Psychopathology in opioid addicts. *Psychiatr Clin North Am* 9:515–532, 1986.

Kotin J, Goodwin FK: Depression during mania: Clinical observations and theoretical implications. *Am J Psychiatry* 129:679–686, 1972.

Kotin J, Post RM, Goodwin FK: Δ9-Tetrahydrocannabinol in depressed patients. *Arch Gen Psychiatry* 28:345–348, 1973a.

Kotin J, Post RM, Goodwin FK: Drug treatment of depressed patients referred for hospitalization. *Am J Psychiatry* 130:1139–1141, 1973b.

Koulu M, Lammintausta R: Effects of L-deprenyl on human growth hormone secretion. *J Neural Transm* 51:223–231, 1981.

Kovacs DA, Zoll JG: Seizure inhibition by median raphe nucleus stimulation in rat. *Brain Res* 70:165–169, 1974.

Kovacs M: Affective disorders in children and adolescents. *Am Psychol* 44:209–215, 1989.

Kovacs M, Feinberg TL, Crouse-Novak M, Paulauskas SL, Pollock M, Finkelstein R: Depressive disorders in childhood: II: A longitudinal study of the risk for a subsequent major depression. *Arch Gen Psychiatry* 41:643–649, 1984.

Koyama T, Lowy MT, Meltzer HY: 5-Hydroxytryptophan-induced cortisol response and CSF 5-HIAA in depressed patients. *Am J Psychiatry* 144:334–337, 1987.

Kraemer BA: Maintenance ECT: A survey of practice. *Convulsive Ther* 3:260–268, 1986.

Kraemer GW, Ebert MH, Lake CR, McKinney WT: Cerebrospinal fluid measures of neurotransmitter changes associated with pharmacological alteration of the despair response to social separation in rhesus monkeys. *Psychiatry Res* 11:303–315, 1984.

Kraepelin E: *Psychiatrie. Ein Lehrbuch für Studirende und Aerzte.* Leipzig: JA Barth, 1896. 8th ed. published in 1913. Reprinted New York: Arno Press, 1976.

Kraepelin E: *Lectures on Clinical Psychiatry.* London: Ballière, Tindall & Cox, 1904a.

Kraepelin E: Vergleichende Psychiatrie. *Z Nervenheilk Psychiatr* 27:433–437, 1904b.

Kraepelin E: *Dementia Praecox and Paraphrenia.* Translated by RM Barclay. Edinburgh: E & S Livingstone, 1919.

Kraepelin E: *Manic-Depressive Insanity and Paranoia.* Translated by RM Barclay, Edited by GM Robertson. Edinburgh: E & S Livingstone, 1921. Reprinted New York: Arno Press, 1976.

Kraines SH: *Mental Depressions and Their Treatment.* New York: Macmillan Co, 1957.

Kramlinger KG, Post RM: Adding lithium carbonate to carbamazepine: Antimanic efficacy in treatment-resistant mania. *Acta Psychiatr Scand* 79:378–385, 1989a.

Kramlinger KG, Post RM: The addition of lithium carbonate to carbamazepine: Antidepressant efficacy in treatment-resistant depression. *Arch Gen Psychiatry* 46:794–800, 1989b.

Krauthammer C, Klerman GL: Secondary mania: Manic syndromes associated with antecedent physical illness or drugs. *Arch Gen Psychiatry* 35:1333–1339, 1978.

Krauthammer C, Klerman GL: The epidemiology of mania. In: B Shopsin, ed: *Manic Illness.* New York: Raven Press, 1979. pp 11–28.

Krebs E, Roubicek J: EEG and clinical profile of a synthetic analogue of methionine-enkephalin FK 33–824. *Pharmakopsychiatr Neuropsychopharmakol* 12:86–93, 1979.

Kretschmer E: *Physique and Character*. New York: Macmillan, 1936.

Krieger DT, Silverberg AI, Rizzo F, Krieger HP: Abolition of circadian periodicity of plasma 17-OHCS levels in the cat. *Am J Physiol* 215:959–967, 1968.

Kripke DF: Phase-advance theories for affective illnesses. In: TA Wehr, FK Goodwin, eds: *Circadian Rhythms in Psychiatry*. Pacific Grove, CA: The Boxwood Press, 1983. pp 41–69.

Kripke DF: Critical interval hypotheses for depression. *Chronobiol Int* 1:73–80, 1984.

Kripke DF: Biological rhythms. In: R Michels, ed: *Psychiatry* Vol 3, Section 2, 59, 1985. pp 1–15.

Kripke DF, Robinson D: Ten years with a lithium group. *McLean Hosp J* 10:1–11, 1985.

Kripke DF, Mullaney DJ, Atkinson M, Wolf S: Circadian rhythm disorders in manic-depressives. *Biol Psychiatry* 13:335–351, 1978.

Kripke DF, Mullaney DJ, Gillin JC, Risch SC, Janowsky DS: Phototherapy of non-seasonal depression. In: C Shagass, RC Josiassen, WH Bridger, KJ Weiss, D Stoff, GM Simpson, eds: *Biological Psychiatry 1985*. New York: Elsevier, 1986. pp. 993–995.

Krishna NR, Taylor MA, Abrams R: Combined haloperidol and lithium carbonate in treating manic patients. *Compr Psychiatry* 19:119–120, 1978.

Krishnan KRR, Swartz MS, Larson MJ, Santoliquido G: Funeral mania in recurrent bipolar affective disorders: Reports of three cases. *J Clin Psychiatry* 45:310–311, 1984.

Krishnan KRR, Goli V, Ellinwood EH, France RD, Blazer DG, Nemeroff CB: Leukoencephalopathy in patients diagnosed as major depressive. *Biol Psychiatry* 23:519–522, 1988a.

Krishnan KR, Manepalli AN, Ritchie JC, Rayasam K, Melville ML, Daughtry G, Thorner MO, Rivier JE, Vale WW, Nemeroff CB, Carroll BJ: Growth hormone-releasing factor stimulation test in depression. *Am J Psychiatry* 145:90–92, 1988b.

Krishnan RR, Maltbie AA, Davidson JRT: Abnormal cortisol suppression in bipolar patients with simultaneous manic and depressive symptoms. *Am J Psychiatry* 140:203–205, 1983.

Kron L, Decina P, Kestenbaum CJ, Farber S, Gargan M, Fieve R: The offspring of bipolar manic-depressives: Clinical features. In: SC Feinstein, JG Looney, AZ Schwartzbert, eds: *Adolescent Psychiatry*. Vol. 10. Chicago: University Press, 1982. pp 273–291

Kronfol Z, House JD: Immune function in mania. *Biol Psychiatry* 24:341–343, 1988.

Kronfol Z, Hamsher K, Digre K, Waziri R: Depression and hemispheric functions: Changes associated with unilateral ECT. *Br J Psychiatry* 132:560–567, 1978.

Kronfol Z, Silva J Jr, Greden J, Dembinski S, Gardner R, Carroll B: Impaired lymphocyte function in depressive illness. *Life Sci* 33:241–247, 1983.

Kronfol Z, Turner R, Nasrallah H, Winokur G: Leukocyte regulation in depression and schizophrenia. *Psychiatry Res* 13:13–18, 1984.

Kronfol Z, Turner R, House JD, Winokur G: Elevated blood neutrophil concentration in mania. *J Clin Psychiatry* 47:63–65, 1986.

Kropf D, Müller-Oerlinghausen B: Changes in learning, memory, and mood during lithium treatment: Approach to a research strategy. *Acta Psychiatr Scand* 59:97–124, 1979.

Kropf D, Müller-Oerlinghausen B: The influence of lithium long-term medication on personality and mood. *Pharmacopsychiatry* 18:104–105, 1985.

Kuchel PW, Hunt GE, Johnson GFS, Beilharz GR, Chapman BE, Jones AJ, Sigh BS: Lithium, red blood cell choline and clinical state: A prospective study in manic-depressive patients. *J Affective Disord* 6:83–94, 1984.

Kuhn R: Über die Behandlung depressiver Zustände mit einem Iminodibenzylderivat (G 22355). [Treatment of depressive states with an iminodibenzyl derivative (G 22355)]. *Schweizerische Medizinische Wochenschrift* 87:1135–1140, 1957.

Kuhn TS: *The Structure of Scientific Revolutions*. 2nd ed, Vol 2, No. 2. Chicago: University of Chicago Press, 1970.

Kuiper NA, Derry PA: Depressed and nondepressed content self-reference in mild depressives. *J Personality* 50:67–80, 1982.

Kukopulos A, Reginaldi D: Does lithium prevent depressions by suppressing manias? *Int Pharmacopsychiatry* 8:152–158, 1973.

Kukopulos A, Tondo L: Lithium non-responders and their treatment. In: FN Johnson, ed: *Handbook of Lithium Therapy*. Baltimore: University Park Press, 1980. pp 143–149.

Kukopulos A, Reginaldi D, Laddomada P, Floris G, Serra G, Tondo L: Course of the manic-depressive cycle and changes caused by treatments. *Pharmakopsychiatr Neuropsychopharmakol* 13:156–167, 1980.

Kukopulos A, Caliari B, Tundo A, Minnai G, Floris G, Reginaldi D, Tondo L: Rapid cyclers, temperament, and antidepressants. *Compr Psychiatry* 24:249–258, 1983.

Kukopulos A, Minnai G, Müller-Oerlinghausen B: The influence of mania and depression on the pharmacokinetics of lithium: A longitudinal single-case study. *J Affective Disord* 8:159–166, 1985.

Kupfer DJ, Detre TP: Tricyclic and monoamine-oxidase-inhibitor antidepressants: Clinical use. In: LL Iversen, SD Iversen, SH Snyder, eds: *Handbook of Psychopharmacology, vol 14. Affective Disorders: Drug Actions in Animals and Man*. New York: Plenum Press, 1978. pp 199–232.

Kupfer DJ, Rush AJ: Recommendations for depression publications. *Psychiatry Res* 8:238–240, 1983.

Kupfer DJ, Spiker DG: Refractory depression: Prediction of non-response by clinical indicators. *J Clin Psychiatry* 42:307–312, 1981.

Kupfer DJ, Himmelhoch JM, Swartzburg M, Anderson C, Byck R, Detre TP: Hypersomnia in manic-depressive disease (a preliminary report). *Dis Nerv Syst* 33:720–724, 1972.

Kupfer DJ, Weiss BL, Foster FG, Detre TP, Delgado J, McPartland R: Psychomotor activity in affective states. *Arch Gen Psychiatry* 30:765–768, 1974.

Kupfer DJ, Pickar D, Himmelhoch JM, Detre TP: Are there two types of unipolar depression? *Arch Gen Psychiatry* 32:866–871, 1975.

Kupfer DJ, Reynolds CF III, Grochocinski VJ, Ulrich RF, McEachran A: Aspects of short REM latency in affective states: A revisit. *Psychiatry Res.* 17:49–59, 1986.

Kupfer DJ, Carpenter LL, Frank E: Is bipolar II a unique disorder? *Compr Psychiatry* 29:228–236, 1988a.

Kupfer DJ, Carpenter LL, Frank E: Possible role of antidepressants in precipitating mania and hypomania in recurrent depression. *Am J Psychiatry* 145:804–808, 1988b.

Kupfer DJ, Frank E, Jarrett DB, Reynolds CF III, Thase ME: Interrelationship of electroencephalographic sleep chronobiology and depression. In: DJ Kupfer, TH Monk, JD Barchas, eds: *Biological Rhythms and Mental Disorders*. New York: Guilford Press, 1988c.

Kupfermann I: Hypothalamus and limbic system I: Peptidergic neurons, homeostasis, and emotional behavior. In: ER Kandel, JH Schwartz, eds: *Principles of Neural Science*. 2nd Ed. New York: Elsevier, 1985a. pp. 611–625.

Kupfermann I: Hypothalamus and limbic system II: Motivation. In: ER Kandel, JH Schwartz, eds: *Principles of Neural Science*. 2nd Ed. New York: Elsevier, 1985b. pp. 626–635.

Kuyler PL: Rapid cycling bipolar II illness in three closely related relatives. *Am J Psychiatry* 145:114–115, 1988.

Kuyler PL, Rosenthal L, Igel G, Dunner DL, Fieve RR: Psychopathology among children of manic-depressive patients. *Biol Psychiatry* 15:589–597, 1980.

Kwentus JA, Silverman JJ, Sprague M: Manic syndrome after metrizamide myelography. *Am J Psychiatry* 141:700–702, 1984.

Labbate LA, Holzgang AJ: Manic syndrome after discontinuation of methyldopa. *Am J Psychiatry* 146:1075–1076, 1989.

Lader M: *The Psychophysiology of Mental Illness*. London: Routledge and Kegan Paul, 1975.

Lake CR, Pickar D, Ziegler MG, Lipper S, Slater S, Murphy DL: High plasma norepinephrine levels in patients with major affective disorder. *Am J Psychiatry* 139:1315–1318, 1982.

Lal S, Martin JB: Neuroanatomy and neuropharmacological regulation of neuroendocrine function. In: HM Van Praag, MH Lader, OJ Rafaelsen, EJ Sachar, eds: *Handbook of Biological Psychiatry,* *Part III: Brain Mechanisms and Abnormal Behavior: Genetics and Neuroendocrinology*. New York: Marcel Dekker, 1980. pp 101–167.

Lalouel JM, Morton NE: Complex segregation analysis with pointers. *Hum Hered* 31:312–321, 1981.

Lalouel JM, Rao DC, Morton NE, Elston RC: A unified model for complex segregation analysis. *Am J Hum Genet* 35:816–826, 1983.

Lamb C: *Elia and the Last Essays of Elia*. New York: Oxford University Press, 1987.

Lambert PA, Venaud G: Utilisation du valpromide en thérapeutique psychiatrique. *L'Encéphale* 13:367–373, 1987.

Lambert PA, Cavaz G, Borselli S, Carrel S: Action neuro-psychotrope d'un nouvel anti-épileptique: Le dépamide. *Ann Med Psychol* 1:707–710, 1966.

Lambert PA, Borselli S, Marcou G, Bouchardy M, Cabrol G: Action thymo-régulatrice à long terme du dépamide dans la psychose maniaco-dépressive. *Ann Med Psychol* 2:442–447, 1971.

Lambert PA, Carraz G, Borselli S, Bouchardy M: [Dipropylacetamide in the treatment of manic-depressive psychosis]. *Encephale* 1:25–31, 1975.

Lambo TA: Neuropsychiatric observations in the western region of Nigeria. *Br Med J* 2:1388–1394, 1956.

Lancet. Editorial, April 5, 1969. pp 709–710.

Lancranjan I, Marbach P: New evidence for growth hormone modulation by the alpha-adrenergic system in man. *Metabolism* 26:1225–1230, 1977.

Landegren U, Kaiser R, Caskey CT, Hood L: DNA diagnostics—molecular techniques and automation. *Science* 242:229–237, 1988.

Lander ES, Botstein D: Strategies for studying heterogeneous genetic traits in humans by using a linkage map of restriction fragment length polymorphisms. *Proc Natl Acad Sci USA* 83:7353–7357, 1986.

Landis C, Page JD: *Modern Society and Mental Disease*. New York: Farrar & Rinehart, Inc. 1938.

Lane JB: Using MMPI lithium response scales [Letter]. *Am J Psychiatry* 142:1388–1389, 1985.

Lange J: *Katatonische Erscheinungen im Rahmen Manischer Erkrankungen* Berlin: Julius Springer, 1922.

Lange J: Die endogenen und reaktiven Gemütserkrankungen und die manisch-depressive konstitution. In: O Bomke, ed: *Geisteskr. VI, Spez. Teil II.* Berlin: Springer, 1928.

Langelüddeke A: Über Lebenserwartung und Rückfallhäufigkeit bei Manisch-Depressiven. *Ztschr Psych Hyg* 14:1–15, 1941.

Langer G, Heinze G, Reim B, Matussek N: Reduced growth hormone responses to amphetamine in "endogenous" depressive patients: Studies in normal, "reactive" and "endogenous" depressive, schizophrenic, and chronic alcoholic subjects. *Arch Gen Psychiatry* 33:1471–1475, 1976.

Langer SZ, Raisman R: Binding of ^{3}H-imipramine and ^{3}H-desipramine as biochemical tool for the studies in depression. *Neuropharmacology* 22:407, 1983.

Langer SZ, Moret C, Raisman R, Dubocovitch ML, Briley M: High-affinity ^{3}H-imipramine binding in rat hypothalamus: Association with uptake of serotonin but not of norepinephrine. *Science* 210:1133–1135, 1980.

Langer SZ, Galzin AM, Lee CR, Schoemaker H: Antidepressant-binding sites in brain and platelets. In: R Porter, G Bock, S Clark, eds: *Antidepressants and Receptor Function.* London: John Wiley & Sons, 1986a. pp 3–29.

Langer SZ, Sechter D, Loo H, Raisman R, Zarifian E: Electroconvulsive shock therapy and maximum binding of platelet tritiated imipramine binding in depression. *Arch Gen Psychiatry* 43:949–952, 1986b.

Langfeldt G: *The Prognosis in Schizophrenia and the Factors Influencing the Course of the Disease: A Katamnestic Study, Including Individual Reexaminations in 1936, With Some Considerations Regarding Diagnosis, Pathogensis, and Therapy.* London: H Milford, Oxford University Press, 1937.

Lansdell H: Laterality of verbal intelligence in the brain. *Science* 135:922–923, 1962.

Lapierre YD, Gagnon A, Kokkinidis L: Rapid recurrence of mania following lithium withdrawal. *Biol Psychiatry* 15:859–864, 1980.

Lapin IP, Oxenkrug GF: Intensification of the central serotoninergic processes as a possible determinant of the thymoleptic effect. *Lancet* 1:132–136, 1969.

LaRoche C, Cheifetz PN, Lester EP: Antecedents of bipolar affective disorders in children. *Am J Psychiatry* 138:986–988, 1981.

LaRoche C, Cheifetz P, Lester EP, Schibuk L, DiTommaso E, Engelsmann F: Psychopathology in the offspring of parents with bipolar affective disorders. *Can J Psychiatry* 30:337–343, 1985.

LaRoche C, Sheiner R, Lester E, Benierakis C, Marrache M, Engelsmann F, Cheifetz P: Children of parents with manic-depressive illness: A follow-up study. *Can J Psychiatry* 32:563–569, 1987.

Laski M: *Ecstasy.* London: Cresset Press, 1961.

Lathrop GM, Lalouel JM, Julier C, Ott J: Strategies for multilocus linkage analysis in humans. *Proc Natl Acad Sci USA* 81:3443–3446, 1984.

Laubscher BJF: *Sex, Custom and Psychopathology: A study of South African Pagan Natives.* London: Routledge and Kegan Paul, 1937.

Laurell B, Ottosson JO: Prophylactic lithium? *Lancet* 2:1245–1246, 1968.

Lavori PW, Keller MB, Roth SL: Affective disorders and ABO blood groups: New data and a reanalysis of the literature using the logistic transformation of proportions. *J Psychiatr Res* 18:119–129, 1984.

Lavori PW, Keller MB, Beardslee WR, Dorer DJ: Affective disorder in childhood: Separating the familial component of risk from individual characteristics of children. *J Affective Disord* 15:303–311, 1988.

Lazare A: Manic behavior. In: A Lazare, ed: *Outpatient Psychiatry: Diagnosis and Treatment.* Baltimore: Williams & Wilkins, 1979. pp. 261–264.

Lazarus JH: *Endocrine and Metabolic Effects of Lithium.* New York: Plenum Publishing, 1986.

Lazarus JH, John R, Bennie EH, Chalmers RJ,

Crockett G: Lithium therapy and thyroid function: A long-term study. *Psychol Med* 11:85–92, 1981.

Lazarus JH, McGregor AM, Ludgate M, Darke C, Creagh FM, Kingswood CJ: Effects of lithium carbonate therapy on thyroid immune status in manic depressive patients: A prospective study. *J Affective Disord* 11:155–160, 1986.

Lebegue B: Mania precipitated by fluoxetine. Letter. *Am J Psychiatry* 144:1620–1621, 1987.

Leber P: "Time-less" risks (A hazard of risk assessment: the example of seizure and antidepressants). *Psychopharmacol Bull* 21:334–338, 1985.

Leckman JF, Maas JW: Plasma MHPG: Relationship to brain noradrenergic systems and emerging clinical applications. In: RM Post, JC Ballenger, eds: *Neurobiology of Mood Disorders.* Baltimore: Williams & Wilkins, 1984. pp 529–538.

Lecrubier Y, Puech AJ, Jouvent R, Simon P, Widlocher D: A beta adrenergic stimulant (salbutamol) versus clomipramine in depression: A controlled study. *Br J Psychiatry* 136:354–358, 1980.

Leff J: International variations in the diagnosis of psychiatric illness. *Br J Psychiatry* 131:329–338, 1977.

Leff JP, Fischer M, Bertelsen AC: A cross-national epidemiological study of mania. *Br J Psychiatry* 129:428–442, 1976.

Legros S, Mendlewicz J, Wybran J: Immunoglobulins, autoantibodies and other serum protein fractions in psychiatric disorders. *Eur Arch Psychiatry Neurol Sci* 235:9–11, 1985.

Lehmann HE, Hanrahan GE: Chlorpromazine: New inhibiting agent for psychomotor excitement and manic states. *Arch Neurol Psychiatry* 71:227–237, 1954.

Leighton AH, Lambo TA, Hughes CC, Leighton DC, Murphy JM, Macklin DB: *Psychiatric Disorder Among the Yoruba: A Report from the Cornell-Aro Mental Health Project in the Western Region, Nigeria.* Ithaca, NY: Cornell University Press, 1963.

Leighton DC, Harding JS, Macklin DB, Macmillan AM, Leighton AH: *The Character of Danger.* New York: Basic Books, 1963.

Lemberger L, Fuller RW, Zerbe RL: Use of specific seotonin uptake inhibitors as antidepressants. *Clin Neuropharmacol* 8:299–317, 1985.

Lemmer B, Jarosch U, Breddin K: Influence of the time interval after venepuncture and the storage temperature on the uptake of ^{14}C-serotonin by human blood platelets. *Life Sci* 21:1665–1674, 1977.

Lenhart RE, Katkin ES: Psychophysiological evidence for cerebral laterality effects in a high-risk sample of students with subsyndromal bipolar depressive disorder. *Am J Psychiatry* 143:602–607, 1986.

Lenox RH, Shipley JE, Peyser JM, Williams JM, Weaver LA: Double-blind comparison of alprazolam versus imipramine in the inpatient treatment of major depressive illness. *Psychopharmacol Bull* 20:79–82, 1984.

Lenox RH, Hitzemann RJ, Richelson E, Kelsoe JR:

Failure to confirm muscarinic receptors on skin fibroblasts [Letter]. *N Engl J Med* 312:861, 1985.

Lenzi A, Lazzerini F, Grossi E, Massimetti G, Placidi GF: Use of carbamazepine in acute psychosis: A controlled study. *J Intl Med Res* 14:78, 1986.

Lenzi A, Lazzerini F, Placidi GF, Cassano, Akiskal HS: Predictors of compliance with lithium and carbamazepine regimens in the long-term treatment of recurrent mood and related psychotic disorders. *Pharmacopsychiatr* 22:34–37, 1989.

Leonhard K: [*The Classification of Endogenous Psychoses.*] 5th ed. Edited by Eli Robins. Translated by Russell Berman. New York: Irvington Publishers, Inc, 1979. *Aufteilung der Endogenen Psychosen*. 1st ed. Berlin: Akademie-Verlag, 1957.

Leonhard K: Cycloid psychoses—endogenous psychoses which are neither schizophrenic nor manic-depressive. *J Ment Sci (Br J Psychiatry)* 107:632–648, 1961.

Lepkifker E, Horesh N, Floru S: Life satisfaction and adjustment in lithium-treated affective patients in remission. *Acta Psychiatr Scand* 78:391–395, 1988.

Lerer B, Stanley M: Does lithium stabilize muscarinic receptors? *Biol Psychiatry* 20:1247–1251, 1985.

Lerer B, Birmacher B, Ebstein RP, Belmaker RH: 48-hour depressive cycling induced by antidepressant. *Br J Psychiatry* 137:183–185, 1980.

Lerer B, Moore N, Meyendorff, Cho SR, Gershon S: Carbamazepine versus lithium in mania: A double-blind study. *J Clin Psychiatry* 48:88–93, 1987.

Lerner P, Goodwin FK, Van Kammen DP, Post RM, Major LF, Ballenger JC, Lovenberg W: Dopamine-beta-hydroxylase in the cerebrospinal fluid of psychiatric patients. *Biol Psychiatry* 13:685–694, 1978.

Lerner Y: The subjective experience of mania. In: RH Belmaker, HM Van Praag, eds: *Mania: An Evolving Concept*. New York: Spectrum Publications, 1980. pp 77–88.

Lesch K-P, Laux G, Erb A, Pfüller H, Beckmann H: Attenuated growth hormone response to growth hormone-releasing hormone in major depressive disorder. *Biol Psychiatry* 22:1495–1499, 1987.

Lesch K-P, Laux G, Erb A, Pfüller H, Beckmann H: Growth hormone (GH) responses to GH-releasing hormone in depression: Correlation with GH release following clonidine. *Psychiatry Res* 25:301–310, 1988a.

Lesch K-P, Laux G, Schulte HM, Pfüller H, Beckmann H: Abnormal responsiveness of growth hormone to human corticotropin-releasing hormone in major depressive disorder. *J Affective Disord* 14:245–250, 1988b.

Lester EP, LaRoche C: Schizophreniform psychosis of childhood: Therapeutic considerations. *Compr Psychiatry* 19:153–159, 1978.

Lettieri DJ, Sayers M, Pearson HW, eds: *Theories on Drug Abuse*. Rockville, MD: National Institute on Drug Abuse, 1980.

Levenson JL: Neuroleptic malignant syndrome. *Am J Psychiatry* 142:1137–1145, 1985.

Leventhal H, Tomarken AJ: Emotion: Today's problems. *Ann Rev Psychol* 37:565–610, 1986.

Levin S, Lipton RB, Holzman PS: Pursuit eye movements in psychopathology: Effects of target characteristics. *Biol Psychiatry* 16:255–267, 1981.

Levine RA, Lovenberg W: CSF tetrahydrobiopterin levels in patients with affective disorders. Letter. *Lancet* 1:283, 1984.

Levinson F, Meyer V: Personality changes in relation to psychiatric status following orbital cortex undercutting. *Br J Psychiatry* 111:207–218, 1965.

Levitan M, Montagu A: *Textbook of Human Genetics*. New York: Oxford University Press, 1971.

Levitt M, Dunner DL, Mendlewicz J, Frewin DB, Lawlor W, Fleiss JL, Stallone F, Fieve RR: Plasma dopamine beta hydroxylase activity in affective disorders. *Psychopharmacologia* 46:205–210, 1976.

Levy AB, Drake ME, Shy KE: EEG evidence for epileptiform paroxysms in rapid cycling bipolar patients. *J Clin Psychiatry* 49:232–234, 1988.

Levy DM, Beck SJ: The Rorschach Test in manic-depressive psychosis. *Am J Orthopsychiatry* 4:31–42, 1934.

Levy MI, DeNigris Y, Davis KL: Rapid antidepressant activity of melanocyte-inhibiting factor: A clinical trial. *Biol Psychiatry* 17:259–263, 1982.

Lewis AJ: Melancholia: A clinical survey of depressive states. *J Ment Sci* 80:277–378, 1934.

Lewis AJ: Prognosis in the manic-depressive psychosis. *Lancet* 2:997–999, 1936.

Lewis CE, Helzer J, Cloninger CR, Croughan J, Whitman BY: Psychiatric diagnosis predispositions to alcoholism. *Compr Psychiatry* 23:451–461, 1982.

Lewis DA, McChesney C: Tritiated imipramine binding distinguishes among subtypes of depression. *Arch Gen Psychiatry* 42:485–488, 1985a.

Lewis DA, McChesney C: Tritiated imipramine binding to platelets in manic subjects. *J Affective Disord* 9:207–211, 1985b.

Lewis DO, Feldman M, Greene M, Martinez-Mustardo Y: Psychomotor epileptic symptoms in six patients with bipolar mood disorders. *Am J Psychiatry* 141:1583–1586, 1984.

Lewis DO, Comite F, Mallouh C, Zadunaisky L, Hutchinson-Williams, K, Cherksey BD, Yeager C: Bipolar mood disorder and endometriosis: preliminary findings. *Am J Psychiatry* 144:1588–1591, 1987.

Lewis JL, Winokur G: The induction of mania: A natural history study with controls. *Arch Gen Psychiatry* 39:303–306, 1982.

Lewis NDC: Mental dynamisms and psychotherapeutic modifications in manic-depressive psychoses. *Res Publ Assoc Res Nerv Ment Dis* 11:754–776, 1931.

Lewis ND, Hubbard LD: Manic-depressive reactions in Negroes. *Res Pub Assoc Res Nerv Ment Dis* 11:779–817, 1931.

Lewis PR, Lobban MC: Dissociation of diurnal rhythms in human subjects living in abnormal time routines. *Quarterly J Exper Physiol Cognate Med Sci* 42:371–386, 1957.

Lewontin RC, Rose S, Kamin LJ: *Not in Our Genes: Biology, Ideology, and Human Nature.* New York: Pantheon Books, 1984.

Lewy AJ: Human melatonin secretion (II): A marker for the circadian system and the effects of light. In: RM Post, JC Ballenger, eds: *Neurobiology of Mood Disorders.* Baltimore: Williams & Wilkins, 1984. pp 215–226.

Lewy AJ, Sack RL: Light therapy and psychiatry. *Proc Soc Exp Biol Med* 183:11–18, 1986.

Lewy AJ, Wehr TA, Gold PW, Goodwin FK: Plasma melatonin in manic-depressive illness. In: E Usdin, IJ Kopin, J Barchas, eds: *Catecholamines: Basic and Clinical Frontiers.* Vol 2. New York: Pergamon Press, 1979. pp 1173–1175.

Lewy AJ, Wehr TA, Goodwin FK, Newsome DA, Markey SP: Light suppresses melatonin secretion in humans. *Science* 210:1267–1269, 1980.

Lewy AJ, Wehr TA, Goodwin FK, Newsome DA, Rosenthal NE: Manic-depressive patients may be supersensitive to light. Letter. *Lancet* 1:383–384, 1981.

Lewy AJ, Kern HA, Rosenthal NE, Wehr TA: Bright artificial light treatment of a manic-depressive patient with a seasonal mood cycle. *Am J Psychiatry* 139:1496–1498, 1982.

Lewy AJ, Nurnberger JI, Wehr TA, Pack D, Becker LE, Powell R-L, Newsome DA: Supersensitivity to light: Possible trait marker for manic-depressive illness. *Am J Psychiatry* 142:725–727, 1985a.

Lewy AJ, Sack RL, Singer CM: Treating phase typed chronobiologic sleep and mood disorders using appropriately timed bright artificial light. *Psychopharmacol Bull* 21:368–372, 1985b.

Lewy AJ, Sack RL, Miller LS, Hoban TM: Antidepressant and circadian phase-shifting effects of light. *Science* 235:352–354, 1987a.

Lewy AJ, Sack RL, Singer CM, White DM: The phase shift hypothesis for bright light's therapeutic mechanism of action: Theoretical considerations and experimental evidence. *Psychopharmacol Bull* 23:349–353, 1987b.

Liberman RP: What is schizophrenia? *Schizophr Bull* 8:435–437, 1982.

Libet JM, Lewinsohn PM: Concept of social skill with special reference to the behavior of depressed persons. *J Consult Clin Psychol* 40:304–312, 1973.

Lieb J, Karmali R, Horrobin D: Elevated levels of prostaglandin E2 and thromboxane B2 in depression. *Prostaglandins Leukotrienes Med* 10:361–367, 1983.

Liebowitz MR, Stallone F, Dunner DL, Fieve RR: Personality features of patients with primary affective disorder. *Acta Psychiatr Scand* 60:214–224, 1979.

Liebowitz MR, Klein DF, Quitkin FM, Stewart JW,

McGrath PJ: Clinical implications of diagnostic subtypes of depression. In: RM Post, JC Ballenger, eds. *Neurobiology of Mood Disorders.* Baltimore: Williams and Wilkins, 1984a. pp. 107–120.

Liebowitz MR, Quitkin FM, Stewart JW, McGrath PJ, Harrison W, Rabkin J, Tricamo E, Markowitz JS, Klein DF: Phenelzine v. imipramine in atypical depression: A preliminary report. *Arch Gen Psychiatry* 41:669–677, 1984b.

Liebowitz MR, Quitkin FM, Stewart JW, McGrath PJ, Harrison WM, Markowitz JS, Rabkin JG, Tricamo E, Goetz DM, Klein DF: Antidepressant specificity in atypical depression. *Arch Gen Psychiatry* 45:129–137, 1988.

Liegghio NE, Yeragani VK: Buspirone-induced hypomania. *J Clin Psychopharmacol* 8:226–227, 1988.

Lin SC, Richelson E: Low levels and lack of function of muscarinic binding sites in human skin fibroblasts from five affectively ill patients and two control subjects. *Am J Psychiatry* 143:658–660, 1986.

Lingjaerde O, Edlund AH, Gormsen CA, Gottfries CG, Haugstad A, Hermann IL, Hollnagel P, Mäkimattilla A, Rasmussen KE, Remvig J, Robak OH: The effect of lithium carbonate in combination with tricyclic antidepressants in endogenous depression: A double-blind, multicenter trial. *Acta Psychiatr Scand* 50:233–242, 1974.

Lingjaerde O, Bratlid T, Hansen T, Gøtestam KG: Seasonal affective disorder and midwinter insomnia in the far north: Studies on two related chronobiological disorders in Norway. *Clin Neuropharmacol* 9(Suppl 4):187–189, 1986.

Linkowski P, de Maertelaer V, Mendlewicz J: Suicidal behaviour in major depressive illness. *Acta Psychiatr Scand* 72:233–238, 1985a.

Linkowski P, Mendlewicz J, LeClercq R, Brasseur M, Hubain P, Golstein J, Copinschi G, Van Cauter E: The 24-hour profile of adrenocorticotropin and cortisol in major depressive illness. *J Clin Endocrinol Metab* 61:429–438, 1985b.

Linkowski P, Van Cauter E, LeClercq R, Desmedt D, Brasseur M, Golstein J, Copinschi G, Mendlewicz J: ACTH, cortisol and growth hormone 24-hour profiles in major depressive illness. *Acta Psychiatr Belg* 85:615–623, 1985c.

Linkowski P, Kerkhofs M, Rielaert C, Mendlewicz J: Sleep during mania in manic-depressive males. *Eur Arch Psychiatr Neurol Sci* 235:339–341, 1986.

Linkowski P, Mendlewicz J, Kerkhofs M, Leclercq R, Golstein J, Brasseur M, Copinschi G, Van Cauter E: 24-hour profiles of adrenocorticotropin, cortisol, and growth hormone in major depressive illness: Effect of antidepressant treatment. *J Clin Endocrinol Metab* 65:141–52, 1987.

Linn MW, Linn BS, Jensen J: Stressful events, dysphoric mood, and immune responsiveness. *Psychol Rep* 54:219–222, 1984.

Linnoila M, Karoum F, Calil HM, Kopin IJ, Potter WZ: Alteration of norepinephrine metabolism with desipramine and zimelidine in depressed patients. *Arch Gen Psychiatry* 39:1025–1028, 1982.

Linnoila M, MacDonald E, Reinila M, Leroy A, Rubinow DR, Goodwin FK: RBC membrane adenosine triphosphatase activities in patients with major affective disorders. *Arch Gen Psychiatry* 40:1021–1026, 1983a.

Linnoila M, Whorton AR, Rubinow DR, Cowdry RW, Ninan PT, Waters RN: CSF prostaglandin levels in depressed and schizophrenic patients. *Arch Gen Psychiatry* 40:405–406, 1983b.

Linnoila M, Litovitz G, Scheinin M, Chang M-D, Cutler NR: Effects of electroconvulsive treatment on monoamine metabolites, growth hormone, and prolactin in plasma. *Biol Psychiatry* 19:79–84, 1984.

Linnoila M, Virkkunen M, Roy A, Potter WZ: Monoamines, glucose metabolism and impulse control. in press.

Lion JR: Conceptual issues in the use of drugs for the treatment of aggression in man. *J Nerv Ment Dis* 160:76–82, 1975.

Lipinski JF, Cohen BM, Frankenburg F, Tohen M, Waternaux C, Altesman R, Jones B, Harris P: Open trial of S-adenosylmethionine for treatment of depression. *Am J Psychiatry* 141:448–450, 1984.

Lipkin KM, Dyrud J, Meyer GG: The many faces of mania: Therapeutic trial of lithium carbonate. *Arch Gen Psychiatry* 22:262–267, 1970.

Lippmann S, Manshadi M, Baldwin H, Drasin G, Rice J, Alrajeh S: Cerebellar vermis dimensions on computerized tomographic scans of schizophrenic and bipolar patients. *Am J Psychiatry* 139:667–668, 1982.

Lipsey JR, Robinson RG, Pearlson GD, Rao K, Price TR: Mood change following bilateral hemisphere brain injury. *Br J Psychiatry* 143:266–273, 1983.

Lipsey JR, Spencer WC, Rabins PV, Robinson RG: Phenomenological comparison of poststroke depression and functional depression. *Am J Psychiatry* 143:527–529, 1986.

Lipton MA, Goodwin FK: A controlled study of thyrotropin releasing hormone in hospitalized depressed patients. *Psychopharmacol Bull* 11:8–29, 1975.

Lipton RB, Levin S, Holzman PS: Horizontal and vertical pursuit eye movements, the oculocephalic reflex, and the functional psychoses. *Psychiatry Res* 3:193–203, 1980.

Lishman WA: Psychiatric disability after head injury: The significance of brain damage. *Proc Royal Soc Med* 59:261–265, 1966.

Lishman WA: Brain damage in relation to psychiatric disability after head injury. *Br J Psychiatry* 114:373–410, 1968.

Lishman WA: *Organic Psychiatry*. Oxford: Blackwell, 1978.

Lishman WA, McMeekan ERL: Hand preference patterns in psychiatric patients. *Br J Psychiatry* 129:158–166, 1976.

Lishman WA, Toone BK, Colbourn CJ, McMeekan ERL, Mance RM: Dichotic listening in psychotic patients. *Br J Psychiatry* 132:333–341, 1978.

Liskow B, Mayfield D, Thiele J: Alcohol and affective disorder: Assessment and treatment. *J Clin Psychiatry* 43:144–147, 1982.

Lloyd C: Life events and depressive disorder reviewed. I. Events as predisposing factors. *Arch Gen Psychiatry* 37:529–535, 1980.

Lloyd GG, Lishman WA: Effect of depression on the speed of recall of pleasant and unpleasant experiences. *Psychol Med* 5:173–180, 1975.

Lloyd KG: Morselli PL: Psychopharmacology of GABAergic drugs. In: HY Meltzer, ed: *Psychopharmacology: The Third Generation of Progress*. New York: Raven Press, 1987. pp 183–195.

Lloyd KG, Farley J, Peck JHN, Hornykiewicz O: Serotonin and 5-hydoxyindoleacetic acid in discrete areas of the brainstem of suicide victims and control patients. *Adv Biochem Psychopharmacol* 11:387–397, 1974.

Lloyd KG, Zivkovic B, Scatton B, Morselli PL, Bartholini G: The GABAergic hypothesis of depression. *Prog Neuro-psychopharmacol Biol Psychiatry* 13:341–351, 1989.

Lloyd KG, Zivkovic B, Sanger D, Depoortere H, Bartholini G: Fengabine, a novel antidepressant GABAergic agent: I. Activity in models for antidepressant drugs and psychopharmacological profile. *J Pharmacol Exp Ther* 241:245–250, 1987.

Lobban MC, Tredre B, Elithorn A, Bridges P: Diurnal rhythms of electrolyte excretion in depressive illness. *Nature* 199:667–669, 1963.

Lobeck F, Nelson MV, Evans RL, Hornstra RK: Evaluation of four methods for predicting lithium dosage. *Clin Pharm* 6:230–233, 1987.

Lobovits DA, Handel PJ: Childhood depression: Prevalence using DSM-III criteria and validity of parent and child depression scales. *J Pediatr Psychol* 10:45–54, 1985.

Lodge Patch IC: Homeless men in London: I: Demographic findings in a lodging house sample. *Br J Psychiatry* 118:313–317, 1971.

Logan J: *Josh: My Up and Down, In and Out Life*. New York: Delacorte Press, 1976.

Loo H, Galinowski A, Boccara I, Richard A: Intérêt de la sismothérapie d'entretien dans les dépressions récurrentes: A propos de 4 observations. *L'Encephale* 14:39–41, 1988.

Loomer HP, Saunders JC, Kline NS: A clinical and pharmacodynamic evaluation of iponiazid as a psychic energizer. *Psychiatr Res Rep Am Psychiatr Assoc* 8:129–141, 1957.

Loosen PT: Thyroid function in affective disorders and alcoholism. *Endocrinol Metab Clin North Am* 17:55–82, 1988.

Loosen PT, Prange AJ Jr, Wilson IC, Lara PP, Pettus C: Thyroid stimulating hormone response after thyrotropin releasing hormone in depressed, schizophrenic and normal women. *Psychoneuroendocrinology* 2:137–148, 1977.

Loosen PT, Wilson IC, Prange AJ Jr: Endocrine and behavioral changes in depression after thyrotropin-releasing hormone (TRH): Alteration by pretreatment with thyroid hormones. *J Affective Disord* 2:267–278, 1980.

Loosen PT, Marciniak R, Thadani K: TRH-induced TSH response in healthy volunteers: Relationship to psychiatric history. *Am J Psychiatry* 144:455–459, 1987.

López-Ibor JJ, Saiz-Ruiz J, Pérez de los Cobos JC: Biological correlations of suicide and aggressivity in major depression (with melancholia): 5-hydroxyindoleacetic acid and cortisol with cerebral spinal fluid, dexamethasone suppression test and therapeutic response to 5-hydroxytryptophan. *Neuropsychobiology* 14:67–74, 1985.

Loranger AW, Levine PM: Age at onset of bipolar affective illness. *Arch Gen Psychiatry* 35:1345–1348, 1978.

Lorenz M, Cobb S: Language behavior in manic patients. *Arch Neurol Psychiatry* 67:763–770, 1952.

Lorimy F, Lôo H, Deniker P: Effets cliniques des traitements prolongés par les sels de lithium sur le sommeil, l'appétit et la sexualité. *L'Encéphale* 3:227–239, 1977.

Lorr M: Assessing psychotic behavior by the IMPS. *Mod Prob Pharmacopsychiat* 7:50–63, 1974.

Los Angeles Times. Interview with Bert Yancey. April 6, 1978.

Loudon JB, Blackburn IM, Ashworth CM: A study of the symptomatology and course of manic illness using a new scale. *Psychol Med* 7:723–729, 1977.

Louie AK, Meltzer HY: Lithium potentiation of antidepressant treatment. *J Clin Psychopharmacol* 4:316–321, 1984.

Louks JL, Smith JR: Homeless: Axis I disorders. *Hosp Community Psychiatry* 39:670–671, 1988.

Love JO: *Virginia Woolf: Sources of Madness and Art.* Berkeley, University of California Press, 1977.

Lovett LM, Shaw DM: Outcome in bipolar affective disorder after stereotactic tractotomy. *Br J Psychiatry* 151:113–116, 1987.

Lowe GR: The phenomenology of hallucinations as an aid to differential diagnosis. *Br J Psychiatry* 123:621–633, 1973.

Lowell R: *For the Union Dead.* New York: Farrar, Straus, 1964.

Lowell R: *Day by Day.* New York: Farrar, Straus and Giroux, 1977.

Lubin B: Adjective checklists for measurement of depression. *Arch Gen Psychiatry* 12:57–62, 1965.

Lucas CP, Rigby JC, Lucas SB: The occurrence of depression following mania: A method of predicting vulnerable cases. *Br J Psychiatry* 154:705–708, 1989.

Luchins DJ, Lewine RR, Meltzer HY: Lateral ventricular size, psychopathology, and medication response in the psychoses. *Biol Psychiatry* 19:29–44, 1984.

Ludwig AM, Ables MF: Mania and marriage: The relationship between biological and behavioral variables. *Comp Psychiatry* 15:411–421, 1974.

Lumry AE, Gottesman II, Tuason VB: MMPI state dependency during the course of bipolar psychosis. *Psychiatry Res* 7:59–67, 1982.

Lund Y, Nissen M, Rafaelson OJ: Long-term lithium treatment and psychological functions. *Acta Psychiatr Scand* 65:233–244, 1982.

Lund R, Kammerloher A, Dirlich G: Body temperature in endogenously depressed patients during depression and remission. In: TA Wehr, FK Goodwin, eds: *Circadian Rhythms in Psychiatry.* Pacific Grove, CA: The Boxwood Press, 1983. pp 77–88.

Lundholm H: Reaction time as an indicator of emotional disturbances in manic-depressive psychoses. *J Abnorm Psychol Soc Psychol* 17:292–318, 1922.

Lundquist G: Prognosis and course in manic-depressive psychoses: A follow-up study of 319 first admissions. *Acta Psychiatr Neurol* (Suppl 35):1–96, 1945.

Luria RE: The validity and reliability of the Visual Analogue Mood Scale. *J Psychiatr Res* 12:51–57, 1975.

Lusznat RM, Murphy DP, Nunn CMH: Carbamazepine vs lithium in the treatment and prophylaxis of mania. *Br J Psychiatry* 153:198–204, 1988.

Luxenburger H: Berufsgliederung und soziale Schichtung in den Familien erblich Geisteskranker. *Eugenik* 3:34–40, 1933.

Lykouras E, Christodoulou GN, Malliaras D: Type and content of delusions in unipolar psychotic depression. *J Affective Disord* 9:249–252, 1985.

Lyskowski J, Nasrallah HA, Dunner FJ, Bucher K: A longitudinal survey of side effects in a lithium clinic. *J Clin Psychiatry* 43:284–286, 1982.

Lyttkens L, Soderberg R, Wetterberg L: Relationship between erythrocyte and plasma lithium concentrations as an index in psychiatric disease. *Ups J Mes Sci* 81:123–128, 1976.

Maany I, Mendels J, Frazer A, Brunswick D: A study of growth hormone release in depression. *Neuropsychobiology* 5:282–289, 1979.

Maarbjerg K, Vestergaard P, Schou M: Changes in serum thyroxine (T4) and serum thyroid stimulating hormone (TSH) during prolonged lithium treatment. *Acta Psychiatr Scand* 75:217–221, 1987.

Maarbjerg K, Aagaard J, Vestergaard P: Adherence to lithium prophylaxis: I. Clinical predictors and patient's reasons for nonadherence. *Pharmacopsychiatry* 21:121–5, 1988.

Maas JW, Fawcett J, Dekirmenjian H: 3-methoxy-4-hydroxyphenylglycol (MHPG) excretion in depressive states. *Arch Gen Psychiatry* 19:129–134, 1968.

Maas JW, Koslow SH, Katz MM, Bowden CL, Gibbons RL, Stokes PE, Robins E, Davis JM: Pretreatment neurotransmitter metabolite levels and response to tricyclic antidepressant drugs. *Am J Psychiatry* 141:1159–1171, 1984.

McCabe MS, Norris B: ECT versus chlorpromazine in mania. *Biol Psychiatry* 12:245–254, 1977.

McCabe MS, Reich T, Winokur G: Methysergide as a treatment for mania. *Am J Psychiatry* 127:354–356, 1970.

McCarley RW, Hobson JA: Neuronal excitability modulation over the sleep cycle: A structural and mathematical model. *Science* 189:58–60, 1975.

McCreadie RG, Farmer JG: Lithium and hair texture. *Acta Psychiatr Scand* 72:387–388, 1985.

McCreadie RG, Morrison DP: The impact of lithium in South-West Scotland: I. Demographic and clinical findings. *Br J Psychiatry* 146:70–74, 1985.

MacDonald E, LeRoy A, Linnoila M: Failure of lithium to counteract vanadate-induced inhibition of red blood cell membrane Na^+, K^+-ATPase. Letter. *Lancet* 2:774, 1982.

MacDonald E, Rubinow D, Linnoila M: Sensitivity of RBC membrane Ca^{2+}-adenosine triphosphatase to calmodulin stimulation. Variations in patients with bipolar affective disorders. *Arch Gen Psychiatry* 41:487–493, 1984.

MacDonald JB: Prognosis in manic-depressive insanity. *J Nerv Ment Dis* 17:20–30, 1918.

McElderry BR Jr, ed: *Shelley's Critical prose.* Lincoln: University of Nebraska Press, 1967.

McElroy SL, Keck PE Jr, Pope HG Jr: Sodium valproate: Its use in primary psychiatric disorders. *J Clin Psychopharmacol* 7:16–24, 1987.

McElroy SL, Keck PE Jr, Pope HG Jr, Hudson JI: Valproate in the treatment of rapid-cycling bipolar disorder. *J Clin Psychopharmacol* 8:275–279, 1988.

McElroy SL, Keck PE Jr, Pope HG Jr, Hudson JI: Valproate in the treatment of rapid-cycling bipolar disorder. *J Clin Psychiatry* 50(Suppl):23–29, 1989.

McGennis AJ: Lithium carbonate and tetracycline interaction. *Br Med J* 1:1183, 1978.

McGlashan TH: The borderline syndrome: II. Is it a variant of schizophrenia or affective disorder? *Arch Gen Psychiatry* 40:1319–1323, 1983.

McGlashan TH: The Chestnut Lodge follow-up study: II. Long-term outcome of schizophrenia and the affective disorders. *Arch Gen Psychiatry* 41:586–601, 1984.

McGlashan TH: Affective disorders and Axis-II comorbidity. Abstract of paper presented at the 139th annual meeting of the American Psychiatric Association, May, 1986.

McGlashan TH: Testing DSM-III symptom criteria for schizotypal and borderline personality disorders. *Arch Gen Psychiatry* 44:143–148, 1987.

McGlashan TH: Adolescent versus adult onset mania. *Am J Psychiatry* 145:221–223, 1988.

McGuire RJ, Mowbray RM, Vallance RC: The Maudsley Personality Inventory used with psychiatric inpatients. *Br J Psychol* 54:157–166, 1963.

McHarg JF: Mania in childhood. AMA *Arch Neurol Psychiatry* 72:531–539, 1954.

McKenna PJ, Kane JM, Parrish K: Psychotic symptoms in epilepsy. *Am J Psychiatry* 142:895–904, 1985.

McKeown SP, Jani CJ: Mania following head injury. *Br J Psychiatry* 151:867–868, 1987.

McKinney WT: Electroconvulsive therapy and animal models of depression. *Ann NY Acad Sci* 462:65–69, 1986.

McKinney WT: *Models of Mental Disorders: A New Comparative Psychiatry.* New York: Plenum Medical Book Co, 1988.

McKinney WT, Young LD, Suomi SJ, Davis JM: Chlorpromazine treatment of disturbed monkeys. *Arch Gen Psychiatry* 29:490–494, 1973.

McKnew DH Jr, Cytryn L, Efron AM, Gershon ES, Bunney WE Jr: Offspring of patients with affective disorders. *Br J Psychiatry* 134:148–152, 1979.

MacLean PD: Some psychiatric implications of physiological studies on frontotemporal portion of limbic system (visceral brain). *Electroencephalogr Clin Neurophysiol* 4:407–418, 1952.

MacLean PD, Ogston K, Grauer L: A behavioral approach to the treatment of depression. *J Behav Ther Exp Psychiatry* 4:323–330, 1973.

McLellan AT, Childress AR, Woody GE: Drug abuse and psychiatric disorders: Role of drug choice. In: AI Alterman, ed: *Substance Abuse and Psychopathology.* New York: Plenum Press, 1985. pp 137–172.

McNair DM: *Profile of Mood States.* San Diego: Educational and Industrial Testing Service, 1971.

McNair DM: Self-evaluations of antidepressants. *Psychopharmacologia* 37:281–302, 1974.

McNamee HB, Moody JP, Naylor GJ: Indoleamine metabolism in affective disorders: Excretion of tryptamine, indoleacetic acid and 5-hydroxy-indoleacetic acid in depressive states. *J Psychosom Res* 16:63–70, 1972.

MacNeil S, Hanson-Novety E, Paschalis C, Eastwood PR, Jenner FA: Diuretics during lithium therapy. *Lancet* 1:1296–1296, 1975.

McNeil TF: Prebirth and postbirth influence on the relationship between creative ability and recorded mental illness. *J Pers* 39:391–406, 1971.

Macphee GJ, McInnes GT, Thompson GG, Brodie MJ: Verapamil potentiates carbamazepine neurotoxicity: A clinically important inhibitory interaction. *Lancet* 1:700–703, 1986.

McPherson FM, Blackburn IM, Draffan JW, McFadyen M: A further study of the grid test of thought disorder. *Br J Soc Clin Psychol* 12:420–427, 1973.

MacVane JR, Lange JD, Brown WA, Zayat M: Psychological functioning of bipolar manic-depressives in remission. *Arch Gen Psychiatry* 35:1351–1354, 1978.

Maggi A, Enna SJ: Regional alterations in rat brain neurotransmitter systems following chronic lithium treatment. *J Neurochem* 34:888–892, 1980.

Maggs R: Treatment of manic illness with lithium carbonate. *Br J Psychiatry* 109:56–65, 1963.

Maguire J: Clonidine: An effective anti-manic agent? *Br J Psychiatry* 150:863–864, 1987.

Maj M: Lithium prophylaxis of schizoaffective disorders: A prospective study. *J Affective Disord* 14:129–135, 1988.

Maj M: A family study of two subgroups of schizo-affective patients. *Br J Psychiatry* 154:640–643, 1989.

Maj M, DelVecchio M, Starace F, Pirozzi R, Kemali D: Prediction of affective psychoses response to lithium prophylaxis. *Acta Psychiatr Scand* 69:37–44, 1984.

Maj M, Starace F, Nolfe G, Kemali D: Minimum plasma lithium levels required for effective prophylaxis in DSM III bipolar disorder: A prospective study. *Pharmacopsychiatry* 19:420–423, 1986.

Maj M, Pirozzi R, Starace F: Previous pattern of course of the illness as a predictor of response to lithium prophylaxis in bipolar patients. *J Affective Disord* 17:237–241, 1989.

Makeeva VL, Gol'davskaia IL, Pozdniakova SL: Somatic changes and side effects from use of lithium salts in prevention of affective-disorders. *Sov Neur R* 7:42–53, 1974.

Makman MH, Brown JH, Mishra RK: Cyclic AMP in retina and caudate nucleus: Influence of dopamine and other agents. *Adv Cyclic Nucleotide Res* 5:661–679, 1975.

Mallinger AG, Hanin I: Membrane Transport processes in affective illness. In: E Usdin, I Hanin, eds: *Biological Markers in Psychiatry and Neurology.* Oxford: Pergamon Press, 1982. pp 137–151.

Mallinger AG, Kopp U, Hanin I: Erythrocyte choline transport in drug-free and lithium-treated individuals. *J Psychiatr Res* 18:107–117, 1984.

Mallinger AG, Edwards DJ, Himmelhoch JM, Knopf S, Ehler J: Pharmacokinetics of tranycypromine in patients who are depressed: Relationship to cardiovascular effects. *Clin Pharmacol Ther* 40:444–450, 1986.

Mallinger AG, Hanin I, Himmelhoch JM, Thase ME, Knopf S: Stimulation of cell membrane sodium transport activity by lithium: Possible relationship to therapeutic action. *Psychiatry Res* 22:49–59, 1987.

Malmgren R, Åsberg M, Olsson P, Tornling G, Unge G: Defective serotonin transport mechanism in platelets from endogenously depressed patients. *Life Sci* 29:2649–2658, 1981.

Malzberg B: *Social and Biological Aspects of Mental Disease.* Utica NY: State Hospitals Press, 1940.

Malzberg B: Mental disease in American Negroes: A statistical analysis. In: O Klineberg, ed: *Characteristics of the American Negro.* New York: Harper, 1944. pp 371–399.

Malzberg B: Mental disease in relation to economic status. *J Nerv Ment Dis* 123:257–261, 1956.

Malzberg B: *Mental Disease Among Jews in New York State.* New York: Intercontinental Medical Book Corp, 1960.

Malzberg B: The distribution of mental disease according to religious affiliation in New York State, 1949–1951. *Mental Hygiene* 46:510–522, 1962.

Malzberg B: Mental disease among native and foreign-born whites in New York State, 1949–1951. *Mental Hygiene* 48:478–499, 1964.

Mandel B, Last U, Belmaker RH, Rosenbaum M: Rorschach markers in euthymic manic-depressive illness. *Neuropsychobiology* 12:96–100, 1984.

Mandel MR, Madsen J, Miller AL, Baldessarini RJ: Intoxication associated with lithium and ECT. *Am J Psychiatry* 137:1107–1109, 1980.

Mandell AJ: From molecular biological simplification to more realistic central nervous system dynamics: An overview. In: R Michels, JO Cavenar Jr, HKH Brodie, AM Cooper, SB Guze, LL Judd, GL Klerman, AJ Solnit, eds: *Psychiatry.* Vol 3. Chapter 72. London: JB Lippincott, 1985.

Mandell AJ: A note on circadian rhythm pathophysiology: Scaling of biological time and the global dynamical stability of nonlinear systems. In: JD Barchas, WE Bunney, eds: *Perspectives in Psychopharmacology: A Collection of Papers in Honor of Earl Usdin.* New York: Alan R. Liss, 1988. pp 99–109.

Mandell AJ, Knapp S: Asymmetry and mood, emergent properties of serotonin regulation. *Arch Gen Psychiatry* 36:909–916, 1979.

Mandell AJ, Knapp S, Ehlers C, Russo PV: The stability of constrained randomness: Lithium prophylaxis at several neurobiological levels. In: RM Post, JC Ballenger, eds: *Neurobiology of Mood Disorders.* Baltimore: Williams & Wilkins, 1984. pp 744–776.

Mander AJ: Is lithium justified after one manic episode? *Acta Psychiatr Scand* 73:60–67, 1986.

Mander AJ: Is there a lithium withdrawal syndrome. *Br J Psychiatry* 150:714, 1987.

Mann AM, Hutchinson JL: Manic reaction associated with procarbazine hydrochloride therapy of Hodgkins' disease. *Can Med Assoc J* 97:1350–1353, 1967.

Mann JJ, Brown RP, Halper JP, Sweeney JA, Kocsis JH, Stokes PE, Bilezikian JP: Reduced sensitivity of lymphocyte beta-adrenergic receptors in patients with endogenous depression and psychomotor agitation. *N Engl J Med* 313:715–720, 1985.

Männistö PT: Endocrine side-effects of lithium. In: FN Johnson, ed: *Handbook of Lithium Therapy.* Baltimore: University Park Press, 1980. pp 310–322.

Marchesi C, De Ferri A, Petrolini N, Govi A, Manzoni GC, Coiro V, De Risio C: Prevalence of migraine and muscle tension headache in depressive disorders. *J Affective Disord* 16:33–36, 1989.

Mardh G: Further studies on 4-hydroxy-3-methoxyphenylglycol oxidation in humans: Effect of pool expansion and stereochemistry. *J Neurochem* 41:299–301, 1983.

Margo A, McMahon P: Lithium withdrawal triggers psychosis. *Br J Psychiatry* 141:407–410, 1982.

Marley E, Wozniak KM: Clinical and experimental aspects of interactions between amine oxidase inhibitors and amine re-uptake inhibitors. *Psychol Med* 13:735–749, 1983.

Marneros A, Tsuang MT, eds: *Schizoaffective Psychoses.* Berlin-Heidelberg: Springer-Verlag, 1986.

Marneros A, Deister A, Rohde A: Syndrome shift in

the long-term course of schizoaffective disorders. *Eur Arch Psychiatry Neurol Sci* 238:97–104, 1988.

Marneros A, Deister A, Rohde A, Steinmeyer EM, Jünemann H: Long-term outcome of schizoaffective and schizophrenic disorders: A comparative study: I. Definitions, methods, psychopathological and social outcome. *Eur Arch Psychiatry Neurol Sci* 238:118–125, 1989.

Maron L, Rechtschaffen A, Wolpert EA: Sleep cycle during napping. *Arch Gen Psychiatry* 11:503–508, 1964.

Marquez C, Taintor Z, Schwartz MA: Diagnosis of manic depressive illness in blacks. *Compr Psychiatry* 26:337–341, 1985.

Marsella AJ, Murray MD: Diagnostic type, gender and consistency vs. specificity in behavior. *J Clin Psychol* 30:484–488, 1975.

Marshall MH, Neumann CP, Robinson M: Lithium, creativity, and manic-depressive illness: Review and prospectus. *Psychosomatics* 11:406–488, 1970.

Martin I, Rees L: Reaction times and somatic reactivity in depressed patients. *J Psychosomatic Res* 9:375–382, 1966.

Martin JB, Reichlin S: *Clinical Neuroendocrinology, 2nd ed.* Philadelphia: Davis Co, 1987.

Martin K: Effects of lithium on choline transport in synaptosomes and human erythrocytes. In: BA Callingham, ed: *Drugs and Transport Processes.* Baltimore: University Park Press, 1974. pp 347–361.

Martin RL, Cloninger R, Guze SB, Clayton PJ: Mortality in a follow-up of 500 psychiatric outpatients: II. Cause-specific mortality. *Arch Gen Psychiatry* 42:58–66, 1985.

Martin-Iverson MT, Leclere JF, Fibiger HC: Cholinergic-dopaminergic interactions and the mechanisms of action of antidepressants. *Eur J Pharmacol* 94:193–201, 1983.

Masala A, Delitala G, Alagna S, Devilla L: Effect of pimozide on levodopa-induced growth hormone release in man. *Clin Endocrinol (Oxf)* 7:253–256, 1977.

Mason CF: Pre-illness intelligence of mental hospital patients. *J Consult Psychol* 20:297–300, 1956.

Mason JW, Giller EL, Kosten TR: Serum testosterone differences between patients with schizophrenia and those with affective disorder. *Biol Psychiatry* 23:357–366, 1988.

Masters AS: The distribution of blood groups in psychiatric illness. *Br J Psychiatry* 113:1309–1315, 1967.

Masterton G, Warner M, Roxburgh B: Supervising lithium: A comparison of a lithium clinic, psychiatric out-patient clinics, and general practice. *Br J Psychiatry* 152:535–538, 1988.

Matarazzo JD: *Wechsler's Measurement and Appraisal of Adult Intelligence.* 5th ed. Baltimore: Williams & Wilkins, 1972.

Mathew RJ, Meyer JS, Francis DJ, Semchuk KM, Mortel K, Claghorn JL: Cerebral blood flow in depression. *Am J Psychiatry* 137:1449–1450, 1980.

Mathew RJ, Ho BT, Khan MM, Perales C, Weinman ML, Claghorn JL: True and pseudo cholinesterases in depression. *Am J Psychiatry* 139:125–127, 1982.

Mathew RJ, Margolin RA, Kessler RM: Cerebral function, blood flow, and metabolism: A new vista in psychiatric research. *Integr Psychiatry* 3:214–225, 1985.

Mattsson A, Seltzer RL: MAOI-induced rapid cycling bipolar affective disorder in an adolescent. *Am J Psychiatry* 138:677–679, 1981.

Matussek N: L-Dopa in the treatment of depression. In: O Vimar, Z Votava, PB Bradley, eds: *Advances in Neuropharmacology.* Amsterdam: North-Holland Publishing Co, 1971. pp 111–119.

Matussek N: Catecholamines and mood: Neuroendocrine aspects. *Current Topics in Neuroendocrinology* 8:141–182, 1980.

Matussek N, Ackenheil M, Hippius H, Müller F, Schröder HT, Schultes H, Wasilewski B: Effect of clonidine on growth hormone release in psychiatric patients and controls. *Psychiatry Res* 2:25–36, 1980.

Matussek P, Feil WB: Personality attributes of depressive patients: Results of group comparisons. *Arch Gen Psychiatry* 40:783–790, 1983.

Maudsley H: *Natural Causes and Supernatural Seemings.* London: Kegan Paul, 1886.

Maugham WS: *Ten Novels and Their Authors.* London: Heinemann, 1954.

Maurizi CP: Influenza and mania: A possible connection with the locus ceruleus. *South Med J* 78:207–209, 1985.

Maxwell MA: *The Alcoholics Anonymous Experience.* New York: McGraw-Hill, 1984.

Maxwell S, Scheftner WA, Kessler HA, Busch K: Manic syndrome associated with zidovudine. *JAMA* 259:3406–3407, 1988.

Mayer-Gross W, Slater E, Roth M: *Clinical Psychiatry.* Baltimore: Williams & Wilkins, 1955.

Mayer-Gross W, Slater E, Roth M: *Clinical Psychiatry.* (2nd Ed.) London: Cassell & Co, 1960.

Mayfield D: Substance abuse in the affective disorders. In: AI Alterman, ed: *Substance Abuse and Psychopathology.* New York: Plenum Press, 1985. pp 69–90.

Mayfield D, Allen D: Alcohol and affect: A psychopharmacological study. *Am J Psychiatry* 123:1346–1351, 1967.

Mayfield DG, Coleman LL: Alcohol use and affective disorder. *Dis Nerv Syst* 29:467–474, 1968.

Mayo JA: Marital therapy with manic-depressive patients treated with lithium. *Comp Psychiatry* 20:419–426, 1979.

Mayo JA, O'Connell RA, O'Brien JD: Families of manic-depressive patients: Effect of treatment. *Am J Psychiatry* 136:1535–1539, 1979.

Mayo PR: Speed and accuracy of depressives on a spiral maze test. *Percept Mot Skills* 23:1034, 1966.

Mazure C, Gershon ES: Blindness and reliability in lifetime psychiatric diagnosis. *Arch Gen Psychiatry* 36:521–525, 1979.

Mazzullo JM, Lasagna L: Take thou. . .But is your patient really taking what you prescribed? *Drug Ther* 2:11–15, 1972.

Mebane AH: L-glutamine and mania. *Am J Psychiatry* 141:1302–1303, 1984.

Meehl PE: Diagnostic taxa as open concepts: Metatheoretical and statistic questions about reliability and construct validity in the grand strategy of nosological revisions. In: T Millon, GL Klerman, eds: *Contemporary Directions in Psychopathology: Toward the DSM-IV.* New York: The Guilford Press, 1986. pp 215–231.

Meijer JW, Binnie CD, Debets RM: Possible hazard of valpromide-carbamazepine combination therapy in epilepsy. *Lancet* 1:802, 1984.

Melia PI: Prophylactic lithium: A double-blind trial in recurrent affective disorders. *Br J Psychiatry* 116:621–624, 1970.

Mellerup ET, Rafaelsen OJ: Electrolyte metabolism and manic-melancholic disorder. In: HM Van Praag, MH Lader, OJ Rafaelsen, EJ Sachar, eds: *Handbook of Biological Psychiatry, Part IV: Brain Mechanisms and Abnormal Behavior Chemistry.* New York: Marcel Dekker, Inc, 1981. pp 207–224.

Mellerup ET, Bech P, Sørensen T, Frederiksen AF, Rafaelsen OJ: Calcium and electroconvulsive therapy of depressed patients. *Biol Psychiatry* 14:711–714, 1979.

Mellerup ET, Plenge P, Rosenberg R: ^{3}H-imipramine binding sites in platelets from psychiatric patients. *Psychiat Res* 7:221–227, 1982.

Mellerup ET, Dam H, Wildschiøtz G, Rafaelsen OJ: Diurnal variation of blood glucose during lithium treatment. *J Affective Disord* 5:341–347, 1983.

Mellerup ET, Plenge P, Rafaelsen OJ: Renal and other controversial adverse effects of lithium. In: HY Meltzer, ed: *Psychopharmacology: The Third Generation of Progress.* New York: Raven Press, 1987. pp 1443–1448.

Meltzer HL, Kassir S: Abnormal Calmodulin-activated CaATPase in manic-depressive subjects. *J Psychiatr Res* 17:29–35, 1983.

Meltzer HL, Kassir S, Goodnick PJ, Fieve RR, Chrisomalis L, Feliciano M, Szypula D: Calmodulin-activated calcium ATPase in bipolar illness. *Neuropsychobiology* 20:169–173, 1988.

Meltzer HY: Creatine kinase and aldolase in serum: Abnormality common to acute psychoses. *Science* 159:1368–1370, 1968.

Meltzer HY: Serum creatine phosphokinase and serum aldolase levels in acutely psychotic patients. In: P Blume, EF Freier, eds: *Enzymology in the Practice of Laboratory Medicine.* New York: Academic Press, 1974. pp 351–379.

Meltzer HY: Neuromuscular abnormalities in the major mental illnesses: I. Serum enzyme studies. In: DX Freedman, ed: *Biology of the Major Psychoses: A Comparative Analysis.* New York: Raven Press, 1975. pp 165–188.

Meltzer HY: What is schizophrenia? *Schizophr Bull* 8:433–435, 1982.

Meltzer HY: Schizoaffective disorder: Is the news of its nonexistence premature? Editor's Introduction. *Schizophr Bull* 10:11–29, 1984.

Meltzer HY, Kupfer DJ, Wyatt R, Snyder F: Sleep disturbance and serum CPK activity in acute psychosis. *Arch Gen Psychiatry* 22:398–405, 1970.

Meltzer HY, Nankin R, Raftery J: Serum creatine phosphokinase activity in newly admitted psychiatric patients: II. *Arch Gen Psychiatry* 24:568–572, 1971.

Meltzer HY, Arora RC, Baber R, Tricou BJ: Serotonin uptake in blood platelets of psychiatric patients. *Arch Gen Psychiatry* 38:1322–1326, 1981.

Meltzer HY, Fang VS, Tricou BJ, Robertson A, Piyaka SK: Effect of dexamethasone on plasma prolactin and cortisol levels in psychiatric patients. *Am J Psychiatry* 139:763–768, 1982.

Meltzer HY, Umberkoman-Wiita B, Robertson A, Tricou BJ, Lowy M, Perline R: Effect of 5-hydroxytryptophan on serum cortisol levels in major affective disorders: I. Enhanced response in depression and mania. *Arch Gen Psychiatry* 41:366–374, 1984a.

Meltzer HY, Perline R, Tricou BJ, Lowy M, Robertson A: Effect of 5-hydroxytryptophan on serum cortisol levels in major affective disorders: II. Relation to suicide, psychosis, and depressive symptoms. *Arch Gen Psychiatry* 41:379–387, 1984b.

Meltzer HY, Lowy M, Robertson A, Goodnick P, Perline R: Effect of 5-hydroxytryptophan on serum cortisol levels in major affective disorders: III. Effect of antidepressants and lithium carbonate. *Arch Gen Psychiatry* 41:391–397, 1984c.

Meltzer HY, Kolakowska T, Fang VS, Fogg L, Robertson A, Levine R, Strahilevitz M, Busch D: Growth hormone and prolactin response to apomorphine in schizophrenia and the major affective disorders. *Arch Gen Psychiatry* 41:512–519, 1984d.

Meltzer HY, Tong C, Luchins DJ: Serum dopamine beta-hydroxylase activity and lateral ventricular size in affective disorders and schizophrenia. *Biol Psychiatry* 19:1395–1402, 1984e.

Meltzer HY, Umberköman-Wiita B, Robertson AG, Tricou BJ, Lowy M: Correction and amplification: Cortisol response to 5-HTP. *Arch Gen Psychiatry* 43:815, 1986.

Mendel E: *Die Manie.* Vienna: Urban and Schwazenberg, 1881.

Mendels J: Lithium in the treatment of depressive states. In: FN Johnson, ed: *Lithium Research and Therapy.* New York: Academic Press, 1975. pp 43–62.

Mendels J: Lithium in the treatment of depression. *Am J Psychiatry* 133:373–378, 1976.

Mendels J, Frazer A: Intracellular lithium concentration and clinical response: Towards a membrane theory of depression. *J Psychiatr Res* 10:9–18, 1973.

Mendels J, Hawkins DR: Longitudinal sleep study in hypomania. *Arch Gen Psychiatry* 25:274–277, 1971.

Mendels J, Secunda SK, Dyson WL: A controlled study of the antidepressant effects of lithium carbonate. *Arch Gen Psychiatry* 26:154–157, 1972a.

Mendels J, Weinstein N, Cochrane C: The relationship between depression and anxiety. *Arch Gen Psychiatry* 27:649–653, 1972b.

Mendelson JH, Mello NK: Experimental analysis of drinking behavior of chronic alcoholics. *Ann NY Acad Sci* 133:828–845, 1966.

Mendelson JH, Mello NK: *The Diagnosis and Treatment of Alcoholism*. New York: McGraw-Hill, 1979.

Mendelson WB, Jacobs LS, Gillin JC: Negative feedback suppression of sleep-related growth hormone secretion. *J Clin Endocrinol Metab* 56:486–488, 1983.

Mendelson WB, Sack DA, James SP, Martin JV, Wagner R, Garnett D, Milton J, Wehr TA: Frequency analysis of the sleep EEG in depression. *Psychiatry Res* 21:89–94, 1987.

Mendlewicz J: The age factor in depressive illness: Some genetic considerations. *J Gerontology* 31:300–303, 1976.

Mendlewicz J: Prediction of treatment outcome: Family and twin studies in lithium prophylaxis and the question of red blood cell/plasma ratios. In: TB Cooper, S Gershon, NS Kline, M Schou, eds: *Lithium: Controversies and Unresolved Issues*. Amsterdam: Excerpta Medica, 1979. pp 226–240.

Mendlewicz J: Biological factors in affective disorders and their relevance to lithium prophylaxis. *Pharmacopsychiatry* 15:11–18, 1982.

Mendlewicz J, Fleiss JL: Linkage studies with X-chromosome markers in bipolar (manic-depressive) and unipolar (depressive) illnesses. *Biol Psychiatry* 9:261–294, 1974.

Mendlewicz J, Gilles C: Growth-hormone stimulation tests in affective-disorders and senile dementia of the Alzheimer type. *Int J Neurs* 31:259, 1986.

Mendlewicz J, Rainer JD: Adoption study supporting genetic transmission in manic-depressive illness. *Nature* 268:327–329, 1977.

Mendlewicz J, Van Praag HM, eds: *Biological Rhythms and Behavior. Advances in Biological Psychiatry*. Vol. 11. Basel: S Karger, 1983.

Mendlewicz J, Youdim MBH: Antidepressant potentiation of 5-hydroxytryptophan by L-deprenil in affective illness. *J Affective Disord* 2:137–146, 1980.

Mendlewicz J, Fieve RR, Rainer J, Fleiss JL: Manic-depressive illness: A comparative study of patients with and without a family history. *Br J Psychiatry* 120:523–530, 1972a.

Mendlewicz J, Fieve RR, Stallone F, Fleiss JL: Genetic history as a predictor of lithium response in manic depressive illness. *Lancet* 1:599–600, 1972b.

Mendlewicz J, Fieve RR, Stallone F: Relationship between effectiveness of lithium therapy and family history. *Am J Psychiatry* 130:1011–1013, 1973.

Mendlewicz J, Massart-Guiot T, Wilmotte J: Blood groups in manic-depressive illness and schizophrenia. *Dis Nerv Syst* 35:39–41, 1974.

Mendlewicz J, Verbanck P, Linkowski P, Wilmotte J: Lithium accumulation in erythrocytes of manic-depressive patients: An *in vivo* twin study. *Br J Psychiatry* 133:436–444, 1978.

Mendlewicz J, Linkowski P, Branchey L, Weinberg U, Weitzman ED, Branchey M: Abnormal 24 hour pattern of melatonin secretion in depression. Letter. *Lancet* 2:1362, 1979a.

Mendlewicz J, Linkowski P, Guroff JJ, Van Praag HM: Color blindness linkage to bipolar manic-depressive illness: New evidence. *Arch Gen Psychiatry* 36:1442–1447, 1979b.

Mendlewicz J, Linkowski P, Wilmotte J: Linkage between glucose-6-phosphate dehydrogenase deficiency and manic-depressive psychosis. *Br J Psychiatry* 137:337–342, 1980a.

Mendlewicz J, Linkowski P, Wilmotte J: Relationship between schizoaffective illness and affective disorders or schizophrenia: Morbidity risk and genetic transmission. *J Affective Disord* 2:289–302, 1980b.

Mendlewicz J, Van Cauter E, Linkowski P, L'Hermite M, Robyn C: The 24-hour profile of prolactin in depression. *Life Sci* 27:2015–2024, 1980c.

Mendlewicz J, Simon P, Sevy S, Charon F, Brocas H, Legros S, Vassart G: Polymorphic DNA marker on X chromosome and manic depression. *Lancet* i:1230–1232, 1987.

Menna-Perper M, Rochford J, Mueller PS, Swartzburg M, Jekelis AW, Manowitz P: Differential response of plasma glucose, amino acids and nonesterified fatty acids to insulin in depressed patients. *Psychoneuroendocrinology* 9:161–171, 1984.

Menninger KA: Influenza and schizophrenia. An Analysis of post influenza dementia praecox as of 1918, and five years later: Further studies of psychiatric aspects of influenza. *Am J Psychiatry* 5:469–529, 1926.

Merikangas KR, Ranella CJ, Kupfer BJ: Marital interaction in hospitalized depressed patients. *J Nerv Ment Dis* 167:689–695, 1979.

Merrin EL: Motor and sighting dominance in schizophrenia and affective disorder: Evidence for right-hand grip strength prominence in paranoid schizophrenia and bipolar illness. *Br J Psychiatry* 146:539–544, 1984.

Merry J, Reynolds C, Bailey J, Coppen A: Prophylactic treatment of alcoholism by lithium carbonate. *Lancet* 2:481–482, 1976.

Messner M, Messner E: Mood disorders following stroke. *Compr Psychiatry* 29:22–27, 1988.

Mestrallet A, Larrivé E: Essai de traitement des accès maniaques par l'hyposulfite de magnésium. *Lyon Med* 149:281–288, 1932.

Mesulam MM, Mufson EJ, Levey AI, Wainer BH: Cholinergic innervation of cortex by the basal forebrain: Cytochemistry and cortical connections of the septal area, diagonal band nuclei, nucleus basalis (substantia innominata), and hypothalamus in the rhesus monkey. *J Comp Neurol* 214:170–197, 1983a.

Mesulam MM, Mufson EJ, Wiener BH, Levey AI:

Central cholinergic pathways in the rat: An overview based on an alternative nomenclature (Ch 1–Ch 6). *Neuroscience* 10:1185–1201, 1983b.

Metcalfe M, Goldman E: Validation of an inventory for measuring depression. *Br J Psychiatry* 111:240–242, 1965.

Metzig E, Rosenberg S, Ast M, Krashen SD: Bipolar manic-depressives and unipolar depressives distinguished by tests of lateral asymmetry. *Biol Psychiatry* 11:313–323, 1976.

Meyer A: *Collected Papers of Adolph Meyer.* EE Winters, ed. Baltimore: Johns Hopkins Press, 1950–1952.

Meyer RE, Hesselbrock MN: Psychopathology and addictive disorders revisited. In: SM Mirin, ed: *Substance Abuse and Psychopathology.* Washington: American Psychiatric Press, 1984. pp 1–18.

Meynert T: [Psychiatry: A clinical treatise on disease of the forebrain based upon a study of its structure, functions, and nutrition.] Translated by B Sachs. [Pt I. *The Anatomy, Physiology, and Chemistry of the Brain.*] New York: GP Putnam, 1885. Originally published in German as Psychiatrie; Klinik der erkrankungen des vorderhirns begründet auf dessen bav, leistungen und ernahrung. Wein: Braumüller, 1884.

Mezzich JE, Raab ES: Depressive symptomatology across the Americas. *Arch Gen Psychiatry* 37:818–823, 1980.

Mezzich JE, Fabrega H, Coffman GA, Haley R: DSM-III disorders in a large sample of psychiatric patients: Frequency and specificity of diagnoses. *Am J Psychiatry* 146:212–219, 1989.

Micciolo R, Zimmermann-Tansella C, Williams P, Tansella M: Seasonal variation in suicide: Is there a sex difference? *Psychol Med* 19:199–203, 1989.

Miccoli L, Porro V, Bertolino A: Comparison between the antidepressant activity and of S-adenosylmethionine (SAMe) and that of some tricyclic drugs. *Acta Neurol (Napoli)* 33:243–255, 1978.

Miklowitz DJ, Goldstein MJ, Nuechterlein KH, Snyder KS, Doane JA: Expressed emotion, affective style, lithium compliance, and relapse in recent onset mania. *Psychopharmacol Bull* 22:628–632, 1986.

Miklowitz DJ, Goldstein MJ, Nuechterlein KH, Snyder KS, Mintz J: Family factors and the course of bipolar affective disorder. *Arch Gen Psychiatry* 45:225–231, 1988.

Milkman H, Frosch WA: On the preferential abuse of heroin and amphetamine. *J Nerv Ment Dis* 156:242–248, 1973.

Miller AH, Silberstein C, Asnis GM, Munk G, Rubinson E, Spigland I, Norin A: Epstein-Barr virus infection and depression. Letter. *J Clin Psychiatry* 47:529–530, 1986.

Miller F, Menninger J: Lithium-neuroleptic neurotoxicity is dose dependent. *J Clin Psychopharmacol* 7:89–91, 1987.

Miller F, Menninger J, Whitcup SM: Lithium-neuroleptic neurotoxicity in the elderly bipolar pa-tient. *J Clin Psychopharmacol* 6:176–178, 1986.

Miller FT, Busch F, Tanenbaum JH: Drug abuse in schizophrenia and bipolar disorder. *Am J Drug Alcohol Abuse* 15:291–295, 1989.

Miller KB, Nelson JC: Dexamethasone nonsuppression and EEG abnormalities. *Biol Psychiatry* 22:1151–1155, 1987.

Miller L: The social psychiatry and epidemiology of mental ill health in Israel. *Topical Probl Psychiatr Neurol* 6:96–137, 1967.

Miller WR: Psychological deficit in depression. *Psychol Bull* 82:238–260, 1975.

Milner B: Discussion of the subject: Experimental analysis of cerebral dominance in man. In: CH Millikan, FL Farley, eds: *Brain Mechanisms Underlying Speech and Language.* New York: Grune and Stratton, 1967. pp 122–145.

Milner P: Theories of reinforcement, drive, and motivation. In: L Iversen, S Iversen, S Snyder, eds: *Handbook of Psychopharmacology.* Vol 7. New York: Liss, 1977. pp 181–200.

Milstein V, Small JG, Shelbourne D, Small IF: Manic depressive illness: Onset, diurnal temperature and season of birth. *Dis Nerv Syst* 37:373–375, 1976.

Milstoc M, Teodoru CV, Fieve RR, Kumbaraci T: Cholinesterase activity and the manic depressive patients. *Dis Nerv Syst* 36:197–199, 1975.

Mineka S, Suomi SJ: Social separation in monkeys. *Psychopharmacol Bull* 85:1376–1400, 1978.

Minors DS, Waterhouse JM: The sleep-wakefulness rhythm, exogenous and endogenous factors (in man). *Experientia* 40:410–416, 1984a.

Minors DS, Waterhouse JM: The use of constant routines in unmasking the endogenous component of human circadian rhythms. *Chronobiol Int* 1:205–216, 1984b.

Minors DS, Waterhouse JM: Circadian rhythms and their mechanisms. *Experientia* 42:1–13, 1986.

Minski L: Mental symptoms associated with 58 cases of cerebral tumors. *J Neurol Psychiatry* 13:330–343, 1933.

Minski L: Psychopathology and psychoses associated with alcohol. *J Ment Sci* 84:985–990, 1938.

Mirin SM, Weiss RD: Affective illness in substance abusers. *Psychiatr Clin North Am* 9:503–514, 1986.

Mirin SM, Schatzberg AF, Creasey DE: Hypomania and mania after withdrawal of tricyclic antidepressants. *Am J Psychiatry* 138:87–89, 1981.

Mirin SM, Weiss RD, Sollogub A, Michael J: Affective illness in substance abusers. In: SM Mirin, ed: *Substance Abuse and Psychopathology.* Washington: American Psychiatric Press, 1984a. pp 57–78.

Mirin SM, Weiss RD, Sollogub A, Michael J: Psychopathology in the families of drug abusers. In: SM Mirin, ed: *Substance Abuse and Psychopathology.* Washington: American Psychiatric Press, 1984b. pp 79–107.

Mirin SM, Weiss RD, Michael J, Griffin ML: Psychopathology in substance abusers: Diagnosis and treatment. *Am J Drug Alcohol Abuse* 14:139–157, 1988.

Mirkin AM, Coppen A: Electrodermal activity in depression: clinical and biochemical correlates. *Br J Psychiatry* 137:93–97, 1980.

Mishra R, Janowsky A, Sulser F: Action of mianserin and zimelidine on the norepinephrine receptor coupled adenylate cyclase system in brain: Subsensitivity without reduction in β-adrenergic receptor binding. *Neuropharmacology* 19:983–987, 1980.

Misiaszek J, Gray F, Yates A: The calming effects of negative air ions on manic patients a pilot study. *Biol Psychiatry* 22:107–110, 1987.

Misra PC, Burns BH: "Lithium non-responders" in a lithium clinic. *Acta Psychiatr Scand* 55:32–40, 1977.

Mitchell JE, MacKenzie TB: Cardiac effects of lithium therapy in man: A review. *J Clin Psychiatry* 43:47–51, 1982.

Mitchell PB, Bearn JA, Corn TH, Checkley SA: Growth hormone response to clonidine after recovery in patients with endogenous depression. *Br J Psychiatry* 152:34–38, 1988.

Mitsuda H: The concept of "atypical psychoses" from the aspect of clinical genetics. *Acta Psychiat Scand* 41:372–377, 1965.

Mitterauer B, Leibetseder M, Pritz WF, Sorgo G: Comparisons of psychopathological phenomena of 422 manic-depressive patients with suicide-positive and suicide-negative family history. *Acta Psychiatr Scand* 77:438–442, 1988.

Modai I, Zemishlany Z, Jerushalmy Z: 5-Hydroxytryptamine uptake by blood platelets of unipolar and bipolar depressed patients. *Neuropsychobiology* 12:93–95, 1984.

Modell JG: Further experience and observations with lorazepam in the management of behavioral agitation. *J Clin Psychiatry* 6:385–387, 1986.

Modell JG, Lenox RH, Weiner S: Inpatient clinical trial of lorazepam for the management of manic agitation. *J Clin Psychopharmacol* 5:109–113, 1985.

Modestin J, Hunger J, Schwartz RB: [Depressive effects of physostigmine]. *Arch Psychiatr Nervenkr* 218:67–77, 1973a.

Modestin J, Schwartz RB, Hunger J: [Investigation about an influence of physostigmine on schizophrenic symptoms (author's transl)]. *Pharmakopsychiatr Neuropsychopharmakol* 6:300–304, 1973b.

Moldin SO, Gottesman II, Erlenmeyer-Kimling L: Psychometric validation of psychiatric diagnoses in the New York high-risk study. *Psychiatry Res* 22:159–177, 1987.

Möller H-J, Von Zerssen D, Emrich HM, Kissling W, Cording C, Schietsch HJ, Riedel E: Action of d-propranolol in manic psychoses. *Arch Psychiatr Nervenkr* 227:301–317, 1979.

Möller H-J, Kissling W, Riehl T, Bäuml J, Binz U, Wendt G: Doubleblind evaluation of the antimanic properties of carbamazepine as a comedication to haloperidol. *Prog Neuro-Psychopharmacol Biol Psychiatry* 13:127–136, 1989.

Moller SE, Kirk L, Fremming KH: Plasma amino acids as an index for subgroups in manic depressive psychosis: correlation to effect of tryptophan. *Psychopharmacology (Berlin)* 49:205–213, 1976.

Molnar GJ, Feeney MG, Mizra M: Terminating lithium therapy in bipolar patients. Abstract of a paper presented at the 142nd Annual Meeting of the American Psychiatric Association, May, 1987. p 234.

Molnar GJ, Feeney MG, Fava GA: Duration and symptoms of bipolar prodromes. *Am J Psychiatry* 145:1576–1578, 1988.

Monnelly EP, Woodruff RA, Robins LN: Manic-depressive illness and social achievement in a public hospital sample. *Acta Psychiatr Scand* 50:318–325, 1974.

Monroe RR: DSM-III style diagnoses of the episodic disorders. *J Nerv Ment Dis* 170:664–669, 1982.

Montgomery SA, Åsberg M: A new depression scale designed to be sensitive to change. *Br J Psychiatry* 134: 382–389, 1979.

Montgomery SA, Åsberg M, Jörnestedt P, Thorén P, Träskman L, McAuley R, Montgomery D, Shaw P: Reliability of the CPRS between the disciplines of psychiatry, general practice, nursing and psychology in depressed patients. *Acta Psychiatr Scand* 271:29–32, 1978a.

Montgomery SA, Åsberg M, Traskman L, Montgomery D: Cross cultural studies on the use of the CPRS in English and Swedish depressed patients. *Acta Psychiatr Scand* 271:33–37, 1978b.

Montgomery SA, Dufour H, Brion S, Gailledreau J, Laqueille X, Ferrey G, Moron P, Parant-Lucena N, Singer L, Danion JM, Beuzen JN, Pierredon MA: The prophylactic efficacy of fluoxetine in unipolar depression. *Br J Psychiatry* 153(Suppl 3):69–76, 1988.

Moore RY: Organization and function of a central nervous system circadian oscillator: The suprachiasmatic hypothalamic nucleus. *Fed Proc* 42:2783–2789, 1983.

Moore RY, Klein DC: Visual pathways and the central neural control of a circadian rhythm in pineal serotonin N-acetyltransferase activity. *Brain Res* 71:17–33, 1974.

Moore-Ede ME, Silzman FM, Fuller CA: *The Clocks That Time Us: Physiology of the Circadian Timing System.* Cambridge, MA: Harvard Press, 1982.

Moran, Lord CMW: *Winston Churchill: The Struggle for Survival, 1940–1965: Taken from the Diaries of Lord Moran.* Boston: Houghton Mifflin, 1966.

Moretti MM, Fine S, Haley G, Marriage K: Childhood and adolescent depression: Child-report versus parent report information. *J Am Acad Child Psychiatry* 24:298–302, 1985.

Morgan HG: The incidence of depressive symptoms during recovery from hypomania. *Br J Psychiatry* 120:537–539, 1972.

Morgan WP: Selected physiological and psychomotor correlates of depression in psychiatric patients. *Dissertation Abstracts* 28:2086-A, 1967.

Mormont C: The influence of age and depression on intellectual and memory performances. *Acta Psychiatr Belg* 84:127–134, 1984.

Morphew JA: Hypomania following complex partial seizures. Letter. *Br J Psychiatry* 152:572, 1988.

Morris JB, Beck AT: The efficacy of antidepressant drugs: A review of research (1958–1972). *Arch Gen Psychiatry* 30:667–674, 1974.

Morrison JR: Bipolar affective disorder and alcoholism. *Am J Psychiatry* 131:1130–1133, 1974.

Morrison JR: The family histories of manic-depressive patients with and without alcoholism. *J Nerv Ment Dis* 160:227–229, 1975.

Morrison J, Winokur G, Crowe R, Clancy J: The Iowa 500: The first follow-up. *Arch Gen Psychiatry* 29:678–682, 1973.

Morselli PL, Bossi L, Musch B: Antidepressant activity of the GABA agonist progabide. *Int J Neurs* 32:907, 1987.

Mortimer PS, Dawber RPR: Hair loss and lithium. *Int J Derm* 23:603–604, 1984.

Morton NE: Sequential tests for the detection of linkage. *Am J Hum Genet* 7:277–318, 1955.

Morton NE, MacLean CH: Analysis of family resemblance. III. Complex segregation of quantitative traits. *Am J Hum Genet* 26:489–503, 1974.

Moscovitch M, Strauss E, Olds J: Handedness and dichotic listening performance in patients with unipolar endogenous depression who received ECT. *Am J Psychiatry* 138:988–990, 1981.

Motto JA: The recognition and management of the suicidal patient. In: FF Flach, SC Draghi, eds: *The Nature and Treatment of Depression*. New York: John Wiley & Sons, 1975. pp 229–254.

Mrosovsky N: Sleep researchers caught napping. (News and views.) *Nature* 319:536–537, 1986.

Mrosovsky N: Phase response curves for social entrainment. *J Comp Physiol [A]* 162:35–46, 1988.

Mrosovsky N: Circadian rhythms: Mutant hamsters in a hurry. (News and views.) *Nature* 337:213–214, 1989.

Mueller PS, Heninger GR, McDonald RK: Insulin tolerance test in depression. *Arch Gen Psychiatry* 21:587–594, 1969.

Mukherjee S, Shukla S, Woodle J, Rosen AM, Olarte S: Misdiagnosis of schizophrenia in bipolar patients: A multiethnic comparison. *Am J Psychiatry* 140:1571–1574, 1983.

Mukherjee S, Shukla S, Rosen A: Neurological abnormalities in patients with bipolar disorder. *Biol Psychiatry* 19:337–345, 1984.

Mukherjee S, Rosen AM, Caracci G, Shukla S: Persistent tardive dyskinesia in bipolar patients. *Arch Gen Psychiatry* 43:342–346, 1986.

Mulginigama LD: Significance of uptake studies with biogenic amines. In: JE Murphy, ed: *Research and Clinical Investigation in Depression*. Northampton: Cambridge Medical, 1976. pp 10–15.

Mullen P: Phenomenology of disordered mental function. In: P Hill, R Murray, G Thorley, eds: *Essentials of Postgraduate Psychiatry*. London: Academic Press, 1979. pp 25–54.

Muller AA, Stoll KD: Carbamazepine and oxcarbazepine in the treatment of manic syndromes: Studies in Germany. In: HM Emrich, T Okuma, AA Muller, eds: *Anticonvulsants in Affective Disorders*. Amsterdam: Excerpta Medica, 1984. pp 139–147.

Muncie W: Postoperative states of excitement. *Arch Neurol Psychiatry* 34:681–703, 1934.

Murphy D, Gardner R, Greden JF, Carroll BJ: Lymphocyte numbers in endogenous depression. *Psychol Med* 17:381–385, 1987.

Murphy DL: Animal models for mania. In: I Hanin, E Usdin, eds: *Animal Models in Psychiatry and Neurology*. New York: Pergamon Press, 1977. pp 211–223.

Murphy DL, Beigel A: Depression, elation, and lithium carbonate responses in manic patient subgroups. *Arch Gen Psychiatry* 31:643–648, 1974.

Murphy DL, Bunney WE Jr: Total body potassium changes during lithium administration. *J Nerv Ment Dis* 152:381–389, 1971.

Murphy DL, Brodie HK, Goodwin FK, Bunney WE Jr: Regular induction of hypomania by L-dopa in "bipolar" manic-depressive patients. *Nature* 229:135–136, 1971a.

Murphy DL, Goodwin FK, Bunney WE: Clinical and pharmacological investigations of the psychobiology of affective disorders. *Int Pharmacopsychiatry* 6:137–146, 1971b.

Murphy DL, Baker M, Goodwin FK, Miller H, Kotin J, Bunney WE Jr: L-tryptophan in affective disorders: Indoleamine changes and differential clinical effects. *Psychopharmacologia* 34:11–20, 1974a.

Murphy DL, Beigel A, Weingartner H, Bunney WE: The quantitation of manic behavior. *Mod Probl Pharmacopsychiatry* 7:203–220, 1974b.

Murphy DL, Donnelly C, Moskowitz J: Catecholamine receptor function in depressed patients. *Am J Psychiatry* 131:1389–1391, 1974c.

Murphy DL, Brand E, Baker M, Van Kammen D, Gordon E: Phenelzine effects in hospitalized unipolar and bipolar depressed patients: Behavioral and biochemical relationships. In: JR Boissier, H Hippius, P Pichot, eds: *Neuropsychopharmacology*. New York: Elsevier, 1975. pp 788–798.

Murphy DL, Lipper S, Campbell IC, Major LF, Slater S, Buchsbaum MS: Comparative studies of MAO-A and MAO-B inhibitors in man. In: TP Singer, RW Von Korff, DL Murphy, eds: *Monoamine Oxidase: Structure, Function, and Altered Functions*. New York: Academic Press, 1979. pp 457–475.

Murphy DL, Coursey RD, Haenel T, Aloi J, Buchsbaum MS: Platelet monoamine oxidase as a biological marker in the affective disorders and alcoholism. In: E Usdin, I Hanin, eds: *Biological Markers in Psychiatry and Neurology*. Oxford: Pergamon Press, 1982a. pp 123–134.

Murphy DL, Pickar D, Alterman IS: Methods for the quantitative assessment of depressive and manic behavior. In: EI Burdock, A Sudilovsky, S Gershon, eds: *The Behavior of Psychiatric Patients: Quantitative Techniques for Evaluation*. New York: Marcel Dekker, 1982b. pp 355–392.

Murphy G: Types of word-association in dementia

praecox, manic-depressives, and normal persons. *Am J Psychiatry* 79:539–571, 1923.

Murphy GE: The physician's responsibility for suicide: I: An error of commission. *Ann Intern Med* 82:301–304, 1975a.

Murphy GE: The physician's responsibility for suicide: II: Errors of omission. *Ann Intern Med* 82:305–309, 1975b.

Murphy GE: Suicide and substance abuse. *Arch Gen Psychiatry* 45:593–594, 1988.

Murphy GE, Simons AD, Wetzel RD, Lustman PJ: Cognitive therapy and pharmacotherapy: Singly and together in the treatment of depression. *Arch Gen Psychiatry* 41:33–41, 1984.

Murphy HBM: Differences between mental disorders of French Canadians and British Canadians. *Can Psychiatr Assoc J* 19:247–257, 1974.

Murphy HBM, Wittkower ED, Fried J, Ellenberger H: A cross-cultural survey of schizophrenic symptomatology. *Int J Soc Psychiatry* 9:237–249, 1963.

Murray LG, Blackburn IM: Personality differences in patients with depressive illness and anxiety neurosis. *Acta Psychiatr Scand* 50:183–191, 1974.

Murray N, Hopwood S, Balfour DJK, Ogston S, Hewick DS: The influence of age on lithium efficacy and side-effects in out-patients. *Psychol Med* 13:53–60, 1983.

Murray RM, Gurling HMD, Bernadt M, Ewusi-Mensah I, Saunders JD, Clifford CA: Do personality and psychiatric disorders predispose to alcoholism? In: G Edwards, J Littleton, eds: *Pharmacological Treatments for Alcoholism*. London: Croon Helm, 1984. pp 445–461.

Muscettola G, Potter WZ, Pickar D, Goodwin FK: Urinary 3-methoxy-4-hydroxyphenylglycol and major affective disorders: A replication and new findings. *Arch Gen Psychiatry* 41:337–342, 1984.

Muscettola G, Di Lauro A, Giannini CP: Platelet ^{3}H-imipramine binding in bipolar patients. *Psychiatry Res* 18:343–353, 1986.

Musch B, Garreau M: The antidepressant activity of SL79.229–00, a new GABA receptor agonist. *Int J Neurosci* 32:907–908, 1986.

Mussini M, Agricola R, Coletti Moia G, Fiore P, Rivolta A: A preliminary study on the use of calcitonin in clinical psychopathology. *J Int Med Res* 12:23–29, 1984.

Myers DH, Davies P: The seasonal incidence of mania and its relationship to climatic variables. *Psychol Med* 8:433–440, 1978.

Myers DH, Neal CD: Suicide in psychiatric patients. *Br J Psychiatry* 133:38–44, 1978.

Myers DH, Carter RA, Burns BH, Armond A, Hussain SB, Chengapa VK: A prospective study of the effects of lithium on thyroid function and on the prevalence of antithyroid antibodies. *Psychol Med* 15:55–61, 1985.

Myers JK, Weissman MM, Tischler GL, Holzer CE, Leaf PJ, Orvaschel H, Anthony JC, Boyd JH, Burke JD, Kramer M, Stoltzman R: Six-month prevalence of psychiatric disorders in three communities: 1980 to 1982. *Arch Gen Psychiatry* 41:959–967, 1984.

Myerson A, Boyle RD: The incidence of manic-depressive psychosis in certain socially important families: Preliminary report. *Am J Psychiatry* 98:11–21, 1941.

Myslobodsky MS, Horesh N: Bilateral electrodermal activity in depressive patients. *Biol Psychol* 6:111–120, 1978.

Nadi NS, Nurnberger JI Jr, Gershon ES: Muscarinic cholinergic receptors on skin fibroblasts in familial affective disorder. *N Engl J Med* 311:225–230, 1984.

Nagatsu T, Yamaguchi T, Kato T, Sugimoto T, Matsuura S, Akino M, Nagatsu I, Iizuka R, Narabayashi H: Biopterin in human brain and urine from controls and parkinsonian patients: Application of a new radioimmunoassay. *Clin Chim Acta* 109:305–11, 1981.

Nähunek K, Svestka J, Kamenická V, Rodová A: Preliminary clinical experience with L-dopa in endogenous depressions. *Act Nerv Super (Praha)* 14:101–102, 1972.

Nankai M, Yoshimoto S, Narita K, Takahashi R: Platelet [^{3}H] imipramine binding in depressed patients and its circadian variations in healthy controls. *J Affective Disord* 11:207–212, 1986.

Narsapur SL, Naylor GJ: Methylene blue: A possible treatment for manic depressive psychosis. *J Affective Disord* 5:155–161, 1983.

Nasr S, Altman EG, Meltzer HY: Concordance of atopic and affective disorders. *J Affective Disord* 3:291–296, 1981.

Nasr SJ, Altman E, Pscheidt G, Meltzer HY: Glucose-6-phosphate dehydrogenase deficiency in a psychiatric population: A preliminary study. *Biol Psychiatry* 17:925–928, 1982.

Nasrallah HA, McCalley-Whitters M: Motor lateralization in manic males. *Br J Psychiatry* 140:521–522, 1982.

Nasrallah HA, Jacoby CG, McCalley-Whitters M: Cerebellar atrophy in schizophrenia and mania. *Lancet* 1:1102, 1981.

Nasrallah HA, Lyskowksi J, Schroeder D: TCA-induced mania: Differences between switchers and nonswitchers. *Biol Psychiatry* 17:271–274, 1982a.

Nasrallah HA, McCalley-Whitters M, Jacoby CG: Cortical atrophy in schizophrenia and mania: A comparative CT study. *J Clin Psychiatry* 43:439–441, 1982b.

Nasrallah HA, Tippin J, McCalley-Whitters M: Neurological soft signs in manic patients: A comparison with schizophrenic and control groups. *J Affective Disord* 5:45–50, 1983.

Nasrallah HA, McCalley-Whitters M, Pfohl B: Clinical significance of large cerebral ventricles in manic males. *Psychiatry Res* 13:151–156, 1984.

Nathan PE, Titler NA, Lowenstein LM, Solomon P, Rossi AM: Behavioral analysis of chronic alcoholism: Interaction of alcohol and human contact. *Arch Gen Psychiatry* 22:419–430, 1970.

Nathan RS, Sachar EJ, Asnis GM, Halbreich U, Halpern FS: Relative insulin insensitivity and cortisol secretion in depressed patients. *Psychiatry Res* 4:291–300, 1981.

Näyhä S: Autumn incidence of suicides re-examined: Data from Finland by sex, age, and occupation. *Br J Psychiatry* 141:512–517, 1982.

Naylor GJ: Vanadium and affective disorders. *Biol Psychiatry* 18:103–112, 1983.

Naylor GJ, Smith AH: Vanadium: A possible aetiological factor in manic depressive illness. *Psychol Med* 11:249–256, 1981.

Naylor GJ, McNamee HB, Moody JP: Changes in erythrocyte sodium and potassium on recovery from a depressive illness. *Br J Psychiatry* 118:219–223, 1971.

Naylor GJ, Dick DAT, Dick EG, LePoidevin D, Whyte SF: Erythrocyte membrane cation carrier in depressive illness. *Psychol Med* 3:502–508, 1973.

Naylor GJ, Dick DA, Dick EG, Moody JP: Lithium therapy and erythrocyte membrane cation carrier. *Psychopharmacologia* 37:81–86, 1974.

Naylor GJ, Watson Y, Stewart M, Worrall EP, Dick P, Peet M: Trial of digoxin in mania. *Lancet* 2:639–640, 1975.

Naylor GJ, Dick DA, Dick EG: Erythrocyte membrane cation carrier, relapse rate of manic-depressive illness and response to lithium. *Psychol Med* 6:257–263, 1976a.

Naylor GJ, Reid AH, Dick DA, Dick EG: A biochemical study of short-cycle manic-depressive psychosis in mental defectives. *Br J Psychiatry* 128:169–180, 1976b.

Naylor GJ, Smith AH, Dick EG, Dick DA, McHarg AM, Chambers CA: Erythrocyte membrane cation carrier in manic-depressive psychosis. *Psychol Med* 10:521–525, 1980.

Naylor GJ, Smith AH, Bryce-Smith D, Ward NI: Tissue vanadium levels in manic-depressive psychosis. *Psychol Med* 14:767–772, 1984.

Naylor GJ, Smith AHW, Bryce-Smith D, Ward NI: Trace elements in manic depressive psychosis. *J Affective Disord* 8:131–136, 1985.

Naylor GJ, Martin B, Hopwood SE, Watson Y: A two-year double-blind crossover trial of the prophylactic effect of methylene blue in manic-depressive psychosis. *Biol Psychiatry* 21:915–920, 1986.

Naylor GJ, Smith AHW, Connelly P: Methylene blue in mania. Letter. *Biol Psychiatry* 24:941–942, 1988.

Neborsky RJ, Janowsky DS, Fann WE: Psychopharmacologic and psychotherapeutic interventions: An integrated treatment approach to depression. *Psychiatr Ann* 10:369–379, 1980.

Negri F, Melica AM, Zuliani R, Smeraldi E: Assortative mating and affective disorders. *J Affective Disord* 1:247–253, 1979.

Nelson JC: Lithium augmentation in refractory depres-
sion. Abstract of paper presented at the 141st annual meeting of the American Psychiatric Association, May, 1988.

Nelson JC, Mazure CM: Lithium augmentation in psychotic depression refractory to combined drug treatment. *Am J Psychiatry* 143:363–366, 1986.

Nelson JC, Schottenfeld RS, Conrad CD: Hypomania after desipramine withdrawal. *Am J Psychiatry* 140:624–625, 1983.

Nelson WH, Khan A, Orr WW: Delusional depression: Phenomenology, neuroendocrine function, and tricyclic antidepressant response. *J Affective Disord* 6:297–306, 1984.

Nemeroff CB, Luttinger D, Hernandez DE, Mailman RB, Mason GA, Davis SD, Widerlöv E, Frye GD, Kilts CA, Beaumont K, Breese GR, Prange AJ Jr: Interactions of neurotensin with brain dopamine systems: Biochemical and behavioral studies. *J Pharmacol Exp Ther* 225:337–345, 1983.

Nemeroff CB, Widerlöv E, Bissette G, Walléus H, Karlsson I, Eklund K, Kilts CD, Loosen PT, Vale W: Elevated concentrations of CSF corticotropin-releasing factor-like immunoreactivity in depressed patients. *Science* 226:1342–1344, 1984.

Nemeroff CB, Simon JS, Haggerty JJ Jr, Evans DL: Antithyroid antibodies in depressed patients. *Am J Psychiatry* 142:840–843, 1985.

Newmark ME, Penry JK: *Genetics of Epilepsy: A Review*. New York: Raven Press, 1980.

Niecks F: *Robert Schumann: A Supplementary and Corrective Biography*. London: JM Dent & Sons, 1925.

Nielsen JA, Biørn-Henriksen T: Prevalence and disease expectancy for depressive psychoses in a geographically delimited Danish rural population. In: M Schou, E Strömgren, eds: *Origin, Prevention and Treatment of Affective Disorders*. London: Academic Press, 1979. pp 199–206.

Nieman GW, DeLong R: Use of the personality inventory for children as an aid in differentiating children with mania from children with attention deficit disorder with hyperactivity. *J Am Acad Child Adolesc Psychiatry* 26:381–8, 1987.

Nieuwenhuys R, Voogd J, Van Huijzen C: *The Human Central Nervous System: A Synopsis and Atlas*. 2nd Revised Ed. Berlin: Springer, 1981.

Niklasson F, Ågren H: Brain energy metabolism and blood-brain barrier permeability in depressive patients: Analyses of creatine, creatinine, urate, and albumin in CSF and blood. *Biol Psychiatry* 19:1183–1206, 1984.

NIMH/NIH Consensus Development Statement: Mood disorders: Pharmacologic prevention of recurrences. *Am J Psychiatry* 142:469–475, 1985.

Nisbit JF: *The Insanity of Genius*. London: Grant Richards, 1900.

Niskanen P, Huttunen M, Tamminen T, Jääskeläinen J: The daily rhythm of plasma tryptophan and tyrosine in depression. *Br J Psychiatry* 128:67–73, 1976.

Nizamie SH, Nizamie A, Borde M, Sharma S: Mania following head injury: Case reports and neuropsychological findings. *Acta Psychiatr Scand* 77:637–639, 1988.

Noack CH, Trautner EM: The lithium treatment of maniacal psychosis. *Med J Aust* 2:219–222, 1951.

Noble AB, McKinney WT, Mohr C, Moran E: Diazepam treatment of socially isolated monkeys. *Am J Psychiatry* 133:1165–1170, 1976.

Noble PJ, Lader MH: Salivary secretion in depressive illness: A physiological and psychometric study. *Psychol Med* 1:372–376, 1971.

Nolen WA, Jansen GS, Broekman M: Measuring plasma levels of carbamazepine: A pharmacokinetic study in patients with affective disorders. *Pharmacopsychiat* 21:252–254, 1988.

Nordin C, Siwers B, Bertilsson L: Bromocriptine treatment of depressive disorders: Clinical and biochemical effects. *Acta Psychiatr Scand* 64:25–33, 1981.

Noreik K, Ödegaard Ö: Psychoses in Norwegians with a background of higher education. *Br J Psychiatry* 112:43–55, 1966.

Norman KP, Cerrone KL, Reus VI: Renal lithium clearance as a rapid and accurate predictor of maintenance dose. *Am J Psychiatry* 139:1625–1626, 1982.

Norman TC, Mathews W, Yohe CD: Effects of strenuous exercise on serum lithium levels. *J Clin Psychopharmacol* 7:434–435, 1987.

Norton B, Whalley LJ: Mortality of a lithium-treated population. *Br J Psychiatry* 145:277–282, 1984.

Norwich JJ: *Christmas Crackers.* Middlesex: Penguin Books, 1982.

Noyes R Jr, Dempsey GM, Blum A, Cavanaugh GL: Lithium treatment of depression. *Compr Psychiatry* 15:187–193, 1974.

Nunes EV, Quitkin FM, Klein DF: Psychiatric diagnosis in cocaine abuse. *Psychiatry Res* 28:105–114, 1989.

Nunn CMH: Mixed affective states and the natural history of manic-depressive psychosis. *Br J Psychiatry* 134:153–160, 1979.

Nurnberg HG: Treatment of mania in the last six months of pregnancy. *Hosp Community Psychiatry* 31:122–126, 1980.

Nurnberg HG, Finkel JA: Carbamazepine in bipolar-depressed disorder complicated by tricyclic antidepressant switching: Case report. *J Clin Psychiatry* 46:487–488, 1985.

Nurnberger JI Jr, Gershon ES: Genetic considerations in the epidemiology of psychoactive drug use. In: G Tognoni, C Bellantuono, M Lader, eds: *Epidemiological Impact of Psychotropic Drugs.* Amsterdam: Elsevier, 1981. pp 19–31.

Nurnberger JI Jr, Gershon ES: Genetics of affective disorders. In: R Post, J Ballenger, eds: *Neurobiology of Mood Disorders.* Baltimore: Williams & Wilkins, 1984. pp 76–101.

Nurnberger JI Jr, Roose SP, Dunner DL, Fieve RR: Unipolar mania: A distinct clinical entity? *Am J Psychiatry* 136:1420–1423, 1979.

Nurnberger JI Jr, Jimerson DC, Allen JR, Simmons S, Gershon E: Red cell ouabain-sensitive Na^+-K^+-adenosine triphosphatase: A state marker in affective disorder inversely related to plasma cortisol. *Biol Psychiatry* 17:981–992, 1982.

Nurnberger JI Jr, Jimerson DC, Simmons-Alling S, Tamminga C, Nadi NS, Lawrence D, Sitaram N, Gillin JC, Gershon ES: Behavioral, physiological, and neuroendocrine responses to arecoline in normal twins and "well state" bipolar patients. *Psychiatry Res* 9:191–200, 1983a.

Nurnberger JI Jr, Pandey G, Gershon ES, Davis JM: Lithium ratio in psychiatric patients: A caveat. *Psychiatry Res* 9:201–206, 1983b.

Nurnberger JI Jr, Sitaram N, Gershon ES, Gillin JC: A twin study of cholinergic REM induction. *Biol Psychiatry* 18:1161–1165, 1983c.

Nurnberger JI Jr, Kessler L, Simmons-Alling S, Gershon ES: Pirbuterol trial as antidepressant. *Biol Psychiatry* 21:565–566, 1986.

Nurnberger JI Jr, Berrettini W, Tamarkin L, Hamovit J, Norton J, Gershon ES: Supersensitivity to melatonin suppression by light in young people at high risk for affective disorder: A preliminary report. *Neuropsychopharmacol* 1:217–223, 1988a.

Nurnberger JI Jr, Guroff JJ, Hamovit J, Berrettini W, Gershon ES: A family study of rapid-cycling bipolar illness. *J Affective Disord* 15:87–91, 1988b.

Nurnberger JI Jr, Berrettini W, Mendelson W, Sack D, Gershon ES: Measuring cholinergic sensitivity: I. Arecoline effects in bipolar patients. *Biol Psychiatry* 25:610–617, 1989.

Nutt DJ, Linnoila M: Neuroreceptor science: A clarification of terms. *J Clin Psychopharm* 8:387–389, 1988.

Oades RD: The role of noradrenaline in tuning and dopamine in switching between signals in the CNS. *Neurosci Biobehav Rev* 9:261–282, 1985.

Oates MR: The treatment of psychiatric disorders in pregnancy and the puerperium. *Clin Ob Gyn* 13:385–395, 1986.

O'Brien CP, DiGiacomo JN, Fahn S: Mental effects of high-dosage levodopa. *Arch Gen Psychiatry* 24:61–64, 1971.

Obrist WD, Thompson HK Jr, King CH, Wang HS: Determination of regional cerebral blood flow by inhalation of 133-Xenon. *Circ Res* 20:124–135, 1967.

O'Connell RA: Psychosocial factors in a model of manic-depressive disease. *Integr Psychiatry* 4:150–161, 1986.

O'Connell RA, Mayo JA: Lithium: A biopsychosocial perspective. *Compr Psychiatry* 22:87–93, 1981.

O'Connell RA, Mayo JA, O'Brien JD, Misrsheidaie F: Children of bipolar manic-depressives. In: J Mendlewicz, B Shopsin, eds: *Genetic Aspects of Affective Illness.* New York: SP Medical and Scientific Books, 1979. pp 55–68.

O'Connell RA, Mayo JA, Eng LK, Jones JS, Gabel RH: Social support and long-term lithium outcome. *Br J Psychiatry* 147:272–275, 1985.

Ödegård Ö: The excess mortality of the insane. *Acta Psychiatr Scand* 27:353–367, 1952.

Ödegård Ö: The incidence of psychoses in various occupations. *Int J Soc Psychiatry* 2:85–104, 1956.

O'Dowd MA, McKegney FP: Manic syndrome associated with zidovudine. *JAMA* 260:3587, 1988.

Oesterreicher W: Peculiarities of Indonesian psychiatry. *Folia Psychiat Neurol Neurochir Neerlandica* 54:431–437, 1951.

Ogborne AC, Glaser FB: Evaluating Alcoholics Anonymous. In: TE Bratter, GG Forrest, eds: *Alcoholism and Substance Abuse.* New York: Free Press, 1985. pp 176–192.

Öhman A: The orienting response, attention, and learning: An information-processing perspective. In: HD Kimmel, EH Van Holst, JF Orlebeke, eds: *The Orienting Response in Humans.* Hillsdale, NJ: Lawrence Earlbaum Associates, 1979. pp 443–471.

Oke A, Keller R, Mefford I, Adams RN: Lateralization of norepinephrine in human thalamus. *Science* 200:1411–1413, 1978.

O'Keeffe R, Brooksbank BW: Determination of 3-methoxy-4-hydroxyphenylethylene glycol, a noradrenaline metabolite, in cerebrospinal fluid and urine. *Clin Chem* 19:1031–1035, 1973.

Okuma T, Shimoyama N: Course of endogenous manic-depressive psychosis, precipitating factors and premorbid personality—A statistical study. *Folia Psychiatr Neurol Japonica* 26:19–33, 1972.

Okuma T, Kishimoto A, Inoue K, Matsumoto H, Ogura A, Matsushita T, Nakao T, Ogura C: Antimanic and prophylactic effects of carbamazepine (Tegretol) on manic depressive psychosis: A preliminary report. *Folia Psychiatr Neurol Jpn* 27:283–297, 1973.

Okuma T, Inanaga K, Otsuki S, Sarai K, Takahashi R, Hazama H, Mori A, Watanabe M: Comparison of the antimanic efficacy of carbamazepine and chlorpromazine: A double-blind controlled study. *Psychopharmacology (Berlin)* 66:211–217, 1979.

Okuma T, Inanaga K, Otsuki S, Sarai K, Takahashi R, Hazama H, Mori A, Watanabe S: A preliminary double-blind study on the efficacy of carbamazepine in prophylaxis of manic-depressive illness. *Psychopharmacoly (Berlin)* 73:95–96, 1981.

Okuma T, Yamashita I, Takahashi R, Itoh H, Kurihara M, Otsuki S, Watanabe S, Sarai K, Hazama H, Inanaga K: Clinical efficacy of carbamazepine in affective, schizoaffective, and schizophrenic disorders. *Pharmacopsychiat* 22:47–53, 1989.

Ollerenshaw DP: The classification of the functional psychoses. *Br J Psychiatry* 122:517–30, 1973.

Olsen T: Follow-up study of manic-depressive patients whose first attack occurred before the age of 19. *Acta Psychiatr Scand* 37(Suppl 162):45–51, 1961.

O'Malley M: Psychoses in the colored race: A study in comparative psychiatry. *Am J Insanity* 71:309–337, 1914.

Oppenheim G: Drug-induced rapid cycling: Possible outcomes and management. *Am J Psychiatry* 139:939–941, 1982.

Oppenheim G, Ebstein RP, Belmaker RH: Effect of lithium on the physostigmine-induced behavioral syndrome and plasma cyclic GMP. *J Psychiatr Res* 15:133–138, 1979.

Oppler W: Manic psychosis in a case of parasagittal meningioma. *Arch Neurol Psychiatry* 64:417–430, 1950.

Oreland L, Wilberg A, Åsberg M, Träskman L, Sjostrand L, Thorén P, Bertilsson L, Tybring G: Platelet MAO activity and monoamine metabolites in cerebrospinal fluid in depressed and suicidal patients and in healthy controls. *Psychiatry Res* 4:21–29, 1981.

O'Rourke D, Wurtman J, Brzezinski A, Abou-Nader T, Marchant P, Wurtman RJ: Treatment of seasonal affective disorder with d-fenfluramine. *Ann NY Acad Sci* 499:329–330, 1987.

Orvaschel H, Weissman MM, Kidd KK: Children and depression; the children of depressed parents: The childhood of depressed parents; depression in children. *J Affective Disord* 2:1–16, 1980.

Orvaschel H, Thompson WD, Belanger A, Prusoff BA, Kidd KK: Comparison of the family history method to direct interview: Factors affecting the diagnosis of depression. *J Affective Disord* 4:45–59, 1982.

O'Shanick GJ, Ellinwood EH Jr: Persistent elevation of thyroid-stimulating hormone in women with bipolar affective disorder. *Am J Psychiatry* 139:513–514, 1982.

Ostenfeld I: Treatment for endogenous depressions: The earliest observations in a Danish mental hospital (1954) and an analysis of the causal mechanism. *Danish Med Bull* 33:45–49, 1986.

Ostow M: The hypomanic personality in history. In: RH Belmaker, HM Van Praag, eds: *Mania: An Evolving Concept.* New York: Spectrum, 1980. pp 387–393.

Ostroff R, Giller E, Bonese K, Ebersole E, Harkness L, Mason J: Neuroendocrine risk factors of suicidal behavior. *Am J Psychiatry* 139:1323–1325, 1982.

Ostroff RB, Giller E, Harkness L, Mason J: The norepinephrine-to-epinephrine ratio in patients with a history of suicide attempts. *Am J Psychiatry* 142:224–227, 1985.

Ostrow DG, Pandey GN, Davis JM, Hurt SW, Tosteson DC: A heritable disorder of lithium transport in erythrocytes of a subpopulation of manic-depressive patients. *Am J Psychiatry* 135:1070–1078, 1978.

Ostrow DG, Trevisan M, Okonek A, Gibbons R, Cooper R, Davis JM: Sodium dependent membrane processes in major affective disorders. In: E Usdin, I Hanin, eds: *Biological Markers in Psychiatry and Neurology.* Oxford: Pergamon Press, 1982. pp 153–168.

Ostrow DG: The new generation antidepressants: Promising innovations or disappointments? *J Clin Psychiatry* 46:25–31, 1985.

Ostwald PF: Robert Schumann and his doctors. *Am J Soc Psychiatry* 3:5–14, 1983.

O'Sullivan K, Whillans P, Daly M, Carroll B, Clare A, Cooney J: A comparison of alcoholics with and without coexisting affective disorder. *Br J Psychiatry* 143:133–138, 1983.

O'Sullivan K, Rynne C, Miller J, O'Sullivan S, Fitzpatrick V, Hux M, Cooney J, Clare A: A follow-up study on alcoholics with and without co-existing affective disorder. *Br J Psychiatry* 152:813–819, 1988.

Oswald I, Brezinova V, Dunleavy DLF: On the slowness of action of tricyclic antidepressant drugs. *Br J Psychiatry* 120:673–677, 1972.

Otto MW, Yeo RA, Dougher MJ: Right hemisphere involvement in depression: Toward a neuropsychological theory of negative affective experiences. *Biol Psychiatry* 22:1201–1215, 1987.

Ottosson J-O: The suicidal patient: Can the psychiatrist prevent his suicide? In: M Schou, E Strömgren, eds: *Origin, Prevention and Treatment of Affective Disorders.* London: Academic Press, 1979. pp 257–267.

Overall JE: The Brief Psychiatric Rating Scale in psychopharmacology research. *Mod Probl Pharmacopsychiat* 7:67–78, 1974.

Overall JE, Gorham DR: The Brief Psychiatric Rating Scale. *Psychol Rep* 10:799–812, 1962.

Overall JE, Hoffmann NG, Levin H: Effects of aging, organicity, alcoholism, and functional psychopathology on WAIS subtest profiles. *J Consult Clin Psychol* 46:1315–1322, 1978.

Overstreet DH: Selective breeding for increased cholingergic function: Development of a new animal model of depression. *Biol Psychiatry* 21:49–58, 1986.

Owen SE, Nurcombe B: The application of the Semantic Differential Test in a case of manic-depressive psychosis. *Austr NZ J Psychiatry* 4:148–154, 1970.

Oxenkrug GF: The content and uptake of 5-HT by blood platelets in depressive patients. *J Neural Transm* 45:285–289, 1979.

Oxenstierna G, Edman G, Iselius L, Oreland L, Ross SB, Sedvall G: Concentrations of monoamine metabolites in the cerebrospinal fluid of twins and unrelated individuals—A genetic study. *J Psychiat Res* 20:19–29, 1986.

Oyama T, Fukushi S, Jin T: Epidural beta-endorphin in treatment of pain. *Can Anaesth Soc J* 29:24–26, 1982.

Oyewumi LK, Lapierre YD: Efficacy of lithium in treating mood disorder occurring after brain stem injury. *Am J Psychiatry* 138:110–112, 1981.

Page C, Benaim S, Lappin F: A long-term retrospective follow-up study of patients treated with prophylactic lithium carbonate. *Br J Psychiatry* 150:175–179, 1987.

Palmai G, Blackwell B: The diurnal pattern of salivary flow in normal and depressed patients. *Br J Psychiatry* 111:334–338, 1965.

Pandey GN, Dorus E, Davis JM, Tosteson DC: Lithium transport in human red blood cells: genetic

and clinical aspects. *Arch Gen Psychiatry* 36:902–908, 1979a.

Pandey GN, Dysken MW, Garver DL, Davis JM: Beta-adrenergic receptor function in affective illness. *Am J Psychiatry* 136:675–678, 1979b.

Pandey GN, Dorus E, Shaughnessy R, Gaviria M, Val E, Davis JM: Reduced platelet MAO activity and vulnerability to psychiatric disorders. *Psychiatry Res* 2:315–321, 1980.

Pandey GN, Janicak PG, Davis JM: Decreased beta-adrenergic receptors in the leukocytes of depressed patients. *Psychiatry Res* 22:265–273, 1987.

Papadimitriou GN, Christodoulou GN, Trikkas GM, Malliaras DE, Lykouras EP, Stefanis CN: Sleep deprivation psychoprophylaxis in recurrent affective disorders. *Bibl Psychiatr* 160:56–61, 1981.

Papeschi R, McClure DJ: Homovanillic and 5-hydroxyindoleacetic acid in the cerebrospinal fluid of depressed patients. *Arch Gen Psychiatry* 25:354–358, 1971.

Papez JW: A proposed mechanism of emotion. *Arch Neurol Psychiatry* 38:725–743, 1937.

Papoušek M: Chronobiologische Aspekte der Zyklothymie. *Fortschritte der Neurologie, Psychiatrie und Ihrer Grenzgebiete* 43:381–440, 1975.

Pare CMB: The present status of monoamine oxidase inhibitors. *Br J Psychiatry* 146:576–584, 1985.

Pare CMB, Sandler M: A clinical and biochemical study of a trial of iproniazid in the treatment of depression. *J Neurol Neurosurg Psychiatry* 22:247–251, 1959.

Pare CMB, Yeung DPH, Price K, Stacey RS: 5-hydroxytryptamine, noradrenaline, and dopamine in brainstem, hypothalamus, and caudate nucleus of controls and of patients committing suicide by coalgas poisoning. *Lancet* 2:133–135, 1969.

Parker CW, Smith JW: Alterations in cyclic adenosine monophosphate metabolism in human bronchial asthma: I. Leukocyte responsiveness to β-adrenergic agents. *J Clin Invest* 52:48–59, 1973.

Parker DC, Rossman LG, Vanderlaan EF: Relation of sleep-entrained human prolactin release to REM-nonREM cycles. *J Clin Endocrinol Metab* 38:646–651, 1974.

Parker DC, Pekary AE, Hershman JM: Effect of normal and reversed sleep-wake cycles upon nyctohemeral rhythmicity of plasma thyrotropin: Evidence suggestive of an inhibitory influence in sleep. *J Clin Endocrinol Metab* 43:318–329, 1976.

Parker G, Walter S: Seasonal variation in depressive disorders and suicidal deaths in New South Wales. *Br J Psychiatry* 140:626–632, 1982.

Parker G, O'Donnell M, Walter S: Changes in the diagnoses of the functional psychoses associated with the introduction of lithium. *Br J Psychiatry* 146:377–382, 1985.

Parker JB, Spielberger CD, Wallace DK, Becker J: Factors in manic-depressive reactions. *Dis Nerv Syst* 20:505–511, 1959.

Parker JB, Meiller RM, Andrews GW: Major psychiatric disorders masquerading as alcoholism. *South Med J* 53:560–564, 1960.

Parker JB, Theilie A, Spielberger CD: Frequency of blood types in a homogeneous group of manic-depressive patients. *J Ment Sci* 107:936–942, 1961.

Parks RW, Loewenstein DA, Dodrill KL, Barker WW, Yoshii F, Chang JY, Emran A, Apicella A, Sheramata WA, Duara R: Cerebral metabolic effects of a verbal fluency test: A PET scan study. *J Clin Exp Neuropsychol* 10:565–575, 1988.

Parry BL: Reproductive factors affecting the course of affective illness in women. *Psychiatr Clin North Am* 12:207–220, 1989.

Parsons PL: Mental health of Swansea's old folk. *Br J Prev Soc Med* 19:43–47, 1965.

Pasamanick B, Roberts DW, Lemkau PV, Krueger DE: A survey of mental disease in an urban population: I: Prevalence by age, sex, and survey of impairment. *Am J Public Health* 47:923–929, 1957.

Paschalis C, Jenner FA, Lee CR: Effects of rubidium chloride on the course of manic-depressive illness. *J R Soc Med* 71:343–352, 1978.

Paul SM, Rehavi M, Skolnick P, Goodwin FK: Demonstration of specific "high affinity" binding sites for [³H] imipramine on human platelets. *Life Sci* 26:953–959, 1980.

Paul SM, Extein I, Calil HM, Potter WZ, Chodoff P, Goodwin FK: Use of ECT with treatment-resistant depressed patients at the National Institute of Mental Health. *Am J Psychiatry* 138:486–489, 1981a.

Paul SM, Rehavi M, Rice KC, Ittah Y, Sholnick P: Does high affinity [³H] imipramine binding label serotonin reuptake sites in brain and platelets. *Life Sci* 28:2753–2760, 1981b.

Paul SM, Rehavi M, Skolnick P, Ballenger JC, Goodwin FK: Depressed patients have decreased binding of tritiated imipramine to platelet serotonin "transporter." *Arch Gen Psychiatry* 38:1315–1317, 1981c.

Paul SM, Rehavi M, Skolnick P, Goodwin FK: [³H]-imipramine binding to the serotonin "transporter" in human brain and platelet: A possible biological marker in depression. In: E Usdin, I Hanin, eds: *Biological Markers in Psychiatry and Neurology.* London: Pergamon Press, 1982. pp 193–204

Pauleikhoff B: Über die seltenheit von alkoholabusus bei zyklothym depressiven. *Nervenzart* 24:445–448, 1953.

Paykel ES, ed: *Handbook of Affective Disorders.* New York: Churchill Livingstone, 1982a.

Paykel ES: Life events and early environment. In: ES Paykel, ed: *Handbook of Affective Disorders.* New York: Churchill Livingstone, 1982b. pp 146–161.

Paykel ES, Prusoff BA: Response set and observer set in the assessment of depressed patients. *Psychol Med* 3:209–216, 1973.

Paykel ES, Weissman MM: Social adjustment and depression: A longitudinal study. *Arch Gen Psychiatry* 28:659–663, 1973.

Paykel ES, Myers JK, Dienelt MN, Klerman GL, Lindenthal JJ, Pepper MP: Life events and depression: A controlled study. *Arch Gen Psychiatry* 21:753–760, 1969.

Payne RW, Hewlett JHG: Thought disorders in psychotic patients. In HJ Eysenck, ed: *Experiments in Personality, Vol 2: Psychodiagnostics and Psychodynamics.* New York: The Humanities Press, 1960. pp 3–104.

Pearlson GD, Veroff AE: Computerised tomographic scan changes in manic-depressive illness. Letter. *Lancet* 2:470, 1981.

Pearlson GD, Garbacz DJ, Tompkins RH, Ahn HS, Gutterman DF, Veroff AE, DePaulo JR: Clinical correlates of lateral ventricular enlargement in bipolar affective disorder. *Am J Psychiatry* 141:253–256, 1984.

Peck AW, Stern WC, Watkinson C: Incidence of seizures during treatment with tricyclic antidepressant drugs and bupropion. *J Clin Psychiatry* 44:197–201, 1983.

Pellegrini D, Kosisky S, Nackman D, Cytryn L, McKnew DH, Gershon E, Hamovit J, Cammuso K: Personal and social resources in children of patients with bipolar affective disorder and children of normal control subjects. *Am J Psychiatry* 143:856–861, 1986.

Penry JK, Daly DD, eds: *Complex Partial Seizures and Their Treatment, Vol 11: Advances in Neurology.* New York: Raven Press, 1975.

Pepper GM, Krieger DT: Hypothalamic-pituitary-adrenal abnormalities in depression: Their possible relation to central mechanisms regulating ACTH release. In: RM Post, JC Ballenger, eds: *Neurobiology of Mood Disorders.* Baltimore: Williams & Wilkins, 1984. pp 245–270.

Perényi A, Rihmer Z, Bánki CM: Parkinsonian symptoms with lithium, lithium-neuroleptic, and lithium-antidepressant treatment. *J Affective Disord* 5:171–177, 1983.

Perényi A, Szücs R, Frecska E: Tardive dyskinesia in patients receiving lithium maintenance therapy. *Biol Psychiatry* 19:1573–1578, 1984.

Perlow MJ, Reppert SM, Artman HA, Fisher DA, Self SM, Robinson AG: Oxytocin, vasopressin, and estrogen-stimulated neurophysin: Daily patterns of concentration in cerebrospinal fluid. *Science* 216:1416–1418, 1982.

Peroutka SJ: 5-Hydroxytryptamine receptor subtypes: Molecular, biochemical and physiological characterization. *Trends Neurs* 11:496–500, 1988.

Perris C, ed: A study of bipolar (manic-depressive) and unipolar recurrent depressive psychoses. *Acta Psychiatr Scand* 42(Suppl 194), 1966a.

Perris C: A study of bipolar (manic-depressive) and unipolar recurrent depressive psychoses: I: Genetic investigation. *Acta Psychiatr Scand* 42(Suppl 194): 15–44, 1966b.

Perris C: A study of bipolar (manic-depressive) and unipolar recurrent depressive psychoses. VI. Studies in perception: a) Colour-form preference. *Acta Psychiatr Scand* 42(Suppl 194):92–101, 1966c.

Perris C: A study of bipolar (manic-depressive) and unipolar recurrent depressive psychoses: VIII. Clinical-electroencephalographic investigation. *Acta Psychiatr Scand* 42(Suppl 194):118–152, 1966d.

Perris C: A study of bipolar (manic-depressive) and unipolar recurrent depressive psychoses, IV: Personality traits. *Acta Psychiatr Scand* (Suppl 194):68–82, 1966e.

Perris C: The course of depressive psychoses. *Acta Psychiatr Scand* 44:238–248, 1968.

Perris C: Personality patterns in patients with affective disorders. *Acta Psychiatr Scand* (Suppl 221):43–51, 1971.

Perris C: A study of cycloid psychoses. *Acta Psychiatr Scand* (Suppl 253):1–75, 1974.

Perris C: Reliability and validity studies of the Comprehensive Psychopathological Rating Scale (CRPS). *Prog Neuropsychopharmacol* 3:413–421, 1979.

Perris C: Central measures of depression. In: HM Van Praag, MH Lader, OJ Rafaelsen, EJ Sachar, eds: *Handbook of Biological Psychiatry Part II: Brain Mechanisms and Abnormal Behavior—Psychophysiology.* New York: Marcel Dekker, Inc, 1980. pp 183–224.

Perris C: The concept of cycloid psychotic disorder. *Psychiatr Dev* 1:37–56, 1988a.

Perris C: Neurophysiological and neuroanatomical studies of depression and mania. In: A Georgotas, R Cancro, eds: *Depression and Mania.* New York: Elsevier, 1988b. pp 213–243.

Perris C, d'Elia G: A study of bipolar (manic-depressive) and unipolar recurrent depressive psychoses: X: Mortality, suicide, and life cycles. *Acta Psychiatr Scand* 42(Suppl 194): 172–183, 1966.

Perris C, Monakhov K, Von Knorring L, Botskarev V, Nikiforov A: Systemic structural analysis of the electroencephalogram of depressed patients: General principles and preliminary results of an international collaborative study. *Neuropsychobiology* 4:207–228, 1978.

Perris C, Maj M, Perris H, Eisemann M: Perceived parental rearing behaviour in unipolar and bipolar depressed patients: A verification study in an Italian sample. *Acta Psychiatr Scand* 72:172–175, 1985.

Perris C, Arrindell WA, Perris H, Eisemann M, Van Der Ende J, Von Knorring L: Perceived depriving parental rearing and depression. *Br J Psychiatry* 148:170–175, 1986.

Perris H: Life events and depression. Part 2. Results in diagnostic subgroups, and in relation to the recurrence of depression. *J Affective Disord* 7:25–36, 1984.

Perry PJ, Alexander B, Dunner FJ, Schoenwald RD, Pfohl B, Miller D: Pharmacokinetic protocol for predicting serum lithium levels. *J Clin Psychopharmacol* 2:114–118, 1982.

Perry PJ, Alexander B, Prince RA, Dunner FJ: Prospective evaluation of two lithium maintenance dose schedules. *J Clin Psychopharmacol* 4:242–246, 1984.

Perry RH, Wilson ID, Bober MJ, Atack J, Blessed G, Tomlinson BE, Perry EK: Plasma and erythrocyte acetylcholinesterase in senile dementia of Alzheimer type. Letter. *Lancet* 1:174–175, 1982.

Pert A, Rosenblatt JE, Sivit C, Pert CB, Bunney WE Jr: Long-term treatment with lithium prevents the development of dopamine receptor supersensitivity. *Science* 201:171–173, 1978.

Pert CB, Snyder SH: Opiate receptor: Demonstration in nervous tissue. *Science* 179:1011–1014, 1973.

Pert CB, Ruff MR, Weber RJ, Herkenham M: Neuropeptides and their receptors: A psychosomatic network. *J Immunol* 135:820s–826s, 1985.

Pervin LA: Affect and addiction. *Addict Behav* 13:83–86, 1988.

Peselow ED, Dunner DL, Fieve RR, Lautin A: Lithium carbonate and weight gain. *J Affective Disord* 2:303–310, 1980.

Peselow ED, Dunner DL, Fieve RR, Deutsch SI, Rubenstein ME: Age of onset of affective illness. *Psychiatr Clin North Am* 15:124–132, 1982a.

Peselow ED, Dunner DL, Fieve RR, Lautin A: Lithium prophylaxis of depression in unipolar, bipolar II, and cyclothymic patients. *Am J Psychiatry* 139:747–752, 1982b.

Pestronk A, Drachman DB: Mechanism of action of lithium on acetylcholine receptor metabolism in skeletal muscle. *Brain Res* 412:302–310, 1987.

Pettegrew JW, Nichols JS, Minshew NJ, Rush AJ, Stewart RM: Membrane biophysical studies of lymphocytes and erythrocytes in manic-depressive illness. *J Affective Disord* 4:237–247, 1982.

Petterson U: Manic-depressive illness: A clinical, social and genetic study. *Acta Psychiatr Scand* (Suppl 269):1–93, 1977a.

Petterson U: Clinical analysis and evaluation of lithium therapy. In: Petterson U: Manic-depressive illness: A clinical, social and genetic study. *Acta Psychiatr Scand* (Suppl 269):23–42, 1977b.

Petterson U, Fyrö B, Sedvall G: A new scale for the longitudinal rating of manic states. *Acta Psychiatr Scand* 49:248–256, 1973.

Pettinati HM, Rosenberg J: Memory self-ratings before and after electroconvulsive therapy: Depression- versus ECT-induced. *Biol Psychiatry* 19:539–548, 1984.

Petty F, Sherman AD: A pharmacologically pertinant animal model of mania. *J Affective Disord* 3:381–387, 1981.

Petty F, Sherman AD: Plasma GABA levels in psychiatric illness. *J Affective Disord* 6:131–138, 1984.

Pfeffer CR, Plutchik R: Co-occurrence of psychiatric disorders in child psychiatric patients and nonpatients: A circumplex model. *Compr Psychiatry* 30:275–282, 1989.

Pfeiffer K, Maltzman I: Warned reaction times of manic-depressive patients with and without lithium. *J Abnorm Psychol* 85:194–200, 1976.

Pfeiffer WM: The symptomatology of depression

viewed transculturally. *Transcul Psychiatr Res Rev* 5:121–124, 1968.

Pflug B, Tölle R: Disturbance of the 24-hour rhythm in endogenous depression and the treatment of endogenous depression by sleep deprivation. *Int Pharmacopsychiatry* 6:187–196, 1971.

Pflug B, Erikson R, Johnsson A: Depression and daily temperature: A long-term study. *Acta Psychiatr Scand* 54:254–266, 1976.

Pflug B, Johnsson A, Ekse AT: Manic-depressive states and daily temperature. *Acta Psychiatr Scand* 63:277–289, 1981.

Pflug B, Johnsson A, Martin W: Alterations in the circadian temperature rhythms in depressed patients. In: TA Wehr, FK Goodwin, eds: *Circadian Rhythms in Psychiatry.* Pacific Grove, CA: The Boxwood Press, 1983. pp 71–76.

Phelps ME, Mazziota JC, Gerner R, Baxter L, Kuhl DE: Human cerebral glucose metabolism in affective disorders: Drug-free states and pharmacologic effects. *J Cereb Blood Flow Metab* 3(Suppl 1):S7–S8, 1983

Phelps ME, Mazziotta JC, Baxter L, Gerner R: Positron emission tomographic study of affective disorders: Problems and strategies. *Ann Neurol* 15(Suppl):S149–S156, 1984.

Phillips L: Case history data and prognosis in schizophrenia. *J Nerv Ment Dis* 117:515–525, 1953.

Physician's Desk Reference. 43rd Ed. Oradell, NJ: Medical Economics Co, 1989.

Pichot P: European perspectives on the classification of depression. *Br J Psychiatry* 153(Suppl 3):11–15, 1988.

Pichot P, Piret J, Clyde DJ: Analyse de la symptomatologie depressive subjective. *Rev Psychologie Appliquée* 2:105–115, 1966.

Pickar D, Sweeney DR, Maas JW, Heninger GR: Primary affective disorder, clinical state change and MHPG excretion: A longitudinal study. *Arch Gen Psychiatry* 35:1378–1383, 1978.

Pickar D, Cohen RM, Murphy DL, Fried D: Tyramine infusions in bipolar illness: Behavioral effects and longitudinal changes in pressor sensitivity. *Am J Psychiatry* 136:1460–1463, 1979.

Pickar D, Davis GC, Schulz SC, Extein I, Wagner R, Naber D, Gold PW, Van Kammen DP, Goodwin FK, Wyatt RJ, Li CH, Bunney WE Jr: Behavioral and biological effects of acute beta-endorphin injection in schizophrenic and depressed patients. *Am J Psychiatry* 138:160–166, 1981.

Pickar D, Extein I, Gold PW, Summers R, Naber D, Goodwin FK: Endorphins and affective illness. In: NS Shah, AG Donald, eds: *Endorphins and Opiate Antagonists in Psychiatric Research: Clinical Implications.* New York: Plenum Medical Book Co, 1982a. pp 375–397.

Pickar D, Vartanian F, Bunney WE Jr, Maier HP, Gastpar MT, Prakash R, Sethi BB, Lideman R, Belyaev BS, Tsutsulkovskaja MV, Jungkunz G, Nedopil N, Verhoeven W, Van Praag H: Short-term naloxone administration in schizophrenic and manic patients: A World Health Organization Collaborative Study. *Arch Gen Psychiatry* 39:313–319, 1982b.

Pickar D, Cowdry RW, Zis AP, Cohen RM, Murphy DL: Mania and hypomania during antidepressant pharmacotherapy: Clinical and research implications. In: RM Post, JC Ballenger, eds. *Neurobiology of Mood Disorders.* Baltimore: Williams & Wilkins, 1984a. pp 836–845.

Pickar D, Dubois M, Cohen MR: Behavioral change in a cancer patient following intrathecal beta-endorphin administration. *Am J Psychiatry* 141:103–104, 1984b.

Pimoule C, Briley MS, Gay C, Loo H, Sechter D, Zarifian E, Raisman R, Langer SZ: ^{3}H-Rauwolscine binding in platelets from depressed patients and healthy volunteers. *Psychopharmacology (Berlin)* 79:308–312, 1983.

Pinard G, Tetreault L: Concerning semantic problems in psychological evaluation. *Mod Prob Pharmacopsychiat* 7:8–22, 1974.

Pinel P: *Traitté Medico-philosophique sur l'Aliénation Mentale.* (1801). Paris: Brosson Translated by DD Davis as *A Treatise on Insanity.* Sheffield: Cadell and Davis (facsimile edition by Hafner, New York, 1962), 1806.

Pines M: *The New Human Genetics: How Gene Splicing Helps Researchers Fight Inherited Disease.* Bethesda, MD: National Institute of General Medical Sciences (NIH Pub. No. 84-662), 1984.

Piotrowski ZA, Lewis ND: An experimental Rorschach diagnostic aid for some forms of schizophrenia. *Am J Psychiatry* 107:360–366, 1950.

Pisciotta AV: Carbamazepine: Hematologic toxicity. In: DM Woodbury, JK Penry, C Pippenger, eds: *Antiepileptic Drugs.* New York: Raven Press, 1982. pp 309–341.

Pittendrigh CS: Circadian systems: General perspective. In: J Aschoff, ed. *Handbook of Behavioral Neurobiology, Vol 4 Biological Rhythms.* New York: Plenum Press, 1981. pp 57–80.

Pittendrigh CS, Daan S: A functional analysis of circadian pacemakers in nocturnal rodents: I: The stability and lability of spontaneous frequency. *J Comp Physiol* 106:223–252, 1976.

Pittman KJ, Jakubovic A, Fibiger HC: The effects of chronic lithium on behavioral and biochemical indices of dopamine receptor supersensitivity in the rat. *Psychopharmacology (Berlin)* 82:371–377, 1984.

Pitts FN, Winokur G: Affective disorder III: Diagnostic correlates and incidence of suicide. *J Nerv Ment Dis* 139:176–181, 1964.

Pitts FN, Winokur G: Affective disorder VII: Alcoholism and affective disorder. *J Psychiat Res* 4:37–50, 1966.

Pitts FN, Allen RE, Allen AD: Systematic immunodeficient Epstein-Barr viral syndrome (SIDES): The most common form of major depression. In press.

Placidi GF, Lenzi A, Lazzerini F, Cassano GB,

Akiskal HS: The comparative efficacy and safety of cabamazepine versus lithium: A randomized, double-blind 3-year trial in 83 patients. *J Clin Psychiatry* 47:490–494, 1986.

Plath S: *The Bell Jar*. New York: Harper & Row, 1971.

Platman SR: A comparison of lithium carbonate and chlorpromazine in mania. *Am J Psychiatry* 127:351–353, 1970.

Platman SR, Plutchik R, Fieve RR, Lawlor WG: Emotion profiles associated with mania and depression. *Arch Gen Psychiatry* 20:210–214, 1969.

Platz C, Kendell RE: A matched-control follow-up and family study of 'puerperal psychoses.' *Br J Psychiatry* 153:90–94, 1988.

Plenge P, Mellerup ET, Bolwig TG: Lithium treatment: Does the kidney prefer one daily dose instead of two? *Acta Psychiatr Scand* 66:121–128, 1982.

Plimpton G, ed: *Writers at Work: The Paris Review Interviews*. New York: Viking Press, 1976.

Plokker JJ: *Art from the Mentally Disturbed, the Scattered Vision of Schizophrenics*. Boston: Little Brown, 1965.

Plutchik R, Platman SR, Fieve RR: Self-concepts associated with mania and depression. *Psychol Rep* 27:399–405, 1970a.

Plutchik R, Platman SR, Tilles R, Fieve RR: Construction and evaluation of a test for measuring mania and depression. *J Clin Psychol* 26:499–503, 1970b.

Poe EA: *The Fall of the House of Usher and Other Writings*. D Galloway, ed. Middlesex: Penguin, 1980.

Pokorny AD, Rawls WE, Adam E, Mefferd RB Jr: Depression, psychopathy, and herpesvirus type I antibodies: Lack of relationship. *Arch Gen Psychiatry* 29:820–822, 1973.

Polatin P, Fieve RR: Patient rejection of lithium carbonate prophylaxis. *JAMA* 218:864–866, 1971.

Pöldinger W: Combined administration of desipramine and reserpine or tetrabenazine in depressive patients. *Psychopharmacologia* 4:308–310, 1963.

Pollock HM: Recurrence of attacks in manic-depressive psychoses. *Am J Psychiatry* 11:568–573, 1931.

Pollock HM: The depression and mental disease in New York State. *Am J Psychiatry* 91:763–771, 1934.

Polsky R, McGuire MT: An ethological analysis of manic-depressive disorder. *J Nerv Ment Dis* 167: 56–65, 1979.

Pons L, Nurberger JI Jr, Murphy DL: Mood-independent aberrancies in associative processes in bipolar affective disorder: An apparent stabilizing effect of lithium. *Psychiatry Res* 14:315–322, 1985.

Pool JL, Correll JV: Psychiatric symptoms masking brain tumors. *J Med Soc New Jersey* 55:4–9, 1958.

Pool R: Is it healthy to be chaotic? *Science* 243:604–607, 1989.

Poole AJ, James HD, Hughes WC: Treatment experiences in the lithium clinic at St. Thomas' Hospital. *J R Soc Med* 71:890–894, 1978.

Poort R: Catamnestic investigations on manic-depressive psychoses with special reference to the prognosis. *Acta Psychiatr Neurol* 20:59–74, 1945.

Pope B, Blass T, Siegman AW, Raher J: Anxiety and depression in speech. *J Consult Clin Psychol* 35:128–133, 1970.

Pope HG Jr: Drug abuse and psychopathology. *N Engl J Med* 301:1341–1343, 1979.

Pope HG Jr: Distinguishing bipolar disorder from schizophrenia in clinical practice: Guidelines and case reports. *Hosp Community Psychiatry* 34:322–328, 1983.

Pope HG, Katz DL: Affective and psychotic symptoms associated with anabolic steroid use. *Am J Psychiatry* 145:487–490, 1988.

Pope HG Jr, Lipinski JS Jr: Diagnosis in schizophrenia and manic-depressive illness: A reassessment of the specificity of "schizophrenic" symptoms in light of current research. *Arch Gen Psychiatry* 35:811–828, 1978.

Pope HG Jr, Ionescu-Pioggia M, Yurgelun-Todd D: Migration and manic-depressive illness. *Compr Psychiatry* 24:158–165, 1983a.

Pope HG Jr, Jonas JM, Hudson JI, Cohen BM, Gunderson JG: The validity of DSM-III borderline personality disorder: A phenomenologic, family history treatment response, and long- term follow-up study. *Arch Gen Psychiatry* 40:23–30, 1983b.

Pope HG Jr, Keck PE, McElroy SL: Frequency and presentation of neuroleptic malignant syndrome in a large psychiatric hospital. *Am J Psychiatry* 143:1227–1233, 1986.

Pope HG Jr, McElroy SL, Satlin A, Hudson JI, Keck PE, Kalish R: Head injury, bipolar disorder, and response to valproate. *Compr Psychiatry* 29:34–38, 1988.

Popescu C, Totoescu A, Christodorescu D, Ionescu R: Personality attributes in unipolar and bipolar affective disorders. *Neurol Psychiatr (Bucur)* 23:231–242, 1985.

Porsolt RD, Anton G, Blavel N, Jalfre M: Depression: A new animal model sensitive to antidepressant treatements. *Nature* 21:730–732, 1977.

Post RD, Clopton JR, Keefer G, Rosenberg D, Blyth LS, Stein M: MMPI predictors of mania among psychiatric inpatients. *J Person Assess* 50:248–256, 1986.

Post RL, Albright CD, Dayani K: Resolution of pump and leak components of sodium and potassium ion transport in human erythrocytes. *J Gen Physiol* 50:1201–1220, 1967.

Post RM: Mechanisms of action of carbamazepine and related anticonvulsants in affective illness. In: HY Meltzer, ed: *Psychopharmacology: The Third Generation of Progress*. New York: Raven Press, 1987. pp 567–576.

Post RM: Time course of clinical effects of carbamazepine: Implications for mechanisms of action. *J Clin Psychiatry* 49(Suppl):35–48, 1988.

Post RM: Mood disorders: Somatic treatment. In: HI Kaplan, BJ Sadock, eds: *Comprehensive Textbook of Psychiatry V*. Baltimore: Williams &

Wilkins, 1989. pp 913–933.

Post RM, Goodwin FK: Approaches to brain amines in psychiatric patients: A reevaluation of cerebrospinal fluid studies. In: LL Iversen, SD Iversen, SH Snyder, eds: *Handbook of Psychopharmacology, Vol 13: Biology of Mood and Antianxiety Drugs.* New York: Plenum Press, 1978. pp 147–185.

Post RM, Kopanda RT: Cocaine, kindling, and psychosis. *Am J Psychiatry* 133:627–634, 1976.

Post RM, Uhde TW: Carbamazepine as a treatment for refractory depressive illness and rapidly cycling manic-depressive illness. In: J Zohar, RH Belmaker, eds: *Special Treatments for Resistant Depression.* New York: Spectrum Press, 1985. 281–288.

Post RM, Uhde TW: Clinical approaches to treatment-resistant bipolar illness. In: RE Hales, AJ Frances, eds: *Psychiatry Update. American Psychiatric Association Annual Review. Vol 6.* Washington, DC: American Psychiatric Press, 1987. pp 125–150.

Post RM, Uhde TW: Refractory manias and alternatives to lithium treatment. In: A Georgotas, R Cancro, eds: *Depression and Mania.* New York: Elsevier, 1988. pp 410–438.

Post RM, Weiss SRB: Non-homologous animal models of affective illness: Clinical relevance of sensitization and kindling. In: G Koob, C Ehlers, DJ Kupfer, eds: *Animal Models of Depression.* Boston: Birkhauser Boston, 1989. pp 30–54.

Post RM, Gordon EK, Goodwin FK, Bunney WE Jr: Central norepinephrine metabolism in affective illness: MHPG in the cerebrospinal fluid. *Science* 179:1002–1003, 1973.

Post RM, Gillin JC, Wyatt RJ, Goodwin FK: The effect of orally administered cocaine on sleep of depressed patients. *Psychopharmacologia (Berlin)* 37:59–66, 1974a.

Post RM, Kotin J, Goodwin, FK: The effects of cocaine on depressed patients. *Am J Psychiatry* 131:511–517, 1974b.

Post RM, Kotin J, Goodwin FK: Effect of sleep deprivation on mood and central amine metabolism in depressed patients. *Arch Gen Psychiatry* 33:627–632, 1976.

Post RM, Stoddard FJ, Gillin JC, Buchsbaum MS, Runkle DC, Black KE, Bunney WE Jr: Alterations in motor activity, sleep, and biochemistry in a cycling manic-depressive patient. *Arch Gen Psychiatry* 34:470–477, 1977.

Post RM, Gerner RH, Carman JS, Gillin JC, Jimerson DC, Goodwin FK, Bunney WE Jr: Effects of a dopamine agonist piribedil in depressed patients: Relationship of pretreatment homovanillic acid to antidepressant response. *Arch Gen Psychiatry* 35:609–615, 1978a.

Post RM, Lake CR, Jimerson DC, Bunney WE, Wood JH, Ziegler MG, Goodwin FK: Cerebrospinal fluid norepinephrine in affective illness. *Am J Psychiatry* 135:907–912, 1978b.

Post RM, Ballenger JC, Goodwin FK: Cerebrospinal fluid studies of neurotransmitter function in manic and depressive illness. In: JH Wood, ed: *The Neurobiology of Cerebrospinal Fluid, Vol 1.* New York: Plenum Press, 1980a. pp 685–717.

Post RM, Ballenger JC, Hare TA, Goodwin FK, Lake CR, Jimerson DC, Bunney WE: Cerebrospinal fluid GABA in normals and patients with affective disorders. *Brain Res Bull* 5(Suppl 2):755–759, 1980b.

Post RM, Jimerson DC, Bunney WE Jr, Goodwin FK: Dopamine and mania: Behavioral and biochemical effects of the dopamine receptor blocker pimozide. *Psychopharmacology (Berlin)* 67:297–305, 1980c.

Post RM, Ballenger JC, Rey AC, Bunney WE Jr: Slow and rapid onset of manic episodes: Implications for underlying biology. *Psychiatry Res* 4:229–237, 1981.

Post RM, Ballenger JC, Uhde TW, Bunney WE Jr: Efficacy of carbamazepine in manic-depressive illness: Implications for underlying mechanisms. In: RM Post, JC Ballenger, eds: *Neurobiology of Mood Disorders.* Baltimore: Williams & Wilkins, 1984a. pp 777–816.

Post RM, Berrettini W, Uhde TW, Kellner C: Selective response to the anticonvulsant carbamazepine in manic-depressive illness: A case study. *J Clin Psychopharmacol* 4:178–185, 1984b.

Post RM, Jimerson DC, Ballenger JC, Lake CR, Uhde TW, Goodwin FK: Cerebrospinal fluid norepinephrine and its metabolites in manic-depressive illness. In: RM Post, JC Ballenger, eds: *Neurobiology of Mood Disorders.* Baltimore: Williams & Wilkins, 1984c. pp 539–553.

Post RM, Putnam F, Contel NR, Goldman B: Electroconvulsive seizures inhibit amygdala kindling: Implications for mechanisms of action in affective illness. *Epilepsia* 25:234–239, 1984d.

Post RM, Rubinow DR, Ballenger JC: Conditioning, sensitization, and kindling: Implications for the course of affective illness. In: RM Post, JC Ballenger, eds: *The Neurobiology of Mood Disorders.* Williams & Wilkins, 1984e. pp 432–466.

Post RM, Weiss SRB, Pert A: Differential effects of carbamazepine and lithium on sensitization and kindling. *Prog Neuropsychopharmacol Biol Psychiat* 8:425–434, 1984f.

Post RM, Uhde TW, Joffe RT, Roy-Byrne PP, Kellner C: Anticonvulsant drugs in psychiatric illness: New treatment alternatives and theoretical implications. In: MR Trimble, ed: *The Psychopharmacology of Epilepsy.* Chichester, England: John Wiley & Sons, 1985. pp 141–171.

Post RM, Rubinow DR, Ballenger JC: Conditioning and sensitization in the longitudinal course of affective illness. *Br J Psychiatry* 149:191–201, 1986a.

Post RM, Uhde TW, Joffe RT, Bierer L: Psychiatric manifestations and implications of seizure disorders. In: IL Extein, ed: *Medical Mimics of Psychiatric Disorders.* Washington, DC: American Psychiatric Press, 1986b. pp 35–76.

Post RM, Uhde TW, Roy-Byrne PP, Joffe RT: Antidepressant effects of carbamazepine. *Am J Psychiatry* 143:29–34, 1986c.

Post RM, Uhde TW, Rubinow DR, Weiss SRB: Antimanic effects of carbamazepine: Mechanisms of action and implications for the biochemistry of manic-depressive illness. In: A Swann, ed: *Mania: New Research and Treatment*. Washington DC: American Psychiatric Press, 1986d. pp 95–176.

Post RM, DeLisi LE, Holcomb HH, Uhde TW, Cohen R, Buchsbaum MS: Glucose utilization in the temporal cortex of affectively ill patients: Positron emission tomography. *Biol Psychiatry* 22:545–553, 1987a.

Post RM, Uhde TW, Roy-Byrne PP, Joffe RT: Correlates of antimanic responses to carbamazepine. *Psychiatry Res* 21:71–83, 1987b.

Post RM, Roy-Byrne PP, Uhde TW: Graphic representation of the life course of illness in patients with affective disorder. *Am J Psychiatry* 145:844–848, 1988a.

Post RM, Weiss SRB, Pert A: Cocaine-induced behavioral sensitization and kindling: Implications for the emergence of psychopathology and seizures. *Ann NY Acad Sci* 537:292–308, 1988b.

Post RM, Weiss SRB, Altshuler L: Changing sensitivity to drugs in bipolar illness. Abstract of paper presented at the 16th CINP Congress, 1988c.

Post RM, Rubinow DR, Uhde TW, Roy-Byrne PP, Linnoila M, Rosoff A, Cowdry R: Dysphoric mania: Clinical and biological correlates. *Arch Gen Psychiatry* 46:353–358, 1989.

Potkin S, Zetin M, Stamenkovic V, Kripke DF, Bunney WE Jr: Seasonal affective disorder: Prevalence varies with latitude and climate. *Clin Neuropharmacol* 9(Suppl 4):181–183, 1986.

Potter WZ: Psychotherapeutic drugs and biogenic amines: Current concepts and therapeutic implications. *Drugs* 28:127–143, 1984.

Potter WZ: Introduction: Norepinephrine as an "umbrella" neuromodulator. *Psychosomatics* 27(Suppl):5–9, 1986.

Potter WZ, Linnoila M: Tricyclic antidepressant concentrations: Clinical and research implications. In: RM Post, JC Ballenger, eds. *Neurobiology of Mood Disorders*. Baltimore: Williams & Wilkins, 1984. pp 698–709.

Potter WZ, Linnoila M: Biochemical classifications of diagnostic subgroups and d-type scores. *Arch Gen Psychiatry* 46:269–271, 1989.

Potter WZ, Murphy DL, Wehr TA, Linnoila M, Goodwin FK: Clorgyline: A new treatment for refractory rapid-cycling disorder. *Arch Gen Psychiatry* 39:505–510, 1982.

Potter WZ, Muscettola G, Goodwin FK: Sources of variance in clinical studies of MHPG. In: JW Maas, ed: *MHPG: Basic Mechanisms and Psychopathology*. New York: Academic Press, 1983. pp 145–165.

Potter WZ, Scheinin M, Golden RN, Rudorfer MV, Cowdry RW, Calil HM, Ross RJ, Linnoila M: Selective antidepressants and cerebrospinal fluid: Lack of specificity on norepinephrine and serotonin metabolites. *Arch Gen Psychiatry* 42:1171–1177, 1985.

Potter WZ, Rudorfer MV, Goodwin FK: Biological findings in bipolar disorders. In: RE Hales, AJ Francis, eds: *American Psychiatric Association Annual Review, vol. 6*. Washington, DC: American Psychiatric Press, Inc, 1987. pp 32–60.

Potter WZ, Rudorfer MV, Linnoila M: New clinical studies support a role of norepinephrine antidepressant action. In: JD Barchas, WE Bunney Jr, eds: *Perspectives in Psychopharmacology: A Collection of Papers in Honor of Earl Usdin*. New York: Alan R. Liss, 1988. pp 495–513.

Poynton A, Bridges PK, Bartlett JR: Resistant bipolar affective disorder treated by stereotactic subcaudate tractotomy. *Br J Psychiatry* 152:354–358, 1988.

Poznanski EO, Israel MG, Grossman J: Hypomania in a four-year-old. *J Am Acad Child Psychiatry* 23:105–110, 1984.

Prange AJ Jr: The pharmacology and biochemistry of depression. *Dis Nerv Syst* 25:217–221, 1964.

Prange AJ Jr, Vitols MM: Cultural aspects of the relatively low incidence of depression in southern Negroes. *Int J Soc Psychiatry* 8:104–112, 1962.

Prange AJ, McCurdy RL, Cochrane CM: The systolic blood pressure response of depressed patients to infused norepinephrine. *J Psychiatr Res* 5:1–13, 1967.

Prange AJ Jr, Wilson IC, Rabon AM, Lipton MA: Enhancement of imipramine antidepressant activity by thyroid hormone. *Am J Psychiatry* 126:457–469, 1969.

Prange AJ Jr, Lara PP, Wilson IC, Alltop LB, Breese GR: Effects of thyrotropin-releasing hormone in depression. *Lancet* 2:999–1002, 1972.

Prange AJ Jr, Breese GR, Cott JM, Martin BR, Cooper BR, Wilson IC, Plotnikoff NP: Thyrotropin releasing hormone: Antagonism of pentobarbital in rodents. *Life Sci* 14:447–455, 1974a.

Prange AJ, Wilson IC, Lara PP, Alltop LB: Effects of thyrotropin-releasing hormone in depression. In: AJ Prange, ed: *The Thyroid Axis, Drugs, and Behavior*. New York: Raven Press, 1974b. pp 135–145.

Prange AJ Jr, Wilson IC, Lynn CW, Alltop LB, Stikeleather RA: L-tryptophan in mania: Contribution to a permissive hypothesis of affective disorders. *Arch Gen Psychiatry* 30:56–62, 1974c.

Prasad AJ: The role of sodium valproate as an antimanic agent. *Pharmatherapeutica* 4:6–8, 1984.

Prescott J, Connolly JF, Gruzelier JH: The augmenting/reducing phenomenon in the auditory evoked potential. *Biol Psychol* 19:31–44, 1984.

Presley AP, Kahn A, Williamson N: Antinuclear antibodies in patients on lithium carbonate. *Br Med J* 2:280–281, 1976.

Pribram KH: The primate frontal cortex. *Neuropsychologia* 7:259–266, 1969.

Price J: Neurotic and endogenous depression: A phylogenetic view. *Br J Psychiatry* 114:119–120, 1968.

Price J, Karim I: Matiruku, A Fijian madness: An initial assessment. *Br J Psychiatry* 133:228–230, 1978.

Price J, O'Kearney R: Changes in hostility during the course of hypomanic illness. *Br J Clin Psychol* 21:103–110, 1982.

Price LH, Nelson JC: Alcoholism and affective disorder. *Am J Psychiatry* 143:1067–1068, 1986.

Price LH, Charney DS, Heninger GR: Manic symptoms following addition of lithium to antidepressant treatment. *J Clin Psychopharmacol* 4:361–362, 1984a.

Price LH, Nelson JC, Charney DS, Quinlan DM: Family history in delusional depression. *J Affective Disord* 6:109–114, 1984b.

Price LH, Charney DS, Heninger GR: Efficacy of lithium-tranylcypromine treatment in refractory depression. *Am J Psychiatry* 142:619–623, 1985.

Price LH, Charney DS, Rubin AL, Heninger GR: Alpha 2-adrenergic receptor function in depression: The cortisol response to yohimbine. *Arch Gen Psychiatry* 43:849–858, 1986.

Price LH, Charney DS, Heninger GR: Reserpine augmentation of desipramine in refractory depression: Clinical and neurobiological effects. *Psychopharmacoloy* 92:431–437, 1987.

Price LH, Charney DS, Delgado PL, Heninger GR: Lithium treatment and serotonergic function: Neuroendocrine and behavioral responses to intravenous tryptophan in affective disorder. *Arch Gen Psychiatry* 46:13–19, 1989.

Price RA, Kidd KK, Pauls DL, Gershon ES, Prussof PA, Weissman MM, Goldin LR: Multiple threshold models for the affective disorders: The Yale-NIMH collaborative family study. *J Psychiat Res* 19:533–546. 1985.

Price RW, Navia BA, Cho ES: AIDS encephalopathy. *Neurol Clin* 4:285–301, 1986.

Price WA, Bielefeld M: Buspirone-induced mania. *J Clin Psychopharmacol* 9:150–151, 1989.

Prichep LS, Lieber AL, John ER, Alper K, Gomez-Mont F, Essig-Peppard T, Flitter M: Quantitative EEG in depressive disorders. In: C Shagass, RC Josiassen, RA Roemer, eds: *Brain Electrical Potentials and Psychopathology*. New York: Elsevier, 1986. pp 223–244.

Prien RF: Long-term prophylactic pharmacologic treatment of bipolar illness. In: L Grinspoon, ed: *Psychiatry Update. The American Psychiatric Association Annual Review, Vol II*. Washington, DC: American Psychiatric Press, 1983. pp 303–318.

Prien RF, Gelenberg AJ: Alternatives to lithium for preventive treatment of bipolar disorder. *Am J Psychiatry* 146:840–848, 1989.

Prien RF, Caffey EM Jr, Klett CJ: Comparison of lithium carbonate and chlorpromazine in the treatment of mania: Report of the Veterans Administration and National Institute of Mental Health Collaborative Study Group. *Arch Gen Psychiatry* 26:146–153, 1972.

Prien RF, Caffey EM Jr, Klett CJ: Prophylactic efficacy of lithium carbonate in manic-depressive illness. *Arch Gen Psychiatry* 28:337–341, 1973a.

Prien RF, Klett CJ, Caffey EM Jr: Lithium carbonate and imipramine in prevention of affective episodes: A comparison in recurrent affective illness. *Arch Gen Psychiatry* 29:420–425, 1973b.

Prien RF, Caffey EM Jr, Klett J: Factors associated with treatment success in lithium carbonate prophylaxis: Report of the Veterans Administration and National Institute of Mental Health Collaborative Study Group. *Arch Gen Psychiatry* 31:189–192, 1974.

Prien RF, Kupfer DJ, Mansky PA, Small JG, Tuason VB, Voss CB, Johnson WE: Drug therapy in the prevention of recurrences in unipolar and bipolar affective disorders: Report of the NIMH Collaborative Study Group comparing lithium carbonate, imipramine, and a lithium carbonate-imipramine combination. *Arch Gen Psychiatry* 41:1096–1104, 1984.

Prien RF, Himmelhoch JM, Kupfer DJ: Treatment of mixed mania. *J Affective Disord* 15:9–15, 1988.

Pringle H: *Theodore Roosevelt: A Biography*. New York: Harcourt, Brace & Co., 1931.

Procci WR: Schizo-affective psychosis: Fact or fiction?: A survey of the literature. *Arch Gen Psychiatry* 33:1167–1178, 1976.

Propping P, Friedl W: Genetic control of adrenergic receptors on human platelets: A twin study. *Hum Genet* 64:105–109, 1983.

Prusoff BA, Klerman GL, Paykel ES: Concordance between clinical assessments and patients' self-report in depression. *Arch Gen Psychiatry* 26:546–552, 1972a.

Prusoff BA, Klerman GL, Paykel ES: Pitfalls in the self-report assessment of depression. *Can Psychiatr Assoc J* 17(Suppl 2):SS101-SS107, 1972b.

Prusoff BA, Merikangas KR, Weissman MM: Lifetime prevalence and age of onset of psychiatric disorders: Recall 4 years later. *J Psychiatr Res* 22:107–117, 1988.

Puig-Antich J, Goetz D, Davies M, Kaplan T, Davies S, Ostrow D, Asnis L, Twomey J, Iyergar S, Ryan ND: A controlled family history study of prepubertal major depressive disorder. *Arch Gen Psychiatry* 46:406–418, 1989.

Purdy RE, Julien RM, Fairhurst AS, Terry MD: Effect of carbamazepine on the in vitro uptake and release of norepinephrine in adrenergic nerves of rabbit aorta and in whole brain synaptosomes. *Epilepsia* 18:251–257, 1977.

Puzynski S, Klosiewicz L: Valproic acid amide in the treatment of affective and schizoaffective disorders. *J Affective Disord* 6:115–121, 1984.

Puzynski S, Rode A, Zaluska M: Studies on biogenic amine metabolizing enzymes (DBH, COMT, MAO) and pathogenesis of affective illness: I. Plasma dopamine-beta-hydroxylase activity in endogenous depression. *Acta Psychiatr Scand* 67:89–95, 1983.

Pycock CJ, Kerwin RW, Carter CJ: Effect of lesion of cortical dopamine terminals on subcortical dopamine receptors in rats. *Nature* 286:74–76, 1980.

Quitkin FM: The importance of dosage in prescribing

antidepressants. *Br J Psychiatry* 147:593–597, 1985.

Quitkin F, Rifkin A, Kane J, Ramos-Lorenzi JR, Klein DF: Prophylactic effect of lithium and imipramine in unipolar and bipolar II patients: A preliminary report. *Am J Psychiatry* 135:570–572, 1978.

Quitkin F, Rifkin A, Klein DF: Monoamine oxidase inhibitors: A review of antidepressant effectiveness. *Arch Gen Psychiatry* 36:749–760, 1979.

Quitkin FM, Kane J, Rifkin A, Ramos-Lorenzi JR, Nayak DV: Prophylactic lithium carbonate with and without imipramine for bipolar 1 patients: A double-blind study. *Arch Gen Psychiatry* 38:902–907, 1981a.

Quitkin FM, Kane JM, Rifkin A, Ramos-Lorenzi JR, Saraf K, Howard A, Klein DF: Lithium and imipramine in the prophylaxis of unipolar and bipolar II depression: A prospective, placebo-controlled comparison. *Psychopharmacol Bull* 17:142–145, 1981b.

Quitkin FM, McGrath P, Liebowitz MR, Stewart J, Howard A: Monoamine oxidase inhibitors in bipolar endogenous depressives. *J Clin Psychopharmacol* 1:70–74, 1981c.

Quitkin FM, Rabkin JG, Ross D, McGrath PJ: Duration of antidepressant drug treatment: What is an adequate trial? *Arch Gen Psychiatry* 41:238–245, 1984.

Quitkin FM, Rabkin JG, Prien RF: Bipolar disorder: Are there manic-prone and depressive-prone forms? *J Clin Psychopharmacol* 6:167–172, 1986.

Racine R, Coscina DV: Effects of midbrain raphe lesions or systematic p-chlorophenylalamine on the development of kindled seizures in rats. *Brain Res Bull* 4:1–7, 1979.

Racy J: Somatization in Saudi women: A therapeutic challenge. *Br J Psychiatry* 137:212–216, 1980.

Radke-Yarrow M, Cummings EM, Kuczynski L, Chapman M: Patterns of attachment in two- and three-year-olds in normal families and families with parental depression. *Child Devel* 56:884–893, 1985.

Rado S: The problem of melancholia. *Int J Psychoanal* 9:420–438, 1928.

Rado S: Psychoanalysis of pharmacothymia. *Psychoanal Q* 2:1–23, 1933.

Rafaelsen OJ, Bolwig TG, Ladefogeol J, Brun C: Kidney function and morphology in long-term treatment. In: TB Cooper, S Gershon, N Kline, M Schou, eds: *Lithium: Controversies and Unresolved Issues*. Amsterdam: Excerpta Medica, 1979. pp 578–583.

Rafaelsen OJ, Bech P, Bolwig TG, Kramp P, Gjerris A: The Bech-Rafaelsen combined rating scale for mania and melancholia. In: K Achté, V Aalberg, J Lönnqvist, eds: *Psychopathology of Depression: Proceedings of the Symposium by the Section of Clinical Psychopathology of the World Psychiatric Association, 1979*. Helsinki: Psychiatric Fennica Supplementum, 1980. pp 327–331.

Ragheb M: Ibuprofen can increase serum lithium level in lithium-treated patients. *J Clin Psychiatry* 48:161–163, 1987.

Ragin AB, Oltmanns TF: Predictability as an index of impaired verbal communication in schizophrenic and affective disorders. *Br J Psychiatry* 143:578–583, 1983.

Ragin AB, Oltmanns TF: Communicability and thought disorder in schizophrenics and other diagnostic groups: A follow-up study. *Br J Psychiatry* 150:494–500, 1987.

Raichle ME, Grubb RL, Gado MH, Eichling JO, Ter-Pogossian MM: Correlation between regional cerebral blood flow and oxidative metabolism: In vivo studies in man. *Arch Neurol* 33:523–526, 1976.

Raisman R, Briley MS, Bouchami F, Sechter D, Zarifian E, Langer SZ: ^{3}H-imipramine binding and serotonin uptake in platelets from untreated depressed patients and control volunteers. *Psychopharmacology* 77:332–335, 1982.

Ralph MR, Menaker M: A mutation of the circadian system in golden hamsters. *Science* 241:1225–1227, 1988.

Ramsey TA, Mendels J: Lithium-responsive depressive illness: Clinical and biological characteristics. In: P Deniker, C Radouco-Thomas, A Villeneuve, D Baronet-Lacroix, F Garein, eds: *Neuropsychopharmacology*. Vol 2. Oxford: Pergamon Press, 1978. pp 1117–1124.

Ramsey TA, Frazer J, Mendels J, Dyson L: The erythrocyte lithium-plasma lithium ratio in patients with primary affective disorders. *Arch Gen Psychiatry* 36:457–461, 1979.

Randall JG: *Lincoln the President: Springfield to Gettysburg*. New York: Dodd, Mead, 1945.

Rangel-Guerra RA, Perez-Payan H, Minikoff L, Todd LE: Nuclear magnetic resonance in bipolar affective disorder. *AJNR* 4:229–231, 1983.

Rao MSS, Socio-economic groups and mental disorders. *Psychiatr Q* 40:677–691, 1966.

Rapaport D: *Diagnostic Psychological Testing: The Theory, Statistical Evaluation, and Diagnostic Application of a Battery of Texts*. Vol 1. Chicago: Yearbook, 1946.

Rapaport D, Gill MM, Schafer R: *Diagnostic Psychological Testing*. New York: International Universities Press, 1968.

Raskin A, Crook TH: Sensitivity of rating-scales completed by psychiatrists, nurses and patients to antidepressant drug effects. *J Psychiatr Res* 13:31–41, 1976.

Raskin A, Schulterbrandt J, Reatig N, Rice CE: Factors of psychopathology in interview, ward behavior, and self-report ratings of hospitalized depressives. *J Consult Psychol* 31:270–278, 1967.

Raskin A, Schulterbrandt J, Reatig N, McKeon JJ: Replication of factors of psychopathology in interview, ward behavior and self-report ratings of hospitalized depressives. *J Nerv Ment Dis* 148:87–98, 1969.

Raskin A, Schulterbrandt JG, Reatig N, McKeon JJ:

Differential response to chlorpromazine, imipramine, and placebo: A study of subgroups of hospitalized depressed patients. *Arch Gen Psychiatry* 23:164–173, 1970.

Raskin A, Friedman AS, DiMascio A: Cognitive and performance deficits in depression. *Psychopharmacol Bull* 18:196–202, 1982.

Rausch JL, Shah NS, Burch EA, Donald AG: Platelet serotonin uptake in depressed patients: Circadian effect. *Biol Psychiatry* 17:121–123, 1982.

Rausch JL, Janowsky DS, Risch SC, Huey LY: A kinetic analysis and replication of decreased platelet serotonin uptake in depressed patients. *Psychiatry Res* 19:105–112, 1986.

Rausch JL, Rich CL, Risch SC: Platelet serotonin transport after a single ECT. *Psychopharmacology (Berlin)* 95:139–141, 1988.

Razani J, White KL, White J, Simpson G, Sloane RB, Rebal R, Palmer R: The safety and efficacy of combined amitriptyline and tranylcypromine antidepressant treatment: A controlled trial. *Arch Gen Psychiatry* 40:657–661, 1983.

Read W: *The Days of Dylan Thomas.* New York: McGraw-Hill, 1964.

Reches A, Wagner HR, Jackson V, Fahn S: Chronic lithium administration has no effect on haloperidol-induced supersensitivity of pre- and postsynaptic dopamine receptors in rat brain. *Brain Res* 246:172–177, 1982.

Reddy PL, Khanna S, Subhash MN, Channabasavanna SM, Rao BSSR: Erythrocyte membrane Na-K ATPase activity in affective disorder. *Biol Psychiatry* 26:533–537, 1989.

Regier DA, Myers JK, Kramer M, Robins LN, Blazer DG, Hough RL, Eaton WW, Locke BZ: The NIMH Epidemiologic Catchment Area Program: Historical context, major objectives, and study population characteristics. *Arch Gen Psychiatry* 41:934–941, 1984.

Regier DA, Boyd JH, Burke JD Jr, Rae DS, Myers JK, Kramer M, Robins LN, George LK, Karno M, Locke BZ: One-month prevalence of mental disorders in the United States: Based on five Epidemiological Catchment Area sites. *Arch Gen Psychiatry* 45:977–986, 1988.

Regier DA, Hirschfeld RMA, Judd LL, Burke JD, Goodwin FK, Lazar JB: The NIMH D/ART Program: Structure, aims, and scientific basis. *Am J Psychiatry* 145:1351–1357, 1988b.

Regier DA, Farmer ME, Raye DS, Locke BZ, Keith SJ, Judd LL, Goodwin FK: Comorbidity of mental disorders with drug and alcohol abuse: Results from the Epidemiologic Catchment Area (ECA) study. *N Engl J Med,* submitted.

Reginaldi D, Tondo L, Floris G, Pignatelli A, Kukopulos A: Poor prophylactic lithium response due to antidepressants. *Int Pharmacopsychiatry* 16:124–128, 1981.

Rego MD, Giller EL: Mania secondary to amantadine treatment of neuroleptic-induced hyperprolactinemia. *J Clin Psychiatry* 50:143–14, 1989.

Rehavi M, Paul SM, Skolnick P, Goodwin FK: Demonstration of specific high affinity binding sites for [^{3}H] imipramine in human brain. *Life Sci* 26:2273–2279, 1980.

Reich LH, Davies RK, Himmelhoch JM: Excessive alcohol use in manic-depressive illness. *Am J Psychiatry* 131:83–86, 1974.

Reich P, Kelly MJ: Suicide attempts by hospitalized medical and surgical patients. *N Engl J Med* 294:298–301, 1976.

Reich T, Winokur G: Postpartum psychoses in patients with manic depressive disease. *J Nerv Ment Dis* 151:60–68, 1970.

Reich T, James JW, Morris CA: The use of multiple thresholds in determining the mode of transmission of semi-continuous traits. *Ann Hum Genetics* 36:163–184, 1972.

Reid AH, Naylor GJ: Short-cycle manic depressive psychosis in mental defectives: A clinical and physiological study. *J Ment Defici Res* 20:67–76, 1976.

Reifman A, Wyatt RJ: Lithium: A brake in the rising cost of mental illness. *Arch Gen Psychiatry* 37:385–388, 1980.

Reimann IW, Diener U, Frölich JC: Indomethacin but not aspirin increases plasma lithium ion levels. *Arch Gen Psychiatry* 40:283–286, 1983.

Reisberg B, Gershon S: Side effects associated with lithium therapy. *Arch Gen Psychiatry* 36:879–887, 1979.

Reisine TD: Cellular mechanisms regulating adrenocorticotropin release. *J Recept Res* 4:291–300, 1984.

Reiss AL: Developmental manifestations in a boy with prepubertal bipolar disorder. *J Clin Psychiatry* 46:441–443, 1985.

Reiss E: *Konstitutionelle Verstimmung und manisch-depressives Irresein: Klinische Untersuchungen über den Zusammenhang von Veranlagung und Psychose.* Berlin: J. Springer, 1910.

Reitan RM: Certain differential effects of left and right cerebral lesions in human adults. *J Comp Physiol Psychol* 48:474–477, 1955.

Reite MZ, Anders TF, Greil W, Hellhammer D, Henn FA, Katz RJ, Kaufman IC, Kraemer GW, Linden M, McGuire MT, McKinney WT, Nissen G, Porsolt RD: Animal models: Group report. In: J Angst, ed: *The Origins of Depression: Current Concepts and Approaches.* Berlin: Springer-Verlag, 1983. pp 405–423.

Reiter RJ, King TS, Richardson BA, Hurlbut EC: Studies on pineal melatonin levels in a diurnal species, the eastern chipmunk (Tamias striatus): Effects of light at night, propranolol administration or superior cervical ganglionectomy. *J Neural Transm* 54:275–284, 1982.

Reitman F: *Psychotic Art.* London: Rutledge and Kegan Paul, 1950.

Rennie TAC: Prognosis in manic-depressive psychoses. *Am J Psychiatry* 98:801–814, 1942.

Reppert SM, Weaver DR, Rivkees SA, Stopa EG: Putative melatonin receptors in a human biological clock. *Science* 242:78–81, 1988.

Resnick HS, Oltmanns TF: Hesitation patterns in the speech of thought-disordered schizophrenic and manic patients. *J Abnorm Psychol* 93:80–86, 1984.

Reus VI: Behavioral aspects of thyroid disease in women. *Psychiatr Clin North Am* 12:153–165, 1989.

Reus VI, Silberman E, Post RM, Weingartner H: d-Amphetamine: Effects on memory in a depressed population. *Biol Psychiatry* 14:345–356, 1979a.

Reus VI, Targum SD, Weingartner H, Post RM: Effect of lithium carbonate on memory processes in bipolar affectively ill patients. *Psychopharmacology (Berlin)* 63:39–42, 1979b.

Reus VI, Joseph M, Dallman M: Regulation of ACTH and cortisol in depression. *Peptides* 4:785–788, 1983.

Reus VI, Peeke HV, Miner C: Habituation and cortisol dysregulation in depression. *Biol Psychiatry* 20:980–989, 1985.

Rey AC, Jimerson DC, Post RM: Lithium and electrolytes in cerebrospinal fluid of affectively ill patients during acute and chronic lithium treatment. *Commun Psychopharmacol* 3:267–278, 1979.

Reynolds CF, Kupfer DJ: Sleep research in affective illness: State of the art circa 1987. *Sleep* 10:199–215, 1987.

Reynolds CF, Gillin JC, Kupfer DJ: Sleep and affective disorders. In: HY Meltzer, ed: *Psychopharmacology: The Third Generation of Progress*. New York: Raven Press, 1987. pp 647–654.

Reynolds EH, Stramentinoli G: Folic acid, S-adenosylmethionine and affective disorder. *Psychol Med* 13:705–710, 1983.

Reynolds EH, Preece JM, Bailey J, Coppen A: Folate deficiency in depressive illness. *Br J Psychiatry* 117:287–292, 1970.

Rice J, McGuffin P, Goldin LR, Shaskan EG, Gershon ES: Platelet monoamine oxidase (MAO) activity: Evidence for a single major locus. *Am J Hum Genet* 36:36–43, 1984.

Rice JP, McDonald-Scott P, Endicott J, Coryell W, Grove WM, Keller MB, Altis D: The stability of diagnosis with an application to bipolar II disorder. *Psychiatry Res* 19:285–296, 1986.

Rice JP, Endicott J, Knesevich MA, Rochberg N: The estimation of diagnostic sensitivity using stability data: An application to major depressive disorder. *J Psychiat Res* 21:337–345, 1987a.

Rice JP, Reich T, Andreasen NC, Endicott J, Van Eerdewegh M, Fishman R, Hirschfeld RMA, Klerman GL: The familial transmission of bipolar illness. *Arch Gen Psychiatry* 44:441–447, 1987b.

Rich CL, Ricketts JE, Fowler RC, Young D: Some differences between men and women who commit suicide. *Am J Psychiatry* 145:718–722, 1988.

Richards RL: Relationships between creativity and psychopathology: An evaluation and interpretation of the evidence. *Genet Psychol Monogr* 103:261–324, 1981.

Richards RL, Kinney DK, Lunde I, Benet M, Merzel AP: Creativity in manic-depressives, cyclothymes, their normal relatives, and control subjects. *J Abnorm Psychol* 97:281–288, 1988.

Richelson E, Snyder K, Carlson J, Johnson M, Turner S, Lumry A, Boerwinkle E, Sing CF: Lithium ion transport by erythrocytes of randomly selected blood donors and manic-depressive patients: Lack of association with affective illness. *Am J Psychiatry* 143:457–462, 1986.

Rickels K, Gordon PE, Meckelnburg R, Sablosky I, Whalen EM, Dion H: Iprindole in neurotic depressed general practice patients: A controlled study. *Psychosomatics* 9:208–214, 1968.

Rickels K, Smith WT, Glaudin V, Amsterdam JB, Weise C, Settle GP: Comparison of two dosage regimens of fluoxetine in major depression. *J Clin Psychiatry* 46:38–41, 1985.

Rieder RO, Gershon ES: Genetic strategies in biological psychiatry. *Arch Gen Psychiatry* 35:866–873, 1978.

Rieder RO, Mann LS, Weinberger DR, Van Kammen DP, Post RM: Computed tomographic scans in patients with schizophrenia, schizoaffective, and bipolar affective disorder. *Arch Gen Psychiatry* 40:735–739, 1983.

Riegel CE, Dailey JW, Jobe PC: The genetically epilepsy-prone rat: An overview of the seizure-prone characteristics and responsiveness to anticonvulsant drugs. *Life Sci* 39:763–774, 1986.

Rigby J, Harvey M, Davies DR: Mania precipitated by benzodiazepine withdrawal. *Acta Psychiatr Scand* 79:406–407, 1989.

Rihmer Z, Arató M: ABO blood groups in manic-depressive patients. *J Affective Disord* 3:1–7, 1981.

Rihmer Z, Bagdy G, Arató M: Serum dopamine-beta-hydroxylase activity and family history of patients with bipolar manic-depressive illness. *Acta Psychiatr Scand* 68:140–141, 1983.

Rimon R, Halonen P: Herpes simplex virus infection and depressive illness. *Dis Nerv Syst* 30:338–340, 1969.

Rimon R, Halonen P, Anttinen E, Evola K: Complement fixing antibody to herpes simplex virus in patients with psychotic depression. *Dis Nerv Syst* 32:822–824, 1971.

Rimón R, Le Grevés P, Nyberg F, Heikkilä L, Salmela L, Terenius L: Elevation of substance P-like peptides in the CSF of psychiatric patients. *Biol Psychiatry* 19:509–516, 1984.

Ringel E: Der Selbstmörd, Abschluss einer krankhaften psychischen Entwicklung: Eine Untersuchung an 745 geretteten Selbstmörden. Wein: W Maudrich, 1953.

Rinieris PM, Stefanis CN, Lykouras EP, Varsou EK: Affective disorders and ABO blood types. *Acta Psychiatr Scand* 60:272–278, 1979.

Risch N, Baron M: X-linkage and genetic heterogeneity in bipolar-related major affective illness: Reanalysis of linkage data. *Ann Hum Genet* 46:153–166, 1982.

Risch N, Baron M, Mendlewicz J: Assessing the role

of X-linked inheritance in bipolar-related major affective disorder. *J Psychiat Res* 20:275–288, 1986.

Risch SC, Janowsky DS: Cholinergic-adrenergic balance in affective illness. In: RM Post, JC Ballenger, ed: *Neurobiology of Mood Disorders*. Baltimore: Williams & Wilkins, 1984. pp 652–663.

Risch SC, Cohen RM, Janowsky DS, Kalin NH, Murphy DL: Mood and behavioral effects of physostigmine on humans are accompanied by elevations in plasma beta-endorphin and cortisol. *Science* 209:1545–1546, 1980.

Risch SC, Cohen RM, Janowsky DS, Kalin NH, Sitaram N, Gillin JC, Murphy DL: Physostigmine induction of depressive symptomatology in normal human subjects. *Psychiatry Res* 4:89–94, 1981a.

Risch SC, Kalin NH, Janowsky DS: Cholinergic challenges in affective illness: Behavioral and neuroendocrine correlates. *J Clin Psychopharm* 1:186–192, 1981b.

Risch SC, Janowsky DS, Judd LL, Huey LY: Elevated plasma beta-endorphin concentrations in depression and cholinergically supersensitive release mechanisms. *Psychopharmacol Bull* 18:211–216, 1982a.

Risch SC, Janowsky DS, Siever LJ, Judd LL, Rausch JL, Huey LY, Beckman KA, Cohen RM, Murphy DL: Cholinomimetic-induced co-release of prolactin and beta-endorphin in man. *Psychopharmacol Bull* 18:21–25, 1982b.

Risch SC, Janowsky DS, Gillin JC: Muscarinic supersensitivity of anterior pituitary ACTH and B-endorphin release in major depressive illness. *Peptides* 4:789–792, 1983a.

Risch SC, Kalin NH, Janowsky DS, Cohen RM, Pickar D, Murphy DL: Co-release of ACTH and beta-endorphin immunoreactivity in human subjects in response to central cholinergic stimulation. *Science* 222:77, 1983b.

Rizzo ND, Fox HM, Laidlaw JC, Thorn GW: Concurrent observations of behavior changes and of adrenocortical variations in a cyclothymic patient during a period of 12 months. *Ann Int Med* 41:798–815, 1954.

Rizzo PA, Amabile G, Caporali M, Pierelli F, Spadaro M, Zanasi M, Morocutti C: A longitudinal CNV study in a group of five bipolar cyclothymic patients. *Biol Psychiatry* 14:581–586, 1979.

Robbins TW, Sahakian BJ: Animal models of mania. In: RH Belmaker, HM Van Praag, eds: *Mania: An Evolving Concept*. Jamaica, NY: Spectrum Publications, 1980. pp 143–216.

Roberts BH, Myers JK: Religion, national origin, immigration, and mental illness. *Am J Psychiatry* 110:759–764, 1954.

Roberts MA, Attah JR: Carbamazepine and ECT. *Br J Psychiatry* 153:418, 1988.

Robertson G, Taylor PJ: Some cognitive correlates of affective disorders. *Psychol Med* 15:297–309, 1985.

Robertson MM, Trimble MR: Depressive illness in patients with epilepsy: A review. *Epilepsia* 24(Suppl 2):S109–S116, 1983.

Robins E, Guze SB: Establishment of diagnostic validity in psychiatric illness: Its application to schizophrenia. *Am J Psychiatry* 126:983–987, 1970.

Robins E, Guze SB: Classification of affective disorders: The primary-secondary, the endogenous-reactive, and the neurotic-psychotic concepts. In: TA Williams, MM Katz, JA Shield Jr, eds: *Recent Advances in the Psychobiology of the Depressive Illnesses*. Washington, DC: US Government Printing Office, 1972. pp 283–293.

Robins E, Gassner S, Kayes J, Wilkinson RH, Murphy GE: The communication of suicidal intent: A study of 134 consecutive cases of successful (completed) suicide. *Am J Psychiatry* 115:724–733, 1959a.

Robins E, Murphy GE, Wilkinson RH, Gassner S, Kayes J: Some clinical considerations in the prevention of suicide based on a study of 134 successful suicides. *Am J Public Health* 49:888–899, 1959b.

Robins E, Gentry KA, Munoz RA, Marten S: A contrast of the three more common illnesses with the ten less common in a study and 18-month follow-up of 314 psychiatric emergency room patients II: Characteristics of patients with the three more common illnesses. *Arch Gen Psychiatry* 34:269–281, 1977.

Robins LN: Epidemiology: Reflections on testing the validity of psychiatric interviews. *Arch Gen Psychiatry* 42:918–924, 1985.

Robins LN, Helzer J, Croughan J: *Renard Diagnostic Interview*. St Louis, Mo: Washington University Medical School, 1977.

Robins LN, Helzer JE, Croughan J, Williams JBW, Spitzer RL: *The NIMH Diagnostic Interview Schedule: Version II*. Rockville, MD: Center for Epidemiologic Studies, NIMH, 1979.

Robins LN, Helzer JE, Croughan J, Ratcliff KS: National Institute of Mental Health Diagnostic Interview Schedule: Its history, characteristics, and validity. *Arch Gen Psychiatry* 38:381–389, 1981.

Robins LN, Helzer JE, Weissman MM, Orvaschel H, Gruenberg E, Burke JD Jr, Regier DA: Lifetime prevalence of specific psychiatric disorders in three sites. *Arch Gen Psychiatry* 41:949–958, 1984.

Robinson RG: Investigating mood disorders following brain injury: An integrative approach using clinical and laboratory studies. *Integr Psychiatry* 1:35–40, 1983.

Robinson RG, Szetela B: Mood change following left hemispheric brain injury. *Ann Neurol* 9:447–453, 1981.

Robinson RG, Kubos KL, Starr LB, Rao K, Price TR: Mood disorders in stroke patients: Importance of location of lesion. *Brain* 107:81–93, 1984.

Robinson RG, Starr LB, Lipsey JR, Rao K, Price TR: A two-year longitudinal study of poststroke mood disorders: In-hospital prognostic factors associated with six-month outcome. *J Nerv Ment Dis* 173:221–226, 1985.

Robinson RG, Lipsey JR, Rao K, Price TR: Two-year longitudinal study of post-stroke mood disorders: Comparison of acute-onset with delayed-onset depression. *Am J Psychiatry* 143:1238–1244, 1986.

Robinson RG, Boston JD, Starkstein SE, Price TR: Comparison of mania and depression after brain injury: Causal factors. *Am J Psychiatry* 145:172–178, 1988a.

Robinson RG, Starkstein SE, Price TR: Post-stroke depression and lesion location. *Stroke* 19:125–126, 1988b.

Roccatagliata G: *A History of Ancient Psychiatry*. New York: Greenwood Press, 1986.

Roe A: The personality of artists. *Educat Psychol Measurement* 6:401–408, 1946.

Roe A: A psychological study of eminent biologists. *Psychol Monogr* 65:1–68, 1951.

Roe A: A psychologist examines sixty-four eminent scientists. *Sci Am* 187:21–25, 1952.

Roos BE, Sjöström R: 5-hydroxyindoleacetic acid (and homovanillic acid) levels in the cerebrospinal fluid after probenecid application in patients with manic-depressive psychosis. *Pharmacologia Clinica* 1:153–155, 1969.

Roose SP, Glassman AH: Delusional depression. In: A Georgotas, R Cancro, eds: *Depression and Mania*. New York: Elsevier, 1988. pp 76–85.

Roose SP, Bone S, Haidorfer C, Dunner DL, Fieve RR: Lithium treatment in older patients. *Am J Psychiatry* 136:843–844, 1979.

Roose SP, Glassman AH, Walsh BT, Woodring S, Vital-Herne J: Depression, delusions, and suicide. *Am J Psychiatry* 140:1159–1162, 1983.

Rorschach H: *Psychodiagnostics: A Diagnostic Test Based on Perception, Including Rorschach's Paper, The Application of the Form Interpretation Test.* (Pub posthumously by E Oberholzer). Trans & English ed. by P Lemkau and B Kronenberg. 3rd ed. Berne: Hans Huber, 1942.

Rosanoff AJ, Handy LH, Plesset IR: The etiology of manic-depressive syndromes with special reference to their occurrence in twins. *Am J Psychiatry* 91:725–740, 1935.

Rose RM, Burt RA, Clayton PJ, Frances A, Friedhoff AJ, Jamison KJ, Janowsky DS, Leff J, Leppick IE, Withrow RP: Consensus Development Conference Statement: Electroconvulsive theapy. *JAMA* 254:2103–2108, 1985.

Rosen AM: Group management of lithium prophylaxis. Abstract of a paper presented at the annual meeting of the American Psychiatric Association, May, 1980.

Rosen AM, Mukherjee S: Long-term lithium outcome and compliance in a community mental health center. Submitted to *Arch Gen Psychiatry*.

Rosen LN, Rosenthal NE, Dunner DL, Fieve RR: Social outcome compared in psychotic and nonpsychotic bipolar I patients. *J Nerv Ment Dis* 171:272–275, 1983a.

Rosen LN, Rosenthal NE, VanDusen PH, Dunner DL, Fieve RR: Age at onset and number of psychotic symptoms in bipolar I and schizoaffective disorder. *Am J Psychiatry* 140:1523–1524, 1983b.

Rosenbaum AH, Barry MJ: Positive therapeutic response to lithium in hypomania secondary to organic brain syndrome. *Am J Psychiatry* 132:1072–1073, 1975.

Rosenberg JD: *The Darkening Glass: A Portrait of Ruskin's Genius*. New York: Columbia University Press, 1986.

Rosenberg JG, Binder RL, Berlant J: Prediction of therapeutic lithium dose: Comparison and improvement of current methods. *J Clin Psychiatry* 48:284–286, 1987.

Rosenblatt S, Gaull GE, Chanley JD, Rosenthal JS, Smith H, Sarkozi L: Amino acids in bipolar affective disorders: Increased glycine levels in erythrocytes. *Am J Psychiatry* 136:672–674, 1979.

Rosenfeld H: Notes on the psychopathology and psychoanalytic treatment of depressive and manic depressive patients. In: H Azima, BC Glueck, eds: *Psychiatric Res Report 17*. Washington, DC: The American Psychiatric Association, 1963. pp 73–83.

Rosenhan DL: On being sane in insane places. *Science* 179:250–258, 1973.

Rosenthal D, Kety SS, eds: *The Transmission of Schizophrenia: Proceedings of the Second Research Conference of the Foundation's Fund for Research in Psychiatry*. Oxford: Pergamon Press, 1968.

Rosenthal J, Strauss A, Minikoff L, Winston A: Identifying lithium-responsive bipolar depressed patients using nuclear magnetic resonance. *Am J Psychiatry* 143:779–780, 1986.

Rosenthal NE, Wehr TA: Seasonal affective disorders. *Psychiatr Ann* 17:670–674, 1987.

Rosenthal NE, Rosenthal LN, Stallone F, Fleiss J, Dunner DL, Fieve RR: Psychosis as a predictor of response to lithium maintenance treatment in bipolar affective disorder. *J Affective Disord* 1:237–245, 1979.

Rosenthal NE, Davenport Y, Cowdry RW, Webster MH, Goodwin FK: Monoamine metabolites in cerebrospinal fluid of depressive subgroups. *Psychiatry Res* 2:113–119, 1980a.

Rosenthal NE, Rosenthal LN, Stallone F, Dunner DL, Fieve RR: Toward the validation of RDC schizoaffective disorder. *Arch Gen Psychiatry* 37:804–810, 1980b.

Rosenthal NE, Lewy AJ, Wehr TA, Kern HE, Goodwin FK: Seasonal cycling in a bipolar patient. *Psychiatry Res* 8:25–31, 1983.

Rosenthal NE, Sack DA, Gillin JC, Lewy AJ, Goodwin FK, Davenport Y, Mueller PS, Newsome DA, Wehr TA: Seasonal affective disorder: A description of the syndrome and preliminary findings with light therapy. *Arch Gen Psychiatry* 41:72–80, 1984.

Rosenthal NE, Sack DA, Carpenter CJ, Parry BL, Mendelson WB, Wehr TA: Antidepressant effects of light in seasonal affective disorder. *Am J Psychiatry* 142:163–170, 1985a.

Rosenthal NE, Sack DA, James SP, Parry BL, Mendelson WB, Tamarkin L, Wehr TA: Seasonal affective disorder and phototherapy. *Ann NY Acad Sci* 453:260–269, 1985b.

Rosenthal NE, Carpenter CJ, James SP, Parry BL, Rogers SLB, Wehr TA: Seasonal affective disorder in children and adolescents. *Am J Psychiatry* 143:356–358, 1986a.

Rosenthal NE, Sack DA, Jacobsen FM, James SP, Parry BL, Arendt J, Tamarkin L, Wehr TA: Melatonin in seasonal affective disorder and phototherapy. *J Neural Transm* (Suppl 21):257–267, 1986b.

Rosenthal NE, Skwerer RG, Sack DA, Duncan CC, Jacobsen FM, Tamarkin L, Wehr TA: Biological effects of morning-plus-evening bright light treatment of seasonal affective disorder. *Psychopharmacol Bull* 23:364–369, 1987.

Rosenthal NE, Jacobsen FM, Sack DA, Arendt J, James SP, Parry BL, Wehr TA: Atenolol in seasonal affective disorder: A test of the melatonin hypothesis. *Am J Psychiatry* 145:52–56, 1988.

Rosenthal NE, Kasper S, Schulz PM, Wehr TA: New concepts and developments in seasonal affective disorder. In: C Thompson, T Silverstone, eds: *Seasonal Affective Disorder*. London: CRC Clinical Neuroscience, in press.

Rosenwasser AM, Adler NT: Structure and function in circadian timing systems: Evidence for multiple coupled circadian oscillators. *Neurosci Biobehav Rev* 10:431–448, 1986.

Ross HE, Glaser FB, Germanson T: The prevalence of psychiatric disorders in patients with alcohol and other drug problems. *Arch Gen Psychiatry* 45:1023–1031, 1988.

Rossi GJ, Rosadini G: Experimental analysis of cerebral dominance in man. In: FL Darley, ed: *Brain Mechanisms Underlying Speech and Language*. New York: Grune and Stratton, 1967. pp 167–184.

Rossi PH, Wright JD, Fisher GA, Willis G: The urban homeless: Estimating composition and size. *Science* 235:1336–1341, 1987.

Roth M: The natural history of mental disorder in old age. *J Ment Sci* 101:281–301, 1955.

Roth M: Depression and affective disorder in later life. In: J Angst, ed: *The Origins of Depression: Current Concepts and Approaches*. Dahlem Konferenzen. Berlin: Springer-Verlag, 1983. pp 39–75.

Roth M, Barnes TRE: The classification of affective disorders: A synthesis of old and new concepts. *Compr Psychiatry* 22:54–77, 1981.

Roth M, Gurney C, Mountjoy CQ: The Newcastle Rating Scales. In: P Pichot, P Berner, R Wolf, K Thau, eds: *Psychiatry: The State of the Art. Vol. 1: Clinical Psychopathology, Nomenclature and Classification*. New York: Plenum, 1985. pp 643–648.

Rothschild AJ: Mania after withdrawal of isocarboxazid. *J Clin Psychopharmacol* 5:340–342, 1985.

Rothschild AJ, Schatzberg AF, Rosenbaum AH, Stahl JB, Cole JO: The dexamethasone suppression test as a discriminator among subtypes of psychotic patients. *Br J Psychiatry* 141:471–474, 1982.

Rotrosen J, Angrist BM, Gershon S, Sachar EJ, Halpern FS: Dopamine receptor alteration in schizophrenia: Neuroendocrine evidence. *Psychopharmacology* 51:1–7, 1976.

Rottanburg D, Robins AH, Ben-Arie O, Teggin A, Elk

R: Cannabis-associated psychosis with hypomanic features. *Lancet* 2:1364–1366, 1982.

Rotter JI, Rimoin DL: Heterogeneity in diabetes mellitus—Update, 1978: Evidence for further genetic heterogeneity within juvenile-onset insulin-dependent diabetes mellitus. *J Am Diabetes Assoc* 27:599–608, 1978.

Rounsaville BJ, Klerman GL, Weissman MM: Do psychotherapy and pharmacotherapy for depression conflict? Empirical evidence from a clinical trial. *Arch Gen Psychiatry* 38:24–29, 1981.

Rounsaville BJ, Weissman MM, Kleber H, Wilber C: Heterogeneity of psychiatric diagnosis in treated opiate addicts. *Arch Gen Psychiatry* 39:161–166, 1982.

Rowe CJ, Daggett DR: Prepsychotic personality traits in manic depressive disease. *J Nerv Ment Dis* 119:412–420, 1954.

Rowitz L, Levy L: Ecological analysis of treated mental disorders in Chicago. *Arch Gen Psychiatry* 19:571–579, 1968.

Rowntree DW, Neven S, Wilson A: The effect of diisopropylfluorophosphonate in schizophrenia and manic depressive psychosis. *J Neurol Neurosurg Psychiatry* 13:47–62, 1950.

Rowse AL: *The Early Churchills*. Middlesex: Penguin Books, 1969.

Roy A: Risk factors for suicide in psychiatric patients. *Arch Gen Psychiatry* 39:1089–1095, 1982.

Roy A: Family history of suicide. *Arch Gen Psychiatry* 40:971–974, 1983.

Roy A: Plasma HVA levels in depressed patients and controls. *J Affective Disord* 14:293–296, 1988.

Roy A, Breier A, Doran AR, Pickar D: Life events in depression. *J Affective Disord* 9:143–148, 1985a.

Roy A, Pickar D, Linnoila M, Doran AR, Ninan P, Paul SM: Cerebrospinal fluid monoamine and monoamine metabolite concentrations in melancholia. *Psychiatry Res* 15:281–292, 1985b.

Roy A, Pickar D, Linnoila M, Potter WZ: Plasma norepinephrine level in affective disorders: Relationship to melancholia. *Arch Gen Psychiatry* 42:1181–1185, 1985c.

Roy A, Jimerson DC, Pickar D: Plasma MHPG in depressive disorders and relationship to the dexamethasone suppression test. *Am J Psychiatry* 143:846–851, 1986.

Roy A, Everett D, Pickar D, Paul SM: Platelet tritiated imipramine binding and serotonin uptake in depressed patients and controls. *Arch Gen Psychiatry* 44:320–327, 1987a.

Roy A, Guthrie S, Pickar D, Linnoila M: Plasma norepinephrine responses to cold challenge in depressed patients and normal controls. *Psychiatry Res* 21:161–168, 1987b.

Roy A, Pickar D, Paul S, Doran A, Chrousos GP, Gold PW: CSF corticotropin-releasing hormone in depressed patients and normal control subjects. *Am J Psychiatry* 144:641–645, 1987c.

Roy A, DeJong J, Linnoila M: Cerebrospinal fluid monoamine metabolites and suicidal behavior in depressed patients: A 5-year follow-up study. *Arch Gen Psychiatry* 46:609–612, 1989.

Roy-Byrne P, Post RM, Rubinow DR, Linnoila M, Savard R, Davis D: CSF 5HIAA and personal and family history of suicide in affectively ill patients: A negative study. *Psychiatry Res* 10:263–274, 1983.

Roy-Byrne P, Uhde TW, Post RM, Joffe RT: Relationship of response to sleep deprivation and carbamazepine in depressed patients. *Acta Psychiatr Scand* 69:379–382, 1984.

Roy-Byrne P, Post RM, Uhde TW, Porcu T, Davis D: The longitudinal course of recurrent affective illness: Life chart data from research patients at the NIMH. *Acta Psychiatr Scand* 71(Suppl 317):1–34, 1985a.

Roy-Byrne PP, Uhde TW, Gold PW, Rubinow DR, Post RM: Neuroendocrine abnormalities in panic disorder. *Psychopharmacol Bull* 21:546–550, 1985b.

Roy-Byrne PP, Weingartner H, Bierer LM, Thompson K, Post RM: Effortful and automatic cognitive processes in depression. *Arch Gen Psychiatry* 43:265–267, 1986.

Roy-Byrne PP, Post RM, Hambrick DD, Leverich GS, Rosoff AS: Suicide and course of illness in major affective disorder. *J Affective Disord* 15:1–8, 1988a.

Roy-Byrne PP, Post RM, Kellner CH, Joffe RT, Uhde TW: Ventricular-brain ratio and life course of illness in patients with affective disorder. *Psychiatry Res* 23:277–284, 1988b.

RS: Pill-Consciousness. *Alcoholics Anonymous Grapevine*. Dec. 1981.

Rubin RT: Multiple biochemical correlates of manic-depressive illness. *J Psychosom Res* 12:171–180, 1968.

Rubin RT: Sex steroid hormone dynamics in endogenous depression: A review. *Int J Ment Health* 10:43–59, 1981.

Rubin RT, Mandell AJ: Adrenal cortical activity in pathological emotional states: A review. *Am J Psychiatry* 123:387–400, 1966.

Rubin RT, Poland RE, Lesser IM, Winston RA, Blodgett AL: Neuroendocrine aspects of primary endogenous depression: I. Cortisol secretory dynamics in patients and matched controls. *Arch Gen Psychiatry* 44:328–336, 1987.

Rubinow DR: Cerebrospinal fluid somatostatin and psychiatric illness. *Biol Psychiatry* 21:341–365, 1986.

Rubinow DR, Gold PW, Post RM, Ballenger JC, Cowdry R, Bollinger J, Reichlin S: CSF somatostatin in affective illness. *Arch Gen Psychiatry* 40:409–12, 1983.

Rubinow DR, Post RM, Gold PW, Ballenger JC, Wolff EA: The relationship between cortisol and clinical phenomenology of affective illness. In: RM Post, JC Ballenger, eds: *Neurobiology of Mood Disorders*. Baltimore: Williams & Wilkins, 1984a. pp 271–289.

Rubinow DR, Post RM, Savard R, Gold PW: Cortisol hypersecretion and cognitive impairment in depression. *Arch Gen Psychiatry* 41:279–283, 1984b.

Rudorfer MV, Linnoila M: Electroconvulsive therapy. In: FN Johnson, ed: *Lithium Therapy Monographs. Vol I: Lithium Combination Treatment*. Basel, Switzerland: Karger, 1986. pp 164–178.

Rudorfer MV, Karoum F, Ross RJ, Potter WZ, Linnoila M: Differences in lithium effects in depressed and healthy subjects. *Clin Pharmacol Ther* 37:66–71, 1985a.

Rudorfer MV, Ross RJ, Linnoila M, Sherer MA, Potter WZ: Exaggerated orthostatic responsivity of plasma norepinephrine in depression. *Arch Gen Psychiatry* 42:1186–1192, 1985b.

Ruestow P, Dunner DL, Bleecker B, Fieve RR: Marital adjustment in primary affective disorder. *Compr Psychiatry* 19:565–571, 1978.

Ruff MR, Sacerdote P, Wiedermann CJ, Pert CB: Neuropeptide receptors are shared components of nervous and immune systems. In: Y Taché, JE Morley, MR Brown, eds: *Neuropeptides and Stress*. New York: Springer-Verlag, 1989.

Runeson B: Mental disorder in youth suicide: DSM-III-R Axes I and II. *Acta Psychiatr Scand* 79:490–497, 1989.

Rusak B, Zucker I: Neural regulation of circadian rhythms. *Physiological Reports* 59:449–526, 1979.

Rush AJ, Schlesser MA, Stokely E, Bonte FR, Altshuller KZ: Cerebral blood flow in depression and mania. *Psychopharmacol Bull* 18:6–8, 1982.

Rush AJ, Schlesser MA, Erman M, Fairchild C: Alprazolam in bipolar-I depressions. *Pharmacotherapy* 4:40–42, 1984.

Rush AJ, Erman MK, Giles DE, Schlesser MA, Carpenter G, Vasavada N, Roffwarg HP: Polysomnographic findings in recently drug-free and clinically remitted depressed patients. *Arch Gen Psychiatry* 43:878–884, 1986a.

Rush AJ, Giles DE, Schlesser MA, Fulton CL, Weissenburger J, Burns C: The Inventory for Depressive Symptomatology (IDS): Preliminary findings. *Psychiatry Res* 18:65–87, 1986b.

Rush B: *Medical Inquiries and Observations Upon the Diseases of the Mind*. Philadelphia: Kimber and Richardson, 1812.

Ruskin J: Mr. Ruskin's illness as described by himself. *Br Med J* 1:225–226, 1900.

Russell GF: Body weight and balance of water, sodium and potassium in depressed patients given electroconvulsive therapy. *Clin Sci* 19:327–336, 1960.

Russell M: The epidemiology of alcoholism. In: NJ Estes, ME Heinemann, eds: *Alcoholism: Development, Consequences, and Interventions*. St. Louis: CV Mosby Co, 1986. pp 31–52.

Rutter M: *Children of Sick Parents: An Environmental and Psychiatric Study*. London: Oxford University Press, 1966.

Rutter M: Childhood schizophrenia reconsidered. *J Autism Childhood Schizophr* 2:315–337, 1972.

Ryan ND, Puig-Antich J: Affective illness in adolescence. In: RE Hales, AJ Frances, eds: *American Psychiatric Association Annual Review, Vol 5*. Washington, DC: American Psychiatric Press, 1986. pp 420–450.

Ryan ND, Puig-Antich J: Pharmacological treatment of adolescent psychiatric disorders. *J Adolesc Health Care* 8:137–142, 1987.

Ryan ND, Puig-Antich J, Ambrosini P, Rabinovich H, Robinson D, Nelson B, Iyengar S, Twomey J: The clinical picture of major depression in children and adolescents. *Arch Gen Psychiatry* 44:854–861, 1987.

Ryback RS, Schwab RS: Manic response to levodopa therapy: Report of a case. *N Engl J Med* 285:788–789, 1971.

Rybakowski J, Chlopocka M, Kapelski Z, Hernacka B, Szajnerman Z, Kasprzak K: Red blood cell lithium index in patients with affective disorders in the course of lithium prophylaxis. *Int Pharmacopsychiatry* 9:166–171, 1974.

Rybakowski J, Frazer A, Mendels J, Ramsey TA: Erythrocyte accumulation of the lithium ion in control subjects and patients with primary affective disorder. *Commun Psychopharmacol* 2:99–104, 1978.

Rybakowski J, Chtopocka-Wozniak M, Kapelski Z, Strzyzewski W: The relative prophylactic efficacy of lithium against mania and depressive recurrences in bipolar patients. *Int Pharmacopsychiatry* 15:86–90, 1980.

Rybakowski J, Potok E, Strzyzewski W: Erythrocyte membrane adenosine triphosphatase activities in patients with endogenous depression and healthy subjects. *Eur J Clin Invest* 11:61–64, 1981.

Rzewuska M, Angst J: Prognosis of periodic bipolar manic depressive and schizo-affective psychoses: A comparison of two studies. *Arch Psychiatr Neurolog Sci* 231:471–486, 1982.

Sabelli HC, Borison RL, Diamond BI, Havdala HS, Narasimhachari N: Phenylethylamine and brain function. *Biochem Pharmacol* 27:1707–1711, 1978.

Sabelli HC, Fawcett J, Gusovsky F, Javaid JI, Wynn P, Edwards J, Jeffriess H, Kravitz H: Clinical studies on the phenylethylamine hypothesis of affective disorder: Urine and blood phenylacetic acid and phenylalanine dietary supplements. *J Clin Psychiatry* 47:66–70, 1986.

Sacchetti E, Vita A, Conte G, Pennati A, Alciati A, Calzerone A, Invernizzi G, Cazzullo CL: Cerebral ventricular size and clinical response to lithium prophylaxis in major affective disorder. *Int J Neurosci* 32:51, 1987.

Sachar EJ, Mushrush G, Perlow M, Weitzman ED, Sassin J: Growth hormone responses to L-dopa in depressed patients. *Science* 178:1304–1305, 1972.

Sachar EJ, Frantz AG, Altman N, Sassin J: Growth hormone and prolactin in unipolar and bipolar depressed patients: Responses to hypoglycemia and L-dopa. *Am J Psychiatry* 130:1362–1367, 1973a.

Sachar EJ, Hellman L, Roffwarg HP, Halpern FS, Fukushima DK, Gallagher TF: Disrupted 24-hour patterns of cortisol secretion in psychotic depression. *Arch Gen Psychiatry* 28:19–24, 1973b.

Sachdev P, Smith JS, Matheson J: Psychosurgery for bipolar affective disorder. *Br J Psychiatry* 153:576, 1988.

Sachs GS: Adjuncts and alternatives to lithium therapy. Abstract of paper presented at the 142nd annual meeting of the American Psychiatric Association, 1989.

Sack DA, Nurnberger J, Rosenthal NE, Ashburn E, Wehr TA: The potentiation of antidepressant medications by phase advance of the sleep-wake cycle. *Am J Psychiatry* 142:606–608, 1985.

Sack DA, Rosenthal NE, Perry BL, Wehr TA: Biological rhythms in psychiatry. In: HY Meltzer, ed: *Psychopharmacology: The Third Generation of Progress*. New York: Raven Press, 1987. pp 669–685.

Sack DA, Duncan W, Rosenthal NE, Mendelson WE, Wehr TA: The timing and duration of sleep in partial sleep deprivation therapy of depression. *Acta Psychiatr Scand* 77:219–224, 1988a.

Sack DA, James SP, Rosenthal NE, Wehr TA: Deficient nocturnal surge of TSH secretion during sleep and sleep deprivation in rapid-cycling bipolar illness. *Psychiatry Res* 23:179–191, 1988b.

Sack RL, Lewy AJ: Desmethylimipramine treatment increases melatonin production in humans. *Biol Psychiatry* 21:406–410, 1986.

Sackeim HA, Steif BL: Neuropsychology of depression and mania. In: A Georgotas and R Cancro, eds: *Depression and Mania*. New York: Elsevier, 1988. pp 265–289.

Sackeim HA, Greenberg MS, Weiman AL, Gur RC, Hungerbuhler JP, Geschwind N: Hemispheric asymmetry in the expression of positive and negative emotions: Neurologic evidence. *Arch Neurol* 39:210–218, 1982.

Sackeim HA, Prohovnik I, Apter S, Lucas L, Decina P, Mukherjee S, Prudic J, Malitz S: Regional cerebral blood flow in affective disorders: Relations to phenomenology and effects of treatment. In: R Takahashi, P Flor-Henry, J Gruzelier, S Niwa, eds: *Cerebral Dynamics, Laterality, and Psychopathology*. New York: Elsevier Science Publishing Co, 1987. pp 477–492.

Sackett DL, Haynes RB, Tugwell P: *Clinical Epidemiology: A Basic Science for Clinical Medicine*. Boston: Little, Brown & Company, 1985.

Safer DJ: Substance abuse by young adult chronic patients. *Hosp Community Psychiatry* 38:511–514, 1987.

Saffer D, Coppen A: Frusemide: A safe diuretic during lithium therapy? *J Affective Disord* 5:289–292, 1983.

Samiy AH, Rosnick PB: Early identification of renal problems in patients receiving chronic lithium treatment. *Am J Psychiatry* 144:670–672, 1987.

Sandler M, Ruthven CR, Goodwin BL, Coppen A:

Decreased cerebrospinal fluid concentration of free phenylacetic acid in depressive illness. *Clin Chim Acta* 93:169–171, 1979a.

Sandler M, Ruthven CR, Goodwin BL, Reynolds GP, Rao VA, Coppen A: Deficient production of tyramine and octopamine in cases of depression. *Nature* 278:357–358, 1979b.

Sandler M, Bonham-Carter SM, Walker PL: Tyramine conjugation deficit as a trait-marker in depression. *Psychopharmacol Bull* 19:501–502, 1983.

Sansone MEG, Ziegler DK: Lithium toxicity: A review of neurologic complications. *Clin Neuropharmacol* 8:242–248, 1985.

Santella RN, Rimmer JM, MacPherson BR: Focal segmental glomerulosclerosis in patients receiving lithium carbonate. *Am J Med* 84:951–954, 1988.

Santos AB, Morton WA: More on clonazepam in manic agitation. *J Clin Psychopharmacol* 7:439–440, 1987.

Sapin LR, Berrettini WH, Nurnberger JI, Rothblat LA: Mediational factors underlying cognitive changes and laterality in affective illness. *Biol Psychiatry* 22:979–986, 1987.

Sapolsky RM, Krey LC, McEwen BS: Stress down-regulates corticosterone receptors in a site-specific manner in the brain. *Endocrinology* 114:287–292, 1984.

Saran BM: The course of recurrent depressive illness in selected patients from a defined population. *Int Pharmacopsychiatry* 5:119–131, 1970.

Sarantidis D, Waters B: A review and controlled study of cutaneous conditions associated with lithium carbonate. *Br J Psychiatry* 143:42–50, 1983.

Sargenti CJ, Rizos AL, Jeste DV: Psychotropic drug interactions in the patient with late-onset psychosis and mood disorder: Part 2. *Psychiatr Clin North Am* 11:235–252, 1988.

Sartorius N: Culture and the epidemiology of depression. *Psychiat Neurol Neurochir (Amst)* 76:479–487, 1973.

Sartorius N, Jablensky A: Towards a public health approach to depression. Abstracts, VI World Congress of Psychiatry, Honolulu, 1977.

Sashidharan SP, McGuire RJ: Recurrence of affective illness after withdrawal of long-term lithium treatment. *Acta Psychiatr Scand* 68:126–133, 1983.

Sashidharan SP, McGuire RJ, Glen AIM: Plasma lithium levels and therapeutic outcome in the prophylaxis of affective disorders: A restrospective study. *Br J Psychiatry* 140:619–622, 1982.

Satel SL, Gawin FH: Seasonal cocaine abuse. *Am J Psychiatry* 146:534–535, 1989.

Satel SL, Nelson JC: Stimulants in the treatment of depression: A critical overview. *J Clin Psychiatry* 50:241–249, 1989.

Satz P: Specific and nonspecific effects of brain lesions in man. *J Abnorm Psychol* 71:65–70, 1966.

Satz P, Richard W, Daniels A: The alteration of intellectual performance after lateralized brain-injury in man. *Psychonomic Sci* 7:369–370, 1967.

Saul RF, Hamburger HA, Selhorst JB: Pseudotumor cerebri secondary to lithium carbonate. *JAMA* 253:2869–2870, 1985.

Savage DD, Reigel CE, Jobe PC: The development of kindled seizures is accelerated in the genetically epilepsy-prone rat. *Life Sci* 39:879–886, 1986.

Savard RJ, Rey AC, Post RM: Halstead-Reitan Category Test in bipolar and unipolar affective disorders: Relationship to age and phase of illness. *J Nerv Ment Dis* 168:297–304, 1980.

Sayed AJ: Mania and bromism: A case report and a look to the future. *Am J Psychiatry* 133:228–229, 1976.

Schaefer A, Brown J, Watson CG, Plemel D, DeMotts J, Howard MT, Petrik N, Balleweg BJ, Anderson D: Comparison of the validities of the Beck, Zung, and MMPI depression scales. *J Consult Clin Psychol* 53:415–418, 1985.

Schaerf FW, Miller R, Pearlson GD, Kaminsky MJ, Weaver D: Manic syndrome associated with zidovudine. *JAMA* 260:3587–3588, 1988.

Schaffer CB, Mungas D, Rockwell E: Successful treatment of psychotic depression with carbamazepine. *J Clin Psychopharmacol* 5:233–235, 1985.

Schalling D, Edman G, Åsberg M: Impulsive cognitive style and inability to tolerate boredom: Psychobiological studies of temperamental vulnerability. In: M Zuckerman, ed: *Biological Bases of Sensation Seeking, Impulsivity and Anxiety.* Hillsdale, NJ: Lawrence Erlbaum Associates, 1983. pp 23–45.

Schatzberg AF, Samson JA, Bloomingdale KL, Orsulak PJ, Gerson B, Kizuka PP, Cole JO, Schildkraut JJ: Toward a biochemical classification of depressive disorders: X: Urinary catecholamines, their metabolites, and d-type scores in subgroups of depressive disorders. *Arch Gen Psychiatry* 46:260–268, 1989.

Schauffler RH: *Florestan: The Life and Work of Robert Schumann.* New York: Henry Holt & Co, 1945.

Schechter MD: Caffeine potentiation of apomorphine discrimination. *Pharmacol Biochem Behav* 13:307–309, 1980.

Scheinin H: Enhanced noradrenergic neuronal activity increases homovanillic acid levels in cerebrospinal fluid. *J Neurochem* 47:665–667, 1986.

Schiffer RB, Wineman NM, Weitkamp LR: Association between bipolar affective disorder and multiple sclerosis. *Am J Psychiatry* 143:94–95, 1986.

Schiffer RB, Weitkamp LR, Wineman NM, Guttormsen S: Multiple sclerosis and affective disorder: Family history, sex, and HLA-DR antigens. *Arch Neurol* 45:1345–1348, 1988.

Schildkraut J: The catecholamine hypothesis of affective disorder: A review of supporting evidence. *Am J Psychiatry* 122:509–522, 1965.

Schildkraut JJ, Keeler BA, Papousek M, Hartmann E: MHPG excretion in depressive disorders: Relation to clinical subtypes and desynchronized sleep. *Science* 181:762–764, 1973.

Schildkraut JJ, Orsulak PJ, LaBrie RA, Schatzberg

AF, Gudeman JE, Cole JO, Rohde WA: Toward a biochemical classification of depressive disorders: II. Application of multivariate discriminant function analysis to data on urinary catecholamines and metabolites. *Arch Gen Psychiatry* 35:1436–1439, 1978.

Schilgen B, Tölle R: Partial sleep deprivation as therapy for depression. *Arch Gen Psychiatry* 37:267–271, 1980.

Schlegel S, Kretzschmar K: Computed tomography in affective disorders: Part I. Ventricular and sulcal measurements. *Biol Psychiatry* 22:4–14, 1987a.

Schlegel S, Kretzschmar K: Computed tomography in affective disorders: Part II. Brain density. *Biol Psychiatry* 22:15–23, 1987b.

Schleifer SJ, Keller SE, Meyerson AT, Raskin MJ, Davis KL, Stein M: Lymphocyte function in major depressive disorder. *Arch Gen Psychiatry* 41:484–486, 1984.

Schleifer SJ, Keller SE, Siris SG, Davis KL, Stein M: Depression and immunity: Lymphocyte function in ambulatory depressed patients, hospitalized schizophrenic patients, and patients hospitalized for herniorrhaphy. *Arch Gen Psychiatry* 42:129–133, 1985.

Schmidt HO, Fonda CP: Rorschach scores in the manic state. *J Psychol* 38:427–437, 1954.

Schmidt U, Miller D: Two cases of hypomania in AIDS. *Br J Psychiatry* 152:839–842, 1988.

Schneider K: *Clinical Psychopathology.* Trans by MW Hamilton. New York: Grune and Stratton, Inc, 1959.

Schneider LS, Severson JA, Sloane RB: Platelet ^{3}H-imipramine binding in depressed elderly patients. *Biol Psychiatry* 20:1234–1237, 1985.

Schneider LS, Severson JA, Sloane B, Fredrickson ER: Decreased platelet ^{3}H-imipramine binding in primary major depression compared with depression secondary to medical illness in elderly outpatients. *J Affective Disord* 15:195–200, 1988.

Scholberg HA, Goodall E: The phosphorus and calcium content of the blood plasma and cerebrospinal fluid in the psychoses. *J Ment Sci* 72:51–74, 1926.

Scholem G: *Sabbatai Sevi: The Mystical Messiah (1626–1676).* Princeton: Princeton University Press, 1973.

Schorer CE: The rediscovery of Kraepelin. *J Operational Psychiatry* 13:73–75, 1982.

Schott A: Klinischer Beitrag zur Lehre von der chronischen Manie. *Monatsschrift für Psychiatrie und Neurologie* 15:1–19, 1904.

Schou M: Normothymotics, "mood-normalizers": Are lithium and the imipramine drugs specific for affective disorders? *Br J Psychiatry* 109:803–809, 1963.

Schou M: Lithium in psychiatric therapy and prophylaxis. *J Psychiatr Res* 6:67–95, 1968.

Schou M: Prophylactic lithium maintenance treatment in recurrent endogenous affective disorder. In: S Gershon, B Shopsin, eds: *Lithium: Its Role in Psychiatric Research and Treatment.* New York: Plenum Press, 1973. pp 269–294.

Schou M: What happened later to the lithium babies? A follow-up study of children born without malformations. *Acta Psychiatr Scand* 54:193–197, 1976.

Schou M: Lithium for the affective disorders: Cost and benefit. In: F Ayd, MA Taylor, eds: *Mood Disorders: The World's Major Public Health Problem.* Baltimore: Ayd Medical Communications, 1978. pp 117–137.

Schou M: Artistic productivity and lithium prophylaxis in manic-depressive illness. *Br J Psychiatry* 135:97–103, 1979a.

Schou M: Lithium as a prophylactic agent in unipolar affective illness: Comparison with cyclic antidepressants. *Arch Gen Psychiatry* 36:849–851, 1979b.

Schou M: Lithium prophylaxis: Is the honeymoon over? *Aust NZ J Psychiatry* 13:109–114, 1979c.

Schou M: Social and psychological implications of lithium therapy. In: FN Johnson, ed: *Handbook of Lithium Therapy.* Baltimore: University Park Press, 1980. pp 378–381.

Schou M: Problems of lithium prophylaxis: Efficacy, serum lithium, selection of patients. *Biblthca Psychiatr* 160:30–37, 1981.

Schou M: Long-lasting neurological sequelae after lithium intoxication. *Acta Psychiatr Scand* 70:594–602, 1984.

Schou M: Lithium prophylaxis: Myths and realities. *Am J Psychiatry* 146:573–576, 1989.

Schou M, Baastrup PC: Personal and social implications of lithium maintenance treatment. In: TA Ban, JR Boissier, GJ Gessa, H Heimann, L Hollister, HE Lehmann, I Munkvad, H Steinberg, F Sulser, A Sundwall, O Vinar, eds: *Psychopharmacology, Sexual Disorders and Drug Abuse.* Amsterdam and London: North-Holland Publishing Co, 1973. pp 65–68.

Schou M, Vestergaard P: Use of propranolol during lithium treatment: An enquiry and a suggestion. *Pharmacopsychiatr* 20:131, 1987.

Schou M, Weeke A: Did manic-depressive patients who committed suicide receive prophylactic or continuation treatment at the time? *Br J Psychiatry* 153:324–327, 1988.

Schou M, Weinstein MR: Problems of lithium maintenance treatment during pregnancy, delivery and lactation. *Agressologie* 21,A:7–9, 1980.

Schou M, Juel-Nielson N, Strömgren E, Voldby H: The treatment of manic psychoses by administration of lithium salts. *J Neurol Neurosurg Psychiatry* 17:250–260, 1954.

Schou M, Amidsen A, Eskjer JS, Olsen T: Occurrence of goitre during lithium treatment. *Br Med J* 3:710–713, 1968.

Schou M, Baastrup PC, Grof P, Weis P, Angst J: Pharmacological and clinical problems of lithium prophylaxis. *Br J Psychiatry* 116:615–619, 1970a.

Schou M, Thomsen K, Baastrup PC: Studies on the course of recurrent endogenous affective disorders.

Int Pharmacopsychiatry 5:100–106, 1970b.

Schou M, Amdisen A, Thomsen K, Vestergaard P, Hetmar O, Mellerup ET, Plenge P, Rafaelsen OJ: Lithium treatment regimen and renal water handling: The significance of dosage pattern and tablet type examined through comparison of results from two clinics with different treatment regimens. *Psychopharmacology (Berlin)* 77:387–90, 1982.

Schou M, Hansen HE, Thomsen K, Vestergaard P: Lithium treatment in Aarhus: 2. Risk of renal failure and of intoxication. *Pharmacopsychiatry* 22:101–103, 1989.

Schuckit MA: Alcoholism and other psychiatric disorders. *Hosp Commun Psychiatry* 34:1022–1027, 1983.

Schuckit MA: *Drug and Alcohol Abuse: Clinical Guide to Diagnosis and Treatment.* New York: Plenum Press, 1984.

Schuckit MA: Studies of populations at high risk for alcoholism. *Psychiatr Dev* 3:31–63, 1985.

Schuckit MA: Genetic and clinical implications of alcoholism and affective disorder. *Am J Psychiatry* 143:140–147, 1986.

Schuckit MA, Pitts FN, Reich T, King LJ, Winokur G: Alcoholism I: Two types of alcoholism in women. *Arch Gen Psychiatry* 20:301–306, 1969.

Schuckit MA, Robins E, Feighner J: Tricyclic antidepressants and monoamine oxidase inhibitors. *Arch Gen Psychiatry* 24:509–514, 1971.

Schulsinger F, Kety SS, Rosenthal D, Wender PH: A family study of suicide. In: M Schou, E Strömgren, eds: *Origin, Prevention, and Treatment of Affective Disorders.* London: Academic Press, 1979. pp 277–287.

Schulte W: Kombinierte psycho- und pharmakotherapie bei melancholikern. In: H Kranz, N Petrillowitsch, eds: *Probleme pharmakopsychiatrischer Kombinations und Langzeitbehandlungen.* Basel, Switzerland: Karger, 1966. pp 150–169.

Schulz B: Sterblichkeit endogen Geisteskranker und ihrer Eltern. *Ztschr Menschl Vererb Konstitutions Lehre* 29:338–367, 1949.

Schulz H, Lund R: Sleep onset REM episodes are associated with circadian parameters of body temperature: A study in depressed patients and normal controls. *Biol Psychiatry* 18:1411–1426, 1983.

Schulz H, Lund R: On the origin of early REM episodes in the sleep of depressed patients: A comparison of three hypotheses. *Psychiatry Res* 16:65–77, 1985.

Schumann RA: *The Letters of Robert Schumann.* Edited by K Storck. London: J Murray, 1907.

Schwab JJ, Bialow MR, Clemmons RS, Holzer CE: Hamilton rating scale for depression with medical in-patients. *Br J Psychiatry* 113:83–88, 1967.

Schwartz DA: Some suggestions for a unitary formulation of the manic-depressive reactions. *Psychiatry* 24:238–245, 1961.

Schwartz GE, For PL, Slat P, Mandel MR, Klerman GL: Facial muscle patterning to affective imagery in depressed and nondepressed subjects. *Science* 192:489–491, 1976.

Schwartz JC, Pollard H, Quach TT: Histamine as a neurotransmitter in mammalian brain: Neurochemical evidence. *J Neurochem* 35:26–33, 1980.

Schwartz JM, Baxter LR Jr, Mazziotta JC, Gerner RH, Phelps ME: The differential diagnosis of depression: Relevance of positron emission tomography studies of cerebral glucose metabolism to the bipolar-unipolar dichotomy. *JAMA* 258:1368–1374, 1987.

Schwartz RB: Manic psychosis in connection with Q fever. *Br J Psychiatry* 124:140–143, 1974.

Schweizer E, Dever A, Clary C: Suicide upon recovery from depression: A clinical note. *J Nerv Ment Dis* 176:633–636, 1988.

Scott M, Reading HW: A comparison of platelet membrane and erythrocyte adenosine triphosphatase specific activities in affective disorders. *Biochem Soc Transactions* 6:642–644, 1978.

Scott M, Reading HW, Loudon JB: Studies on human blood platelets in affective disorder. *Psychopharmacology (Berlin)* 60:131–135, 1979.

Scott ML, Golden CJ, Ruedrich SL, Bishop RJ: Ventricular enlargement in major depression. *Psychiatry Res* 8:91–93, 1983.

Seager CP: Controlled trial of straight and modified electroplexy. *J Ment Sci* 105:1022–1028, 1959.

Secunda SK, Katz MM, Swann A, Koslow SH, Maas JW, Chuang S, Croughan J: Mania: Diagnosis, state measurement and prediction of treatment response. *J Affective Disord* 8:113–121, 1985.

Secunda SK, Swann A, Katz MM, Koslow SH, Croughan J, Chang S: Diagnosis and treatment of mixed mania. *Am J Psychiatry* 144:96–98, 1987.

Sedivec V: [Effect of seasons of year on the development of pathological mood phases of affective melancholia.] *Ceskoslovenska Psychiatrie* 72:98–103, 1976.

Sedler MJ: Falret's discovery: The origin of the concept of bipolar affective illness. *Am J Psychiatry* 140:1127–1133, 1983.

Seggie J, Canny C, Mai F, McCrank E, Waring E: Antidepressant medication reverses increased sensitivity to light in depression: Preliminary report. *Prog Neuropsychopharmacol Biol Psychiatry* 13:537–541, 1989a.

Seggie J, Carney PA, Parker J, Grof E, Grof P: Effect of chronic lithium on sensitivity to light in male and female bipolar patients. *Prog Neuropsychopharmacol Biol Psychiatry* 13:543–549, 1989b.

Seligman MEP, Maier SF: Failure to escape traumatic shock. *J Exper Psychol* 74:1–9, 1967.

Selye H: The evolution of the stress concept. *Am Sci* 61:692–699, 1973.

Semba JI, Nankai M, Maruyama Y, Kaneno S, Watanabe A, Takahashi R: Increase in urinary β-phenylethylamine preceding the switch from mania to depression: A "rapid cycler." *J Nerv Ment Dis* 176:116–119, 1988.

Sengar DPS, Waters BGH, Dunne JV, Bouer IM: Lymphocyte subpopulations and mitogenic responses to lymphocytes in manic-depressive disorders. *Biol Psychiatry* 17:1017–1022, 1982.

Sengupta N, Datta SC, Sengupta D, Bal S: Platelet and erythrocyte-membrane adenosine triphosphatase activity in depressive and manic-depressive illness. *Psychiatry Res* 3:337–344, 1980.

Serry M: The lithium excretion test I: Clinical application and interpretation. *Aust NZ J Psychiatry* 3:390–394, 1969.

Sethy VH, Harris DW: Role of beta-adrenergic receptors in the mechanism of action of second-generation antidepressants. *Drug Dev Res* 2:403–406, 1982.

Settle EC, Settle GP: A case of mania associated with fluoxetine. *Am J Psychiatry* 141:280–281, 1984.

Sexton LG, Ames L, eds: *Anne Sexton: A Self-Portrait in Letters*. Boston: Houghton Mifflin, 1977.

Shagass C: EEG and evoked potentials in the psychoses. In: DX Freedman, ed: *Biology of the Major Psychoses: A Comparative Analysis*. Research Publications: Association for Research in Nervous and Mental Disease. Vol 54. New York: Raven Press, 1975. pp 101–127.

Shagass C, Amadeo M, Overton DA: Eye-tracking performance in psychiatric patients. *Biol Psychiatry* 9:245–260, 1974.

Shagass C, Roemer RA, Straumanis JJ Jr, Amadeo M: Topography of sensory evoked potentials in depressive disorders. *Biol Psychiatry* 15:183–207, 1980.

Shakir SA, Volkmar FR, Bacon S, Pfefferbaum A: Group psychotherapy as an adjunct to lithium maintenance. *Am J Psychiatry* 136:455–456, 1979.

Shan-Ming Y, Luxi X: Early- and late-onset bipolar affective disorder: A study of heterogeneity. *IRCS Med Sci* 13:328–329, 1985.

Shan-Ming Y, Deyi C, Zhen CY, Jingsu J, Taylor MA: Prevalence and characteristics of mania in Chinese inpatients: A prospective study. *Am J Psychiatry* 139:1150–1153, 1982.

Shan-Ming Y, Flor-Henry P, Dayi C, Tiangi L, Shuguang Q, Zenxiang M: Imbalance of hemispheric functions in the major psychoses: A study of handedness in the People's Republic of China. *Biol Psychiatry* 20:906–917, 1985.

Shapira B, Oppenheim G, Zohar J, Segal M, Malach D, Belmaker RH: Lack of efficacy of estrogen supplementation to imipramine in resistant female depressives. *Biol Psychiatry* 20:576–579, 1985.

Shapiro DR, Quitkin FM, Fleiss JL, Response to maintenance therapy in bipolar illness: Effect of index episode. *Arch Gen Psychiatry* 46:401–405, 1989.

Shapiro MB, Nelson EH: An investigation of the nature of cognitive impairment in co-operative psychiatric patients. *Br J Med Psychol* 28:239–256, 1955.

Shapiro RW, Rafaelsen OJ, Ryder LP, Svejgaard A, Sørensen H: ABO blood groups in unipolar and bipolar manic-depressive patients. *Am J Psychiatry* 134:197–200, 1977.

Shapiro S, Skinner EA, Kessler LG, Von Korff M, German PS, Tischler GL, Leaf PJ, Benham L, Cottler L, Regier DA: Utilization of health and mental health services: Three Epidemiologic Catchment Area sites. *Arch Gen Psychiatry* 41:971–978, 1984.

Shaughnessy R, Greene SC, Pandey GN, Dorus E: Red-cell lithium transport and affective disorders in a multigeneration pedigree: Evidence for genetic transmission of affective disorders. *Biol Psychiatry* 20:451–460, 1985.

Shaw DM, Camps FE, Eccleston EG: 5-hydroxytryptamine in the hind brain of depressive suicides. *Br J Psychiatry* 113:1407–1411, 1967.

Shaw DM, MacSweeney DA, Woolcock N, Bevan-Jones AB: Uptake and release of 14 C-5-hydroxytryptamine by platelets in affective illness. *J Neurol Neurosurg Psychiatry* 34:224–225, 1971.

Shaw DM, O'Keeffe R, MacSweeny DA, Brooksbank BWL, Noguera R, Coppen A: 3-methoxy-4-hydroxyphenylglycol in depression. *Psychol Med* 3:333–336, 1973.

Shaw ED, Mann JJ, Stokes PE, Manevitz AZ: Effects of lithium carbonate on associative productivity and idiosyncrasy in bipolar outpatients. *Am J Psychiatry* 143:1166–1169, 1986.

Shaw ED, Stokes PE, Mann JJ, Manevitz AZA: Effects of lithium carbonate on the memory and motor speed of bipolar outpatients. *J Abnorm Psychol* 96:64–69, 1987.

Shea PA, Small JG, Hendrie HC: Elevation of choline and glycine in red blood cells of psychiatric patients due to lithium treatment. *Biol Psychiatry* 16:825–830, 1981.

Sheard MH: Effect of lithium on human aggression. *Nature* 230:113–114, 1971.

Sheard MH: Lithium in the treatment of aggression. *J Nerv Ment Dis* 160:108–118, 1975.

Shenton ME, Solovay MR, Holzman P: Comparative studies of thought disorders: II. Schizoaffective disorder. *Arch Gen Psychiatry* 44:21–30, 1987.

Sherfey MJ: Psychopathology and character structure in chronic alcoholism. In: O Diethelm, ed: *Etiology of Chronic Alcoholism*. Springfield, IL: Charles C. Thomas, 1955. pp 16–42.

Sherman AD, Petty F: Learned helplessness decreases [^{3}H] imipramine binding in rat cortex. *J Affective Disord* 6:25–32, 1984.

Sherrington R, Brynjolfsson J, Petursson H, Potter M, Dudleston K, Barraclough B, Wasmuth J, Dobbs M, Gurling H: Location of a susceptibility locus for schizophrenia on chromosome 5. *Nature* 336:164–167, 1988.

Shima S, Shikano T, Kitamura T, Masuda Y, Tsukumo T, Kanba S, Asai M: Depression and ventricular enlargement. *Acta Psychiatr Scand* 70:275–277, 1984.

Shneidman ES: Suicide. In: AM Freedman, HI Kaplan, BJ Sadock, eds: *Comprehensive Textbook of Psychiatry*. Vol 2, 2nd ed. Baltimore: Williams & Wilkins, 1975. pp 1774–1785.

Shobe FO, Brion P: Long-term prognosis in manic-depressive illness: A follow-up investigation of 111 patients. *Arch Gen Psychiatry* 25:334–337, 1971.

Shopsin B: Part 1: Mania: Clinical aspects, rating scales and incidence of manic-depressive illness. In:

B Shopsin, ed: *Manic Illness*. New York: Raven Press, 1979. pp 57–74.

Shopsin B: Bupropion's prophylactic efficacy in bipolar affective illness. *J Clin Psychiatry* 44:163–169, 1983.

Shopsin B, Gershon S: Cogwheel rigidity related to lithium maintenance. *Am J Psychiatry* 132:536–538, 1975.

Shopsin B, Gershon S: Dopamine receptor stimulation in the treatment of depression: Piribedil (ET-495). *Neuropsychobiology* 4:1–14, 1978.

Shopsin B, Stern S, Gershon S: Altered carbohydrate metabolism during treatment with lithium carbonate: Absence of diagnostic specificity in hospitalized psychiatric patients. *Arch Gen Psychiatry* 26:566–571, 1972.

Shopsin B, Wilk S, Sathananthan G, Gershon S, Davis K: Catecholamine and affective disorders revised: A critical assessment. *J Nerv Ment Dis* 158:369–383, 1974.

Shopsin B, Gershon S, Thompson H, Collins P: Psychoactive drugs in mania: A controlled comparison of lithium carbonate, chlorpromazine, and haloperidol. *Arch Gen Psychiatry* 32:34–42, 1975a.

Shopsin B, Janowsky D, Davis J, Gershon S: Rebound phenomena in manic patients following physostigmine: Preliminary observations. *Neuropsychobiology* 1:180–187, 1975b.

Shopsin B, Georgotas A, Kane S: Psychopharmacology of mania. In: B Shopsin, ed: *Manic Illness*. New York: Raven Press, 1979. pp 177–218.

Shukla S, Godwin CD, Long LEB, Miller MG: Lithium-carbamazepine neurotoxicity and risk factors. *Am J Psychiatry* 141:1604–1606, 1984.

Shukla S, Cook BL, Mukherjee S, Godwin C, Miller MG: Mania following head trauma. *Am J Psychiatry* 144:93–96, 1987.

Shukla S, Cook BL, Hoff AL, Aronson TA: Failure to detect organic factors in mania. *J Affective Disord* 15:17–20, 1988a.

Shukla S, Mukherjee S, Decina P: Lithium in the treatment of bipolar disorders associated with epilepsy: An open study. *J Clin Psychopharmacol* 8:201–204, 1988b.

Shukla VR, Borison RL: Lithium and lupuslike syndrome. *JAMA* 248:921–922, 1982.

Shulgin A: Profiles of psychedelic drugs: 10. DOB. *J Psychoactive Drugs* 13:99, 1981.

Shulman K, Post F: Bipolar affective disorder in old age. *Br J Psychiatry* 136:26–32, 1980.

Shulman KI, Mackenzie S, Hardy B: The clinical use of lithium carbonate in old age: A review. *Prog Neuropsychopharmacol Biol Psychiatry* 11:159–164, 1987.

Siegel J, Murphy GJ: Serotonergic inhibition of amygdala-kindled seizures in cats. *Brain Res* 174:337–340, 1979.

Siegel RK: Cocaine: Recreational use and intoxication. In: RC Petersen, RC Stillman, eds: *Cocaine*. Washington, DC: US Government Printing Office, 1977. pp 119–136.

Siegel RK: Cocaine smoking. *J Psychoactive Drugs* 14:321–337, 1982.

Siever LJ, Uhde TW: New studies and perspectives on the noradrenergic receptor system in depression: Effects of the alpha 2-adrenergic agonist clonidine. *Biol Psychiatry* 19:131–156, 1984.

Siever LJ, Uhde TW, Insel TR, Roy BF, Murphy DL: Growth hormone response to clonidine unchanged by chronic clorgyline treatment. *Psychiatry Res* 7:139–144, 1982a.

Siever LJ, Uhde TW, Murphy DL: Possible subsensitization of alpha 2-adrenergic receptors by chronic monoamine oxidase inhibitor treatment in psychiatric patients. *Psychiatry Res* 6:293–302, 1982b.

Siever LJ, Uhde TW, Silberman EK, Jimerson DC, Aloi JA, Post RM, Murphy DL: Growth hormone response to clonidine as a probe of noradrenergic receptor responsiveness in affective disorder patients and controls. *Psychiatry Res* 6:171–183, 1982c.

Siever LJ, Uhde TW, Silberman EK, Lake CR, Jimerson DC, Risch SC, Kalin NH, Murphy DL: Evaluation of alpha-adrenergic responsiveness to clonidine challenge and noradrenergic metabolism in the affective disorders and their treatment. *Psychopharmacol Bull* 18:118–119, 1982d.

Siever LJ, Kafka MS, Targum S, Lake CR: Platelet alpha-adrenergic binding and biochemical responsiveness in depressed patients and controls. *Psychiatry Res* 11:287–302, 1984a.

Siever LJ, Murphy DL, Slater S, de la Vega E, Lipper S: Plasma prolactin changes following fenfluramine in depressed patients compared to controls: An evaluation of central serotonergic responsivity in depression. *Life Sci* 34:1029–1039, 1984b.

Siever LJ, Uhde TW, Jimerson DC, Post RM, Lake CR, Murphy DL: Plasma cortisol responses to clonidine in depressed patients and controls: Evidence for a possible alteration in noradrenergic-neuroendocrine relationships. *Arch Gen Psychiatry* 41:63–68, 1984c.

Siever LJ, Uhde TW, Jimerson DC, Lake CR, Kopin IJ, Murphy DL: Indices of noradrenergic output in depression. *Psychiatry Res* 19:59–73, 1986.

Siever LJ, Coccaro EF, Davis KL: Chronobiologic instability of the noradrenergic system in depression. In: A Halaris, ed: *Chronobiology and Psychiatric Disorders*. New York: Elsevier, 1987. pp 1–21.

Siffre M: Six months alone in a cave. *Natl Geographic* 147:426–435, 1975.

Sigal JJ, Star KH, Franks CM: Hysterics and dysthymics as criterion groups in the study of introversion-extraversion. *J Abnorm Soc Psychol* 57:143–148, 1958.

Silberman EK, Reus VI, Jimerson DC, Lynott AM, Post RM: Heterogeneity of amphetamine response in depressed patients. *Am J Psychiatry* 138:1302–1307, 1981.

Silberman EK, Weingartner H, Post RM: Thinking disorder in depression: Logic and strategy in an abstract reasoning task. *Arch Gen Psychiatry* 40:775–

780, 1983.

Silberman EK, Post RM, Nurnberger J, Theodore W, Boulenger J-P: Transient sensory, cognitive and affective phenomena in affective illness: A comparison with complex partial epilepsy. *Br J Psychiatry* 146:81–89, 1985.

Silfverskiöld P, Risberg J: Regional cerebral blood flow in depression and mania. *Arch Gen Psychiatry* 46:253–259, 1989.

Silverstein ML, Warren RA, Harrow M, Grinker RR, and Pawelski T: Changes in diagnosis from *DSM-II* to the Research Diagnostic Criteria and DSM-III. *Am J Psychiatry* 139:366–368, 1982.

Silverstone T: Dopamine, mood and manic-depressive psychosis. In: S Garattini, ed: *Depressive Disorders*. Stuttgart: FK Schattauer Verlag, 1978. pp 419–430.

Silverstone T: Response to bromocriptine distinguishes bipolar from unipolar depression. Letter. *Lancet* 1:903–904, 1984.

Silverstone T, Romans-Clarkson S: Bipolar affective disorder: Causes and prevention of relapse. *Br J Psychiatry* 154:321–335, 1989.

Silvestri A, Santonastaso P, Paggiarin D: Alopecia areata during lithium therpy: A case report. *Gen Hosp Psychiatry* 10:46–48, 1988.

Simon P, Lecrubier Y, Jouvent R, Puech AJ, Allilaire JF, Widlöcher D: Experimental and clinical evidence of the antidepressant effect of a beta-adrenergic stimulant. *Psychol Med* 8:335–338, 1978.

Simon RI: Involutional psychosis in Negroes: A report and discussion of low incidence. *Arch Gen Psychiatry* 13:148–154, 1965.

Simon RJ, Fleiss JL, Gurland BJ, Stiller PR, Sharpe L: Depression and schizophrenia in hospitalized black and white mental patients. *Arch Gen Psychiatry* 28:509–512, 1973.

Simons AD, Garfield SL, Murphy GE: The process of change in cognitive therapy and pharmacotherapy for depression: Changes in mood and cognition. *Arch Gen Psychiatry* 41:45–51, 1984.

Simpson CD, Vega A: Unilateral brain damage and patterns of age-corrected WAIS Subtest Scores. *J Clin Psychology* 27:204–208, 1971.

Simpson DM, Davis GC: Measuring thought disorder with clinical rating scales in schizophrenic and non-schizophrenic patients. *Psychiatry Res* 15:313–318, 1985.

Singer K: Depressive disorders from a transcultural perspective. *Soc Science Med* 9:289–301, 1975.

Siris SG, Chertoff HR, Perel JM: Rapid-cycling affective disorders during imipramine treatment: A case report. *Am J Psychiatry* 136:341–342, 1979.

Sitaram N, Gillin JC: Development and use of pharmacological probes of the CNS in man: Evidence of cholinergic abnormality in primary affective illness. *Biol Psychiatry* 15:925–955, 1980.

Sitaram N, Nurnberger JI Jr, Gershon ES, Gillin JC: Faster cholinergic REM sleep induction in euthymic patients with primary affective illness. *Science* 208:200–202, 1980.

Sitaram N, Nurnberger JI Jr, Gershon ES, Gillin JC: Cholinergic regulation of mood and REM sleep: Potential model and marker of vulnerability to affective disorder. *Am J Psychiatry* 139:571–576, 1982.

Sitaram N, Gillin JC, Bunney WE Jr: Cholinergic and catecholaminergic receptor sensitivity in affective illness: Strategy and theory. In: RM Post, JC Ballenger, eds: *Neurobiology of Mood Disorders*. Baltimore: Williams & Wilkins, 1984. pp 629–651.

Sitaram N, Jones D, Dube S, Bell J, Rivard P: Supersensitive ACH REM-induction as a genetic vulnerability marker of MDD. Abstract of paper presented at IVth World Congress of Biological Psychiatry, Philadelphia, 1986.

Sitaram N, Dube S, Keshavan M, Davies A, Reynal P: The association of supersensitive cholinergic REM-induction and affective illness within pedigrees. *J Psychiat Res* 21:487–497, 1987.

Sitland-Marken PA, Rickman LA, Wells BG, Mabie WC: Pharmacologic management of acute mania in pregnancy. *J Clin Psychopharmacol* 9:78–87, 1989.

Sjoestedt ML: *Gods and Heroes of the Celts*. Trans by M. Dillon. Berkeley: Turtle Island Foundation, 1982.

Sjöström R: 5-Hydroxyindole acetic acid and homovanillic acid in cerebrospinal fluid in manic-depressive psychosis and the effect of probenecid treatment. *Eur J Clin Pharmacol* 6:75–80, 1973.

Skarda CA, Freeman WJ: How brains make chaos in order to make sense of the world. *Behav Brain Sci* 10:161–195, 1987.

Skoven I, Thormann J: Lithium compound treatment and psoriasis. *Arch Dermatol* 115:1185–1187, 1979.

Skwerer RG, Jacobsen FM, Duncan CC, Kelly KA, Sack DA, Tamarkin L, Gaist PA, Kasper S, Rosenthal NE: Neurobiology of seasonal affective disorder and phototherapy. *J Biol Rhy* 3:135–154, 1988.

Slater E: The creative personality. In: M Roth, V Cowie, eds: *Psychiatry, Genetics and Pathography: A Tribute to Eliot Slater*. London: Gaskell Press, 1979. pp 89–103.

Slater E: Zur periodik des manische-depressiven irreseins. *Ztschr Neurol Psychiatr* 162:794–801, 1938a.

Slater E: Zur Erbpathologie des Manische-Depressive Irreseins: Die Eltern und Kinder von Manische-Depressiven. *Ztschr Neurol Psychiatr* 163:1–47, 1938b.

Slater E, Meyer A: Contributions to a pathography of the musicians: 1. Robert Schumann. *Confin Psychiat* 2:65–94, 1959.

Slater E, Meyer A: Contributions to a pathography of the musicians: 2. Organic and psychotic disorders. *Confin Psychiat* 3:129–145, 1960.

Slater E, Roth M: *Clinical Psychiatry*. (3rd ed, Mayer-Gross, Slater, and Roth). Baltimore: Williams & Wilkins, 1969.

Slater S, de La Vega CE, Skyler J, Murphy DL: Plasma prolactin stimulation by fenfluramine and amphetamine. *Psychopharmacol Bull* 12:26–27, 1976.

Slife BD, Miura S, Thompson LW, Shapiro JL, Gallagher D: Differential recall as a function of mood disorder in clinically depressed patients: Between- and within-subject differences. *J Abnorm Psychol* 93:391–400, 1984.

Small JG, Small IF: Pharmacology—neurophysiology of lithium. In: S Gershon, B Shopsin, eds: *Lithium: Its Role in Psychiatric Research and Treatment.* New York: Plenum Press, 1973. pp 83–106.

Small JG, Small IF, Moore DF: Experimental withdrawal of lithium in recovered manic-depressive patients: A report of five cases. *Am J Psychiatry* 127:1555–1558, 1971a.

Small JG, Small IF, Perez HC: EEG, evoked potential, and contingent negative variations with lithium in manic depressive disease. *Biol Psychiatry* 3:47–58, 1971b.

Small JG, Small IF, Milstein V, Moore DF: Familial associations with EEG variants in manic-depressive disease. *Arch Gen Psychiatry* 32:43–48, 1975.

Small JG, Kellams JJ, Milstein V, Small IF: Complications with electroconvulsive treatment combined with lithium. *Biol Psychiatry* 15:103–112, 1980.

Small JG, Small IF, Milstein V, Kellams JJ, Klapper MH: Manic symptoms: An indication for bilateral ECT. *Biol Psychiatry* 20:125–134, 1985.

Small JG, Milstein V, Klapper MH, Kellams JJ, Miller MJ, Small IF: Electroconvulsive therapy in the treatment of manic episodes. *Ann NY Acad Sci* 462:37–49, 1986.

Small JG, Klapper MH, Kellams JJ, Miller MJ, Milstein V, Sharpley PH, Small IF: Electroconvulsive treatment compared with lithium in the management of manic states. *Arch Gen Psychiatry* 45:727–732, 1988.

Smallwood RG, Avery DH, Pascualy RA, Prinz PN: Circadian temperature rhythms in primary depression. *Sleep Res* 12:215 , 1983.

Smart C: A song to David (1763). In: *A Translation of the Psalms of David, Attempted in the Spirit of Christianity, and Adapted to the Divine Service.* London: Dryden Leach, 1765.

Smeraldi E, Negri F, Melica AM, Scorza-Smeraldi R: HLA system and affective disorders: A sibship study. *Tissue Antigens* 12:270–274, 1978.

Smeraldi E, Petroccione A, Gasperini M, Macciardi F, Orsini A, Kidd KK: Outcomes on lithium treatment as a tool for genetic studies in affective disorders. *J Affective Disord* 6:139–151, 1984.

Smigan L: Long-term lithium treatment: Some clinical, psychological and biological aspects. *Acta Psychiatr Scand* 71:160–170, 1985.

Smigan L, Bucht G, Von Knorring L, Perris C, Wahlin A: Long-term lithium treatment and renal functions: A prospective study. *Neuropsychobiology* 11:33–38, 1984.

Smith AD, Winkler H: Fundamental mechanisms in the release of catecholamines. In: H Blaschko, E Muscholl, eds: *Handbook of Experimental Pharmacology, Vol. 33 Catecholamines.* Berlin: Springer-Verlag, 1972. pp 538–617.

Smith AH, Chambers C, Naylor GJ: Bromocriptine in mania: A placebo-controlled double-blind trial. *Br Med J* 280:86, 1980.

Smith JH: The metaphor of the manic-depressive. *Psychiatry* 123:375–383, 1960.

Smith RE, Helms PM: Adverse effects of lithium therapy in the acutely ill elderly patient. *J Clin Psychiatry* 43:94–99, 1982.

Smith WT, Glaudin V: Double-blind efficacy and safety study comparing adinazolam mesylate and placebo in depressed inpatients. *Acta Psychiatr Scand* 74:238–245, 1986.

Smithberg M, Dixit PK: Teratogenic effects of lithium in mice. *Teratology* 26:239–246, 1982.

Smouse PE, Feinberg M, Carroll BJ: The Carroll Rating Scale for Depression: II. Factor analyses of the feature profiles. *Br J Psychiatry* 138:201–204, 1981.

Snaith RP: Rating scales. *Br J Psychiatry* 138:512–514, 1981.

Snaith RP, Ahmed SN, Mehta S, Hamilton M: Assessment of the severity of primary depressive illness: Wakefield self-assessment depression inventory. *Psychol Med* 1:143–149, 1971.

Snaith RP, Bridge GWK, Hamilton M: The Leeds Scales for the self-assessment of anxiety and depression. *Br J Psychiatry* 128:156–165, 1976.

Snow DA, Baker SG, Anderson L, Martin M: The myth of pervasive mental illness among the homeless. *Social Problems* 33:407–423, 1986.

Snyder F: NIH studies of EEG sleep in affective illness. In: TA Williams, MM Katz, JA Shield Jr, eds: *Recent Advances in the Psychobiology of Depressive Illness.* Washington, DC: US Government Printing Office, 1972. pp 171–192.

Solomon MI, Hellon CP: Suicide and age in Alberta, Canada, 1951 to 1977: A cohort analysis. *Arch Gen Psychiatry* 37:511–513, 1980.

Solovay MR, Shenton ME, Holzman PS: Comparative studies of thought disorders: I. Mania and schizophrenia. *Arch Gen Psychiatry* 44:13–20, 1987.

Sørensen PS, Gjerris A, Hammer M: Cerebrospinal fluid vasopressin in neurological and psychiatric disorders. *J Neurol Neurosurg Psychiatry* 48:50–57, 1985.

Sørensen R, Svendsen K, Schou M: T.R.H. in depression. *Lancet* 1:865–866, 1974.

Sotsky SM, Tossell JW: Tolmetin induction of mania. *Psychosomatics* 25:626–628, 1984.

Soubrie P, Blas C, Ferron A, Glowinski J: Chlordiazepoxide reduces in vivo serotonin release in the basal ganglia of encéphale isolé but not anesthetized cats: Evidence for a dorsal raphe site of action. *J Pharmacol Exp Ther* 226:526–532, 1983.

Soucek K, Zjolsky R, Krulik K, Filip V, Vinarova E, Dostal T: The levels of lithium in serum and red blood cells and its ratios in manic-depression patients. *Act Nerv Super (Praha)* 16:193–194, 1974.

Souêtre E, Pringuey D, Salvati E, Robert P, Darcourt G: Rythmes circadiens de la température centrale et de la cortisolémie dans les dépressions endogènes. *L'Encéphale* 11:185–198, 1985.

Souêtre E, Salvati E, Pringuey D, Krebs B, Plasse Y, Darcourt G: The circadian rhythm of plasma thyrotropin in depression and recovery. *Chronobiol Int* 3:197–205, 1986.

Souêtre E, Salvati E, Pringuey D, Plasse Y, Savelli M, Darcourt G: Antidepressant effects of the sleep/wake cycle phase advance: Preliminary report. *J Affective Disord* 12:41–46, 1987a.

Souêtre E, Salvati E, Belugou JJL, Douillet P, Braccini T, Darcourt G: Seasonality of suicides: Environmental, sociological and biological covariations. *J Affective Disord* 13:215–225, 1987b.

Souêtre E, Salvati E, Wehr TA, Sack DA, Krebs B, Darcourt G: Twenty-four-hour profiles of body temperature and plasma TSH in bipolar patients during depression and during remission and in normal control subjects. *Am J Psychiatry* 145:1133–1137, 1988.

Souêtre E, Salvati E, Belugou J-L, Pringuey D, Candito M, Krebs B, Ardisson J-L, Darcourt G: Circadian rhythms in depression and recovery: Evidence for blunted amplitude as the main chronobiological abnormality. *Psychiatry Res* 28:263–278, 1989.

Souêtre E, Rosenthal NE, Wehr TA: Biological clocks, depression and environment. *Arch Gen Psychiatry*, in press.

Spalt L: Sexual behavior and affective disorders. *Dis Nerv Syst* 36:974–977, 1975.

Spar JE, Ford CV, Liston EH: Bipolar affective disorder in aged patients. *J Clin Psychiatry* 40:504–507, 1979.

Spencer JH, Glick ID, Haas GL, Clarkin JF, Lewis AB, Peyser J, DeMane N, Good-Ellis M, Harris E, Lestelle V: A randomized clinical trial of inpatient family intervention, III: Effects at 6-month and 18-month follow-ups. *Am J Psychiatry* 145:1115–1121, 1988.

Spensley J: A useful adjunct in the treatment of heroin addicts in a methadone program. *Int J Addict* 11:191–197, 1976.

Sperry RW: Hemisphere deconnection and unity in conscious awareness. *Am Psychol* 23:723–733, 1968.

Spicer CC, Hare EH, Slater E: Neurotic and psychotic forms of depressive illness: Evidence from age-incidence in a national sample. *Br J Psychiatry* 123:535–541, 1973.

Spielberger CD, Borgman R, Becker J, Parker JB: Affective expression in manic-depressive reactions. *J Nerv Ment Dis* 141:664–669, 1966.

Spiker DG, Pugh DD: Combining tricyclic and monoamine oxidase inhibitor antidepressants. *Arch Gen Psychiatry* 33:828–830, 1976.

Spiker DG, Weiss JC, Dealy RS, Griffin SJ, Hanin I, Neil JF, Perel JM, Rossi AJ, Soloff PH: The pharmacological treatment of delusional depression. *Am J Psychiatry* 142:430–436, 1985.

Spinedi E, Negro-Vilar A: Serotonin and adrenocorticotropin (ACTH) release: Direct effects at the anterior pituitary level and potentiation of arginine vasopressin-induced ACTH release. *Endocrinology* 112:1217–1223, 1983.

Spitz RA: Anaclitic depresssion: An inquiry into the genesis of psychiatric conditions in early childhood, II. *Psychoanal Study Child* 2:313–347, 1946.

Spitzer RL, Endicott J: *Schedule for Affective Disorders and Schizophrenia*. New York: Biometrics Research, Evaluation Section, New York State Psychiatric Institute, 1978.

Spitzer RL, Endicott J, Robins E: *Research Diagnostic Criteria*. New York: Biometrics Research, Evaluation Section, New York State Psychiatric Institute, 1978a.

Spitzer RL, Endicott J, Robins E: Research diagnostic criteria: Rationale and reliability. *Arch Gen Psychiatry* 35:773–782, 1978b.

Spitzer RL, Williams JBW, Gibbon M: *Structured Clinical Interview for DSM-III*. New York State Psychiatric Institute. New York: Biometrics Research, 1984.

Spring G, Schweid D, Gray C, Steinberg J, Horwitz M: A double-blind comparison of lithium and chlorpromazine in the treatment of manic states. *Am J Psychiatry* 126:1306–1310, 1970.

Squillace K, Post RM, Savard R, Erwin-Gorman M: Life charting of the longitudinal course of recurrent affective illness. In: RM Post, JC Ballenger, eds: *Neurobiology of Mood Disorders*. Baltimore: Williams & Wilkins, 1984. pp 38–59

Squire LR: Memory functions as affected by electroconvulsive therapy. *Ann NY Acad Sci* 462:307–314, 1986.

Squire LR, Chace PM: Memory functions six to nine months after electroconvulsive therapy. *Arch Gen Psychiatry* 32:1557–1564, 1975.

Squire LR, Slater PC: Bilateral and unilateral ECT: Effects on verbal and nonverbal memory. *Am J Psychiatry* 135:1316–1320, 1978.

Squire LR, Slater PC, Miller PL: Retrograde amnesia and bilateral electroconvulsive therapy: Long-term follow-up. *Arch Gen Psychiatry* 38:89–95, 1981.

Srole L, Langner TS, Michael ST, Opler MK, Rennie TAC: *Mental Health in the Metropolis: The midtown Manhattan Study*. New York: McGraw-Hill, 1962.

Stahl SM: The human platelet: A diagnostic and research tool for the study of biogenic amines in psychiatric and neurologic disorders. *Arch Gen Psychiatry* 34:509–516, 1977.

Stahl SM, Meltzer HY: A kinetic and pharmacologic analysis of 5-hydroxytryptamine transport by human platelets and platelet storage granules: Comparison with central serotonergic neurons. *J Pharmacol Exp Ther* 205:118–132, 1978.

Stahl SM, Woo DJ, Mefford IN, Berger PA, Ciaranello RD: Hyperserotonemia and platelet serotonin uptake and release in schizophrenia and affective disorders. *Am J Psychiatry* 140:26–30, 1983.

Stallone F, Shelley E, Mendlewicz J, Fieve RR: The use of lithium in affective disorders: III: A double blind study of prophylaxis in bipolar illness. *Am J Psychiatry* 130:1006–1010, 1973.

Stallone F, Dunner DL, Ahearn J, Fieve RR: Statistical predictions of suicide in depressives. *Compr Psychiatry* 21:381–387, 1980.

Stancer HC, Forbath N: Hyperparathyroidism, hypothyroidism, and impaired renal function after 10 to 20 years of lithium treatment. *Arch Int Med* 149:1042–1045, 1989.

Stancer HC, Persad E: Treatment of intractable rapid-cycling manic-depressive disorder with levothyroxine: Clinical observations. *Arch Gen Psychiatry* 39:311–312, 1982.

Stancer HC, Furlong FW, Godse DD: A longitudinal investigation of lithium as a prophylactic agent for recurrent depressions. *Can Med Assoc J* 15:29–40, 1970.

Stancer HC, Persad E, Wagener DK, Jorna T: Evidence for homogeneity of major depression and bipolar affective disorder. *J Psychiatr Res* 21:37–53, 1987.

Standish-Barry HMAS, Bouras N, Hale AS, Bridges PK, Bartlett JR: Ventricular size and CSF transmitter metabolite concentrations in severe endogenous depression. *Br J Psychiatry* 148:386–392, 1986.

Stanhope PHS: *Notes of Conversations With the Duke of Wellington 1831–1835*. November 2, 1831. London: J Murray, 1988.

Stanton TL, Beckman AL, Winokur A: Thyrotropin-releasing-hormone effects in the central nervous system: Dependence on arousal state. *Science* 214:678–681, 1981.

Stanton TL, Winokur A, Beckman AL: Seasonal variation in thyrotropin-releasing-hormone (TRH) content of different brain regions and the pineal in the mammalian hibernator, Citellus Lateralis. *Regul Pept* 3:135–144, 1982.

Stapleton M: *The Cambridge Guide to English Literature*. Cambridge: Cambridge University Press, 1983.

Starkstein SE, Robinson RG: Affective disorders and cerebral vascular disease. *Br J Psychiatry* 154:170–182, 1989.

Starkstein SE, Pearlson GD, Boston J, Robinson RG: Mania after brain injury: A controlled study of causative factors. *Arch Neurol* 44:1069–1073, 1987.

Starkstein SE, Boston JD, Robinson RGG: Mechanisms of mania after brain injury: 12 case reports and review of the literature. *J Nerv Ment Dis* 176:87–100, 1988a.

Starkstein SE, Robinson RG, Price TR: Comparison of patients with and without poststroke major depression matched for size and location of lesion. *Arch Gen Psychiatry* 45:247- 252, 1988b.

Starkstein SE, Robinson RG, Honig MA, Parikh RM, Joselyn J, Price TR: Mood changes after right-hemisphere lesions. *Br J Psychiatry* 155:79–85, 1989.

Stasiek C, Zetin M: Organic manic disorders. *Psychosomatics* 26:394–402, 1985.

Staton RD, Wilson H, Brumback RA: Cognitive improvement associated with tricyclic antidepressant treatment of childhood major depressive illness. *Percept Mot Skills* 53:219–234, 1981.

Staunton DA, Magistretti PJ, Shoemaker WJ, Bloom FE: Effects of chronic lithium treatment on dopamine receptors in the rat corpus striatum: I. Locomotor activity and behavioral supersensitivity. *Brain Res* 232:391–400, 1982.

Steer RA, Kotzker E: Affective changes in male and female methadone patients. *Drug Alcohol Depend* 5:115–122, 1980.

Stefanis CN, Kokkevi A: Depression and drug use. *Psychopathology* 19(Suppl 2):124–131, 1986.

Steif B, Sackeim H, Portnoy S, Decina P, Malitz S: Effects of depression and ECT on short-term visual memory. Abstract of paper presented at the Fourth World Congress of Biological Psychiatry, Philadelphia, 1986a.

Steif BL, Sackeim HA, Portnoy S, Decina P, Malitz S: Effects of depression and ECT on anterograde memory. *Biol Psychiatry* 21:921–930, 1986b.

Steiger A, Von Bardeleben U, Herth T, Holsboer F: Sleep EEG and nocturnal secretion of cortisol and growth hormone in male patients with endogenous depression before treatment and after recovery. *J Affective Disord* 16:189–195, 1989.

Stein L: Effects and interactions of imipramine, chlorpromazine, reserpine and amphetamine on self-stimulation: Possible neurophysiological basis of depression. In: J Wortis, ed: *Recent Advances in Biological Psychiatry Vol 4*. New York: Plenum Press, 1962. pp 288–309.

Stein L: Self-stimulation of the brain and central stimulant action of amphetamine. *Fed Proc* 23:117–119, 1964.

Stein M, Schleifer SJ, Keller SE: Psychoimmunology in clinical psychiatry. In: RE Hales, AJ Frances, eds: *American Psychiatric Association Annual Review Vol 5*. Washington, DC: American Psychiatric Press, 1987. pp 210–234.

Steinberg D, Hirsch SR, Marston SD, Reynolds K, Sutton RN: Influenza infection causing manic psychosis. *Br J Psychiatry* 120:531–535, 1972.

Steinbrook RM, Chapman AB: Lithium responders: An evaluation of psychological test characteristics. *Compr Psychiatry* 11:524–530, 1970.

Steiner M, Seggie J, Martin J, Fairman M, Simpson J: ECT reduces sensitivity to light. Abstract of paper presented at the 27th annual meeting of the American College of Neuropsychopharmacologists, December, 1988.

Stenbäck A, Achté KA: Hospital first admissions and social class. *Acta Psychiatr Scand* 42:113–124, 1966.

Stengaard-Pedersen K, Schou M: *In vitro* and *in vivo* inhibition by lithium of enkephalin binding to opiate receptors in rat brain. *Neuropharmacology* 21:817–823, 1982.

Stenstedt Å: A study in manic-depressive psychosis: Clinical, social, and genetic investigations. *Acta Psychiatr et Neurol* (Suppl 79):1–111, 1952.

Stern K, Dancey T: Glioma of the diencephalon in a

manic patient. *Am J Psychiatry* 98:716, 1942.

Stern L: Kulturkreis und form der geistigen erkrankung. *Nerven- und Geisteskrankheiten* 10:1–61, 1913.

Stern SL, Brandt JT, Hurley RS, Stagno SJ, Stern MG, Smeltzer DJ: Serum and red cell folate concentrations in outpatients receiving lithium carbonate. *Int Clin Psychopharmacol* 3:49–52, 1988.

Stern-Piper L: Der psychopathologische index der kultur. *Arch Psychiatr Nervenkr* 74:514–525, 1925.

Sternberg DE, Jarvik ME: Memory functions in depression: Improvement with antidepressant medication. *Arch Gen Psychiatry* 33:219–224, 1976.

Stevens JR, Mark VH, Erwin F, Pacheco P, Suematsu K: Deep temporal stimulation in man: Long latency, long lasting psychological changes. *Arch Neurol* 21:157–169, 1969.

Stewart DE: Prophylactic lithium in postpartum affective psychosis. *J Nerv Ment Dis* 176:485–489, 1988.

Stockmeier CA, Kellar KJ: In vivo regulation of the serotonin–2 receptor in rat brain. *Life Sci* 38:117–127, 1986.

Stoddard FJ, Post RM, Bunney WE: Slow and rapid psychobiological alterations in a manic-depressive patient: Clinical phenomenology. *Br J Psychiatry* 130:72–78, 1977.

Stokes PE, Sikes CR: The hypothalamic-pituitary-adrenocortical axis in major depression. *Endocrinol Metab Clin North Am* 17:1–19, 1988.

Stokes PE, Shamoian CA, Stoll PM, Patton MJ: Efficacy of lithium as acute treatment of manic-depressive illness. *Lancet* 1:1319–1325, 1971.

Stokes PE, Pick GR, Stoll PM, Nunn WD: Pituitary-adrenal function in depressed patients: Resistance to dexamethasone suppression. *J Psychiat Res* 12:271–281, 1975.

Stokes PE, Kocsis JH, Arcuni OJ: Relationship of lithium chloride dose to treatment response in acute mania. *Arch Gen Psychiatry* 33:1080–1084, 1976.

Stokes PE, Stoll PM, Koslow SH, Maas JW, Davis JM, Swann AC, Robins E: Pretreatment DST and hypothalamic-pituitary-adrenocortical function in depressed patients and comparison groups: A multi-center study. *Arch Gen Psychiatry* 41:257–267, 1984.

Stone EA: Adaptation to stress and brain noradrenergic receptors. *Neurosci Biobehav Rev* 7:503–509, 1983a.

Stone EA: Problems with current catecholamine hypotheses of antidepressant agents: Speculations toward a new hypothesis. *Behav Brain Sci* 6:535–577, 1983b.

Stone K: Mania in the elderly. *Br J Psychiatry* 155:220–224, 1989.

Stone MH: Toward early detection of manic-depressive illness in psychoanalytic patients: I: Patients who later develop a manic illness. *Am J Psychother* 32:427–439, 1978.

Stone MH: *The Borderline Syndromes: Constitution, Personality, and Adaptation.* New York:

McGraw-Hill, 1980.

Storr A: *The Dynamics of Creation.* London: Secker & Warburg, 1972.

Storr A: Churchill: The man. (1968) In: A Storr: *Churchill's Black Dog, Kafka's Mice, and Other Phenomena of the Human Mind.* New York: Grove Press, 1988.

Storr A: *The Sanity of True Genius.* Unpublished manuscript.

Strack S, Coyne JC: Social confirmation of dysphoria: Shared and private reactions to depression. *J Pers Soc Psychol* 44:798–806, 1983.

Strandman E: "Psychogenic needs" in patients with affective disorders. *Acta Psychiatr Scand* 58:16–29, 1978.

Strandman E, Wetterberg L, Perris C, Ross SB: Serum dopamine-beta-hydroxylase in affective disorders. *Neuropsychobiology* 4:248–255, 1978.

Strauss H, Keschner M: Mental symptoms in cases of tumour of the frontal lobe. *Arch Neurol Psychiatry* 33:986–1105, 1935.

Strauss JS: Hallucinations and delusions as points on continua function: Rating scale evidence. *Arch Gen Psychiatry* 21:581–586, 1969.

Strayhorn JM, Nash JL: Severe neurotoxicity despite "therapeutic" serum lithium levels. *Dis Nerv Syst* 38:107–111, 1977.

Strik WK, La Malfa G, Cabras P: A bidimensional model for diagnosis and classification of functional psychoses. *Compr Psychiatry* 30:313–319, 1989.

Strober M: Familial aspects of depressive disorder in early adolescence In: EB Weller, RA Weller, eds: *Current Perspectives on Major Depressive Disorders in Children.* Washington, DC: American Psychiatric Press, 1984. pp. 38–48.

Strober M, Carlson G: Bipolar illness in adolescents with major depression: Clinical, genetic, and psychopharmacologic predictors in a three- to four-year prospective follow-up investigation. *Arch Gen Psychiatry* 39:549–555, 1982.

Strober M, Green J, Carlson G: Phenomenology and subtypes of major depressive disorder in adolescence. *J Affective Disord* 3:281–290, 1981.

Strober M, Morrell W, Burroughs J, Lampert C, Danforth H, Freeman R: A family study of bipolar I disorder in adolescence: Early onset of symptoms linked to increased familial loading and lithium resistance. *J Affective Disord* 15:255–268, 1988.

Strober M, Hanna G, McCracken J: Bipolar disorder. In: CG Last, M Hersen, eds: *Handbook of Child Psychiatric Diagnosis.* New York: John Wiley and Sons, 1989. pp 299–319.

Strober M, Burroughs J, Salkin B, Green J: Ancestral secondary cases of psychiatric illness in adolescents with mania, depression, schizophrenia, and conduct disorder. *Biol Psychiatry* in press.

Strober M, Morrell W, Lampert C, Burroughs: Lithium carbonate in the prophylactic treatment of bipolar I illness in adolescents: A naturalistic study. *Am J Psychiatry* submitted.

Stroebel CF: Biologic rhythm correlates of disturbed

behavior in the rhesus monkey. *Bibl Primat* 9:91–105, 1969.

Strömgren LS: Unilateral versus bilateral electroconvulsive therapy: Investigations into the therapeutic effect in endogenous depression. *Acta Psychiatr Scand* (Suppl 240):8–65, 1973.

Strömgren LS: The influence of depression on memory. *Acta Psychiatr Scand* 56:109–128, 1977.

Strömgren LS, Boller S: Carbamazepine in treatment and prophylaxis of manic-depressive disorder. *Psychiatr Dev* 4:349–367, 1985.

Strongin EI, Hinsie LE: Parotid gland secretion in manic-depressive patients. *Am J Psychiatry* 94:1459–1462, 1938.

Strongin EI, Hinsie LE: A method for differentiating manic-depressive depressions from other depressions by means of parotid secretions. *Psychiatr Q* 13:697–704, 1939.

Suarez BK, Croughan J: Is the major histocompatibility complex linked to genes that increase susceptibility to affective disorders? A critical appraisal. *Psychiat Res* 7:19–27, 1982.

Suarez BK, Reich T: HLA and major affective disorders. *Arch Gen Psychiatry* 41:22–27, 1984.

Subrahmanyam S: Role of biogenic amines in certain pathological conditions. *Brain Res* 87:355–362, 1975.

Sugrue MF: Chronic antidepressant therapy and associated changes in central monoaminergic receptor functioning. *Pharmacol Ther* 21:1–33, 1983.

Sultzer DL, Cummings JL: Drug-induced mania—Causative agents, clinical characteristics and management: A retrospective analysis of the literature. *Med Toxicol Adverse Drug Exper* 4:127–143, 1989.

Sundby P, Nyhus P: Major and minor psychiatric disorders in males in Oslo. *Acta Psychiatr Scand* 39:519–547, 1963.

Suomi SJ: Relevance of animal models for clinical psychology. In: PC Kendell, JN Butcher, eds: *Handbook of Research Methods in Clinical Psychology*. New York: Wiley, 1982. pp 249–271.

Suomi SJ, Delizio RD, McKinney WT: Effects of imipramine treatment of separation induced social disorders in rhesus monkeys. *Arch Gen Psychiatry* 35:321–325, 1978.

Suranyi-Cadotte BE, Wood PL, Nair NPV, Schwartz G: Normalization of platelet [³H]imipramine binding in depressed patients during remission. *Eur J Pharmacol* 85:357–358, 1982.

Suranyi-Cadotte BE, Wood PL, Schwartz G, Nair NPV: Altered ³H-imipramine binding in schizoaffective and depressive disorders. *Biol Psychiatry* 18:923–927, 1983.

Swann AC, Maas JW, Hattox SE, Landis H: Catecholamine metabolites in human plasma as indices of brain function: Effects of debrisoquin. *Life Sci* 27:1857–1862, 1980.

Swann AC, Secunda S, Davis JM, Robins E, Hanin I, Koslow SH, Maas JW: CSF monoamine metabolites in mania. *Am J Psychiatry* 140:396–400, 1983.

Swann AC, Secunda SK, Katz MM, Koslow SH, Maas JW, Chang S, Robins E: Lithium treatment of mania: Clinical characteristics, specificity of symptom change, and outcome. *Psychiatry Res* 18:127–141, 1986.

Swazey JP: *Chlorpromazine in Psychiatry: A Study of Therapeutic Innovation*. Cambridge, MA: MIT Press, 1974.

Swift HM: The prognosis of recurrent insanity of manic-depressive type. *Am J Insanity* 64:311–326, 1907.

Sylvester CE, Burke PM, McCauley EA, Clark CJ: Manic psychosis in childhood: Report of two cases. *J Nerv Ment Dis* 172:12–15, 1984.

Symonds RL, Williams P: Seasonal variation in the incidence of mania. *Br J Psychiatry* 129:45–48, 1976.

Symonds RL, Williams P: Lithium and the changing incidence of mania. *Psychol Med* 11:193–196. 1981.

Syrett H: *Interview at Weehawken: The Burr-Hamilton Duel as Told in Original Documents*. Middleton, CN: Wesleyan University Press, 1960.

Szabadi E, Bradshaw CM, Besson JAO: Elongation of pause-time in speech: A simple, objective measure of motor retardation in depression. *Br J Psychiatry* 129:592–597, 1976.

Szabo KT: Teratogenic effect of lithium carbonate in the foetal mouse. *Nature* 225:73–75, 1970.

Szádóczky E, Falus A, Arató M, Németh A, Teszéri G, Moussong-Kovács E: Phototherapy increases platelet ³H-imipramine binding in patients with winter depression. *J Affective Disord* 16:121–125, 1989.

Szentistvanyi I, Janka Z: Correlation between the lithium ratio and Na-dependent Li transport of red blood cells during lithium prophylaxis. *Biol Psychiatry* 14:973–977, 1979.

Szentistvanyi I, Janka Z, Rimanoczy A: Alteration of erythrocyte phosphate transport in primary depressive disorders. *J Affective Disord* 2:229–238, 1980.

Tagliamonte A, Tagliamonte P, Perez-Cruet J, Gessa GL: Increase in brain tryptophan caused by drugs which stimulate serotonin synthesis. *Nature New Biol* 229:125–126, 1971.

Takahashi E: Seasonal variation of conception and suicide. *Tohoku J Exp Med* 84:215–227, 1964.

Takahashi R, Sakuma A, Itoh K, Itoh H, Kurihara M: Comparison of efficacy of lithium carbonate and chlorpromazine in mania: Report of collaborative study group on treatment of mania in Japan. *Arch Gen Psychiatry* 32:1310–1318, 1975.

Takahashi SH, Kondo H, Yoshimura M, Ochi Y: Antidepressant effect of thyrotropin releasing hormone (TRH) and the plasma thyrotropin levels in depression. *Folia Psychiatr Neurol Jpn* 27:305–314, 1973.

Takahashi SH, Yamane H, Kondo H, Tani N, Kato N: CSF monoamine metabolites in alcoholism: A comparative study with depression. *Folia Psychiatr Neurol Jpn* 28:347–354, 1974.

Takahashi Y, Kipnis DM, Daughaday WH: Growth hormone secretion during sleep. *J Clin Invest* 47:2079–2090, 1968.

Takazawa N, Kimura T, Nanko S: Blood groups and affective disorders. *Jpn J Psychiatr Neurol* 42:753–758, 1988.

Tamarkin L, Craig CJ, Garrick NA, Wehr TA: Effect of clorgyline (a MAO type A inhibitor) on locomotor activity in the syrian hamster. *Am J Physiol* 245:R215–R221, 1983.

Tan ES: The presentation of affective symptoms in non-western countries. In: GD Burrows, ed: *Handbook of Studies on Depression*. Amsterdam: Excerpta Medica, 1977. pp 121–133.

Tanaka Y, Hazama H, Fukuhara T, Tsutui T: Computerized tomography of the brain in manic-depressive patients: A controlled study. *Folia Psychiatr Neurol Jpn* 36:137–144, 1982.

Tandon R, Flegel P, Greden JF: Carroll and Hamilton rating scales for depression. Abstract of paper presented at the American Psychiatric Association, May, 1986.

Tandon R, Channabasavanna SM, Greden JF: CSF biochemical correlates of mixed affective states. *Acta Psychiatr Scand* 78:289–297, 1988.

Tanna VL, Winokur G: A study of association and linkage of ABO blood types and primary affective disorder. *Br J Psychiatry* 114:1175–1181, 1968.

Targum SD, Gershon ES: Pregnancy, genetic counseling, and the major psychiatric disorders. In: JD Schulman, JL Simpson, eds: *Genetic Diseases in Pregnancy: Maternal Effects and Fetal Outcome*. New York: Academic Press, 1981. pp. 413–438.

Targum SD, Davenport YB, Webster MJ: Postpartum mania in bipolar manic-depressive patients withdrawn from lithium carbonate. *J Nerv Ment Dis* 167:572–574, 1979a.

Targum SD, Gershon ES, Van Eerdewegh M, Rogentine N: Human leukocyte antigen system not closely linked to or associated with bipolar manic-depressive illness. *Biol Psychiatry* 14:615–636, 1979b.

Targum SD, Dibble ED, Davenport YB, Gershon ES: The Family Attitudes Questionnaire: Patients' and spouses' views of bipolar illness. *Arch Gen Psychiatry* 38:562–568, 1981.

Targum SD, Rosen LR, DeLisi LE, Weinberger DR, Citrin CM: Cerebral ventricular size in major depressive disorder: Association with delusional symptoms. *Biol Psychiatry* 18:329–336, 1983.

Targum SD, Greenberg RD, Harmon RL, Kessler K, Salerian AJ, Fram DH: Thyroid hormone and the TRH stimulation test in refractory depression. *J Clin Psychiatry* 45:345–346, 1984.

Taschev T: The course and prognosis of depression on the basis of 652 patients deceased. In: J Angst, ed: *Classification and Prediction of Outcome of Depression*. Symposium Schloss Reinhartshausen/Rhein. Symposia Medica Hoechst 8. Stuttgart: FK Schattauer, 1974. pp 157–172.

Taub JM, Hawkins DR, Van de Castle RL: Electrographic analysis of the sleep cycle in young depressed patients. *Biol Psychol* 7:203–214, 1978.

Taube SL, Kirstein LS, Sweeney DR, Heninger GR, Maas JW: Urinary 3-methoxy-4-hydroxyphenylglycol and psychiatric diagnosis. *Am J Psychiatry* 135:78–82, 1978.

Taylor MA: Schizoaffective and allied disorders. In: RM Post and JC Ballenger, eds: *Neurobiology of Mood Disorders*. Baltimore: Williams & Wilkins, 1984. pp 136–156.

Taylor MA, Abrams R: Manic states: A genetic study of early and late onset affective disorders. *Arch Gen Psychiatry* 28:656–658, 1973a.

Taylor MA, Abrams R: The phenomenology of mania: A new look at some old patients. *Arch of Gen Psychiatry* 29:520–522, 1973b.

Taylor MA, Abrams R: Acute mania: Clinical and genetic study of responders and nonresponders to treatment. *Arch Gen Psychiatry* 32:863–865, 1975.

Taylor MA, Abrams R: Catatonia: Prevalence and importance in the manic phase of manic-depressive illness. *Arch Gen Psychiatry* 34:1223–1225, 1977.

Taylor MA, Abrams R: Familial and non-familial mania. *J Affective Disord* 2:111–118, 1980.

Taylor MA, Abrams R: Early- and late-onset bipolar illness. *Arch Gen Psychiatry* 38:58–61, 1981a.

Taylor MA, Abrams R: Prediction of treatment response in mania. *Arch Gen Psychiatry* 38:800–803, 1981b.

Taylor MA, Abrams R: Cerebral hemisphere dysfunction in the major psychoses. In: P Flor-Henry, J Gruzelier, eds: *Laterality and Psychopathology*. Amsterdam: Elsevier, 1983. pp 153–162.

Taylor MA, Abrams R: Mania and DSM-III schizophreniform disorder. *J Affective Disord* 6:19–24, 1984.

Taylor MA, Abrams R, Gaztanaga P: Manic-depressive illness and schizophrenia: A partial validation of research diagnostic criteria utilizing neuropsychological testing. *Compr Psychiatry* 16:91–96, 1975.

Taylor MA, Greenspan B, Abrams R: Lateralized neuropsychological dysfunction in affective disorder and schizophrenia. *Am J Psychiatry* 136:1031–1034, 1979.

Taylor MA, Abrams R, Hayman MA: The classification of affective disorders: A reassessment of the bipolar-unipolar dichotomy: A clinical, laboratory, and family study. *J Affective Disord* 2:95–109, 1980.

Taylor MA, Redfield J, Abrams R: Neuropsychological dysfunction in schizophrenia and affective disease. *Biol Psychiatry* 16:467–478, 1981.

Taylor R: *Robert Schumann: His Life and Work*. London: Granada, 1982.

Tchaikovsky MI: *The Life and Letters of Peter Il'ich Tchaikovsky*. Edited and translated by R Newmarch. London: John Lane, 1906.

Teasdale JD, Bancroft J: Manipulation of thought content as a determinant of mood and corrugator electromyographic activity in depressed patients. *J Ab-*

norm Psychol 86:235–241, 1977.

Teasdale JD, Fogarty SJ: Differential effects of induced mood on retrieval of pleasant and unpleasant events from episodic memory. J Abnorm Psychol 88:248–258, 1979.

Teja JS, Narang RL, Aggarwal AK: Depression across cultures. Br J Psychiatry 119:253–260, 1971.

Telford R, Worrall EP: Cognitive functions in manic-depressives: Effects of lithium and physostigamine. Br J Psychiatry 133:424–428, 1978.

Telner JI, Lapierre YD, Horn E, Browne M: Rapid reduction of mania by means of reserpine therapy. Am J Psychiatry 143:1058, 1986.

Terenius L, Wahlström A, Lindström L, Widerlöv E: Increased CSF levels of endorphins in chronic psychosis. Neurosci Lett 3:157–162, 1976.

Terenius L, Wahlström A, Ågren H: Naloxone (Narcan) treatment in depression: Clinical observations and effects on CSF endorphins and monoamine metabolites. Psychopharmacology (Berlin) 54:31–33, 1977.

Terman M: On the question of mechanism in phototherapy for seasonal affective disorder: Considerations of clinical efficacy and epidemiology. J Biol Rhythms 3:155–172, 1988.

Terman M, Quitkin FM, Terman JS, Stewart JW, McGrath PJ: The timing of phototherapy: Effects on clinical response and the melatonin cycle. Psychopharmacol Bull 23:354–357, 1987.

Terzian H: Behavioral and EEG effects of intracarotid sodium amytal injection. Acta Neurochir (Wien) 12:230–239, 1964.

Thakar JH, Lapierre YD, Waters BG: Erythrocyte membrane sodium-potassium and magnesium ATPase in primary affective disorder. Biol Psychiatry 20:734–740, 1985.

Thase ME, Hersen M, Bellack AS, Himmelhoch JM, Kupfer DJ: Validation of a Hamilton subscale for endogenomorphic depression. J Affective Disord 5:267–278, 1983.

Thase ME, Kupfer DJ, Ulrich RF: Electroencephalographic sleep in psychotic depression: A valid subtype? Arch Gen Psychiatry 43:886–893, 1986.

Thase ME, Himmelhoch JM, Mallinger AG: Tranylcypromine vs. imipramine in anergic bipolar depression. Abstract of paper presented at the 43rd annual meeting of the Society for Biological Psychiatry, May, 1988.

Thase ME, Himmelhoch JM, Mallinger AG, Jarrett DB, Kupfer DJ: Sleep EEG and DST findings in anergic bipolar depression. Am J Psychiatry 146:329–333, 1989.

Thoits PA: Dimensions of life events that influence psychological distress: An evaluation and synthesis of the literature. In: HB Kaplan, ed: Psychosocial Stress: Trends in Theory and Research. New York: Academic Press, 1983. pp 33–103.

Thomas A, Sillen A: Racism and Psychiatry. New York: Brunner/Mazel, 1972.

Thomas L: The wonderful mistake. The Medusa and the Snail: More Notes of a Biology Watcher. New York: The Viking Press, 1979. pp 27–30.

Thomas R, Beer R, Harris B, John R, Scanlon M: GH responses to growth hormone releasing factor in depression. J Affective Disord 16:133–137, 1989.

Thompson C, Franey C, Arendt J, Checkley SA: A comparison of melatonin secretion in depressed patients and normal subjects. Br J Psychiatry 152:260–265, 1988.

Thompson CC, Weinberger C, Lebo R, Evans RM: Identification of a novel thyroid hormone receptor expressed in the mammalian central nervous system. Science 237:1610–1614, 1987.

Thomsen KC, Hendrie HC: Environmental stress in primary depressive illness. Arch Gen Psychiatry 26:130–132, 1972.

Thysell H, Brante G, Sjöstedt L, Lindergard B, Lindholm T, Franzén G, Rorsman B: Glomerular filtration rate and calcium metabolism in long-term lithium treatment. Neuropsychobiology 7:105–111, 1981.

Tietze C, Lemkau P, Cooper M: Schizophrenia, manic-depressive psychosis and social-economic status. Am J Sociology 47:167–175, 1941.

Tilkian AG, Schroder JS, Kao J, Hultgren H: Effect of lithium on cardiovascular performance: Report on extended ambulatory monitoring and exercise testing before and during lithium therapy. Am J Cardiol 38:701–708, 1976.

Till E, Vuckovic S: Uber den Einfluss der thymoleptischen behandlung auf den verlauf endogener deprssionen. Int Pharmacopsychiatry 4:210–219, 1970.

Tillotson KJ, Fleming R: Personality and sociologic factors in the prognosis and treatment of chronic alcoholism. N Engl J Med 217:611–615, 1937.

Timsit-Berthier M, Gerono A, Rousseau JC, Mantanus H, Abraham P, Verhey FH, Lamers T, Emonds P: An international pilot study of CNV in mental illness. Second report. Ann NY Acad Sci 425:629–637, 1984.

Tompson T: Interdosage fluctuations in plasma carbamazepine concentration determine intermittent side effects. Arch Neurol 41:830–834, 1984.

Toone BK, Cooke E, Lader MH: Electrodermal activity in the affective disorders and schizophrenia. Psychol Med 11:497–508, 1981.

Tooth G: Studies in Mental Health in the Gold Coast. London: Colonial Research Publications, 1950.

Torrey EF, Yolken RH, Winfrey CJ: Cytomegalovirus antibody in cerebrospinal fluid of schizophrenic patients detected by enzyme immunoassay. Science 216:892–894, 1982.

Tow PM: Personality Change Following Frontal Leukotomy. London: Oxford University Press, 1955.

Transbøl I, Christiansen C, Baastrup PC: Endocrine effects of lithium: I. Hypothyroidism, its prevalence in long-term treated patients. Acta Endocrinol (Copenh) 87:759–767, 1978.

Träskman L, Tybring G, Åsberg M, Bertilsson L, Lantto O, Schalling D: Cortisol in the CSF of depressed and suicidal patients. *Arch Gen Psychiatry* 37:761–767, 1980.

Träskman L, Åsberg M, Bertilsson L, Sjöstrand L: Monoamine metabolites in CSF and suicidal behavior. *Arch Gen Psychiatry* 38:631–636, 1981.

Trautner EM, Morris R, Noack CH, Gershon S: The excretion and retention of ingested lithium and its effect on the ionic balance of man. *Med J Aust* 2:280–291, 1955.

Tredgold R, Wolff H: *U.C.H. Handbook of Psychiatry: For Students and General Practitioners.* London: Duckworth, 1975.

Treiser SL, Cascio CS, O'Donohue TL, Thoa NB, Jacobowitz DM, Kellar KJ: Lithium increases serotonin release and decreases serotonin receptors in the hippocampus. *Science* 213:1529–1531, 1981.

Trimble M: Anticonvulsant drugs, behavior and cognitive abilities. *Curr Dev Psychopharmacol* 6:65–91, 1981.

Trimble MR, Cummings JL: Neuropsychiatric disturbances following brainstem lesions. *Br J Psychiatry* 138:56–59, 1981.

Trulson ME, Sampson HW: Ultrastructural changes of the liver following L-tryptophan ingestion in rats. *J Nutr* 116:1109–1115, 1986.

Tsai LY, Nasrallah HA, Jacoby CG: Hemispheric asymmetries on computed tomographic scans in schizophrenia and mania. *Arch Gen Psychiatry* 40:1286–1289, 1983.

Tsuang MT: Suicide in schizophrenics, manics, depressives and surgical controls: A comparison with general suicide mortality. *Arch Gen Psychiatry* 35:153–155, 1978.

Tsuang MT, Simpson JC: Schizoaffective disorder: Concept and reality. *Schizophr Bull* 10:14–25, 1984.

Tsuang MT, Winokur G: The Iowa 500: Field work in a 35-year follow-up of depression, mania, and schizophrenia. *Can Psychiatr Assoc J* 20:359–365, 1975.

Tsuang MT, Woolson RF: Mortality in patients with schizophrenia, mania, depression and surgical conditions. *Br J Psychiatry* 130:162–166, 1977.

Tsuang MT, Woolson R, Fleming JA: Long-term outcome of major psychoses: I. Schizophrenia and affective disorders compared with psychiatrically symptom-free surgical conditions. *Arch Gen Psychiatry* 36:1295–1301, 1979.

Tsuang MT, Woolson R, Fleming JA: Causes of death in schizophrenia and manic-depression. *Br J Psychiatry* 136:239–242, 1980.

Tsuang MT, Woolson RF, Simpson JC: An evaluation of the Feighner criteria for schizophrenia and affective disorders using long-term outcome data. *Psychol Med* 11:281–287, 1981.

Tsuang MT, Faraone SV, Fleming JA: Familial transmission of major affective disorders: Is there evidence supporting the distinction between unipolar and bipolar disorders? *Br J Psychiatry* 146:268–271, 1985.

Tsuang MT, Lyons MJ, Faraone SV: Problems of diagnoses in family studies. *J Psychiat Res* 21:391–399, 1987.

Tucker DM: Lateral brain function, emotion, and conceptualization. *Psychol Bull* 89:19–46, 1981.

Tucker DM, Stenslie CE, Roth RS, Shearer SL: Right frontal lobe activation and right hemisphere performance: Decrement during a depressed mood. *Arch Gen Psychiatry* 38:169–174, 1981.

Tuomisto J, Tukiainen E: Decreased uptake of 5-hydroxytryptamine in blood platelets from depressed patients. *Nature* 262:596–598, 1976.

Tuomisto J, Tukiainen E, Ahlfors UG: Decreased uptake of 5-hydroxytryptamine in blood platelets from patients with endogenous depression. *Psychopharmacology (Berlin)* 65:141–147, 1979.

Turek FW: Circadian neural rhythms in mammals. *Ann Rev Physiol* 47:49–64, 1985.

Turner SM, Jacob RG, Beidel DC, Griffin S: A second case of mania associated with fluoxetine. *Am J Psychiatry* 142:274–275, 1985.

Turner WJ, King S: Two genetically distinct forms of bipolar affective disorder? *Biol Psychiatry* 16:417–439, 1981.

Turns D: The epidemiology of major affective disorders. *Am J Psychother* 32:5–19, 1978.

Tyrer SP: Lithium in the treatment of mania. *J Affective Disord* 8:251–257, 1985.

Tyrer SP, Shopsin B: Symptoms and assessment of mania. In: ES Paykel, ed: *Handbook of Affective Disorders.* Edinburgh: Churchill Livingstone, 1982. pp 12–23.

Tyrer SP, Schacht RG, McCarthy MJ, Menard KN, Leong S, Shopsin B: The effect of lithium on renal haemodynamic function. *Psychol Med* 13:61–69, 1983.

U'Prichard DC, Daiguji M, Tong C, Mitrius JC, Meltzer HY: α_2-adrenergic receptors: Comparative biochemistry of neural and non-neural receptors, and in vitro analysis in psychiatric patients. In: E Usdin, I Hanin, eds: *Biological Markers in Psychiatry and Neurology.* Oxford: Pergamon Press, 1982. pp 205–217.

U'Prichard DC, Mitrius JC, Kahn DJ, Perry BD: The alpha 2-adrenergic receptor: Multiple affinity states and regulation of a receptor inversely coupled to adenylate cyclase. *Adv Biochem Psychopharmacol* 36:53–72, 1983.

Ueno Y, Aoki N, Yabuki T, Kuraishi F: Electrolyte metabolism in blood and cerebrospinal fluid in psychoses. *Folia Psychiatr Neurol Jap* 15:304–326, 1961.

Uhde TW, Bierer LM, Post RM: Caffeine-induced escape from dexamethasone suppression. Letter. *Arch Gen Psychiatry* 42:737–738, 1985.

Untermeyer L: Rebel against reality: Percy Bysshe Shelley. In: *Lives of the Poets.* New York: Simon and Schuster, 1959.

Usdin E, Åsberg M, Bertilsson L, Sjöqvist F: *Frontiers in Biochemical and Pharmacological Research in Depression.* New York: Raven Press, 1984.

Uytdenhoef P, Portelange P, Jacquy J, Charles G, Linkowski P, Mendlewicz J: Regional cerebral blood flow and lateralized hemispheric dysfunction in depression. *Br J Psychiatry* 143:128–132, 1983.

Vaillant GE: Alcoholism and drug dependence. In: AM Nicholi, ed: *The Harvard Guide to Modern Psychiatry*. Cambridge, MA: Belknap Press, 1978. pp 567–577.

Val ER, Nasr SJ, Gaviria FM, Prasad RB: Depression, borderline disorder, and the DST. *Am J Psychiatry* 140:819, 1983.

Vale W, Spiess J, Rivier C, Rivier J: Characterization of a 41-residue ovine hypothalamic peptide that stimulates secretion of corticotropin and beta-endorphin. *Science* 213:1394–1397, 1981.

Van Brunt N: The clinical utility of tricyclic antidepressant blood levels: A review of the literature. *Ther Drug Monit* 5:1–10, 1983.

Van Cauter E, Turek FW: Depression: A disorder of timekeeping? *Pers Biol Med* 29:510-5-9, 1986.

Van den Hoofdakker RH, Beersma DGM: On the explanation of short REM latencies in depression. *Psychiatry Res* 16:155–163, 1985.

Van den Hoofdakker RH, Beersma DG, Dijk DJ, Bouhuys AL, Dols LCW: Effects of total sleep deprivation on mood and chronophysiology in depression. In: C Shagass, RC Josiassen, WH Bridger, KJ Weiss, D Stoff, GM Simpson, eds: *Biological Psychiatry 1985: Proceedings of the IVth World Congress of Biological Psychiatry*. New York: Elsevier, 1986. pp. 969–971.

Van der Velde CD: Effectiveness of lithium carbonate in the treatment of manic-depressive illness. *Am J Psychiatry* 127:345–351, 1970.

Van der Velde CD: Rapid clinical effectiveness of MIF-I in the treatment of major depressive illness. *Peptides* 4:297–300, 1983.

Van Dyke C, McDaniel K, Reus V, Kaufman IC: Immune responses in depression and Cushing's Disease. Abstract of paper presented at the 137th annual meeting of the American Psychiatric Association. May, 1984.

van Gogh V: Introduction to *The Complete Letters of Vincent van Gogh*. Vol 1. Boston: New York Graphic Society, 1958.

Van Hiele LJ: L-5-Hydroxytryptophan in depression: The first substitution therapy in psychiatry? The treatment of 99 out-patients with "therapy-resistant" depressions. *Neuropsychobiology* 6:230–240, 1980.

Van Kammen DP, Levine R, Sternberg D: Preliminary evaluation of hydroxylase cofactor in human spinal fluid: Potential biochemical and clinical relevance for psychiatric disorders. *Psychopharmacol Bull* 14:51–52, 1978.

Van Praag HM: A transatlantic view of the diagnosis of depressions according to the DSM III: I. Controversies and misunderstandings in depression diagnosis. *Compr Psychiatry* 23:315–329, 1982a.

Van Praag HM: A transatlantic view of the diagnosis of depressions according to the DSM III: II. Did the DSM III solve the problem of depression diagnosis? *Compr Psychiatry* 23:330–338, 1982b.

Van Praag HM: In search of the mode of action of antidepressants: 5-HTP/tyrosine mixtures in depressions. *Neuropharmacology* 22:433–440, 1983.

Van Praag HM: Depression, suicide, and serotonin metabolism in the brain. In: RM Post, JC Ballenger, eds. *Neurobiology of Mood Disorders*. Baltimore: Williams & Wilkins, 1984. pp 601–618.

Van Praag HM, De Haan S: Central serotonin metabolism and frequency of depression. *Psychiatry Res* 1:219–224, 1979.

Van Praag H, De Haan S: Depression vulnerability and 5-hydroxytrytophan prophylaxis. *Psychiatry Res* 3:75–83, 1980.

Van Praag HM, Korf J: Endogenous depression with and without disturbances in 5-hydroxytryptamine metabolism: A biochemical classification? *Psychopharmacologia* 19:148–152, 1971.

Van Praag HM, Korf J: Central monoamine deficiency in depressions: Causative of secondary phenomenon? *Pharmakopsychiatr Neuropsychopharmakol* 8:322–326, 1975.

Van Praag HM, Korf J, Schut D: Cerebral monoamine and depression. *Arch Gen Psychiatry* 28:827–831, 1973.

Van Putten T: Why do patients with manic-depressive illness stop their lithium? *Compr Psychiatry* 16:179–183, 1975.

Van Putten T, Crumpton E, Yale C: Drug refusal in schizophrenia and the wish to be crazy. *Arch Gen Psychiatry* 33:1443–1446, 1976.

Van Riper DA, Absher MP, Lenox RH: Muscarinic receptors on intact human fibroblasts: Absence of receptor activity in adult skin cells. *J Clin Invest* 76:882–886, 1985.

Van Royen EA, de Bruíne JF, Hill TC, Vyth A, Limburg M, Byse BL, O'Leary DH, de Jong JM, Hijdra A, Van der Schoot JB: Cerebral blood flow imaging with thallium–201 diethyldithiocarbamate SPECT. *J Nucl Med* 28:178–183, 1987.

Van Scheyen JD: Recurrent vital depression. *Psychiatr Neurol Neurochir* 76:93–112, 1973.

Van Sweden B: Disturbed vigilance in mania. *Biol Psychiatry* 21:311–313, 1986.

Van Woert MH, Ambani LM, Weintraub MI: Manic behavior and levodopa. *N Engl J Med* 285:1326, 1971.

Van Wulfften-Palthe PM: Psychiatry and neurology in the tropics. In: CD deLangen, A Lichtenstein, eds: *A Clinical Textbook of Tropical Medicine*. Batavia: G Kloff and Co, 1936. pp 525–547.

Varanka TM, Weller EB, Weller RA, Fristad MA: Lithium treatment of psychotic features in prepubertal children. *Am J Psychiatry* 145:1557–1559, 1988.

Vasile RG, Samson JA, Bemporad J, Bloomingdale KL, Creasey D, Fenton BT, Gudeman JE, Schildkraut JJ: A biopsychosocial approach to treating patients with affective disorders. *Am J Psychiatry* 144:341–344, 1987.

Veith RC, Raskind MA, Barnes RF, Gumbrecht G, Ritchie JL, Halter JB: Tricyclic antidepressants and supine, standing, and exercise plasma nor-epinephrine levels. *Clin Pharmacol Ther* 33:763–769, 1983.

Venables PH: A short scale for rating "activity-withdrawal" in schizophrenics. *J Ment Sci* 103:197–199, 1957.

Vencovsky E, Soucek K, Kabes J: Prophylactic effect of dipopylacetamide in patients with bipolar affective disorder. In: HM Emrich, T Okuma, AA Müller, eds: *Anticonvulsants in Affective Disorders*. New York: Elsevier, 1984. pp 66–67.

Venkatarangam SHM, Kutcher SP, Notkin RM: Secondary mania with steroid withdrawal. *Can J Psychiatry* 33:631–632, 1988.

Verbanck PM, Lotstra F, Gilles C, Linkowski P, Mendlewicz J, Vanderhaeghen JJ: Reduced cholecystokinin immunoreactivity in the cerebrospinal fluid of patients with psychiatric disorders. *Life Sci* 34:67–72, 1984.

Vergnes M, Kiesmann M, Marescaux C, DePaulis A, Micheletti G, Warter J-M: Kindling of audiogenic seizures in the rat. *Int J Neurosci* 36:167–176, 1987.

Vestergaard P: Clinically important side effects of long-term lithium treatment: A review. *Acta Psychiatr Scand* 67(Suppl 305):11–33, 1983.

Vestergaard P, Amdisen A: Patient attitudes towards lithium. *Acta Psychiatr Scand* 67:8–12, 1983.

Vestergaard P, Schou M: The effect of age on lithium dosage requirements. *Pharmacopsychiatry* 17:199–201, 1984.

Vestergaard P, Schou M: Does long-term lithium treatment induce diabetes mellitus? *Neuropsychobiology* 17:130–132, 1987.

Vestergaard P, Schou M: Prospective studies on a lithium cohort. I. General features. *Acta Psychiatr Scand* 78:421–426, 1988.

Vestergaard P, Sørensen T, Hoppe E, Rafaelsen OJ, Yates CM, Nicolaou N: Biogenic amine metabolites in cerebrospinal fluid of patients with affective disorders. *Acta Psychiatr Scand* 58:88–96, 1978.

Vestergaard P, Amdisen A, Schou M: Clinically significant side effects of lithium treatment: A survey of 237 patients in long-term treatment. *Acta Psychiatr Scand* 62:193–200, 1980.

Vestergaard P, Poulstrup I, Schou M: Prospective studies on a lithium cohort 3: Tremor, weight gain, diarrhea, psychological complaints. *Acta Psychiatr Scand* 78:434–441, 1988.

Viamontes JA: Review of drug effectiveness in the treatment of alcoholism. *Am J Psychiatry* 128:1570–1571, 1972.

Viberti GC, Keen H, Mackintosh D: Beta 2-microglobulinaemia: A sensitive index of diminishing renal function in diabetics. *Br Med J* 282:95–98, 1981.

Victor BS, Link NA, Binder RL, Bell IR: Use of clonazepam in mania and schizoaffective disorders. *Am J Psychiatry* 141:1111–1112, 1984.

Viswanathan R, Glickman L: Clonazepam in the treatment of steroid-induced mania in a patient after renal transplantation. *N Engl J Med* 320:319–320, 1989.

Vogel F: Research strategies in human behavior genetics. *J Med Genetics* 24:129–138, 1987.

Vogel F, Motulsky AG: *Human Genetics*. Berlin: Springer-Verlag, 1986.

Vogel GW, Vogel F, McAbee RS, Thurmond AJ: Improvement of depression by REM sleep deprivation: New findings and a theory. *Arch Gen Psychiatry* 37:247–253, 1980.

Vogel W, Klaiber EL, Broverman DM: A comparison of the antidepressant effects of a synthetic androgen (mesterolone) and amitriptyline in depressed men. *J Clin Psychiatry* 46:6–8, 1985.

Vojtechovsky M: *Ploblemy psychiatrie v proxi a ve vyzkumu*. Prague: Czechoslovak Medical Press, 1957.

Volk W, Bier W, Braun JP, Grüter W, Spiegelberg U: Behandlung von erregten psychosen mit einem beta-rezeptoren-blocker (Oxprenolol) in hoher dosierung. *Nervenarzt* 43:491–492, 1972.

Volkmar FR, Shakir SA, Bacon S, Pfefferbaum A: Group therapy in the management of manic-depressive illness. *Am J Psychotherapy* 35:226–234, 1981.

Von Euler US, Gaddum JH: An unidentified depressor substance in certain tissue extracts. *J Physiol (Lond)* 72:74–87, 1931.

Von Gall M, Becker H: Zur Anwendung der computer-tomographie (CT) in der klinischen psychiatrie. *Fortschr Neurol Psychiatr* 17:381–386, 1978.

Von Knorring A-L, Cloninger CR, Bohman M, Sigvardsson S: An adoption study of depressive disorders and substance abuse. *Arch Gen Psychiatry* 40:943–950, 1983.

Von Knorring L: Visual averaged evoked responses in patients with bipolar affective disorders. *Neuropsychobiology* 4:314–320, 1978.

Von Knorring L, Johansson F: Visual evoked potentials as a predictor of reported side effects during a trial of zimelidine vs. placebo in chronic pain patients. *Psychiatry Res* 1:225–230, 1979.

Von Knorring L, Espvall M, Perris C: Average evoked responses, pain measures, and personality variables in patients with depressive disorders. *Acta Psychiatr Scand* 255:99–108, 1974.

Von Knorring L, Smigan L, Perris C, Oreland L: Lithium and neuroleptic drugs in combination: Effect on lithium RBC/plasma ratio. *Int Pharmacopsychiatry* 17:287–292, 1982.

Von Zerssen D: Beta-adrenergic blocking agents in the treatment of psychoses: A report on 17 cases. In: C Carlsson, J Engel, L Hanson, eds: *Neuro-Psychiatric Effects of Adrenergic Beta-Receptor Blocking Agents*. Munich: Urban and Scwarzenberg, 1976. pp 105–115.

Von Zerssen D: Premorbid personality and affective psychoses. In: GD Burrows, ed: *Handbook of Studies on Depression*. Amsterdam: Excerpta Medica, 1977. pp 79–103.

Von Zerssen D: Personality and affective disorders. In: ES Paykel, ed. *Handbook of Affective Disorders*.

New York: Guilford Press, 1982. pp 212–228.

Von Zerssen D, Cording C: The measurement of change in endogenous affective disorders. *Arch Psychiatr Nervenkr* 226:95–112, 1978.

Waddington JL, Youssef HA: Tardive dyskinesia in bipolar affective disorder: Aging, cognitive dysfunction, course of illness, and exposure to neuroleptics and lithium. *Am J Psychiatry* 145:613–616, 1988.

Wade JB, Hart R, Lehman L, Hamer R: Neuropsychological dysfunction in schizophrenia and bipolar disorder. *J Clin Exper Neuropsychol* 10:71, 1988.

Wadeson HS, Bunney WE Jr: Manic-depressive art: A systematic study of differences in a 48-hour cyclic patient. *J Nerv Ment Dis* 150:215–231, 1970.

Wadeson HS, Carpenter WT Jr: A comparative study of art expression of schizophrenic, unipolar depressive, and bipolar manic-depressive patients. *J Nerv Ment Dis* 162:334–344, 1976.

Waehrens J, Gerlach J: Bromocriptine and imipramine in endogenous depression: A double-blind controlled trial in out-patients. *J Affective Disord* 3:193–202, 1981.

Wägner A, Aberg-Wistedt A, Åsberg M, Eqvist B, Martensson B, Montero D: Lower ³H-imipramine binding in platelets from untreated depressed patients compared to healthy controls. *Psychiatry Res* 16:131–139, 1985.

Wagner HN Jr, Burns HD, Dannals RF, Wong DF, Langstrom B, Duelfer T, Frost JJ, Ravert HT, Links JM, Rosenbloom SB, Lukas SE, Kramer AV, Kuhar MJ: Imaging dopamine receptors in the human brain by positron tomography. *Science* 221:1264–1266, 1983.

Wagner PS: A comparative study of Negro and white admissions to the Psychiatric Pavilion of the Cincinnati General Hospital. *Am J Psychother* 95:167–183, 1938.

Wakoh H, Hatotani N: Endocrinological treatment of psychoses. In: K Lissák, ed: *Hormones and Brain Function*. New York: Plenum Press, 1973. pp 491–498.

Waldfogel S, Guy W: Wechsler-Bellevue subtest scatter in the affective disorders. *J Clin Psychol* 7:135–139, 1951.

Walinder J, Skott A, Carlsson A, Nagy A, Roos BE: Potentiation of the antidepressant action of clomipramine by tryphtophan. *Arch Gen Psychiatry* 33:1384–1389, 1976.

Walker E, Green M: Soft signs of neurological dysfunction in schizophrenia: An investigation of lateral performance. *Biol Psychiatry* 17:381–386, 1982.

Walker F: *Hugo Wolf: A Biography*. London: JM Dent & Sons, 1968.

Walsh D: Mental illness in Dublin: First admissions. *Br J Psychiatry* 115:449–456, 1969a.

Walsh D: Social class and mental illness in Dublin. *Br J Psychiatry* 115:1151–1161, 1969b.

Walsh K: *Neuropsychology: A Clinical Approach*. 2nd ed. Edinburgh: Churchill Livingstone, 1987.

Walter SD: Seasonality of mania: A reappraisal. *Br J Psychiatry* 131:345–350, 1977.

Walters GD, Greene RL: Differentiating between schizophrenic and manic inpatients by means of the MMPI. *J Person Assess* 52:91–95, 1988.

Walton RG: Seizure and mania after high intake of aspartame. *Psychosomatics* 27:218–220, 1986.

Wang YC, Pandey GN, Mendels J, Frazer A: Platelet adenylate cyclase responses in depression: Implications for a receptor defect. *Psychopharmacologia* 36:291–300, 1974.

Ward NG, Doerr HO, Storrie MC: Skin conductance: A potentially sensitive test for depression. *Psychiatry Res* 10:295–302, 1983.

Warheit GJ, Holzer CE, Arey SA: Race and mental illness: An epidemiologic update. *J Health Soc Behav* 16:243–256, 1975.

Warren EW, Groome DH: Memory test performance under three different waveforms of ECT for depression. *Br J Psychiatry* 144:370–375, 1984.

Warren LR, Butler RW, Katholi CR, McFarland CE, Crews EL, Halsey JH Jr: Focal changes in cerebral blood flow produced by monetary incentive during a mental mathematics task in normal and depressed subjects. *Brain Cogn* 3:71–85, 1984.

Warren M, Bick PA: Two case reports of trazodone-induced mania. *Am J Psychiatry* 141:1103–1104, 1984.

Watanabe S, Ishino H, Otsuki S: Double-blind comparison of lithium carbonate and imipramine in treatment of depression. *Arch Gen Psychiatry* 32:659–668, 1975.

Waters BGH: Early symptoms of bipolar affective psychosis: Research and clinical implications. *Can Psychiatr Assoc J* 2:55–60, 1979.

Waters BGH, Lapierre YD: Secondary mania associated with sympathomimetic drug use. *Am J Psychiatry* 138:837–838, 1981.

Waters BGH, Marchenko-Bouer I: Psychiatric illness in the adult offspring of bipolar manic-depressives. *J Affective Disord* 2:119–126, 1980.

Waters B, Marchenko I, Abrams N, Smiley D, Kalin D: Assortative mating for major affective disorders. *J Affective Disord* 5:9–17, 1983a.

Waters BGH, Marchenko I, Smiley D: Affective disorder, paranatal and educational factors in the offspring of bipolar manic-depressives. *Can J Psychiatry* 28:527–531, 1983b.

Waters BGH, Thakar J, Lapierre Y: Erythrocyte lithium transport variables as a marker for manic-depressive disorder. *Neuropsychobiology* 9:94–98, 1983c.

Watkins JG, Stauffacher JC: An index of pathological thinking in the Rorschach. *J Projective Techniques* 16:276–286, 1952.

Watkins SE, Callender K, Thomas DR, Tidmarsh SF, Shaw DM: The effect of carbamazepine and lithium on remission from affective illness. *Br J Psychiatry* 150:180–182, 1987.

Watts CAH: The incidence and prognosis of endogenous depression. *Br Med J* 1:1392–1397, 1956.

Waziri R, Wilcox J, Sherman AD, Mott J: Serine metabolism and psychosis. *Psychiatry Res* 12:121–

136, 1984.

Weber G, Simon FB, Stierlin H, Schmidt G: Therapy for families manifesting manic-depressive behavior. *Fam Proc* 27:33–49, 1988.

Weeke A: Causes of death in manic-depressives. In: M Schou, E Strömgren, eds: *Origin, Prevention and Treatment of Affective Disorders*. London: Academic Press, 1979. pp 289–299.

Weeke A: Admission pattern and diagnostic stability among unipolar and bipolar manic-depressive patients. *Acta Psychiatr Scand* 70:603–613, 1984.

Weeke A, Vaeth M: Excess mortality of bipolar and unipolar manic-depressive patients. *J Affective Disord* 11:227–234, 1986.

Weeke A, Weeke J: Disturbed circadian variation of serum thyrotropin in patients with endogenous depression. *Acta Psychiatr Scand* 57:281–289, 1978.

Weeke A, Bille M, Videbech Th, Dupont A, Juel-Nielsen N: Incidence of depressive syndromes in a Danish county. The Aarhus County investigation. *Acta Psychiatr Scand* 51:28–41, 1975.

Weeke J: Circadian variation of the serum thyrotropin level in normal subjects. *Scand J Clin Lab Invest* 31:337–342, 1973.

Weetman AP, McGregor AM, Lazarus JH, Smith BR, Hall R: The enhancement of immunoglobulin synthesis by human lymphocytes with lithium. *Clin Immunol Immunopathol* 22:400–407, 1982.

Wehr TA: Phase and biorhythm studies of affective illness. pp.321–324. In: WE Bunney Jr, moderator: The switch process in manic-depressive psychosis. *Ann Intern Med* 87:319–335, 1977.

Wehr TA: A brain heating function for REM sleep. Submitted

Wehr TA: Effects of wakefulness and sleep on depression and mania. In: J Montplaisir, Godbout R, eds: *Sleep and Biological Rhythms*. London: Oxford Press, in press.

Wehr T, Goodwin FK: Catecholamines in depression. In: GD Burrows, ed: *Handbook of Studies on Depression*. Amsterdam: Excerpta Medica, 1977. pp 283–303.

Wehr TA, Goodwin FK: Rapid cycling in manic-depressives induced by tricyclic antidepressants. *Arch Gen Psychiatry* 36:555–559, 1979.

Wehr TA, Goodwin FK: Biological rhythms and psychiatry. In: S Arieti, HKH Brodie, eds: *American Handbook of Psychiatry: Vol. 7, Advance and New Directions*. 2nd ed. New York: Basic Books, 1981. pp 46–74.

Wehr TA, Goodwin FK: Stress, circadian rhythms and affective disorders. *Stress and Coping*. Unit I: Psychophysiology. Philadelphia: SmithKline Corp., 1981a.

Wehr TA, Goodwin FK, eds: *Circadian Rhythms in Psychiatry*. Pacific Grove, CA: The Boxwood Press, 1983a.

Wehr TA, Goodwin FK: Introduction. In: TA Wehr, FK Goodwin, eds: *Circadian Rhythms in Psychiatry*. Pacific Grove, CA: The Boxwood Press, 1983b. pp 1–15.

Wehr TA, Goodwin FK: Biological rhythms in manic-depressive illness. In: TA Wehr, FK Goodwin, eds: *Circadian Rhythms in Psychiatry*. Pacific Grove, CA: The Boxwood Press, 1983c. pp 129–184.

Wehr TA, Goodwin FK: Can antidepressants cause mania and worsen the course of affective illness? *Am J Psychiatry* 144:1403–1411, 1987a.

Wehr TA, Goodwin FK: Do antidepressants cause mania? *Psychopharmacol Bull* 23:61–65, 1987b.

Wehr TA, Goodwin FK: Reply: Antidepressants and mania. *Am J Psychiatry* 145:906–907, 1988.

Wehr TA, Rosenthal NE: Seasonality and affective illness. *Am J Psychiatry* 146:829–839, 1989.

Wehr TA, Sack DA: The relevance of sleep research to affective illness. In: WP Koella, F Obál, H Schulz, P Visser: *Sleep '86*. New York: Gustav Fischer Verlag, 1988. pp 207–211.

Wehr TA, Wirz-Justice A: Internal coincidence model for sleep deprivation and depression. In WP Koella, ed: *Sleep 80* Basel: Karger, 1981. pp 26–33.

Wehr TA, Wirz-Justice A: Circadian rhythm mechanisms in affective illness and in antidepressant drug action. *Pharmacopsychiatry* 15:31–39, 1982.

Wehr TA, Wirz-Justice A, Goodwin FK, Duncan W, Gillin JC: Phase advance of the circadian sleep-wake cycle as an antidepressant. *Science* 206:710–713, 1979.

Wehr TA, Muscettola G, Goodwin FK: Urinary 3-methoxy-4-hydroxyphenylglycol circadian rhythm: Early timing (phase-advance) in manic-depressives compared with normal subjects. *Arch Gen Psychiatry* 37:257–263, 1980.

Wehr TA, Goodwin FK, Wirz-Justice A, Breitmeier J, Craig C: 48-hour sleep-wake cycles in manic-depressive illness: Naturalistic observations and sleep-deprivation experiments. *Arch Gen Psychiatry* 39:559–565, 1982.

Wehr TA, Rosenthal NE, Sack DA, Gillin JC: Antidepressant effects of sleep deprivation in bright and dim light. *Acta Psychiatr Scand* 72:161–165, 1985a.

Wehr TA, Sack DA, Duncan WC, Mendelson WB, Rosenthal NE, Gillin JC, Goodwin FK: Sleep and circadian rhythms in affective patients isolated from external time cues. *Psychiatry Res* 15:327–339, 1985b.

Wehr TA, Jacobsen FM, Sack DA, Arendt J, Tamarkin L, Rosenthal NE: Phototherapy of seasonal affective disorder: Time of day and suppression of melatonin are not critical for antidepressant effects. *Arch Gen Psychiatry* 43:870–875, 1986.

Wehr TA, Sack DA, Rosenthal NE: Sleep reduction as a final common pathway in the genesis of mania. *Am J Psychiatry* 144:201–204, 1987a.

Wehr TA, Sack DA, Rosenthal NE: Seasonal affective disorder with summer depression and winter hypomania. *Am J Psychiatry* 144:1602–1603, 1987b.

Wehr TA, Sack DA, Rosenthal NE, Goodwin FK: Sleep and biological rhythms in bipolar illness. In: RE Hales, A Francis AJ, eds: *Psychiatry Update*. Vol. 6. Washington, DC, 1987c. pp 61–80.

Wehr TA, Skwerer RG, Jacobsen FM, Sack DA, Rosenthal NE: Eye versus skin phototherapy of seasonal affective disorder. *Am J Psychiatry* 144:753–757, 1987d.

Wehr TA, Sack DA, Rosenthal NE, Cowdry RW: Rapid cycling affective disorder: Contributing factors and treatment responses in 51 patients. *Am J Psychiatry* 145:179-184, 1988.

Wehr TA, Geisen H, Schulz PM, Joseph-Vanderpool JR, Kasper S, Kelly K, Rosenthal NE: Summer depression: Description of the syndrome and comparison with winter depression. In: NE Rosenthal, MC Blehar, eds: *Seasonal Affective Disorders and Phototherapy*. New York: Guilford Press, 1989. pp. 55–63.

Weilburg JB, Sachs G, Falk WE: Triazolam-induced brief episodes of secondary mania in a depressed patient. 48:492–493, 1987.

Weinberg WA, Brumback RA: Mania in childhood: Case studies and literature review. *Am J Diseases of Child* 130:380–385, 1976.

Weinberger DR, Kleinman JE: Observations on the brain in schizophrenia. In: AJ Frances, RE Hales, eds: *American Psychiatric Association Annual Review, Vol 5*. Washington, DC: American Psychiatric Press, 1986. pp 42–67.

Weinberger DR, DeLisi LE, Perman GP, Targum S, Wyatt RJ: Computed tomography in schizophreniform disorder and other acute psychiatric disorders. *Arch Gen Psychiatry* 39:778–783, 1982.

Weiner IB, Del Gaudio AC: Psychopathology in adolescence. *Arch Gen Psychiatry* 33:187–193, 1976.

Weiner M, Chausow A, Wolpert E, Addington W, Szidon P: Effect of lithium on the responses to added respiratory resistances. *N Engl J Med* 308:319–322, 1983.

Weiner RD: Does electroconvulsive therapy cause brain damage? *Behav Brain Sci* 7:1–53, 1984.

Weiner RD, Whanger AD, Erwin CW, Wilson WP: Prolonged confusional state and EEG seizure activity following concurrent ECT and lithium use. *Am J Psychiatry* 137:1452–1453, 1980.

Weingartner H, Silberman E: Cognitive changes in depression. In: RM Post, JC Ballenger, eds. *Neurobiology of Mood Disorders*. Baltimore: Williams & Wilkins, 1984. pp 121–135.

Weingartner H, Miller H, Murphy DL: Mood-state-dependent retrieval of verbal associations. *J Abnorm Psychol* 86:276–284, 1977.

Weingartner H, Cohen RM, Murphy DL, Martello J, Gerdt C: Cognitive processes in depression. *Arch Gen Psychiatry* 38:42–47, 1981a.

Weingartner H, Gold P, Ballenger JC, Smallberg SA, Summers R, Rubinow DR, Post RM, Goodwin FK: Effects of vasopressin on human memory functions. *Science* 211:601–603, 1981b.

Weingartner H, Grafman J, Boutelle W, Kaye W, Martin P: Forms of memory failure. *Science* 221:380–382, 1983a.

Weingartner H, Rudorfer MV, Buchsbaum MS, Linnoila M: Effects of serotonin on memory impairments produced by ethanol. *Science* 221:472–474, 1983b.

Weingartner H, Rudorfer MV, Linnoila M: Cognitive effects of lithium treatment in normal volunteers. *Psychopharmacology (Berlin)* 86:472–474, 1985.

Weisert KN, Hendrie HC: Secondary mania? A case report. *Am J Psychiatry* 134:929–930, 1977.

Weiss BL, Foster FG, Reynolds CF, Kupfer DJ: Psychomotor activity in mania. *Arch Gen Psychiatry* 31:379–383, 1974.

Weiss JM, Bailey WH, Goodman PA, Hoffammn LJ, Ambrose MJ, Salman S, Charry JM: A model for neurochemical study of depression. In: MY Spiegelstein, A Levy, eds: *Behavioral Models and the Analysis of Drug Action*. Amsterdam: Elsevier, 1982. pp 195–223.

Weiss JM, Goodman P, Ambrose MJ, Webster A, Hoffman LJ: Neurochemical basis of behavioral depression. In: E Katkin, S Manuck, eds: *Advances in Behavioral Medicine*. Vol. 1. Greenwich, Conn: JAI Press, 1984. pp 233–276.

Weiss RD, Mirin SM: Drug, host, and environmental factors in the development of chronic cocaine abuse. In: SM Mirin, ed: *Substance Abuse and Psychopathology*. Washington: American Psychiatric Press, 1984. pp 41–56.

Weiss RD, Mirin SM: Subtypes of cocaine abusers. *Psychiatr Clin North Am* 9:491–501, 1986.

Weiss RD, Mirin SM: Substance abuse as an attempt at self-medication. *Psychiatr Med* 3:357–367, 1987.

Weiss RD, Mirin SM, Michael JL, Sollogub AC: Psychopathology in chronic cocaine abusers. *Am J Drug Alcohol Abuse* 12:17–29, 1986.

Weiss RD, Mirin SM, Griffin ML, Michael JL: Psychopathology in cocaine abusers: Changing trends. *J Nerv Ment Dis* 176:719–725, 1988.

Weissman MM: Psychotherapy and its relevance to the pharmacotherapy of affective disorders: From ideology to evidence. In: MA Lipton, A DiMascio, KF Killam, eds: *Psychopharmacology: A Generation of Progress*. New York: Raven Press, 1978. pp 1313–1321.

Weissman MM: The psychological treatment of depression: Evidence for the efficacy of psychotherapy alone, in comparison with, and in combination with pharmacotherapy. *Arch Gen Psychiatry* 36:1261–1269, 1979.

Weissman MM, Boyd JH: The epidemiology of mental disorders. In: RM Post, JC Ballenger, eds: *Neurobiology of Mood Disorders*. Baltimore: Williams & Wilkins, 1984. pp 60–75.

Weissman MM, Klerman GL: Psychotherapy with depressed women: An empirical study of content themes and reflection. *Br J Psychiatry* 123:55–61, 1973.

Weissman MM, Klerman GL: Sex differences and the epidemiology of depression. *Arch Gen Psychiatry* 34:98–111, 1977.

Weissman MM, Klerman GL: Epidemiology of mental disorders: Emerging trends in the United States. *Arch Gen Psychiatry* 35:705–712, 1978.

Weissman MM, Myers JK: Affective disorders in a US

urban community: The use of Research Diagnostic Criteria in an epidemiological survey. *Arch Gen Psychiatry* 35:1304–1311, 1978.

Weissman MM, Myers JK: Clinical depression in alcoholism. *Am J Psychiatry* 137:372–373, 1980.

Weissman MM, Paykel ES: *The Depressed Woman: A Study of Social Relationships.* Chicago: University of Chicago Press, 1974.

Weissman MM, Paykel ES, Siegel R, Klerman GL: The social role performance of depressed women: Comparisons with a normal group. *Am J Orthopsychiatry* 41:390–405, 1971.

Weissman MM, Paykel ES, Klerman GL: The depressed woman as a mother. *Soc Psychiatry* 7:98–108, 1972.

Weissman MM, Sholomskas D, Pottenger M, Prusoff BA, Locke BZ: Assessing depressive symptoms in five psychiatric populations: A validation study. *Am J Epidemiology* 106:203–214, 1977.

Weissman MM, Prusoff BA, DiMascio A, Neu C, Goklaney M, Klerman GL: The efficacy of drugs and psychotherapy in the treatment of acute depressive episodes. *Am J Psychiatry* 136:555–558, 1979.

Weissman MM, Gershon ES, Kidd KK, Prusoff BA, Leckman JF, Dibble E, Hamovit J, Thompson WD, Pauls DL, Guroff, JJ Psychiatric disorders in the relatives of probands with affective disorders: The Yale-National Institute of Mental Health collaborative study. *Arch Gen Psychiatry* 41:13–21, 1984a.

Weissman MM, Prusoff BA, Merikangas KR: Is delusional depression related to bipolar disorder? *Am J Psychiatry* 141:892–893, 1984b.

Weissman MM, Wickramaratne P, Merikangas KR, Leckman JF, Prusoff BA, Caruso KA, Kidd KK, Gammon D: Onset of major depression in early adulthood: Increased familial loading and specificity. *Arch Gen Psychiatry* 41: 1136–1143, 1984c.

Weissman MM, Merikangas KR, Boyd JH: Epidemiology of affective disorders. In: R Michels, JO Cavenar, HKH Brodie, AM Cooper, SB Guze, LL Judd, GL Klerman, AJ Solnit, eds: *Psychiatry, Vol 1.* Philadelphia: JB Lippincott, 1985. Ch 60. pp 1–14.

Weissman MM, Jarrett RB, Rush JA: Psychotherapy and its relevance to the pharmacotherapy of major depression: A decade later (1976–1985). In: HY Meltzer, ed: *Psychopharmacology: The Third Generation of Progress.* New York: Raven Press, 1987a. pp 1059–1069.

Weissman MM, Wickramaratne P, Warner V, John K, Prusoff BA, Merikangas KR, Gammon GD: Assessing psychiatric disorders in children: Discrepancies between mothers' and children's reports. *Arch Gen Psychiatry* 44:747–753, 1987b.

Weissman MM, Leaf PJ, Tischler GL, Blazer DG, Karno M, Bruce ML, Florio LP: Affective disorders in five United States communities. *Psychol Med* 18:141–153, 1988a.

Weissman MM, Warner V, John K, Prusoff BA, Merikangas KR, Wickramaratne P, Gammon GD: Delusional depression and bipolar spectrum: Evidence for a possible association from a family study of children. *Neuropsychopharm* 1:257–264, 1988b.

Weissman MM, Warner V, Wickramaratne P, Prusoff BA: Early-onset major depression in parents and their children. *J Affective Disord* 15:269–77, 1988c.

Weitkamp LR, Stancer HC, Persad E, Flood C, Guttormsen S: Depressive disorders and HLA: A gene on chromosome 6 that can affect behavior. *N Engl J Med* 305:1301–1306, 1981.

Weitzman ED, Nogeire C, Perlow M, Fukushima D, Sassin J, McGregor P, Gallagher TF, Hellman L: Effects of a prolonged 3-hour sleep-wake cycle on sleep stages, plasma cortisol, growth hormone and body temperature in man. *J Clin Endocrinol Metab* 38:1018–1030, 1974.

Weitzman ED, Czeisler CA, Zimmerman JC, Ronda JM: The sleep-wake pattern of cortisol and growth hormone secretion during non-entrained (free-running) conditions in man. In: E Van Cauter, G Copinschi, eds: *Human Pituitary Hormones: Circadian and Episodic Variations.* The Hague: Martinus Nijhoff, 1981. pp. 29–41.

Weller EB, Weller RA: Neuroendocrine changes in affectively ill children and adolescents. *Endocrinol Metab Clin North Am* 17:41–53, 1988.

Weller EB, Weller RA, Fristad MA: Lithium dosage guide for prepubertal children: A preliminary report. *J Am Acad Child Psychiatry* 25:92–95, 1986.

Weller EB, Weller RA, Fristad MA, Cantwell M, Tucker S: Saliva lithium monitoring in prepubertal children. *J Am Acad Child Adolesc Psychiatry* 26:173–175, 1987.

Weller MPI, Ang PC, Latimer-Sayer DT, Zachary A: Drug abuse and mental illness. *Lancet* 1:997, 1988.

Weller RA, Weller EB, Tucker SG, Fristad MA: Mania in prepubertal children: Has it been underdiagnosed? *J Affective Disord* 11:151–154, 1986.

Wellner J, Marstal HB: Symptoms in mania, an analysis of 279 attacks of manic depressive elation. In: B Jansson, ed: Report on the Fourteenth Congress of Scandanavian Psychiatrist. *Acta Psychiatr Scand* 40(Supp 180):175–176, 1964.

Wells CE: Organic mental disorders. In: HI Kaplan, BJ Sadock, eds: *Comprehensive Textbook of Psychiatry/IV.* Vol 1. Baltimore: Williams & Wilkins, 1985. pp 834–882.

Wells EL, Kelley CM: Intelligence and psychosis. *Am J Insanity* 77:17–45, 1920.

Welner A, Liss JL, Robins E: Psychiatric symptoms in white and black inpatients: II: Follow-up study. *Compr Psychiatry* 14:483–488, 1973.

Welner A, Welner Z, Leonard A: Bipolar manic-depressive disorder: A reassessment of course and outcome. *Compr Psychiatry* 18:327–332, 1977.

Welner Z, Rice J: School-aged children of depressed parents: a blind and controlled study. *J Affective Disord* 15:291–302, 1988.

Welsh DK, Nino-Murcia G, Gander PH, Keenan S, Dement WC: Regular 48-hour cycling of sleep duration and mood in a 35-year-old woman: Use of lithium in time isolation. *Biol Psychiatry* 21:527–

537, 1986.

Wender PH, Kety SS, Rosenthal D, Schulsinger F, Ortmann J, Lunde I: Psychiatric disorders in the biological and adoptive families of adopted individuals with affective disorders. *Arch Gen Psychiatry* 43:923–929, 1986.

Wernicke C: *Grundriss der Psychiatrie in Klinischen Vorlesungen.* Leipzig: Georg Thieme, 1900.

Wertham FI: A group of benign psychoses: Prolonged manic excitements: With a statistical study of age, duration and frequency in 2000 manic attacks. *Am J Psychiatry* 9:17–78, 1929.

West AP, Meltzer HY: Paradoxical lithium neurotoxicity: A report of five cases and a hypothesis about risk for neurotoxicity. *Am J Psychiatry* 136:963–966, 1979.

West LJ: Integrative psychotherapy of deprssive illness. In: FF Flach, SC Draghi, eds: *The Nature and Treatment of Depression.* New York: John Wiley and Sons, 1975.

Westenberg HG, Van Praag HM, de Jong JT, Thijssen JH: Postsynaptic serotonergic activity in depressive patients: Evaluation of the neuroendocrine strategy. *Psychiatry Res* 7:361–371, 1982.

Westermeyer J: Resuming social approaches to psychiatric disorder: A critical contemporary need. *J Nerv Ment Dis* 176:703–706, 1988.

Weston PG, Howard MQ: The determination of Na, K, Ca, and Mg in the blood and spinal fluid of patients suffering from manic-depressive insanity. *Arch Neurol Psychiatry* 8:179–183, 1922.

Wever R: The effects of electric fields on circadian rhythmicity in men. *Life Sciences and Space Res* 8:177–187, 1970.

Wever R: Human circadian rhythms under the influence of weak electric fields and the different aspects of these studies. *Int J Biometeorol* 17:227–232, 1973.

Wever R: Quantitative studies of the interaction between different circadian oscillators within the human multi-oscillator system. *International Society for Chronobiology: XII International Conference Proceedings.* Il Ponte, Milan: The Publishing House, 1977. p 525.

Wever RA: *The Circadian System of Man: Results of Experiments Under Temporal Isolation.* New York: Springer-Verlag, 1979.

Wever RA: Phase shifts of human circadian rhythms due to shifts of artificial Zeitgebers. *Chronobiologia* 7:303–327, 1980.

Wever RA: Organization of the human circadian system: Internal interations. In: TA Wehr, FK Goodwin, eds: *Circadian Rhythms in Psychiatry.* Pacific Grove, CA: The Boxwood Press, 1983. pp 17–32.

Wexler BE: A Model of brain function: Its implications for psychiatric research. *Br J Psychiatry* 148:357–362, 1986.

Wexler BE, Heninger GR: Alterations in cerebral laterality during acute psychotic illness. *Arch Gen Psychiatry* 36:278–284, 1979.

Whalley LJ, Scott M, Reading HW, Christie JE: Effect of electroconvulsive therapy on erythrocyte adenosine triphosphatase activity in depressive illness. *Br J Psychiatry* 137:343–345, 1980.

Wheatley D: Potentiation of amitriptyline by thyroid hormone. *Arch Gen Psychiatry* 26:229–233, 1972.

Whitaker PM, Warsh JJ, Stancer HC, Persad E, Vint CK: Seasonal variation in platelet ^{3}H-imipramine bindings: Comparable values in control and depressed populations. *Psychiatry Res* 11:127–131, 1984.

White K, Simpson G: Combined MAOI-tricyclic antidepressant treatment: A reevaluation. *J Clin Psychiatry* 1:264–282, 1981.

White K, Simpson G: Should the use of MAO inhibitors be abandoned? *Integr Psychiatry* 3:34–45, 1985.

White K, Bohart R, Whipple K, Boyd J: Lithium effects on normal subjects: Relationships to plasma and RBC lithium levels. *Int Pharmacopsychiatry* 14:176–183, 1979.

White R, Lalouel J: Chromosome mapping with DNA markers. *Sci Am* 258:40–48, 1988.

Whitehead A: Verbal learning and memory in elderly depressives. *Br J Psychiatry* 123:203–208, 1973.

Whiteley JS: Down and out in London: Mental illness in the lower social groups. *Lancet* 2:608–610, 1955.

Whitwell JR: *Historical Notes on Psychiatry (Early Times—End of 16th Century).* London: HK Lewis & Co, 1936.

Whybrow PC, Mendels J: Toward a biology of depression: Some suggestions from neurophysiology. *Am J Psychiatry* 125:1491–1500, 1969.

Whybrow PC, Prange AJ, Treadway CR: Mental changes accompanying thyroid gland dysfunction. *Arch Gen Psychiatry* 20:48–63, 1969.

Whybrow PC, Akiskal HS, McKinney WT: *Mood Disorders: Toward a New Psychobiology.* New York: Plenum Press, 1984.

Whyte A: Vanadate and manic-depressive illness. Letter. *Lancet* 2:865, 1981.

Widerlöv E, Bissette G, Nemeroff CB: Monoamine metabolites, corticotropin releasing factor and somatostatin as CSF markers in depressed patients. *J Affective Disord* 14:99–107, 1988a.

Widerlöv E, Lindström LH, Wahlestest C, Ekman R: Neuropeptide Y and Peptide YY as possible cerebrospinal fluid markers for major depression and schizophrenia, respectively. *J Psychiatr Res* 22:69–79, 1988b.

Widlöcher DJ: Psychomotor retardation: Clinical, theoretical, and psychometric aspects. *Psychiatr Clin North Am* 6:27–40, 1983.

Wiegand M, Berger M, Zulley J, Lauer C, Von Zerssen D: The influence of daytime naps on the therapeutic effect of sleep deprivation. *Biol Psychiatry* 22:389–392, 1986.

Wightman WPD: *The Emergence of Scientific Medicine.* Edinburgh: Oliver & Boyd, 1971.

Wikler A: Psychodynamic study of a patient during experimental self-regulated readdiction of morphine. *Psychiatr Q* 26:270–293, 1952.

Wilenski RH: *John Ruskin: An Introduction to Further Study of His Life and Work.* London: Faber & Faber, 1933.

Wilk S, Shopsin B, Gershon S, Suhl M: Cerebrospinal fluid levels of MHPG in affective disorders. *Nature* 235:440–441, 1972.

Wilkinson DM, Halpern LM: The role of biogenic amines in amygdalar kindling: I. Local amygdalar afterdischarge. *J Pharmacol Exp Ther* 211:151–158, 1979.

Wilkinson M: *The Way of the Makers.* New York: MacMillan, 1925.

Willcox DRC, Gillan R, Hare EH: Do psychiatric outpatients take their drugs? *Br Med J* 2:790–792, 1965.

Williams JBW: A structured interview guide for the Hamilton Depression Rating Scale. *Arch Gen Psychiatry* 45:742–747, 1988.

Williams JBW, Link MJ, Rosenthal NE, Terman M: Hypomania interview guide (including hyperthymia) for seasonal affective disorder. Personal communication, 1987.

Williams KM, Iacono WG, Remick RA: Electrodermal activity among subtypes of depression. *Biol Psychiatry* 20:158–162, 1985.

Willner P: Dopamine and depression: A review of recent evidence: III. The effects of antidepressant treatments. *Brain Res* 287:237–246, 1983.

Willner P: The validity of animal models of depression. *Psychopharmacology* 83:1–16, 1984.

Willner P: *Depression: A Psychobiological Synthesis.* New York: John Wiley & Sons, 1985.

Wilson BW: Chronic exposure to ELF fields may induce depression. *Bioelectromagnetics* 9:195–205, 1988.

Wilson DC: Families of manic depressives. *Dis Nerv Syst* 12:362–369, 1951.

Wilson M: *The Life of William Blake.* Edited by G Keynes. London: Oxford University Press, 1971.

Wilson S: *What Shall We Wear to This Party? The Man in the Gray Flannel Suit; Twenty Years Before and After.* New York: Arbor House, 1976.

Wing JK, Birley JLT, Cooper JE, Graham P, Isaacs AD: Reliability of a procedure for measuring and classifying "present psychiatric state." *Br J Psychiatry* 113:499–515, 1967.

Wing JK, Cooper JE, Sartorius N: *The Measurement and Classification of Psychiatric Symptoms: An Instruction Maniual for the PSE and CATEGO Program.* London: Cambridge University Press, 1974.

Wing JK, Mann SA, Leff JP, Nixon JM: The concept of a "case" in psychiatric population surveys. *Psychol Med* 8:203–217, 1978.

Winokur A, March V, Mendels J: Primary affective disorder in relatives of patients with anorexia nervosa. *Am J Psychiatry* 137:695–698, 1980.

Winokur G: The Iowa 500: Heterogeneity and course of manic-depressive illness (bipolar). *Compr Psychiatry* 16:125–131, 1975.

Winokur G: Duration of illness prior to hospitalization (onset) in the affective disorders. *Neuropsychobiology* 2:87–93, 1976.

Winokur G: Studies in psychiatry: Unipolar depression. In: XO Breakfield, ed: *Neurogenetics: Genetic Approaches to the Nervous System.* New York: Elsevier, 1979a.

Winokur G: Unipolar depression: Is it divisible into autonomous subtypes? *Arch Gen Psychiatry* 36:47–52, 1979b.

Winokur G: Is there a common genetic factor in bipolar and unipolar affective disorder? *Compr Psychiatry* 21:460–468, 1980a.

Winokur G: What to do?, or What do we owe our residents? *Biol Psychiatry* 15:599–611, 1980b.

Winokur G: Alcoholism and depression. *Substance and Alcohol Actions/Misuse* 4:111–119, 1983.

Winokur G: Psychosis in bipolar and unipolar affective illness with special reference to schizo-affective disorder. *Br J Psychiatry* 145:236–242, 1984.

Winokur G, Clayton P: Family history studies: I. Two types of affective disorders separated according to genetic and clinical factors. In: J Wortis, ed: *Recent Advances in Biological Psychiatry.* Vol. 10. New York: Plenum, 1967. pp 35–50.

Winokur G, Kadrmas A: A polyepisodic course in bipolar illness: Possible clinical relationships. *Compr Psychiatry* 30:121–127, 1989.

Winokur G, Tsuang MT: Elation versus irritability in mania. *Compr Psychiatry* 16:435–436, 1975a.

Winokur G, Tsuang MT: The Iowa 500: Suicide in mania, depression, and schizophrenia. *Am J Psychiatry* 132:650–651, 1975b.

Winokur G, Tsuang M: Expectancy of alcoholism in a midwestern population. *J Stud Alcohol* 39:1964–1967, 1978.

Winokur G, Clayton PJ, Reich T: *Manic Depressive Illness.* St. Louis: CV Mosby, 1969.

Winokur G, Reich T, Rimmer J, Pitts FN: Alcoholism III. Diagnosis and familial psychiatric illness in 259 alcoholic probands. *Arch Gen Psychiatry* 23:104–111, 1970.

Winokur G, Rimmer J, Reich T: Alcoholism IV. Is there more than one type of alcoholism? *Br J Psychiatry* 118:525–531, 1971.

Winters KC, Neale JM: Mania and low self-esteem. *J Abnorm Psychol* 94:282–290, 1985.

Winters KC, Stone AA, Weintraub S, Neale JM: Cognitive and attentional deficits in children vulnerable to psychopathology. *J Abnorm Child Psychol* 9:435–453, 1981.

Wirz-Justice A: Antidepressant drugs: Effects on the circadian system. In: TA Wehr, FK Goodwin, eds: *Circadian Rhythms and Psychiatry.* Pacific Grove, CA: The Boxwood Press, 1983. pp 235–264.

Wirz-Justice A, Pühringer W: Seasonal incidence of an altered diurnal rhythm of platelet serotonin in unipolar depression. *J Neural Transm* 42:45–53, 1978.

Wirz-Justice A, Richter R: Seasonality in biochemical determinations: A source of variance and a clue to the temporal incidence of affective illness. *Psychiatry Res* 1:53–60, 1979.

Wirz-Justice A, Pühringer W, Hole G, Menzi R: Monoamine oxidase and free tryptophan in human plasma: Normal variations and their implications for biochemical research in affective disorders. *Pharmakopsychiatr Neuropsychopharmakol* 8:310–317, 1975.

Wirz-Justice A, Pühringer W, Hole G: Response to sleep deprivation as a predictor of therapeutic results with antidepressant drugs. *Am J Psychiatry* 136:1222–1223, 1979.

Wirz-Justice A, Bucheli Ch, Graw P, Fisch H-U, Woggon B, Kielholz P: The Swiss SAD study: Incidence of seasonal depression and light therapy. Abstract, IVth World Congress of Biological Psychiatry, Philadelphia 1985.

Wirz-Justice A, Bucheli C, Graw P, Kielholz P, Fisch H-U, Woggon B: Light treatment of seasonal affective disorder in Switzerland *Acta Psychiatr Scand* 74:193–204, 1986.

Wirz-Justice A, Graw P, Bucheli Ch, Schmid AC, Gisin B, Jochum A, Poldiner W: Seasonal affective disorder in Switzerland: A clinical perspective. In: C Thompson, T Silverstone, eds: *Seasonal Affective Disorder*. London: CRC Clinical Neuroscience, in press.

Wittenborn JR, Kiremitci N, Weber ESP: The choice of alternative antidepressants. *J Nerv Ment Dis* 156:97–108, 1973.

Wittkower ED, Rin H: Transcultural psychiatry. *Arch Gen Psychiatry* 13:387–394, 1965.

Wittman P: The Babcock deterioration test in state hospital practice. *J Abnorm Soc Psychol* 28:70–83, 1933.

Wodehouse PG: *The Code of the Woosters*. New York: Random House, 1975.

Woggon B: Untersuchung zur validität der übergeordneter AMP-Skalen durch Vergleiche mit Hamilton-Depressions-Skala, BPRS, und IMPS. *Int Pharmacopsychiat* 14:338–349, 1979.

Woggon B, Dittrich A: Konstruktion übergeordneter AMP-Skalen: "manische-depressives" und "schizophrenes Syndrom." *Int Pharmacopsychiat* 14:325–337, 1979.

Wolfe J, Granholm E, Butters N, Saunders E, Janowsky D: Verbal memory deficits associated with major affective disorders: A comparison of unipolar and bipolar patients. *J Affective Disord* 13:83–92, 1987.

Wolff EA, Putnam FW, Post RM: Motor activity and affective illness: The relationship of amplitude and temporal distribution to changes in affective state. *Arch Gen Psychiatry* 42:288–294, 1985.

Wolff J: The endocrine effects of lithium. In: JR Boissier, H Hippius, P Pichot, eds: *Proceedings of the IX Congress of the Collegium Internationale Neuropsychopharmacologicum*. New York: Elsevier, 1974. pp 621–628.

Wolkowitz OM, Doran AR, Breier A, Roy A, Jimerson DC, Sutton ME, Golden RN, Paul SM, Pickar D: The effects of dexamethasone on plasma homovanillic acid and 3-methoxy–4-hydroxyphenylglycol: Evidence for abnormal corticosteroid-catecholamine interactions in major depression. *Arch Gen Psychiatry* 44:782–789, 1987.

Wolpert E, Chausow A, Szidon JP: Respiratory failure and lithium. *Psychiatry Res* 15:249–252, 1985.

Wong DF, Pearlson G, Tune L, Villemagne V, Ross C, Dannals RF, Links J, Ravert H, Wilson A, Wagner HN, Gjedde A: *In vivo* measurement of D2 dopamine receptor abnormalities in drug naive and treated manic-depressive patients. *J Nucl Med* 28:611, 1987.

Wood JH, Hare TA, Enna SJ, Manyam NVB: Sites of origin and rostrocaudal gradients of GABA in cerebrospinal fluid. *Brain Res Bull* 5(Suppl 2):111–114, 1980.

Wood K, Coppen A: Prophylactic lithium treatment of patients with affective disorders is associated with decreased platelet [H-3]dihydroergocryptine binding. *J Affective Disord* 5:253–258, 1983.

Wood K, Harwood J, Coppen A: Platelet accumulation of histamine in depression. Letter. *Lancet* 2:519–520, 1983.

Wood K, Harwood J, Coppen A: Platelet accumulation of histamine in controls, depressed and lithium-treated patients. *J Affective Disord* 7:149–158, 1984.

Wood K, Harwood J, Coppen J: Plasma immunoglobulins in depressed and lithium-treated patients. *Br J Psychiatry* 147:581–582, 1986.

Woodruff RA Jr, Robins LN, Winokur G, Walbran B: Educational and occupational achievement in primary affective disorder. *Am J Psychiatry* 124(Suppl): 7–64, 1968.

Woodruff RA Jr, Guze SB, Clayton PJ: Unipolar and bipolar primary affective disorder. *Br J Psychiatry* 119:33–38, 1971a.

Woodruff RA Jr, Robins LN, Winokur G, Reich T: Manic depressive illness and social achievement. *Acta Psychiatr Scand* 47:237–249, 1971b.

Woodruff RA Jr, Guze SB, Clayton PJ: Alcoholics who see a psychiatrist compared with those who do not. *Q J Studies Alcohol* 34:1162–1171, 1973.

Woodruff RA Jr, Guze SB, Clayton PJ, Carr D: Alcoholism and depression. In: DW Goodwin, CK Erickson, eds: *Alcoholism and Affective Disorders: Clinical, Genetic, and Biochemical Studies*. New York: SP Medical and Scientific Books, 1979. pp 39–48.

Woods JW, Parker JC, Watson BS: Perturbation of sodium-lithium countertransport in red cells. *N Engl J Med* 308:1258–1261, 1983.

Woodside B, Zilli C, Fisman S: Biologic markers and bipolar disease in children. *Can J Psychiatry* 34:128–131, 1989.

Woodward DJ, Moises HC, Waterhouse BD, Hoffer BJ, Freedman R: Modulatory actions of norepinephrine in the central nervous system. *Fed Proc*

38:2109–2116, 1979.

Woody GE, O'Brien CP, Rickels K: Depression and anxiety in heroin addicts: A placebo-controlled study of doxepin in combination with methadone. *Am J Psychiatry* 132:447–450, 1975.

Woody GE, O'Brien CP, McLellan AT, Marcovici M, Evans BD: The use of antidepressants with methadone in depressed maintenance patients. *Ann NY Acad Sci* 398:120–127, 1982.

Woolf L: *Beginning Again: An Autobiography of the Years 1911 to 1918.* New York: Harcourt, 1964.

Woolf V: *The Letters of Virginia Woolf.* N Nicholson, J Trautman, eds. Six volumes. New York: Harcourt, 1975–1980.

Worden FG, Childs B, Matthysse S, Gershon ES, eds: Frontiers of psychiatric genetics. *Neurosci Res Prog Bull* 14:1–107, 1976.

Worland J: Rorschach developmental level in the offspring of patients with schizophrenia and manic-depressive illness. *J Personal Assess* 43:591–594, 1979.

Worland J, Lander H, Hesselbrock V: Psychological evaluation of clinical disturbance in children at risk for psychopathology. *J Abnorm Psychol* 88:13–26, 1979.

World Health Organization: *Manual of the International Statistical Classification of Diseases, Injuries, and Causes of Death, 9th Revision.* vol. 1. Geneva: WHO, 1977.

Worrall EP, Moody JP, Peet M, Dick P, Smith A, Chambers C, Adams M, Naylor GJ: Controlled studies of the acute antidepressant effects of lithium. *Br J Psychiatry* 135:255–262, 1979.

Wright AF, Crichton DN, Loudon JB, Morten JEN, Steel CM: β-adrenoceptor binding defects in cell lines from families with manic-depressive disorder. *Ann Hum Genet* 48:201–214, 1984.

Wright G, Galloway L, Kim J, Dalton M, Miller L, Stern W: Bupropion in the long-term treatment of cyclic mood disorders: Mood stabilizing effects. *J Clin Psychiatry* 46:22–25, 1985.

Wright JM, Sachdev PS, Perkins RJ, Rodriguez P: Zidovudine-related mania. *Med J Aust* 150:339–341, 1989.

Wulsin L, Bachop M, Hoffman D: Group therapy in manic- depressive illness. *Am J Psychother* 42:263–271, 1988.

Wurmser L: Psychoanalytic considerations of the etiology of compulsive drug use. *J Am Psychoanal Assoc* 22:820–843, 1974.

Wyatt RJ: *Practical Psychiatric Practice: Forms and Protocols for Clinical Use.* American Psychiatric Press, in press.

Wyatt RJ, Portnoy B, Kupfer DJ, Snyder F, Engelman K: Resting plasma catecholamine concentrations in patients with depression and anxiety. *Arch Gen Psychiatry* 24:65–70, 1971.

Wyatt RJ, Alexander RC, Egan MF, Kirch DG: Schizophrenia: just the facts: What do we know, how well do we know it? *Schizophr Res* 1:3–18, 1988.

Yamaguchi N, Maeda K, Kuromaru S: The effects of sleep deprivation on the circadian rhythm of plasma cortisol levels in depressive patients. *Folia Psychiatr Neurolog Japonica* 32:479–487, 1978.

Yamamoto H, Nagai K, Nakagawa H: Additional evidence that the suprachiasmatic nucleus is the center for regulation of insulin secretion and glucose homeostasis. *Brain Res* 304:237–21, 1984.

Yap PM: Phenomenology of affective disorder in Chinese and other cultures. In: AVS de Reuck, R Porter, eds: *Transcultural Psychiatry: A Ciba Foundation Symposium.* London: J & A Churchill, 1965. pp 84–105.

Yassa R, Nair NPV, Iskandar H: Late-onset bipolar disorder. *Psychiatr Clin North Am* 11:117–131, 1988a.

Yassa R, Saunders A, Nastase C, Camille Y: Lithium-induced thyroid disorders: A prevalence study. *J Clin Psychiatry* 49:14–16, 1988b.

Yates WR, Jacoby CG, Andreasen NC: Cerebellar atrophy in schizophrenia and affective disorder. *Am J Psychiatry* 144:465–467, 1987.

Yatham LN, Benbow JC, Jeffers AM: Mania following head injury. *Acta Psychiatr Scand* 77:359–360, 1988.

Yeats WB: A remonstrance with Scotsmen for having soured the dispositions of their ghosts and faeries. (1893) *The Celtic Twilight and a Selection of Early Poems.* New York: Signet Classics, 1962.

Yeats WB: *The Celtic Twilight.* New York: Signet Classics, 1962.

Yerevanian BI: Treatment of seasonal affective disorder with bright incandescent light: Is timing of treatment important? Abstract of paper presented at the 140th annual meeting of the American Psychiatric Association, May, 1987.

Yerevanian BI, Anderson JL, Grota LJ, Bray M: Effects of bright incandescent light on seasonal and nonseasonal major depressive disorder. *Psychiatry Res* 18:355–364, 1986.

Younes RP, DeLong GR, Neiman G, Rosner B: Manic-depressive illness in children: Treatment with lithium carbonate. *J Child Neurology* 1:364–368, 1986.

Young MA, Abrams R, Taylor MA, Meltzer HY: Establishing diagnostic criteria for mania. *J Nerv Ment Dis* 171:676–682, 1983.

Young PM: *Handel.* London: JM Dent, 1975.

Young RC, Biggs JT, Ziegler VE, Meyer DA: A rating scale for mania: Reliability, validity and sensitivity. *Br J Psychiatry* 133:429–435, 1978.

Young RC, Schreiber MT, Nysewander RW: Psychotic mania. *Biol Psychiatry* 18:1167–1173, 1983.

Youngerman J, Canino IA: Lithium carbonate use in children and adolescents. *Arch Gen Psychiatry* 35:216–224, 1978.

Youngren MA, Lewinsohn PM: The functional relationship between depression and problematic interpersonal behavior. *J Abnorm Psychol* 89:333–341, 1980.

Yozawitz A, Bruder G, Sutton S, Sharpe L, Gurland

B, Fleiss J, Costa L: Dichotic perception: Evidence for right hemisphere dysfunction in affective psychosis. *Br J Psychiatry* 135:224–237, 1979.

Zacharski LR, Hill RW, Maldonado JE: The lymphocyte. *Mayo Clinic Proc* 42:431–451, 1967.

Zahn TP: Psychophysiological approaches to psychopathology. In: MGH Coles, E Donchin, SW Porges, eds: *Psychophysiology: Systems, Processes and Applications.* New York: Gilford Press, 1986.

Zahn TP, Nurnberger JI Jr, Berrettini WH: Electrodermal activity in young adults at genetic risk for affective disorder. *Arch Gen Psychiatry* 46:1120–1124, 1989.

Zahn-Waxler C, Chapman M, Cummings EM: Cognitive and social development in infants and toddlers with a bipolar parent. *Child Psychiatr Hum Devel* 15:75–85, 1984a.

Zahn-Waxler C, Cummings EM, Iannotti RJ, Radke-Yarrow M: Young offspring of depressed parents: A population at risk for affective problems. In: D Cicchetti, K Schneider-Rosen, eds: *Childhood Depression.* New Directions for Child Development Series, No. 26. San Francisco: Jossey-Bass, 1984b. pp. 81–105.

Zahn-Waxler C, McKnew DH, Cummings EM, Davenport YB, Radke-Yarrow M: Problem behaviors and peer interactions of young children with a manic-depressive parent. *Am J Psychiatry* 141:236–240, 1984c.

Zahn-Waxler C, Mayfield A, Radke-Yarrow M, McKnew DH, Cytryn L, Davenport YB: A followup investigation of offspring of parents with bipolar disorder. *Am J Psychiatry* 145:506–509, 1988.

Zakowska-Dabrowska T, Rybakowski J: Lithium-induced EEG changes: Relation to lithium levels in serum and red blood cells. *Acta Psychiatr Scand* 49:457–465, 1973.

Zaremba D, Rybakowski J: Erythrocyte lithium transport during lithium treatment in patients with affective disorders. *Pharmacopsychiatry* 19:63–67, 1986.

Zarin DA, Pass TM: Lithium and the single episode: When to begin long-term prophylaxis for bipolar disorder. *Medical Care* 25:S76–S84, 1987.

Zatz M, Brownstein MJ: Injection of alpha-bungarotoxin near the suprachiasmatic nucleus blocks the effects of light on nocturnal pineal enzyme activity. *Brain Res* 213:438–442, 1981.

Zealley AK, Aitken RCB: Measurement of mood. *Proc Roy Soc Med* 62:993–996, 1969.

Zemishlany Z, Munitz H, Rotman A, Wijsenbeek H: Increased uptake of serotonin by blood platelets from patients with bipolar primary affective disorder-bipolar type. *Psychopharmacology (Berlin)* 77:175–178, 1982.

Zetin M, Garber D, De Antonio M, Schlegel A, Feureisen S, Fieve R, Jewett C, Reus V, Huey LY: Prediction of lithium dose: A mathematical alternative to the test-dose method. *J Clin Psychiatry* 47:175–178, 1986.

Zhang Y, Meltzer HL: Increased content of a minor ankyrin in erythrocyte membranes of bipolar subjects. *Psychiatry Res* 27:267–275, 1989.

Zhang M, Xu S: *Current Practice of Psychotropic Drugs in China: Seminar on Psychopharmacology.* Shanghai: World Health Organization, 1980.

Zhou D, Shen Y, Shu L, Lo H: Dexamethasone suppression test and urinary MHPG·SO$_4$ determination in depressive disorders. *Biol Psychiatry* 22:883–891, 1987.

Zilboorg G: *A History of Medical Psychology.* New York: WW Norton, 1941.

Zimmerman J, Garfinkle L: Preliminary study of the art productions of the adult psychotic. *Psychiatr Q* 16:313–318, 1942.

Zimmerman M, Coryell W, Corenthal C, Wilson S: A self-report scale to diagnose major depressive disorder. *Arch Gen Psychiatry* 43:1076–1081, 1986.

Zimmerman SF, Whitmyre JW, Fieldo FRJ: Factor analytic structure of the Wechsler Adult Intelligence Scale in patients with diffuse and lateralized cerebral dysfunction. *J Clin Psychol* 26:462–465, 1970.

Zis AP, Goodwin FK: Major affective disorder as a recurrent illness: A critical review. *Arch Gen Psychiatry* 36:835–839, 1979.

Zis AP, Grof P, Goodwin FK: The natural course of affective disorders: Implications for lithium prophylaxis. In: TB Cooper, S Gershon, NS Kline, M Schou, eds: *Lithium: Controversies and Unresolved Issues.* Amsterdam: Exerpta Medica, 1979. pp 381–398.

Zis AP, Grof P, Webster M, Goodwin FK: Prediction of relapse in recurrent affective disorder. *Psychopharmacol Bull* 16:47–49, 1980.

Ziskind E, Somerfeid-Ziskind E, Ziskind L: Metrazol and electric convulsive therapy of the affective psychoses. *Arch Psychiatr Neurol* 53:212–217, 1945.

Zisook S: Cyclic 48-hour unipolar depression. *J Nerv Ment Dis* 176:53–56, 1988.

Zisook S, Schuckit MA: Male primary alcoholics with and without family histories of affective disorder. *J Stud Alcohol* 48:337–344, 1987.

Zohar J, Drummer D, Edelstein ED, Kaiser N, Belmaker RH, Nir I: Effect of lysine vasopressin in depressed patients on mood and 24-hour rhythm of growth hormone, cortisol, melatonin and prolactin. *Psychoneuroendocrinology* 10:273–279, 1985.

Zubenko GS, Nixon RA: Mood-elevating effect of captopril in depressed patients. *Am J Psychiatry* 141:110–111, 1984.

Zubenko GS, Cohen BM, Lipinski JF, Jonas JM: Clonidine in the treatment of mania and mixed bipolar disorder. *Am J Psychiatry* 141:1617–1618, 1984.

Zuckerman M, Lubin B: *Multiple Affect Adjective Checklists.* San Diego: Educational and Industrial Testing Service, 1967.

Zung WWK: A self-rating depression scale. *Arch Gen Psychiatry* 12:63–70, 1965.

Zung WWK: The measurement of affects: Depression and anxiety. *Mod Prob Pharmacopsychiat* 7:170–188, 1974.

Zung WWK, Green RL: Seasonal variation of suicide and depression. *Arch Gen Psychiatry* 30:89–91, 1974.

Credits

General Psychiatry 39:665–671. Copyright 1982 by the American Medical Association; and from: Harrow M, et al.: A longitudinal study of thought pathology in manic patients. *Archives of General Psychiatry* 43:781–785. Copyright 1986 by the American Medical Association.

Figure 11-3 reprinted by permission of the publisher from: Hoffman RE, et al.: A comparative study of manic vs schizophrenic thought disorganization. *Archives of General Psychiatry* 43:831–838. Copyright 1986 by the American Medical Association.

Figure 11-4 reprinted by permission of the publisher from: Gruzelier J, et al.: Impairments on neuropsychologic tests of temporohippocampal and frontohippocampal functions and word fluency in remitting schizophrenia and affective disorders. *Archives of General Psychiatry* 45:623–629. Copyright 1988 by the American Medical Association.

Figure 12-1 reprinted by permission of the publisher from: Owen SE & Nurcombe B: The application of the Semantic Differential Test in a case of manic-depressive psychosis. *Australia and New Zealand Journal of Psychiatry* 4:149–154. Copyright 1970 by the Australia and New Zealand Journal of Psychiatry.

Figure 12-2 reprinted by permission of the publisher from: Donnelly ET, et al.: Cross-sectional and longitudinal comparisons of bipolar and unipolar depressed groups on the MMPI. *Journal of Consulting and Clinical Psychology* 44:233–237. Copyright 1976 by the American Psychological Association.

Figure 12-3 reprinted by permission of the publisher from: Lumry AE, et al.: MMPI state dependency during the course of bipolar psychosis. *Psychiatry Research* 7:59–67. Copyright 1982 by Elsevier Science Publishers.

Table 13-1 reprinted by permission of the authors from: Beigel A, et al.: The manic-state rating scale: Scale construction, reliability, and validity. *Archives of General Psychiatry* 25:256–262, 1971.

Table 13-2 reprinted by permission of the publisher from: Depue RA, et al.: A behavioral paradigm for identifying persons at risk for bipolar depressive disorder: A conceptual framework and five validation studies. *Journal of Abnormal Psychology* 90:381–437. Copyright 1981 by the American Psychological Association.

Figure 13-1 reprinted by permission of the publisher from: Zealley AK & Aitken RCB: Measurement of mood. *Proceedings of the Royal Society of Medicine* 62:993–996. Copyright 1969 by the Royal Society of Medicine.

Table 14-1 reprinted by permission of the publisher from: the *Diagnostic and Statistical Manual of Mental Disorders: Third Edition.* Copyright 1980 by the American Psychiatric Association Press, Inc.

Tables 14-3 and 14-4 reprinted by permission of the publisher from: Andreasen NC: Creativity and mental illness: Prevalence rates in writers and their first-degree relatives. *American Journal of Psychiatry* 144:1288–1292. Copyright 1987 by the American Psychiatric Association.

Table 14-5 reprinted by permission of the publisher from: Richards R, et al.: Creativity in manic-depressives, cyclothymes, their normal relatives, and control subjects. *Journal of Abnormal Psychology* 97:281–288. Copyright 1988 by the American Psychological Association.

Figure 14-1 reprinted by permission of the publisher from: Slater E & Meyer A: Contributions to a pathography of musicians: 1. Robert Schumann. *Confina Psychiatria* 2:65–94. Copyright 1959 by S Karger AG.

Figure 14-2 reprinted by permission of the publisher from: Richards R, et al.: Creativity in manic-depressives, cyclothymes, their normal relatives, and control subjects. *Journal of Abnormal Psychology* 97:281–288. Copyright 1988 by the American Psychological Association.

Figures 14-3 and 14-4 reprinted by permission of the publisher from: Jamison KR: Mood disorders and patterns of creativity in British writers and artists. *Psychiatry* 52:125–134. Copyright 1989 by the Washington School of Psychiatry.

Figures 14-5, 14-6, and 14-7 reprinted by permission of the publisher from: Jamison KR: Mood disorders and patterns of creativity in British writers and artists. *Psychiatry* 52:125–134. Copyright 1989 by the Washington School of Psychiatry.

Tables 15-2 and 15-6 reprinted by permission of the publisher from: Gershon ES, et al.: Genetics of affective illness. *Psychopharmacology: The Third Generation of Progress.* (HY Meltzer, ed). Copyright 1987 by Raven Press.

Tables 15-3 and 15-4 reprinted by permission of the authors from: Gershon ES, et al.: A controlled family study of chronic psychoses: Schizophrenia and schizoaffective disorder. *Archives of General Psychiatry* 45:328–336, 1988.

Figure 15-1 reprinted by permission of the authors from: Gershon ES, et al.: Birth-cohort changes in manic and depressive disorders in relatives of bipolar and schizoaffective patients. *Archives of General Psychiatry* 44:314–319, 1987.

Figure 15-2 reprinted by permission of the publisher from: Gershon ES, et al.: Genetics of affective illness. *Psychopharmacology: The Third Generation of Progress.* (HY Meltzer, ed). Copyright 1987 by Raven Press.

Figure 15-3 reprinted by permission of the publisher from: White R & Lalouel J-M: Chromosome mapping with DNA markers. *Scientific American* 258:40–48. Copyright 1988 by Scientific American, Inc.

Figure 16-2 reprinted by permission of the publisher from: Kelly JP: Principles of the functional and anatomical organization of the nervous system. *Principles of Neural Science.* 2nd Edition. (ER Kandel & JH Schwartz, eds). Copyright 1985 by Elsevier Scientific Publishing Co.

Figures 16-3a,b reprinted by permission of the publisher from: Kupfermann I: Hypothalamus and limbic

Psychiatry 13:109–114. Copyright 1979 by the Australia and New Zealand Journal of Psychiatry.

Table 23-16 reprinted by permission of the publisher from: Kukopulos A, et al.: Course of manic-depressive cycle and changes caused by treatments. *Pharmakopsychiatrie Neuro-psychopharmakologie* 13:156–167. Copyright 1980 by George Thieme Verlag.

Figure 23-4 reprinted by permission of the publisher from: Post RM, Uhde TW: Clinical approaches to treatment-resistant bipolar illness. *Psychiatry Update: Annual Review, Vol. 6*. (RE Hales & AJ Frances, eds). Copyright 1987 by the American Psychiatric Association Press, Inc.

Table 24-1 reprinted by permission of the publisher from: Jamison KR & Goodwin FK: Psychotherapeutic issues in bipolar illness. *Psychiatry Update: Annual Review, Vol II*. (L Grinspoon, ed). Copyright 1983 by the American Psychiatric Association Press, Inc.

Figure 24-2 reprinted by permission of the authors from: Squillace K, et al.: Life-charting of the longitudinal course of recurrent affective illness. *Neurobiology of Mood Disorders*. (RM Post & JC Ballenger, eds), 1984. pp. 38–59.

Figure 24-3 reprinted by permission of the publisher from: Baastrup PC & Schou M: Lithium as a prophylactic agent: Its effects against recurrent depressions and manic-depressive psychosis. *Archives of General Psychiatry* 16:162–172. Copyright 1967 by the American Medical Association.

Table 25-6 reprinted by permission of the authors from: Jamison KR, et al.: Patient and physician attitudes toward lithium: Relationship to compliance. *Archives of General Psychiatry* 36:866–869, 1979.

Table 27-3 reprinted by permission of the publisher from: Jamison KR: Suicide prevention in depressed women. *Journal of Clinical Psychiatry* 49(Suppl):42–45. Copyright 1988 by Physicians Postgraduate Press, Inc.

Case report on page 93 reprinted by permission of the authors from: Bunney WE Jr, et al.: A behavioral-biochemical study of lithium treatment. *American Journal of Psychiatry* 125:499–512, 1968.

Case reports on pages 100, 105–106 and 105, note 15 reprinted by permission of the publisher from: Akiskal HS & Puzantian VR: Psychotic forms of depression and mania. *Psychiatric Clinics of North America* 2:419–439. Copyright 1979 by W.B. Saunders Company.

Case report page 105 reprinted by permission of the publisher from: Pope HG: Distinguishing bipolar disorder from schizophrenia in general practice: Guidelines and case reports. *Hospital and Community Psychiatry* 34:322–328. Copyright 1983 by the American Psychiatric Association Press, Inc.

Case report pages 113–115 reprinted by permission of the publisher from: Cowdry RW & Goodwin FK: Dementia of bipolar illness: Diagnosis and response to lithium. *American Journal of Psychiatry* 138:1118–1119. Copyright 1981 by the American Psychiatric Association.

Case report pages 118–119 reprinted by permission of the publisher from: Himmelhoch JM: Major mood disorders related to epileptic changes. *Psychiatric Aspects of Epilepsy*. (D Blumer, ed). Copyright 1984 by the American Psychiatric Association Press, Inc.

Case report page 194 reprinted by permission of the publisher from: Akiskal HS, et al.: Affective disorders in referred children and younger siblings of manic-depressives: Mode of onset and prospective course. *Archives of General Psychiatry* 42:996–1003. Copyright 1985 by the American Medical Association.

Case report page 260 reprinted by permission of the publisher from: Hoffman RE, et al.: A comparative study of manic and schizophrenic speech disorganization. *Archives of General Psychiatry* 43:831–835. Copyright 1986 by the American Medical Association.

Case report page 765 reprinted by permission of the publisher from: Akiskal HS, et al.: Cyclothymic temperamental disorders. *Psychiatric Clinics of North America* 2:527–554. Copyright 1979 by W.B. Saunders Company.

Quoted material pages 17, 22–24, 36–38, 45, and 50 reprinted by permission of the publisher from: Campbell JD: *Manic-Depressive Disease: Clinical and Psychiatric Significance*. Copyright 1953 by J.B. Lippincott, Co.

Quoted material page 20 reprinted by permission of the publisher from: Endler NS: *Holiday of Darkness: A Psychologist's Personal Journey Out of His Depression*. (1982). Copyright 1990 by Wall & Emerson, Inc.

Quoted material pages 20–21, 25–29, 41–42, and 253 reprinted by permission of the publisher from: Custance J: *Wisdom, Madness, and Folly: The Philosophy of a Lunatic*. Copyright 1952 by Farrar, Straus, & Giroux, Inc.

Quoted material pages 23 and 40 reprinted by permission of the publisher from: Henderson D & Gillespie RD: *A Text-book of Psychiatry for Students and Practitioners*. 7th ed. Copyright 1950 by Oxford University Press.

Quoted material pages 57–58 reprinted by permission of the publisher from: Roccatagliata G: *A History of Ancient Psychiatry*. Copyright 1986 by Greenwood Press, Inc.

Quoted material page 186, note 1 reprinted by permission of the publisher from: Norwich JJ: *Christmas Crackers*. Copyright 1982 by Penguin Books.

Quoted material pages 235–236 reprinted by permission of the publisher from: Alvarez A: *The Savage God: A Study of Suicide*. Copyright 1973 by Weidenfeld and Nicholson.

Quoted material page 264 reprinted by permission of the publisher from: Kendler KS, et al.: Dimensions of delusional experience. *American Journal of Psychiatry* 140:466–469. Copyright 1983 by the American Psychiatric Association.

INDEX

Italicized entries are used to denote terms used in formal diagnostic systems or to describe forms of illness with specific characteristics.

ABO blood groups, 484
Accomplishment and achievement, 167, 169, 173, 336–42
Acetylcholine (ACh), 423–24
  CRF, stimulation of release, 449, 452
  drug effects on, 423–24, 445–47
  genetic predisposition, role in, 445
  levels in affective illness, 423–24
  receptors and, 423
  somatostatin and, 462
  see also Cholinergic–noradrenergic balance hypothesis
Acetylcholinesterase (AChE)
  bipolar–unipolar difference in, 441
  physostigmine and, 452
Acquired immune deficiency syndrome (AIDS), 112
  AIDS dementia, 115
Acrophase, 555, 571
ACTH. *See* Adrenocorticotropin hormone
Activity
  in bipolar depression, description, 38, 42
  in hypomania, 23
  in mania, 24–25, 35–37
  see also Behavioral symptoms; Energy levels
Activity–Withdrawal Scale, 104
Addison's disease, 112
Adolescent-onset illness, 186–96
  adult onset, compared, 191–94
  alcohol abuse in, 764
  borderline personality disorder and, 110
  clinical description of, 191–94
  cyclothymia, diagnostic criteria, 97
  developmental task problems, 732
  diagnosis, differential, 189–91
  DSM-III-R criteria, 189–91, 195, 197, 208
  early vs late onset, 33, 195–96, 380–81
  lithium compliance in, 723
  prediction of bipolarity in, 194–95
  prognosis, 186, 194–95, 208
  prophylactic treatment in, 668, 671–72, 691–92
  seasonal affective disorder in, 194
  signs and symptoms of, 188–89, 196, 208
  substance abuse, association with, 190
  suicide in, 186, 201, 233
  treatment of acute mania in, 612, 614, 627–28
  type II alcoholism in, 764
  see also Early-onset illness

Adrenal cortex, cortisol and, 449, 451
Adrenergic agents
  in treatment of bipolar depression, 654
  see also Clonidine; Idazoxan; Pirbuterol; Salbutamol; Receptors
Adrenocorticotropin hormone (ACTH)
  cortisol and 451–53
  CRF, 448–49, 451, 489
  drug effects on, 452–53
  serotonin and, 452
  somatostatin and, 462
  VIP (agonist), 466
  in well interval 487
ADRS. *See* Affective Disorder Rating Scale
Advanced instruction. *See* Informed consent
Affect reaction, 377
Affective Disorder Rating Scale (ADRS), 322, 329–31
Affective–schizophrenic continuum, 102–3, 583–84
  genetic evidence for, 381
Age and illness prevalence, 165–68, 174, 185
  see also Demographic correlates of illness; Epidemiologic Catchment Area program; Epidemiology
Age of onset, 128–32
  alcohol abuse and, 764
  bipolar–unipolar differences in, 64, 399, 580
  criteria for determining, 128, 154
  early vs late, 128, 140–41, 186–88, 195–96
  epidemiology of, 167
  episode characteristics and, 134–37, 140
  gender differences, 132
  genetic risk and early onset, 381, 386
  kindling–sensitization and, 406, 408
  late, in women, 129
  in offspring of patients, 385
  prepubertal, 129, 186–88
  prophylactic response and, 697, 700
  psychotic features and, 33, 129
  schizoaffective features and, 129
  treatment factors and, 632
  see also Adolescent-onset illness; Early-onset illness
Aggression/impulsivity, 93, 286
  bipolar–unipolar differences in, 234
  carbamazepine and, 778
  in childhood and adolescence, 190, 197, 208
  CSF 5-HIAA levels and, 426, 489, 492–93
  5-HT and, 483, 492–95
  in mania, 290, 292
  suicide and, 489, 492–93